Measuring Immunity:
Basic Biology and Clinical Assessment

To the Institute and Departmental leaders at the University of Pittsburgh: Richard Simmons, Thomas Starzl, Timothy Billiar, Joseph Glorioso, Ronald Herbman and Arthur Levine who have all supported our work both in the laboratory and the clinic.

Measuring Immunity:
Basic Biology and Clinical Assessment

Edited by Michael T. Lotze and Angus W. Thomson

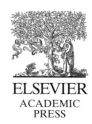

ELSEVIER
ACADEMIC
PRESS

AMSTERDAM • BOSTON • HEIDELBERG • LONDON • NEW YORK • OXFORD
PARIS • SAN DIEGO • SAN FRANCISCO • SINGAPORE • SYDNEY • TOKYO

Elsevier Academic Press
525 B Street, Suite 1900, San Diego, California 92101-4495, USA
http://www.elsevier.com

Elsevier Academic Press
84 Theobald's Road, London WC1X 8RR, UK
http://www.elsevier.com

British Library Cataloguing in Publication Data
A catalogue record for this book is available from the British Library

Library of Congress Control Number: 2004116778

ISBN 0-12-455900-X

For information on all Elsevier Academic Press publications
visit our website at http://www.books.elsevier.com

Typeset by Newgen Imaging Systems (P) Ltd., Chennai, India
Printed and bound in Great Britain
05 06 07 08 9 8 7 6 5 4 3 2 1

Contents

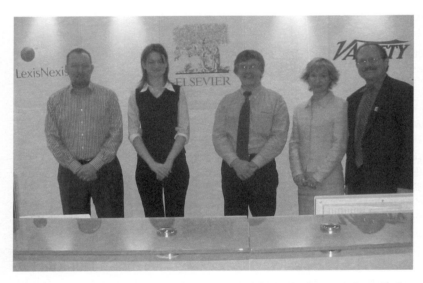

Christopher Gibson (Publishing Director, Elsevier), Victoria Lebedeva (Developmental Editor, Elsevier), Angus W. Thomson (Editor), Tessa Picknett (Senior Publisher, Elsevier) and Michael T. Lotze (Editor).

Foreword

THE BEDSIDE IS THE BENCH

Jeffrey A. Bluestone[1] and Vicki Seyfert-Margolis[2]

[1]*Director, Immune Tolerance Network, Director and Professor, UCSF Diabetes Center and the Department of Medicine, University of California, San Francisco, San Francisco, CA;* [2]*Executive Director, Tolerance Assay Group, Immune Tolerance Network and Assistant Professor, UCSF Diabetes Center and the Department of Medicine, University of California, San Francisco, San Francisco, CA, USA*

A young woman confronted with a diagnosis of systemic lupus erythematosus (SLE) can expect lifelong complications arising from the disease itself, as well as the therapies used to treat this condition. About 50–70 per cent of SLE patients experience inflammation of the kidneys. As such, the young woman can expect to be treated with high doses of corticosteroids, often accompanied by the alkylating agent cyclophosphamide. Unfortunately, the prednisone and cyclophosphamide treatment often results in an initial improvement, but more than 50 per cent of SLE patients will experience a disease flare again within 2 years. Moreover, serious complications of high-dose corticosteroid and cytoxan therapy in SLE patients include osteoporosis, aseptic necrosis, hypertension, diabetes, opportunistic infection, and cataracts as well as gonadal failure, hemorrhagic cystitis and cancer. Clearly, safer and more effective therapies are needed for SLE. Most importantly, there is no way to predict the flares or remission using immunological analyses in affected patients.

Practically speaking, treatment of SLE and other autoimmune diseases remains similar to the therapies used 10 years ago. However, years of elegant work studying immunity and immune-mediated diseases in animal models combined with recent advances in human immunology and genomics offers an unprecedented opportunity to develop new therapies. There is, arguably, no more important concern in moving forward in the development of new immunotherapies than the measurement and quantification of the human immune response. Indeed, with the observed increase in immune-mediated disease and an ever-growing stable of immunomodulatory agents reaching clinical stages of development, the need for reliable indicators of the state of the human immune system has never been greater. The editors of this guide should therefore be congratulated for assembling a highly relevant, and indeed, very timely portrait of our current abilities and future prospects in this respect.

Importantly, if perhaps not unexpectedly, we have come to discover that the human immune system differs in many significant ways from the preclinical animal models used as justification for pursuing new therapies in human studies. A growing body of literature detailing the many examples of therapies that work well in mice but fail to generate similar efficacy in humans (Mestas and Hughes, 2004) underscores the divide between our respective understanding of mouse and human immunology. The scarcity of hard human data on immune mechanisms is truly the Achilles heel of immune-based therapeutic development. Typically, immune-based diseases are diagnosed by measuring a pathological process that has already taken place. This means that the destruction by the immune system is already well underway. Effective monitoring and early detection of these diseases is challenging at many levels, unlike preclinical efforts which can sample the immune response at the site of immune attack (e.g. graft, draining lymph node or inflamed tissue); human sampling is relegated often to the peripheral blood far away from where the action is and rarely before the immune response is already damaging to the target tissue.

Take for example, the case of organ transplantation, where the key clinical challenges are to combat both acute and chronic rejection. At present, the gold standard for diagnosis of organ dysfunction is biopsy, which while accurate, provides its diagnosis only after significant organ damage has occurred. Immunological methods that detect events occurring upstream of the pathology would provide a welcome window of opportunity for earlier intervention. A related issue in organ transplantation is that of clinical tolerance induction. New potential tolerogenic strategies are now entering the clinic, many with the goal of complete immunosuppressive therapy withdrawal. Immunosuppressive withdrawal, however, is more than just the objective of these studies; rather it has been elevated to the status of an endpoint for these trials. Until have a clear description of the immunological properties of tolerance in humans, we are left with only an operational, rather than mechanistic definition of tolerance in humans.

Achieving a therapeutic benefit is the goal of all phase II and III trials and is currently measured using clinical endpoints. Clinical indicators, as currently measured, often do not offer objective quantitative markers for assessments of drug actions. Thus clinical endpoints will greatly benefit from the addition of studies designed to measure human immunity qualitatively and quantitatively. There is a pressing need for new surrogate markers for measuring changes in the immune system.

A case demonstrating the problems associated with relying on clinical endpoints can be made by looking at the history of immunologic therapies for HIV infection. Antiretroviral therapy has effectively reduced the rate of progression of HIV-infected patients to AIDS to ~2 per cent per year. Thus, trials of additional therapies require large patient populations and/or many years of treatment in order to obtain statistically significant proof of improved efficacy. Furthermore, studies of early HIV infection are virtually impossible without some alternative marker for disease progression because of the long time it takes (up to 10 years or more) for many patients to get sick. Similarly, in the case of cancer, current therapeutic inventions rely on clinical endpoints such as disease progression and death to determine efficacy. These endpoints, although a fair assessment of the clinical efficacy of the therapy, do not provide insights in the immune manifestations of therapy. Is the immune system activated by the therapy, is the tumor resistant to the therapy or does it escape immune surveillance by mutating target antigens?

But perhaps the clinical settings that most appropriately illustrate the need for new technologies and data that allow us to characterize the human immune system are the autoimmune diseases. The diagnosis of specific autoimmune diseases is often problematic due to overlapping pathologies and a lack of clearly distinguishable clinical features between the various diseases. American College of Rheumatology (ACR) diagnostic guidelines rely upon primarily pathologic criteria that, similar to the diagnosis of allograft rejection, present well into disease development – features such as clinical and radiological evidence of tissue damage. The prognostication of specific autoimmune diseases presents an even greater challenge, given that the etiology of many of these diseases remains unclear. In fact, one of the most fundamental questions in autoimmunity remains unanswered: what are the immunological characteristics that distinguish a healthy patient from one with an underlying autoimmune disorder? At present, there are no reliable laboratory-based immunologic methods that are capable of discriminating between a rheumatoid arthritis patient from a healthy control and a multiple sclerosis patient from the same. This 'readout' problem is so severe that in diseases such as type 1 diabetes, current therapeutic interventions rely on clinical endpoints such as hemoglobin A1c to determine efficacy. This metabolic parameter can be influenced by the rigor of glucose control, diet and environmental factors not the quintessential immunology of autoimmune disease. If we have no measurable description of the immunological hallmarks of the disease itself, how then can we begin to assess the efficacy of one therapy over another?

Clearly, our potential for success in the clinic is now limited by our inability to assess the immunological impact of our interventions. Throughout the field of immunology, it is therefore imperative that we develop new biological assays that allow precise and reliable measures of human immunity. The benefits will be enormous: surrogate markers for clinical efficacy providing more relevant, accurate and ethically justified means of assessing new therapeutics; new diagnostic tools that would permit earlier intervention and perhaps even preventative therapies; the ability to move beyond 'one size fits all' medicine towards more individualized therapy; and a wealth of new, direct knowledge of the human clinical experience that will pave the way for improved, second generation therapies. Much of the research elegantly summarized in this book reflects the growing efforts to identify specialized markers that can be used in individual disease settings to distinguish the patient from normal individuals, the responder from the non-responders.

Thus, the papers presented within this volume are a testament to the grand opportunity that lies before us. They serve not only to highlight the progress already achieved towards this goal, but present us with a series of difficult challenges as we move forward. Together they suggest that we have moved into a new phase of development in measuring immunity, one where old approaches might be best discarded in favor of a new paradigm for assay development.

In fact, this new paradigm may be best summed up by the multiple efforts emerging in the academic community, with the primary goal to develop robust standardized assays for measuring human immunity. These efforts include various workshops, as well as the emergence of several large clinical trials consortiums such as the

Immune Tolerance Network (ITN) whose philosophy is 'The bedside *is* the bench'. These consortiums have created organizations with the infrastructure necessary to become the perfect testing ground for many of the assays described within this text, performed in a real-world environment to produce data and ultimately, new tools of extraordinary clinical relevance. And with a growing list of immunologically active agents destined for clinical evaluation, the timing for such a fresh approach is ideal.

Indeed, the emergence of new and improved methodologies provides a solid foundation for the development of new clinically focused immunoassays. High throughput genomics assays, for example, offer exciting new opportunities for identifying new biomarkers and many investigators have already taken up this challenge, with more sure to join them. Federal funding agencies have recognized the import of this approach.

New models are developed, like the ITN, to perform clinical studies on a much grander scale than has likely ever been attempted previously. Infrastructures consisting of core facilities, large relational databases and a combination of mechanistic and discovery efforts will allow comparison studies across diseases, therapies and patient populations under highly standardized protocols and analysis methods in order to answer the simple question – can we distinguish immunologically the diseased from the normal individual as well as the patient that has benefited by the immunotherapy?

Although the development of this infrastructure is an enormous undertaking, emphasis on cooperation and working together to create a whole that is greater than the sum of its parts are vital. The time spent in developing rigorously standardized procedures for each assay and meticulously performing routine quality assurance testing will bring enormous benefits in terms of the knowledge gained from this effort: pooling of assay data will be possible between multiple clinical sites operating within the same trial to increase the statistical resolution; assay data can be analyzed in the context of the related clinical information in a multiparametric fashion; longitudinal studies can be carried out with built-in normalization; and as yet undiscovered assays can be applied to archived specimens for cross-analysis at a later time.

The editors of this book have done a remarkably thorough job of covering all the emerging techniques and principles of measuring immunity and they should be congratulated and thanked for what has surely been a tremendous undertaking. The techniques and concepts described in the pages of this book will provide the insights that large networks will apply to the clinical trial setting. I believe that a volume such as this is just what is needed to capture the imagination of the immunology community and may ultimately serve as a fine starting point towards a new paradigm for direct and coordinated investigation of the mechanisms inherent in human immunological diseases.

Acknowledgements

The authors wish to thank Jeffrey Mathews for his extensive editorial assistance and the rest of the Immune Tolerance Network staff for their important contributions and dedicated support of this effort.

REFERENCE

Mestas, J. and Hughes, C.C.W. (2004). Of mice and not men: differences between mouse and human immunology. J Immunol *172*, 2731–2738.

Preface

Michael T. Lotze and Angus W. Thomson

An Acte against conjuration Witchcrafte and dealinge with evill and wicked Spirits. BE it enacted by the King our Sovraigne Lorde the Lordes Spirituall and Temporall and the Comons in this p'sent Parliment assembled, and by the authoritie of the same, That the Statute made in the fifte yeere of the Raigne of our late Sov'aigne Ladie of the most famous and happy memorie Queene Elizabeth, intituled An Acte againste Conjurations Inchantments and witchcraftes, be from the Feaste of St. Michaell the Archangell nexte cominge, for and concerninge all Offences to be comitted after the same Feaste, utterlie repealed. AND for the better restrayning of saide Offenses, and more severe punishinge the same, be it further enacted by the authoritie aforesaide, That if any pson or persons after the saide Feaste of Saint Michaell the Archangell next comeing, shall use practise or exercsise any Invocation or Conjuration of any evill and spirit, or shall consult covenant with entertaine employ feede or rewarde any evill and wicked Spirit to or for any intent or pupose; or take any dead man woman or child out of his her or theire grave or any other place where the dead body resteth, or the skin, bone or any other parte of any dead person, to be imployed or used in any manner of Witchecrafte, Sorcerie, Charme or Inchantment; or shall use practise or exercise any Witchcrafte Sorcerie, Charme or Incantment wherebie any pson shall be killed destroyed wasted consumed pined or lamed in his or her bodie, or any parte therof ; then that everie such Offendor or Offendors theire Ayders Abettors and Counsellors, being of the saide Offences dulie and lawfullie convicted and attainted, shall suffer pains of deathe as a Felon or Felons, and shall loose the priviledge and benefit of Cleargie and Sanctuarie …

Witchcraft Act of 1604 – 1 Jas. I, c. 12

We have come quite a long way in the four centuries since the Witchcraft Act was passed during the end of the Elizabethan Age, which limited access to the parts of any body, dead or alive to be used in any 'witchcrafte, sorcerie, charme, or inchantment'. Clearly many of the practices employed and recommended by the strong coterie of authors brought together in this volume would have offended some Elizabethan audiences in 1604! In the same year London was just hearing Shakespeare's Measure for Measure performed on stage for the first time and enabling a 26-year-old William Harvey, who discerned how blood circulates, by admitting him as a candidate to the Royal College of Physicians. Considering the cells and the serologic components circulating within the blood as migratory biosensors and potential measures of immune function within the tissues is a modern interpretation provided by the current retinue of clinical immunologists and pathologists assembled here. A century ago in 1904, Paul Ehrlich published three articles in the New England Journal of Medicine (then the Boston Medical and Surgical Journal), detailing his work in immunochemistry, the mechanism of immune hemolysis and the sidechain theory of antibodies, work which subsequently served as a basis for winning the Nobel Prize along with Elie Metchinikoff. We have since substantially applied measures of the serologic response to pathogens and immunogens but the integration of multiple other assays, particularly cellular assays championed by Metchinikoff, many of them only appreciated and developed in the last decade, into a single readable text has not been previously carried out. The central goal of Measuring Immunity is to define which assays of immune function, largely based on ready and repeated access to the blood compartment, are helpful in the assessment of a myriad of clinical disorders involving inflammation and immunity, arguably the central problems of citizens of the modern world. This is not a methods manual and should not be perceived as such. Authors were given broad scope and freedom in integrating and assessing the clinical evidence that polymorphisms in genes regulating immune function (Section I), the actual assays themselves (Sections II–V) and how they were applied in clinical conditions (Section VI) might be best illustrated and championed. We are also particularly pleased that new measures and methods, not yet fully realized, are detailed here in Section VII. The greatest value from this work, we believe, is the juxtaposition in one place of the basic science foundations as well as the approaches currently applied and found valuable in the disparate and inchoate regions of clinical medicine.

As always the 'conjurations, inchantments and witchcraftes' of our colleagues are what make this volume a ready sanctuary for those seeking enlightenment. The dedication and craftsmanship in their work as well as the exposition here is gratifying to both us and the publishers. Indeed, we recently met with the publishers in London to discuss this work and those planned for the future and considered under the Academic Press/Elsevier banner of 'Building Insights; Breaking Boundaries', particularly reflecting on what the role of the 'Book' was and how it might be more useful for us and our colleagues. Isaac Elsevier first used the Elsevier corporate logo in 1620, just after the Witchcraft Act, as a printer's mark. It shows an elm, its trunk entwined by the tendrils of a vine.

A solitary man stands beside the tree, which supports a banner bearing the Latin motto *Non Solus* (not alone). Elsevier published books by outstanding scholars of the day, including Scaliger, Galileo, Erasmus and Descartes. Indeed the contemporary multiauthor authoritative text honors that history and provides a suitable reason for scholarly books. As a given, we believe that there is still substantial value in books, that they provide an authoritative and tightly edited source of integrated information, not easily assessed by perusing the modern literature. By constraining authors to formulate their work in a bounded space with common goals and deliverables, we enable them to indeed build new insights and cross boundaries usually maintained in academic circles, not so different from a Shakespearian drama, distilling human experience derived from a changing world.

Acknowledgements

The editors and publisher would like to thank Farzad Alemi, Minnie Sarwal and Elaine Mansfield for creating and allowing the use of an illustration that inspired the front cover artwork of this book (**Figure 60.3**) that we have entitled 'Molecular Tartan'.

Outstanding, dedicated and highly professional interactions of Victoria Lebedeva, Pauline Sones and Tessa Picknett are gratefully acknowledged.

Michael T. Lotze, MD
Angus W. Thomson, PhD
Pittsburgh
April 2004

Contributors

Joseph M. Ahearn (Chapters 10 and 11)
Division of Rheumatology and Clinical Immunology,
University of Pittsburgh School of Medicine,
Pittsburgh, PA, USA

Matthew L. Albert (Chapter 32)
Laboratory of Dendritic Cell Immunobiology,
Pasteur Institute, Paris, France

Farzad Alemi (Chapter 60)
Lucile Salter Packard Children's Hospital Nephrology,
Stanford, California, CA, USA

Rachel Allen (Chapter 8)
University of Cambridge,
Tennis Court Road, Cambridge, UK

Beatriz Garcia Alvarez (Chapter 54)
Servicio de Cirugia Vascular y Endovascular,
Hospital Universitario Vall d'Hebron,
Barcelona, Spain

Daniel R. Ambruso (Chapter 36)
Department of Pediatrics,
University of Colorado School of Medicine,
Denver, Colorado, CO, USA

Beau M. Ances (Chapter 45)
Department of Neurology,
Hospital of the University of Pennsylvania, PA, USA

Donald D. Anthony (Chapter 33)
Departments of Medicine and Pathology,
Case Western Reserve University,
The Cleveland Clinic Foundation,
Cleveland, OH, USA

Philip E. Auron (Chapter 7)
University of Pittsburgh School of Medicine,
University of Pittsburgh, Pittsburgh, PA, USA

Laura J. Balcer (Chapter 45)
Department of Neurology, Hospital of the
University of Pennsylvania, PA, USA

Edward D. Ball (Chapter 41)
Blood and Bone Marrow Transplantation Program
and Division, University of California,
San Diego, CA, USA

Penelope A. Bedford (Chapter 30)
Antigen Presentation Research Group,
Northwick Park Institute for Medical Research,
Imperial College Faculty of Medicine, London, UK

Jeff L Bidwell (Chapter 4)
University of Bristol, Department of Pathology, Bristol, UK

Jeffrey A. Bluestone (Foreword)
Immune Tolerance Network, UCSF Diabetes
Center and the Department of Medicine,
University of California,
San Francisco, CA, USA

Ezio Bonifacio (Chapter 15)
Immunology of Diabetes Unit and Diagnostica e
Ricerca San Raffaele, San Raffaele Scientific Institute,
Milan, Italy

Franklin A. Bontempo (Chapter 37)
University of Pittsburgh School of Medicine,
Pittsburgh, PA, USA

Deborah Braun (Chapter 32)
Laboratory of Dendritic Cell Immunobiology,
Pasteur Institute, Paris, France

William J. Burlingham (Chapter 35)
Department of Surgery/Transplant,
The Ohio State University College of Medicine,
Columbus, Ohio, USA

Sharon Chambers (Chapter 44)
Centre for Rheumatology, Department of Medicine,
London, UK

Amy Y. Chow (Chapter 2)
Department of Cell Biology and Section of
Immunobiology, Ludwig Institute for Cancer
Research, Yale University School of Medicine,
New Haven, Connecticut, USA

Timothy M. Clay (Chapter 28)
Departments of Surgery, Pathology, Immunology and
Medicine, Duke University Medical Center,
Durham, USA

Jan Willem Cohen Tervaert (Chapter 48)
Departments of Medical Microbiology,
Neurology, Pathology and Internal Medicine,
Academic Hospital Maastricht, Maastricht,
The Netherlands

Bonnie A. Colleton (Chapter 50)
Department of Pathology, University of Pittsburgh,
PA, USA

Anne Cooke (Chapter 8)
University of Cambridge, Tennis Court Road,
Cambridge, UK

Darshana Dadhania (Chapter 49)
Department of Transplantation Medicine,
The New York Presbyterian Hospital,
Weill Cornell Medical Center,
New York, NY, USA

Jan Damoiseaux (Chapter 48)
Departments of Medical Microbiology, Neurology,
Pathology and Internal Medicine, Academic Hospital
Maastricht, Maastricht, The Netherlands

Richard DeMarco (Chapters 19 and 29)
University of Pittsburgh School of Medicine,
Pittsburgh, PA, USA

Mary L. Disis (Chapter 40)
UW Medical Center, Seattle, WA, USA

Manuel Matas Docampo (Chapter 54)
Servicio de Cirugia Vascular y Endovascular, Hospital
Universitario Vall d'Hebron, Barcelona, Spain

Albert D. Donnenberg (Chapter 20)
Departments of Medicine, Infectious Disease and
Microbiology, University of Pittsburgh Schools of
Medicine, Graduate School of Public Health,
Pittsburgh, PA, USA

Vera S. Donnenberg (Chapter 20)
Departments of Surgery and Pharmaceutical Sciences,
University of Pittsburgh Schools of Medicine and
Pharmacy, Pittsburgh, PA, USA

Diane Dubois (Chapter 12)
Department of Pathology, Division of Clinical
Immunopathology, University of Pittsburgh Medical
Center, Pittsburgh, PA, USA

Clemens Esche (Chapter 53)
Johns Hopkins University, Baltimore, MD, USA

Joyce Eskdale (Chapter 4)
Department of Oral Biology, University of Medicine and
Dentistry of New Jersey, Newark, New Jersey, USA

Zoltán Fehérvari (Chapter 27)
Department of Experimental Pathology, Institute for
Frontier Medical Sciences, Kyoto University, Sakyo-ku,
Kyoto, Japan

Jennifer E. Fenner (Chapter 5)
Centre for Functional Genomics and Human Disease,
Monash Institute of Reproduction and Development,
Monash University, Clayton, Victoria, Australia

Kenneth Field (Chapter 24)
Department of Microbiology and Immunology,
University of Melbourne, Royal Parade, Parkville,
Victoria, Australia

Kenneth A. Foon (Chapter 13)
Division of Hematology-Oncology, University of
Pittsburgh Cancer Institute, Pittsburgh, PA, USA

Grant Gallagher (Chapter 4)
Department of Oral Biology, University of Medicine
and Dentistry of New Jersey, Newark,
New Jersey, USA

Dmitriy W. Gutkin (Chapter 9)
VA Pittsburgh Healthcare System,
Pittsburgh, PA, USA

Derek N.J. Hart (Chapter 24)
Mater Medical Research Institute, Aubigny Place,
South Brisbane, Australia

Choli Hartono (Chapter 49)
Department of Transplanation Medicine,
The New York Presbyterian Hospital,
Weill Cornell Medical Center,
New York, NY, USA

Milos Hauskrecht (Chapter 57)
Department of Computer Science, University of
Pittsburgh, PA, USA

Thomas Hawn (Chapter 6)
Division of Infectious Diseases, University of Washington
Medical Center, Seattle, WA, USA

Theodore L. Hazlett (Chapter 16)
Laboratory for Fluorescence Dynamics,
University of Illinois at Urbana-Champaign,
Urbana, IL, USA

Peter S. Heeger (Chapter 33)
Department of Immunology, The Cleveland Clinic
Foundation, Cleveland, OH, USA

Paul J. Hertzog (Chapter 5)
Centre for Functional Genomics and Human Disease,
Monash Institute of Reproduction and Development,
Monash University, Clayton, Victoria, Australia

Gottfried Himmler (Chapter 26)
IGENEON Krebs-Immuntherapie, Forschungs- und
Entwicklungs-AG, Vienna, Austria

Amy C. Hobeika (Chapter 28)
Departments of Surgery, Pathology, Immunology and
Medicine, Duke University Medical Center, Durham, USA

Peter Holman (Chapter 41)
University of California, La Jolla, USA

Donald E. Hricik (Chapter 33)
Departments of Medicine and Pathology, Case Western
Reserve University, The Cleveland Clinic Foundation,
Cleveland, OH, USA

David A. Isenberg (Chapter 44)
Centre for Rheumatology, Department of Medicine,
London, UK

Ewa Jankowska-Gan (Chapter 35)
Department of Surgery and Transplantation,
The Ohio State University College of Medicine,
Columbus, Ohio, USA

Kenneth Kalunian (Chapter 17)
UCLA Medical Plaza, Los Angeles, CA, USA

Tatsuya Kanto (Chapter 52)
Department of Molecular Therapeutics, Department of
Dendritic Cell Biology and Clinical Application, Osaka
University Graduate School of Medicine, Osaka, Japan

Sirid-Aimée Kellermann (Chapter 13)
Abgenix, Inc., USA

Stella C. Knight (Chapter 30)
Antigen Presentation Research Group,
Northwick Park Institute for Medical Research,
Imperial College Faculty of Medicine, UK

Andres Kriete (Chapter 61)
School of Biomedical Engineering Science and
Health Systems, Drexel University,
Philadelphia, PA, USA

Martin A.F.J. van de Laar (Chapter 14)
Department for Rheumatology, Medisch Spectrum
Twente & University Twente, The Netherlands

Vito Lampasona (Chapter 15)
Immunology of Diabetes Unit and Diagnostica e Ricerca
San Raffaele, San Raffaele Scientific Institute, Milan, Italy

Peter P. Lee (Chapter 22)
Department of Medicine, Division of Hematology,
Stanford University School of Medicine, Stanford, CA,
USA

Chau-Ching Liu (Chapters 10 and 11)
Division of Rheumatology and Clinical Immunology,
University of Pittsburgh School of Medicine, Pittsburgh,
PA, USA

Hans Loibner (Chapter 26)
IGENEON Krebs-Immuntherapie, Forschungs- und
Entwicklungs-AG, Vienna, Austria

Anna Lokshin (Chapter 18)
Department of Obstetrics/Gynecology and
Reproductive Sciences, University of Pittsburgh,
Pittsburgh, PA, USA

Brian J. Lopresti (Chapter 39)
Department of Radiology, University of Pittsburgh,
Pittsburgh, PA, USA

Michael T. Lotze (Preface, Chapters 19, 29, 57 and 58)
Director, Translational Research, Molecular Medicine
Institute, University of Pittsburgh School of Medicine,
Pittsburgh, PA, USA

Matthew J. Loza (Chapter 21)
Jefferson Medical College, Department of
Microbiology and Immunology, Kimmel Cancer Center,
Philadelphia, PA, USA

Lina Lu (Chapter 58)
Starzl Transplantation Institute, Pittsburgh School of
Medicine, Pittsburgh, PA, USA

Patrizia Luppi (Chapter 43)
Division of Immunogenetics, Children's Hospital of
Pittsburgh, Pittsburgh, PA, USA

H. Kim Lyerly (Chapter 28)
Departments of Surgery, Pathology, Immunology and
Medicine, Duke University Medical Center,
Durham, USA

James Lyons-Weiler (Chapter 57)
Department of Computer Science, University of
Pittsburgh, PA, USA

David Malehorn (Chapter 57)
Department of Computer Science, University of
Pittsburgh, PA, USA

Ashley Mansell (Chapter 5)
Centre for Functional Genomics and Human Disease,
Monash Institute of Reproduction and Development,
Monash University, Clayton,
Victoria, Australia

Francesco M. Marincola (Chapter 59)
Immunogenetics Section Department of Transfusion
Medicine, Clinical Center, National Institutes of Health,
Bethesda, Maryland, USA

N. Scott Mason (Chapter 39)
Department of Radiology, University of Pittsburgh,
Pittsburgh, PA, USA

Chester A. Mathis (Chapter 39)
Department of Radiology, University of Pittsburgh,
Pittsburgh, PA, USA

David H. McDermott (Chapter 3)
Laboratory of Host Defenses, National Institute of
Allergy and Infectious Diseases, NIH,
Bethesda, MD, USA

Maureen McMahon (Chapter 17)
UCLA Medical Plaza, Los Angeles, CA, USA

Ira Mellman (Chapter 2)
Department of Cell Biology and Section of
Immunobiology, Ludwig Institute for Cancer Research,
Yale University School of Medicine, New Haven,
Connecticut, USA

Diana Metes (Chapter 9)
Department of Surgery, Division of Clinical
Immunopathology, Pittsburgh, PA, USA

Michael A. Morse (Chapter 28)
Departments of Surgery, Pathology, Immunology and
Medicine, Duke University Medical Center,
Durham, USA

Paul J. Mosca (Chapter 28)
Departments of Surgery, Pathology, Immunology and
Medicine, Duke University Medical Center, Durham, USA

Salvador Nares (Chapter 25)
Oral Infection and Immunity Branch,
National Institute of Dental and Craniofacial Research,
NIH, Bethesda, MD, USA

Nancy J. Newman (Chapter 45)
Department of Neurology, Emory School of Medicine,
Emory University, Atlanta, GA, USA

Andreas Obwaller (Chapter 26)
IGENEON Krebs-Immuntherapie, Forschungs- und
Entwicklungs-AG, Vienna, Austria

Charles G. Orosz (Chapter 35)
Department of Surgery/Transplant, The Ohio State
University College of Medicine, Columbus, Ohio, USA

Takuya Osada (Chapter 28)
Departments of Surgery, Pathology, Immunology and
Medicine, Duke University Medical Center,
Durham, USA

Monica C. Panelli (Chapter 59)
Immunogenetics Section Department of Transfusion
Medicine, Clinical Center, National Institutes of Health,
Bethesda, Maryland, USA

Robertson Parkman (Chapter 55)
Division of Research Immunology/Bone Marrow
Transplantation and The Saban Research Institute,
Children's Hospital Los Angeles, Los Angeles, CA, USA

Patricia Paukovits (Chapter 26)
IGENEON Krebs-Immuntherapie, Forschungs- und
Entwicklungs-AG, Vienna, Austria

Richard Pelikan (Chapter 57)
Department of Computer Science, University of
Pittsburgh, Pittsburgh, PA, USA

Ronald P. Pelletier (Chapter 35)
Department of Surgical Oncology, The Ohio State
University College of Medicine, Columbus,
Ohio, USA

Bice Perussia (Chapter 21)
Jefferson Medical College, Department of Microbiology
and Immunology, Kimmel Cancer Center, Philadelphia,
PA, USA

Popovic Petar (Chapter 12)
Department of Surgery, University of Pittsburgh
School of Medicine, Pittsburgh, PA, USA

Paolo Piazza (Chapter 50)
Department of Pathology, University of Pittsburgh, PA, USA

Scott E. Plevy (Chapter 46)
Division of Gastroenterology, Hepatology and Nutrition
Inflammatory Bowel Disease Center, Pittsburgh,
PA, USA

Jillian A. Poole (Chapter 56)
University of Colorado Health Science Center and
the Division of Allergy and Clinical Immunology,
National Jewish Medical and Research
Center, Denver, CO, USA

Bruce S. Rabin (Chapter 12)
Department of Pathology, Division of Clinical
Immunopathology, University of Pittsburgh Medical
Center, Pittsburgh, PA, USA

Miguel Reguiero (Chapter 46)
Division of Gastroenterology, Hepatology and Nutrition
Co-Director, Inflammatory Bowel Disease Center,
Pittsburgh, PA, USA

Charles R. Rinaldo Jr (Chapter 50)
Department of Pathology
University of Pittsburgh, PA, USA

Lanny J. Rosenwasser (Chapter 56)
University of Colorado Health Science Center and the
Division of Allergy and Clinical Immunology, National
Jewish Medical and Research Center, Denver, CO, USA

Lorin K. Roskos (Chapter 13)
Abgenix, Inc., USA

David Rowe (Chapter 51)
Department of Infectious Diseases and Microbiology,
Graduate School of Public Health, Pittsburgh, PA, USA

Shimon Sakaguchi (Chapter 27)
Department of Experimental Pathology, Institute for
Frontier Medical Sciences, Kyoto University, Sakyo-ku,
Kyoto, Japan

Russell D. Salter (Chapter 1)
University of Pittsburgh School of Medicine,
Pittsburgh, PA, USA

Minnie Sarwal (Chapter 60)
Lucile Salter Packard Children's Hospital Nephrology,
Stanford, California, CA, USA

Vicki Seyfert-Margolis (Foreword)
Immune Tolerance Network, UCSF Diabetes Center and
the Department of Medicine, University of California,
San Francisco, CA, USA

Michael R. Shurin (Chapters 9 and 12)
Department of Pathology, Division of Clinical
Immunopathology, University of Pittsburgh Medical
Center, Pittsburgh, PA, USA

Craig L. Slingluff, Jr (Chapter 38)
Department of Surgery, University of Virginia,
Charlottesville, USA

Andrew J. Stagg (Chapter 30)
Antigen Presentation Research Group, Northwick Park
Institute for Medical Research, Imperial College Faculty
of Medicine, UK

Michael T. Stang (Chapter 47)
Department of Surgery, University of Pittsburgh
School of Medicine, Pittsburgh, PA, USA

Manikkam Suthanthiran (Chapter 49)
Division of Nephrology, Departments of Medicine and
Transplantation Medicine, Weill Medical College of
Cornell University, New York, NY, USA

D. Lansing Taylor (Chapter 58)
Chairman and CEO, Cellomics Inc.,
Pittsburgh, PA, USA

Peter C. Taylor (Chapter 42)
The Kennedy Institute of Rheumatology Division, Faculty
of Medicine, Imperial College London, London, UK

Sergey Y. Tetin (Chapter 16)
Abbott Laboratories, Abbott Diagnostics Division,
Abbott Park, IL, USA

Angus W. Thomson (Preface)
Director of Transplant Immunology
University of Pittsburgh, Pittsburgh, PA, USA

Massimo Trucco (Chapter 43)
Division of Immunogenetics, Children's Hospital of
Pittsburgh, Pittsburgh, PA, USA

David M. Underhill (Chapter 6)
Institute for Systems Biology, Seattle, WA, USA

Julia J. Unternaehrer (Chapter 2)
Department of Cell Biology and Section of
Immunobiology, Ludwig Institute for Cancer
Research, Yale University School of Medicine,
New Haven, Connecticut, USA

Anne M. VanBuskirk (Chapter 35)
Department of Surgery, The Ohio State University
College of Medicine, Columbus, Ohio, USA

Jean-Pierre Vendrell (Chapter 23)
Centre Hospitalier Régional et Universitaire de
Montpellier, Institut National de la Santé et de la
Recherche Médicale, France

Slavica Vuckovic (Chapter 24)
Mater Medical Research Institute, Aubigny Place, South
Brisbane, Australia

Nikola L. Vujanovic (Chapter 34)
University of Pittsburgh Cancer Institute, Hillman Cancer
Center, Pittsburgh, PA, USA

Sharon M. Wahl (Chapter 25)
Oral Infection and Immunity Branch, National Institute of
Dental and Craniofacial Research, NIH, Bethesda, MD,
USA

Theresa L. Whiteside (Chapter 31)
University of Pittsburgh Cancer Institute, Research
Pavilion at the Hillman Cancer Center, Pittsburgh, PA,
USA

Stephen E. Winikoff (Chapters 19 and 29)
University of Pittsburgh School of Medicine, Pittsburgh,
PA, USA

Galina V. Yamshchikov (Chapter 38)
Department of Surgery, University of Virginia,
Charlottesville, USA

John H. Yim (Chapter 47)
Department of Surgery, University of Pittsburgh School of
Medicine, Pittsburgh, PA, USA

Herbert J. Zeh (Chapters 19 and 29)
University of Pittsburgh School of Medicine, Pittsburgh,
PA, USA

Section I

Fundamentals of the immune response

MHC Class I

Chapter
1

Russell D. Salter

Department of Immunology, University of Pittsburgh School of Medicine, Pittsburgh, PA USA

Self-defence is nature's eldest law.

John Dryden

INTRODUCTION

Although class I MHC proteins were first identified over 50 years ago, their function has only been understood in detail in the past two decades. The three-dimensional structure of the human class I molecule HLA-A2 represented a landmark achievement in the field (Bjorkman et al., 1987a,b). The structure revealed the presence of a binding cleft suggesting antigen binding capability and offered tantalizing evidence of the nature of peptides bound. Shortly thereafter, bacterially produced recombinant class I proteins were re-folded with synthetic peptides which, upon crystallographic analysis, elucidated the molecular details of peptide binding in the cleft (Garrett et al., 1989). In addition to their importance for understanding T-cell recognition, these studies formed the basis for developing class I MHC tetramers, reagents with widespread current use in identifying antigen-specific CD8+ T cells, as will be discussed elsewhere in this volume.

A further seminal discovery was made by Rammensee and coworkers and Van Bleek and Nathenson who first developed methods for extracting peptides from the class I binding cleft (Van Bleek and Nathenson, 1990; Falk et al., 1991). These pooled peptides were analyzed by Edman degradation, resulting in mixed sequences which,

nonetheless, revealed some very important properties of class I MHC-binding peptides. The presence of relatively conserved residues at certain positions of all peptides bound to a single type of class I molecule was noted. These were designated anchor residues, based on their role in stabilizing peptide binding. In a leap of insight, highly variable positions within the peptide were proposed to potentially interact with T cell receptors (TCR) and this was later confirmed by crystallographic analyses (Garboczi et al., 1996). The identities and positions of the anchor residues when summarized for an individual class I MHC protein represented its 'peptide binding motif'. This concept has been invaluable for prediction of possible MHC binding peptides within a protein of interest, since without this information, sets of peptides covering the entire protein would need to be tested as potential epitopes. It is now commonplace to use computer-based algorithms, many available on the world wide web, to interrogate protein sequences for sequences corresponding to binding motifs of interest and to base epitope discovery strategies upon such information (Papassavas and Stavropoulos-Giokas, 2002; Hebart et al., 2003; Peters et al., 2003; Saxova et al., 2003).

In this chapter, our current knowledge of class I MHC biology and how this may impact treatment of diseases that involve CD8+ T cell responses will be reviewed. In addition, the importance of the high degree of allelic polymorphism present in class I MHC heavy chains will be discussed. How processing of antigens for class I MHC presentation influences the immune response to be

Measuring Immunity, edited by Michael T. Lotze and Angus W. Thomson
ISBN 0-12-455900-X, London

generated will also be explored, with emphasis on the molecular mechanisms involved.

CLASS I GENES WITHIN THE MHC REGION

Genetic and physical mapping analyses by many laboratories culminated several years ago in publication of the complete sequence of the human MHC region (Beck and Trowsdale, 2000). The presence of dozens of class I loci, including the well known HLA-A, B and C loci, as well as a number of other class I genes, both functional and nonfunctional, were revealed. Of these, only HLA-A, B and C have been shown definitively to present peptide antigens to CD8+ T cells. HLA-C may have as its primary role interaction with receptors on NK cells that either inhibit or activate lytic function (Fan et al., 1996; Snyder et al., 1999). In contrast, the best known function of HLA-A and -B molecules is to present peptide antigens to CD8+ T cells.

POLYMORPHISM IN CLASS I MHC HEAVY CHAINS

Class I HLA alleles were first identified using antibodies generated in multiparous or transfused individuals and then later using monoclonal antibodies developed by immunizing mice with human cells or purified HLA proteins (Parham, 1983). Serological definition resulted in designation of class molecules such as HLA-A2 or -B7, with numerical names assigned for each locus roughly in their order of discovery. Biochemical analyses using isoelectric focusing revealed additional heterogeneity within the serologic designations and many specificities were divided further into subtypes based on differences in electrophoretic charge (Neefjes et al., 1986). With the advent of widespread DNA sequencing, definitive analyses were soon possible, leading to a great expansion of the number of alleles identified at each locus. For example, HLA-A2, a specificity defined on the basis of antibody reactivity, has been subdivided into 15 alleles as defined by DNA sequencing (Parham et al., 1989). Although some of these alleles are distinguished by non-coding substitutions, others differ at nucleotides that result in amino acid differences, some of which demonstrably alter peptide binding or T-cell recognition.

There are currently identified over 200 alleles at HLA-A and about 400 at HLA-B, with most of the variation in amino acid sequence between alleles present in residues in the peptide binding cleft (Parham et al., 1989). This strongly supports the hypothesis that sequence diversification is driven by the requirement for broad antigen presentation capability, particularly in pathogen-laden environments. Examples of class I alleles that are associated with resistance to certain diseases have been identified, such as that observed in West Africa, where HLA-B53 has been associated with resistance to severe malaria (Hill et al., 1992).

MOLECULAR TYPING OF CLASS I HLA ALLELES

A review of the technical aspects of MHC typing is beyond the scope of this chapter, but some of the principles will be discussed briefly. Primer sets are designed and used for PCR amplification of cDNA to obtain fragments of class I genes, typically those encoding the α1 and α2 domains, where most of the polymorphism resides. After the amplified fragments are applied to a membrane, labeled oligonucleotide probes that can anneal to specific regions of individual class I genes are used in liquid hybridization to detect alleles. Alternatively, additional allele-specific primers are used in a second round of PCR amplification to generate DNA fragments that allow for allele assignment. For both approaches, prior knowledge of class I sequences is necessary and novel or unknown alleles cannot be identified. In the research laboratory setting, it is typically more efficient to identify class I alleles from unknown cells using DNA sequencing of the primary PCR product, rather than establishing secondary screening procedures mentioned above. In a clinical testing laboratory, where multiple samples will be routinely analyzed, the use of secondary screening assays, such as filter hybridization, is more common. There are a number of technologies that are being currently developed to reduce the expense or effort required for molecular HLA testing. Some of these involve the development of membrane or bead arrays that allow for automation of these processes (Guo et al., 1999; Balazs et al., 2001).

CLASS I MHC ANTIGEN PROCESSING PATHWAY

How peptides are generated from protein antigens in the cytosol for delivery to class I molecules has been studied intensively in the past decade. At the forefront in this process is the proteasome, a large organelle with multiple proteolytic activities. Rock and Goldberg and their coworkers first demonstrated that proteasome inhibitors could inhibit class I MHC antigen processing and presentation to T cells (Michalek et al., 1993; Goldberg et al., 2002). This was due to blocking generation of the major supply of peptides required for stabilization of class I molecules and the lack of this peptide pool resulted in their retention in the endoplasmic reticulum (ER). This phenotype was similar to that seen in mutant cell lines that lack the proteins TAP (transporter of antigenic peptides) or tapasin (DeMars et al., 1985; Salter and Cresswell, 1986; Ortmann et al., 1997). These latter proteins are required to facilitate peptide transport into the ER and subsequent class I loading.

The class I biosynthetic pathway can be summarized as follows (Table 1.1). Class I heavy chains are inserted into the lumen of the ER and associate cotranslationally with a second subunit, β_2-microglobulin (β_2m) and with

Table 1.1 Antigen processing machinery associated with class I MHC proteins

Accessory protein(s)	Molecular weight (kDa)	Family	Binds to:	Binding site on class I molecule	Polymorphic
Calnexin	65	Lectin-type chaperone	Newly synthesized heavy (H) chain	N-linked glycan at asparagine 86 in α1; also sites on protein	No
ER$_p$57	57	Thiolreductase	Calnexin-associated H chain	Sulfhydryl group in α3	No
Calreticulin	46	Lectin-type chaperone	H chain-β_2m complex	N-linked glycan at asparagine 86 in α1	No
Tapasin	48	Ig superfamily	H chain-β_2m-calreticulin complex	Loop in α2 residues 128–136, α3 residues 219–233	No
TAP1 TAP2	72	ABC-transporter	H chain-β_2m-calreticulin-tapasin complex	None (associates with class I complex via tapasin)	Yes; allelic differences in rat, mouse and human; functional differences between allelic forms in rat

calnexin, a molecular chaperone that binds to N-glycans and protein elements of substrate proteins (Jackson et al., 1994; Tector and Salter, 1995; Zhang et al., 1995; Diedrich et al., 2001; Paquet and Williams, 2002). ERp57, which promotes protein folding through formation and disruption of disulfide bonds, also associates with the class I dimer (Radcliffe et al., 2002). As conformational stability is attained, another N-glycan-recognizing chaperone, calreticulin, binds thereby displacing calnexin from human class I molecules (Sadasivan et al., 1996). At this stage, class I molecules associate with at least two additional molecules, tapasin and TAP, which have specific roles in facilitating peptide loading (Sadasivan et al., 1996; Zarling et al., 2003). Tapasin binds to class I heavy chains via residues in the α2 and α3 domains and also interacts with TAP (Paquet and Williams, 2002). TAP is the transporter of antigenic peptides that has been shown to translocate peptides from the cytosol into the ER lumen (Androlewicz et al., 1994). Class I dimers in the fully constituted peptide loading complex described above undergo a conformational change that increases their receptivity to peptides (Suh et al., 1999; Reits et al., 2000). The local concentration of peptides imported by TAP is likely to be relatively high in the vicinity of the complex, which may explain why most class I molecules are able to bind appropriate peptides even when the motifs recognized are relatively uncommon.

PROTEOLYTIC PROCESSING OF PROTEINS BY PROTEASOMES TO GENERATE CLASS I-BINDING PEPTIDES

The proteasome plays a central role in degradation of proteins within all cells, including bacteria and all higher life forms. Thus it is clear that class I MHC molecules evolved at a much later stage to survey intracellular peptides derived from proteasome and that class I presented epitopes are necessarily related to their cleavage specificity. Proteasomes are highly complex structures, consisting of more than a dozen individual subunits, and can be categorized as either regulatory or catalytic in activity (DeMartino and Slaughter, 1999). These are arranged in four stacks of seven membered rings to constitute the core or 20S proteasome, which has a central pore through which protein substrates pass to undergo cleavage (Figure 1.1). The diameter of the pore is such that globular proteins would usually need to become unfolded to allow for threading through the central passage. An additional protein complex, PA700, binds to each end of the structure to generate the 26S proteasome. PA700 consists of ~20 subunits and has the capacity to bind to ubiquinated substrates, which imparts selectivity for unfolded proteins that have become modified through recognition by ubiquitin-conjugating enzymes (Strickland et al., 2000). In several cases, ubiquination of antigens has been shown to increase their degradation and presentation by class I MHC molecules, presumably by this mechanism. An additional regulator of proteasome activity, consisting of members of the PA28 family, can be upregulated by IFNγ, but does not recognize ubiquinated substrates. There is evidence suggesting that PA28 modified proteasome may be able to generate some epitopes that bind to class I MHC with high efficiency (Preckel et al., 1999).

Further modifications of the proteasome are also possible by incorporation of MHC-encoded subunits, such as LMP-2 and LMP-7, and also the subunit MECL (Griffin et al., 1998). Expression of these proteins is induced by IFNγ and in the case of LMP-2, also IFNα, and the subunits replace catalytic subunits of the core proteasome. These modifications result in generation of

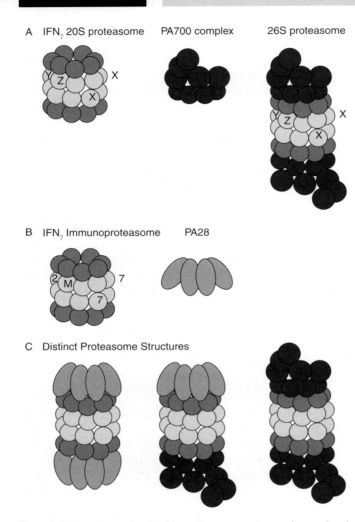

A   IFN$_\gamma$ 20S proteasome   PA700 complex   26S proteasome

B   IFN$_\gamma$ Immunoproteasome   PA28

C   Distinct Proteasome Structures

Figure 1.1 Proteasomes involved in antigen processing can be regulated by IFNγ. In A, the structure of the 20S constitutive proteasome is shown, with α subunits dark gray and β subunits in light gray. Addition of the PA700 complex results in 26S proteasome. In B, subunits X, Y and Z are replaced by LMP-2 (2), MECL (M) and LMP-7 (7) to generate immunoproteasome following stimulation by IFNγ, which also induces the PA28 complex. In C, possible combined proteasomes are shown (figure modified from Fruh and Yang, 1999).

immunoproteasomes, which have properties distinct from constitutive 26S proteasomes, including increased cleavage of substrates at sites with certain amino acid residues, such as positively charged residues lysine or arginine or hydrophobic residues such as valine, isoleucine or leucine when activated via PA28γ (Fruh and Yang, 1999). Decreased cleavage capacity after negatively charged residues such as glutamic or aspartic acids is also seen. These observations can be interpreted in a satisfying way by noting that the C-terminal positions of many class I binding peptides are constrained to be positively charged or hydrophobic residues, but rarely are negatively charged acidic residues. This suggests that immunoproteasomes are particularly equipped to generate the C-terminal end of the potential class I binding peptides.

AMINOPEPTIDASES IN CLASS I ANTIGEN PROCESSING

In contrast to constraints at the C-terminus of peptides, there is no indication that proteasomes of any type are able to tailor peptides with appropriate amino termini for binding class I MHC, or that cleavage is precisely controlled to generate the 8–9 amino acid long peptides that are typically bound to class I molecules. This suggests that further trimming of the amino terminus might be required to generate many peptide epitopes. Rock and co-workers and Shastri and coworkers have identified aminopeptidases that fulfil such a role in the ER (ERAP1 or ERAAP, ER-associated aminopeptidase) (Serwold et al., 2002; York et al., 2002). There is strong evidence that these latter enzymes are necessary to generate at least a subset of peptides that can bind efficiently to class I MHC.

DRIPS AS SOURCE OF CLASS I MHC BINDING PEPTIDES

Jonathan Yewdell and coworkers several years ago demonstrated that protein biosynthesis within cells is far less efficient than had previously been presumed. By careful measurements using metabolic radiolabeling, it was shown that a major fraction of newly synthesized proteins is rapidly degraded, due to defects that prevent polypeptides from attaining their final conformation, including mis-translation, mis-folding and truncation (Schubert et al., 2000). These products, called defective ribosomal initiation products (DRiPs), have particular importance for class I MHC antigen processing, since they are substrates for processing by proteasomes and subsequent TAP transport. The most convincing evidence that DRiPs form an important source of class I-bound peptides derives from experiments measuring the kinetics of presentation with protein antigens of well-characterized stability. In experiments where protein synthesis could be tightly regulated temporally, class I presentation clearly depended on the presence of newly synthesized antigen and did not require 'aging' of intact protein to allow for its degradation after unfolding (Princiotta et al., 2003). This demonstrates that the class I antigen processing pathway can respond more rapidly to antigenic challenge than was previously believed during intracellular infections where endogenously synthesized antigens are presented, as represented in Figure 1.2.

ANOTHER POSSIBILITY: PEPTIDE SPLICING

Although the previous sections have documented several ways in which potential epitopes are generated, there may exist still another possibility. Hanada and coworkers recently showed that a tumor antigen, fibroblast growth

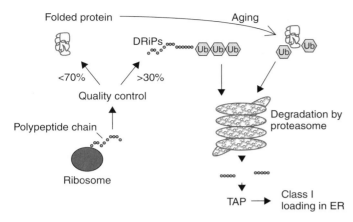

Figure 1.2 Generation of class I binding peptides either from the DRiPs (defective ribosomal initiation products) pathway or from the conventional pathway by which cytosolic proteins that unfold are degraded. Both pathways involve proteasomal degradation as shown to generate short peptides that are transported into the ER lumen by TAP.

factor-5, could provide an epitope that binds to HLA-A3 (Hanada et al., 2004). What was unusual about this epitope was that the residues were not contiguous within the protein sequence, but instead were a patchwork consisting of five residues from one region of the protein and four residues from a region located more than 20 positions closer to the C′ terminus. Although it must be stated that this isolated example does not allow an estimate of how often this type of splicing occurs, it has interesting implications for antigen processing, particularly in the area of autoimmunity, where splicing of peptides in the periphery but not in the thymus could generate unique autoantigens. So far, novel enzymes capable of splicing peptides have been identified in some plants, but not in animal cells.

AN ADDITIONAL INTRACELLULAR SITE FOR CLASS I ANTIGEN PROCESSING AND LOADING IN DENDRITIC CELLS

There is intense interest in how dendritic cells process and present exogenous antigens via class I molecules, as discussed elsewhere in this book. This process is called cross-presentation and is critical for generation of CD8+ T cell responses in infectious diseases and cancer. Particulate antigens are typically quite efficient at inducing cross-presentation, suggesting that dendritic cells might have unique pathways for inducing their loading into class I MHC (Kovacsovics-Bankowski and Rock, 1995). There have now been several reports demonstrating that components of the ER, including class I MHC dimers and the associated processing components, TAP, tapasin, calreticulin, ERp57 and also ERAP, are present within latex bead-containing phagosomes (Garin et al., 2001; Ackerman et al., 2003; Guermonprez et al., 2003). This suggests that phagosomes are fully competent for processing antigens from

particulates for class I loading. The additional presence of SEC61 in the phagosome would allow for export of antigen out of the phagosome and into the cytosol where processing by proteasomes could occur, followed by import by TAP back into the phagosome. If the export and import processes are tightly coupled or linked by peptide carriers that allow for the continued association of antigen with an individual vesicle, processing of such antigens could take place entirely within the phagosome. It is also possible that exported antigen would be processed and then delivered to other sites within the ER where nascent class I complexes are present. A final possibility, which might be important for some epitopes, involves processing entirely within the phagosome by lysosomal hydrolases, without any contribution from proteasomes. This may explain TAP-independent presentation of some epitopes from particulates. How efficient and/or epitope-dependent each of these processes might be has not been established.

ALLELIC POLYMORPHISMS IN ANTIGEN PROCESSING ASSOCIATED MOLECULES

Given the large number of components needed for generation or loading of peptides into class I MHC molecules, heterogeneity in some or all of these components could presumably impact the process of antigen presentation in major ways. As will be discussed below, allelic polymorphism plays a relatively small role here, while regulation of expression and its dysregulation under some disease conditions appears more important in this regard.

Calnexin, calreticulin and ERp57 all are important for the folding of proteins in addition to class I MHC and thus allelic polymorphisms in these genes might affect a number of cellular processes in addition to antigen presentation. The same logic would apply to subunits of the proteasome, which plays a critical role in degradation of many cellular proteins. There have not been reports of allelic polymorphism in these proteins that impact the function of class I MHC. In contrast, tapasin and TAP function solely within the class I pathway. Allelic polymorphism within TAP has been identified. A particularly striking example was first reported in rats, where cimA and cimB, representing two allelic forms of TAP, were shown to differ dramatically in ability to transport peptides across membranes (Powis et al., 1996). This resulted in very different sets of peptides bound to the class I molecule RT-1A. In mice and humans, however, the allelic forms of TAP that have been identified differ in fairly minor ways and there is little evidence that this impacts peptide transport in a significant way (Heemels et al., 1993; Schumacher et al., 1994). TAP-1 polymorphism may play a bigger role than TAP-2 in this regard (Quadri and Singal, 1998). Although there have been a few conflicting reports, it is generally accepted that human and mouse TAP do not select peptides for transport based upon their sequence or amino acid composition to a great extent. However, there are constraints on peptide length as indicated by a preference for peptides between 7 and 15 amino acids (Androlewicz et al., 1994).

REGULATION OF CLASS I MHC ANTIGEN PROCESSING COMPONENTS

In contrast to allelic polymorphism, alterations in expression of many of the individual components mentioned above can dramatically impact antigen processing and T-cell recognition. The normal regulation of the class I antigen processing components has been studied to some extent, but there is clearly much work left to be done here, particularly in cell types such as dendritic cells that are of critical importance.

The promoter regions of class I genes and many associated processing components contain type I interferon (IFN) responsive elements and also IFNγ responsive elements. This can explain the observed upregulation of class I MHC in many different cell types following treatment with these IFN (Sugita et al., 1987). Upregulation of class I MHC would help to promote CD8+ T-cell-mediated immune responses during viral or other intracellular infections that have been shown to trigger IFNα production.

A less well understood process of class I MHC regulation is seen in dendritic cells during their maturation. Increases in surface class I MHC levels during maturation have been reported, although most groups find that this is somewhat variable and not always very large in magnitude. There are striking changes in TAP and proteasome subunits however, and, interestingly, these occur with maturation induced by toll-like receptor (TLR) ligands that are not known to cause a strong IFN response (Li et al., 2001; Gil-Torregrosa et al., 2004). The significance of these alterations is not well understood, but they presumably are important for processing of antigens that have been internalized. Thus the timing of the changes in expression of antigen processing components is likely to be critical and it will be important to understand the signaling pathways involved, as well as defining what may be novel regulatory elements in the promoters of genes involved in antigen processing that allow their upregulation in response to maturational stimuli.

DYSREGULATION OF CLASS I MHC ANTIGEN PROCESSING COMPONENTS

While an extensive review of this topic is beyond the scope of this chapter, it is well recognized that pathogens have developed strategies to subvert the immune response that include disruption of the class I MHC processing machinery. Herpes viruses in particular have a number of different proteins that can interact with class I heavy chains in the ER, resulting in their retention or degradation, in inhibition of

TAP function (ICP 47) or in altered antigen proteolysis (Jugovic et al., 1998; Petersen et al., 2003). Since the antigen processing machinery is highly interdependent, loss of one component often results in a global defect in class I MHC expression in infected cells.

In tumors that lose expression of class I MHC as a result of immune selective pressure, many of the same principles are observed. Loss of one or more of the antigen processing components can result in an overall decrease in class I levels (Kamarashev et al., 2001). Selective loss of individual alleles at class I loci has also been observed however, and the mechanism responsible for this is not always clear. In many tumors, downregulation of TAP or β_2m has been observed, while in others mutations in individual class I heavy chain genes have been reported. Loss of class I expression is often reversible and apparently due to transient selective pressure exerted by the immune response (Giorda et al., 2003).

FUTURE DIRECTIONS FOR CLASS I MHC RESEARCH AND CLINICAL APPLICATIONS

Towards better epitope prediction

The use of algorithms to predict MHC-binding peptides within antigens of interest is now routine and allows for more efficient experimental design (Papassavas and Stavropoulos-Giokas, 2002; Hebart et al., 2003; Peters et al., 2003; Saxova et al., 2003). However, typically only about 20–30 per cent of predicted binding peptides can be confirmed using experimental assays to measure binding. This may be due to the rudimentary state of early class I binding motifs, since more refined motifs incorporating secondary anchor positions have been developed for some class I molecules and shown to have greater predictive value. It will be also be necessary to determine whether splicing to generate peptide epitopes occurs frequently enough to warrant consideration in designing improved predictive algorithms. It has become apparent that affinity of peptide binding to class I MHC does not correlate with the likelihood that the peptide is an epitope and, in fact, there may be an optimal affinity of binding that characterizes agonist peptides. Some predictive algorithms incorporate this concept, but there does not seem to be general agreement upon how best to use affinity measurements of peptide binding to increase the overall success rate. Proteasomal cleavage sites have also been incorporated into some algorithms to increase the likelihood that predicted epitopes could be generated inside cells during antigen processing, as referenced above. Finally, it should be noted that peptide binding algorithms do not directly identify T cell epitopes, only predict MHC binding and this clearly remains a major obstacle to epitope mapping studies. The ability truly to predict epitopes would represent a quantum leap in the field, but it is unclear at this stage how this might be accomplished.

Detection of epitopes on the surface of antigen presenting cells

T cells have been used traditionally to detect the presence of processed antigen on the surface of cells and are very sensitive to small numbers of copies of an epitope. They usually do not allow for direct measurement of antigen processing efficiency however, since their stimulation depends upon factors in addition to MHC-antigen complex, including co-stimulation and cytokine production, during T cell priming at least. It would be desirable to quantitate the number of copies of epitopes presented on antigen presenting cells (APCs) in many situations and this has been accomplished using a monoclonal antibody that recognizes the OVA-derived SIINFEKL epitope bound to H-2K[b] (Porgador et al., 1997). The production of other such antibodies has been very difficult and the lack of reagents for important epitope-class I complexes in humans imposes a bottleneck for experiments related to vaccine design and immune evasion, where direct quantitation of antigen processing efficiency would be desirable. The development of additional such reagents through the use of synthetic antibody libraries may speed their design and production.

Subunit vaccine design

An important vaccine strategy for generation of CD8+ T cell responses against intracellular pathogens or tumors involves the use of genetic vectors that induce antigen expression in dendritic cells. Both viral (e.g. adenovirus, retrovirus) and bacterial (e.g. *Salmonella, Listeria*) vehicles have been used with some success by incorporation of cDNA encoding the antigen of interest (Darji et al., 2003; Nakamura et al., 2003; Russmann et al., 2003; Jaffray et al., 2004; Patterson et al., 2004; Worgall et al., 2004). Given our current understanding of class I antigen processing, it will be important to evaluate the potential of novel methods for antigen delivery, for example those that accentuate DRiP formation, as a way of promoting antigen presentation. These may provide superior means for stimulating CD8+ T cells if they promote epitope formation beyond that seen with processing of full length protein antigen.

Can antigen processing pathways in dendritic cells suggest strategies for improved vaccine development?

It is clear that dendritic cells (DC) have numerous adaptations that enhance their ability to stimulate both CD4 and CD8 T cell responses. What is less clear is how class I antigen processing is regulated in DC. Maturation induced by TLR ligands or cytokine mixes increases the antigen processing machinery within these cells and certainly they become more potent APC under these conditions (Gil-Torregrosa et al., 2004). However, it is difficult to separate these effects from those that accompany maturation such as increases in co-stimulation or cytokine production.

Since dendritic cells are now known to have specialized phagocytic compartments containing the class I antigen processing machinery (Ackerman et al., 2003), new strategies for vaccine delivery might take advantage of these observations, once we obtain a more complete understanding of the biology of the system.

REFERENCES

Ackerman, A.L., Kyritsis, C., Tampe, R. and Cresswell, P. (2003). Early phagosomes in dendritic cells form a cellular compartment sufficient for cross presentation of exogenous antigens. PNAS *100*, 12889–12894.

Androlewicz, M., Ortmann, B., Endert, P., Spies, T. and Cresswell, P. (1994). Characteristics of peptide and major histocompatibility complex class I/{beta}2-microglobulin binding to the transporters associated with antigen processing (TAP1 and TAP2). PNAS *91*, 12716–12720.

Balazs, I., Beekman, J., Neuweiler, J., Liu, H., Watson, E. and Ray, B. (2001). Molecular typing of HLA-A, -B, and DRB using a high throughput micro array format. Hum Immunol *62*, 850–857.

Beck, S. and Trowsdale, J. (2000). The human major histocompatability complex: lessons from the DNA sequence. Annu Rev Genomics Hum Genet *1*, 117–137.

Bjorkman, P., Saper, M., Samraoui, B., Bennett, W., Strominger, J. and Wiley, D. (1987a). The foreign antigen binding site and T cell recognition regions of class I histocompatibility antigens. Nature *329*, 512–518.

Bjorkman, P., Saper, M., Samraoui, B., Bennett, W., Strominger, J. and Wiley, D. (1987b). Structure of the human class I histocompatibility antigen, HLA-A2. Nature *329*, 506–512.

Darji, A., Mohamed, W., Domann, E. and Chakraborty, T. (2003). Induction of immune responses by attenuated isogenic mutant strains of Listeria monocytogenes. Vaccine *21*, S102–S109.

DeMars, R., Rudersdorf, R., Chang, C. et al. (1985). Mutations that impair a posttranscriptional step in expression of HLA-A and -B antigens. Proc Natl Acad Sci USA *82*, 8183–8187.

DeMartino, G.N. and Slaughter, C.A. (1999). The proteasome, a novel protease regulated by multiple mechanisms. J Biol Chem *274*, 22123–22126.

Diedrich, G., Bangia, N., Pan, M. and Cresswell, P. (2001). A role for calnexin in the assembly of the MHC class I loading complex in the endoplasmic reticulum. J Immunol *166*, 1703–1709.

Falk, K., Rotzschke, O., Stevanovic, S., Jung, G. and Rammensee, H. (1991). Allele-specific motifs revealed by sequencing of self-peptides eluted from MHC molecules. Nature *351*, 290–296.

Fan, Q.R., Garboczi, D.N., Winter, C.C., Wagtmann, N., Long, E.O. and Wiley, D.C. (1996). Direct binding of a soluble natural killer cell inhibitory receptor to a soluble human leukocyte antigen-Cw4 class I major histocompatibility complex molecule. PNAS *93*, 7178–7183.

Fruh, K. and Yang, Y. (1999). Antigen presentation by MHC class I and its regulation by interferon gamma. Curr Opin Immunol *11*, 76–81.

Garboczi, D., Ghosh, P., Utz, U. et al. (1996). Structure of the complex between human T-cell receptor, viral peptide and HLA-A2. Nature *384*, 134–141.

Garin, J., Diez, R., Kieffer, S. et al. (2001). The phagosome proteome: insight into phagosome functions. J Cell Biol *152*, 165–180.

Garrett, T., Saper, M., Bjorkman, P. et al. (1989). Specificity pockets for the side chains of peptide antigens in HLA-Aw68. Nature *342*, 692–696.

Gil-Torregrosa, B., Lennon-Dumenil, A., Kessler, B. et al. (2004). Control of cross-presentation during dendritic cell maturation. Eur J Immunol *34*, 398–407.

Giorda, E., Sibilio, L., Martayan, A. et al. (2003). The antigen processing machinery of class I human leukocyte antigens: linked patterns of gene expression in neoplastic cells. Cancer Res *63*, 4119–4127.

Goldberg, A.L., Cascio, P., Saric, T. and Rock, K.L. (2002). The importance of the proteasome and subsequent proteolytic steps in the generation of antigenic peptides. Mol Immunol *39*, 147–164.

Griffin, T.A., Nandi, D., Cruz, M. et al. (1998). Immunoproteasome assembly: cooperative incorporation of interferon gamma (IFN-gamma)-inducible subunits. J Exp Med *187*, 97–104.

Guermonprez, P., Saveanu, L., Kleijmeer, M., Davoust, J., Van Endert, P. and Amigorena, S. (2003). ER-phagosome fusion defines an MHC class I cross-presentation compartment in dendritic cells. Nature *425*, 397–402.

Guo, Z., Hood, L. and Petersdorf, E. (1999). Oligonucleotide arrays for high resolution HLA typing. Rev Immunogenet *1*, 220–230.

Hanada, K., Yewdell, J. and Yang, J. (2004). Immune recognition of a human renal cancer antigen through post-translational protein splicing. Nature *427*, 252–256.

Hebart, H., Rauser, G., Stevanovic, S. et al. (2003). A CTL epitope from human cytomegalovirus IE1 defined by combining prediction of HLA binding and proteasomal processing is the target of dominant immune responses in patients after allogeneic stem cell transplantation*1. Exp Hematol *31*, 966–973.

Heemels, M., Schumacher, T., Wonigeit, K. and Ploegh, H. (1993). Peptide translocation by variants of the transporter associated with antigen processing. Science *262*, 2059–2063.

Hill, A., Elvin, J., Willis, A. et al. (1992). Molecular analysis of the association of HLA-B53 and resistance to severe malaria. Nature *360*, 434–439.

Jackson, M., Cohen-Doyle, M., Peterson, P. and Williams, D. (1994). Regulation of MHC class I transport by the molecular chaperone, calnexin (p88, IP90). Science *263*, 384–387.

Jaffray, A., Shephard, E., van Harmelen, J., Williamson, C., Williamson, A.-L. and Rybicki, E.P. (2004). Human immunodeficiency virus type 1 subtype C Gag virus-like particle boost substantially improves the immune response to a subtype C gag DNA vaccine in mice. J Gen Virol *85*, 409–413.

Jugovic, P., Hill, A.M., Tomazin, R., Ploegh, H. and Johnson, D.C. (1998). Inhibition of major histocompatibility complex class I antigen presentation in pig and primate cells by herpes simplex virus type 1 and 2 ICP47. J Virol *72*, 5076–5084.

Kamarashev, J., Ferrone, S., Seifert, B. et al. (2001). TAP1 downregulation in primary melanoma lesions: an independent marker of poor prognosis. Int J Cancer *95*, 23–28.

Kovacsovics-Bankowski, M. and Rock, K. (1995). A phagosome-to-cytosol pathway for exogenous antigens presented on MHC class I molecules. Science *267*, 243–246.

Li, J., Schuler-Thurner, B., Schuler, G., Huber, C. and Seliger, B. (2001). Bipartite regulation of different components of the MHC class I antigen-processing machinery during dendritic cell maturation. Int Immunol *13*, 1515–1523.

Michalek, M., Grant, E., Gramm, C., Goldberg, A.L. and Rock, K. (1993). A role for the ubiquitin-dependent proteolytic pathway in MHC class I-restricted antigen presentation. Nature *363*, 552–554.

Nakamura, Y., Suda, T., Nagata, T. et al. (2003). Induction of protective immunity to Listeria monocytogenes with dendritic cells retrovirally transduced with a cytotoxic T lymphocyte epitope minigene. Infect Immun *71*, 1748–1754.

Neefjes, J., Breur-Vriesendorp, B., van Seventer, G., Ivanyi, P. and Ploegh, H. (1986). An improved biochemical method for the analysis of HLA-class I antigens. Definition of new HLA-class I subtypes. Hum Immunol *16*, 169–181.

Ortmann, B., Copeman, J., Lehner, P. et al. (1997). A critical role for tapasin in the assembly and function of multimeric MHC class I-TAP complexes. Science *277*, 1306–1309.

Papassavas, A.C. and Stavropoulos-Giokas, C. (2002). Definition of the immunogenic HLA epitopes based on an epitope prediction algorithm. Transplant Proc *34*, 2049–2052.

Paquet, M.-E. and Williams, D.B. (2002). Mutant MHC class I molecules define interactions between components of the peptide-loading complex. Int Immunol *14*, 347–358.

Parham, P. (1983). Monoclonal antibodies against HLA products and their use in immunoaffinity purification. Methods Enzymol *92*, 110–138.

Parham, P., Lawlor, D., Lomen, C. and Ennis, P. (1989). Diversity and diversification of HLA-A,B,C alleles. J Immunol *142*, 3937–3950.

Patterson, L.J., Malkevitch, N., Venzon, D. et al. (2004). Protection against mucosal Simian immunodeficiency virus SIVmac251 challenge by using replicating adenovirus-SIV multigene vaccine priming and subunit boosting. J Virol *78*, 2212–2221.

Peters, B., Tong, W., Sidney, J., Sette, A. and Weng, Z. (2003). Examining the independent binding assumption for binding of peptide epitopes to MHC-I molecules. Bioinformatics *19*, 1765–1772.

Petersen, J.L., Morris, C.R. and Solheim, J.C. (2003). Virus evasion of MHC Class I molecule presentation. J Immunol *171*, 4473–4478.

Porgador, A., Yewdell, J., Deng, Y., Bennink, J. and Germain, R. (1997). Localization, quantitation, and in situ detection of specific peptide-MHC class I complexes using a monoclonal antibody. Immunity *6*, 715–726.

Powis, S., Young, L., Joly, E. et al. (1996). The rat cim effect: TAP allele-dependent changes in a class I MHC anchor motif and evidence against C-terminal trimming of peptides in the ER. Immunity *4*, 159–165.

Preckel, T., Fung-Leung, W.-P., Cai, Z. et al. (1999). Impaired immunoproteasome assembly and immune responses in PA28/ mice. Science *286*, 2162–2165.

Princiotta, M., Finzi, D. et al. (2003). Quantitating protein synthesis, degradation, and endogenous antigen processing. Immunity *18*, 343–354.

Quadri, S. and Singal, D. (1998). Peptide transport in human lymphoblastoid and tumor cells: effect of transporter associated with antigen presentation (TAP) polymorphism. Immunol Lett *61*, 25–31.

Radcliffe, C.M., Diedrich, G., Harvey, D.J., Dwek, R.A., Cresswell, P. and Rudd, P.M. (2002). Identification of specific glycoforms of major histocompatibility complex class I heavy chains suggests that class I peptide loading is an adaptation of the quality control pathway involving calreticulin and ERp57. J Biol Chem *277*, 46415–46423.

Reits, E., Vos, J., Gromme, M. and Neefjes, J. (2000). The major substrates for TAP in vivo are derived from newly synthesized proteins. Nature *404*, 774–778.

Russmann, H., Gerdemann, U., Igwe, E.I. et al. (2003). Attenuated Yersinia pseudotuberculosis carrier vaccine for simultaneous antigen-specific CD4 and CD8 T-cell induction. Infect Immun 71, 3463–3472.

Sadasivan, B., Lehner, P., Ortmann, B., Spies, T. and Cresswell, P. (1996). Roles for calreticulin and a novel glycoprotein, tapasin, in the interaction of MHC class I molecules with TAP. Immunity 5, 103–114.

Salter, R. and Cresswell, P. (1986). Impaired assembly and transport of HLA-A and -B antigens in a mutant TxB cell hybrid. EMBO J 5, 934–939.

Saxova, P., Buus, S., Brunak, S. and Kesmir, C. (2003). Predicting proteasomal cleavage sites: a comparison of available methods. Int Immunol 15, 781–787.

Schubert, U., Anton, L., Gibbs, J., Norbury, C., Yewdell, J. and Bennink, J. (2000). Rapid degradation of a large fraction of newly synthesized proteins by proteasomes. Nature 404, 770–774.

Schumacher, T., Kantesaria, D., Serreze, D., Roopenian, D. and Ploegh, H. (1994). Transporters from H-2b, H-2d, H-2s, H-2k, and H-2g7 (NOD/Lt) haplotype translocate similar sets of peptides. Proc Natl Acad Sci USA 91, 13004–13008.

Serwold, T., Gonzalez, F., Kim, J., Jacob, R. and Shastri, N. (2002). ERAAP customizes peptides for MHC class I molecules in the endoplasmic reticulum. Nature 419, 480–483.

Snyder, GA., Brooks, A.G. and Sun, P.D. (1999). Crystal structure of the HLA-Cw3 allotype-specific killer cell inhibitory receptor KIR2DL2. PNAS 96, 3864–3869.

Strickland, E., Hakala, K., Thomas, P.J. and DeMartino, G.N. (2000). Recognition of misfolding proteins by PA700, the regulatory subcomplex of the 26 S proteasome. J Biol Chem 275, 5565–5572.

Sugita, K., Miyazaki, J., Appella, E. and Ozato, K. (1987). Interferons increase transcription of a major histocompatibility class I gene via a 5′ interferon consensus sequence. Mol Cell Biol 7, 2625–2630.

Suh, W.K., Derby, M.A., Cohen-Doyle, M.F. et al. (1999). Interaction of murine MHC class I molecules with tapasin and TAP enhances peptide loading and involves the heavy chain {alpha}3 Domain. J Immunol 162, 1530–1540.

Tector, M. and Salter, R.D. (1995). Calnexin influences folding of human class I histocompatibility proteins but not their assembly with beta(2)-microglobulin. J Biol Chem 270, 19638–19642.

Van Bleek, G. and Nathenson, S. (1990). Isolation of an endogenously processed immunodominant viral peptide from the class I H-2Kb molecule. Nature 348, 213–216.

Worgall, S., Busch, A., Rivara, M. et al. (2004). Modification to the capsid of the adenovirus vector that enhances dendritic cell infection and transgene-specific cellular immune responses. J Virol 78, 2572–2580.

York, I., Chang, S., Saric, T. et al. (2002). The ER aminopeptidase ERAP1 enhances or limits antigen presentation by trimming epitopes to 8-9 residues. Nat Immunol 3, 1177–1184.

Zarling, A.L., Luckey, C.J., Marto, J.A. et al. (2003). Tapasin is a facilitator, not an editor, of class I MHC peptide binding J Immunol 171, 5287–5295.

Zhang, Q., Tector, M. and Salter, R.D. (1995). Calnexin recognizes carbohydrate and protein determinants of class I major histocompatibility complex molecules. J Biol Chem 270, 3944–3948.

MHC Class II

Chapter 2

Amy Y. Chow*, Julia J. Unternaehrer* and Ira Mellman
Department of Cell Biology and Section of Immunobiology, Ludwig Institute for Cancer Research, Yale University School of Medicine, New Haven, CT, USA
* Contributed equally

It is most urgent that the skin homograft problem should be settled once for all – not merely because it is of immediate practical importance, but also because some surgeons still use homografts, apparently with the hope 'that a natural law will be suspended in their favour.

(Medawar, 1943)

INTRODUCTION

Major histocompatibility complex class II molecules (MHCII) serve to bind antigenic peptides and engage CD4 T cell receptors in order to initiate an immune response. MHCII is both polygenic and polymorphic. In the mouse, two genes – I-E and I-A – code for MHCII and in the human, three genes – HLA-DP, -DQ, and -DR – are present. For each copy of each gene, any of a large number (>200 in some cases) of alleles can be expressed which results in the polymorphic nature of MHCII. Alleles differ from one another by up to 20 amino acids and, as such, are the most highly polymorphic genes known. Polymorphisms, most of which are on the exposed surfaces including the peptide-binding groove, account for critical diversity within the population and are the cause for restriction (Janeway et al., 2001).

Early studies of tissue transplantation and immunization by P. Gorer led toward the formation of the concept of MHC antigens. He transferred tumors between strains of mice, noting absence of growth in allogeneic mice, growth followed by regression in hybrid animals, or unrestricted growth in syngeneic animals (Gorer, 1937). P. Medawar greatly assisted in the previously abysmal

success rate of human skin grafts, noting that nearly all initially appeared to 'take', then several weeks later almost as many began a process of 'melting away'. He proposed a theory of active, transferable immunity, noting that the recipient had to have the same genetic makeup as the donor (Medawar, 1943). Immune response (Ir) gene defects provided clues to the antigen presentation function of MHC molecules; since inbred mice express only one MHC molecule from each locus, there are many peptides they cannot present and they therefore have Ir defects (Janeway et al., 2001). McDevitt and colleagues established that the Ir gene products were responsible for the variations in responsiveness to synthetic peptides and eventually came to the conclusion that they were one and the same as the Ia or MHCII antigens (McDevitt, 2000). MHC restriction was discovered by Zinkernagel and Doherty and for this insight they received the Nobel Prize in Physiology or Medicine in 1996. Their studies showed that CTLs could kill cells of the same haplotype infected with virus, but not cells of a different haplotype, though also infected with virus (Zinkernagel and Doherty, 1997). These and countless other scientists provide the foundation upon which current MHCII studies are based, with applications in areas as diverse as immunity to pathogens, autoimmune disease and tumor immunology.

REGULATION OF MHCII EXPRESSION

Constitutive expression of MHC class II molecules (MHCII) is limited to cells specialized for the function

Measuring Immunity, edited by Michael T. Lotze and Angus W. Thomson
ISBN 0-12-455900-X, London

Copyright © 2005, Elsevier. All rights reserved.

of antigen presentation to CD4 T lymphocytes. These so-called 'antigen presenting cells' typically include dendritic cells (DCs), B lymphocytes, macrophages and certain populations of epithelial cells, particularly at sites of inflammation. Macrophages also express MHCII at a low level until induced by interferon-γ. This cytokine can also induce MHCII expression in certain otherwise non-expressing cell types. Both constitutive and regulated expression of MHCII requires activity of the transcriptional transactivator CIITA (Steimle et al., 1994).

Levels of MHCII expression in antigen presenting cells are also regulated in a temporal fashion. In B cells, initiation of MHCII expression coincides with an early stage of B cell development; i.e. shortly after commitment to the B lymphocytic lineage. Expression is highest in the mature, active B cell and declines as differentiation to the plasma cell stage occurs (Boss, 1997). Dendritic cells, the most potent antigen presenting cell type, exist in distinct functional and phenotypic stages referred to as immature and mature. In DCs, *de novo* synthesis of MHCII occurs at a high level early on even while the cell is in the immature stage, is transiently accelerated following maturational stimulation by inflammatory factors (Cella et al., 1997), but is turned off some time after the DC matures (Landmann et al., 2001). From a functional standpoint, MHCII surface arrival in DCs is developmentally regulated at the level of intracellular transport. The immature DC is optimized for antigen accumulation and therefore has no need for surface expression of MHCII; as a result, its MHCII molecules are primarily accumulated in lysosomes where they reside together with endocytosed antigen. It is the role of the mature DC to present antigen to naïve T cells; as such, it transports its MHCII to the cell surface (Pierre et al., 1997).

INTRACELLULAR EVENTS

Assembly and transport

MHCII is composed of two type I transmembrane glycoproteins, α and β, which are assembled into a complex together with a third glycoprotein known as invariant chain (Ii) following synthesis in the endoplasmic reticulum (ER) (Figure 2.1). As its name implies, Ii is non-polymorphic but is able to associate with highly polymorphic alpha and beta subunits of MHCII. It can be expressed in alternatively spliced forms commonly referred to as p31 and p41. In humans, alternatively translated forms known as p35 and p43 have 16 amino acid N-terminal extensions added to p31 and p41, respectively. Ii is a type II transmembrane protein which trimerizes prior to association with the MHCII subunits. Each of the Ii forms can be incorporated into trimers, though the p31 (and p35) form predominates. A portion of Ii known as CLIP (for class II-associated invariant chain peptide) mediates the association between Ii and each MHCII dimer by binding in the MHCII peptide binding groove (Cresswell, 1994). The resulting nonameric complex, comprised of three Ii chains, each with an associated MHCII α β dimer (Roche et al., 1991), is transported from the Golgi directly to the endocytic pathway, apparently by means of a dileucine signal in the cytoplasmic tail of Ii (Bakke and Dobberstein, 1990; Pieters et al., 1993; Odorizzi et al., 1994).

Thus, Ii serves several functions: it occludes the peptide binding groove in the ER such that peptides do not prematurely bind, it stabilizes the nonameric complex and it mediates transport from the Golgi to the endocytic pathway. Though the general mechanism for MHCII transport to late endosomes and lysosomes follows the pathway outlined above, allelic differences exist which result in variation of the dependence of MHCII transport on invariant chain. In particular, I-A^b α β dimers in mice cannot assemble properly without invariant chain, whereas k and d haplotypes assemble and traffic appropriately (Bikoff et al., 1991).

Once in the endocytic pathway, MHCII transport varies slightly in different cell types. Localization of MHCII in B cells by electron microscopy (Peters et al., 1991), subcellular fractionation (Amigorena et al., 1994; Tulp et al., 1994) and immunofluorescence studies (Salamero et al., 1990; Benaroch et al., 1995) has identified compartments all along the endocytic pathway, from early endosomes to lysosomes and possibly in specialized structures termed CIIV (Amigorena et al., 1994). In general, however, MHCII in B cells accumulates in organelles that are otherwise indistinguishable from their counterparts in cells that are not antigen presenting cells (Pierre et al., 1996; Kleijmeer et al., 1997). MHCII is also found to recycle from the plasma membrane through recycling endosomes in these cells (Pinet et al., 1995). Similarly, in macrophages, MHCII was co-localized with internalized heat-killed *Listeria monocytogenes* (Harding and Geuze, 1992). DCs are able to control MHCII transport in a highly synchronous nature not seen in the other cell types. The immature DC accumulates the majority of its MHCII molecules in lysosomes. Only following stimulation with inflammatory stimuli are these molecules mobilized *en masse* to the cell surface (Cella et al., 1997; Pierre et al., 1997; Turley et al., 2000).

While some of these studies have simply localized accumulated pools of MHCII in different cell types, some also attempted to identify the more relevant compartment in which peptide loading occurs by biochemical detection of the SDS-stable dimer, a MHCII conformation that is thought to be indicative of an antigenic peptide-loaded form (Tulp et al., 1994; Amigorena et al., 1995). Other studies have made use of antibodies that more directly recognize the peptide loaded form of MHCII (Inaba et al., 2000).

Recent investigations in DCs have analyzed the transport of MHCII from its site of storage in lysosomes to the cell surface. These studies have shown that transport occurs from lysosomes directly to the plasma membrane (Turley et al., 2000; Chow et al., 2002) and is mediated by compartments of a tubular morphology (Kleijmeer et al., 2001; Boes et al., 2002; Chow et al., 2002).

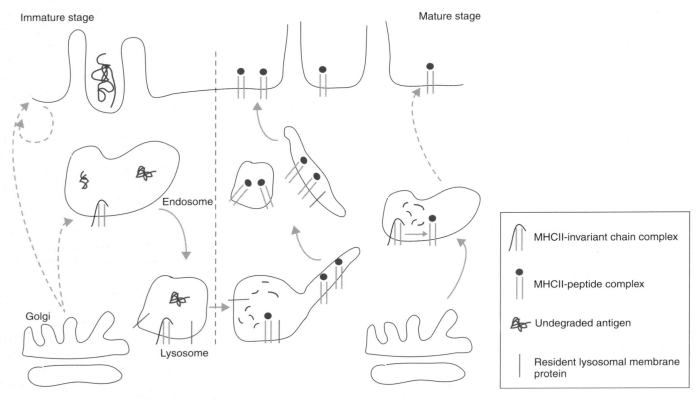

Immature stage   Mature stage

Golgi

Endosome

Lysosome

⊓ MHCII-invariant chain complex

●┃ MHCII-peptide complex

🦋 Undegraded antigen

┃ Resident lysosomal membrane protein

Figure 2.1 In dendritic cells, MHCII transport and function is regulated according to maturation state.

Not only have studies of MHCII transport been useful for the basic understanding of MHCII antigen presentation, they have also been applicable towards designing strategies for effective loading of antigen for the purpose of generating a specific immune response. These strategies include engineering antigens expressed within antigen presenting cells that contain targeting signals similar to those of lysosomal membrane proteins or invariant chain, so that the antigen is assured of entering the same compartment containing MHCII (Koch et al., 2000). Similar strategies include targeting antigen to specific receptors for increasing the efficiency of endocytosis and subsquent encounter between MHCII and antigen (Mahnke et al., 2000; Hawiger, 2001).

Such attempts to selectively enhance antigen processing are applicable specifically in recent efforts involving the use of dendritic cells for cancer immunotherapy. Dendritic cells have been singled out as a potential cancer vaccine agent since their potency of antigen presentation and interaction with a number of immune cell types make them central to focusing the character of an immune response (Nestle et al., 2001). Protocols for the use of DCs in cancer immunotherapy involve expanding DCs either *ex vivo* or *in vivo* and loading them with antigen either by endogenous (self-expressed) or exogenous (external administration) means (Guermonprez et al., 2002). Clinical trials using DCs in cancer patients have sought to treat tumors as wide ranging as melanoma,

lymphoma, myeloma and those in prostate and renal cancer (Zitvogel et al., 2000).

Characteristics of peptides that bind MHCII molecules

Initial understanding of the characteristics of MHCII-binding peptides came from studies which eluted these peptides from affinity purified MHCII molecules of B cell lines. Results showed that the peptides were longer (13–17 amino acids) than those that had been similarly isolated from MHCI (9–11 amino acids). The cleavage ends did not reveal a pattern indicative of a specific protease responsible for generating the peptide. The identity of the peptides confirmed that MHCII is responsible for presenting exogenous peptides since they were all derived from proteins which were accessible to the endocytic pathway. Interestingly, a prominently isolated peptide was one derived from an MHCII molecule. This finding made mechanistic sense since there would obviously be MHCII derivatives in the MHCII peptide loading compartment within the cell and it also had important implications for presentation of self-peptides.

The studies also implied that the peptide binding groove was less conformationally restrictive than MHCI since the length of the peptides indicated that their ends would protrude from the MHCII molecule and, also contrary to MHCI, there appeared to be less rigid patterns in the peptide sequences that indicated pockets within the

MHCII molecule that would bind specific types of amino acids (Rudensky et al., 1991, 1992).

Further understanding of the interaction between peptides and MHCII came from solving crystal structures of the molecules. In these analyses, binding pockets were identified which mediated the sequestering of peptide anchor residues as well as high affinity binding between peptides and MHCII molecules. As a result, allele-specific peptide sequence motifs were identified which explained the tendency of certain peptide epitopes to associate with specific MHCII molecules (Fremont et al., 1996, 1998, 2002).

Peptide generation

The generation of peptides has been elucidated in studies on the proteases involved in antigen processing. Those expressed in antigen presenting cells include the cysteine proteases cathepsins B, H, L, S, F, Z, V, O, C and possibly K. Aspartic proteases expressed in antigen presenting cells include cathepsins D and E and asparaginyl endopeptidase (Watts, 2001). The variety of proteases available is consistent with the diversity of peptides found to bind MHCII molecules. Even so, few protease processing sites on native proteins have been identified which explain the generation of a particular epitope. Cathepsin D has been shown to be necessary for the processing of exogenous glutamate decarboxylase, a target autoantigen in diabetes mellitus (Lich et al., 2000). Cathepsin S is required for Ii (more about this below) (Riese et al., 1996) and type II collagen processing (Nakagawa et al., 1999). Asparaginyl endopeptidase (AEP) was found to be necessary for the initiation of processing of tetanus toxin antigen (Antoniou et al., 2000). Despite these examples, in the vast majority of cases it is likely that there is considerable redundancy and plasticity in terms of the proteases that can produce antigenic epitopes.

In addition to the cleaving between amino acids which is necessary for the generation of peptides, some antigens require disulfide bond reduction for unfolding before the proteases will have access to cleavage sites. GILT, an IFNγ-inducible lysosomal thiol reductase, is present in MHCII containing compartments and seems to be involved in antigen processing (Arunachalam et al., 2000; Phan et al., 2000; Maric et al., 2001).

Since invariant chain occludes the peptide binding groove of MHCII, it must be cleaved and removed in order for efficient loading of peptide antigens to occur. The cleavage has been shown to occur in a stepwise fashion involving a series of proteases. Cleavage of the intact protein to a 22/23 kDa fragment (p22/p23) is not inhibited by leupeptin, a cysteine protease inhibitor, and may be mediated by AEP or other proteases providing redundant activity (Manoury et al., 2003). The formation of a 10 kDa amino-terminal Ii fragment (p10) from p22/p23 is leupeptin-sensitive but the proteases involved are not yet fully understood. The formation of CLIP from p10 involves the activity of cathepsin S in antigen presenting cells such as B cells and DCs and cathepsin L in cortical thymic epithelial cells in mice (Nakagawa et al., 1998). In humans, cathepsin S may perform this function even in thymic epithelium (Bania et al., 2003). Removal of CLIP and exchange for an antigenic peptide is mediated by an MHC related molecule, HLA-DM (H2-M in mice) and is modulated by the activity of HLA-DO (Denzin and Cresswell, 1995; Denzin et al., 1997).

Exquisite timing of these processes has been shown to be developmentally regulated in DCs at a number of different levels. Using antibodies that detect the MHCII-peptide conformation, investigators have shown that complex formation does not occur until an inflammatory stimulus has been detected by the cell (Inaba et al., 2000). This regulation may be due in part to the control of Ii cleavage in developing DCs. The activity of cathepsin S has been shown to be altered by levels of cystatin C, a natural inhibitor of cathepsin S, which varies depending on the maturation state of the DC (Pierre and Mellman, 1998). More recently, developmentally controlled acidification of lysosomes has been shown to occur in DCs (Trombetta et al., 2003), a finding which has important implications for the overall digestive capacity of the lysosomal compartment and for the activity of proteases and other enzymes involved in antigen processing, as many of them act optimally only at low pH.

Conventionally, MHCII antigen processing and peptide loading has been assumed to happen in stepwise order: protein antigens are first cleaved into peptides of appropriate lengths followed by binding to MHCII. However, an alternative view supports the hypothesis that MHCII binds longer peptides or native (or unfolded) protein forms and then proteases trim away that which is not protected by the MHCII molecule (Sercarz and Maverakis, 2003). Detection of longer forms of antigens bound to MHCII provide some support for this model (Castellino et al., 1998) as do studies on the competition of binding of overlapping peptide sequences to their respective MHCII alleles (Deng et al., 1993). Theories based on fragmentary or anecdotal evidence will not suffice however, and further studies will be required to clarify this most fundamental of problems in antigen processing.

MHCII-peptide binding

Binding of peptides to the MHCII antigen-binding groove has been characterized as of relatively low affinity (low μM), due to slow association rates. Once they are formed, however, these complexes are very stable (Busch and Rothbard, 1990). Peptides compete for antigen presentation and the consequences for immunity are significant: presentation of particular epitopes is associated with autoimmune disease; blocking via competition is one strategy for treatment of certain autoimmune pathology (Adorini and Nagy, 1990). Indeed, the incidence and severity of EAE, a mouse model of MS, has been greatly decreased using this approach (Smilek et al., 1991).

Exosomes

Though not the main pathway by which MHCII is transported out of the cell, another possibly biologically and clinically relevant process is the release of exosomes. Exosomes are small vesicles released into the extracellular space when multivesicular bodies (i.e. late endosomes and lysosomes) derived from the endocytic pathway fuse with the plasma membrane. The release of exosomes has been shown to occur in many cell types, but only in MHCII expressing cells do the exosomes carry MHCII on their surface (Raposo et al., 1996). The exosomes express MHCII due to a poorly understood process by which MHCII is concentrated on the internal vesicles of multivesicular bodies (Kleijmeer et al., 2001). Exosomes have been found to contain not only MHCII but also other immunostimulatory molecules and therefore have been purported to be capable of stimulating an immune response. Some reports show this immunostimulatory capacity to be indirect (requiring the presence of certain cell types) and some direct (Zitvogel et al., 1998). Recent efforts have sought to use exosomes as immunotherapy for cancer (Thery et al., 2002; Chaput et al., 2003).

SURFACE EXPRESSION AND FUNCTION

Interaction of T cell receptors with peptide-MHCII

Once peptide-loaded MHCII arrives at the cell surface, it is then able to accomplish the function for which APCs were named. Early interactions between T cells and APCs, mediated by adhesion molecules such as LFA-1 with ICAM-1 and -3, and CD2 with LFA-3, allow the prolonged cell contact necessary for the T cell to scan for the TCR ligand in the form of MHCII-peptide complexes (Hauss et al., 1995; Inaba and Steinman, 1987). The presence of abundant large adhesion and signaling molecules (whose extracellular domains span 45 nm) on the surface of both T cell and APC is assumed to impede interaction of the smaller (<10 nm) TCR and MHCII molecules (Shaw and Dustin, 1997). The affinity of TCR-MHCII-peptide interactions is low, in the low micromolar range, with a slow association rate; additionally, the off-rate for this receptor–ligand pair is high, all combining to make for exceptionally challenging binding. Notwithstanding these significant barriers to TCR/MHCII-peptide binding and further the odds of the TCR encountering a rare MHCII-peptide complex, when these molecules do interact, the TCR is aligned diagonally over the peptide and binding groove, with TCR α over the $\alpha2$ domain of MHCII and the amino terminus of the peptide and the CDR3 loops of TCR α and β meeting over the central amino acids of the peptide (Janeway et al., 2001). Upon MHCII/TCR interaction, signaling through the TCR complex delivers a stop signal to migrating lymphocytes and triggers an increase in avidity of LFA-1/ICAM-1 interactions (Dustin and Springer, 1989; Dustin et al., 1997), as well as many other downstream events. TCR binding to MHCII may also have an effect on TCR conformation, and/or cause a more ordered state of TCRs and their binding sites. Many studies have shown the necessity of cross-linking, oligomerizing, or dimerizing the TCR for full activation; T cell stimulation by antibodies that cannot cross-link the TCR can result in T cell inactivation (Lake et al., 1999). How this TCR clustering is mediated in physiological interactions with APCs such as DC will be discussed below.

MHCII coreceptor interactions

CD4 binds invariant sites on the $\beta2$ domain of MHCII, allowing for simultaneous TCR/MHCII interactions (Janeway et al., 2001). Binding appears to occur after TCR/MHCII oligomerization and functions to amplify the dose response of the T cell 10–100 fold; it may also stabilize clusters of TCR/ligand (Hampl et al., 1997; Reich et al., 1997; Krummel et al., 2000). Clustering of MHCII is not mediated by CD4 (Wulfing et al., 2002).

MHCII surface distribution

MHCII surface distribution may affect the efficiency with which the APC is able to stimulate T cells and several studies have shown higher-order interactions of MHCII molecules. MHCII molecules have been observed to cluster with each other and with MHC-I by scanning force microscopy and EM (Setum et al., 1993; Jenei et al., 1997). 'Superdimers' of MHCII were observed in the original three-dimensional crystal structure of human MHCII (Brown et al., 1993) and, although it is not clear whether this represented an artifact of the crystallization conditions, some further evidence for dimers of dimers in B lymphocytes has been presented, although evidence for function is lacking (Schafer and Pierce, 1994; Roucard et al., 1996; Cherry et al., 1998). A fraction of MHC-II has been observed to be localized to glycolipid rafts and, at low antigen concentration, rafts have been shown to be important for antigen presentation in B lymphocyte lines (Anderson et al., 2000; Hiltbold et al., 2003). Several reports have demonstrated association of MHCII molecules with members of the tetraspanin family, possibly serving to connect them to each other or to other molecules important for antigen presentation (Schick and Levy, 1993; Angelisova et al., 1994; Rubinstein et al., 1996; Szollosi et al., 1996; Kropshofer et al., 2002). Coordinated interactions with specific tetraspanins at intercellular or plasma membrane locations have been proposed to be involved in MHCII distribution and function (Engering and Pieters, 2001). In developing DCs MHCII is present in a punctuate distribution, to some extent colocalizing with the costimulatory molecule CD86 (Turley et al., 2000); possibly these domains are important for improving the strength of T cell stimulation.

MHCII rearrangements upon T cell interaction

Studies of the immunological synapse (IS) showed moderate enrichment of endogenous MHCII at the contact zone of antigen-specific B cell/T cell conjugates at low antigen dose, with accumulations in the center of the synapse, as expected by virtue of its interaction with the TCR (which also clusters there) (Monks et al., 1998; Hiltbold et al., 2003). In MHCII-transfected fibroblasts, invariant chain knockout DCs and B lymphoma cells, similar MHCII clustering was seen (Chmielowski et al., 2002; Wetzel et al., 2002; Wulfing et al., 2002). Several of these studies addressed the presence of non-specific MHCII complexes in the IS, finding predominantly the specific complexes remaining in the central supramolecular activation cluster (c-SMAC) over time in naïve T cell conjugates. In one study, tubules containing MHCII expressed as a knock-in were directed toward sites of T cell contact (Boes et al., 2002).

These and other findings challenge the notion that MHCII is the passive player in MHC/TCR interactions. Rather, the APC (notably the DC) appears to play a role in pre-clustering its MHCII molecules and targeting them to sites of T cell contact (rather than being dragged there by TCR interactions).

MHCII signaling

Signaling through MHCII molecules leads to effects as diverse as proliferation, activation/maturation, chemokine secretion and induction of cell death. An MHCII ligand, LAG (lymphocyte-activating gene)-3, has recently been identified and is produced by activated T cells or NK cells, resulting in maturation and chemokine secretion (Triebel, 2003); as such, it is probably not critical in the initiation of primary immune responses (Al-Daccak et al., 2004). In DCs, MHCII ligation has different effects, depending upon the stage of the cells: in immature DCs it results in Syk (a protein tyrosine kinase) activation and maturation (Andreae et al., 2003), while in mature DCs it induces caspase-independent cell death probably mediated by PKCδ, which could serve to limit the extent of the immune response (Bertho et al., 2002). Tyrosine phosphorylation downstream of MHCII signaling results in IgM production in B cells (Tabata et al., 2000) and MHCII signals have also been shown to result in death in B cell lines. Thus MHCII signals can activate either the tyrosine kinase pathways linked to cytokine production, differentiation and maturation, or the PKC pathway leading to cell death (Al-Daccak et al., 2004).

Since MHCII molecules have only short cytoplasmic tails with no known signaling motifs, some of their downstream effects are thought to be mediated by associated molecules. Examples of signal transducers include HLA-DR-induced CD20 activation of Lyn in B cells and HLA-DR/β2 integrin complex involvement in the death pathway (Al-Daccak et al., 2004). MHCII raft localization has also been proposed to facilitate signaling, though many signaling activities have been found to be independent of rafts (Huby et al., 2001; Bouillon et al., 2003; Al-Daccak et al., 2004).

MHCII polymorphisms appear to play roles in signaling, as DR ligation stimulates monocyte IL-1β secretion, while DQ and DP induce IL-10 production (Al-Daccak et al., 2004).

Surface peptide loading and recycling

Surface-expressed MHCII can be loaded with exogenously applied peptide at the plasma membrane. Although many can be directly exchanged, selected peptides require an internalization step (Roosnek et al., 1988; Busch and Rothbard, 1990; Davidson et al., 1991; Watts, 1997; Pathak and Blum, 2000). MHCII molecules can recycle through endocytic compartments, a process that requires the α and β chain cytoplasmic tails. Presentation of some T cell epitopes does not require extensive processing and thus could be accomplished in early endosomes (Watts, 1997).

ALTERNATIVE ANTIGEN PRESENTATION PATHWAYS

As described in this section, MHCII is classically thought to be specialized for presenting antigens from exogenous sources. MHC class I, on the other hand, is responsible for presenting endogenous antigens. In some circumstances, however, MHCII is able to present endogenous antigens and, likewise, exogenous antigens can be presented on MHC class I. The former situation is known as the endogenous pathway of antigen presention by MHCII (Lechler et al., 1996). This process has been shown to occur for the priming of CD4+ T cells with cytotoxic activity towards measles virus-infected cells. Moreover, in some studies analyzing peptides eluted from MHCII, peptides derived from cytosolic proteins were identified. These observations may simply reflect the internalization of proteins released from dead cells, but they also raise the possibility of an alternative pathway of MHCII presentation in which endogenous proteins either reach the endocytic pathway or are anomalously loaded onto MHCII during its synthesis in the ER (Lechler et al., 1996).

A much better characterized and more likely physiologically relevant alternative antigen processing pathway is commonly known as cross-presentation, whereby exogenous antigens are presented on MHC I molecules (Belz et al., 2002). Such a process would be deemed necessary under conditions in which MHC class I restricted activation of CD8+ T cells occurs by professional antigen presenting cells that have not themselves been virally infected. Indeed, DCs have been shown to be particularly adept at cross-presentation and, as another example, are capable of presenting tumor antigens derived from endocytosed tumor cells on MHC I (Mellman and Steinman, 2001). In cross-presentation, the internalized antigen reaches the MHC I pathway by gaining access to the cytosol from an endocytic compartment. It then follows the conventional MHC I antigen processing pathway in which degradation is carried out by the proteasome, peptides are transported through the TAP transporters into the ER for loading onto MHC I and peptide-MHC I complexes traffic through the normal secretory pathway to the cell surface (Mellman and Steinman, 2001).

It has also been proposed that cross-presentation can occur within endocytic vesicles such as phagosomes (Ackerman et al., 2003; Guermonprez et al., 2003; Houde et al., 2003). In macrophages (which do not efficiently cross-present) and dendritic cells (which do) certain phagosomes may contain TAP and possibly other ER components that could work together to load exogenous antigen onto MHCI in a fashion that avoids a cytosolic intermediate and translocation into the ER. Although a fascinating possibility, it is controversial since the origin or function of ER components in phagosomes remains uncertain.

T CELL SELECTION

During thymocyte development, MHCII on thymic cortical epithelium mediates engagement of the T-cell receptor (TCR) on CD4+ cells thereby promoting selection. Negative selection, or the elimination of thymocytes, occurs when a high affinity interaction occurs between MHCII-peptide and the TCR and prevents the T cell repertoire from containing self-reactive, possibly autoimmunity-promoting cells. Positive selection, or stimulation through the TCR allowing for survival, occurs when a moderate to low affinity interaction occurs allowing thymocytes which recognize self-MHCII to live. Death by neglect occurs when a thymocyte is not at all reactive to a given MHCII-peptide complex. The resulting T cell repertoire contains cells, in principle therefore, which are restricted to recognizing self-MHCII but not self-peptide complexed to self-MHCII (Fink and Bevan, 1995).

TRANSPLANTATION

Since self is defined during the process of selection as described above, transplantation of tissues between individuals is complicated in outbred populations. Host T cells recognize the MHC molecules of the allograft (often on donor DCs, but also on endothelial cells) as foreign causing rejection often mediated by CTL cytotoxicity.

Donor DCs can migrate to draining lymph nodes, where their surface MHC molecules activate an allo response ('direct' recognition) (Gould and Auchincloss, 1999), or alternatively host APCs can migrate into the graft and endocytose and present alloantigens, again

activating host T cells ('indirect' recognition). Donor T cells (if not depleted) recognize the MHC molecules of the host as foreign and mediate graft versus host disease (Kuby, 1997). These pathologies can only be completely avoided when donor and recipient are identical at MHC and minor histocompatibility antigen loci, which is only the case in monozygotic twins. Some differences can be tolerated through the use of immunosuppressive drugs, although outcomes are better the more closely matched donor and recipient are. Liver allografts provide an interesting exception: in this case HLA compatibility is not definitively associated with long-term survival (Dausset and Rapaport, 1996). Hepatic grafts are often tolerogenic, the mechanism of which is under study, but is hypothesized to be the high number of passenger leukocytes, the most important of which are thought to be dendritic cells (Starzl et al., 2003); donor stem cells may also play a role (Starzl et al., 2000). This, along with pregnancy, points to mechanisms allowing host tolerance of a donated organ or fetus with HLA discrepancy (Dausset and Rapaport, 1996).

DISEASE ASSOCIATIONS

Disease linkage studies utilizing gene probes allow rapid, definite detection of genetic identification and have proven to be a great improvement over the cellular or serotyping methods of the past. Many diseases have apparent MHC linkage, but these may be overestimated due to linkage disequilibrium, whereby HLA genes are linked to non-MHC genes. In some cases the cause of the disease is the gene to which the HLA gene is linked, which can be on the same haplotype, but unrelated to MHCII (Nepom and Erlich, 1991). In most if not all cases, many other factors besides MHCII haplotype play roles; even in individuals with the highest disease association, pathology is not 100 per cent penetrant.

Autoimmune diseases

MHCII polymorphisms control whether key antigenic determinants will be presented, in development (influencing central tolerance) and later in life (affecting activation of self-reactive T cell clones). Genes affecting the transcriptional regulation of HLA genes may also play a role; polymorphisms in promoter elements can lead to altered MHCII expression levels, a factor in immune responses including autoimmunity. One model proposes that MHCII molecules compete for binding of specific peptides and if the susceptibility gene outcompetes other MHCII molecules, based on affinities and relative abundance, disease may ensue (Nepom and Erlich, 1991).

Type I diabetes

Insulin-dependent diabetes mellitus (IDDM) is a very well-studied example of a disease with HLA-linked genetic influence. In man, HLA-DQ0302, DQ8, DR4, DR3, and to a lesser extent DR1 and DR8 are susceptible, while DQ0602, DR2 and DR5, DR6 are dominantly negatively associated. The mechanism for protection is unknown, but possibly certain haplotypes more efficiently delete self-reactive T cells in development, or, as alluded to above, outcompete the susceptibility allele for peptide binding. The NOD mouse I-A^{g7} confers susceptibility, but I-E^{g7} is protective. These associations are complex; for example, DR3/DR4 heterozygotes are at the highest risk, but different combinations appear to be synergistic with regard to disease risk (Nepom and Erlich, 1991). Some alleles conferring protection in Caucasians, but not people of Asian descent, contain an Asp at position 57 of the β chain (as opposed to a Ser in other alleles), which forms an interdimer salt bridge, thought to impart the observed high degree of SDS stability (McFarland and Beeson, 2002). Whether this increased stability is involved in protection is controversial, but many patients with IDDM also have an Asp at this position, as do both the susceptible and the non-diabetes prone strain of rat (Nepom and Erlich, 1991).

Rheumatoid arthritis

Rheumatoid arthritis (RA) has also been extensively studied; 65–80 per cent of RA patients are HLA-DR4, especially subtypes Dw4 and Dw14. The DR4 negative patients are usually DR1, with a Dw14-like epitope, pointing to this region as generally immunologically significant. The pauciarticular form of juvenile RA shows synergistic risk with several alleles (DR5, 6, 8 and DPw2) (Nepom and Erlich, 1991).

Other diseases

Two more diseases should be mentioned. Celiac disease, marked by inflammation and malabsorption in the small intestine, has been linked to HLA-DR3 and DR7. Pemphigus vulgaris is caused by the presence of autoantibodies in the epidermis and is associated with DR4, Dw10 and DR6, Dw9, possibly representing independent pathways to this disease (Nepom and Erlich, 1991).

Other pathology and disease resistance

Atopy is described as inappropriate IgE production in response to particular allergens, predisposing a strong Th2 response. For example, ragweed allergy is associated with DRB1*1501. In West Africa, HLA-B53 is associated with recovery from a potentially lethal malaria (Janeway et al., 2001).

CONCLUDING REMARKS

In recent years, it has become widely appreciated that most of the action in initiating and promulgating MHCII-dependent immune responses depends on the activities of dendritic cells. Their ability to process and present a wide range of antigens to even immunologically naïve T cells is exceptional if not unique. As a result, all considerations of how MHCII-restricted presentation works in health and disease must take into account the participation of dendritic cells at one stage or another. Indeed, the fact that dendritic cells are increasingly associated with maintaining peripheral tolerance to self antigens strongly suggests that they are also somehow responsible for breakdowns in regulation of the immune response resulting in autoimmune or chronic inflammatory disorders.

REFERENCES

Ackerman, A.L., Kyritsis, C., Tampe, R. and Cresswell, P. (2003). Early phagosomes in dendritic cells form a cellular compartment sufficient for cross presentation of exogenous antigens. Proc Natl Acad Sci USA 100, 12889–12894.

Adorini, L. and Nagy, Z.A. (1990). Peptide competition for antigen presentation. Immunol Today 11, 21–24.

Al-Daccak, R., Mooney, N. and Charron, D. (2004). MHC class II signaling in antigen-presenting cells. Curr Opin Immunol 16, 108–113.

Amigorena, S., Drake, J.R., Webster, P. and Mellman, I. (1994). Transient accumulation of new class II MHC molecules in a novel endocytic compartment in B lymphocytes. Nature 369, 113–120.

Amigorena, S., Webster, P., Drake, J., Newcomb, J., Cresswell, P. and Mellman, I. (1995). Invariant chain cleavage and peptide loading in major histocompatibility complex class II vesicles. J Exp Med 181, 1729–1741.

Anderson, H., Hiltbold, E. and Roche, P. (2000). Concentration of MHC class II molecules in lipid rafts facilitates antigen presentation. Nat Immunol 1, 156–162.

Andreae, S., Buisson, S. and Triebel, F. (2003). MHC class II signal transduction in human dendritic cells induced by a natural ligand, the LAG-3 protein (CD223). Blood 102, 2130–2137.

Angelisova, P., Hilgert, I. and Horejsi, V. (1994). Association of four antigens of the tetraspans family (CD37, CD53, TAPA-1, and R2/C33) with MHC class II glycoproteins. Immunogenetics 39, 249–256.

Antoniou, A.N., Blackwood, S.L., Mazzeo, D. and Watts, C. (2000). Control of antigen presentation by a single protease cleavage site. Immunity 12, 391–398.

Arunachalam, B., Phan, U.T., Geuze, H.J. and Cresswell, P. (2000). Enzymatic reduction of disulfide bonds in lysosomes: characterization of a gamma-interferon-inducible lysosomal thiol reductase (GILT). Proc Natl Acad Sci USA 97, 745–750.

Bakke, O. and Dobberstein, B. (1990). MHC class II-associated invariant chain contains a sorting signal for endosomal compartments. Cell 63, 707–716.

Bania, J., Gatti, E., Lelouard, H. et al. (2003). Human cathepsin S, but not cathepsin L, degrades efficiently MHC class II-associated invariant chain in nonprofessional APCs. Proc Natl Acad Sci USA 100, 6664–6669.

Belz, G.T., Carbone, F.R. and Heath, W.R. (2002). Cross-presentation of antigens by dendritic cells. Crit Rev Immunol 22, 439–448.

Benaroch, P., Yilla, M., Raposo, G. et al. (1995). How MHC class II molecules reach the endocytic pathway. EMBO J 14, 37–49.

Bertho, N., Blancheteau, V.M., Setterblad, N. et al. (2002). MHC class II-mediated apoptosis of mature dendritic cells proceeds by activation of the protein kinase C-delta isoenzyme. Int Immunol 14, 935–942.

Bikoff, E.K., Jaffe, L., Ribaudo, R.K., Otten, G.R., Germain, R.N. and Robertson, E.J. (1991). MHC class I surface expression in embryo-derived cell lines inducible with peptide or interferon. Nature 354, 235–238.

Boes, M., Cerny, J., Massol, R. et al. (2002). T-cell engagement of dendritic cells rapidly rearranges MHC class II transport. Nature 418, 983–988.

Boss, J.M. (1997). Regulation of transcription of MHC class II genes. Curr Opin Immunol 9, 107–113.

Bouillon, M., El Fakhry, Y., Girouard, J., Khalil, H., Thibodeau, J. and Mourad, W. (2003). Lipid raft-dependent and -independent signaling through HLA-DR molecules. J Biol Chem 278, 7099–7107.

Brown, J.H., Jardetzky, T.S., Gorga, J.C. et al. (1993). Three-dimensional structure of the human class II histocompatibility antigen HLA-DR1 (see comments). Nature 364, 33–39.

Busch, R. and Rothbard, J.B. (1990). Detection of peptide-MHC class II complexes on the surface of intact cells. J Immunol Methods 134, 1–22.

Castellino, F., Zappacosta, F., Coligan, J.E. and Germain, R.N. (1998). Large protein fragments as substrates for endocytic antigen capture by MHC class II molecules. J Immunol 161, 4048–4057.

Cella, M., Engering, A., Pinet, V., Pieters, J. and Lanzavecchia, A. (1997). Inflammatory stimuli induce accumulation of MHC class II complexes on dendritic cells. Nature 388, 782–787.

Chaput, N., Schartz, N.E., Andre, F. and Zitvogel, L. (2003). Exosomes for immunotherapy of cancer. Adv Exp Med Biol 532, 215–221.

Cherry, R.J., Wilson, K.M., Triantafilou, K. et al. (1998). Detection of dimers of dimers of human leukocyte antigen (HLA)-DR on the surface of living cells by single-particle fluorescence imaging. J Cell Biol 140, 71–79.

Chmielowski, B., Pacholczyk, R., Kraj, P., Kisielow, P. and Ignatowicz, L. (2002). Presentation of antagonist peptides to naive CD4+ T cells abrogates spatial reorganization of class II MHC peptide complexes on the surface of dendritic cells. Proc Natl Acad Sci USA 99, 15012–15017.

Chow, A., Toomre, D., Garrett, W. and Mellman, I. (2002). Dendritic cell maturation triggers retrograde MHC class II transport from lysosomes to the plasma membrane. Nature 418, 988–994.

Cresswell, P. (1994). Assembly, transport, and function of MHC class II molecules. Ann Rev Immunol 12, 259–293.

Dausset, J. and Rapaport, F. (1996). Transplantation Biology: Cellular and Molecular Aspects. Philadelphia, New York: Lippincott-Raven Publishers.

Davidson, H.W., Reid, P.A., Lanzavecchia, A. and Watts, C. (1991). Processed antigen binds to newly synthesized MHC class II molecules in antigen-specific B lymphocytes. Cell 67, 105–116.

Deng, H., Apple, R., Clare-Salzler, M. et al. (1993). Determinant capture as a possible mechanism of protection afforded by major histocompatibility complex class II molecules in autoimmune disease. J Exp Med 178, 1675–1680.

Denzin, L.K. and Cresswell, P. (1995). HLA-DM induces CLIP dissociation from MHC class II alpha beta dimers and facilitates peptide loading. Cell 82, 155–165.

Denzin, L.K., Sant'Angelo, D.B., Hammond, C., Surman, M.J. and Cresswell, P. (1997). Negative regulation by HLA-DO of MHC class II-restricted antigen processing. Science 278, 106–109.

Dustin, M.L., Bromley, S.K., Kan, Z., Peterson, D.A. and Unanue, E.R. (1997). Antigen receptor engagement delivers a stop signal to migrating T lymphocytes. Proc Natl Acad Sci USA 94, 3909–3913.

Dustin, M.L. and Springer, T.A. (1989). T-cell receptor cross-linking transiently stimulates adhesiveness through LFA-1. Nature 341, 619–624.

Engering, A. and Pieters, J. (2001). Association of distinct tetraspanins with MHC class II molecules at different subcellular locations in human immature dendritic cells. Int Immunol 13, 127–134.

Fink, P.J. and Bevan, M.J. (1995). Positive selection of thymocytes. Adv Immunol 59, 99–133.

Fremont, D.H., Dai, S., Chiang, H., Crawford, F., Marrack, P. and Kappler, J. (2002). Structural basis of cytochrome c presentation by IE(k). J Exp Med 195, 1043–1052.

Fremont, D.H., Hendrickson, W.A., Marrack, P. and Kappler, J. (1996). Structures of an MHC class II molecule with covalently bound single peptides. Science 272, 1001–1004.

Fremont, D.H., Monnaie, D., Nelson, C.A., Hendrickson, W.A. and Unanue, E.R. (1998). Crystal structure of I-Ak in complex with a dominant epitope of lysozyme. Immunity 8, 305–317.

Gorer, P.A. (1937). The genetic and antigenic basis of tumour transplantation. J Pathol of Bacterial 44, 691–697.

Gould, D.S. and Auchincloss, H., Jr. (1999). Direct and indirect recognition: the role of MHC antigens in graft rejection. Immunol Today 20, 77–82.

Guermonprez, P., Saveanu, L., Kleijmeer, M., Davoust, J., Van Endert, P. and Amigorena, S. (2003). ER-phagosome fusion defines an MHC class I cross-presentation compartment in dendritic cells. Nature 425, 397–402.

Guermonprez, P., Valladeau, J., Zitvogel, L., Thery, C. and Amigorena, S. (2002). Antigen presentation and T cell stimulation by dendritic cells. Annu Rev Immunol 20, 621–667.

Hampl, J., Chien, Y.H. and Davis, M.M. (1997). CD4 augments the response of a T cell to agonist but not to antagonist ligands. Immunity 7, 379–385.

Harding, C.V. and Geuze, H.J. (1992). Class II MHC molecules are present in macrophage lysosomes and phagolysosomes that function in the phagocytic processing of Listeria monocytogenes for presentation to T cells. J Cell Biol 119, 531–542.

Hauss, P., Selz, F., Cavazzana-Calvo, M. and Fischer, A. (1995). Characteristics of antigen-independent and antigen-dependent interaction of dendritic cells with CD4+ T cells. Eur J Immunol 25, 2285–2294.

Hawiger, D., Inaba, K., Dorsett, Y., et al. (2001). Dendritic cells induce peripheral T cell unresponsiveness under steady state conditions in vivo. J Exp Med 194, 769–79.

Hiltbold, E.M., Poloso, N.J. and Roche, P.A. (2003). MHC class II-peptide complexes and APC lipid rafts accumulate at the immunological synapse. J Immunol 170, 1329–1338.

Houde, M., Bertholet, S., Gagnon, E. et al. (2003). Phagosomes are competent organelles for antigen cross-presentation. Nature 425, 402–406.

Huby, R. Chowdhury, F. and Lombardi, G. (2001). Rafts for antigen presentation? Nat Immunol 2, 3.

Inaba, K. and Steinman, R.M. (1987). Monoclonal antibodies to LFA-1 and to CD4 inhibit the mixed leukocyte reaction after the antigen-dependent clustering of dendritic cells and T lymphocytes. J Exp Med 165, 1403–1417.

Inaba, K., Turley, S., Iyoda, T. et al. (2000). The formation of immunogenic major histocompatibility complex class II-peptide ligands in lysosomal compartments of dendritic cells is regulated by inflammatory stimuli. J Exp Med 191, 927–936.

Janeway, C.A., Jr., Travers, P., Walport, M. and Shlomchik, M. (2001). Immunobiology: The Immune System in Health and Disease, 5th edn. New York and London: Garland Publishing.

Jenei, A., Varga, S., Bene, L. et al. (1997). HLA class I and II antigens are partially co-clustered in the plasma membrane of human lymphoblastoid cells. Proc Natl Acad Sci USA 94, 7269–7274.

Kleijmeer, M.J., Morkowski, S., Griffith, J.M., Rudensky, A.Y. and Geuze, H. J. (1997). Major histocompatibility complex class II compartments in human and mouse B lymphoblasts represent conventional endocytic compartments. J Cell Biol 139, 639–649.

Kleijmeer, M., Ramm, G., Schuurhuis, D. et al. (2001). Reorganization of multivesicular bodies regulates MHC class II antigen presentation by dendritic cells. J Cell Biol 155, 53–63.

Koch, N., van Driel, I.R. and Gleeson, P.A. (2000). Hijacking a chaperone: manipulation of the MHC class II presentation pathway. Immunol Today 21, 546–550.

Kropshofer, H., Spindeldreher, S., Rohn, T.A. et al. (2002). Tetraspan microdomains distinct from lipid rafts enrich select peptide- MHC class II complexes. Nat Immunol 3, 61–68.

Krummel, M., Wulfing, C., Sumen, C. and Davis, M.M. (2000). Thirty-six views of T-cell recognition. Philos Trans R Soc Lond B Biol Sci 355, 1071–1076.

Kuby, J. (1997). Immunology. New York: W.H. Freeman and Company.

Lake, R.A., Robinson, B.W. and Hayball, J.D. (1999). MHC multimerization, antigen expression and the induction of APC amnesia in the developing immune response. Immunol Cell Biol 77, 99–104.

Landmann, S., Muhlethaler-Mottet, A., Bernasconi, L. et al. (2001). Maturation of dendritic cells is accompanied by rapid transcriptional silencing of class II transactivator (CIITA) expression. J Exp Med 194, 379–391.

Lechler, R., Aichinger, G. and Lightstone, L. (1996). The endogenous pathway of MHC class II antigen presentation. Immunol Rev 151, 51–79.

Lich, J.D., Elliott, J.F. and Blum, J.S. (2000). Cytoplasmic processing is a prerequisite for presentation of an endogenous antigen by major histocompatibility complex class II proteins. J Exp Med 191, 1513–1524.

Mahnke, K., Guo, M., Lee, S. et al. (2000). The dendritic cell receptor for endocytosis, DEC-205, can recycle and enhance antigen presentation via major histocompatibility complex class II-positive lysosomal compartments. J Cell Biol 151, 673–684.

Manoury, B., Mazzeo, D., Li, D.N. et al. (2003). Asparagine endopeptidase can initiate the removal of the MHC class II invariant chain chaperone. Immunity 18, 489–498.

Maric, M., Arunachalam, B., Phan, U.T. et al. (2001). Defective antigen processing in GILT-free mice. Science 294, 1361–1365.

McDevitt, H.O. (2000). Discovering the role of the major histocompatibility complex in the immune response. Annu Rev Immunol 18, 1–17.

McFarland, B.J. and Beeson, C. (2002). Binding interactions between peptides and proteins of the class II major histocompatibility complex. Med Res Rev 22, 168–203.

Medawar, P.B. (1943). Notes on the problem of skin homografts. Bull War Med 4, 1–4.

Mellman, I. and Steinman, R.M. (2001). Dendritic cells: specialized and regulated antigen processing machines. Cell 106, 255–258.

Monks, C.R., Freiberg, B.A., Kupfer, H., Sciaky, N. and Kupfer, A. (1998). Three-dimensional segregation of supramolecular activation clusters in T cells. Nature 395, 82–86.

Nakagawa, T., Roth, W., Wong, P. et al. (1998). Cathepsin L: critical role in Ii degradation and CD4 T cell selection in the thymus. Science 280, 450–453.

Nakagawa, T.Y., Brissette, W.H., Lira, P.D. et al. (1999). Impaired invariant chain degradation and antigen presentation and diminished collagen-induced arthritis in cathepsin S null mice. Immunity 10, 207–217.

Nepom, G.T. and Erlich, H. (1991). MHC class-II molecules and autoimmunity. Annu Rev Immunol 9, 493–525.

Nestle, F.O., Banchereau, J. and Hart, D. (2001). Dendritic cells: On the move from bench to bedside. Nat Med 7, 761–765.

Odorizzi, C.G., Trowbridge, I.S., Xue, L., Hopkins, C.R., Davis, C.D. and Collawn, J.F. (1994). Sorting signals in the MHC class II invariant chain cytoplasmic tail and transmembrane region determine trafficking to an endocytic processing compartment. J Cell Biol 126, 317–330.

Pathak, S.S. and Blum, J.S. (2000). Endocytic recycling is required for the presentation of an exogenous peptide via MHC class II molecules. Traffic 1, 561–569.

Peters, P.J., Neefjes, J.J., Oorschot, V., Ploegh, H.L. and Geuze, H.J. (1991). Segregation of MHC class II molecules from MHC class I molecules in the Golgi complex for transport to lysosomal compartments. Nature 349, 669–676.

Phan, U.T., Arunachalam, B. and Cresswell, P. (2000). Gamma-interferon-inducible lysosomal thiol reductase (GILT). Maturation, activity, and mechanism of action. J Biol Chem 275, 25907–25914.

Pierre, P., Denzin, L.K., Hammond, C. et al. (1996). HLA-DM is localized to conventional and unconventional MHC class II-containing endocytic compartments. Immunity 4, 229–239.

Pierre, P. and Mellman, I. (1998). Developmental regulation of invariant chain proteolysis controls MHC class II trafficking in mouse dendritic cells. Cell 93, 1135–1145.

Pierre, P., Turley, S.J., Gatti, E. et al. (1997). Developmental regulation of MHC class II transport in mouse dendritic cells. Nature 388, 787–792.

Pieters, J., Bakke, O. and Dobberstein, B. (1993). The MHC class II-associated invariant chain contains two endosomal targeting signals within its cytoplasmic tail. J Cell Sci 106, 831–846.

Pinet, V., Vergelli, M., Martin, R., Bakke, O. and Long, E. O. (1995). Antigen presentation mediated by recycling of surface HLA-DR molecules. Nature 375, 603–606.

Raposo, G., Nijman, H.W., Stoorvogel, W. et al. (1996). B lymphocytes secrete antigen-presenting vesicles. J Exp Med 183, 1161–1172.

Reich, Z., Altman, J.D., Boniface, J.J. et al. (1997). Stability of empty and peptide-loaded class II major histocompatibility complex molecules at neutral and endosomal pH: comparison to class I proteins. Proc Natl Acad Sci USA 94, 2495–2500.

Riese, R.J., Wolf, P.R., Bromme, D. et al. (1996). Essential role for cathepsin S in MHC class II-associated invariant chain processing and peptide loading. Immunity 4, 357–366.

Roche, P.A., Marks, M.S. and Cresswell, P. (1991). Formation of a nine-subunit complex by HLA class II glycoproteins and the invariant chain. Nature 354, 392–394.

Roosnek, E., Demotz, S., Corradin, G. and Lanzavecchia, A. (1988). Kinetics of MHC-antigen complex formation on antigen-presenting cells. J Immunol 140, 4079–4082.

Roucard, C., Garban, F., Mooney, N.A., Charron, D.J. and Ericson, M.L. (1996). Conformation of human leukocyte antigen class II molecules. Evidence for superdimers and empty molecules on human antigen presenting cells. J Biol Chem 271, 13993–14000.

Rubinstein, E., Le Naour, F., Lagaudriere-Gesbert, C., Billard, M., Conjeaud, H. and Boucheix, C. (1996). CD9, CD63, CD81, and CD82 are components of a surface tetraspan network connected to HLA-DR and VLA integrins. Eur J Immunol 26, 2657–2665.

Rudensky, A., Preston-Hurlburt, P., Hong, S.C., Barlow, A. and Janeway, C.A. Jr (1991). Sequence analysis of peptides bound to MHC class II molecules. Nature 353, 622–627.

Salamero, J., Humbert, M., Cosson, P. and Davoust, J. (1990). Mouse B lymphocyte specific endocytosis and recycling of MHC class II molecules. EMBO J 9, 3489–3496.

Schafer, P.H. and Pierce, S.K. (1994). Evidence for dimers of MHC class II molecules in B lymphocytes and their role in low affinity T cell responses. Immunity 1, 699–707.

Schick, M.R. and Levy, S. (1993). The TAPA-1 molecule is associated on the surface of B cells with HLA-DR molecules. J Immunol 151, 4090–4097.

Sercarz, E.E. and Maverakis, E. (2003). Mhc-guided processing: binding of large antigen fragments. Nat Rev Immunol 3, 621–629.

Setum, C.M., Serie, J.R. and Hegre, O.D. (1993). Dendritic cell/lymphocyte clustering: morphologic analysis by transmission electron microscopy and distribution of gold-labeled MHC class II antigens by high-resolution scanning electron microscopy. Anat Rec 235, 285–295.

Shaw, A.S. and Dustin, M.L. (1997). Making the T cell receptor go the distance: a topological view of T cell activation. Immunity 6, 361–369.

Smilek, D.E., Wraith, D.C., Hodgkinson, S., Dwivedy, S., Steinman, L. and McDevitt, H.O. (1991). A single amino acid change in a myelin basic protein peptide confers the capacity to prevent rather than induce experimental autoimmune encephalomyelitis. Proc Natl Acad Sci USA 88, 9633–9637.

Starzl, T.E., Murase, N., Demetris, A., Trucco, M. and Fung, J. (2000). The mystique of hepatic tolerogenicity. Semin Liver Dis 20, 497–510.

Starzl, T.E., Murase, N., Abu-Elmagd, K., et al. (2003). Tolerogenic immunosuppression for organ transplantation. 361, 1502–1510.

Steimle, V., Siegrist, C.A., Mottet, A., Lisowska-Grospierre, B. and Mach, B. (1994). Regulation of MHC class II expression by interferon-gamma mediated by the transactivator gene CIITA. Science 265, 106–109.

Szollosi, J., Horejsi, V., Bene, L., Angelisova, P. and Damjanovich, S. (1996). Supramolecular complexes of MHC class I, MHC class II, CD20, and tetraspan molecules (CD53, CD81, and CD82) at the surface of a B cell line JY. J Immunol 157, 2939–2946.

Tabata, H., Matsuoka, T., Endo, F., Nishimura, Y. and Matsushita, S. (2000). Ligation of HLA-DR molecules on B cells induces enhanced expression of IgM heavy chain genes in association with Syk activation. J Biol Chem 275, 34998–35005.

Thery, C., Zitvogel, L. and Amigorena, S. (2002). Exosomes: composition, biogenesis and function. Nat Rev Immunol 2, 569–579.

Triebel, F. (2003). LAG-3: a regulator of T-cell and DC responses and its use in therapeutic vaccination. Trends Immunol 24, 619–622.

Trombetta, E.S., Ebersold, M., Garrett, W., Pypaert, M. and Mellman, I. (2003). Activation of lysosomal function during dendritic cell maturation. Science 299, 1400–1403.

Tulp, A., Verwoerd, D., Dobberstein, B., Ploegh, H.L. and Pieters, J. (1994). Isolation and characterization of the intracellular MHC class II compartment. Nature 369, 120–126.

Turley, S.J., Inaba, K., Garrett, W.S. et al. (2000). Transport of peptide-MHC class II complexes in developing dendritic cells. Science 288, 522–527.

Watts, C. (1997). Capture and processing of exogenous antigens for presentation on MHC molecules. Ann Rev Immunol 15, 821–850.

Watts, C. (2001). Antigen processing in the endocytic compartment. Curr Opin Immunol 13, 26–31.

Wetzel, S.A., McKeithan, T.W. and Parker, D.C. (2002). Live-cell dynamics and the role of costimulation in immunological synapse formation. J Immunol 169, 6092–6101.

Wulfing, C., Sumen, C., Sjaastad, M.D., Wu, L.C., Dustin, M.L. and Davis, M.M. (2002). Costimulation and endogenous MHC ligands contribute to T cell recognition. Nat Immunol 3, 42–47.

Zinkernagel, R.M. and Doherty, P.C. (1997). The discovery of MHC restriction. Immunol Today 18, 14–17.

Zitvogel, L., Angevin, E. and Tursz, T. (2000). Dendritic cell-based immunotherapy of cancer. Ann Oncol 11 Suppl 3, 199–205.

Zitvogel, L., Regnault, A., Lozier, A. et al. (1998). Eradication of established murine tumors using a novel cell-free vaccine: dendritic cell-derived exosomes. Nat Med 4, 594–600.

Cytokine Receptor Heterogeneity

Chapter 3

David H. McDermott

Molecular Signaling Section, Laboratory of Host Defenses, National Institute of Allergy and Infectious Diseases, National Institutes of Health, Bethesda, USA

There is no need to be a doctor or scientist to wonder why the human body is capable of resisting so many harmful agents in the course of everyday life … Disease does not strike everyone indifferently. For some individuals who go down at the attack, there are others who have immunity to a greater or lesser extent … Whenever the organism enjoys immunity, the introduction of infectious microbes is followed by the accumulation of mobile cells, of white corpuscles of the blood in particular which absorb the microbes and destroy them … We thus have the right to hope that for the future, medicine will find more than one way to bring phagocytosis into play for the benefit of health.

> Ilya Mechnikov Nobel Lecture, December 11, 1908, From *Nobel Lectures*, Physiology or Medicine 1901–1921, Elsevier Publishing Company, Amsterdam.

INTRODUCTION

Over 100 years ago the Russian scientist, Ilya Mechnikov recognized the importance of the human cellular immune system at fighting off invading microorganisms, but he also noted that there was great individual heterogeneity in the response. Now, 50 years after the discovery of the structure of DNA and in the year of the completion of the sequencing of the human genome, we are poised to begin to truly understand the heterogeneity of the immune response at the molecular level. Mechnikov also recognized that leukocytes were capable of 'sensing the chemical composition of the surrounding medium' and that 'this form of sensitiveness is a condition indispensable

to a state of immunity and to the disappearance of microorganisms' (Mechnikov, 1905). We now call these small molecules that influence leukocytes, cytokines.

Among these proteins are molecular distress signals that control the development and activation of the humoral and cellular arms of the immune system. They act by binding to sensitive receptors on the cell surface that activate intracellular signaling pathways resulting in a variety of cell responses such as locomotion, proliferation and modulation of gene expression. With regard to locomotion, a human leukocyte like a neutrophil (PMN) can sense a cytokine concentration difference of less than 2 per cent across its length (Zigmond, 1977). This small difference in concentration gradient then causes the PMN to stick to the area of inflamed endothelium where the cytokine signal originated. Resisting the force of blood flow, the PMN then crawls between two blood vessel lining endothelial cells thereby exiting the circulation. Once in the subendothelial space, the PMN may completely envelope (phagocytose) the invading pathogen and kill the invader. Further release of cytokines by the PMN and surrounding cells may cause the immune response to evolve over time, bringing more or different types of effector cells from the circulation to the site of injury or infection. With some infectious agents, processing of the pathogen leads to stimulation of an adaptive immune response and creation of the specific memory cells that provide long-term protection against future attacks (Figure 3.1). However, the system must be carefully controlled because too little immune response will allow the

Measuring Immunity, edited by Michael T. Lotze and Angus W. Thomson
ISBN 0-12-455900-X, London

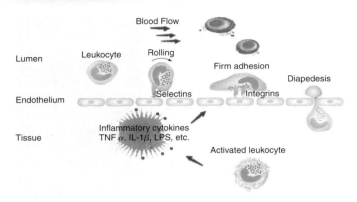

Figure 3.1 Inflammatory cytokines cause the vascular endothelium to express adhesion molecules and chemokines that result in the recruitment of leukocytes from the circulation to sites of injury where they become activated for host defense or tissue repair.

pathogen to overwhelm the host and too much response will damage uninfected tissue creating long-term disability or even death for the host. Misrecognition of host molecules as pathogens or a failure to limit the response after a true challenge can result in dysregulation of the system and autoimmune diseases.

Thus, there is a constant struggle of the immune system to recognize and destroy true invaders and ignore benign or beneficial colonization of microorganisms as well as self molecules. In evolutionary terms there is also a constant potential of pathogens to exploit host defenses. Like in modern warfare, for every new weapon developed there is a countermeasure. Viruses have evolved to take over the host cellular protein manufacturing machinery and pathogenic bacteria, parasites and fungi have evolved mechanisms to protect themselves from being phagocytosed and killed by the immune response. Since cytokine receptors are key molecules in controlling the immune response, they are a favorite target of opportunity in the evolution of pathogens. Through molecular mimicry, some pathogens have developed both binding proteins to block the action of cytokines to silence the alarm and molecules that behave like cytokines or mimic their receptors to control the immune response (McFadden and Murphy, 2000; McDermott and Murphy, 2000; Liston and McColl, 2003). In some cases, as we shall see below, pathogens have exploited human cytokine receptors to gain entry into immune system cells. When and how this panoply of countermeasures is deployed is specific to each pathogen. However, it is this constant struggle between man and pathogen and between protective controlled response and autoimmunity that has created rapid evolution of the immune system. By studying a variety of immune system proteins, it has been estimated that the immune system is evolving at about three times the rate of other host proteins (Murphy, 1993). On a molecular level, natural selection is manifested as frequent polymorphisms or mutations in the genes encoding cytokines and cytokine receptors. These genetic variants occur both in the regulatory regions

to affect the amount or timing of cytokine/cytokine receptor expression and in the protein coding regions to affect cytokine/cytokine receptor function.

This chapter will review a few major examples of cytokine receptor heterogeneity that alter disease susceptibility in man. These findings have provided important insights into disease pathogenesis and have pointed to new therapeutic targets. In some cases the discovery of these inflammatory pathways has already led to the development of novel therapeutics currently finding their niche in modern medicine. Ultimately if we can improve our ability to recognize the key molecules that control the immune system and find ways to safely regulate their expression or function, we will be able to ameliorate many diseases. Also by measuring levels of key biomarkers or finding the genotypes that control those levels, we may be able to predict who is susceptible to a particular disease and offer preventive therapies with fewer side effects to a more refined population where the benefits will outweigh the risks.

CHEMOKINE RECEPTORS

One class of cytokine receptor is the *chemo*tactic cyto*kine* or chemokine receptor. Chemokines are 8–12 kDa proteins that can be secreted from or displayed on the cell surface of almost all somatic cells (Dong et al., 2003). They can bind to and activate specific receptors on the surface of leukocytes. Most chemokines also have the ability to bind to glycosoaminoglycans and this aids in their ability to coat endothelial surfaces and be presented to leukocytes that are moving through the circulation or lymphatics. In addition to inflammatory roles, chemokines are also integrally involved in the development and maintenance of the human immune system by helping immature hematopoietic cells move from the bone marrow to the thymus, spleen, lymph nodes and secondary lymphoid tissues. Chemokines are also important in stimulating the chemotaxis of antigen presenting cells like dendritic cells to the lymph nodes and in shaping the quality of the immune response to pathogens.

More than 40 human chemokines and 18 signaling receptors have been discovered to date and a systematic classification of both has been endorsed by the IUIS/WHO Subcommittee on Chemokine Nomenclature that simplifies the naming of these molecules (2003). The human chemokines are classified structurally by the number and position of four conserved cysteines into four subfamilies: CC, CXC, CX3C and XC (where X indicates any amino acid in the first three subfamilies so that none, one, or three residues separate the first two cysteines respectively; XC chemokines lack both the first and third cysteines). Human chemokines of a particular structural subfamily generally bind only to that subfamily of receptor, although there are numerous exceptions in the pathogen encoded chemokine receptor binding proteins. For example, vMIP-II encoded by human herpesvirus 8, the causative agent of Kaposi's sarcoma, is capable of binding to a variety of both CC and CXC receptors to act as a chemokine antagonist (Kledal et al., 1997). In the human system, there is also considerable overlap in binding of a particular chemokine to multiple receptors and in most cases each receptor can signal in response to more than one chemokine. This has created a certain redundancy in the system but, nonetheless, the loss of a particular member can create specific susceptibilities which, in some cases, can be lethal as demonstrated by animal models (Gao et al., 1997; Zou et al., 1998).

The Duffy antigen and *Plasmodium vivax* infection

In the 1970s, Miller and coworkers discovered that individuals who did not express the Duffy blood group antigen, a phenotype nearly universal in West Africans, were resistant to malaria caused by the parasite *Plasmodium vivax* (Miller et al., 1976). The Duffy antigen was subsequently identified as a non-signaling chemokine binding protein that facilitates an initial binding of the parasite to red blood cells (RBCs) (Horuk et al., 1993). The Duffy negative phenotype was found to be due in most cases to a single nucleotide polymorphism (SNP) in the promoter region of the gene that blocks expression only in (RBCs) (Tournamille et al., 1995). Presumably this SNP has been selected for by improving the genetic fitness of the individuals who lack RBC Duffy expression and are thereby less susceptible to *P. vivax* malaria. Thus, the parasite has exploited Duffy to infect RBCs, and this in turn appears to have provided strong selection pressure for fixation of an allele that is no longer expressed in RBCs.

Chemokine receptors and HIV

In the mid 1990s, several key discoveries resulted in a better understanding of the pathogenesis of HIV infection. It was well known that CD4 was necessary for cell entry but it was not sufficient since different HIV-1 strains were restricted to a subset of CD4+ cells. A functional cloning strategy was used to identify the chemokine receptor CXCR4 as a coreceptor able to complement CD4 for T cell line infection (Feng et al., 1996). The discovery that the same chemokines that bind to the chemokine receptor CCR5 could suppress HIV infection of monocytes resulted in identification of CCR5 as an HIV coreceptor (Cocchi et al., 1995; Alkhatib et al., 1996; Choe et al., 1996; Deng et al., 1996; Doranz et al., 1996; Dragic et al., 1996). This led to replacement of previous cytotropism- and cytopathicity-based classification schemes for HIV by a more precise molecular classification scheme, whereby HIV strains are defined as X4, R5 or R5X4 (those that are capable of using CXCR4, CCR5 or both for cell entry) (Berger et al., 1998). Since then, it has become apparent that a variety of chemokine and related receptors can serve as HIV coreceptors in transfected cells *in vitro*; but for most their significance *in vivo* is not yet clear (Table 3.1).

Further crystallographic and antibody blocking studies have revealed that the HIV envelope protein, gp120 first binds to CD4 and that subsequent binding to a chemokine receptor results in another HIV envelope protein, gp41, springing forward to spear the host cell membrane causing membrane fusion of the virus with the host cell (Moore and Doms, 2003). Thus binding of gp120 to the chemokine receptor and CD4 acts as a molecular trigger to allow HIV to gain entry into cells. Animal and *in vitro* studies have revealed that the coreceptor expression levels are critically important to the efficiency of HIV entry (Picchio et al., 1997; Wu et al., 1997; Naif et al., 1998).

Analogous to the inactivating polymorphism in Duffy described above, the discovery of CCR5Δ32 proved the importance of functional CCR5 to HIV disease. The CCR5Δ32 mutant allele results from a 32 base pair deletion in the open reading frame. This results in a non-functional truncated receptor that is not expressed on the cell surface and thus cannot function as an HIV coreceptor. In addition, the CCR5Δ32 gene product appears to

Table 3.1 HIV coreceptors that permit infection of CD4+ cell lines *in vitro*

Coreceptor	Ligands	Isolate usage	References
CCR2	MCP-1, MCP-2, MCP-3	+	(Doranz et al., 1996)
CCR3	Eotaxin, eotaxin-2, MCP-3, MCP-4, RANTES	++	(Doranz et al., 1996; Choe et al., 1996)
CCR5	MIP-1a/B, RANTES, MCP-2	++++	(Alkhatib et al., 1996; Deng et al., 1996; Dragic et al., 1996)
CCR8	I-309	++	(Rucker et al., 1997)
CCR9	TECK	+	(Choe et al., 1998)
CXCR4	SDF-1	+++	(Feng et al., 1996)
CXCR6	Bonzo ligand	+	(Liao et al., 1997; Deng et al., 1997)
CX3CR1	Fractalkine	+	(Combadiere et al., 1998)
APJ	Apelin	+	(Choe et al., 1998; Edinger et al., 1998b)
ChemR23	Chemerin	+	(Samson et al., 1998)
GPR1	?	+	(Edinger et al., 1998a)
GPR15/Bob	?	+	(Edinger et al., 1998a)
RDC1	?	+	(Shimizu et al., 2000)

interfere with normal CCR5 and CXCR4 receptor function through homo/heterodimerization (Benkirane et al., 1997; Mellado et al., 1999). The homozygous CCR5Δ32 genotype is found at much lower than expected frequency among HIV+ individuals, and heterozygotes exhibit slowed progression to AIDS (Liu et al., 1996; Samson et al., 1996; Dean et al., 1996; Huang et al., 1996; Zimmerman et al., 1997).

The CCR5Δ32 mutation is found at an allele frequency of 10 per cent in North American Caucasians, but is absent in other races. In Europe there is a higher allele frequency in the north which declines steadily as one moves south and by comparison to adjacent genetic markers the mutation is estimated to have arisen approximately 1000 years ago (Libert et al., 1998; Stephens et al., 1998). In a possible example of convergent evolution, two other rarer human mutations that cause a truncated form of the receptor have also been identified, CCR5m303 and CCR5-894(-) (Ansari-Lari et al., 1997; Quillent et al., 1998). Likewise a more evolutionarily ancient 24 base pair deletion of CCR5 that interferes with function has been found in sooty mangabey monkeys (Palacios et al., 1998; Chen et al., 1998). Since HIV is a relatively recent human affliction, it is not thought to be the factor responsible for fixation of the CCR5Δ32 allele at such high levels so quickly. Therefore speculation has focused on another ancestral epidemic in which CCR5 function was important. The finding that myxoma virus, a poxvirus of rabbits, can cause CCR5 signaling that affects its replication, has fueled speculation that CCR5 may also be a virulence factor for variola and that CCR5Δ32 may have been selected for by smallpox epidemics (Lalani et al., 1999; Masters et al., 2001). Individuals lacking CCR5 have no known health problems (Nguyen et al., 1999). Likewise, CCR5 -/- mice are normal, unless stressed. However, if human CCR5Δ32 homozygotes like CCR5 -/- mice are more susceptible to listeria, cryptococcus, cerebral malaria or other infections, this may provide a balancing positive selection pressure to retain CCR5 (Zhou et al., 1998; Huffnagle et al., 1999; Belnoue et al., 2003).

The CCR5 promoter is highly polymorphic, which could account for the wide variation in CCR5 expression that has been reported and at least one of these polymorphisms (59029-A, also called 303A, and −2459A) or the haplotype it is found on (P1 or HHE) has been associated with increased rate of progression to AIDS in multiple studies (McDermott et al., 1998; Martin et al., 1998; Gonzalez et al., 1999; Clegg et al., 2000; Ometto et al., 2001; Singh et al., 2003) and is associated with increased production of CCR5 in an in vitro promoter assay and increased CCR5 expression and HIV infectability of macrophages (McDermott et al., 1998; Salkowitz et al., 2003). A chemokine ligand for CCR5 called RANTES has two common promoter SNPs called RANTES-403A and -28G that have been associated with both the risk of HIV transmission and progression (Liu et al., 1999; McDermott et al., 2000a; Gonzalez et al., 2001).

Genetic studies have also implicated other chemokine receptors in HIV pathogenesis. These include a common SNP in the CCR2 gene called CCR2–64I associated with slower progression to AIDS (Smith et al., 1997; Kostrikis et al., 1998; Mummidi et al., 1998; Easterbrook et al., 1999; Mangano et al., 2000); however, the mechanism of how this polymorphism affects progression is unknown. A SNP in the promoter of the gene for the chemokine ligand of CCR2, MCP-1-2578G, has also been associated with decreased risk of HIV transmission, but increased risk of HIV progression and AIDS dementia (Gonzalez et al., 2002). The findings of altered HIV progression in SDF1-3′α and CX3CR1 M280 homozygotes by Winkler et al. (1998) and Faure et al. (2000) have not been confirmed by other studies (Winkler et al., 1998; Faure et al., 2000; McDermott et al., 2000b; Ioannidis et al., 2001).

Chemokine receptor polymorphisms may also affect response to antiretroviral therapy by influencing coreceptor availability or function. In particular, a number of studies have found that CCR5Δ32 heterozygotes are more likely to respond fully to antiretroviral therapy (Valdez et al., 1999; O'Brien et al., 2000; Guerin et al., 2000; Kasten et al., 2000); however, this has not been seen in several other studies (Brumme et al., 2001; Wit et al., 2002). A study has found that the effect of the currently approved drug Enfuvirtide (T-20) in vitro is dependent on HIV coreceptor levels suggesting that this new agent may also be influenced by chemokine receptor levels in clinical practice (Reeves et al., 2002). Another study has found that in HIV patients treated with the cytokine IL-2, there was a more robust increase in CD4+ cells in the CCR5Δ32 heterozygotes (Clegg et al., 2003). Taken together, these findings indicate that host genetic testing may have prognostic significance in the treatment of HIV similar to that now being done in clinical practice to genotype HIV itself. In addition, the finding that HIV coreceptors are essential for viral entry has led to the development of a whole new class of cytokine receptor blocking agents to inhibit fusion and viral entry (Este, 2003; Moore and Doms, 2003). Most of these target the chemokine receptors CCR5 and CXCR4. While none has yet been approved, several orally bioavailable small molecule inhibitors are in clinical testing.

Chemokine receptors and atherosclerosis

Atherosclerosis, the underlying mechanism of peripheral vascular disease, coronary artery disease and strokes, is increasingly being understood to be an inflammatory disease of the arteries. Leukocytes, primarily monocytes and lymphocytes, migrate into the vessel wall at sites of vascular injury and lipid deposition. Activated, lipid laden, monocyte-derived macrophages called foam cells are believed to play a key role in lesions by secreting cytokines like vascular endothelial growth factor (VEGF) that stimulate the growth of other cell types such as smooth muscle. At least three chemokine receptors

(CXCR2, CCR2 and CX3CR1) have been implicated in playing a proinflammatory role in atherosclerosis in susceptible animal models such as LDLR or apo-E deficient mice. Genetic targeting of these receptors has resulted in less atherosclerosis in susceptible mouse models (Boisvert et al., 1998; Boring et al., 1998; Gu et al., 1998; Lesnik et al., 2003; Combadiere et al., 2003). Human genetic association studies have further supported CCR2 and CX3CR1 playing a significant role in disease (McDermott et al., 2001, 2003; Moatti et al., 2001; Szalai et al., 2001; Ortlepp et al., 2003). Clinical trials with chemokine receptor blocking agents have not been reported; however, in a primate model, an antibody that blocks CCR2 was able to prevent neo-intimal hyperplasia (restenosis) following vascular stenting and another directed against CX3CR1 was able to block cardiac transplant rejection (Horvath et al., 2000; Robinson et al., 2000).

TUMOR NECROSIS FACTOR RECEPTORS

The first of the tumor necrosis factor (TNF) receptors was cloned in 1990 (Loetscher et al., 1990; Schall et al., 1990), but in the past two decades the TNF receptor superfamily has grown to 30 members (see http://www.gene.ucl. ac.uk/nomenclature/genefamily/tnftop.html). Both the ligands and receptors share structural similarities and the mature ligands all form trimers (Hehlgans and Mannel, 2002). This review will focus on TNF and the TNF receptors themselves because of space considerations although this family includes a variety of very interesting receptors such as the costimulatory receptor that plays a critical role in antibody isotype class switching, CD40 (TNFRSF5), a herpes virus entry mediator, HVEM (TNFRSF14), and a receptor important for lymphocyte apoptosis, FAS (TNFRSF6).

TNF is synthesized as a membrane-bound protein that can be cleaved by a specific metalloproteinase called TACE (for TNF-α converting enzyme) to form a soluble protein that is also biologically active (Black et al., 1997). TNF acts by binding to two different membrane bound receptors termed TNFRSF1A and TNFRSF1B which can also both be cleaved from the cell surface to form nonsignaling TNF binding (decoy) receptors. TNFRSF1A is expressed on many cell types and mediates both apoptosis by activation of caspases thru death domain signaling and nuclear factor kappa B (NFκB) activation of proinflammatory cytokine transcription; whereas, TNFRSF1B is primarily expressed on leukocytes and endothelial cells and acts to stimulate transcription thru NFκB but lacks a death domain (Smith et al., 1990; Grell et al., 1995). In addition to having a membrane bound and soluble cleaved form, the TNFRSF1B gene also has an intracellular isoform resulting from alternative splicing termed icp75TNFR that can also activate NFκB in an autocrine manner in cells that make TNF (Seitz et al., 2001). In a final

complexity, both of the TNF receptors can also bind trimers of a closely related family member called lymphotoxin-α either secreted by activated lymphocytes or cell-surface bound with lymphotoxin-β (McDermott, 2001).

TNFRSF1A knockout mice are less susceptible to endotoxin induced shock, TNF induced skin necrosis, experimental autoimmune encephalitis (EAE) and graft versus host disease, but demonstrate greatly increased mortality to L. monocytogenes, T. gondii and M. tuberculosis (Pfeffer et al., 1993; Flynn et al., 1995; Amar et al., 1995; Speiser et al., 1997; Deckert-Schluter et al., 1998; Suvannavejh et al., 2000). TNFRSF1B knockout mice on the other hand are more susceptible to EAE and hypersensitivity pneumonitis, show reduced CD8+ T cell activation and less Fas/Fas ligand induced apoptosis (Peschon et al., 1998; Teh et al., 2000; Kim and Teh, 2001), but are protected from cerebral malaria (Lucas et al., 1997). A transgenic TNF producing mouse develops arthritis which is diminished by removing either TNF receptor (Keffer et al., 1991; Alexopoulou et al., 1997).

TNF receptors and human disease

The development of TNF inhibitors has been a very active area of drug development in the past decade. The above animal studies and the recognition that TNF and its receptors were markedly upregulated in rheumatoid arthritis (RA) in the inflamed synovium led to the hypothesis that TNF receptor signaling played a pathogenic role (Feldmann et al., 1996). In the USA three inhibitors of TNF have been approved for treatment of RA. The first of these to show clinical efficacy was infliximab (Remicade), a chimeric (mouse/human) monoclonal anti-TNF antibody (Knight et al., 1993). The second is etanercept (Enbrel) which is a TNFRSF1B dimer linked to the Fc portion of human IgG (Mohler et al., 1993). Lenercept, a similar dimer of TNFRSF1A linked to Fc showed promise in animal models but was not as effective in human clinical trials possibly due to its immunogenicity and is no longer in development (Taylor, 2003). The third agent, adalimumab (Humira), is a fully human anti-TNF monoclonal antibody (Bain and Brazil, 2003). A variety of other antibodies directed against TNF and a PEGylated TNF receptor are in development (Taylor, 2003). Infliximab has also been approved for the treatment of Crohn's disease, an inflammatory disease of the gastrointestinal tract, based on efficacy in a multicenter, double-blinded and placebo controlled study (Targan et al., 1997).

Since these agents are not small molecules they require parenteral administration and maintenance of an effect requires continued treatment. With repeated injections, anti-therapeutic molecule antibodies may develop that limit the efficacy of further therapy and/or cause injection reactions. In addition, all approved therapies have been associated with reactivation of latent M. tuberculosis infection, lupus-like autoimmune disease and a potentially increased risk of lymphoma (Palladino et al., 2003).

Case reports of opportunistic infections occurring in those on anti-TNF therapy such as listeriosis, histoplasmosis and pneumocystis have also been published (Sfikakis and Kollias, 2003). This points to the key role that TNF plays in host defense against intracellular bacteria and in lymphocyte apoptosis. Oral bioavailability and greater efficacy with fewer side effects are goals in the further development of these inhibitors.

A rare hereditary periodic fever syndrome named TRAPS for TNF receptor-associated periodic syndrome has been found to result from functional mutations in the TNFRSF1A receptor (McDermott et al., 1999; Aksentijevich et al., 2001). This syndrome is characterized by recurrent attacks of fever, abdominal, muscle and joint pains, and skin and eye inflammation that last for more than a week. Attacks respond to corticosteroid therapy and etanercept. In about 25 per cent of cases systemic amyloidosis, which can result in renal failure, is also seen in affected family members (Drenth and van der Meer, 2001). Several of the TNFRSF1A mutations (C52F, T50M and C33Y) that cause TRAPS appear to reduce receptor cleavage and thus demonstrate the normal immune system downmodulatory effect of the soluble form of the receptor which no longer signals but can still bind free TNF (McDermott, 2001).

A variety of common TNF (- 308A, - 238A) and TNFRSF1B (M196R) polymorphisms have been identified, but associations with disease have been inconsistent (Baugh and Bucala, 2001). A recent study, yet to be confirmed, has found an association between TNFRSF1B haplotype as determined by four common SNPs and femoral neck bone mineral density (Spotila et al., 2003). Since TNF has previously been shown to be involved in osteoclast differentiation and migration, this provides additional biological evidence that TNF receptor heterogeneity may be important in osteoporosis.

INTERFERON RECEPTORS

Interferons (IFN) are cytokines critical to host defense against intracellular bacteria and viruses. They were named because of their capability of interfering with viral replication (Nagano and Kojima, 1954; Isaacs and Lindenmann, 1957). They act by regulating the transcription of many inflammatory genes. The type I interferon genes (IFNα, IFNβ, and IFNω are clustered on chromosome 9p22 and signal through a receptor which is heterodimeric with IFNαRα and IFNαRβ chains encoded by genes clustered on chromosome 21q22 (Fountain et al., 1992; Diaz et al., 1996). Mice deficient in either IFNα or the type I interferon receptors fail to control the replication of many viruses and exhibit increased mortality (Muller et al., 1994; van den Broek et al., 1995; Weck et al., 1997). Presumably to reduce the host inflammatory response, poxviruses such as vaccinia secrete a soluble type I IFN receptor that binds IFNα (Symons et al., 1995). Humans with mutations resulting in non-functional type I

interferon receptor have not been found to date possibly because of the strong selection against these mutations or lethality in fetal development/infancy. IFNα/ribavirin combination therapy is now the standard of care for treating chronic hepatitis C infection and IFNα is also widely used in chronic myelogenous leukemia (Lipman and Cotler, 2003; Druker et al., 2001). Clinical trials are currently studying the efficacy of PEGylated IFNα/lamivudine combination therapy to treat chronic hepatitis B and IFNβ is widely used in multiple sclerosis (Chofflon, 2000).

Type II IFN, IFNγ is encoded by a single gene on chromosome 12q14 and its receptor is heterodimeric with IFNγR1 and IFNγR2 chains encoded on chromosome 6q24 and 21q22 respectively. IFNγ-deficient and IFN-γR deficient mice have demonstrated deficiency of host defense against the intracellular bacteria *L. monocytogenes*, mycobacteria like *M. tuberculosis*, *M. avium*, and *M. bovis*, the parasite *T. gondii* and some viruses such as vaccinia, Theiler's and γHV 68 (Kamijo et al., 1993; Dalton et al., 1993; Huang et al., 1993; Muller et al., 1994; van den Broek et al., 1995; Yap and Sher, 1999). In humans various rare functional defects in both IFNγR1 and IFNγR2 have been identified (Dorman and Holland, 2000; Ottenhoff et al., 2003). Phenotypically these result in severe recurrent infections with non-tuberculous mycobacteria, salmonella and various viruses. Detection of one of these mutations in several different unrelated families who have affected family members has identified a so-called mutational hotspot present in IFNγR1 at basepair 818 where a 4 bp deletion results in accumulation of non-signaling IFNγ binding receptors on the cell surface (Jouanguy et al., 1999). A second hotspot associated with a 4 bp deletion at basepair 561 has recently been found in the IFNγR1 (Rosenzweig et al., 2002). Each of these mutations that interfere with receptor function appears to be quite rare in the general population, however. A more common polymorphism of the IFNγR2 gene (Arg64Gln) has been associated with the autoimmune disease, systemic lupus erythematosus when found in combination with a polymorphism in IFNγR1 (G88A) in a Japanese cohort but this has yet to be confirmed (Nakashima et al., 1999). An intronic dinucleotide repeat microsatellite (CA)$_n$ of the gene encoding IFNγR1 has been reported to be associated with risk of tuberculosis but another study was unable to replicate this (Fraser et al., 2003; Newport et al., 2003).

IFNγ is used therapeutically to prevent infections in the rare genetic immunodeficiency, chronic granulomatous disease based on an international, double-blinded, placebo-controlled trial performed by The International Chronic Granulomatous Disease Cooperative Study Group (ICGDC, 1991). It is also used in the rare genetic bone disease, osteopetrosis where it increases bone resorption and decreases infections and anemia (Key et al., 1995). IFNγ potently reduces collagen synthesis and thus may have use in autoimmune diseases where fibrosis is a major problem like progressive systemic sclerosis (scleroderma) or idiopathic pulmonary fibrosis (Freundlich et al., 1992; Grassegger et al., 1998; Ziesche et al., 1999). IFNγ may have a role in the treatment of the parasitic disease, visceral leishmaniasis, where several small studies have shown a beneficial role using combination IFNγ/antimonial treatment (Badaro and Johnson, 1993; Sundar et al., 1997). Finally, IFNγ may have a therapeutic role in the treatment of the mycobacterial diseases caused by *M. leprae*, *M. avium* complex, and *M. tuberculosis* when used in combination with anti-mycobacterials (Squires et al., 1989; Sampaio et al., 1992; Holland et al., 1994; Chatte et al., 1995; Condos et al., 1997).

CONCLUSION

Since the pioneering work of Edward Jenner and Louis Pasteur on early vaccines, medicine has sought to control and direct the immune response to protect against pathogens. Cytokine receptors are a clear pharmaceutical target that are already being utilized for therapeutic intervention in a variety of infectious, inflammatory and malignant diseases. Because of their cell surface location and structural properties many of these receptors are very amenable to specific blockade by orally active compounds, i.e. they are very druggable. Many of the cytokine receptors also exhibit mutations or polymorphisms that may affect the response to or complications from such therapies. As genotyping and DNA sequencing become less expensive, it may be possible to determine each individual's genomic profile to identify propensity to various diseases and likely reactions to treatments allowing custom-tailored therapy and personalized medicine. In addition, cytokine or cytokine receptor based biomarkers like TNF/TNF receptor levels may help to monitor the response to treatment. However, the sheer complexity of the cytokine network and the delicate balancing needed to optimize the immune response for each individual will continue to challenge investigators for the next century if not longer.

REFERENCES

Aksentijevich, I., Galon, J., Soares, M. et al. (2001). The tumor-necrosis-factor receptor-associated periodic syndrome: new mutations in TNFRSF1A, ancestral origins, genotype-phenotype studies, and evidence for further genetic heterogeneity of periodic fevers. Am J Hum Genet 69, 301–314.

Alexopoulou, L., Pasparakis, M. and Kollias, G. (1997). A murine transmembrane tumor necrosis factor (TNF) transgene induces arthritis by cooperative p55/p75 TNF receptor signaling. Eur J Immunol 27, 2588–2592.

Alkhatib, G., Combadiere, C., Broder, C.C. et al. (1996). CC CKR5: a RANTES, MIP-1alpha, MIP-1beta receptor as a fusion cofactor for macrophage-tropic HIV-1. Science 272, 1955–1958.

Amar, S., Van Dyke, T.E., Eugster, H.P., Schultze, N., Koebel, P. and Bluethmann, H. (1995). Tumor necrosis factor (TNF)-induced cutaneous necrosis is mediated by TNF receptor 1. J Inflamm 47, 180–189.

Ansari-Lari, M.A., Liu, X.M., Metzker, M.L., Rut, A.R. and Gibbs, R.A. (1997). The extent of genetic variation in the CCR5 gene. Nat Genet 16, 221–222.

Badaro, R. and Johnson, W.D. Jr (1993). The role of interferon-gamma in the treatment of visceral and diffuse cutaneous leishmaniasis. J Infect Dis 167 Suppl 1, S13–17.

Bain, B. and Brazil, M. (2003). Adalimumab. Nat Rev Drug Discov 2, 693–694.

Baugh, J.A. and Bucala, R. (2001). Mechanisms for modulating TNF alpha in immune and inflammatory disease. Curr Opin Drug Discov Devel 4, 635–650.

Belnoue, E., Kayibanda, M., Deschemin, J.C. et al. (2003). CCR5 deficiency decreases susceptibility to experimental cerebral malaria. Blood 101, 4253–4259.

Benkirane, M., Jin, D.Y., Chun, R.F., Koup, R.A. and Jeang, K.T. (1997). Mechanism of transdominant inhibition of CCR5-mediated HIV-1 infection by ccr5delta32. J Biol Chem 272, 30603–30606.

Berger, E.A., Doms, R.W., Fenyo, E.M. et al. (1998). A new classification for HIV-1 (letter). Nature 391, 240.

Black, R.A., Rauch, C.T., Kozlosky, C.J. et al. (1997). A metalloproteinase disintegrin that releases tumour-necrosis factor-alpha from cells. Nature 385, 729–733.

Boisvert, W.A., Santiago, R., Curtiss, L.K. and Terkeltaub, R.A. (1998). A leukocyte homologue of the IL-8 receptor CXCR-2 mediates the accumulation of macrophages in atherosclerotic lesions of LDL receptor-deficient mice. J Clin Invest 101, 353–363.

Boring, L., Gosling, J., Cleary, M. and Charo, I.F. (1998). Decreased lesion formation in CCR2-/- mice reveals a role for chemokines in the initiation of atherosclerosis. Nature 394, 894–897.

Brumme, Z.L., Chan, K.J., Dong, W. et al. (2001). CCR5Delta32 and promoter polymorphisms are not correlated with initial virological or immunological treatment response. AIDS 15, 2259–2266.

Chatte, G., Panteix, G., Perrin-Fayolle, M. and Pacheco, Y. (1995). Aerosolized interferon gamma for Mycobacterium avium-complex lung disease. Am J Respir Crit Care Med 152, 1094–1096.

Chen, Z., Kwon, D., Jin, Z. et al. (1998). Natural infection of a homozygous delta24 CCR5 red-capped mangabey with an R2b-tropic simian immunodeficiency virus. J Exp Med 188, 2057–2065.

Choe, H., Farzan, M., Konkel, M. et al. (1998). The orphan seven-transmembrane receptor apj supports the entry of primary T-cell-line-tropic and dualtropic human immunodeficiency virus type 1. J Virol 72, 6113–6118.

Choe, H., Farzan, M., Sun, Y. et al. (1996). The beta-chemokine receptors CCR3 and CCR5 facilitate infection by primary HIV-1 isolates. Cell 85, 1135–1148.

Chofflon, M. (2000). Recombinant human interferon beta in relapsing-remitting multiple sclerosis: a review of the major clinical trials. Eur J Neurol 7, 369–380.

Clegg, A.O., Ashton, L.J., Biti, R.A. et al. (2000). CCR5 promoter polymorphisms, CCR5 59029A and CCR5 59353C, are under represented in HIV-1-infected long-term non-progressors. The Australian Long-Term Non-Progressor Study Group. AIDS 14, 103–108.

Clegg, A., Williamson, P., Biti, R. et al. (2003). Chemokine receptor genotype and response to interleukin-2 therapy in HIV-1-infected individuals. Clin Immunol 106, 36–40.

Cocchi, F., DeVico, A.L., Garzino-Demo, A., Arya, S.K., Gallo, R.C. and Lusso, P. (1995). Identification of RANTES, MIP-1 alpha, and MIP-1 beta as the major HIV-suppressive factors produced by CD8+ T cells (see comments). Science 270, 1811–1815.

Combadiere, C., Potteaux, S., Gao, J.L. et al. (2003). Decreased atherosclerotic lesion formation in CX3CR1/apolipoprotein E double knockout mice. Circulation 107, 1009–1016.

Combadiere, C., Salzwedel, K., Smith, E.D. et al. (1998). Identification of CX3CR1. A chemotactic receptor for the human CX3C chemokine fractalkine and a fusion coreceptor for HIV-1. J Biol Chem 273, 23799–23804.

Condos, R., Rom, W.N. and Schluger, N.W. (1997). Treatment of multidrug-resistant pulmonary tuberculosis with interferon-gamma via aerosol. Lancet 349, 1513–1515.

Dalton, D.K., Pitts-Meek, S., Keshav, S., Figari, I.S., Bradley, A. and Stewart, T.A. (1993). Multiple defects of immune cell function in mice with disrupted interferon-gamma genes. Science 259, 1739–1742.

Dean, M., Carrington, M., Winkler, C. et al. (1996). Genetic restriction of HIV-1 infection and progression to AIDS by a deletion allele of the CKR5 structural gene. Hemophilia Growth and Development Study, Multicenter AIDS Cohort Study, Multicenter Hemophilia Cohort Study, San Francisco City Cohort, ALIVE Study (see comments) (published erratum appears in Science 1996 Nov 15;274(5290):1069). Science 273, 1856–1862.

Deckert-Schluter, M., Bluethmann, H., Rang, A., Hof, H. and Schluter, D. (1998). Crucial role of TNF receptor type 1 (p55), but not of TNF receptor type 2 (p75), in murine toxoplasmosis. J Immunol 160, 3427–3436.

Deng, H., Liu, R., Ellmeier, W. et al. (1996). Identification of a major co-receptor for primary isolates of HIV-1 (see comments). Nature 381, 661–666.

Deng, H.K., Unutmaz, D., KewalRamani, V.N. and Littman, D.R. (1997). Expression cloning of new receptors used by simian and human immunodeficiency viruses (see comments). Nature 388, 296–300.

Diaz, M.O., Bohlander, S. and Allen, G. (1996). Nomenclature of the human interferon genes. J Interferon Cytokine Res 16, 179–180.

Dong, V.M., McDermott, D.H. and Abdi, R. (2003). Chemokines and diseases. Eur J Dermatol 13, 224–230.

Doranz, B.J., Rucker, J., Yi, Y. et al. (1996). A dual-tropic primary HIV-1 isolate that uses fusin and the beta-chemokine receptors CKR-5, CKR-3, and CKR-2b as fusion cofactors. Cell 85, 1149–1158.

Dorman, S.E. and Holland, S.M. (2000). Interferon-gamma and interleukin-12 pathway defects and human disease. Cytokine Growth Factor Rev 11, 321–333.

Dragic, T., Litwin, V., Allaway, G.P. et al. (1996). HIV-1 entry into CD4+ cells is mediated by the chemokine receptor CC-CKR-5 (see comments). Nature 381, 667–673.

Drenth, J.P. and van der Meer, J.W. (2001). Hereditary periodic fever. N Engl J Med 345, 1748–1757.

Druker, B.J., Sawyers, C.L., Capdeville, R., Ford, J.M., Baccarani, M. and Goldman, J.M. (2001). Chronic myelogenous leukemia. Hematology (Am Soc Hematol Educ Program) 87–112.

Easterbrook, P.J., Rostron, T., Ives, N., Troop, M., Gazzard, B.G. and Rowland-Jones, S.L. (1999). Chemokine receptor polymorphisms and human immunodeficiency virus disease progression. J Infect Dis 180, 1096–1105.

Edinger, A.L., Hoffman, T.L., Sharron, M., Lee, B., O'Dowd, B. and Doms, R.W. (1998a). Use of GPR1, GPR15, and STRL33 as coreceptors by diverse human immunodeficiency virus type 1 and simian immunodeficiency virus envelope proteins. Virology 249, 367–378.

Edinger, A.L., Hoffman, T.L., Sharron, M. et al. (1998b). An orphan seven-transmembrane domain receptor expressed widely in the brain functions as a coreceptor for human immunodeficiency virus type 1 and simian immunodeficiency virus. J Virol 72, 7934–7940.

Este, J.A. (2003). Virus entry as a target for anti-HIV intervention. Curr Med Chem 10, 1617–1632.

Faure, S., Meyer, L., Costagliola, D. et al. (2000). Rapid progression to AIDS in HIV+ individuals with a structural variant of the chemokine receptor CX3CR1. Science 287, 2274–2277.

Feldmann, M., Brennan, F.M. and Maini, R.N. (1996). Role of cytokines in rheumatoid arthritis. Annu Rev Immunol 14, 397–440.

Feng, Y., Broder, C.C., Kennedy, P.E. and Berger, E.A. (1996). HIV-1 entry cofactor: functional cDNA cloning of a seven-transmembrane, G protein-coupled receptor (see comments). Science 272, 872–877.

Flynn, J.L., Goldstein, M.M., Chan, J. et al. (1995). Tumor necrosis factor-alpha is required in the protective immune response against Mycobacterium tuberculosis in mice. Immunity 2, 561–572.

Fountain, J.W., Karayiorgou, M., Taruscio, D. et al. (1992). Genetic and physical map of the interferon region on chromosome 9p. Genomics 14, 105–112.

Fraser, D.A., Bulat-Kardum, L., Knezevic, J. et al. (2003). Interferon-gamma receptor-1 gene polymorphism in tuberculosis patients from Croatia. Scand J Immunol 57, 480–484.

Freundlich, B., Jimenez, S.A., Steen, V.D., Medsger, T.A., Jr., Szkolnicki, M. and Jaffe, H.S. (1992). Treatment of systemic sclerosis with recombinant interferon-gamma. A phase I/II clinical trial. Arthritis Rheum 35, 1134–1142.

Gao, J.L., Wynn, T.A., Chang, Y. et al. (1997). Impaired host defense, hematopoiesis, granulomatous inflammation and type 1-type 2 cytokine balance in mice lacking CC chemokine receptor 1. J Exp Med 185, 1959–1968.

Gonzalez, E., Bamshad, M., Sato, N. et al. (1999). Race-specific HIV-1 disease-modifying effects associated with CCR5 haplotypes. Proc Natl Acad Sci USA 96, 12004–12009.

Gonzalez, E., Dhanda, R., Bamshad, M. et al. (2001). Global survey of genetic variation in CCR5, RANTES, and MIP-1alpha: impact on the epidemiology of the HIV-1 pandemic. Proc Natl Acad Sci USA 98, 5199–5204.

Gonzalez, E., Rovin, B.H., Sen, L. et al. (2002). HIV-1 infection and AIDS dementia are influenced by a mutant MCP-1 allele linked to increased monocyte infiltration of tissues and MCP-1 levels. Proc Natl Acad Sci USA 99, 13795–13800.

Grassegger, A., Schuler, G., Hessenberger, G. et al. (1998). Interferon-gamma in the treatment of systemic sclerosis: a randomized controlled multicentre trial. Br J Dermatol 139, 639–648.

Grell, M., Douni, E., Wajant, H. et al. (1995). The transmembrane form of tumor necrosis factor is the prime activating ligand of the 80 kDa tumor necrosis factor receptor. Cell 83, 793–802.

Gu, L., Okada, Y., Clinton, S.K. et al. (1998). Absence of monocyte chemoattractant protein-1 reduces atherosclerosis in low density lipoprotein receptor-deficient mice. Mol Cell *2*, 275–281.

Guerin, S., Meyer, L., Theodorou, I. et al. (2000). CCR5 delta32 deletion and response to highly active antiretroviral therapy in HIV-1-infected patients. AIDS *14*, 2788–2790.

Hehlgans, T. and Mannel, D.N. (2002). The TNF-TNF receptor system. Biol Chem *383*, 1581–1585.

Holland, S.M., Eisenstein, E.M., Kuhns, D.B. et al. (1994). Treatment of refractory disseminated nontuberculous mycobacterial infection with interferon gamma. A preliminary report. N Engl J Med *330*, 1348–1355.

Horuk, R., Chitnis, C.E., Darbonne, W.C. et al. (1993). A receptor for the malarial parasite Plasmodium vivax: the erythrocyte chemokine receptor. Science *261*, 1182–1184.

Horvath, R., Cerny, J., Benedik, J., Hokl, J. and Jelinkova, I. (2000). The possible role of human cytomegalovirus (HCMV) in the origin of atherosclerosis. J Clin Virol *16*, 17–24.

Huang, S., Hendriks, W., Althage, A. et al. (1993). Immune response in mice that lack the interferon-gamma receptor. Science *259*, 1742–1745.

Huang, Y., Paxton, W.A., Wolinsky, S.M. et al. (1996). The role of a mutant CCR5 allele in HIV-1 transmission and disease progression (see comments). Nat Med *2*, 1240–1243.

Huffnagle, G.B., McNeil, L.K., McDonald, R.A. et al. (1999). Cutting edge: Role of C-C chemokine receptor 5 in organspecific and innate immunity to *Cryptococcus neoformans*. J Immunol *163*, 4642–4646.

I C G D C study group (1991). A controlled trial of interferon gamma to prevent infection in chronic granulomatous disease. N Engl J Med *324*, 509–516.

Ioannidis, J.P., Rosenberg, P.S., Goedert, J.J. et al. (2001). Effects of CCR5-Delta32, CCR2-64I, and SDF-1 3′A alleles on HIV-1 disease progression: An international meta-analysis of individual-patient data. Ann Intern Med *135*, 782–795.

Isaacs, A. and Lindenmann, J. (1957). Virus interference. I. The interferon. Proc R Soc Lond B Biol Sci *147*, 258–267.

IUIS/WHO Subcommittee on Chemokine Nomenclature (2003). Chemokine/chemokine receptor nomenclature. Cytokine *21*, 48–49.

Jouanguy, E., Lamhamedi-Cherradi, S., Lammas, D. et al. (1999). A human IFNGR1 small deletion hotspot associated with dominant susceptibility to mycobacterial infection. Nat Genet *21*, 370–378.

Kamijo, R., Le, J., Shapiro, D. et al. (1993). Mice that lack the interferon-gamma receptor have profoundly altered responses to infection with Bacillus Calmette-Guerin and subsequent challenge with lipopolysaccharide. J Exp Med *178*, 1435–1440.

Kasten, S., Goldwich, A., Schmitt, M. et al. (2000). Positive influence of the Delta32CCR5 allele on response to highly active antiretroviral therapy (HAART) in HIV-1 infected patients. Eur J Med Res *5*, 323–328.

Keffer, J., Probert, L., Cazlaris, H. et al. (1991). Transgenic mice expressing human tumour necrosis factor: a predictive genetic model of arthritis. EMBO J *10*, 4025–4031.

Key, L.L., Jr, Rodriguiz, R.M., Willi, S.M. et al. (1995). Long-term treatment of osteopetrosis with recombinant human interferon gamma. N Engl J Med *332*, 1594–1599.

Kim, E.Y. and Teh, H.S. (2001). TNF type 2 receptor (p75) lowers the threshold of T cell activation. J Immunol *167*, 6812–6820.

Kledal, T.N., Rosenkilde, M.M., Coulin, F. et al. (1997). A broadspectrum chemokine antagonist encoded by Kaposi's sarcoma-associated herpesvirus. Science *277*, 1656–1659.

Knight, D.M., Trinh, H., Le, J. et al. (1993). Construction and initial characterization of a mouse-human chimeric anti-TNF antibody. Mol Immunol *30*, 1443–1453.

Kostrikis, L.G., Huang, Y., Moore, J.P et al. (1998). A chemokine receptor CCR2 allele delays HIV-1 disease progression and is associated with a CCR5 promoter mutation (see comments). Nat Med *4*, 350–353.

Lalani, A.S., Masters, J., Zeng, W. et al. (1999). Use of chemokine receptors by poxviruses. Science *286*, 1968–1971.

Lesnik, P., Haskell, C.A. and Charo, I.F. (2003). Decreased atherosclerosis in CX3CR1-/- mice reveals a role for fractalkine in atherogenesis. J Clin Invest *111*, 333–340.

Liao, F., Alkhatib, G., Peden, K.W., Sharma, G., Berger, E.A. and Farber, J.M. (1997). STRL33, a novel chemokine receptorlike protein, functions as a fusion cofactor for both macrophage-tropic and T cell line-tropic HIV-1. J Exp Med *185*, 2015–2023.

Libert, F., Cochaux, P., Beckman, G. et al. (1998). The deltaccr5 mutation conferring protection against HIV-1 in Caucasian populations has a single and recent origin in Northeastern Europe. Hum Mol Genet *7*, 399–406.

Lipman, M.M. and Cotler, S.J. (2003). Antiviral therapy for hepatitis C. Curr Treat Options Gastroenterol *6*, 445–453.

Liston, A. and McColl, S. (2003). Subversion of the chemokine world by microbial pathogens. Bioessays *25*, 478–488.

Liu, H., Chao, D., Nakayama, E.E. et al. (1999). Polymorphism in RANTES chemokine promoter affects HIV-1 disease progression. Proc Natl Acad Sci USA *96*, 4581–4585.

Liu, R., Paxton, W.A., Choe, S. et al. (1996). Homozygous defect in HIV-1 coreceptor accounts for resistance of some multiplyexposed individuals to HIV-1 infection. Cell *86*, 367–377.

Loetscher, H., Pan, Y.C., Lahm, H.W. et al. (1990). Molecular cloning and expression of the human 55 kd tumor necrosis factor receptor. Cell *61*, 351–359.

Lucas, R., Juillard, P., Decoster, E. et al. (1997). Crucial role of tumor necrosis factor (TNF) receptor 2 and membrane-bound TNF in experimental cerebral malaria. Eur J Immunol *27*, 1719–1725.

Mangano, A., Kopka, J., Batalla, M., Bologna, R. and Sen, L. (2000). Protective effect of CCR2-64I and not of CCR5-delta32 and SDF1-3′A in pediatric HIV-1 infection. J Acquir Immune Defic Syndr *23*, 52–57.

Martin, M.P., Dean, M., Smith, M.W. et al. (1998). Genetic acceleration of AIDS progression by a promoter variant of CCR5. Science *282*, 1907–1911.

Masters, J., Hinek, A.A., Uddin, S. et al. (2001). Poxvirus infection rapidly activates tyrosine kinase signal transduction. J Biol Chem *276*, 48371–48375.

McDermott, D.H., Beecroft, M.J., Kleeberger, C.A. et al. (2000a). Chemokine RANTES promoter polymorphism affects risk of both HIV infection and disease progression in the Multicenter AIDS Cohort Study. Aids *14*, 2671–2678.

McDermott, D.H., Colla, J.S., Kleeberger, C.A. et al. (2000b). Genetic polymorphism in CX3CR1 and risk of HIV disease. Science *290*, 2031.

McDermott, D.H., Fong, A.M., Yang, Q. et al. (2003). Chemokine receptor mutant CX3CR1-M280 has impaired adhesive function and correlates with protection from cardiovascular disease in humans. J Clin Invest *111*, 1241–1250.

McDermott, D.H., Halcox, J.P., Schenke, W.H. et al. (2001). Association between polymorphism in the chemokine receptor CX3CR1 and coronary vascular endothelial dysfunction and atherosclerosis. Circ Res 89, 401–407.

McDermott, D.H. and Murphy, P. (2000). Chemokines and their receptors in infectious disease. Springer Semin Immunopathol 22, 393–415.

McDermott, D.H., Zimmerman, P.A., Guignard, F., Kleeberger, C.A., Leitman, S.F. and Murphy, P.M. (1998). CCR5 promoter polymorphism and HIV-1 disease progression. Multicenter AIDS Cohort Study (MACS). Lancet 352, 866–870.

McDermott, M.F. (2001). TNF and TNFR biology in health and disease. Cell Mol Biol (Noisy-le-grand) 47, 619–635.

McDermott, M.F., Aksentijevich, I., Galon, J. et al. (1999). Germline mutations in the extracellular domains of the 55 kDa TNF receptor, TNFR1, define a family of dominantly inherited autoinflammatory syndromes. Cell 97, 133–144.

McFadden, G. and Murphy, P.M. (2000). Host-related immunomodulators encoded by poxviruses and herpesviruses. Curr Opin Microbiol 3, 371–378.

Mechnikov, I. (1905). In Immunity in Infectious Diseases. Cambridge University Press.

Mellado, M., Rodriguez-Frade, J.M., Vila-Coro, A.J., de Ana, A.M. and Martinez, A. (1999). Chemokine control of HIV-1 infection (letter). Nature 400, 723–724.

Miller, L.H., Mason, S.J., Clyde, D.F. and McGinniss, M.H. (1976). The resistance factor to Plasmodium vivax in blacks. The Duffy-blood- group genotype, FyFy. N Engl J Med 295, 302–304.

Moatti, D., Faure, S., Fumeron, F. et al. (2001). Polymorphism in the fractalkine receptor CX3CR1 as a genetic risk factor for coronary artery disease. Blood 97, 1925–1928.

Mohler, K.M., Torrance, D.S., Smith, C.A. et al. (1993). Soluble tumor necrosis factor (TNF) receptors are effective therapeutic agents in lethal endotoxemia and function simultaneously as both TNF carriers and TNF antagonists. J Immunol 151, 1548–1561.

Moore, J. and Doms, R.W. (2003). The entry of entry inhibitors: a fusion of science and medicine. Proc Natl Acad Sci USA 100, 10598–10602.

Muller, U., Steinhoff, U., Reis, L.F. et al. (1994). Functional role of type I and type II interferons in antiviral defense. Science 264, 1918–1921.

Mummidi, S., Ahuja, S.S., Gonzalez, E. et al. (1998). Genealogy of the CCR5 locus and chemokine system gene variants associated with altered rates of HIV-1 disease progression. Nat Med 4, 786–793.

Murphy, P.M. (1993). Molecular mimicry and the generation of host defense protein diversity. Cell 72, 823–826.

Nagano, Y. and Kojima, Y. (1954). [Immunizing property of vaccinia virus inactivated by ultraviolets rays.] C R Seances Soc Biol Fil 148, 1700–1702.

Naif, H.M., Li, S., Alali, M. et al. (1998). CCR5 expression correlates with susceptibility of maturing monocytes to human immunodeficiency virus type 1 infection. J Virol, 72, 830–836.

Nakashima, H., Inoue, H., Akahoshi, M. et al. (1999). The combination of polymorphisms within interferon-gamma receptor 1 and receptor 2 associated with the risk of systemic lupus erythematosus. FEBS Lett 453, 187–190.

Newport, M.J., Awomoyi, A.A. and Blackwell, J.M. (2003). Polymorphism in the interferon-gamma receptor-1 gene and susceptibility to pulmonary tuberculosis in The Gambia. Scand J Immunol 58, 383–385.

Nguyen, G.T., Carrington, M., Beeler, J.A. et al. (1999). Phenotypic expressions of CCR5-delta32/delta32 homozygosity. J Acquir Immune Defic Syndr 22, 75–82.

O'Brien, T.R., McDermott, D.H., Ioannidis, J.P. et al. (2000). Effect of chemokine receptor gene polymorphisms on the response to potent antiretroviral therapy. AIDS 14, 821–826.

Ometto, L., Bertorelle, R., Mainardi, M. et al. (2001). Polymorphisms in the CCR5 promoter region influence disease progression in perinatally human immunodeficiency virus type 1-infected children. J Infect Dis 183, 814–818.

Ortlepp, J.R., Vesper, K., Mevissen, V. et al. (2003). Chemokine receptor (CCR2) genotype is associated with myocardial infarction and heart failure in patients under 65 years of age. J Mol Med 81, 363–367.

Ottenhoff, T.H., De Boer, T., van Dissel, J.T. and Verreck, F.A. (2003). Human deficiencies in type-1 cytokine receptors reveal the essential role of type-1 cytokines in immunity to intracellular bacteria. Adv Exp Med Biol 531, 279–294.

Palacios, E., Digilio, L., McClure, H.M. et al. (1998). Parallel evolution of CCR5-null phenotypes in humans and in a natural host of simian immunodeficiency virus. Curr Biol 8, 943–946.

Palladino, M.A., Bahjat, F.R., Theodorakis, E.A. and Moldawer, L.L. (2003). Anti-TNF-alpha therapies: the next generation. Nat Rev Drug Discov 2, 736–746.

Peschon, J.J., Torrance, D.S., Stocking, K.L. et al. (1998). TNF receptor-deficient mice reveal divergent roles for p55 and p75 in several models of inflammation. J Immunol 160, 943–952.

Pfeffer, K., Matsuyama, T., Kundig, T.M. et al. (1993). Mice deficient for the 55 kd tumor necrosis factor receptor are resistant to endotoxic shock, yet succumb to L. monocytogenes infection. Cell 73, 457–467.

Picchio, G.R., Gulizia, R.J. and Mosier, D.E. (1997). Chemokine receptor CCR5 genotype influences the kinetics of human immunodeficiency virus type 1 infection in human PBL-SCID mice. J Virol 71, 7124–7127.

Quillent, C., Oberlin, E., Braun, J. et al. (1998). HIV-1-resistance phenotype conferred by combination of two separate inherited mutations of CCR5 gene (see comments). Lancet 351, 14–18.

Reeves, J.D., Gallo, S.A., Ahmad, N. et al. (2002). Sensitivity of HIV-1 to entry inhibitors correlates with envelope/coreceptor affinity, receptor density, and fusion kinetics. Proc Natl Acad Sci USA 99, 16249–16254.

Robinson, L.A., Nataraj, C., Thomas, D.W. et al. (2000). A role for fractalkine and its receptor (CX3CR1) in cardiac allograft rejection. J Immunol 165, 6067–6072.

Rosenzweig, S., Dorman, S.E., Roesler, J., Palacios, J., Zelazko, M. and Holland, S.M. (2002). 561del4 defines a novel small deletion hotspot in the interferon-gamma receptor 1 chain. Clin Immunol 102, 25–27.

Rucker, J., Edinger, A.L., Sharron, M. et al. (1997). Utilization of chemokine receptors, orphan receptors, and herpesvirus-encoded receptors by diverse human and simian immunodeficiency viruses. J Virol 71, 8999–9007.

Salkowitz, J.R., Bruse, S.E., Meyerson, H. et al. (2003). CCR5 promoter polymorphism determines macrophage CCR5 density and magnitude of HIV-1 propagation in vitro. Clin Immunol 108, 234–240.

Sampaio, E.P., Moreira, A.L., Sarno, E.N., Malta, A.M. and Kaplan, G. (1992). Prolonged treatment with recombinant interferon gamma induces erythema nodosum leprosum in lepromatous leprosy patients. J Exp Med 175, 1729–1737.

Samson, M., Edinger, A.L., Stordeur, P. et al. (1998). ChemR23, a putative chemoattractant receptor, is expressed in monocyte-derived dendritic cells and macrophages and is a coreceptor for SIV and some primary HIV-1 strains. Eur J Immunol 28, 1689–1700.

Samson, M., Libert, F., Doranz, B.J. et al. (1996). Resistance to HIV-1 infection in caucasian individuals bearing mutant alleles of the CCR-5 chemokine receptor gene (see comments). Nature 382, 722–725.

Schall, T.J., Lewis, M., Koller, K.J. et al. (1990). Molecular cloning and expression of a receptor for human tumor necrosis factor. Cell 61, 361–370.

Seitz, C., Muller, P., Krieg, R.C., Mannel, D.N. and Hehlgans, T. (2001). A novel p75TNF receptor isoform mediating NFkappa B activation. J Biol Chem 276, 19390–19395.

Sfikakis, P.P. and Kollias, G. (2003). Tumor necrosis factor biology in experimental and clinical arthritis. Curr Opin Rheumatol 15, 380–386.

Shimizu, N., Soda, Y., Kanbe, K. et al. (2000). A putative G protein-coupled receptor, RDC1, is a novel coreceptor for human and simian immunodeficiency viruses. J Virol 74, 619–626.

Singh, K.K., Barroga, C.F., Hughes, M.D. et al. (2003). Genetic influence of CCR5, CCR2, and SDF1 variants on human immunodeficiency virus 1 (HIV-1)-related disease progression and neurological impairment, in children with symptomatic HIV-1 infection. J Infect Dis 188, 1461–1472.

Smith, C.A., Davis, T., Anderson, D. et al. (1990). A receptor for tumor necrosis factor defines an unusual family of cellular and viral proteins. Science 248, 1019–1023.

Smith, M.W., Dean, M., Carrington, M. et al. (1997). Contrasting genetic influence of CCR2 and CCR5 variants on HIV-1 infection and disease progression. Hemophilia Growth and Development Study (HGDS), Multicenter AIDS Cohort Study (MACS), Multicenter Hemophilia Cohort Study (MHCS), San Francisco City Cohort (SFCC), ALIVE Study. Science 277, 959–965.

Speiser, D E., Bachmann, M.F., Frick, T.W. et al. (1997). TNF receptor p55 controls early acute graft-versus-host disease. J Immunol 158, 5185–5190.

Spotila, L.D., Rodriguez, H., Koch, M. et al. (2003). Association analysis of bone mineral density and single nucleotide polymorphisms in two candidate genes on chromosome 1p36. Calcif Tissue Int 73, 140–146.

Squires, K.E., Murphy, W.F., Madoff, L.C. and Murray, H.W. (1989). Interferon-gamma and Mycobacterium avium-intracellulare infection. J Infect Dis 159, 599–600.

Stephens, J.C., Reich, D.E., Goldstein, D.B. et al. (1998). Dating the origin of the CCR5-Delta32 AIDS-resistance allele by the coalescence of haplotypes. Am J Hum Genet 62, 1507–1515.

Sundar, S., Singh, V.P., Sharma, S., Makharia, M.K. and Murray, H.W. (1997). Response to interferon-gamma plus pentavalent antimony in Indian visceral leishmaniasis. J Infect Dis 176, 1117–1119.

Suvannavejh, G.C., Lee, H.O., Padilla, J., Dal Canto, M.C., Barrett, T.A. and Miller, S.D. (2000). Divergent roles for p55 and p75 tumor necrosis factor receptors in the pathogenesis of MOG(35-55)-induced experimental autoimmune encephalomyelitis. Cell Immunol 205, 24–33.

Symons, J.A., Alcami, A. and Smith, G.L. (1995). Vaccinia virus encodes a soluble type I interferon receptor of novel structure and broad species specificity. Cell 81, 551–560.

Szalai, C., Duba, J., Prohaszka, Z. et al. (2001). Involvement of polymorphisms in the chemokine system in the susceptibility for coronary artery disease (CAD). Coincidence of elevated Lp(a) and MCP-1 -2518 G/G genotype in CAD patients. Atherosclerosis 158, 233–239.

Targan, S.R., Hanauer, S.B., van Deventer, S.J. et al. (1997). A short-term study of chimeric monoclonal antibody cA2 to tumor necrosis factor alpha for Crohn's disease. Crohn's Disease cA2 Study Group. N Engl J Med 337, 1029–1035.

Taylor, P.C. (2003). Anti-cytokines and cytokines in the treatment of rheumatoid arthritis. Curr Pharm Des 9, 1095–1106.

Teh, H.S., Seebaran, A. and Teh, S.J. (2000). TNF receptor 2-deficient CD8 T cells are resistant to Fas/Fas ligand-induced cell death. J Immunol 165, 4814–4821.

Tournamille, C., Colin, Y., Cartron, J.P. and Le Van Kim, C. (1995). Disruption of a GATA motif in the Duffy gene promoter abolishes erythroid gene expression in Duffy-negative individuals. Nat Genet 10, 224–228.

Valdez, H., Purvis, S.F., Lederman, M.M., Fillingame, M. and Zimmerman, P.A. (1999). Association of the CCR5delta32 mutation with improved response to antiretroviral therapy (letter). J Am Med Assoc 282, 734.

van den Broek, M.F., Muller, U., Huang, S., Zinkernagel, R.M. and Aguet, M. (1995). Immune defence in mice lacking type I and/or type II interferon receptors. Immunol Rev 148, 5–18.

Weck, K.E., Dal Canto, A.J., Gould, J.D. et al. (1997). Murine gamma-herpesvirus 68 causes severe large-vessel arteritis in mice lacking interferon-gamma responsiveness: a new model for virus-induced vascular disease. Nat Med 3, 1346–1353.

Winkler, C., Modi, W., Smith, M.W et al. (1998). Genetic restriction of AIDS pathogenesis by an SDF-1 chemokine gene variant. ALIVE Study, Hemophilia Growth and Development Study (HGDS), Multicenter AIDS Cohort Study (MACS), Multicenter Hemophilia Cohort Study (MHCS), San Francisco City Cohort (SFCC). Science 279, 389–393.

Wit, F.W., van Rij, R.P., Weverling, G.J., Lange, J.M. and Schuitemaker, H. (2002). CC chemokine receptor 5 delta32 and CC chemokine receptor 2 64I polymorphisms do not influence the virologic and immunologic response to anti-retroviral combination therapy in human immunodeficiency virus type 1-infected patients. J Infect Dis 186, 1726–1732.

Wu, L., Paxton, W.A., Kassam, N. et al. (1997). CCR5 levels and expression pattern correlate with infectability by macrophage-tropic HIV-1, in vitro. J Exp Med 185, 1681–1691.

Yap, G.S. and Sher, A. (1999). Effector cells of both nonhemopoietic and hemopoietic origin are required for interferon (IFN)-gamma- and tumor necrosis factor (TNF)-alpha-dependent host resistance to the intracellular pathogen, Toxoplasma gondii. J Exp Med 189, 1083–1092.

Zhou, Y., Kurihara, T., Ryseck, R.P. et al. (1998). Impaired macrophage function and enhanced T cell-dependent immune response in mice lacking CCR5, the mouse homologue of the major HIV-1 coreceptor. J Immunol 160, 4018–4025.

Ziesche, R., Hofbauer, E., Wittmann, K., Petkov, V. and Block, L. H. (1999). A preliminary study of long-term treatment with interferon gamma-1b and low-dose prednisolone in patients with idiopathic pulmonary fibrosis. N Engl J Med *341*, 1264–1269.

Zigmond, S.H. (1977). Ability of polymorphonuclear leukocytes to orient in gradients of chemotactic factors. J Cell Biol *75*, 606–616.

Zimmerman, P.A., Buckler, W.A., Alkhatib, G. et al. (1997). Inherited resistance to HIV-1 conferred by an inactivating mutation in CC chemokine receptor 5: studies in populations with contrasting clinical phenotypes, defined racial background, and quantified risk. Mol Med *3*, 23–36.

Zou, Y.R., Kottmann, A.H., Kuroda, M., Taniuchi, I. and Littman, D.R. (1998). Function of the chemokine receptor CXCR4 in haematopoiesis and in cerebellar development. Nature *393*, 595–599.

Genetic Diversity at Human Cytokine Loci in Health and Disease

Chapter 4

Grant Gallagher[1], Joyce Eskdale[1] and Jeff L Bidwell[2]

[1]*Department of Oral Biology, University of Medicine and Dentistry of New Jersey, Newark, NJ, USA;* [2]*Department of Pathology, University of Bristol, UK*

Oh wad some power the giftie gie us to see oursels as ithers see us! It wad frae monie a blunder free us, an' foolish notion.

To a Louse, Robert Burns (1786)

INTRODUCTION

The degree to which antigens induce an immune response varies markedly between individuals. Much of this variation is determined by the combination of antigen presenting molecules, both class I and class II MHC, that the individual is expressing and the range of T-cell receptor structures that have accumulated. Together, these determine whether and how well that individual's immune system will see any given antigen and it will be apparent that the random nature of T cell and B cell receptor construction means that even monozygotic twins will show variation in this respect, or at least have this potential. These aspects of the immune system have formed the backbone of the science of immunogenetics and continue to do so. Immunology, and particularly immunogenetics, continues to be an expanding field. First, as sequence differences are discovered in promoters and coding regions of immunologically relevant genes – such as cytokines and their receptors – the breadth of immune variation between individuals has become apparent. Second, as genome scans of autoimmune, infectious and malignant diseases define loci of pathogenic importance, specific genomic regions automatically become of interest in immunogenetics, even though they may not contain any 'obviously' immunological candidate genes. Third, although normal variation in the immune system can be important in disease development in the presence of contributing factors, certain rare mutations can themselves be fundamental in causing disease. Such variations may be associated with susceptibility to certain diseases or contribute to severity and progression. In addition, the same disease may have different contributing actions in one ethnic group compared with another and, of course, certain polymorphisms may exist only in one ethnic group (or be absent from that group).

CYTOKINES, CHEMOKINES AND IMMUNE RECEPTORS REGULATE IMMUNITY

Over the last 10 years then, it has become obvious that aspects of the immune system other than the MHC also show genetic variation. These variations have been noted in the whole range of immunologically important molecules, from adhesion molecules and other cell-surface structures to cytokines and other soluble signals. Thus, the science of immunogenetics has moved into a new 'post-HLA' phase and it is clear that the vast variation of the immune system must impact on all theatres of immunological activity, from the daily response to minor environmental antigens, through infectious and autoimmune diseases to malignancy and man-made immunological insults, such as vaccination and transplantation. The importance of cytokines to the immune system cannot be understated: they are soluble immuno-modulatory proteins which are

Copyright © 2005, Elsevier. All rights reserved.

active on a vast array of target cells, generally, but not wholly, within the immune and hematopoietic systems. Their actions are mediated through highly specific cell-surface receptors and usually result in gene activation with subsequent mitotic, activation, suppression or differentiation effects. Often they act in concert or in complex interactive loops, which can be positive or negative and, furthermore, these effects may differ with the target cell. It is small wonder then, that cytokines and particularly inflammatory cytokines, have received the lion's share of attention and much of our work has focused on these molecules.

Cytokines are produced by a wide range of cell types and have often been broadly classified as 'monokines' (produces by cells of the monocyte lineage) or 'lymphokines' (produced by cells of the lymphocye lineages). This simplistic classification has been variously replaced (e.g. Th1 and Th2 cytokines), but any classification belies the highly complex network in which cytokines always seem to work. For example, they may induce or repress their own expression as well as that of other cytokines. In addition, many are pleiotropic, affecting several cell types and there is a poorly understood functional redundancy between individual cytokines which, nonetheless, can have individual functions. These properties of cytokines continue to complicate efforts to analyze both the function of individual cytokines and the influence of cytokine gene polymorphisms on gene expression and disease.

As will be seen by the tables presented in this chapter (Bidwell et al., 1999, 2001; Haukim et al., 2002), a significant amount of work has been conducted in the field of cytokine genetics. There are below several examples of cytokine genetic studies in human disease. Broadly speaking, however, the rationale for studying cytokine gene polymorphisms is as follows:

- to improve our understanding of the origin and mechanism of human disease
- to identify novel diagnostic markers of susceptibility, severity and outcome
- to identify novel therapeutic targets and suitable patients for immunomodulatory treatments
- to identify novel intervention strategies, (enhanced vaccination, for example).

Such examples are predicated upon the assumption that cytokine levels do vary between individuals, so it is worthwhile to ask if this is the case and if, being so, diseases are affected. The question of whether a person's genetic makeup or living environment contributes more to their risk of disease has been an important one for some time. In 1988 Sorensen and colleagues (Sorensen et al., 1988) demonstrated clearly that adopted individuals carried a risk of death from infectious causes that was equivalent to that of their natural, rather than adoptive parents. In so doing they established unequivocally that premature death in adults from infectious causes had a strong

genetic background. This is seen in the context of the wide genetic variation known to exist in the immune system, manifested in the mundane including individuals with few upper respiratory infections and those who have them frequently. Recently, the expansion of the known receptors for exogenous pathogens, including viruses, parasites and bacteria interacting with toll-like receptors, to at least 11 (Zhang et al., 2004), suggests that analysis of polymorphisms in these genes will be informative (see Chapter 6).

INFECTIOUS DISEASES

Tumor necrosis factor (TNF) and most recently interleukin 10 (IL-10), have received particular attention in infectious disease. A range of experiments in murine models, together with studies on human material *in vitro*, demonstrate that variations in IL-10 production can profoundly alter response to, and outcome from, infectious disease. In the mouse, experimental diminution or removal of IL-10 has been achieved by the administration of monoclonal antibodies which neutralize IL-10, or by genetically knocking out the IL-10 gene. The complementary augmentation of IL-10 levels has been accomplished by injecting recombinant IL-10 or by using IL-10 transgenic mice. Such experiments are designed to explore the extremes of IL-10 levels (i.e. none, or receptor-saturating) and are therefore models for trends in immune responses that might be expected to result from natural, genetically defined differences in cytokine levels. In these contexts, a range of bacterial and other infections have been studied. Typical results include studies on *Lysteria monocytogenes* which demonstrated that withdrawing IL-10 by antibody neutralization (Wagner et al., 1994) or by genetic knockout (Dai et al., 1997) led to marked increase in disease resistance and improved outcome while increasing the amount of IL-10 present during an infection, either by rIL-10 administration (Kelly and Bancroft, 1996) or in IL-10 transgenic animals (Groux et al., 1999), led to worse disease and poorer outcome. Similar results exist for experimental infection with *Streptococcus pneumoniae* with high levels of IL-10 supporting increased disease development in mice and IL-10 absence allowing the mice to resist infection (van der Poll et al., 1996). IL-10 also affects responses to mycobacterial infections (Murray et al., 1997). Although responses to viruses have been less frequently studied, vaccinia virus replication was dramatically impaired in IL-10 knock-out animals (van den Broek et al., 2000) and herpes simplex associated skin pathology is ameliorated by application of IL-10 topically (Tumpey et al., 1994). A more complete summary of these experiments is described in the review of Moore et al. (2001), but in general, these experiments suggest that bacterial infections are worse in the context of high IL-10 levels and less severe in a relative absence of IL-10, while the opposite may be true of viral infections.

Similar work has been done for TNF. TNF is considered to be an important mediator of protection from parasitic, bacterial and viral infection (Vassalli, 1992). Once again using *Lysteria monocytogenes* as a model organism, it has been shown that withdrawing TNF with neutralizing monoclonal antibodies is extremely detrimental (Havell, 1989). However, the effects of high or low TNF are not clear cut and appear to vary with the infection – for example, withdrawing TNF protects from endotoxemic death (Buetler et al., 1985) while elevated TNF levels are associated with a much poorer outcome in human malaria (Kwiatowski et al., 1990). Conversly, TNF knock-out mice are completely susceptible to mycobacterial infections, developing uncontrolled, fatal infections (Jacobs et al, 2000). These experimental studies come together to show clearly that levels of both IL-10 and TNF are important in determining the course and outcome of infectious disease.

Even as recently as 1995, genetic studies had demonstrated that markers existed which could be related to differential TNF levels (e.g. Pociot et al., 1992) and many studies had also looked closely at IL-1; these have been extensively reviewed elsewhere and will not be discussed in detail here. No such markers existed for IL-10 and indeed it was not widely accepted that cytokines in general would display genetically defined intra-individual differences. Clearly, however, a wealth of experimental evidence supported the concept that differences in susceptibility to and severity of diseases might well have their roots in genetically defined differences in the ability to produce important cytokines. Parallel studies in human infection supported this concept. These are perhaps best demonstrated by the elegant studies of Westendorp et al. (1997a, 1997b; van Dissel et al., 1998). They showed that low TNF production was associated with a 10-fold risk of fatal outcome from meningococcal meningitis, while high IL-10 levels were associated with a 20-fold risk of fatality. Despite the recognized ability of TNF to induce IL-10 levels from monocytes and IL-10 to downregulate TNF, these two factors were independent, that is the levels of one cytokine were not dependent upon those of the other. These studies complemented earlier reports of high IL-10 levels being associated with fatal bacterial infections in man. Recently, it has been shown to affect macrophage responses during mycobacterial infections (Murray et al., 1997). Furthermore, the severity to which meningitis progresses is associated with serum IL-10 levels, such that high serum IL-10 was observed in patients with a poor or fatal outcome, while patients who had mild disease and a good prognosis had lower serum IL-10 levels (e.g. Lehmann et al., 1995).

Recent studies have demonstrated clearly that levels of TNF and IL-10 vary between individuals in this way and that highly informative genetic markers exist with which to examine the heritable basis of this. In the TNF locus, a complex pattern of microsatellite alleles and single nucleotide polymorphism (SNP) alleles form a system which demonstrates that three families of haplotypes exist, associated with TNF secretion (Weissensteiner and Lanchbury, 1997). Notwithstanding the relationship between the TNF locus and the class I and class II MHC alleles (Gallagher et al., 1997), TNF genetics are not merely a subset of the greater MHC. TNF secretion following LPS stimulation has been shown clearly to vary independently of the MHC (Pociot et al., 1992) and it can be demonstrated that disease associations which involve the TNF locus are independent of (although complementary to) the MHC (Rood et al., 2000; Caballero et al., 2000). While many studies examine the SNP alleles (Wilson et al., 1995; Majetschak et al., 1999; Negoro et al., 1999), in fact, microsatellite alleles or combinations thereof, may provide more accurate information. Thus, the TNFd4 microsatellite allele (Weissensteiner and Lanchbury, 1997) and the TNFa2 microsatellite allele (Pociot et al., 1992) offer excellent resolution of the bewildering array of SNP allelic possibilities. Indeed, the TNFa2d4 haplotype has been associated with a range of chronic inflammatory disorders against disparate MHC backgrounds (Plevy et al., 1996; Mattey et al., 1999).

While much work has concentrated on TNF and IL-10, other studies have demonstrated functional genetic variation in other cytokines. The range of genetic markers in human cytokine genes is very large and these have been used to study functional or disease associations, but only in single populations (Bidwell et al., 1999, 2001; Mullighan et al., 1999). Some of the better studies are on genes with relevance to infection. For example, a promoter polymorphism in the IL-6 gene defines high or low producers in both resting and stimulated conditions (Fishman et al., 1998). In addition, chemokines and their receptors (Gonzalez et al., 2001; Paxton et al., 2001) have also been studied recently and proven to be both polymorphic and informative. These studies have been accompanied by a very small number of reports which specifically address the question of ethnic variation within the distribution of polymorphic elements in cytokine (and related) genes. These studies have shown that the geographic/ethnic distribution of alleles in a number of genes does in fact vary (Cox et al., 2001; Gonzalez et al., 2001; Padyukov et al., 2000). Thus, early studies which concentrated on demonstrating individual differences in cytokine production, or the association of higher (or lower) cytokine production with disease have in more recent years developed to confirm these differences and indicate their genetic origins.

CYTOKINE POLYMORPHISMS IN THE UNDERSTANDING OF HUMAN DISEASE

The influence of cytokine gene polymorphisms on gene expression and disease has largely been addressed as two separate subjects and only a few studies have integrated the two. Two excellent examples come in atopy/ asthma. A number of SNPs exist in the IL-13 promoter (Pantelidis et al., 2000), at least one of which (C-T at -1055; van der Pouw Kraan et al., 1999) affects the binding of a specific transcription factor to the IL-13 promoter, altering its function such that the TT genotype is associated with increased levels of IL-13 production in allergic asthma patients (Ahmed et al., 2000; Liu et al., 2000; Howard et al., 2001). Asthma provides an additional example of where functional cytokine genetics studies have been fruitful in man and mouse (Webb et al., 2004). In the promoter of RANTES, lies a G-A SNP at position -403. The -403.A allele is associated with increased susceptibility to both atopy and asthma, with homozygosity for -403.A being associated with a 6.5-fold increase in prevalence of responsive airway obstruction (Fryer et al., 2000). In a parallel study, it was shown to produce/destroy a GATA site and in the presence of the GATA site not only was RANTES promoter activity increased in transfection studies but the extra GATA site was strongly associated with atopy in general, supporting the previous asthma study (Nickel et al., 2000). The RANTES gene locus is also associated with rates of HIV progression (Paxton et al., 2001). TARC, a chemokine, is associated with atopic dermatitis, but not the polymorphisms which have been identified (Morita et al., 2004).

One of the most interesting series of studies in human cytokine genetics has involved the autoimmune disease systemic lupus erythematosus (SLE) and the cytokine IL-10. One of the earliest observations following the discovery of IL-10 was that it appeared to be over-produced in SLE. While many symptoms can come together to provide a diagnosis of SLE, it is usually held to be a disease characterized by autoantibody production. IL-10 is recognized to stimulate the proliferation of human B cells and their secretion of all classes of immunoglobulin (Rousset et al., 1992). IL-10 was originally defined as a cytokine able to alter the balance of murine Th1/Th2 activity, in favor of the Th2-type response (Fiorentino et al., 1991) and it has several properties which would appear to encourage lupus autoimmunity. One critical aspect of this is its ability to diminish macrophage activation and antigen presentation, thereby directly and indirectly inhibiting T cell function (Enk, 1993; de Waal Malefyt, 1993). In particular, IL-10 can function as a negative autocrine regulator of TNF production (Wanidworanun and Strober, 1993). IL-10 may also promote inflammatory responses through its potent stimulation of Bcell proliferation and differentiation (Rousset et al., 1992). Raised IL-10 levels have been reported in several autoimmune states (Llorente et al., 1994), originating from both B cells and monocytes. Also, in vitro studies have shown that hypergammaglobulinemia in SLE is IL-10 dependent (Llorente et al., 1995) and it has been reported to protect B cells from apoptosis (Levy et al., 1994). In addition, the ability of IL-10 to induce anergy in T cells (Taga et al., 1993) may relieve some elements of the normal control over B cell function, if suppression is reduced. (It may be of interest that, conversely, IL-10 can function as a growth factor for gamma/delta-positive human T cells (Pawelec et al., 1995). Increased IL-10 production may therefore contribute to SLE by direct effects on B cell autoantibody production and survival and it is of interest

that a recent study has suggested that the region of IL-10: IFNγ secreting cells in SLE is an indicator of disease severity (Hagiwara et al., 1996). Administration of anti-IL-10 antibodies slows the development of murine autoimmunity (Ishida et al., 1994). This may well be through a mechanism which prevents the activation to autoreactivity of Ly-1 (i.e. CD5) positive B cells (Ishida et al., 1992), themselves thought to be a major source of B cell-derived IL-10 (O'Garra et al., 1992). In addition, the lingering question of whether lupus is a TNF-deficiency disorder is supported by anecdotal reports that rheumatoid arthritis patients receiving anti-TNF therapy may, in exceptional circumstances, develop autoantibody specificities characteristic of lupus; there have also been reports that experimental lupus can be treated in some respects by the administration of TNF. Thus, the well-characterized ability of IL-10 to directly downregulate TNF production (Wanidworanun and Strober, 1993) is also implicated as a mechanism by which high levels of IL-10 could be permissive for lupus development.

IL-10 secretion levels do vary between indivduals and this can be associated with disease outcome. Most dramatically, this has been shown in studies on meningitis patients (Westendorp et al., 1997a), where individuals with genetically high IL-10 secretion fared very poorly in comparison to those patients with low IL-10 secretion. Increased levels of IL-10 in mononuclear cells from lupus patients has been demonstrated in a number of studies (Llorente et al., 1993, 1994; Houssiau et al., 1995; Al-Janadi et al., 1996; Hagiwara et al., 1996). Indeed, unaffected primary and secondary family members of lupus patients produce over five times as much IL-10 than do control subjects (Llorente et al., 1997). Taken together, these findings are consistent with high production of IL-10 functioning as one of a limited number of primary genetic defects which are permissive for lupus, but it also clearly demonstrates that high IL-10 secretion is not in itself causative of this condition. Certainly, all of the molecular abnormalities that have been described in lupus patients could not be directly the consequence of alleles in the gene of the gene product being assayed. The most parsimonious model is that most of the cytokine abnormalities are secondary, meaning that the observed abnormality is the result of something else that is causing them. A few, however, represent intrinsic abnormalities that predispose to lupus and 'cause' the others. IL-10 level is a good candidate for such an intrinsic abnormality. Having been found in family members suggests that it would also have been found in the lupus patients before disease onset and part of the milieu which governs the immune response to the putative 'lupus causing' environmental factor toward lupus autoimmunity.

The region immediately upstream of the human IL-10 gene is highly polymorphic, with two dinucleotide repeats and many single base substitutions. The interest in this gene is such that several groups of workers have investigated these polymorphic elements independently. The two microsatellites were described first in the literature by Eskdale and co-workers (Eskdale and Gallagher, 1995; Eskdale et al., 1996), while Fabio Cominelli's group first described the -1082 A/G substitution marker (Tountas and Cominelli, 1996). The two additional single base substitutions were first described by Turner and colleagues (1997) and independently characterized by Eskdale et al. (Eskdale et al., 1997a); Turner et al. also independently identified the Cominelli A/G SNP, now often referred to as 'IL10 -1082'. One of these microsatellite loci (IL10.G) has shown an altered distribution of allele frequencies in lupus patients in comparison to controls (Eskdale et al., 1997b), with evidence that associations between microsatellite alleles and the class of autoantibody present also exist. While this latter observation remains to be verified, several groups have followed and confirmed the basic association between the IL10.G microsatellite and the presence of SLE (Mehrian et al., 1998; D'Alfonso et al., 2000). A follow-up study in SLE families, which would have the potential to reveal linkage, is still awaited, but it is of interest that one recent study also finds association between this microsatellite and Sjogren's syndome, which shares many lupus-like features with SLE (Hulkkonen et al., 2001). Polymorphisms of the IL-1β gene in Japanese patients with primary and secondary Sjogren's syndrome (Muraki et al., 2004) have also been observed, perhaps reflecting the multigenic nature of these disorders. SNPs studied in IL-10 have also proved informative in lupus (Lazarus et al., 1997; Mok et al., 1998; Gibson et al,. 2001) and further more distal markers continue to be discovered (Kube et al., 2001). The intrinsic susceptibility to atherosclerotic disease as manifested by renovascular disease also appears to be dependent on IL-10 low producer genotype, more frequent in patients with renal artery stenosis (George et al., 2004).

Thus, there is ample evidence that an enormous genetic variation occurs in human cytokine genes, but only a small proportion of the studies carried out have demonstrated a functional role for these markers. A similar small proportion of the disease association studies carried out have been confirmed in independent, replicate populations and in only a few cases have disease-associated SNPs also been shown to exert a functional effect – so far! This should encourage us, rather than discourage us, to continue as a research community to use and investigate these markers and to consider cytokine genes as highly informative reservoirs of genetic variation in the immune system.

But these exciting developments in the understanding of cytokine genetics should be interepreted with a note of caution, to prevent us from being seduced into thinking that only markers within individual cytokine genes can control differences in inter-individual cytokine secretion. This is not so. Other elements which can influence the expression of cytokine (and other?) genes should not be forgotten. For example, the rigor with which

Fishman et al. (1998) approached the measurement of IL-6 production in their control subjects, demonstrates the importance of the natural metabolic variation which occurs daily. This supported earlier studies, for example that of Petrovsky and Harrison (1997a) who showed that the LPS induction of IL-10 and IFN-gamma varied throughout the day, observing that the IFN-gamma/IL-10 ratio peaked early in the morning and concluding that both cortisol and melatonin could regulate diurnal immune variation. Much has been made of the requirement for caution when interpreting genetic data from the TNF cluster without due consideration of the MHC and linkage disequilibrium; MHC effects on cytokines off chromosome 6 have not been so well documented. The evidence has begun to emerge, however, to define the relevant factors. A study in 1997 (Petrovsky and Harrison, 1997b) demonstrated that secreted levels of IFN-gamma varied markedly with class-II alleles, in an MLR. DR1, DR2 and DR6 were associated with high IFN-gamma secretion while DR3, DR4 and DR7 were associated with lower IFN-gamma production. Similar conclusions were drawn for those DQ alleles in linkage disequilibrium with the DR alleles noted above. This pattern was reversed for TNF secretion (i.e. DR3 was high TNF and so on), mirroring earlier work by Pociot et al. (1992) who demonstrated a DR-based hierarchy of TNF secretion which was of greater magnitude than the TNF-allele results for which they are more usually remembered. Similar data are available for other aspects of the immune system, for example antibody production (Mineta et al., 1996) and response to vaccination (Wang et al., 2004). In this regard, DR3 has received the greatest attention. T cell activation varies in DR3-positive individuals, perhaps because of diminished CD69 expression (Candore et al., 1995), as do cytokines themselves (Caruso et al., 1996) particularly in regard to autoimmune DR3-positive subjects (Lio et al., 1997). Apoptosis may differ because these individuals have diminished expression of CD95/FAS (Stassi et al., 1997) and indeed lower total lymphocyte counts have been described in association with B8-DR3 (Caruso et al., 1997). Extent of colitis may vary based on polymorphisms in chemokine genes such as macrophage migration inhibitory factor (Nohara et al., 2004), suggesting that natural variants in diseases may themselves be driven by such polymorphisms, confounding low powered analyses even in relatively homogeneous people such as the Japanese. Little insight to the mechanism of the various effects of class II on immune function was available until recently, when it was demonstrated that different class II molecules varied in the efficiency with which they transduce signals from CD4 across the cell membrane, and that this variation is carried with the intracellular portion of the class II molecule (Fleury et al., 1995). As if this were not confusing enough, the age of the donors themselves has been shown to affect T cell activation (Lio et al., 1996) through various mechanisms. In conclusion, the genetic effect seen to be acting on cytokine production and

Table 4.1 List of human cytokine gene polymorphisms.

Gene	Polymorphism	First author, year[1]
GM-CSF	codon 117 C→T	Tagiev, 1995
GM-CSF-Rα	nt1148 G→A	Wagner, 1994
GM-CSF-Rα	nt199 C→G	Wagner, 1994
GM-CSF-Rα	nt428 A→G	Wagner, 1994
GM-CSF-Rα	nt640 A→G	Wagner, 1994
GM-CSF-Rα	nt824 C→T	Wagner, 1994
GM-CSF-Rβ	nt1306 C→T (Ser426)	Freeburn, 1996
		Freeburn, 1998
GM-CSF-Rβ	nt1835 C→A	Freeburn, 1996
GM-CSF-Rβ	nt1968 G→T	Freeburn, 1996
GM-CSF-Rβ	nt1972 G→A	Freeburn, 1996
GM-CSF-Rβ	nt1982 G→A	Freeburn, 1996
GM-CSF-Rβ	nt2427 G→A	Freeburn, 1996
GM-CSF-Rβ	nt301 C→T (Cys91)	Freeburn, 1998
GM-CSF-Rβ	nt773 G→C (Glu249Glu)	Freeburn, 1998
GM-CSF-Rβ	nt962 G→A (Asp312Asn)	Freeburn, 1998
IFNγ	Exon 4, 5199 A→T	Iwasaki, 2001
IFNγ	Exon 4, 5272 A→G	Iwasaki, 2001
IFNγ	Intron 3, 2459 A→G	Iwasaki, 2001
IFNγ	Intron 3, 2671 T→C	Iwasaki, 2001
IFNγ	Intron 3, 3177 T→C	Iwasaki, 2001
IFNγ	Intron 3, 3273 G→A	Iwasaki, 2001
IFNαR	−18G→A	Muldoon, 2001
IFNαR	−408C→T	Muldoon, 2001
IFNα	Dinucleotide repeat	Kwiatkowski, 1992
IFNα (IFNA10)	nt1265 A→C	Golovleva, 1996
IFNα (IFNA10)	nt991 (60*) T→A Cys20Stop (Sau3A I)	Golovleva, 1996 Miterski, 1999
IFNα (IFNA17)	nt1101 (170*) A→C	Golovleva, 1996 unconfirmed Miterski, 1999
IFNα (IFNA17)	nt1453 C→T	Golovleva, 1996
IFNα (IFNA17)	nt1482 (551*) T→G Ile184Arg (Ssp I RFLP)	Golovleva, 1996 Miterski, 1999
IFNα (IFNA17)	nt171insA (Nla III RFLP)	Miterski, 1999
IFNα (IFNA2)	nt1068 G→A	Golovleva, 1996 unconfirmed Miterski, 1999
IFNα (IFNA2)	nt1101 G→A	Golovleva, 1996 unconfirmed Miterski, 1999
IFNαR	HindIII RFLP	Vielh, 1990
IFNβ	3′ MspI RFLP	Riggin, 1982
IFNβ	nt153 C→T	Miterski, 1999
IFNγ	−333 C→T	Giedraitis, 1999
IFNγ	Intron 1, (CA) repeat	Gray, 1983; Ruiz-Linares, 1993
IFNγRI	TaqI RFLP	Hauptschein, 1992
IL-10	−1082 G→A	Tounas, 1996 Turner, 1997
IL-10	−1255 C→T	D'Alfonso, 2000
IL-10	−1349 A→G	D'Alfonso, 2000
IL-10	−2013 A→G	D'Alfonso, 2000
IL-10	−2050 G→A	Gibson, 2001
IL-10	−2100 C→A	Gibson, 2001
IL-10	−2739 A→G	D'Alfonso, 2000
IL-10	−2763 C→A	Gibson, 2001
IL-10	−2769 A→G	D'Alfonso, 2000
IL-10	−2776 A→G	Gibson, 2001
IL-10	−2849 G→A	Gibson, 2001
IL-10	3′ flanking region, +117 after stop codon C→T	Donger, 2001
IL-10	−3533 A→T	D'Alfonso, 2000
IL-10	−3575 T→A	Gibson, 2001

Table 4.1 (*Continued*)

Gene	Polymorphism	First author, year[1]
IL-10	−3715 A→T	Gibson, 2001
IL-10	5′ distal (CA) repeat (IL10.R)	Eskdale, 1996
IL-10	5′ proximal (CA) repeat (IL10.G)	Eskdale, 1995
IL-10	−5402 C→G	Kube, 2001
IL-10	−592 C→A	Eskdale, 1997 Turner, 1997
IL-10	−6208 G→C	Kube, 2001
IL-10	−657 A→G	D'Alfonso, 2000
IL-10	−6752 A→T	Kube, 2001
IL-10	−7400 (3 bp deletion)	Kube, 2001
IL-10	−819 C→T	Eskdale, 1997 Turner, 1997
IL-10	−851 A→G	D'Alfonso, 2000
IL-10	−8531 G→A	Kube, 2001
IL-10	−8571 C→T	Kube, 2001
IL-10	Exon 1, +78 G→A (Gly15→Arg)	Donger, 2001
IL-10	Intron 3, +19 C→T	Donger, 2001
IL-10	Intron 3, +953 T→C	Donger, 2001
IL-11	5′ dinucleotide repeat	Bellingham, 1998
IL-12 (p35)	−916 C → T	Pravica, 2000
IL-12 (p35)	−916 C→T	Pravica, 2000
IL-12 (p40)	−1287 G → T	Pravica, 2000
IL-12 (p40)	−1287 G→T	Pravica, 2000
IL-12 (p40)	Exon 7, +16117 G→C	Huang, 2000
IL-12 (p40)	Exon 8, +16974 A→C	Huang, 2000
IL-12 (p40)	Intron 1, +3696 A→G	Huang, 2000
IL-12 (p40)	Intron 1, +3757 T→C	Huang, 2000
IL-12 (p40)	Intron 1, +4572, TG insertion	Huang, 2000
IL-12 (p40)	Intron 1, +4793 C→G	Huang, 2000
IL-12 (p40)	Intron 2, +8798 TAA repeat	Huang, 2000
IL-12 (p40)	Intron 2, +8930 A→G	Huang, 2000
IL-12 (p40)	Intron 2, +8944 A→G	Huang, 2000
IL-12 (p40)	Intron 3, +9910 G→A	Huang, 2000
IL-12 (p40)	Intron 4, +11244 A→T	Huang, 2000
IL-12 (p40)	Intron 4, +11563 AT repeat	Huang, 2000
IL-12 (p40)	Intron 7, +16521 A→C	Huang, 2000
IL-12 (p40)	nt1188 (5′UTR) A→C	Hall, 2000
IL-13	−1055 C→T	van der Pouw Kraan, 1999 Laundy, 2000
IL-13	3′ UTR, +2525 G A	Graves, 2000
IL-13	3′ UTR, +2749	Graves, 2000
IL-13	3′UTR, +2580 C A	Graves, 2000
IL-13	3′-UTR, nt2043 G→A	Pantelidis, 2000
IL-13	3′-UTR, nt2579 C→A	Pantelidis, 2000
IL-13	5′ promoter, −1512 A C	Graves, 2000
IL-13	additional Gln residue, position 98	McKenzie, 1993
IL-13	Exon 4, +2044 G A	Graves, 2000
IL-13	Intron 1, nt543 G→C	Pantelidis, 2000
IL-13	Intron 3, +1923 C T	Graves, 2000
IL-13	Intron 3, nt1922 C→T	Pantelidis, 2000
IL-13	nt 4257, G→A	Liu, 2000
IL-13Rα	nt1050 C→T	Ahmed, 2000
IL-13Rα	+1050 C→T	Ahmed, 2000
IL-16	−295 T→C	Nakayama, 2000
IL-18	+113 T→G	Giedraitis, 2001
IL-18	+127 C→T	Giedraitis, 2001
IL-18	−137 G→C	Giedraitis, 2001
IL-18	−607 C→A	Giedraitis, 2001
IL-18	−656 G→T	Giedraitis, 2001
IL-1Ra	+2016 T→C	Kornman, 1998
IL-1Ra	Intron 2 86bp VNTR	Tarlow, 1993

Table 4.1 (*Continued*)

Gene	Polymorphism	First author, year[1]
IL-1Ra	nt11100 T→C (MspA1I)	Guasch, 1996
IL-1Ra	nt1731 G→A	Langdahl, 2000
IL-1Ra	nt1821 G→A	Langdahl, 2000
IL-1Ra	nt1868 A→G	Langdahl, 2000
IL-1Ra	nt1887 G→C	Langdahl, 2000
IL-1Ra	nt1934 T→C	Langdahl, 2000
IL-1Ra	nt8006 T→C (MspI)	Guasch, 1996
IL-1Ra	nt8061 C→T (MwoI)	Guasch, 1996
IL-1Ra	nt9589 A→T (SspI)	Guasch, 1996
IL-1RI	2 PstI RFLPs	Bergholdt, 1995
IL-1RI	Exon 1C, +140 A→T	Sitara, 1999
IL-1RI	Exon 1C, +52 C→A (BsrB I)	Sitara, 2000
IL-1RI	Exon 1C, +97 G→A (Sty I)	Sitara, 2000
IL-1RI	Intron 1A, +1622 (of AF302042) G→A (Hinf I)	Bergholdt, 2000
IL-1RI	Intron 1A, +701 (of AF302042) G→A (Pst I)	Bergholdt, 2000
IL-1RI	Intron 1B, +52 (of AF146426) A→G (Msp I)	Sitara, 1999
IL-1RI	Intron 1C, +1498 (of AF302043) T→C (Alu I)	Bergholdt, 2000
IL-1RI	Intron 1C, +976 (of AF302043) T→C (BstF5 I)	Bergholdt, 2000
IL-1α	(TTA) repeat	Zuliani, 1990
IL-1α	+4345 T→G	Kornman, 1998
IL-1α	−889	Kornman, 1998
IL-1α	Dinucleotide repeat	Todd, 1991 Epplen, 1994
IL-1α	Intron 6, 46bp VNTR	Bailly, 1993
IL-1β	+3953 (nt5887) C→T (Taql)	Pociot, 1992
IL-1β	−35 T→C (AluI)	Guasch, 1996
IL-1β	−511 G→A (Aval)	di Giovine, 1992
IL-1β	nt3263 C→T	Langdahl, 2000
IL-1β	nt5810 A→T (BsoFI)	Guasch, 1996
IL-2	+166	John, 1998
IL-2	−330	John, 1998
IL-2	Allele A: 122bp dinucleotide repeat	Khani-Hanjani, 2001
IL-2	Dinucleotide repeat	Epplen, 1994
IL-2	exon 1 nt742 T→G	Denny, 1997
IL-2R	Allele 0: 165 bp dinucleotide repeat	Khani-Hanjani, 2001
IL-2R	Allele 2: 169 bp dinucleotide repeat	Khani-Hanjani, 2001
IL-2R	Allele 9: 147 bp dinucleotide repeat	Khani-Hanjani, 2001
IL-2Rα	Taql RFLP	Cottrell, 1994
IL-2Rβ	Dinucleotide repeat	Brewster, 1991
IL-3	+131 C→T	Jeong, 1998
IL-3	+5 C→T	Jeong, 1998
IL-3	−16 C→T	Jeong, 1998
IL-3	−211 C→A	Jeong, 1998
IL-3	BglII RFLP	Jaquet, 1989
IL-3	Enhancer nt232	Jeong, 1998
IL-3	Enhancer nt236	Jeong, 1998
IL-3	Enhancer nt283	Jeong, 1998
IL-4	+33 C→T	Suzuki, 1999
IL-4	−34 C→T	Takabayashi, 1999
IL-4	−524 C→T	Borish, 1994
IL-4	−590 C→T (BsmFI)	Walley, 1996
IL-4	intron 2 dinucleotide repeat	Marsh, 1994
IL-4	Intron 2, 70bp VNTR	Mout, 1991
IL-4	Intron 3, (GT) repeat	Mout, 1991
IL-4R	nt1124 A→C	Deichmann, 1997
IL-4R	nt1167 G→T	Deichmann, 1997

Table 4.1 (*Continued*)

Gene	Polymorphism	First author, year[1]
IL-4R	nt1216 T→C	Deichmann, 1997
IL-4R	nt1218 C→T	Deichmann, 1997
IL-4R	nt1224 T→C	Deichmann, 1997
IL-4R	nt1232 C→T	Deichmann, 1997
IL-4R	nt148 A→G	Deichmann, 1997
IL-4R	nt1902 G→A (R576Q)	Hershey, 1997
IL-4R	nt2281 T→C	Deichmann, 1997
IL-4R	nt426 C→T	Deichmann, 1997
IL-4R	nt747 C→G	Deichmann, 1997
IL-4R	nt864 T→C	Deichmann, 1997
IL-4Rα	−1914 T→C	Hackstein, 2001
IL-4Rα	−3223 C→T	Hackstein, 2001
IL-4Rα	−890 T→C	Hackstein, 2001
IL-4Rα	CAAAA repeat (5–7)	Hackstein, 2001
IL-4Rα	Exon 11, +1654 G→A (V554→I)	Lozano, 2001
IL-4Rα	nt1124 A→C (E375A)	Deichmann, 1997 Deichmann, 1999
IL-4Rα	nt1216 T→C (C406R)	Deichmann, 1997 Deichmann, 1999
IL-4Rα	nt148 A→G (I50V)	Deichmann, 1997 Deichmann, 1999
IL-4Rα	nt1682 T→C (S478P) (previously S503P)	Deichmann, 1997 Deichmann, 1999 Kruse, 1999
IL-4Rα	nt1902 G→A (R551Q) (previously R576Q)	Hershey, 1997 Deichmann, 1999
IL-4Rα	nt2281 T→C (S761P)	Deichmann, 1997 Deichmann, 1999
IL-5Rα	−80 G→A (MaeIII)	Kollintza, 1998 Kollintza, 1998
IL-5Rα	Dinucleotide repeat	Epplen, 1994
IL-6	(CA)n repeat	Tsukamoto, 1998
IL-6	−174 G→C (NlaIII)	Olomolaiye, 1997 Olomolaiye, 1998 Fishman, 1998
IL-6	3' (AT)-rich minisatellite	Bowcock, 1989 Murray, 1997
IL-6	5' (AT)-tract (5 alleles)	Fishman, 1998
IL-6	−572 G→C	Terry, 2000
IL-6	−597 G→A	Terry, 2000
IL-6	BglII RFLP	Fugger, 1989 Blankenstein, 1989
IL-6	MspI RFLP	Fugger, 1989
IL-6	nt565 G→A (FokI)	Fishman, 1998
IL-6	XbaI RFLP	Linker-Israeli, 1996
IL-6R	(CA)n repeat	Tsukamoto, 1998
IL-8	HindIII RFLP	Fey, 1993
IL-9	Dinucleotide repeat	Polymeropoulos, 1991
LTα (TNFβ)	AspHI RFLP	Ferencik, 1992
LTα (TNFβ)	Intron 1, NcoI RFLP (Thr26Asn) (TNFB*1 = Asn26; TNFB*2 = Thr26)	Messer, 1991 Rink, 1996
RANTES	−109 T→C	Azzawi, 2001
RANTES	−28 C→G	al Sharif, 1999
RANTES	−403 A→G	Hajeer, 1999
TGFα	Taql RFLP	Hayward, 1987
TGFβ1	−509	Cambien, 1996 Awad, 1998
TGFβ	−800	Cambien, 1996 Awad, 1998
TGβ1	−988	Cambien, 1996
TGFβ1	nt713–8delC	Langdahl, 1997

Table 4.1 (*Continued*)

Gene	Polymorphism	First author, year[1]
TGFβ1	nt72 unspecified	Awad, 1998
TGFβ1	nt788 C→T	Langdahl, 1997
TGFβ1	nt869 (Leu10Pro)	Cambien, 1996 Awad, 1998
TGFβ1	nt915 (Arg25Pro)	Cambien, 1996 Awad, 1998
TGFβ1	R124S	Stewart, 1999
TGFβ2	4 RFLPs, SSCPs	Nishimura, 1993
TGFβ2	5′UTR (4 bp insertion–ACCA)	Alansari, 2001
TGFβ2	Exon 1 (SNP G→A)	Alansari, 2001
TNFRSF1A (p55)	−383 A→C (BglII)	Pitts, 1998
TNFRSF1A (p55)	nt36 A→G (MspA1 I)	Pitts, 1998
TNFRSF1A (p55)	Intron 1, 11-allele polymorphic microsatellite marker	Eskdale, 2000
TNFRSF1B (p75)	3′-UTR SSCP '5/6'	Kaufman, 1994
TNFRSF1B (p75)	3′-UTR SSCP '7/8'	Kaufman, 1994
TNFRSF1B (p75)	exon 10, nt1663 A→G	Pantelidis, 1999
TNFRSF1B (p75)	exon 10, nt1668 T→G	Pantelidis, 1999

Table 4.1 (*Continued*)

Gene	Polymorphism	First author, year[1]
TNFRSF1B (p75)	exon 10, nt1690 C→T	Pantelidis, 1999
TNFRSF1B (p75)	exon 6, M196R	Komata, 1999
TNFRSF1B (p75)	exon 6, nt676 C→T	Pantelidis, 1999
TNFα	+70 G→A	Brinkman, 1997
TNFα	TNFα	TNFα
TNFα	−163 G→A	Brinkman, 1997
TNFα	−238 G→A	D'Alfonso, 1994
TNFα	−308 G→A (TNF1 = G; TNF2 = A)	Wilson, 1993 Wilson, 1997
TNFα	−376 G→A	Brinkman, 1997
TNFα	−574	Uglialoro, 1998
TNFα	−856 (*− 857)	Uglialoro, 1998 *Higuchi, 1998
TNFα	−862 (*− 863)	Uglialoro, 1998 *Higuchi, 1998
TNF	TNFa, b, c, d, e microsatellites	Nedospasov, 1991 Udalova, 1993

[1] Full references are provided in the appropriate Genes and Immunity reviews and supplements (references 1–3) and in the references found here.

Table 4.2 *In vitro* expression studies in various cytokine polymorphisms

Gene	Polymorphism and allele (or haplotype)	Expression	First author, year[1]
IFNγ	(CA)n intron 1 (all alleles)	No effect	Cartwright, 1999
IFNγ	(CA)n intron 1 (allele 2)	Increased	Pravica, 1999
IL-10	−1082 A, −819 C, −592 C	Decreased	Turner, 1997
IL-10	−1082 A, −819 T, −592 A	Decreased	Turner, 1997
IL-10	−1082 G, −819 C, −592 C	Increased	Turner, 1997
IL-10	−1082 A, −819 T, −592 A	Decreased	Crawley, 1999
IL-10	−1082 G, −819 C, −592 C	Increased	Crawley, 1999; Maurer, 2000
IL-10	R 2, G 14	Increased	Eskdale, 1998
IL-10	R 3	Decreased	Eskdale, 1998
IL-10	R 3, G 7	Decreased	Eskdale, 1998
IL-13	−1055 T	Increased	van der Pouw Kraan, 1999
IL-18	−607 homozygous for C, −137 homozygous for G	Increased (not statistically significant)	Giedraitis, 2001
IL-1Ra	intron 2 86bp VNTR (allele 2)	Decreased	Tountas, 1999
IL-1Ra	Intron 2 86bp VNTR, (allele 2)	Increased	Tarlow, 1993; Danis, 1995; Hurme, 1998
IL-1α	Intron 6, 46bp VNTR	Related To VNTR allele	Bailly, 1993 Bailly, 1993
IL-1β	+3953 (nt5887) T	Increased	Pociot, 1992
IL-4Rα	3223 C→T	Reduced sIL-4R	Hackstein, 2001
IL-6	−174 G	Increased	Fishman, 1998
IL-6	3′ (AT)-rich minisatellite (790, 792, 808 and 820bp alleles)	Increased	Linker-Israeli, 1999
IL-6	−597A, −572G, −373A8/T12, −174G haplotype	Decreased	Terry, 2000
IL-6	−597G, −572G, −373A9/T11, −174G haplotype	Increased	Terry, 2000
IL-6	IL-6 −174 G→C (NlaIII)	Increased in neonates, not in adults	Kilpinen, 2001
LT	Intron 1, NcoI RFLP	No effect on LT secretion	Pociot, 1993
LT	Intron 1, NcoI RFLP: TNFB*1 (Asn26)	Increased	Messer, 1991
LT	Intron 1, NcoI RFLP: TNFB*2 (Thr26)	Decreased	Messer, 1991
LT + TNFα	Intron 1, NcoI RFLP: TNFB*1 (Asn26), TNFa6	Decreased	Pociot, 1993
LT + TNFα	Intron 1, NcoI RFLP: TNFB*2 (Thr26), TNFa2	Increased	Pociot, 1993
TGFβ1	nt915 (Arg25)	Increased	Awad, 1998; Awad, 1998
TNFα	+489, −308, −1031, −863, −857	No difference	Kaijzel, 2001
TNFα	+70 G→A	No effect	Uglialoro, 1998
TNFα	−1031	Increased	Higuchi, 1998
TNFα	−238 A	Increased	Grove, 1997
TNFα	−238 G→A	No effect	Pociot, 1995; Huizinga, 1997; Kaijzel, 1998; Uglialoro, 1998
TNFα	−238, allele 2	Decreased	Kaluza, 2000
TNFα	−244, −238	Increase (in certain cell lines)	Bayley, 2001
TNFα	−308	No effect	Pociot, 1993; Turner, 1995; Huizinga, 1997; Uglialoro, 1998

Table 4.2 (*Continued*)

Gene	Polymorphism and allele (or haplotype)	Expression	First author, year[1]
TNFα	−308 (TNF2)	Increased	Huang, 1999; Kroeger, 2000; Maurer, 1999
TNFα	−308 (TNF2)	Increased	Wilson, 1997; Galbraith, 1998
TNFα	−308 (TNF2)	No effect	Sotgiu, 1999
TNFα	−308, − 376	No effect	Bayley, 2001
TNFα	−376 G→A	No effect	Huizinga, 1997; Kaijzel, 1998
TNFα	−509 T	Increased	Luedecking, 2000
TNFα	−574	No effect	Uglialoro, 1998
TNFα	−856 (*−857)	Increased	Higuchi, 1998
TNFα	−856 (*−857)	No effect	Uglialoro, 1998
TNFα	−857T	Increased	Hohjoh, 2001
TNFα	−862 (*−863)	Increased	Higuchi, 1998
TNFα	−862 (*−863)	No effect	Uglialoro, 1998
TNFα	−863 A	Decreased (31%)	Skoog, 1999
TNFα	−863 A	Increased	Hohjoh, 2001
TNF	a	No effect on LT secretion	Pociot, 1993
TNF	a2	Decreased	Derkx, 1995
TNF	c	No effect on LT secretion	Pociot, 1993
TNF	d3	Increased	Turner, 1995
TNF	a13	Decreased	Obayashi, 1999
TNF	a2 and a9	Increased	Obayashi, 1999

[1] Full references are provided in the appropriate Genes and Immunity reviews and supplements (references 1–3) and in the references found here.

Table 4.3 *In vivo* disease association studies with cytokine polymorphisms

Cytokine and polymorphism	Disease	Association	First author, year[1]
EPO-R nt5964 C→G	Primary familial and congenital polycythemia	Yes	Kralovics, 1998
FGF1-α (GT)n 5′-UTR	Early-onset pauciarticular juvenile chronic arthritis	No	Epplen, 1995
FGF1-α (GT)n 5′-UTR	Multiple sclerosis	No	Epplen, 1997
GM-CSF-Rβ nt1306 C→T (Ser426)	Acute myeloid leukemia	No	Freeburn, 1998
GM-CSF-Rβ nt301 C→T (Cys91)	Acute myeloid leukemia	No	Freeburn, 1998
GM-CSF-Rβ nt773 G→C (Glu249Glu)	Acute myeloid leukemia	No	Freeburn, 1998
GM-CSF-Rβ nt962 G→A (Asp312Asn)	Acute myeloid leukemia	No	Freeburn, 1998
IFNα (CA)n intron 1	Early-onset pauciarticular juvenile chronic arthritis	No	Epplen, 1995
IFNα (GT)n allele 02	Multiple sclerosis	Yes (protection)	Miterski, 1999
IFNα (GT)n allele 07	Multiple sclerosis	Yes (susceptibility)	Miterski, 1999
IFNα (IFNA10) nt991 (60*) T → A Cys20Stop (Sau3A I)	Multiple sclerosis	No	Miterski, 1999
IFNα (IFNA17) nt1482 (551*) T→ G Ile184Arg (Ssp I RFLP)	Multiple sclerosis	No	Miterski, 1999
IFNα (IFNA17) nt171insA (Nla III RFLP)	Multiple sclerosis	Yes (susceptibility)	Miterski, 1999
IFNβ nt153 C→T	Multiple sclerosis	No	Miterski, 1999
IFNγ CA(13) intron A microsatellite	Rheumatoid arthritis	No	Pokorny, 2001
IFNγ (CA)n intron 1	Atopic asthma	Yes (Japanese children)	Nakao, 2001
IFNγ (CA)n intron 1	Graft-versus-host disease	Yes (increased severity)	Cavet, 2001
IFNγ (CA)n intron 1	Graves' disease	Yes (increased frequency of allele 5; decreased frequency of allele 2)	Siegmund, 1998
IFNγ (CA)n intron 1	Hay fever	Yes (in conjunction with TNF widtype)	Nieters, 2001
IFNγ (CA)n intron 1	Insulin-dependent diabetes mellitus	No	Pociot, 1997
IFNγ (CA)n intron 1	Insulin-dependent diabetes mellitus	Yes	Awata, 1994
IFNγ (CA)n Intron 1	Insulin-dependent diabetes mellitus	Yes	Jahromi, 2000
IFNγ (CA)n intron 1	Lung allograft fibrosis	Yes	Awad, 1998
IFNγ (CA)n intron 1	Multiple sclerosis	No	Epplen, 1997 Wansen, 1997 He, 1998
IFNγ (CA)n intron 1	Multiple sclerosis	No	Dai, 2001
IFNγ (CA)n Intron 1	Multiple sclerosis	No (Europeans)	Goris, 1999
IFNγ (CA)n Intron 1	Rejection of renal transplant	No	Pelletier, 2000
IFNγ (CA)n intron 1	Systemic lupus erythematosus	No	Lee, 2001

Table 4.3 (*Continued*)

Cytokine and polymorphism	Disease	Association	First author, year[1]
IFNγ (CA)n Intron 1 (126 bp repeat)	Rheumatoid arthritis	Yes (susceptibility and severity)	Khani-Hanjani, 2000
IFNγ (CA)n Intron 1 and IL-10 −−1082 G→A	Renal transplant rejection	Yes	Asderakis, 1998
IFNγ −333 C→T	Multiple sclerosis	No	Giedraitis, 1999
IFNγ-R1 (Val14Met)	Systemic lupus erythematosus	Yes	Tanaka, 1999
IFNγ-R1 (Val14Met), IFNγ-R2 Gln64/Arg64	Atopic asthma	No (Japanese children)	Nakao, 2001
IFNγ-R1 Met14/Val14 genotype and IFNγ-R2 Gln64/Gln64 genotype	Systemic lupus erythematosus	Yes (development)	Nakashima, 1999
IFNγ−R Val14Met	Systemic lupus erythematosus	Yes	Tanaka, 1999
IL-10 (IL10.G)	Chronic graft-versus-host disease	Yes	Takahashi, 2000
IL-10 (IL10.G)	Early-onset periodontal disease	No	Hennig, 2000
IL-10 (IL10.G)	Inflammatory bowel disease and ulcerative colitis	No	Parkes, 1998
IL-10 (IL10.G)	Multiple sclerosis	No	He, 1998
IL-10 (IL10.G)	Psoriasis	Yes	Asadullah, 2001
IL-10 (IL10.G)	Systemic lupus erythematosus	Yes	Eskdale, 1997 Mehrian, 1998
IL-10 (IL10.G)	UVB-induced immunosuppression	No	Allen, 1998
IL-10 (IL10.G10 and G12)	Reactive arthritis	Yes (protective)	Kaluza, 2001
IL-10 (IL10.G12-G15)	Graft-versus-host disease in allogeneic bone marrow transplantation	Yes	Middleton, 1998
IL-10 (IL10.G12-G15)	HLA-identical bone marrow	Yes (increased graft-versus-host disease)	Cavet, 1999
IL-10 (R2-G-C-C)	Unrelated bone marrow transplantation	Yes (increased mortality)	Keen, 2004
IL-10 (IL10.R)	Rheumatoid arthritis	Yes	Eskdale, 1998
IL-10 (IL10.R)	Systemic lupus erythematosus	No	Eskdale, 1997
IL-10 +571 C→A	Asthma (elevated IgE)	Yes	Hobbs, 1998
IL-10 −1082	Acute rejection in orthotopic liver transplantation	No	Bathgate, 2000
IL-10 −1082	Asthma severity	Yes	Lim, 1998
IL-10 −1082	End-stage liver disease	No	Bathgate, 2000
IL-10 −1082	Multiple sclerosis	No	Maurer, 2000
IL-10 −1082	Psoriasis	No	Reich, 1999
IL-10 −1082	Rheumatoid arthritis	No	Hajeer, 1998
IL-10 −1082	Rheumatoid arthritis	No	Cantagrel, 1999
IL-10 −1082	Type I autoimmune hepatitis	No	Cookson, 1999 Czaja, 1999
IL-10 −1082 A	Epstein-Barr virus infection	Yes (susceptibility)	Helminen, 1999
IL-10 −1082 A	Joint destruction	Yes	Huizinga, 2000
IL-10 −1082 A	Recurrence of hepatitis C in liver transplant recipients	Yes	Tambur, 2001
IL-10 −1082 A	Recurrent spontaneous abortions	No	Karhukorpi, 2001
IL-10 −1082 A	Cutaneous malignant melanoma	Yes	Howell, 2001
IL-10 −1082 A	Renal transplant rejection	No	Marshall, 2000
IL-10 −1082 G	Inflammatory bowel disease	Yes (decreased frequency)	Tagore, 1999
IL-10 −1082 G	Rejection of renal transplant	Yes	Pelletier, 2000
IL-10 −1082 G	Ulcerative colitis	Yes (decreased frequency)	Tagore, 1999
IL-10 −1082 G/A	Renal transplantation outcome	Yes	Poole, 2001
IL-10 −1082, −819, −592 haplotype	Chronic cutaneous lupus erythematosus	No	van der Linden, 2000
IL-10 −1082, −819, −592 haplotype	Multiple sclerosis	No	Pickard, 1999 Maurer, 2000
IL-10 −1082, −819, −592 haplotype	Rejection of pediatric heart transplant	Yes (high IL-10 production is protective)	Awad, 2001
IL-10 −1082, −819, −592 haplotype	Rheumatoid arthritis and Felty's syndrome	No	Coakley, 1998
IL-10 −1082A, −592A	Inflammatory bowel disease	No	Klein, 2000
IL-10 −1082A, −819C, −592C haplotype	Primary sclerosing cholangitis	No	Donaldson, 2000
IL-10 −1082A, −819C, −592C haplotype	Rheumatoid arthritis (IgA RF+ve, IgG RF−ve)	Yes	Hajeer, 1998
IL-10 −1082A, −819T, −592A haplotype	Coronary artery disease and myocardial Infarction	No	Koch, 2001
IL-10 −1082A, −819T, −592A haplotype	EBV infection	Yes (protective)	Helminen, 2001

Table 4.3 (*Continued*)

Cytokine and polymorphism	Disease	Association	First author, year[1]
IL-10 −1082A, −819T, −592A haplotype	Juvenile rheumatoid arthritis	Yes (involvement of >4 joints)	Crawley, 1999
IL-10 −1082A, −819T, −592A haplotype	Response of chronic hepatitis C to IFNα therapy	Yes (improved response)	Edwards-Smith, 1999
IL-10 −1082A, −819T, −592A haplotype	Systemic lupus erythematosus nephritis (Chinese)	Yes	Mok, 1998
IL-10 −1082G, −819C, −592C haplotype	Systemic lupus erythematosus	Yes (Ro+)	Lazarus, 1997
IL-10 −1082G, −819C, −592C haplotype, also occurs in combination with IL-10 −1082A, −819T, −592A haplotype	Primary Sjogren's syndrome	Yes (susceptibility)	Hulkkonen, 2001
IL-10 1082 G-allele	Mortality in acute renal failure	Yes	Jaber, 2004
IL-10 −592	Primary biliary cirrhosis	No	Zappala, 1998
IL-10 −592	Type I autoimmune hepatitis	No	Cookson, 1999 Czaja, 1999
IL-10 −592 C→A	Sudden infant death syndrome	Yes	Summers, 2000
IL-10 −627 C→A	Advanced liver disease	Yes	Grove, 2000
IL-10 −627 C→A	Primary sclerosing cholangitis	Yes	Mitchell, 2001
IL-10 −627, −1117	Inflammatory bowel diseases	No	Aithal, 2001
IL-10 −819	Type I autoimmune hepatitis	No	Cookson, 1999 Czaja, 1999
IL-10 Exon 1, +78 G→A (Gly15→Arg) IL-10 Intron 3, +19 C→T IL-10 Intron 3, +953 T→C IL-10 3' flanking region, +117 after stop codon C→T	Myocardial infarction	No	Donger, 2001
IL-12 (p40) 3'UTR nt1188 A→C	Rheumatoid arthritis, multiple sclerosis	No	Hall, 2000
IL-13 −1055 C→T	Asthma	Yes	van der Pouw Kraan, 1999
IL-13, nt 4257 G→A	Atopic dermatitis	Yes	Liu, 2000
IL-13Rα 1050 C→T	Atopic asthma	No (Japanese population)	Ahmed, 2000
IL-13R130Q	Asthma	No	Leung, 2001
IL-18 −607, −137	Multiple sclerosis	No	Giedraitis, 2001
IL-18 −607, −137	Type I diabetes mellitus	Yes (association with CTLA-4)	Ide, 2004
IL-1R1 Pst I-A	Insulin-dependent diabetes mellitus	No	Kristiansen, 2000
IL-1Ra (240 bp allele)	Bone loss in inflammatory bowel disease	Yes (protective)	Schulte, 2000
IL-1Ra intron 2 86bp VNTR	Acute myeloid leukemia (secondary)	No	Langabeer, 1998
IL-1Ra intron 2 86bp VNTR	Acute myocardial infarction	No	Iacoviello, 2000
IL-1Ra intron 2 86bp VNTR	Alcoholic hepatic fibrosis (Japanese)	Yes	Takamatsu, 1998
IL-1Ra intron 2 86bp VNTR	Alopecia areata	Yes (severity)	Tarlow, 1994 Cork, 1995
IL-1Ra intron 2 86bp VNTR	Bone loss (early postmenopausal)	Yes	Keen, 1998
IL-1Ra intron 2 86bp VNTR	Corneal melting in systemic vasculitis	No	McKibbin, 2000
IL-1Ra intron 2 86bp VNTR	EBV seronegativity	Weak	Hurme, 1998
IL-1Ra intron 2 86bp VNTR	Graft-versus-host disease	Yes (protective)	Cullup, 2001
IL-1Ra intron 2 86bp VNTR	Graves' disease	Yes	Blakemore, 1995
IL-1Ra intron 2 86bp VNTR	Graves' disease and Graves' ophthalmopathy	No	Mühlberg, 1998 Cuddihy, 1996
IL-1Ra intron 2 86bp VNTR	Helicobacter pylori	No (susceptibility)	Hamajima, 2001
IL-1Ra intron 2 86bp VNTR	Henoch-Schonlein nephritis	Yes	Liu, 1997
IL-1Ra intron 2 86bp VNTR	Inflammatory bowel disease	No	Hacker, 1997 Hacker, 1998
IL-1Ra intron 2 86bp VNTR	Inflammatory bowel disease	Yes	Mansfield, 1994 Bioque, 1996 Louis, 1996
IL-1Ra intron 2 86bp VNTR	Insulin-dependent diabetes mellitus	No	Kristiansen, 2000
IL-1Ra intron 2 86bp VNTR	Insulin-dependent diabetes mellitus	Yes	Pociot, 1994
IL-1Ra intron 2 86bp VNTR	Insulin-dependent diabetes mellitus, Non-insulin-dependent diabetes mellitus nephropathy	Yes	Blakemore, 1996
IL-1Ra intron 2 86bp VNTR	Lichen sclerosis	Yes	Clay, 1994
IL-1Ra intron 2 86bp VNTR	Malaria (*Plasmodium falciparum*): severity	No	Bellamy, 1998

Table 4.3 (*Continued*)

Cytokine and polymorphism	Disease	Association	First author, year[1]
IL-1Ra intron 2 86bp VNTR	Multiple sclerosis	No	Huang, 1996 Epplen, 1997 Semana, 1997 Wansen, 1997
IL-1Ra intron 2 86bp VNTR	Multiple sclerosis	No	Feakes, 2000
IL-1Ra intron 2 86bp VNTR	Multiple sclerosis	Yes	Crusius, 1995 de la Concha, 1997
IL-1Ra intron 2 86bp VNTR	Myasthenia gravis	No	Huang, 1996
IL-1Ra intron 2 86bp VNTR	Osteoporosis	No	Bajnok, 2000
IL-1Ra intron 2 86bp VNTR (A1/A2 genotype)	Perinuclear ANCA Ulcerative colitis	Yes	Papo, 1999
IL-1Ra intron 2 86bp VNTR	Polymyositis and dermatomyositis	No	Son, 2000
IL-1Ra intron 2 86bp VNTR	Rheumatoid arthritis	No	Cantagrel, 1999
IL-1Ra intron 2 86bp VNTR	Rheumatoid arthritis	No	Perrier, 1998
IL-1Ra intron 2 86bp VNTR	Single vessel coronary disease	Yes	Francis, 1999
IL-1Ra intron 2 86bp VNTR	Sjögren's syndrome	Yes	Perrier, 1998
IL-1Ra intron 2 86bp VNTR	Spondylarthropathies	No	Djouadi, 2001
IL-1Ra intron 2 86bp VNTR	Systemic lupus erythematosus	No	Danis, 1995
IL-1Ra intron 2 86bp VNTR	Systemic lupus erythematosus	Yes	Blakemore, 1994 Suzuki, 1997
IL-1Ra intron 2 86bp VNTR	Type I autoimmune hepatitis	No	Cookson, 1999 Czaja, 1999
IL-1Ra intron 2 86bp VNTR	Ulcerative colitis	No	Bouma, 1999
IL-1Ra intron 2 86bp VNTR & IL-1β + 3953 exon 5	Myasthenia gravis	Yes	Huang, 1998
IL-1Ra intron 2 86bp VNTR (A1 allele)	Alcoholism	Yes (Spanish)	Pastor, 2000
IL-1Ra intron 2 86bp VNTR (A1 allele)	Juvenile idiopathic inflammatory myopathies	Yes (Caucasians)	Rider, 2000
IL-1Ra intron 2 86bp VNTR (A1 allele)	Multiple sclerosis	Yes	Sciacca, 1999
IL-1Ra intron 2 86bp VNTR (A1 allele)	Primary biliary cirrhosis	Yes (homozygotes)	Arkwright, 2001
IL-1Ra intron 2	HCV-induced cirrhosis	Yes (low impact)	Bahr, 2003
IL-1Ra intron 2 86bp VNTR (A1/A2/A3 alleles)	Corneal melting in vasculitis	No	McKibbin, 2000
IL-1Ra intron 2 86bp VNTR (A1A1/A3 alleles)	Multiple myeloma	No	Zheng, 2000
IL-1Ra intron 2 86bp VNTR (A1A1/A3 alleles)	Osteoporosis	Yes	Langdahl, 2000
IL-1Ra intron 2 86bp VNTR (A1A1/A3 alleles)	Osteoporotic fractures	Yes	Langdahl, 2000
IL-1Ra intron 2 86bp VNTR (A2 allele)	CD4 count in HIV	No	Witkin, 2001
IL-1Ra intron 2 86bp VNTR (A2 allele)	Chronic obstructive pulmonary disease	No	Ishii, 2000
IL-1Ra intron 2 86bp VNTR (A2 allele)	Early-onset sporadic Alzheimer's disease	Yes	Rebeck, 2000
IL-1Ra intron 2 86bp VNTR (A2 allele)	Gastric cancer	Yes	Machado, 2001
IL-1Ra intron 2 86bp VNTR (A2 allele)	Gastric cancer from *H. pylori*	Yes	El-Omar, 2001
IL-1Ra intron 2 86bp VNTR (A2 allele)	Idiopathic recurrent miscarriage	Yes	Tempfer, 2001, Unfried, 2001
IL-1Ra intron 2 86bp VNTR (A2 allele)	IgA nephropathy	Yes	Shu, 2000
IL-1Ra intron 2 86bp VNTR (A2 allele)	Ischemic heart disease	No	Manzoli, 1999
IL-1Ra intron 2 86bp VNTR (A2 allele)	Juvenile idiopathic arthritis	Yes	Vencovsky, 2001
IL-1Ra intron 2 86bp VNTR (A2 allele)	Multivessel coronary disease	No	Francis, 1999
IL-1Ra intron 2 86bp VNTR (A2 allele)	Nephropathia epidemica	Yes (protective)	Makela, 2001
IL-1Ra intron 2 86bp VNTR (A2 allele)	Polymyalgia rheumatica	Yes (with susceptibility, not severity)	Boiardi, 2000
IL-1Ra intron 2 86bp VNTR (A2 allele)	Primary sclerosing cholangitis	No	Donaldson, 2000
IL-1Ra intron 2 86bp VNTR (A2 allele)	Severe sepsis	Yes	Fang, 1999
IL-1Ra intron 2 86bp VNTR (A2 allele)	Single-vessel coronary disease	Yes	Francis, 1999
IL-1Ra intron 2 86bp VNTR (A2 allele)	Stenosis after angioplasty	Yes (protective)	Francis, 2001
IL-1Ra intron 2 86bp VNTR (A2 allele)	Systemic lupus erythematosus	Yes (in LD with HLA DR17, DQ2)	Tjernstrom, 1999
IL-1Ra intron 2 86bp VNTR (A2 allele)	Tuberculin (Mantoux) reactivity	Yes (reduced)	Wilkinson, 1999
IL-1Ra intron 2 86bp VNTR (A2 allele)	Ulcerative colitis	No (Spaniards)	Gonzalez Sarmiento, 1999
IL-1Ra intron 2 86bp VNTR (A2 allele)	Ulcerative colitis	Yes	Tountas, 1999
IL-1Ra intron 2 86bp VNTR (A2 allele)	*Ureaplasma urealyticum* vaginal colonization	Yes (negative association)	Jeremias, 1999

Table 4.3 (*Continued*)

Cytokine and polymorphism	Disease	Association	First author, year[1]
IL-1Ra intron 2 86bp VNTR (A2 allele)	Vulvar vestibulitis	Yes	Jeremias, 2000
IL-1Ra intron 2 86bp VNTR (A2 allele)	Vulvar vestibulitis	Yes	Jeremias, 2000
IL-1Ra intron 2 86bp VNTR (A2 allele) and IL-1β C511T haplotype	Decline in lung function	Yes	Joos, 2001
IL-1Ra intron 2 86bp VNTR (A2 allele) and IL-1β +3953 (allele 2)	Early-onset periodontitis	Yes (combined genotypes increase risk for smokers)	Parkhill, 2000
IL-1Ra intron 2 86bp VNTR (A2 allele) and IL-1β +3953 (allele 2)	Multiple sclerosis	Yes (progression)	Schrijver, 1999
IL-1Ra intron 2 86bp VNTR (A3 allele)	Juvenile idiopathic inflammatory myopathies	Yes (African-Americans)	Rider, 2000
IL-1Ra intron 2 86bp VNTR A2(-)/ IL-1β + 3953 A1(+)	Tuberculous pleurisy	Yes	Wilkinson, 1999
IL-1Ra nt8061 C→T (Mwol)	Ulcerative colitis	Yes	Stokkers, 1998
IL-1Ra, +2018 (allele 2)	Fibrosing alveolitis	Yes	Whyte, 2000
IL-1Ra, +2018 (allele 2)	Pouchitis following ileal pouch-anal anastomosis	Yes	Carter, 2001
IL-1Ra, +2018 (allele 2)	Restenosis after coronary stenting	Yes (protective)	Kastrati, 2000
IL-1RI	Insulin-dependent diabetes mellitus	Yes	Pociot, 1994; Metcalfe, 1996
IL-1RI RFLP-A	Insulin-dependent diabetes mellitus	Yes	Bergholdt, 1995
IL-1α (CA)n intron 5	Early-onset pauciarticular juvenile chronic arthritis	No	Epplen, 1995
IL-1α (CA)n intron 5	Juvenile chronic arthritis	No	Donn, 1999
IL-1α (CA)n intron 5	Multiple sclerosis	No	Epplen, 1997
IL-1α (CA)n intron 5	Rheumatoid arthritis	No	Gomolka, 1995
IL-1α −889	Alzheimer's disease	Yes	Du, 2000
IL-1α −889	Early-onset Alzheimer's disease	Yes	Grimaldi, 2000
IL-1α −889	Juvenile chronic arthritis	No	Donn, 1999
IL-1α −889	Juvenile rheumatoid arthritis	Yes	McDowell, 1995
IL-1α −889	Multiple sclerosis	No	Ferri, 2000
IL-1α −889	Periodontal disease	Yes	Shirodaria, 2000
IL-1α −889	Single and multivessel coronary disease	No	Francis, 1999
IL-1α −889 (T allele)	Alzheimer's disease	Yes	Nicoll, 2000
IL-1α −889 (T allele)	Systemic sclerosis	Yes	Hutyrova, 2004
IL-1α −889 T→C	*H. pylori* infection	No	Hamajima, 2001
IL-1α intron 6	Rheumatoid arthritis	No	Bailly, 1995
IL-1α +4845, IL-1β +3953	Periodontitis	Yes	McDevitt, 2000
IL-1α +4845, IL-1β +3953	Severity of periodontitis and antibody response to microbiota	Yes	Papapanou, 2001
IL-1β	Periodontitis	Yes	Kornman, 1997; Kornman, 1998
IL-1β	Non-small cell lung cancer	Yes	Zienolddiny, 2004
IL-1β +IL-1Ra	Inflammatory bowel disease	Yes	Bioque, 1995; Heresbach, 1997
IL-1β +3953 (nt5887) C→T	Multiple sclerosis	No	Kantarci, 2000
IL-1β +3953 (nt5887) C→T (Taql)	Adult periodontitis	Yes	Galbraith, 1999
IL-1β +3953 (nt5887) C→T (Taql)	Alopecia areata	Yes (in combination with KM loci)	Galbraith, 1999
IL-1β +3953 (nt5887) C→T (Taql)	Alzheimer's disease	Yes (in conjunction with a T,T genotype in ACT gene)	Licastro, 2000
IL-1β +3953 (nt5887) C→T (Taql)	Inflammatory bowel disease	Yes (white South Africans)	Mwantembe, 2001
IL-1β +3953 (nt5887) C→T (Taql)	Pancreatic cancer	Yes (shortened survival)	Barber, 2000
IL-1β +3953 (nt5887) C→T (Taql)	Polymyalgia rheumatica	No	Boiardi, 2000
IL-1β +3953 (nt5887) C→T (Taql)	Severe sepsis	No	Fang, 1999
IL-1β +3953 (nt5887) C→T (Taql)	Silicosis	No	Yucesoy, 2001
IL-1β +3953 (nt5887) C→T (Taql)	Single and multivessel coronary disease	No	Francis, 1999
IL-1β +3953 (nt5887) C→T (Taql)	Spondylarthropathies	No	Djouadi, 2001
IL-1β +3953 (nt5887) C→T (Taql)	Type I autoimmune hepatitis	No	Cookson, 1999; Czaja, 1999
IL-1β +3953 (nt5887) C→T (Taql)	Wegener's granulomatosis	No	Huang, 2000
IL-1β +3953 (nt5887) C→T (Taql): allele 1,1 (homozygous)	Primary biliary cirrhosis	Yes	Arkwright, 2001
IL-1β +3953 (nt5887) C→T (Taql): T allele	Idiopathic recurrent miscarriage	No	Hefler, 2001
IL-1β +3953 (nt5887) C→T (Taql): T allele	Inflammatory bowel disease	No	Hacker, 1998
IL-1β +3953 (nt5887) C→T (Taql): T allele	Insulin-dependent diabetes mellitus	No	Lanng, 1993
IL-1β +3953 (nt5887) C→T (Taql): T allele	Insulin-dependent diabetes mellitus	No	Kristiansen, 2000
IL-1β +3953 (nt5887) C→T (Taql): T allele	Insulin-dependent diabetes mellitus (DR3-/DR4-)	Yes	Pociot, 1992

Table 4.3 (*Continued*)

Cytokine and polymorphism	Disease	Association	First author, year[1]
IL-1β +3953 (nt5887) C→T (TaqI): T allele	Insulin-dependent diabetes mellitus (with nephropathy)	Yes	Loughrey, 1998
IL-1β +3953 (nt5887) C→T (TaqI): T allele	Joint destruction in rheumatoid arthritis	Yes (increased)	Buchs, 2001
IL-1β +3953 (nt5887) C→T (TaqI): T allele	Localized juvenile periodontitis	No (African-Americans)	Walker, 2000
IL-1β +3953 (nt5887) C→T (TaqI): T allele	Low-grade squamous intraepithelial lesions	Yes	Majeed, 1999
IL-1β +3953 (nt5887) C→T (TaqI): T allele	Multiple myeloma	No	Zheng, 2000
IL-1β +3953 (nt5887) C→T (TaqI): T allele	Multiple sclerosis	No	Wansen, 1997
IL-1β +3953 (nt5887) C→T (TaqI): T allele	Myasthenia gravis	Yes	Huang, 1998
IL-1β +3953 (nt5887) C→T (TaqI): T allele, IL-1RN VNTR	Peptic ulcer disease	Yes (severity)	Garcia-Gonzalez, 2001
IL-1β +3953 (nt5887) C→T (TaqI): T allele	Periodontitis	No (in population of Chinese heritage)	Armitage, 2000
IL-1β +3953 (nt5887) C→T (TaqI): T allele	Periodontitis	Yes	Gore, 1998
IL-1β +3953 (nt5887) C→T (TaqI): T allele and IL-1α +4845	Periodontitis	Yes	Socransky, 2000
IL-1β +3953 (nt5887) C→T (TaqI): T allele	Primary sclerosing cholangitis	No	Donaldson, 2000
IL-1β +3953 (nt5887) C→T (TaqI): T allele	Rheumatoid arthritis	Yes (predictive of erosive disease)	Cantagrel, 1999
IL-1β +3953 (nt5887) C→T (TaqI): T allele	Ulcerative colitis	No	Bouma, 1999
IL-1β +3953 (nt5887) C→T (TaqI): T allele	Ulcerative colitis	Yes	Stokkers, 1998
IL-1β +3953 (nt5887) C→T (TaqI): T allele	Wegener's granulomatosis	No	Huang, 2000
IL-1β −511 C→T	Gastric cancer	No	Kato, 2001
IL-1β −511 C→T	Gastric cancer	Yes	Machado, 2001
IL-1β −511 C→T	Multiple sclerosis	No	Ferri, 2000
IL-1β −511 C→T	Temporal lobe epilepsy	No	Buono, 2001
IL-1β −511 G→A (AvaI) and +3953 (nt5887) C→T (TaqI)	Alcoholic liver disease	Yes (in Japanese alcoholics)	Takamatsu, 2000
IL-1β −511 G→A (AvaI) and +3953 (nt5887) C→T (TaqI)	Inflammatory bowel disease	Yes	Nemetz, 1999
IL-1β −511 G→A (AvaI), +3953 (nt5887) C→T (TaqI), +3877 G→A	Osteoporotic fractures	No	Langdahl, 2000
IL-1β −511 G→A	Brain alterations in schizophrenics	Yes	Meisenzahl, 2001
IL-1β −511 G→A	Early onset of Parkinson's disease	Increased severity for homozygotes of allele 1	Nishimura, 2000
IL-1β −511 G→A	Localization related epilepsy	Yes	Peltola, 2001
IL-1β −511 G→A	Low bone mass in inflammatory bowel disease	Yes	Muldoon, 2001
IL-1β −511 G→A (AvaI)	Chronic obstructive pulmonary disease	No	Ishii, 2000
IL-1β −511 G→A (AvaI)	EBV seronegativity	Yes	Hurme, 1998
IL-1β −511 G→A (AvaI)	Hippocampal sclerosis	Possible association in Japanese study	Kanemoto, 2000
IL-1β −511 G→A (AvaI)	Insulin-dependent diabetes mellitus	No	Kristiansen, 2000
IL-1β −511 G→A (AvaI)	Meningococcal disease	Increased severity for homozygotes with either allele	Read, 2000
IL-1β −511 G→A (AvaI)	Nephropathia epidemica	Yes (protective)	Makela, 2001
IL-1β −511 G→A (AvaI)	Parkinson's disease	No (although age of onset in homozygotes was lower)	Nishimura, 2001
IL-1β −511 G→A (AvaI)	Polymyalgia rheumatica	No	Boiardi, 2000
IL-1β −511 G→A (AvaI)	Rheumatoid arthritis	No	Cantagrel, 1999
IL-1β −511 G→A (AvaI)	Single and multivessel coronary disease	No	Francis, 1999
IL-1β −511 G→A (AvaI)	Temporal lobe epilepsy with hippocampal	Possible association for A homozygotes	Kanemoto, 2000

Table 4.3 (*Continued*)

Cytokine and polymorphism	Disease	Association	First author, year[1]
IL-1β −511 G→A (Aval), IL-1α −889, +3953 C→T, IL-1Ra VNTR	Multiple sclerosis	No	Luomala, 2001
IL-1β −511 G→A (Aval), IL-1α −889, IL-1Ra VNTR	Schizophrenia	Yes	Katila, 1999
IL-1β 31 C→T	Gastric cancer from *H. pylori*	Yes	El-Omar, 2001
IL-1β 31 C→T	*H. pylori* infection	Yes (susceptibility)	Hamajima, 2001
IL-2 (CA)n 3'-flanking region	Early-onset pauciarticular juvenile chronic arthritis	No	Epplen, 1995
IL-2 (CA)n 3'-flanking region	Inflammatory bowel disease	No	Parkes, 1998
IL-2 (CA)n 3'-flanking region	Multiple sclerosis	No	Epplen, 1997 He, 1998
IL-2 (CA)n 3'-flanking region	Rheumatoid arthritis	No	Gomolka, 1995
IL-2 (CA)n 3'-flanking region	Ulcerative colitis	Weak	Parkes, 1998
IL-2Rβ (GT)n 5'-UTR	Multiple sclerosis	No	Epplen, 1997
IL-2Rβ dinucleotide repeat	Schizophrenia	No	Nimgaonkar, 1995 Tatsumi, 1997
IL-2Rγ	Severe combined immunodeficiency disease*	Yes	Clark, 1995 Pepper, 1995 Puck, 1995 O'Marcaigh, 1997 Puck, 1997 Puck, 1997 Wengler, 1998 Fugmann, 1998
IL-3 −16 C→T	Rheumatoid arthritis	Yes	Yamada, 2001
IL-4 −34 C→T	Atopic eczema	No	Elliott, 2001
IL-4 −590 C→T (BsmFI)	Asthma and atopy	Weak	Walley, 1996
IL-4 −590 C→T (BsmFI)	Asthma and atopy (Japanese)	Yes	Noguchi, 1998 Kawashima, 1998
IL-4 −590 C→T (BsmFI)	Autoimmune thyroid disease	Yes	Hunt, 2000
IL-4 −590 C→T (BsmFI)	Renal allograft rejection	No	Cartwright, 2001
IL-4 −590 C→T (BsmFI)	Acquisition of syncytium-inducing variants of HIV-1 in patients	Increased (In Japanese HIV-1+ patients)	Nakayama, 2000
IL-4 −590 C→T (BsmFI)	Asthma	Increased in fatal/near fatal asthma	Sandford, 2000
IL-4 −590 C→T (BsmFI)	Asthma	No (Kuwaiti Arabs) Yes (in US and Japanese)	Hijazi, 2000
IL-4 −590 C→T (BsmFI)	Atopic eczema	No	Elliott, 2001
IL-4 −590 C→T (BsmFI)	Atopy, asthma, rhinitis	Yes (Japanese infant population)	Zhu, 2000
IL-4 −590 C→T (BsmFI)	Childhood atopic asthma	No (Japanese population)	Takabayashi, 2000
IL-4 −590 C→T (BsmFI)	Crohn's disease	Yes	Klein, 2001
IL-4 −590 C→T (BsmFI)	IgE levels	No	Dizier, 1999
IL-4 −590 C→T (BsmFI)	Insulin-dependent diabetes mellitus	No	Jahromi, 2000
IL-4 −590 C→T (BsmFI)	Renal transplantation outcome	Yes	Poole, 2001
IL-4 −590 C→T (BsmFI)	Rheumatoid arthritis	No	Cantagrel, 1999
IL-4 intron 2 dinucleotide repeat	IgE levels	No	Dizier, 1999
IL-4 intron 2 dinucleotide repeat	Minimal change nephropathy	No	Parry, 1999
IL-4 Intron 2, 70bp VNTR	Multiple sclerosis	Yes	Vandenbroeck, 1997
IL-4 Intron 2, 70bp VNTR	Myasthenia gravis	No	Huang, 1998
IL-4 Intron 3, (GT) repeat	Chronic polyarthritis	Yes (protective)	Buchs, 2000
IL-4 Intron 3, (GT) repeat	Multiple sclerosis	No	He, 1998
IL-4 Intron 3, (GT) repeat	Myasthenia gravis	No	Huang, 1998
IL-4 Intron 3, 70bp VNTR (RP1 allele)	Rheumatoid arthritis	Yes	Cantagrel, 1999
IL-4Rα nt148 A→G (I50V)	Atopy/asthma	No	Noguchi, 1999
IL-4Rα nt148 A→G (I50V)	Childhood atopic asthma	Yes	Takabayashi, 2000
IL-4Rα nt148 A→G (I50V)	Atopic disease	Yes	Mitsuyasu, 1998 Izuhara, 1999
IL-4Rα nt1902 G→A (R576Q)	Asthma	No effect on severity	Sandford, 2000
IL-4Rα nt1902 G→A (R576Q)	Atopic disease	Yes	Hershey, 1997
IL-4Rα nt1902 G→A (R576Q)	Chronic polyarthritis	No	Buchs, 2000
IL-4Rα nt1902 G→A (R551Q, previously R576Q)	Atopic disease/asthma	No (Japanese)	Noguchi, 1999

Table 4.3 (*Continued*)

Cytokine and polymorphism	Disease	Association	First author, year[1]
IL-4Rα nt1902 G→A (R551Q, previously R576Q)	Childhood atopic asthma	No	Takabayashi, 2000
IL-4Rα val50ile, gln576arg, A3044G, G3289A	Inflammatory bowel disease	No	Olavesen, 2000
IL-4Rα nt1682 T→C (S478P) (previously S503P)	Atopy/asthma	Yes	Kruse, 1999
IL-4Rα nt1902 G→A (R551Q) (previously R576Q)	Atopy/asthma	Yes	Kruse, 1999 Rosa-Rosa, 1999
IL-4Rα nt1902 G→A (R551Q) (previously R576Q), IL-4 −34 C→T	Crohn's disease	Yes	Aithal, 2001
IL-4Rα nt1902 G→A (R551Q, previously R576Q)	Adult atopic dermatitis	Yes	Oiso, 2000
IL-4Rα nt1902 G→A (R551Q, previously R576Q)	Minimal change nephropathy	No	Parry, 1999
IL-4Rα, Q576R	Mastocytosis	Yes (protective)	Daley, 2001
IL-4Rα, S786P	Asthma	No	Andrews, 2001
IL-5Rα (GA)n 3′-UTR	Early-onset pauciarticular juvenile chronic arthritis	No	Epplen, 1995
IL-5Rα (GA)n 3′-UTR	Multiple sclerosis	No	Epplen, 1997
IL-5Rα (GA)n 3′-UTR	Rheumatoid arthritis	No	Gomolka, 1995
IL-6 (130 bp allele)	Bone loss in inflammatory bowel disease	Yes	Schulte, 2000
IL-6 (CA)n repeat (allele 1)	Female menopause	Yes (bone mineral density)	Tsukamoto, 1999
IL-6 (intron 4G) and TNF-R2 1690 C allele	Idiopathic pulmonary fibrosis	Yes	Pantelidis, 2001
IL-6 −174, −597	Multiple sclerosis	No	Fedetz, 2001
IL-6 −174 C→G	Insulin-dependent diabetes mellitus	Yes	Jahromi, 2000
IL-6 −174 C→G	Lipid abnormalities	Yes	Fernandez-Real, 2000
IL-6 −174 C→G	Rejection of renal transplant	Yes	Reviron, 2001
IL-6 −174 C→G	Asymptomatic carotid artery atherosclerosis	Yes	Rauramaa, 2000
IL-6 −174 C→G (NlaIII)	Kaposi sarcoma	Yes (increased susceptibility in HIV-infected men)	Foster, 2000
IL-6 −174 C→G (NlaIII)	Systemic-onset juvenile chronic arthritis	Yes	Fishman, 1998
IL-6 −174 G→C (NlaIII)	Abdominal aortic aneurysms	Predictor of future cardiovascular mortality	Jones, 2001
IL-6 −174 G→C (NlaIII)	Alzheimer's disease	No	Bagli, 2000
IL-6 −174 G→C (NlaIII)	Alzheimer's disease	No	Bagli, 2000
IL-6 −174 G→C (NlaIII)	Ankylosing spondylitis	No	Collado-Escobar, 2000
IL-6 −174 G→C (NlaIII)	Breast cancer (aggressive)	Yes	Iacopetta, 2004
IL-6 −174 G→C (NlaIII)	Graft-versus-host disease	Yes (increased severity)	Cavet, 2001
IL-6 −174 G→C (NlaIII)	Inflammatory bowel disease	No	Klein, 2001
IL-6 −174 G→C (NlaIII)	Multiple myeloma	No	Zheng, 2000
IL-6 −174 G→C (NlaIII)	Myasthenia gravis	No	Huang, 1999
IL-6 −174 G→C (NlaIII)	Osteoporosis	Yes (susceptibility)	Ferrari, 2001
IL-6 −174 G→C (NlaIII)	Primary Sjogren's syndrome	No	Hulkkonen, 2001
IL-6 −174 G→C (NlaIII)	Renal allograft rejection	No	Cartwright, 2001
IL-6 −174 G→C (NlaIII)	Renal allograft rejection	Yes	Marshall, 2001
IL-6 −174 G→C (NlaIII)	Systemic lupus erythematosus	No	Linker-Israeli, 1999
IL-6 −174 G→C (NlaIII)	Systemic lupus erythematosus	Yes (clinical features)	Schotte, 2001
IL-6 −174 G→C (NlaIII) G allele	Lipid abnormalities	Yes	Fernandez-Real, 2000
IL-6 3′ (AT)-rich minisatellite	Bone loss (bone mineral density)	Yes	Murray, 1997
IL-6 3′ (AT)-rich minisatellite	Myasthenia gravis	No	Huang, 1999
IL-6 3′ (AT)-rich minisatellite	Systemic lupus erythematosus	Yes	Linker-Israeli, 1996
IL-6 3′ (AT)-rich minisatellite (792bp allele)	Systemic lupus erythematosus	Yes (susceptibility: Caucasians and African-Americans)	Linker-Israeli, 1999
IL-6 3′ (AT)-rich minisatellite (796bp and 828bp alleles)	Systemic lupus erythematosus	Yes (protection: Caucasians)	Linker-Israeli, 1999
IL-6 3′ (AT)-rich minisatellite (808bp and 820bp alleles)	Systemic lupus erythematosus	Yes (susceptibility: Caucasians)	Linker-Israeli, 1999
IL-6 3′ (AT)-rich minisatellite (828bp allele)	Systemic lupus erythematosus	Yes (protection: African-Americans)	Linker-Israeli, 1999

Table 4.3 (*Continued*)

Cytokine and polymorphism	Disease	Association	First author, year[1]
IL-6 3' (AT)-rich minisatellite and IL-6174 G→C (NIaIII) haplotype	Alzheimer's disease	Yes	Bagli, 2000
IL-6 3' flanking region (9 alleles)	Multiple sclerosis	Yes (allele determines course and onset)	Vandenbroeck, 2000
IL-6 3' flanking region (C allele)	Multiple sclerosis	No	Schmidt, 2000
IL-6 3' UTR	Low bone mineral density	No	Takacs, 2000
IL-6 BgIII	Rheumatoid arthritis	No	Blankenstein, 1989
IL-6 MspI & BgIII	Rheumatoid arthritis, pauciarticular juvenile rheumatoid arthritis, systemic lupus erythematosus	No	Fugger, 1989
IL-6: − 174, − 622	Mean age of onset of rheumatoid arthritis	Yes	Pascual, 2000
IRF-1 (GT)n intron 7	Multiple sclerosis	No	Epplen, 1997
LTα (TNFβ) Asp HI	Cardiac transplant rejection	No	Abdallah, 1999
LTα (TNFβ) intron 1 NcoI RFLP	Ankylosing spondylitis	No	Verjans, 1991
LTα (TNFβ) intron 1 NcoI RFLP	Ankylosing spondylitis	Yes	Fraile, 1998
LTα (TNFβ) intron 1 NcoI RFLP (2/2 genotype)	Atopic asthma	Yes (females)	Trabetti, 1999
LTα (TNFβ) intron 1 NcoI RFLP	Atopy	No	Castro, 2000
LTα (TNFβ) intron 1 NcoI RFLP	Autoimmune thyroiditis	No	Chung, 1994
LTα (TNFβ) intron 1 NcoI RFLP	Bronchial hyperreactivity in asthma	No	Li Kam Wa, 1999
LTα (TNFβ) intron 1 NcoI RFLP	Cardiac transplant rejection	No	Abdallah, 1999
LTα (TNFβ) intron 1 NcoI RFLP	Chronic lymphocytic leukemia	Yes (advanced stage)	Demeter, 1997
LTα (TNFβ) intron 1 NcoI RFLP	Disease progression in sepsis (neonates)	No	Weitkamp, 2000
LTα (TNFβ) intron 1 NcoI RFLP	Gastric cancer	Yes (survival)	Shimura, 1995
LTα (TNFβ) intron 1 NcoI RFLP	Graves' disease	via LD with HLA?	Badenhoop, 1992
LTα (TNFβ) intron 1 NcoI RFLP	Hashimoto's disease	No	Badenhoop, 1990
LTα (TNFβ) intron 1 NcoI RFLP	Hyperinsulinemia in coronary artery disease	Yes	Braun, 1998
LTα (TNFβ) intron 1 NcoI RFLP	Idiopathic membranous nephropathy	via LD with HLA?	Medcraft, 1993
LTα (TNFβ) intron 1 NcoI RFLP	Inflammatory bowel disease	No	Xia, 1995
LTα (TNFβ) intron 1 NcoI RFLP	Insulin resistance	Yes (decreases)	Hayakawa, 2000
LTα (TNFβ) intron 1 NcoI RFLP	Insulin-dependent diabetes mellitus	via LD with HLA?	Badenhoop, 1989 Badenhoop, 1989 Badenhoop, 1990 Jenkins, 1991 Pociot, 1991 Yamagata, 1991 Ilonen, 1992 Feugeas, 1993 Pociot, 1993 Vendrell, 1994 Whichelow, 1996
LTα (TNFβ) intron 1 NcoI RFLP	Lung cancer	Yes (survival)	Shimura, 1994 Hagihara, 1995
LTα (TNFβ) intron 1 NcoI RFLP	Multiple sclerosis and optic neuritis	No	Fugger, 1990 He, 1995
LTα (TNFβ) intron 1 NcoI RFLP	Myasthenia gravis	Yes	Zelano, 1998
LTα (TNFβ) intron 1 NcoI RFLP	Non-insulin-dependent diabetes mellitus (hypertriglyceridemia)	Yes	Vendrell, 1995
LTα (TNFβ) intron 1 NcoI RFLP	Pancreatic cancer	No	Barber, 1999
LTα (TNFβ) intron 1 NcoI RFLP	Primary biliary cirrhosis	No	Messer, 1991
LTα (TNFβ) intron 1 NcoI RFLP	Primary biliary cirrhosis	via LD with HLA?	Fugger, 1989
LTα (TNFβ) intron 1 NcoI RFLP	Primary sclerosing cholangitis	No	Bernal, 1999
LTα (TNFβ) intron 1 NcoI RFLP	Proliferative diabetic retinopathy	Yes	Kankova, 2001
LTα (TNFβ) intron 1 NcoI RFLP	Rheumatoid arthritis	No	Vinasco, 1997
LTα (TNFβ) intron 1 NcoI RFLP	Rheumatoid arthritis, pauciarticular juvenile rheumatoid arthritis, systemic lupus erythematosus, Sjogren's syndrome	via LD with HLA?	Fugger, 1989 Atsumi, 1992 Bettinotti, 1993 Campbell, 1994 Vandevyver, 1994
LTα (TNFβ) intron 1 NcoI RFLP	Sarcoidosis	No	Somoskovi, 1999
LTα (TNFβ) intron 1 NcoI RFLP	Severe posttraumatic sepsis	Yes	Majetschak, 1999
LTα (TNFβ) intron 1 NcoI RFLP	Severe sepsis	Yes	Stuber, 1995
LTα (TNFβ) intron 1 NcoI RFLP	Severe sepsis	Yes (non-survival)	Fang, 1999
LTα (TNFβ) intron 1 NcoI RFLP	Spontaneous abortion	No	Laitinen, 1992

Table 4.3 (*Continued*)

Cytokine and polymorphism	Disease	Association	First author, year[1]
LTα (TNFβ) intron 1 Ncol RFLP	Systemic scleroderma	Yes	Pandey, 1999
LTα (TNFβ) intron 1 Ncol RFLP	Type 1 respiratory failure	Yes (in homozygotes)	Waterer, 2001
LTα (TNFβ) intron 1 Ncol RFLP	Wegener's granulomatosis	No	Huang, 2000
LTα (TNFβ) intron 1 Ncol RFLP & EcoRI	Behcet's disease	Yes (Ncol)	Mizuki, 1992
LTα (TNFβ) intron 1 Ncol RFLP (Allele 1)	Alcoholic brain atrophy	Yes	Yamauchi, 2001
LTα (TNFβ) intron 1 Ncol RFLP (Allele 1)	Myasthenia gravis (early onset)	Yes	Skeie, 1999
LTα (TNFβ) intron 1 Ncol RFLP (Allele 1)	Prolonged clinical course of sarcoidosis	Yes	Yamaguchi, 2001
LTα (TNFβ) intron 1 Ncol RFLP (Allele 2)	Childhood immune thrombocytopenia	Yes (as part of haplotype with FCGR3B)	Foster, 2001
LTα (TNFβ) intron 1 Ncol RFLP (rare B1 allele)	Plaque psoriasis	Yes	Vasku, 2000
LTα (TNFβ) intron 1 Ncol RFLP, TNFa, b, c	Multiple sclerosis	No	Roth, 1994 Vandevyver, 1994
NFa11	Proliferative diabetic retinopathy	Yes (high risk allele)	Kumaramanickavel, 2001
RANTES −403 G→A	Atopy and asthma	Yes	Fryer, 2000
RANTES −403 G→A	HIV and asthma	Yes	Marshall, 2001
RANTES −403 G→A	HIV transmission	Yes	McDermott, 2000
TGFα Allele 4, TGFβ Allele 2	Cleft lip and cleft palate	Yes	Tanabe, 2000
TGFα TaqI RFLP	Cleft lip	No	Scapoli, 1998
TGFβ1 −509 C→T	Multiple sclerosis	Yes (with HLA-DR2)	Green, 2001
TGFβ1 −509 C→T, −800 G →A	Systemic sclerosis	No	Zhou, 2000
TGFβ1 −800, −509, nt788 C→T (T263I)	Alzheimer's disease	No	Luedecking, 2000
TGFβ1 nt509 C→T	Asthma (elevated IgE)	Yes	Hobbs, 1998
TGFβ1 nt509 C→T	Coronary artery disease and hypertension	No	Syrris, 1998
TGFβ1 nt509 C→T	Plasma levels of TGFβ1	Yes	Grainger, 1999
TGFβ1 nt509 C→T and/or TGFβ1 nt 869 T→C	Susceptibility to osteoporosis	Yes (Japanese)	Yamada, 2001
TGFβ1 nt713–8delC	Diabetic nephropathy	No	Pociot, 1998
TGFβ1 nt713–8delC	Insulin-dependent diabetes mellitus	No	Pociot, 1998
TGFβ1 nt713–8delC	Osteoporosis	Yes	Langdahl, 1997
TGFβ1 nt713–8delC	Osteoporosis	Yes	Bertoldo, 2000
TGFβ1 nt713–8delC	Osteoporosis in beta-thalassemia patients	No	Perrotta, 2000
TGFβ1 nt788 C→T (T263I)	Coronary artery disease and hypertension	No	Syrris, 1998
TGFβ1 nt788 C→T (T263I)	Diabetic nephropathy	Yes	Pociot, 1998
TGFβ1 nt788 C→T (T263I)	Insulin-dependent diabetes mellitus	No	Pociot, 1998
TGFβ1 nt800 G→A	Coronary artery disease and hypertension	No	Syrris, 1998
TGFβ1 nt800 G→A	Plasma levels of TGFβ1	Yes	Grainger, 1999
TGFβ1 nt869 (Leu10Pro)	Bone mineral density	Yes	Yamada, 2001
TGFβ1 nt869 (Leu10Pro)	Coronary artery disease and hypertension	No	Syrris, 1998
TGFβ1 nt869 (Leu10Pro)	End-stage heart failure due to cardiomyopathy	Yes	Holgate, 2001
TGFβ1 nt869 (Leu10Pro)	Graft vascular disease (in recipient)	Yes	Holweg, 2001
TGFβ1 nt869 (Leu10Pro)	Multiple sclerosis	Yes (in association with HLA-DR2)	
TGFβ1 nt869 (Leu10Pro)	Ossification of the posterior longitudinal ligament	Yes (Japanese patients)	Kamiya, 2001
TGFβ1 nt869 (Leu10Pro)	Osteoporosis and spinal osteoarthritis	Yes	Yamada, 2000
TGFβ1 nt869 (Leu10Pro)	Postmenopausal osteoporosis (Japanese)	Yes	Yamada, 1998
TGFβ1 nt869 (Leu10Pro)	Recurrence of hepatitis C in liver transplant recipients	Yes	Tambur, 2001
TGFβ1 nt869 (Leu10Pro), TGFβ1 nt915 (Arg25Pro)	Acute rejection in orthotopic liver transplantation	No	Bathgate, 2000
TGFβ1 nt869 (Leu10Pro), TGFβ1 nt915 (Arg25Pro)	End-stage liver disease	No	Bathgate, 2000
TGFβ1 nt915 (Arg25Pro)	Atopic dermatitis	Yes	Arkwright, 2001
TGFβ1 nt915 (Arg25Pro)	Coronary artery disease and hypertension	No	Syrris, 1998
TGFβ1 nt915 (Arg25Pro)	Fibrotic lung disease and lung allograft fibrosis	Yes	Awad, 1998 Awad, 1998
TGFβ1 nt915 (Arg25Pro)	Hypertension	Yes	Li, 1999
TGFβ1 nt915 (Arg25Pro)	Idiopathic dilated cardiomyopathy	No	Tiret, 2000
TGFβ1 nt915 (Arg25Pro)	Renal failure after clinical heart transplantation	Yes	Baan, 2000
TGFβ1 nt915 (Arg25Pro) (homozygous for G)	Cardiac transplant vasculopathy	Yes	Densem, 2000
TGFβ1 T29C (Leu10Pro)	Severity of diabetic nephropathy	No	Akai, 2001
TGFβ1 T29C (Leu10Pro)	Spinal osteophytosis	Yes	Yamada, 2000

Table 4.3 (*Continued*)

Cytokine and polymorphism	Disease	Association	First author, year[1]
TGFβ−RI missense mutations in exons 2,3,4 and 6	Ovarian carcinogenesis	Yes	Chen, 2001
TGFβ−RI, exon 5 (frameshift mutation at codons 276–277)	Ovarian carcinogenesis	Yes	Wang, 2000
TGFβ−RII codon 389 C→T	Early onset colorectal cancer	Yes	Shin, 2000
TGFβ 1T29C (Leu10Pro)	Breast cancer	Yes (elderly white and Chinese)	Ziv, 2001; Shu, 2004
TGFβ 1T29C (Leu10Pro)	Myocardial infarction	Yes (males)	Yokota, 2000
TNFα −1031, −863 and TNFRSF1A −383	Human T-cell lymphotropic virus-1 associated myelopathy	No (Japanese patients)	Nishimura, 2000
TNFa	Cardiac transplant rejection	No	Abdallah, 1999
TNFa	Multiple sclerosis	Yes (118bp allele)	McDonnell, 1999
TNFa, TNFb	Multiple sclerosis	Yes, via LD with HLA?	Sandberg-Wollheim, 1995
TNFa, TNFb, TNFc, TNFd	Pharyngeal cancer	No	Matthias, 1998
TNFa/b	Rheumatoid arthritis	Yes	Martinez, 2000
TNFa1 and a7	Basal cell carcinoma	Yes	Hajeer, 2000
TNFa10	*Helicobacter pylori*-associated duodenal ulcers	Yes (males: negative association)	Kunstmann, 1999
TNFa10	IgA deficiency	Yes (protective)	De la Concha, 2000
TNFa10b4	Multiple sclerosis	Yes	Allcock, 1999
TNFa11	Cervical cancer	Yes (in association with HLA)	Ghaderi, 2001 Ghaderi, 2000
TNFa11	Multiple sclerosis	Yes	Lucotte, 2000
TNFa11	Rheumatoid arthritis (severity)	Yes (in LD with HLA-DRB1)	Mu, 1999
TNFa11, b4	Multiple sclerosis	Yes	Allcock, 1999
TNFa12	Progression to type-1 diabetes form adult-onset diabetes	Yes	Obayashi, 2000
TNFa13	Systemic sclerosis	Yes (Japan)	Takeuchi, 2000
TNFa1b5	Multiple sclerosis	Yes	Allcock, 1999
TNFa1b5, a2b1, a2b3, a7b4, a6b5	Insulin-dependent diabetes mellitus	via LD with HLA?	Monos, 1995 Hajeer, 1996
TNFa2	*Campylobacter jejuni*-related Guillain-Barre syndrome	Yes	Ma, 1998
TNFa2	Celiac disease	Yes	Metcalfe, 1996
TNFa2	Colorectal cancer	Yes	Gallagher, 1998
TNFa2	IgA deficiency	No	De la Concha, 2000
TNFa2	Multiple sclerosis	Yes, via LD with HLA?	Epplen, 1997
TNFa2	Myasthenia gravis	Yes	Hjelmstrom, 1998
TNFa2	Rheumatoid arthritis	Yes	Gomolka, 1995
TNFa2 and TNF −238 (G allele)	Alzheimer's disease	Yes (later onset)	Perry, 2001
TNFa2, a6	Insulin-dependent diabetes mellitus	Yes	Pociot, 1993
TNFa2, b3	Celiac disease	via LD with HLA-DQ2 + haplotypes	Polvi, 1998
TNFa2, b3	Giant cell arteritis and polymyalgia rheumatica	Yes	Mattey, 2000
TNFa2, b4, d5	Basal cell carcinoma	Yes	Hajeer, 2000
TNFa2, b4, d5	Basal cell carcinoma	Yes	Hajeer, 2000
TNFa3	Gastric cancer	Yes	Saito, 2001
TNFa4	Proliferative diabetic retinopathy	Yes (low risk allele)	Kumaramanickavel, 2001
TNFa6	Early-onset pauciarticular juvenile chronic arthritis	Yes	Epplen, 1995
TNFa6	*Helicobacter pylori*-associated gastric ulcers	Yes (females: negative association)	Kunstmann, 1999
TNFa6	Rheumatoid arthritis	Yes (Peru)	Castro, 2001
TNFa6	Rheumatoid arthritis	Yes (with HLA-DRB1 shared epitope)	Mattey, 1999
TNFa6, b5, c1, d3, e3	Rheumatoid arthritis	Yes	Mulcahy, 1996
TNFa7, a11	Early onset of multiple sclerosis	Yes	Boiko, 2000
TNFa9	Insulin-dependent diabetes mellitus (early onset)	Yes	Obayashi, 1999
TNFa9	Renal transplant rejection	Yes	Asano, 1997
TNFb2	Parkinson's disease	Yes (reduced risk of disease)	Kruger, 2000
TNFb3	Laryngeal cancer	Yes	Matthias, 1998
TNFb3, d4, d5	Clozapine-induced agranulocytosis	Yes	Turbay, 1997
TNFc	Rheumatoid arthritis	Yes	Bali, 1999

Table 4.3 (*Continued*)

Cytokine and polymorphism	Disease	Association	First author, year[1]
TNFc	Ulcerative colitis (progression)	Yes	Bouma, 1999
TNFc1	Rheumatoid arthritis	Yes	Mulcahy, 1996
TNFc2	HIV disease progression	Yes	Khoo, 1997
TNFd	Multiple sclerosis	No	McDonnell, 1999
TNFd3	Cardiac transplant rejection	Yes	Turner, 1995
TNFd3	Graft-versus-host disease in allogeneic bone marrow transplantation	Yes	Middleton, 1998
TNFd3d3	HLA-identical bone marrow transplantation	Yes (early mortality)	Cavet, 1999
TNFd4	Renal transplant rejection	Yes	Asano, 1997
TNFd4 and d6	Basal cell carcinoma	Yes	Hajeer, 2000
TNFd4 and d6	Basal cell carcinomas	Yes	Hajeer, 2000
TNFd4 and TNF 1031C allele	Unrelated donor stem cell transplantation	Yes (increased mortality)	Keen, 2004
TNFd7	Colorectal cancer	Yes	Saito, 2001
TNFRSF1A (p55) C52F	TNF receptor-associated periodic syndromes	Yes	McDermott, 1999
TNFRSF1B	Schizophrenia	No	Wassink, 2000
TNFRSF1B (p75) exon 6, M196R	Crohn's disease	No	Kawasaki, 2000
TNFRSF1B (p75) exon 6, M196R	Narcolepsy	No	Hohjoh, 2000
TNFRSF1B (p75) exon 6, M196R	Rheumatoid arthritis	No	Shibue, 2000
TNFRSF1B (p75) exon 6, M196R	Rheumatoid arthritis	Yes	Barton, 2001
TNFRSF1B (p75) exon 6, M196R	SLE (Japanese)	Yes	Komata, 1999
TNFRSF1B (p75) exon 6, M196R	Systemic lupus erythematosus	No	Al-Ansari, 2000 Sullivan, 2000
TNFRSF1B (p75) exon 6, M196R	Systemic lupus erythematosus	No	Lee, 2001
TNFRSF1B (p75) exon 6, M196R	Thai adult malaria sensitivity	No	Hananantachai, 2001
TNFRSF1B 3'-UTR SSCP "7/8"	Graves' disease	No	Rau, 1997
TNFRSF1B 3'-UTR SSCP "7/8"	Insulin-dependent diabetes mellitus	No	Rau, 1997
TNFRSF1B 3'-UTR SSCP "7/8"	Systemic lupus erythematosus	No	Sullivan, 2000
TNFRSF1B Intron 4 (CA repeat)	Familial combined hyperlipidemia	Yes	Geurts, 2000
TNFRSF1B (p75) exon 6, M196R	Autoimmune diseases accompanied by vasculitis	No	Takahashi, 2001
TNFRSF1B, Intron 4 (CA16 allele in microsatellite)	Coronary artery disease	Yes	Benjafield, 2001
TNFRSF1B, nt168 (K56K)	Systemic lupus erythematosus	No	Tsuchiya, 2000
TNFα −863C/A and −308G/A	Coronary artery disease and myocardial infarction	No	Koch, 2001
TNFα +488A	Common variable immunodeficiency	Yes	Mullighan, 1997
TNFα −1031	HTLV-1 uveitis	Yes	Seki, 1999
TNFα −1031	Kawasaki disease	No	Kamizono, 1999
TNFα −1031 (C allele)	Crohn's disease	Yes	Negoro, 1999
TNFα −1031 (C allele)	Ophthalmopathy in Graves' disease	Yes	Kamizono, 2000
TNFα −1031 (C allele)	Parkinson's disease	Yes (early onset)	Nishimura, 2001
TNFα −1031 (C allele)	Systemic juvenile chronic arthritis	Yes	Date, 1999
TNFα −1031, −863, −857, −308, −238	Psoriatic arthritis	No	Hamamoto, 2000
TNFα −1031C, −863A haplotype	Insulin-dependent diabetes mellitus	No	Hamaguchi, 2000
TNFα −1031C, −863A, −857C	Crohn's disease	Yes	Kawasaki, 2000
TNFα −163	Non-insulin-dependent diabetes mellitus	No	Hamann, 1995
TNFα −238	Alcoholic steatohepatitis	Yes	Grove, 1997
TNFα −238	Ankylosing spondylitis	No (German populations)	Milicic, 2000
TNFα −238	Ankylosing spondylitis	Yes (in HLA-B27 negative patients)	Gonzalez, 2001
TNFα −238	Antiphospholipid syndrome	No	Bertolaccini, 2001
TNFα −238	Antiphospholipid syndrome	No	Bertolaccini, 2001
TNFα −238	Brucellosis	No	Caballero, 2000
TNFα −238	Cancers (gastric, uterine, renal and cervical)	Yes (protective)	Jang, 2001
TNFα −238	Cardiac transplant rejection	No	Abdallah, 1999
TNFα −238	Chronic active hepatitis C	Yes	Höhler, 1998
TNFα −238	Chronic hepatitis B	Yes	Höhler, 1998
TNFα −238	Early-onset pauciarticular juvenile chronic arthritis	No	Epplen, 1995
TNFα −238	Early-onset psoriasis	No	Jacob, 1999
TNFα −238	Insulin resistance (decreased)	Yes	Day, 1998
TNFα −238	Kawasaki disease	No	Kamizono, 1999
TNFα −238	Multiple sclerosis	No	Epplen, 1997
TNFα −238	Multiple sclerosis	Yes	Huizinga, 1997

Table 4.3 (*Continued*)

Cytokine and polymorphism	Disease	Association	First author, year[1]
TNFα −238	Non-insulin-dependent diabetes mellitus	No	Hamann, 1995
TNFα −238	Periodontitis (adult)	No	Galbraith, 1998
TNFα −238	Primary sclerosing cholangitis	No	Bernal, 1999
TNFα −238	Psoriasis	Yes (males)	Reich, 1999
TNFα −238	Rheumatoid arthritis	No	Vinasco, 1997
TNFα −238	Rheumatoid arthritis	Yes (erosion)	Brinkman, 1997
TNFα −238	Rheumatoid arthritis	Yes (joint destruction)	Kaijzel, 1998
TNFα −238	Scarring trachoma (chlamydial)	No	Conway, 1997
TNFα −238	Silicosis	Higher for severe form, lower for moderate form	Yucesoy, 2001
TNFα −238	Type I autoimmune hepatitis	No	Cookson, 1999 Czaja, 1999
TNFα −238 (A allele)	Ankylosing spondylitis	Yes (via LD with HLA-B27)	Kaijzel, 1999
TNFα −238 (G/A), −308 (G/A)	Insulin resistance syndrome	No (Danish populations)	Rasmussen, 2000
TNFα −238, −244, −308	Chagas' disease	No	Beraun, 1998
TNFα −238, −308	Ankylosing spondylitis	No	Fraile, 1998
TNFα −238, −308	Carbamazepine hypersensitivity reactions	Yes, via LD with HLA	Pirmohamed, 2001
TNFα −238, −308	Hepatitis C-induced cirrhosis	Yes (histological severity)	Yee, 2000
TNFα −238, −308	Meningococcal disease	No	Westendorp, 1997
TNFα −238, −308	Multiple sclerosis	No	Lucotte, 2000 Anlar, 2001
TNFα −238, −308	Pneumoconiosis	Yes (TNFα −308)	Zhai, 1998
TNFα −238, −308	Systemic lupus erythematosus (Whites and Black S. Africans)	No, via LD with HLA?	Rudwaleit, 1996
TNFα −238, TNFa	Systemic lupus erythematosus (Italians)	No	D'Alfonso, 1996
TNFα −308	Actinic prurigo	No	Carey, 1998
TNFα −308	Acute rejection in orthotopic liver transplantation	Yes	Bathgate, 2000
TNFα −308	Adult asthma	No	Louis, 2000
TNFα −308	Adult asthma	Yes (but no phenotypic difference)	Thomas, 2001
TNFα −308	Alcoholic steatohepatitis	No	Grove, 1997
TNFα −308	Ankylosing spondylitis	No	Verjans, 1994
TNFα −308	Atherosclerosis	No	Keso, 2001
TNFα −308	Atherosclerosis	No	Wang, 2000
TNFα −308	Atopic asthma	No	Trabetti, 1999
TNFα −308	Atopy, asthma, rhinitis	No	Zhu, 2000
TNFα −308	Bipolar affective puerperal psychosis	No	Middle, 2000
TNFα −308	Body fat content	Yes (AA genotype)	Hoffstedt, 2000
TNFα −308	Bronchial hyperreactivity in asthma	Yes, via LD with HLA?	Li Kam Wa, 1999
TNFα −308	Brucellosis	Yes (1/2 genotype)	Caballero, 2000
TNFα −308	Cardiac transplant rejection	No	Turner, 1995
TNFα −308	Cardiac transplant rejection	No	Abdallah, 1999
TNFα −308	Celiac disease	via LD with HLA?	Manus, 1996
TNFα −308	Celiac disease	Yes	de la Concha, 2000
TNFα −308	Cerebral malaria	Yes	McGuire, 1994
TNFα −308	Chronic active hepatitis C	No	Höhler, 1998
TNFα −308	Chronic hepatitis B	No	Höhler, 1998
TNFα −308	Chronic lymphocytic leukemia	No	Wihlborg, 1999
TNFα −308	Chronic lymphocytic leukemia	Yes	Demeter, 1997
TNFα −308	Chronic obstructive pulmonary disease	No	Higham, 2000
TNFα −308	Chronic obstructive pulmonary disease	No	Higham, 2000 Ishii, 2000
TNFα −308	Chronic obstructive pulmonary disease	Yes (homozygous for A allele)	Keatings, 2000
TNFα −308	Corneal melting in systemic vasculitis	No	McKibbin, 2000
TNFα −308	Coronary heart disease	No	Herrmann, 1998
TNFα −308	Dermatitis herpetiformis	via LD with HLA?	Wilson, 1995
TNFα −308	Early-onset pauciarticular juvenile chronic arthritis	No	Epplen, 1995
TNFα −308	Graft-versus-host disease in allogeneic bone marrow transplantation	No	Mayer, 1996 Middleton, 1998
TNFα −308	Hepatitis C-related liver failure	Yes (TNF2)	Rosen, 1999
TNFα −308	HIV-encephalitis	No	Sato-Matsumura, 1998
TNFα −308	Hodgkin's disease	No	Wihlborg, 1999

Table 4.3 (*Continued*)

Cytokine and polymorphism	Disease	Association	First author, year[1]
TNFα −308	Idiopathic dilated cardiomyopathy	No (TNF2)	Tiret, 2000
TNFα −308	Infant malarial infection and morbidity	No	Stirnadel, 1999
TNFα −308	Inflammatory bowel disease	Trend	Louis, 1996
TNFα −308	Insulin resistance	No	Day, 1998
TNFα −308	Insulin resistance and obesity	No	Lee, 2000
TNFα −308	Insulin resistance syndrome	No	da Sliva, 2000
TNFα −308	Insulin-dependent diabetes mellitus	No, via LD with HLA?	Pociot, 1993
			Wilson, 1993
			Deng, 1996
TNFα −308	Irritant contact dermatitis	Yes	Allen, 2000
TNFα −308	Kawasaki disease	No	Kamizono, 1999
TNFα −308	Leprosy	No (tuberculoid)	Roy, 1997
TNFα −308	Leprosy	Yes (lepromatous)	Roy, 1997
TNFα −308	Lichen sclerosus	No	Clay, 1996
TNFα −308	Liver damage in hereditary hemochromatosis	Yes (protective)	Fargion, 2001
TNFα −308	Metabolic syndrome	No	Lee, 2000
TNFα −308	Multiple myeloma	No	Zheng, 2000
TNFα −308	Multiple sclerosis	No	He, 1995
			Epplen, 1997
			Wingerchuck, 1997
			Huizinga, 1997
TNFα −308	Nephropathia epidemica	Yes	Kanerva, 1998
TNFα −308	Non-insulin-dependent diabetes mellitus	No	Hamann, 1995
TNFα −308	Obesity	Yes	Herrmann, 1998
TNFα −308	Pancreatic cancer	No	Barber, 1999
TNFα −308	Periodontitis (adult)	No	Galbraith, 1998
TNFα −308	Polycystic ovaries	No	Milner, 1999
TNFα −308	Primary sclerosing cholangitis	Yes	Bernal, 1999
TNFα −308	Rejection of pediatric heart transplant	Yes (low TNF is protective)	Awad, 2001
TNFα −308	Renal allograft rejection	No	Cartwright, 2001
TNFα −308	Renal failure, acute mortality	Yes	Jaber, 2004
TNFα −308	Rheumatoid arthritis	No	Lacki, 2000
TNFα −308	Rheumatoid arthritis	Yes (Nodular disease)	Vinasco, 1997
TNFα −308	Rheumatoid arthritis, systemic lupus erythematosus	Yes, via LD with HLA?	Wilson, 1994
			Danis, 1995
TNFα −308	Sarcoidosis	No	Somoskovi, 1999
TNFα −308	Scarring trachoma	Yes	Conway, 1997
TNFα −308	Schizophrenia	Yes	Boin, 2001
TNFα −308	Sclerosing cholangitis	Yes	Bathgate, 2000
TNFα −308	Septic shock	Yes	Mira, 1999
TNFα −308	Severe malarial and other infections	Yes	Wattavidanage, 1999
TNFα −308	Severe sepsis	No	Stuber, 1995
TNFα −308	Silicosis	Yes	Yucesoy, 2001
TNFα −308	Subacute systemic lupus erythematosus	Yes	Werth, 2000
TNF α−308	Systemic lupus erythematosus	Yes (TNF2+ genotypes independent of DR3)	Rood, 2000
TNFα −308	Systemic lupus erythematosus and nephritis (Koreans)	Yes, via LD with HLA?	Kim, 1995
			Kim, 1996
TNFα−308	Systemic lupus erythematosus (African-Americans)	Yes	Sullivan, 1997
TNFα −308	Systemic lupus erythematosus (Chinese)	No, via LD with HLA?	Fong, 1996
TNFα −308	Type 1 autoimmune hepatitis	Yes, via LD with HLA?	Cookson, 1999
			Czaja, 1999
TNFα −308	UVB-induced immunosuppression	No	Allen, 1998
TNFα −308	Venous thromboembolism	No	Brown, 1998
TNFα −308	Wegener's granulomatosis	No	Huang, 2000
TNFα −308 (G→A) and LTα (TNFβ NcoI (A→G)	Coronary atherothrombotic disease	Possible	Padovani, 2000
TNFα −308 (G/A or A/A)	Rejection in renal transplants	Yes	Reviron, 2001
TNFα −308 (TNF1)	Adult periodontitis	Yes (advanced disease)	Galbraith, 1999
TNFα −308 (TNF1)	Ankylosing spondylitis	Yes	McGarry, 1999
TNFα −308 (TNF1)	Childhood immune thrombocytopenia	Yes (as part of haplotype with FCGR3A)	Foster, 2001
TNFα −308 (TNF1)	*Helicobacter pylori*-associated duodenal ulcers	Yes (females) (increased risk)	Kunstmann, 1999

Table 4.3 (*Continued*)

Cytokine and polymorphism	Disease	Association	First author, year[1]
TNFα −308 (TNF1)	Idiopathic dilated cardiomyopathy	No	Tiret, 2000
TNFα −308 (TNF1) and LTα (allele 2) haplotype	Leprosy	Yes (susceptibility)	Shaw, 2001
TNFα −308 (TNF1/1)	Primary biliary cirrhosis	Yes (late stage disease)	Jones, 1999
TNFα −308 (TNF1/2)	Chronic obstructive pulmonary disease	No	Higham, 2000 Teramoto, 2001
TNFα −308 (TNF1/2)	Chronic obstructive pulmonary disease	Yes	Sakao, 2001
TNFα −308 (TNF1/2)	Corneal melting in vasculitis	No	McKibbin, 2000
TNFα −308 (TNF1/2)	Parkinson's disease	Yes	Kruger, 2000
TNFα −308 (TNF1/2)	Thai adult malaria severity	No	Hananantachai, 2001
TNFα −308 (TNF2)	Acute graft-versus-host disease	Yes	Takahashi, 2000
TNFα −308 (TNF2)	Alveolitis in farmers' lung	Yes	Schaaf, 2001
TNFα −308 (TNF2)	Ankylosing spondylitis	No (protective haplotype in HLA-B27 positives)	Rudwaleit, 2001
TNFα −308 (TNF2)	Ankylosing spondylitis	Yes (German populations)	Milicic, 2000
TNFα −308 (TNF2)	Asthma	Yes	Chagani, 1999
TNFα −308 (TNF2)	Atopy	Yes	Castro, 2000
TNFα −308 (TNF2)	Bone cancer	No (in children)	Patio-Garcia, 2000
TNFα −308 (TNF2)	Breast carcinoma	Yes	Mestiri, 2001
TNFα −308 (TNF2)	Cardiac sarcoidosis	Yes	Takashige, 1999
TNFα −308 (TNF2)	Childhood asthma	Yes (UK/Irish populations)	Winchester, 2000
TNFα −308 (TNF2)	Chronic beryllium disease	Yes	Maier, 2001
TNFα −308 (TNF2)	Crohn's disease (steroid-dependent)	Yes	Louis, 2000
TNFα −308 (TNF2)	Delayed-type hypersensitivity reaction in the skin of borderline tuberculoid leprosy patients	Yes	Moraes, 2001
TNFα −308 (TNF2)	Erythema nodosum	Yes	Labunski, 2001
TNFα −308 (TNF2)	Excessive fat accumulation (females)	Yes (TNF2 homozygotes)	Hoffstedt, 2000
TNFα −308 (TNF2)	Fibrosing alveolitis	Yes	Whyte, 2000
TNFα −308 (TNF2)	Infection with *H. pylori* caga	Yes	Yea, 2001
TNFα −308 (TNF2)	Leprosy	Yes (protective)	Santos, 2000
TNFα −308 (TNF2)	Malaria morbidity and childhood morbidity	Yes	Aidoo, 2001
TNFα −308 (TNF2)	Meliodosis	Yes	Nuntayanuwat, 1999
TNFα −308 (TNF2)	Mortality from septic shock	Yes	Tang, 2000
TNFα −308 (TNF2)	Multiple sclerosis	No	Maurer, 1999
TNFα −308 (TNF2)	Myasthenia gravis	Yes (in LD with HLA?)	Huang, 1999
TNFα −308 (TNF2)	Myasthenia gravis (early onset)	Yes	Skeie, 1999
TNFα −308 (TNF2)	Neuritis in leprosy	Yes (heterozygotes)	Sarno, 2000
TNFα −308 (TNF2)	Obesity	Yes (Caucasian populations)	Brand, 2001
TNFα −308 (TNF2)	Primary biliary cirrhosis	Yes	Tanaka, 1999
TNFα −308 (TNF2)	Primary biliary cirrhosis	Yes (negative association)	Gordon, 1999
TNFα −308 (TNF2)	Primary sclerosing cholangitis	Yes	Mitchell, 2001
TNFα −308 (TNF2)	Pulmonary sarcoidosis (Lofgren)	Yes (in LD with HLA?)	Swider, 1999
TNFα −308 (TNF2)	Recurrent pregnancy loss	Yes	Reid, 2001
TNFα −308 (TNF2)	Rejection of renal transplant	Yes	Pelletier, 2000
TNFα −308 (TNF2)	Spontaneous preterm birth	Yes	Roberts, 1999
TNFα −308 (TNF2)	Subacute cutaneous lupus erythematosus	Yes	Millard, 2001
TNFα −308 (TNF2)	Systemic lupus erythematosus	Yes	Rood, 2000
TNFα −308 (TNF2)	Ulcerative colitis	Yes	Hirv, 1999
TNFα −308 (TNF2) −1031, −863, −857 and −237	Palmoplantar pustulosis	No	Niizeki, 2000
TNFα −308 (TNF2) and LTα (allele2) haplotype	Leprosy	Yes (protective)	Shaw, 2001
TNFα −308 (TNF2) and LTα (TNFβ) NcoI	Chronic obstructive pulmonary disease	No (in Caucasoid individuals)	Patuzzo, 2000
TNFα −308 (TNF2) and LTα G allele	Septic shock	Yes	Waterer, 2001
TNFα −308 (TNF2), TNF −238	Ankylosing spondylitis	No (English populations)	Milicic, 2000
TNFα −308 and IL-10 −1082 G→A	Cardiac transplant rejection	Yes	Turner, 1997
TNFα −308 and IL-10 −1082 G→A	Renal transplant rejection	Yes, TNFα − 308 alone	Sankaran, 1998 Sankaran, 1998
TNFα −308 and LTα (TNFβ) NcoI	Asthma	Yes	Moffatt, 1997
TNFα −308 and LTα (TNFβ) NcoI	Asthma (childhood)	Yes	Albuquerque, 1998
TNFα −308 and LTα (TNFβ) NcoI	Asthma and atopy (Italians)	Yes (LTα (TNFβ) NcoI only)	Trabetti, 1999

Table 4.3 (*Continued*)

Cytokine and polymorphism	Disease	Association	First author, year[1]
TNFα −308 and LTα (TNFβ) NcoI	Colorectal cancer	Yes (β NcoI only)	Park, 1998
TNFα −308 and LTα (TNFβ) NcoI	Congestive heart failure	No	Kubota, 1998
TNFα −308 and LTα (TNFβ) NcoI	Dermatitis herpetiformis	Yes	Messer, 1994
TNFα −308 and LTα (TNFβ) NcoI	Hairy cell leukemia	No	Demeter, 1997
TNFα −308 and LTα (TNFβ) NcoI	Mucocutaneous leishmaniaisis	Yes	Cabrera, 1995
TNFα −308 and LTα (TNFβ) NcoI	Multiple sclerosis	Yes (development)	Mycko, 1998
TNFα −308 and LTα (TNFβ) NcoI	Non-Hodgkin's lymphoma (outcome)	Yes	Warzocha, 1998
TNFα −308 G/A	Early-onset periodontitis	No	Shapira, 2001
TNFα −308 G/A	Obesity and insulin resistance	No	Romeo, 2001
TNFα −308, −238, TNFa2 (2-1-2 haplotype)	Alzheimer's disease	Yes	Collins, 2000
TNFα −308, TNF B	Acute pancreatitis	No	Powell, 2001
TNFα −376 G→A	Ankylosing spondylitis	No	Kaijzel, 1999
TNFα −376 G→A	Cardiac transplant rejection	No	Abdallah, 1999
TNFα −376 G→A	Multiple sclerosis	No	Huizinga, 1997
TNFα −376 G→A	Multiple sclerosis	Yes (HLA-independent)	Fernandez-Arquero, 1999
TNFα −376 G→A	Non-insulin-dependent diabetes mellitus	No	Hamann, 1995
TNFα −850	Narcolepsy	No	Kato, 1999
TNFα −850 C→T	Alzheimer's disease	Yes (with apolipoprotein E)	McCusker, 2001
TNFα −850 C→T	Vascular dementia	Yes	McCusker, 2001
TNFα −857	Kawasaki disease	No	Kamizono, 1999
TNFα −857 (T allele)	Crohn's disease	Yes	Negoro, 1999
TNFα −857 (T allele)	Insulin-dependent diabetes mellitus	No	Hamaguchi, 2000
TNFα −857 (T allele)	Insulin-dependent diabetes mellitus	No	Hamaguchi, 2000
TNFα −857 (T allele)	Narcolepsy	Yes	Hohjoh, 1999
TNFα −857 (T allele)	Non-insulin-dependent diabetes mellitus	Possible association for obese −857 T homozygotes	Kamizono, 2000
TNFα −857 (T allele)	Progression to adult T cell leukemia from human T cell lymphotropic virus-1	Yes	Tsukasaki, 2001
TNFα −857 (T allele)	Rheumatoid arthritis	Yes	Seki, 1999
TNFα −857 (T allele)	Systemic juvenile chronic arthritis	Yes	Date, 1999
TNFα −857 (T allele), TNFRSF1B (exon 6, T→G), LTα (TNFβ) NcoI	Human T cell lymphotropic virus-1 associated myelopathy	Yes (Japanese patients)	Nishimura, 2000
TNFα −863	HTLV-1 uveitis	Yes	Seki, 1999
TNFα −863	Kawasaki disease	No	Kamizono, 1999
TNFα −863 (A allele)	Crohn's disease	Yes	Negoro, 1999
TNFα −863 (A allele)	Ophthalmopathy in Graves' disease	Yes	Kamizono, 2000
TNFα −863 (A allele)	Systemic juvenile chronic arthritis	Yes	Date, 1999
TNFα −863 (A allele)	Clearance of hepatitis C virus	Yes, varying by race	Thio, 2004
TNFα −863 (A allele),	Diabetes	No	Hamaguchi, 2000
TNFα −1031 (C allele)	Diabetes	No	Kamizono, 2000

[1] Full references are provided in the appropriate Genes and Immunity reviews and supplements (references 1–3) and in the references found here.

implicating them as disease-associated loci in their own right, is complicated by the MHC and age and likely other genetic and environmental factors. How well we as a research community deal with these complications will determine how efficiently the influence of cytokine immunogenetics on disease is elucidated.

REFERENCES

Ahmed, S., Ihara, K., Sasaki, Y. et al. (2000). Novel polymorphism in the coding region of the IL-13 receptor alpha' gene: association study with atopic asthma in the Japanese population. Exp Clin Immunogenet *17*, 18–22.

Al-Janadi, M., Al-Dalaan, A., Al-Balla, S., Al-Humaidi, M. and Raziuddin S. (1996). Interleukin-10 secretion in systemic lupus erythematosus and rheumatoid arthritis: IL-10-dependent CD4+ CD45RO+ T cell-B-cell antibody synthesis. J Clin Immunol *16*, 145–150.

Bahr, M.J., el Menuawy, M., Boeker, K.H., Musholt, P.B., Manns, M.P. and Lichtinghagen, R. (2003). Cytokine gene polymorphisms and the susceptibility to liver cirrhosis in patients with chronic hepatitis C. Liver Int *23*, 420–425.

Bidwell, J., Keen, L., Gallagher, G. et al. (1999). Cytokine gene polymorphism in human disease: on-line databases. Genes Immun *1*, 3–19.

Bidwell, J., Keen, L., Gallagher, G. et al. (2001). Cytokine gene polymorphism in human disease: on-line databases, supplement 1. Genes Immun *2*, 61–70.

Buetler, B., Milsark, I.W. and Cerami, A.C. (1985). Passive immunisation against cachectin/tumor necrosis factor protects mice from the lethal effects of endotoxin. Science 229, 869–871.

Caballero, A., Bravo, M.J., Nieto, A., Colmenero, J.D., ALonso, A. and Martin, J. (2000). TNF-A promoter polymorphis and susceptibility to brucellosis. Clin Expl Immunol 12, 480–483.

Candore, G., Cigna, D. and Todaro, M. (1995). T-cell activation in HLA-B8, DR3-positive individuals. Early antigen expression defect in vitro. Hum Immunol 42, 289–294.

Caruso, C., Bongiardina, C. and Candore, G. (1997). HLA-B8, DR3 haplotype affects lymphocyte blood levels. Immunol Invest 26, 333–340.

Caruso, C., Candore, G. and Modica, M.A. (1996). Major histocompatibility complex regulation of cytokine production. J Interferon Cytokine Res 16, 983–988.

Cox, E.D., Hoffmann, S.C., DiMercurio, B.S. et al. (2001). Cytokine polymorphic analyses indicate ethnic differences in the allelic distribution of interleukin-2 and interleukin-6. Transplantation 72, 720–726.

Dai, W.J., Kohler, G. and Brombascher, F. (1997). Both innate and acquired immunity to Lysteria monocytogenes infection are increased in IL-10 deficient mice. J Immunol 158, 2259–2267.

D'Alfonso, S., Rampi, M., Bocchio, D., Colombo, G., Scorza-Smeraldi, R. and Momigliano-Richardi, P. (2000). Systemic lupus erythematosus candidate genes in the Italian population: evidence for a significant association with interleukin-10. Arthritis Rheum 43, 120–128.

de Waal Malefyt, R., Yssel, H. and de Vries, J.E. (1993). Direct effect of IL-10 on subsets of human CD4+ T cell clones and resting T cells: Specific inhibition of IL-2 production and proliferation. J Immunol 150, 4754–4765.

Enk, A.H., Angeloni, V.T., Udey, M.C. and Katz, S.I. (1993). Inhibition of Langerhans cell antigen-presenting function by IL-10: a role for IL-10 in induction of tolerance. J Immunol 151, 2390–2398.

Eskdale, J. and Gallagher, G. (1995). A polymorphic dinucleotide repeat in the human IL-10 promoter. Immunogenetics 42, 444–445.

Eskdale, J., Kube, D. and Gallagher, G. (1996). A second polymorphic dinucleotide repeat in the 5′ flanking region of the human IL10 gene. Immunogenetics 45, 82–83.

Eskdale, J., Kube, D., Tesch, H. and Gallagher, G. (1997a). Mapping of the human IL10 gene and further characterization of the 5′ flanking sequence. Immunogenetics 46, 120–128.

Eskdale, J., Wordsworth, P., Bowman, S., Field, M. and Gallagher, G. (1997b). Association between polymorphisms at the human IL-10 locus and systemic lupus erythematosus. Tissue Antigens 49, 635–639.

Fiorentino, D.F., Zlotnic, A., Viera, P. et al. (1991). IL-10 acts on the antigen presenting cell to inhibit cytokine production by Th1 cells. J Immunol 146, 3444–3451.

Fishman, D., Faulds, G., Jeffery, R. et al. (1998). The effect of novel polymorphisms in the interleukin-6 (IL-6) gene on IL-6 transcription and plasma IL-6 levels, and an association with systemic-onset juvenile chronic arthritis. J Clin Inv 102, 1369–1376.

Fleury, S., Thibodeau, J. and Croteau, G. (1995). HLA-DR polymorphism affects the interaction with DR4. J Exp Med 182, 733–741.

Fryer, A.A., Spiteri, M.A., Bianco, A. et al. (2000). The -403G—>A promoter polymorphism in the RANTES gene is associated with atopy and asthma.Genes Immunol 1, 509–514.

Gallagher, G., Eskdale, J., Oh, H.H., Richards, S.D., Campbell, D.A. and Field, M. (1997). Polymorphisms in the TNF gene cluster and MHC serotypes in the West of Scotland. Immunogenetics 45, 188–194.

George, S., Ruan, X.Z., Navarrete, C. et al. (2004). Renovascular disease is associated with low producer genotypes of the anti-inflammatory cytokine interleukin-10 Tissue Antigens 63, 470–475.

Gibson, A.W., Edberg, J.C., Wu, J,. Westendorp, R.G., Huizinga, T.W. and Kimberly, R.P. (2001). Novel single nucleotide polymorphisms in the distal IL-10 promoter affect IL-10 production and enhance the risk of systemic lupus erythematosus. J Immunol 166, 3915–3922.

Gonzalez, E., Dhanda, R., Bamshad, M. et al. (2001). Global survey of genetic variation in CCR5, RANTES, and MIP-1 aplha: impact on the epidemiology of the HIV-1 pandemic. Proc Natl Acad Sci USA 98, 5199–5204.

Groux, H., Cottrez, F., Rouleau, M. et al. (1999). A transgenic model to analyse the immunoregulatory role of IL-10 secreted by antigen-presenting cells. J Immunol 162, 1723–1729.

Hagiwara, E., Gourley, M.F., Lee, S. and Klinman, D.M. (1996). Disease severity in systemic lupus erythematosus correlates with an increased ratio of interleukin-10: interferon-(gamma)-secreting cells in the peripheral blood. Arthritis Rheum 39, 370–385.

Haukim, N., Bidwell, J.L., Smith, A.J. et al. (2002). Cytokine gene polymorphism in human disease: on-line databases, supplement 2. Genes Immun 3, 313–330.

Havell, E.A. (1989). Evidence that tumor necrosis factor has an important role in antibacterial resistance. J Immunol 143, 2894–2899.

Houssiau, F.A., Lefebvre, C., van den Berghe, M., Lambert, M., Devogelaer, J.-P., Renauld, J.-J. (1995). Serum interleukin 10 titers in systemic lupus erythematosus reflect disease activity. Lupus 4, 393–395.

Howard, T.D., Whittaker, P.A., Zaiman, A.L. et al. (2001). Identification and association of polymorphisms in the interleukin-13 gene with asthma and atopy in a Dutch population. Am J Respir Cell Mol Biol 25, 377–384.

Hulkkonen, J., Pertovaara, M., Antonen, J., Lahdenpohja, N., Pasternack, A. and Hurme, M. (2001). Genetic association between interleukin-10 promoter region polymorphisms and primary Sjogren's syndrome. Arthritis Rheum 44, 176–179.

Hutyrova, B., Lukac, J., Bosak, V., Buc, M., du Bois, R. and Petrek, M. (2004). Interleukin 1α single-nucleotide polymorphism associated with systemic sclerosis. J Rheumatol 31, 81–84.

Iacopetta, B., Grieu, F. and Joseph, D. (2004). The -174 G/C gene polymorphism in interleukin-6 is associated with an aggressive breast cancer phenotype. Br J Cancer 90, 419–422.

Ide, A., Kawasaki, E., Abiru, N. et al. (2004). Association between IL-18 gene promoter polymorphisms and CTLA-4 gene 49A/G polymorphism in Japanese patients with type 1 diabetes. J Autoimmun 22, 73–78.

Ishida, H., Hastings, R., Kearney, J. and Howard, M. (1992). Continuous anti-interleukin-10 antibody administration depletes mice of Ly-1 B-cells but not conventional B-cells. J Exp. Med 175, 1213–1220.

Ishida, H., Muchamunl, T., Sakaguchi, S., Andrade, S., Menon, S. and Howard, M. (1994). Continuous administration of anti-interleukin-10 antibodies delays the onset of autoimmunity in NZB/W F1 mice. J Expl Med 179, 305–310.

Jaber, B.L., Rao, M., Guo, D. et al. (2004). Cytokine gene promoter polymorphisms and mortality in acute renal failure. Cytokine 25, 212–219.

Jacobs, M., Brown, N., Allie, N. and Ryffel B. (2000). Fatal Mycobacterium bovis BCG infection in TNF-LT-alpha-deficient mice. Clin Immunol 94, 192–199.

Keen, L.J., DeFor, T.E., Bidwell, J.L., Davies, S.M., Bradley, B.A. and Hows, J.M. (2004). Interleukin-10 and tumor necrosis factor alpha region haplotypes predict transplant-related mortality after unrelated donor stem cell transplantation. Blood 103, 3599–3602.

Kelly, J.P. and Bancroft, G.J. (1996). Administration of interleukin-10 abolishes innate resistance to Listeria monocytogenes. J Immunol 26, 356–364.

Kube, D., Rieth, H., Eskdale, J., Kremsner, P.G. and Gallagher, G. (2001). Structural characterisation of the distal 5' flanking region of the human interleukin-10 gene. Genes Immun 2, 181–190.

Kwiatowski, D., Hill, A.V.S., Sambou, I. et al. (1990). TNF concentrations in fatal cerebral, non-fatal cerebral, and uncomplicated Plasmodium falciparum malaria. Lancet 336, 1201–1204.

Lazarus, M., Hajeer, A.H., Turner, D. et al. (1997). Genetic variation in the Interleukin-10 gene promoter and systemic lupus erythematosus. J Rheumatol 24, 2314–2317.

Lehmann, A.K., Halstenen, A., Sornes, S., Rokke, O. and Waage, A. (1995). High levels of interleukin-10 in serum are associated with fatality in meningococcal disease. Infect Immun 63, 2109–2115.

Levy, Y. and Brouet, J.-C. (1994). Interleukin-10 prevents spontaneous cell death of germinal centre B-cells by induction of the Bcl-2 protein. J Clin Invest 93, 424–428.

Lio, D., Candore, G. and Cigna, D. (1996). In vitro T-cell activation in elderly individuals: failure in CD69 and CD71 expression. Mech Ageing Dev 89, 51–58.

Lio, D., Candore, G. and Romano, G.C. (1997). Modification of cytokine secretion patterns in subjects bearing the HLA-B8, DR3 phenotype: implications for autoimmunity. Cytokines Cell Mol Ther 3, 217–224.

Liu, X., Nickel, R., Beyer, K. et al. (2000). An IL13 coding region variant is associated with a high total serum IgE level and atopic dermatitis in the German multicenter atopy study (MAS-90). J Allergy Clin Immunol 106, 167–170.

Llorente, L., Richaud-Patin, Y., Couderc, J. et al. (1997). Dysregulation of interleukin-10 production in relatives of patients with systemic lupus erythematosus. Arthrit Rheum 40, 1429–1435.

Llorente, L., Richaud-Patin, Y., Fior, R. et al. (1994). In vivo production of Interleukin-10 by non-T cells in rheumatoid arthritis, Sjogren's syndrome, and systemic lupus erythematosus: a potential mechanism of B lymphocyte hyperactivity and autoimmunity. Arthrit Rheum 37, 1647–1655.

Llorente, L., Richaud-Patin, Y., Wijdenes, J. et al. (1993). Spontaneous production of Interleukin-10 by B lymphocytes and monocytes in systemic lupus erythematosus. Eur Cytokine Newt 4, 421–430.

Llorente, L., Zou, W., Levy, Y. et al. (1995). Role of Interleukin 10 in the B cell lymphocyte hyperactivity and autoantibody production of human systemic lupus erythematosus. J Exp Med 181, 839–844.

Majetschak, M., Floche, S., Obertacke, U. et al. (1999). Relation of a TNF gene polymorphism to severe sepsis in trauma patients. Ann Surg 230, 207–214.

Mattey, D.L., Hassell, A.B., Dawes, P.T., Ollier, W.E. and Hajeer, A. (1999). Interaction between tumor necrosis factor microsatellite polymorphisms and the HLA-DRB1 shared epitope in rheumatoid arthritis: influence on disease outcome. Arthrit Rheum 42, 2698–2704.

Mehrian, R., Quismorio, F.P. Jr, Strassmann, G. et al. (1998). Synergistic effect between IL-10 and bcl-2 genotypes in determining susceptibility to systemic lupus erythematosus. Arthritis Rheum 41, 596–602.

Mineta, M., Tanimura, M., Tana, T. et al. (1996). Contribution of HLA class I and class II alleles to the regulation of antibody production to hepatitis B surface antigen in humans. Int Immunol 8, 525–531.

Mok, C.C., Lanchbury, J.S., Chan, D.W. and Lau, C.S. (1998). Interleukin-10 promoter polymorphisms in Southern Chinese patients with systemic lupus erythematosus. Arthrit Rheum 41, 1090–1095.

Moore, K.W., de Waal Malefyt, R., Coffman, R.L. and O'Garra, A. (2001). Interleukin-10 and the Interleukin-10 receptor. Ann Rev Immunol 19, 683–765.

Morita, E., Hiragun, T., Mihara, S. (2004). Determination of thymus and activation-regulated chemokine (TARC)-contents in scales of atopic dermatitis. J Dermatol Sci 34, 237–240.

Mulligan, C.G., Marshall, S.E., Bunce, M. and Welsh, K.I. (1999). Variation in immunoregulatory genes determines the clinical phenotype of common variable immunodeficiency. Genes Immun 1, 137–148.

Muraki, Y., Tsutsumi, A., Takahashi, R. et al. (2004). Polymorphisms of IL-1 β gene in Japanese patients with Sjogren's syndrome and systemic lupus erythematosus. J Rheumatol 31, 720–725.

Murray, P.J., Wang, L., Onufry, R.C., Tepper, R.I. and Young, R.A. (1997). T-cell derived IL-10 antagonises macrophage function in mycobacterial infection. J Immunol 158, 315–321.

Negoro, K., Kinouchi, Y., Hiwatashi, N. et al. (1999). Crohn's disease is associated with novel polymorphisms in the 5'-flanking region of the tumor necrosis factor gene. Gastroenterology 117, 1062–1068.

Nickel, R.G., Casolaro, V., Wahn, U. et al. (2000). Atopic dermatitis is associated with a functional mutation in the promoter of the C-C chemokine RANTES. J Immunol 164, 1612–1616.

Nohara, H., Okayama, N., Inoue, N. et al. (2004). Association of the -173G/C polymorphism of the macrophage migration inhibitory factor gene with ulcerative colitis. J Gastroenterol 39, 242–246.

O'Garra, A., Chang, R., Go, N., Hastings, R., Haughton, G. and Howard, M. (1992). Ly-1 (B-1) B-cells are the main source of B-cell derived interleukin-10. Eur J Immunol 22, 711–717.

Padyukov, L., Hahn-Zoric, M., Lau, Y.L. and Hanson, L.A. (2000). Different allelic frequencies of several cytokine genes in Hong-Kong Chinese and Swedish Caucasians. Genes Immun 2, 280–283.

Pantelidis, P., Jones, M.G., Welsh, K.I., Taylor, A.N. and du Bois, R.M. (2000). Identification of four novel interleukin-13 gene polymorphisms. Genes Immun 1, 341–345.

Pawalec, G., Pohla, H., Scholtz, E. et al. (1995). Interleukin-10 is a human T-cell growth factor in-vitro. Cytokine 7, 355–363.

Paxton, W.A., Neumann, A.U., Kang, S. et al. (2001). RANTES production from CD4+ lymphocytes correlates with host genotype and rates of human immunodeficiency virus type 1 disease progression. J Infect Dis 183, 1678–1681.

Petrovsky, N. and Harrison, L.C. (1997a). Diurnal rhythmicity of human cytokine production – A dynamic disequilibrium in T helper cell type 1/T helper cell type 2 balance? J Immunol *158*, 5163–5168.

Petrovsky, N. and Harrison, L.C. (1997b). HLA-class 11-associated polymorphism of interferon-gamma production. Implications for HLA disease association. Hum Immunol *53*, 12–16.

Plevy, S.E., Targan, S.R., Yang, H., Fernandez, D., Rotter, J.I. and Toyoda, H. (1996). Tumor necrosis factor microsatellites define a Crohn's disease-associated haplotype on chromosome 6. Gastroenterology *110*, 1053–1060.

Pociot, F., Briant, L., Jongeneel, C.V. et al. (1992). Association of tumor necrosis factor (TNF) and class II major histocompatibility complex alleles with the secretion of TNF-alpha and TNF-beta by human mononuclear cells: a possible link to insulin-dependent diabetes mellitus. Eur J Immunol *23*, 224–231.

Rood, M.J., van Krugten, M.V., Zanelli, E. et al. (2000). TNF-308A and HLA-DR3 alleles contribute independently to susceptibility in systemic lupus erythematosus. Arthrit Rheum *43*, 129–134.

Rousset, F., Garcia, E., Defrance, T. et al. (1992). IL-10 is a potent growth and differentiation factor for human B-cells. Proc Natl Acad Sci USA *89*, 1890–1893.

Shu, X.O., Gao, Y.T., Cai, Q. (2004). Genetic polymorphisms in the TGF-β 1 gene and breast cancer survival: a report from the Shanghai Breast Cancer Study. Cancer Res *64*, 836–839.

Sorensen, T.T., Nielsen, G.G., Andersen, P.K. and Teasdale, T.W. (1988). Genetic and environmental influences on premature death in adult adoptees. N Engl J Med *318*, 727–732.

Stassi, G., Todaro, M. and De Maria, R. (1997). Defective expression of CD95 (FAS/APO-1) molecule suggests apoptosis impairment of T and B cells in HLA-B8, DR3-positive individuals. Hum Immunol *55*, 39–45.

Taga, K., Mostowski, H. and Tosado, G. (1993). Human interleukin-10 can directly inhibit T-cell growth. Blood *81*, 2964–2971.

Thio, C.L., Goedert, J.J., Mosbruger, T. et al. (2004). An analysis of tumor necrosis factor alpha gene polymorphisms and haplotypes with natural clearance of hepatitis C virus infection. Genes Immun.

Tountas, N.A. and Cominelli, F. (1996). Identification and initial characterisation of two polymorphisms in the human interleukin-10 promoter (Abstract). Eur Cytokine Netw *7*, 578.

Tumpey, T.M., Elner, V.M., Chen, S.H., Oakes, J.E. and Lausch, R.N. (1994). Interleukin-10 treatment can suppress stromal keratitis induced by herpes simplex virus type 1. J Immunol *153*, 2258–2265.

Turner, D.M., Williams, D.M., Sankaran, D., Lazarus, M., Sinnott, P.J. and Hutchinson, I.V. (1997). An investigation of polymorphism in the interleukin-10 gene promoter. Eur J Immunogenetics *24*, 1–8.

van den Broek, M., Bachmann, M.F., Kohler, G. et al. (2000). IL-4 and IL-10 antagonise IL-12 mediated protection against acute Vaccinia virus infection with a limited role of IFN-gamma and nitric oxide synthetase 2. J Immunol *164*, 371–37.

van der Poll, T., Marchant, A., Keogh, C.V., Goldman, M. and Lowry, S.F. (1996). Interleukin-10 impairs host defence in murine pneumococcal pneumonia. J Infect Dis *174*, 994–1000.

van der Pouw Kraan, T.C., van Veen, A., Boeije, L.C. et al. (1999). An IL-13 promoter polymorphism associated with increased risk of allergic asthma. Genes Immun *1*, 61–65.

van Dissel, J.T., van Langevelde, P., Westendorp, R.G., Kwappenberg, K. and Frolich, M. (1998). Anti-inflammatory cytokine profile and mortality in febrile patients. Lancet *351*, 950–953.

Vassalli, P. (1992). The pathophysiology of tumor necrosis factor. Annu Rev Immunol *10*, 411–452.

Wagner, R.D., Maroushek, N.M., Brown, J.F. and Czuprynski, C.J. (1994). Treatment with anti-Interleukin-10 monoclonal antibody enhances early resistance to but impairs complete clearance of *Listeria monocytogenes* infection in mice. Infect Immun *62*, 2345–2353.

Wang, C., Tang, J., Song, W., Lobashevsky, E., Wilson, C.M. and Kaslow, R.A. (2004). HLA and cytokine gene polymorphisms are independently associated with responses to hepatitis B vaccination. Hepatology *39*, 978–988.

Wanidworanun, C. and Strober, W. (1993). Predominant role of tumour necrosis factor-alpha in human monocyte IL-10 synthesis. J Immunol *151*, 6853–6861.

Webb, D.C., Matthaei, K.I., Cai, Y., McKenzie, A.N. and Foster, P.S. (2004). Polymorphisms in IL-4R alpha correlate with airways hyperreactivity, eosinophilia, and Ym protein expression in allergic IL-13-/- mice. J Immunol *172*, 1092–1098.

Weissensteiner, T. and Lanchbury, J.S. (1997). TNFB polymorphisms characterize three lineages of TNF region microsatellite haplotypes. Immunogenetics *47*, 6–16.

Westendorp, R.G.J., Langermans, J.A.M., Huizinga, T.W.J. et al. (1997a). Genetic influence on cytokine production in fatal meningococcal disease. Lancet *349*, 170–173.

Westendorp, R.G., Langermans, J.A., Huizinga, T.W., Verweij, C.L. and Sturk, A. (1997b). Genetic influence on cytokine production in meningococcal disease. *Lancet, 349:* 1912–1913.

Wilson, A.G., di Giovine, F.S. and Duff, G.W. (1995). Genetics of tumour-necrosis factor-a in autoimmune, infectious and neoplastic disease. J Inflamm *45*, 1–12.

Zhang, D., Zhang, G., Hayden, M.S. et al. (2004). A toll-like receptor that prevents infection by uropathogenic bacteria. Science *303*, 1522–1526.

Zienolddiny, S., Ryberg, D., Maggini, V., Skaug, V., Canzian, F. and Haugen, A. (2004). Polymorphisms of the interleukin-1 β gene are associated with increased risk of non-small cell lung cancer. Int J Cancer *109*, 353–356.

Signaling Molecules Affecting Immune Response

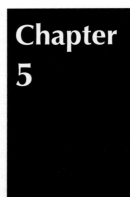

Chapter 5

Paul J. Hertzog, Jennifer E. Fenner and Ashley Mansell
Centre for Functional Genomics and Human Disease, Monash Institute of Reproduction and Development, Monash University, Clayton, Victoria, Australia

Don't shoot the messenger.

INTRODUCTION

Signal transducing molecules are the intracellular *messengers* necessary for generating the immune response. 'Shooting the messenger' or inactivation of signal transducing molecules by genetic mutation or by products of invading microorganisms results in immunodeficiency disease or infection.

Immune responses are driven by stimulation of immune cells from pathogens, antigens, cytokines and factors affecting growth or survival. These stimuli trigger responses via cellular receptors; signals are transduced by protein adapters and enzymes leading to modification, cleavage or release of proteins, activation and nuclear translocation of transcription factors and up or down modulation of expression of genes whose products are responsible for generating biological responses.

The immune response is complex and diverse because it involves many cell types, principally macrophages, natural killer cells and dendritic cells of the innate immune system and T and B cells of the adaptive immune system. These cells have specialized functions in immunity designed to elicit specific actions in response to specific stimuli. In keeping with this, the signal transduction systems utilized are often cell specific or unique either individually or in combination. It is not possible to comprehensively cover this entire field in one chapter in

a book. Therefore in this chapter, we present broad concepts referenced to recent reviews and examples of signaling molecules that are relevant to each branch of the immune response to different stimuli and examples that are important to human disease.

All cells of the immune system receive signals that orchestrate their development, maintenance, growth, proliferation, survival or death. This review will focus on signaling in response to 'activation' stimuli that constitute an immune response, but it is important to remember that these responses are intimately related to these 'maintenance' or developmental signals. For example, the deletion of autoreactive T cells that recognize 'self' antigens during the development of an immune response utilizes the same T cell receptor that will be later used to generate an antigen-specific immune response to foreign antigen. The difference, it seems, is that ligand engagement at low versus high affinity with the same receptor can activate different signals that mediate the opposite effects of cell death by apoptosis, versus survival and proliferation. This is one example of the subtlety of signaling in the immune system.

The first thing that the developed immune system 'sees' is foreign material, whether it be pathogen or antigen. The first line of defense, the innate immune response is now realized to contain a sensing system called the toll-like receptors (TLR). The 11 characterized members of this receptor family recognize the so-called pathogen associated molecular patterns (PAMPs) of infectious organisms including bacteria, viruses, flagellates, parasites and

Measuring Immunity, edited by Michael T. Lotze and Angus W. Thomson
ISBN 0-12-455900-X, London

Table 5.1 Extracellular signals affecting immune cells

Cell type	Activation stimulus		Maintenance stimulus
Macrophage	PAMP cytokines, chemotaxis	cell contacts	growth, survival, death
Dendritic cell	PAMP, cytokines, chemotaxis	cell contacts	growth, survival, death
NK cell	Cell, cytokines, chemotaxis	cell contacts	growth, survival, death
NKT cell	Cell, cytokines, chemotaxis	cell contacts	growth, survival, death
B cell	antigen, cytokines, chemotaxis	cell contacts	growth, survival, death
T cell	antigen, cytokines, chemotaxis	cell contacts	growth, survival, death

potential 'endogenous' ligands (Janeway and Medzhitov, 2002). Activation of these receptors in cells of the innate immune system such as macrophages and dendritic cells (DC), result in the production of cytokines and chemokines that orchestrate the subsequent phase of the host response, including an inflammatory response through cytokines such as IL-6, TNFα and IL-1, and immune activation through IL-12, IFNα, β and γ and cytokines. Cytokines such as interferon (IFN) have many specific functions, such as protection of exposed cells from viral infection, activation of NK and other cells, and survival of memory T cells (Hertzog et al., 2003). Once the innate immune system is activated, the cytokines generated either by pathogen recognition by the innate immune system or antigen stimulation of DC, B or T cells act further on the immune cells to generate specific responses. In addition to soluble or humoral stimuli, immune cells also receive signals directly from cells with which they are in contact. The classic example of this is the coreceptor signals activated by antigen presenting cells when engaged with T cells. Aspects of T and B cell signaling, receptors and transcription factors will be discussed elsewhere in this book. Therefore, signaling by the T cell and B cell receptors of the adaptive immune response and chemokines that signal for the recruitment of immune cells to the appropriate tissue compartment – a lesion, lymph node or central immune organ – will not be covered in this chapter. Nevertheless it is noteworthy that many signaling factors are common to the multiple arms of the immune system, particularly MAP kinases, PI3 kinase and CD45; whereas others such as src family kinases are better characterized in the adaptive immune response (Mustelin and Tasken, 2003). The focus of signaling in this chapter will therefore be on intracellular proteins involved in the initial phase of TLR activation and the secondary phase of cytokine action.

TLR SIGNALING MOLECULES IN RESPONSE TO PATHOGENS

The toll-like receptor family currently comprises 11 transmembrane receptors characterized by an extracellular domain with leucine rich repeats and a cytosolic toll-IL-1 receptor (TIR) signaling domain that shares homology with the IL-1 receptor family (Janeway and Medzhitov, 2002; O'Neill, 2004). Ex vivo studies and knockout mice

have been widely used to determine the microbial product specificities of various TLRs. These studies have shown that TLR2 is activated primarily by lipoproteins in conjunction with TLR1, TLR3 recognizes viral dsRNA/polyI:C, TLR4 is predominantly activated by LPS, TLR5 recognizes bacterial flagellin, TLR6 recognizes MALP-2 from mycobacteria in conjunction with TLR2, TLR7 and TLR8 recognize imidazoquinoline compounds and viral single-stranded RNA, TLR9 responds to unmethylated bacterial CpG DNA, and the recently described TLR 11 recognizes uropathogenic bacteria (O'Neill 2004; Diebold et al., 2004; Heil et al., 2004; Takeda and Akira, 2004; Zhang et al., 2004).

The TIR domain is found not only in transmembrane receptors, but also in several key cytosolic signaling adapters involved in TLR signaling termed MyD88, Mal, TRIF and the recently described TRAM (Takeda and Akira, 2004). These adaptors assemble signal transduction complexes that contain adaptor molecules and kinases including IRAK-1, IRAK-4 and TRAF6, which subsequently activate the IKK signalsome leading to activation of the prototypic inflammatory transcription factor, NF-κB, MAP kinases and IRF3 which culminates in pro-inflammatory cytokine production and subsequent immune responses. These responses will either successfully remove the threat to the host, or if this response recurs through dysregulation, will eventuate in chronic inflammation and possibly septic shock.

TIR-containing adapters

MyD88

MyD88 is a common TIR-containing adaptor protein recruited to all ligand-activated TLR and IL-1 receptor family members allowing the proximal recruitment and subsequent activation of IRAK-1/4 and TRAF6 (see below). Activation of this complex leads to phosphorylation of the IKK signalsome, culminating in nuclear translocation of NF-κB. MyD88 is a 296 amino acid protein, consisting of a TIR domain (159–296) and an N-terminal death domain (54–109) responsible for homotypic death domain recruitment of proteins such as IRAK-1 (Akira et al., 2001). A critical role for MyD88 in TLR and IL-1 signaling was found with the generation of MyD88-deficient mice (MyD88-/-) mice. These mice displayed a normal response to non-TLR-mediated signaling (TNF, IL-2), whereas their response to IL-1β (IL-1R), LPS (TLR4), MALP2 (TLR2), CpG-DNA (TLR9) and pI:C (TLR3) was severely impaired. This supported the role of MyD88 as a universal adapter for TIR-containing receptors. However, NF-κB nuclear translocation by LPS and poly I:C signaling was delayed, but not inhibited (Kawai et al.,1999). Furthermore, the induction of interferon (IFN) β and IFN-regulated genes (IRGs) were found to be unimpaired in LPS-treated MyD88-/- cells, suggesting the presence of an 'MyD88-independent' signaling pathway (Kawai et al., 2001) responsible for the detection and response to the two major activators of innate immunity, bacteria and viruses. These data support earlier reports of the importance of activation of the IFN system in response to LPS (Hwang et al., 1995; Hamilton et al., 1996; Hertzog et al., 2003).

Mal/TIRAP

Mal/TIRAP was the second TIR-containing adaptor protein to be identified. Mal consists of 235 amino acids, constituting a TIR domain (84–235), and an N-terminal domain (1–83) of no known function. Mal was found to inhibit TLR4-induced activation of NF-κB, but had no effect upon TLR-9- or IL-1R-mediated activation (Fitzgerald et al., 2001). These results suggested Mal to be an adaptor for TLR4-mediated signaling. Mal dimerized with both MyD88 and TLR4. Ectopic expression data also suggested a role for Mal in LPS-induced apoptosis, and activation of IRF-3 leading to the expression of IFNβ (Shinobu et al., 2002). Mal-/- mice were more resistant to the toxic effects of LPS and Mal-/- macrophages resembled MyD88-/-derived macrophages, in that there is no LPS-induced expression of IL-6, TNF or IL-12p40, while LPS-mediated activation of NF-κB and JNK was delayed, but not inhibited (Hornig et al., 2002; Yamamoto et al., 2002a). The activation of IRF-3 by LPS and the regulation of IRF-3-dependent genes such as IP-10 and IFNβ were apparently intact, suggesting that Mal was not the missing adaptor responsible for the 'MyD88-independent' pathway. Furthermore, double knockout mice that are deficient in both Mal and MyD88 were still responsive to LPS-induced activation of IRF-3 and the induction of CD80/CD86, confirming that the 'MyD88-independent' signaling pathway was intact and that neither Mal nor MyD88 compensated for the other (Yamamoto et al., 2002a). The response of Mal-/- cells to TLR2 ligands was totally abolished, as was found with MyD88-/- mice. This finding implicates Mal and MyD88 as essential adaptors for TLR2-mediated signaling. These studies therefore failed to identify a specific role for Mal in TLR4-mediated signaling; however, it clearly showed the implicit role of Mal in TLR4-mediated NF-κB-dependent gene expression.

TRIF and TRAM

A combination of overexpression experiments and gene-deficient mice has found that TIR-domain-containing adaptor inducing IFNβ (TRIF) and TRIF-related adaptor molecule (TRAM) appear to regulate this 'MyD88-independent' pathway. Overexpressed TRIF in vitro activated an IFNβ promoter, but only weakly activated NF-κB. Truncated forms of TRIF suggested the C-terminus mediates IFNβ promoter activation and the TIR-containing N-terminal mediates NF-κB activation (Yamamoto et al., 2002b; Oshiumi et al., 2003). Two independent studies found TRIF-deficient and TRIF-mutated mice defective in both TLR3- and TLR4-mediated expression of IFNβ and activation of IRF3. Furthermore, LPS-induced cytokine production was severely impaired and MyD88/TRIF double knockouts displayed complete loss of NF-κB nuclear translocation. The MAP kinase pathway however was found to be unaffected (Yamamoto et al., 2003a; Hoebe et al., 2003). TRAM overexpression also activates IRF3 leading to IFNβ production, but unlike the other adaptors, appears to be specific for the TLR4 pathway (Fitzgerald et al., 2003; Bin et al., 2003). Crucially, TRAM-deficient mice showed defects in cytokine production in response to TLR4 ligand, but not other TLR ligands, and importantly, TLR4- but not TLR3-mediated MyD88-independent IFNβ production and activation of signaling pathways were abolished (Yamamoto et al., 2003b). Furthermore, TRAM was found to act upstream of TRIF in TLR4-mediated signaling.

IRAKS 1, 2, M and 4

IRAK-1 is a serine/threonine kinase that is recruited by MyD88 to the signaling complex, then undergoes phosphorylation, dissociates from the complex and initiates downstream signaling events by associating with TRAF6 (Cao et al., 1996). Further studies have shown that the phosphorylation of IRAK-1 induces polyubiquitination, thereby targeting IRAK-1 for degradation by the 26S proteasome. However, it was found that NF-κB activation, and the cytokine and stress response in IRAK-1 deficient mice were reduced, but not abolished, on challenge with IL-1, IL-18 and LPS (Kanakaraj et al., 1998,1999; Thomas et al., 1999; Swantek et al., 2000). These results suggested that while IRAK-1 may be crucial for an optimal response to TIR-mediated signaling, there is considerable redundancy within IRAK function (Medzhitov et al., 1998).

Perhaps the most important member of the IRAK family is IRAK-4. In IRAK-4-deficient mice IL-1 responses were completely inhibited, there being no residual NF-κB activation, nor cytokine production, in contrast to that seen in the IRAK-1-/- mice (Suzuki et al., 2002b). IRAK-4-/- mice were also highly resistant to LPS-induced septic shock and unable to clear *Staphylococcus aureus* infections. Interestingly however, LPS-induced NF-κB activation and stress responses were still detected in IRAK-4-/- cells, but with delayed kinetics. These results suggest that IRAK-4 plays a non-redundant role in TIR-mediated signaling and may affect the stability or activation of components of the TIR-signaling complex. *In vitro* kinase assays have demonstrated that IRAK-4 can induce the phosphorylation of IRAK-1 and data indicate that IRAK-4 likely functions upstream of IRAK-1 and may activate IRAK-1 such that it can then undergo autophosphorylation, signal complex disengagement and subsequent degradation (Suzuki et al., 2002a).

The remaining members of the IRAK family, namely IRAK-M (Wesche et al., 1999) and IRAK-2 (Muzio et al., 1997), have been suggested to act as negative regulators of TIR signaling. Both are capable of activating NF-κB activation when overexpressed. It has been proposed that IRAK-M functions in a regulatory role by inhibiting dissociation of the IRAK-1/IRAK-4 complex from ligand-induced TIR dimerization by either effecting the stabilization of the IRAK complex, or inhibiting the phosphorylation of IRAK-1 and IRAK-4. Indeed, cells stimulated with LPS show increased expression of IRAK-M, thereby increasing this inhibitory effect and further suggesting a regulatory role for this protein. IRAK-M deficient mice (IRAK-M-/-) show enhanced TLR signaling, exhibiting enhanced cytokine production, increased intestinal inflammatory responses and enlarged and inflamed Peyer's patches when challenged with bacteria (Kobayashi et al., 2002).

TRAF6/TAB1/TAB2/TAK1

TRAF6 belongs to a family of proteins first described to participate in TNF signaling, however a physiological role for TRAF6 was initially described, as a signal mediator in IL-1 signaling. Characteristics of the family include a C-terminal region of homology known as the TRAF domain, which facilitates TRAF protein oligomerization and interaction with other signaling proteins. TRAF6 is unique among the TRAF protein family in that it is the only protein member that does not directly interact with the receptor complex (Cao et al.,1996). Overexpression of TRAF6 was shown to activate NF-κB and JNK and p38, MAP kinases, suggesting that TRAF6 may be the point of divergence for NF-κB and MAPK kinase activation. However, Wang et al. (2001) found that oligomerization of TRAF6, in the presence or absence of signaling from the IL-1R complex, triggers its ubiquitination through the action of TRAF6-regulated IKK activator 1 (TRIKA1). This is an example of ubiquitination not targeting a protein for proteasomal degradation, but promoting signal transduction. They also purified TRIKA2, which was found to comprise TAK1, TAB1 and TAB2. It was found that ubiquitinated TRAF6 directly activates TAK1, which recruits TAB2 from the cell membrane to the cytoplasm. TAK1 is then able to activate IKK through an as yet unknown mechanism. The dissociation of the TRAF6/TAK1/TAB1/TAB2 complex from the membrane-bound TIR/IRAK-1 complex allows the ubiquitination and degradation of IRAK-1. The translocation of this complex to the cytosol and subsequent interaction with additional signaling mediators, induces the phosphorylation of TAK1 and the activation of both JNK and NF-κB.

IκB and IKK and NF-κB activation

NF-κB is sequestered in the cytoplasm of unstimulated cells comprising a transcriptionally active dimer bound to the inhibitory protein IκB (Ghosh and Baltimore, 1990). Upon stimulation with potent activators of NF-κB, such as the IL-1 or LPS, activation of the large molecular weight, serine specific IκB kinase (IKK) complex rapidly phosphorylates IκB. This targets the inhibitor protein for ubiquitination and subsequent degradation (Karin, 1999). As with the NF-κB protein family, there are several isoforms of IκB protein (including IκBα, IκBβ and IκBε) that bind with varying affinities to a variety of NF-κB complexes, thus conferring different regulation on NF-κB translocation in a tissue specific manner. In all members of the IκB family, two serine residues (Ser^{32}, Ser^{36}) are crucial as important sites of phosphorylation by IKKs, and one tyrosine residue (Tyr^{42}) also undergoes phosphorylation (202, 236). Biochemical and structural analysis has also shown that IκBα has multiple interactions with individual NF-κB complexes concealing the DNA localization domain (Chen and Ghosh, 1999). IκBα, β and ε have been demonstrated to preferentially target p65 and cRel containing complexes, masking their nuclear localization sequence and thus preventing nuclear translocation. IκBα, IκBβ and ε become inducibly phosphorylated on serine residues which target them for ubiquitination subsequent proteolytic degradation (Karin, 1999). The selective targeting of particular IκB proteins by various stimuli increases the means by which NF-κB activation is regulated. For example, IL-1, TNF, LPS and the phorbol ester PMA target IκBα, whereas IκBβ is only responsive to IL-1 and LPS, presumably via a TIR specific pathway.

A high molecular weight multiprotein complex termed the signalsome with IκB kinase activity was isolated from TNF-treated HeLa cells. Purification of this 900 kDa multiprotein complex identified two proteins of 85 and 87 kDa that demonstrated IκB kinase activity (Mercurio et al., 1997). Microsequencing demonstrated that active IKK is a complex consisting of the initial formation of IKKα (IKK1) and IKKβ (IKK2) as a heterodimer, followed by the subsequent addition of either a dimer or trimer of IKKγ (also known as NEMO) proteins. IKKα and IKKβ have similar primary structures with a 52 per cent overall homology, containing N-terminal kinase domains, leucine zippers and helix-loop-helix motifs in the C-terminus. The degree of homology between the IKKs suggests that the two kinases may have functionally redundant roles in the cell. IKKα-/- mice have been found to die within 4 h after birth and show severe developmental defects consistent with a role for IKKα in regulating epidermal differentiation. In addition, studies on these mice showed that IKKα was not essential for IKK complex activation by pro-inflammatory stimuli (Hu et al.,1999; Takeda et al.,1999). In contrast, IKKβ deficient mice are embryonically lethal as a result of massive liver apoptosis, exhibiting a phenotype similar to p65 knockout mice (Li et al., 1999a). They also demonstrate very little NF-κB activation in response to IL-1 or TNF, indicating that IKKβ is predominantly responsible for regulating IKK complex activation in response to IL-1. It has been found that IKKα and IKKβ act as the catalytic subunits of the kinase complex. IKKγ has no identifiable catalytic domain, but contains a leucine zipper inserted in helix-loop-helix motifs acting as the regulatory subunit (Karin, 1999).

Other signaling factors in TLR signaling

There are more signaling pathways activated by TLR engagement than those which activate the NFκB and IRF3 pathways. Other major pathways that are currently receiving less focus than the above include the MAP kinases, p38, JNK and ERK (Fig. 5.1).

SIGNALING MOLECULES MEDIATING CYTOKINE RESPONSES

The cytokine family is extensive, being composed of interleukins, IL-1 to -27, colony stimulating factors (CSFs) and interferons (IFNs) among many others. Despite the diversity of this family of protein ligands and their

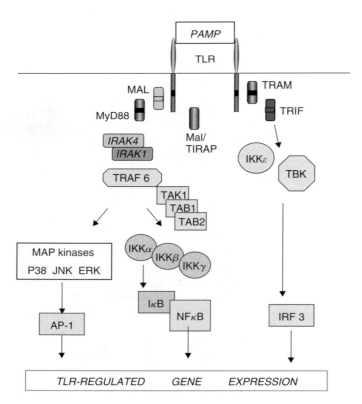

Figure 5.1 TLR-regulated gene expression. TLR signaling involves a cascade of distal events leading to gene regulation. Following interaction with a PAMP (pathogen associated molecular patterns) usually derived from a pathogen or occasionally endogenous ligands, downstream signaling results in activation and translocation of regulatory factors to the nucleus including AP1, NF-κB, and IRF3.

receptors, the signal transduction has common patterns (Boulay et al., 2001). This is largely due to the family of JAK kinases and signal transducers and activators of transcription (STATs) that are involved in signaling in all cases.

JAK family kinases

In the mammalian system, there are four JAKs, including JAK1, JAK2, JAK3 and TYK2 that preferentially preassociate with cytokine receptors.

TYK2 was the first to be discovered in a screen of a T cell cDNA library with c-fms catalytic domain (Krolewski et al., 1990), while JAK1, JAK2 and JAK3 were cloned utilizing a PCR strategy using primers corresponding to conserved motifs within the catalytic domain of Tyk2 (Wilks, 1991; Harpur et al., 1992). Once activated by ligand binding and subsequent trans-phosphorylation, the JAKs have three functions; first, they phosphorylate their associated receptors on tyrosine residues (Colamonici et al., 1994) which become STAT docking sites (see below). The second function of JAKs is the subsequent phosphorylation of tyrosine residue on the STAT proteins (Darnell et al., 1994). Thirdly, JAKs are able to assist in the formation/stability of the receptor complex in the membrane, generating the highest affinity for its respective ligand, as TYK2 does for IFNAR1 (Velazquez et al., 1995). While most of the literature discusses the JAKs in terms of phophorylating STAT proteins, they also associate or activate GRB2, SHP2, VAV and STAM resulting in the activation of multiple pathways (Yin et al., 1997; Chauhan et al., 1995; Matsuguchi et al., 1995; Takeshita et al., 1997). Activated JAKs have also been shown to bind to SOCS family members which target proteins for proteasomal degradation (Yasukawa et al., 1999; Nicholson et al., 1999) (see below).

JAK proteins range in size from 110 kDa to 140 kDa, possess a C-terminal protein kinase domain (JH1), an adjacent kinase or kinase-related domain (JH2) plus a further five domains extending towards the N-terminus (JH3–7) (Harpur et al., 1992). The JH1 domain, which is the tyrosine kinase domain, has been reported to require the pseudo-domain JH2, in order to elicit its catalytic activity (Velazquez et al., 1995). The remaining five domains, JH3–7, have been implicated in receptor association. The chromosomal locations of each of the JAKs have been identified in humans as chromosomes 1 for JAK1, 9 for JAK2 and 19 for JAK3 and TYK2 (Krowlewski et al., 1990; Pritchard et al., 1992; Riedy et al., 1996). In mice, Jak1, Jak2, Jak3 and Tyk2 localize to chromosome 4, 19, 8 and 9 respectively (Gough et al., 1995; Kono et al., 1996; Mouse Genome Informatics Scientific Curators, 2002). JAK1, JAK2 and TYK2 are expressed ubiquitously and bind to numerous cytokine receptor subunits, whereas JAK3 appears to be restricted to cells of hematopoietic origin (Ihle, 1995).

JAK1

JAK1 is activated by the cytokines type I IFN and IFNγ, IL-10 and -13, the γ common chain-utilizing cytokines such

Table 5.2 JAK family kinase usage by cytokines

JAK1	IFNα	IFNγ	IL-10		IL-13		γc Cytokines[a]	gp130 Cytokines[c]
JAK2	IFNγ		IL-12	IL-13	EPO		βcom Cytokines[b]	gp130 Cytokines[c]
JAK3							γc Cytokines[a]	
Tyk2	IFNα	IL-10	IL-12	IL-13				gp130 Cytokines[c]

[a] γc utilizing cytokines = IL-2, IL-4, IL-7, IL-4, IL-9, IL-15
[b] β common utilizing cytokines = IL-3, IL-5, GM-CSF
[c] gp130 utilizing cytokines = IL-6, IL-11, oncostatin M, CNTF, LIF

as IL-2 and IL-15 and the gp130-utilizing cytokines such as IL-6. It was demonstrated using *Jak1* mutant cells (U4A) that JAK-1 was essential for signaling *in vitro* (Müller et al., 1993). The *Jak1-/-* mice exhibited perinatal lethality from both defective neural function and lymphoid development consistent with the necessity for this kinase in CNTF signaling in neurons and γ common chain signaling in immune cells (Rodig et al., 1998).

JAK2

JAK2 is activated by cytokines IFNγ, IL-12 and -13, erythropoietin, cytokines GM-CSF, IL-3 and IL-5 that signal via the β-common chain and the gp130 utilizing cytokines. A *Jak2* mutant cell line (γ1A) failed to respond to IFNγ (Neubauer et al., 1998) but responded normally to IFNα/β (Watling et al., 1993) indicating that JAK2 was not involved in type I IFN signaling. The *Jak2-/-* mutation causes embryonic lethality in mice resulting from the absence of erythropoiesis and anemia due to the failure of erythropoietin signaling (Neubauer et al., 1998; Parganas et al., 1998; Aringer et al., 1999). These data, along with the *Jak1* mutant studies, indicated that although sequence/structural similarity exists between these proteins, there is little functional redundancy within this family.

JAK3

JAK3 specifically interacts with the γ common chain in response to IL-2, IL-4, IL-7, IL-9 and IL-15 signaling. Cells deficient for *Jak3* are therefore deficient in γ common chain signaling, especially in response to IL-2 (Oakes et al., 1996). Therefore it is not surprising that JAK3 plays an essential role in γ common chain dependent lymphoid development (Di Santo et al., 1995; Cao et al., 1995; Thomis et al., 1995; Nosaka et al., 1995; Park et al., 1995). *Jak3-/-* mice suffer from severe immunodeficiency due to a marked reduction in the number of T and B cells (Nosaka et al., 1995; Park et al., 1995; Thomis et al., 1995) and exhibit a phenotype similar to human severe combined immunodeficiency (SCID) resulting from *JAK3* mutations (Macchi et al., 1995; Russell et al., 1995). Unlike JAK1, JAK2 and TYK2, JAK3 appears to have little or no effect on the IFN system.

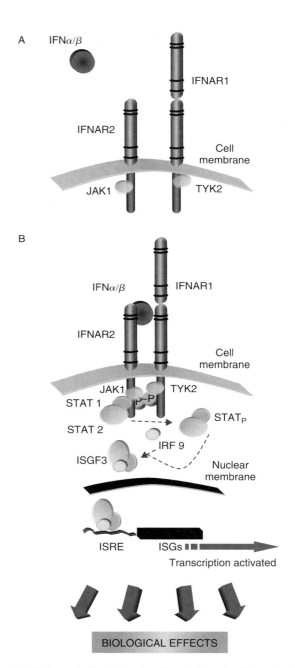

Figure 5.2 Biological effects. Paradigm for cytokine signal transduction. Following interaction of a prototypic type 1 interferon with its receptor, JAK1 and Tyk2 drive stat phosphorylation, heterodimerization and ultimately targeting of interferon stimulated response elements (ISRE) driving expression of interferon stimulated genes (ISG).

TYK2

Tyk2 is activated by type I IFN, IL-10, 12 and 13 and gp130 utilizing cytokines. In the IFN system, TYK2 associates with IFNAR1 (Uze et al., 1990; Yang et al., 1996) and positively influences ligand binding, perhaps by stabilizing the receptor in the plasma membrane. TYK2-deficient cells (11,1) do not respond to IFNα, but residual responses to IFNβ were detected (Velazquez et al., 1995). *Tyk2-/-* mice display no overt developmental abnormalities, but demonstrated suboptimal responses to type I IFNs and have a defect in IL-12 induced T cell function (Shimoda et al., 2000). The fact that there is residual signaling occurring in response to type I IFNs in *Tyk2* deficient cells suggests that unlike the other JAK proteins there may be some TYK2 functional redundancy, as IFN signaling is not dependent on fully functional TYK2. Recent studies have demonstrated that *Tyk2-/-* mice are resistant to septic shock induced by LPS treatment, making *Tyk2* a component of the LPS signaling pathway (Karaghiosoff et al., 2003).

SIGNAL TRANSDUCERS AND ACTIVATORS OF TRANSCRIPTION (STATs)

The STAT proteins, which form an integral part of the majority of cytokine signaling, were first discovered through investigations into transcription factors which bound to promoter regions of IFN stimulated genes (ISGs) (Darnell et al., 1994). Subsequently, seven structurally and functionally related STATs have been identified, including STAT1, STAT2, STAT3, STAT4, STAT5a, STAT5b and STAT6. All STATs are expressed ubiquitously, with the exception of STAT4, which is expressed only in the brain, heart, spleen, blood cells and testis (Fu et al., 1992; Zhong et al., 1994; Akira et al., 1994; Yamamoto et al., 1994; Wakao et al., 1994; Hou et al., 1994; Mui et al., 1995; Azam et al., 1995; Lin et al., 1996). Generally, STATs are involved in signaling from the cell membrane receptors following recruitment to activated receptor complexes to the nucleus. Once in the nucleus, they mediate transcriptional regulation in response to numerous growth factor and cytokine families (Darnell et al., 1994; Darnell, 1997).

Genetic mapping of the STAT gene family has demonstrated that in both human and mouse, the *STAT/Stat* genes localize to three separate clusters on different chromosomes. Both *STAT1/Stat1* and *STAT4/Stat4* cluster together on human chromosome 2 and mouse chromosome 1. *STAT2/Stat2* and *STAT6/Stat6* make up the second group localized to human chromosome 12 and mouse chromosome 10, with the remaining *STAT3/Stat3*, *STAT5a/Stat5a* and *STAT5b/Stat5b* localized to human chromosome 17 and mouse chromosome 11 (Copeland et al., 1995; Lin et al., 1995). The similarities in the clustering and structure of both human and mouse *STAT/Stat* genes, suggest that each of the STATs has evolved from a

number of tandem duplications during the evolution of multicellular organisms (Hou et al., 1996).

The STAT proteins range in size from 750 to 850 amino acids with six functional domains. The domains include the *amino terminal domain* (NH2) which has been implicated in interactions with receptor domains and other transcription factors such as CBP/p300 and PIAS proteins (Horvath, 2000; Shuai, 2000). The *coiled-coiled domain* (CCD) forms an interactive surface to which other helical proteins such as IRF9 are able to bind (Horvath and Darnell, 1996). The *DNA binding domain* (DBD) makes up the region that recognizes DNA sequences within promoter regions of STAT induced genes. STAT1 dimers can interact with *gamma activated sequence* (GAS) elements in both IFNγ and IFNα/β signaling. STAT2 is the only STAT that does not interact directly with DNA (Qureshi et al., 1995). *The linker domain* connects the DBD to the SH2 domain and has been implicated in transcriptional regulation through interactions with the SH2 domain, which is a docking site for interaction with other transcription factors (Chen et al., 1998; Yang et al., 1996). *The SH2 domain* contains the tyrosine activation motif that is integral in signaling. The SH2 domain plays an important role in recruitment to the receptor chain, interaction with the activated JAKs and the subsequent hetero- or homo-dimerization (Shuai et al., 1994; Gupta et al., 1996; Barahmand-Pour et al., 1998). The *transcriptional activation domain* (TAD) located at the carboxyl terminus is poorly conserved between the STAT proteins and thus gives each of the STATs some specificity. Each of the STATs harbors conserved domains as discussed which suggests that they each carry out similar functions albeit within different signaling pathways activated by numerous stimuli.

The STATs are predominantly involved in pathways that utilize receptor subunits lacking in intrinsic kinase activity and hence recruit JAKs. However, STATs have been shown to be activated by receptor tyrosine kinases EGF-R and CSF1-R (Leonard and O'Shea, 1998; Schindler and Strehlow, 2000) as well as non-receptor kinases such as src and abl (Bromberg and Darnell, 2000).

STAT1

Studies using mutant *STAT1* cells (U3A) (McKendry et al., 1991) have demonstrated that STAT1 is required for both type I and II IFN signaling, evidence which was supported by data resulting from the generation of the *Stat1-/-* mouse (Durbin et al., 1996). Numerous ligands activate STAT1 *in vitro*, however, the *Stat1-/-* mouse developed normally and demonstrated a lack of type I and II IFN signaling, in particular immune responses to viruses and bacteria (Durbin et al., 1996; Meraz et al., 1996). Surprisingly, these mice still respond normally to other cytokines and growth factors which activate STAT1 *in vitro* (Larner et al., 1993; Fu and Zhang, 1993; Finbloom and Winestock, 1995; Wen et al., 1995).

STAT2

STAT2 is only known to be activated by type I IFNs. Mutant cell lines lacking functional STAT2 (U6A) were used to discover that STAT2 is required for ISGF3 formation in response to IFNα/β and there was a lack of STAT1 homodimer formation in response to IFNα/β in the *Stat2* deficient cells (Leung et al., 1995). The phenotype exhibited by *Stat2-/-* mice involves unresponsiveness to type I IFN, a high susceptibility to viral infection and defects in macrophages and T cell responses. This evidence supported a role for IFNs in innate and acquired immune responses. Type I IFNs were unable to induce ISGF3 driven or GAS driven genes in *Stat2-/-* mice (Park et al., 2000).

STAT3

STAT3 is activated primarily by cytokines that act through the gp130 receptor subunit (Gadina et al., 2001), as well as type I IFNs (Owczarek et al., 1997) and IL-10. *Stat3-/-* mice are embryonic lethal, perhaps due to a defect in LIF signaling and conditionally targeted mice demonstrate a role for STAT3 in myeloid cell inflammatory responses via IL-10 signaling, G-CSF signaling and mammary gland epithelial function.

STAT4

STAT4 is expressed at high levels in thymus, spleen and activated T cells and is activated by IL-12. Accordingly, *Stat4*-deficient mice have defective Th1 differentiation due to deficient IL-12 signaling (Kaplan et al., 1996; Thierfelder et al., 1996). Type I IFNs can activate STAT4 in human but not murine cells via STAT2. A microsatellite insertion in the murine Stat2 prevents this interaction (Farrar et al., 2000). This result represents an important example of different immune responses between species, which might explain why type I IFNs can induce Th1 differentiation in humans but not in mice.

STAT5

There are two STAT5 genes, 5a and 5b, which are activated by prolactin, growth hormone and IL-2 (Gadina et al., 2001). *Stat5a* deficient mice have impaired mammary gland development and lactation (Liu et al., 1997). *Stat5b* deficient mice exhibit defects in sex gland development and growth hormone signaling (Udy et al., 1997). Immune defects are also evident in *Stat5* null mice. These include aberrant NK cell development and T cell responses to IL-2.

STAT6

STAT6 activation by IL-4 is well characterized and by IL-13 less so. *Stat6-/-* mice fail to develop Th2 responses due to the deficiency in IL-4 signaling (Takeda et al., 1996;

Shimoda et al., 1996) and are more susceptible to allergic and asthmatic disease (Miyata et al., 1999).

Non-JAK/STAT cytokine signaling

While the discovery of the JAK/STAT signaling pathways and the elucidation of their role in cytokine signaling has revolutionized our understanding of signal transduction and generation of immune responses, it has become clear that additional pathways are necessary to generate the diversity of responses of which cytokines are capable. This is best characterized in the interferon system where the JAK/STAT pathway was first described and most extensively studied. For example, the IFNα growth inhibitory signal in lymphocytes requires the expression and association to IFNAR of phosphatase CD45 and tyrosine kinases LCK and ZAP70, signaling proteins that have best been characterized for their role in T cell receptor signaling (Petricoin et al., 1997). Activation of the type I IFN complex can result in the engagement of multiple proteins including insulin receptor substrate 1 (IRS1) and IRS2 (Uddin et al., 1995; Platanias et al., 1996), the regulatory p85 subunit of phosphatidylinositol 3-kinase (PI3kinase) (Pfeffer et al., 1997) and activation of MAP kinases (Platanias, 2003). As genome-wide technologies enable a more thorough analysis of gene expression, so the complexity of signal transduction pathways is becoming evident. For example STAT independent signaling in response to IFNs results in the altered expression of many genes with potentially important biological consequences (Ramana et al., 2002).

INTERFERON REGULATORY FACTORS (IRFs)

The IFN regulatory factor (IRF) family of nine transcription factors (IRF1–9) are not only involved in the production and responses to cytokines, but some are also involved in TLR responses to PAMPs (see above). Furthermore, not only do they function as transcription factors, but as binding partners to form signaling complexes such as the IRF9, which binds to STAT1 and STAT2 to form the ISGF3 signaling complex. The IRF family have been extensively characterized for their role in IFN signal transduction and IFN production, but also have important roles in signaling for other cytokines such as IL-6 and IL-15, in immune functions and cell growth (Nguyen et al., 1997; Taniguchi et al., 2001). The multiple members of this family all share 125 amino acid homology at the N-terminal region which encodes the DNA binding domain that binds to IFN response elements (IREs) within promoter regions of ISGs and IFN genes. The more divergent C-terminal domain serves as the regulatory domain and aids in the classification of the IRFs into three groups. The three groups include activators (IRF1, IRF3, IRF7 and IRF9/ISGF 3γ/p48), repressors (IRF2 and IRF8/ICSBP) and lastly those that can behave as either activators or repressors (IRF2 and IRF4/LSIRF/Pip) (Taniguchi et al., 2001). Generally, IRFs are capable of interacting with other IRF proteins and also with members of other transcription factor families to modify translocation, binding to their cognate IRE elements in target gene promoters and in transactivation.

IRF1

IRF1 was discovered as a transcription activator of type I IFNs, but subsequently found also to function in signaling in response to type I and II IFNs as well as other cytokines. The *Irf1-/-* mice were immunodeficient, lacking the expression of gene products involved in antigen presentation, Th1 and NK cell responses (Matsuyama et al., 1993; Duncan et al., 1996; White et al., 1996).

IRF2

IRF2 is a transcriptional repressor of cytokine signaling, like IRF1, identified for its role in regulation of IFN production (in this case repression) and response. The generation of the *Irf2-/-* mouse supported the importance of IRF2 as a regulator of IFN signaling. The responses to type I IFNs were uncontrolled which leads to abnormal CD8+ T cell activation (Hida et al., 2000). These mice were also unable to respond to IL-12 and therefore failed to induce Th1 cell differentiation and NK cell development (Lohoff et al., 2000) which made them susceptible to viral infection. The *Irf2* deficient mice develop an inflammatory skin disease caused by a continual low level of ISGF3 induction, suggesting that IRF2 is required to keep a balance between the beneficial and harmful effects of the type I IFNs (Hida et al., 2000).

IRF3

IRF3 is activated downstream of TLR3, recognition of virus, and TLR4, recognition of LPS, which through the adapter molecule TRIF/TICAM1 activate the kinases IKKϵ and TBK1 (Fitzgerald et al., 2003). Once IRF3 is activated it plays a very important role in the induction of IFN genes following viral infection, being directly responsible for the activation of IFNβ and IFNα4 expression (Marie et al., 1998; Yoneyama et al., 1998; Noah et al., 1999).

IRF4

IRF4 induces immunoglobulin gene expression and is essential for maturation and homeostasis of lymphocytes. Expression of IRF4 is limited to T and B cell lineages (Eisenbeis et al., 1995; Matsuyama et al., 1995). *Irf4-/-* mice are immunodeficient with defects in both B and T cell proliferation resulting in an imbalance in lymphocyte homeostasis (Mittrucker et al., 1997).

IRF5 and 6

IRF5 and 6 are the least characterized. Both IRF5 and 6 are structurally related and IRF5 is induced by IFNα/β; however, how IRF6 is induced is unknown (Taniguchi et al., 2001).

IRF7

IRF7 was originally cloned as a factor that bound to a promoter region in the Epstein-Barr virus using a yeast one-hybrid system (Zhang and Pagano, 1997). IRF7, once induced, is present in the cytoplasm as an inactive protein that is also phosphorylated on specific C-terminal residues by TBK1 and/or possibly IKKϵ kinases (Fitzgerald et al., 2003; Sharma et al., 2003). IRF7 has an important role in the regulation of *IFNA* genes other than A4. Human cells deficient for *IRF7* are unable to induce the expression of these genes (Yeow et al., 2000). Therefore it appears that both IRF3 and IRF7 together are responsible for the induction of the full spectrum of the type I IFN genes in response to viral infection, but the priming action of IRF3 on the production of IFNs *B* and A4 is necessary for the secondary production of the remaining IFNα genes driven by IRF7.

IRF8

The *IFN consensus sequence binding protein* (ICSBP)/ IRF8 was originally identified as a protein that bound to ISREs in the promoter region of MHC class I (Driggers et al., 1990; Weiz et al., 1992). Expression of IRF8 is induced by IFNγ, not IFNα/β and is restricted to myeloid and lymphoid cell lines (Driggers et al., 1990). The function of IRF8 is similar to that of IRF2 in that it represses ISG expression (Nelson et al., 1993). *Irf8-/-* mice have been generated and present with chronic myelogenous leukemia (CML)-like disease and immunodeficiency (Holtschke et al., 1996). Interestingly, patients who suffer from CML have suppressed IRF8 expression. When these patients are administered IFNα, IRF8 expression is restored, suggesting that *IRF8* may act as a tumor suppressor (Schmidt et al., 1998).

IRF9

IRF9 was previously known as p48 or ISGF3γ as it was IFNγ inducible (Levy et al., 1990; Matsumoto et al., 1999) and forms a heterotrimeric transcription factor, binding to the STAT1:STAT2 heterodimer through its carboxyl-terminal domain termed as *IFN stimulated gene factor 3* (ISGF3). This transcriptional activation complex is then able to cross the nuclear membrane where IRF9 and STAT1 are able to bind to the DNA in specific regions termed ISREs (Horvath and Darnell, 1996; Martinez-Moczygemba et al., 1997). Mice deficient for *Irf9* fail to survive viral infection, which is not surprising as no ISGF3 dependent genes are able to be induced in response to IFN (Kimura et al.,

1996). Human cells which lack *IRF9* are unable to express IRF7, therefore no *IFNA* genes are able to be induced (Sato et al., 1998).

NEGATIVE REGULATION OF SIGNALING

An important advance in our understanding of the fine-tuning of signaling responses is the discovery of negative regulators. These occur at all levels of responses: extracellular through soluble receptors and binding proteins, intracellular as negative regulators of signal transduction, transcriptional repressors and products of gene expression with negative effects on biological functions. Just as tumor suppressor genes are essential for keeping cancer development in check by opposing the effects of oncogenes so the negative regulators of immune responses are necessary to prevent the consequences of unchecked immune stimulation which can result in chronic disease including autoimmunity and even death. Well characterized negative regulators of cytokine signaling include phosphatases, PIAS proteins and SOCS proteins (see below). A more recent type of negative regulation includes conjugation to ISG15, a member of a ubiquitin-like protein family. This 'ISGylation' targets JAK, STAT and other cellular proteins for degradation (Malakhov et al., 2003).

Phosphatases

The tyrosine phosphatase SHP1 is a protein tyrosine phosphatase (PTP) that contains an SH2 domain and is expressed primarily in hemopoietic cells. The 'moth-eaten' mice, which are *Shp1* deficient, suffer from multiple hemopoietic abnormalities including autoimmunity and macrophage hyperactivation, indicative of a malfunction in negative regulation (Shultz et al., 1993, 1997; Tsui et al., 1993). In *Shp1-/-* macrophages stimulated with IFNα, an increase in the amplitude of JAK1 phosphorylation is observed (David et al., 1995). The recruitment of SHP1 to the receptor complex results in the dephosphorylation of the receptor associated JAK1 (Haque et al., 1998; Migone et al., 1998; Weiss and Schlessinger, 1998); but interestingly the levels of phosphorylated TYK2 were no different from the wild-type macrophages implying that there was some specificity in the target substrates of SHP1 (David et al., 1995). Other receptor complexes sensitive to SHP1 include the IL3 receptor, erythropoietin (Epo) receptor, steel factor and colony stimulating factor 1 (CSF1) (Yi et al., 1993; David et al., 1995; Klingmuller et al., 1995; Chen et al., 1996; Paulson et al., 1996). CD45 was discovered as the first transmembrane PTP (Charbonneau et al., 1988) which differs from SHP1 in that it contains two PTPase domains with one lacking enzyme activity. CD45 has been demonstrated to be a JAK phosphatase in cells of hematopoietic lineage in response to a variety of cytokines including IL-3, IL-4, EPO and IFNα (Irie-Sasaki

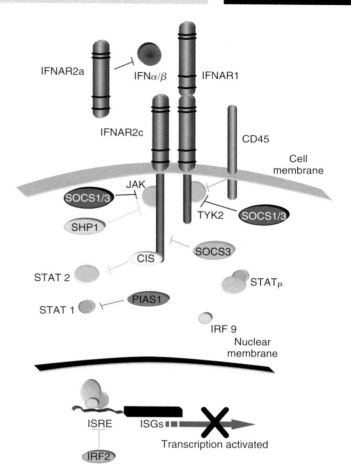

Figure 5.3 Negative regulation of signaling. Numerous proteins mediate negative effects on individual components of the JAK/STAT pathway induced by type I interferons. Factors involved include the phosphatases SHP1 and CD45, PIAS, SOCS1, SOCS3, CIS and IRF2.

et al., 2001; Penninger et al., 2001). *Cd45-/-* mice have defects in thymic development due to enhanced apoptosis, and dysfunctional TCR signaling and are more resistant to lethal coxsackie viral infection due to amplified IFNα antiviral activity (Irie-Sasaki et al., 2001). Interestingly CD45 also has the ability to function in a positive capacity in T cell antiproliferative activities in response to IFNα/β (Petricoin et al., 1997). It has also been found through the use of *Cd45-/-* cells that CD45 is a critical positive regulator of the T cell receptor and the B cell receptor in the activation and development of lymphocytes (Kishihara et al., 1993; Byth et al., 1996).

Protein inhibitors of activated STATs (PIAS)

Activated STAT molecules are a target for negative regulation of signal transduction by a family of proteins comprising five structurally related members PIAS1/GBP, PIAS3, PIASxα, PIASxβ and PIASγ (Chung et al., 1997; Liu et al., 1998). Each of the PIAS proteins contains a central zinc finger and an acidic transactivation domain at the C-terminal (Chung et al., 1997; Liu et al., 1998). These proteins prevent DNA recognition by binding to phosphorylated STAT dimers, thus inhibiting STAT mediated signaling cascades (Shuai, 2000). PIAS1 was discovered as a specific binding partner of activated STAT1, but not of STAT2 or STAT3 in vivo (Liu et al., 1998). PIAS3 (Chung et al., 1997) interacts with phosphorylated STAT3 and not STAT1 (Liu et al., 1998). The in vivo impact of PIAS proteins has not yet been investigated.

Suppressors of cytokine signaling (SOCS)

Socs1 was the first member of this family to be discovered, by three independent groups, as an inhibitor of IL-6 function (Starr et al., 1997), as JAB using a yeast two hybrid screen for JAK2-binding proteins (Endo et al., 1997), and as SSI1 with homology to the SH2 domain of STAT3 and termed STAT induced STAT inhibitor (SSI-1) (Naka et al., 1997). Subsequently, database searches have revealed a family of SOCS proteins including CIS and SOCS1-7. Each SOCS family member contains a conserved SH2 domain and a 40 amino acid C-terminal region of homology termed the 'SOCS box' which targets bound proteins for ubiquitin-mediated degradation via binding to Elongin BC complex.

SOCS1

SOCS 1 is rapidly induced by cytokines including types I and II IFNs, IL-2, IL-4, IL-6, GH, G-CSF and LIF as well as LPS (Naka et al., 1997; Endo et al., 1997; Starr et al., 1997; Adams et al., 1998; Sakamoto et al., 1998; Song and Shuai, 1998; Losman et al., 1999; Stoiber et al., 1999). SOCS1 binds to JAK1 and 2 and Tyk2 via its SH2 domain to inhibit kinase activity and cytokine signaling. SOCS1-/- mice die as neonates with severe multiorgan leukocyte infiltration and necrosis due to a hypersensitivity to IFNγ signaling. Thus, this phenotype can be rescued by crossing mice to IFNγ null mice or by injection of neutralizing antibodies to IFNγ. Subsequent studies have demonstrated that the SOCS1 deficient mice demonstrate more subtle but important roles in regulating other aspects of the immune response via IL-12, IL-2, IL-4, IL-7, IL-15 (Eyles et al., 2002; Chong et al., 2003; Cornish et al., 2003). Our own studies further demonstrate that when challenged with viral infection, an essential role of SOCS1 in regulating type I IFN responses in vivo is uncovered (Alexander et al., 1999; Fenner et al., 2004).

SOCS3

SOCS3 is the other member of this family that has been shown to have immunoregulatory roles. SOCS3 is also induced by many cytokines including IL-6, type I and II IFNs, GH, EPO, GM-CSF, LIF (Gadina et al., 2001). However, unlike SOCS1, it binds to the activated receptors to inhibit JAKs. Socs3-/- mice die during embryogenesis,

between E11.5 and E16.5. Recently, conditional SOCS3 targeting has demonstrated its importance in regulating IL-6 signaling via STAT3 in macrophages (Marine et al., 1999). Furthermore, elegant microarray experiments have demonstrated that the gene expression profile of IL-6 treated cells in Socs3 deficient hepatocytes is similar to that induced by IFNγ, thus implying that normally, SOCS3 acts to prevent IFNγ responses in IL-6 stimulated cells (Croker et al., 2003).

Other SOCS

CIS and SOCS2, unlike SOCS1 and 3, are not induced by cytokines such as type I and II IFNs, IL-6 and similarly do not inhibit their actions in vitro or in vivo. The lack of an obvious phenotype in Cis-/- mice suggests that it might be functionally redundant (Gadina et al., 2001). Mice that are deficient for Socs2 are larger in size compared to their wild-type littermates due to a hyperresponsiveness to GH and insulin-like growth factor 1 (IGF1) (Metcalf et al., 2000).

Non-cytokine interaction of SOCS

LPS and CpG DNA acting through TLR4 and TLR9 in macrophages respectively induce both Socs1 and 3 (Stoiber et al., 1999; Crespo et al., 2000; Dalpke et al., 2001; Kinjyo et al., 2002). Then, similarly to other factors that induce Socs1 and 3, the proteins are capable of acting in a negative feedback loop to switch off LPS signaling through both direct and indirect mechanisms (Nakagawa et al., 2002). Mice deficient in Socs-1 were hypersensitive to LPS-induced shock. Socs-1-/- macrophages were also refractory to LPS-induced tolerance which is a transient state of LPS non-responsiveness following initial LPS exposure, preventing excessive or prolonged pro-inflammatory response to continued LPS exposure. These studies thus demonstrate that SOCS1 is a key regulatory component of the innate immune system (Kinjyo et al., 2002).

The phenotype of the Socs1-/- mice illustrates the importance of keeping cytokine signaling in check by negative regulation; too much IFNγ signaling is lethal!

SIGNALING MOLECULES IN HUMAN DISEASES

Aberrations in the activity or levels of signaling molecules are features of certain human immune diseases and often are the underlying cause of disease. For example, there are immunodeficiency disorders that are caused by mutation in the gene encoding a signaling molecule.

Mutations in genes encoding signaling molecules in the TLR/NF-κB pathway including IKKγ, IKBα and IRAK4 (Picard et al., 2004) give rise to a variety of immunodeficiency disorders. For example children with inherited IRAK4 mutations develop infections caused by pyogenic bacteria and cells from these patients do not activate NF-κB or MAP kinase pathways or inflammatory cytokines in response to TLR activation (Picard et al., 2003). These findings highlight the importance of dissecting the TLR mediated immunity in humans.

Mutations in components of the cytokine signal transduction pathway also result in immunodeficiency diseases in humans. Interestingly, different mutations in STAT1 that affect type I and II IFN signaling give rise to susceptibility to viral infection and mycobacterial infection; the latter is similar to patients with mutations in the IFNγ receptor gene (Dupuis et al., 2003). However, mutations in STAT 1 that affect IFNγ signaling specifically give rise to a susceptibility to mycobacterial infection (not viral infection) (Dupuis et al., 2001). Unsurprisingly from the lethality of the mouse gene targeting studies, mutations in the ubiquitously expressed JAKs 1 and 2 have not been found in humans. However, patients deficient in JAK3, which is mainly expressed in hemopoietic cells, present with severe combined immunodeficiency diseases (SCID), which is more severe than patients with the more common genetic mutations in the X chromosome-located γ common chain gene associated with IL-2, 4, 7, 9 and 15 signaling (Aringer et al., 1999).

Not only can signaling molecules involved in immune responses contribute to the pathogenesis of disease, but they are also candidates for targeting by immunosuppressive therapeutic drugs. Since JAK 3 is necessary for signaling in response to many immunomodulatory cytokines, it is a prime target for immunosuppressive therapy. Indeed, Changelian et al. (2003) recently reported the prevention of organ allograft rejection using a specific JAK3 inhibitor.

Cytokine signaling molecules are frequently present in immune diseases in an activated state. For example, markedly increased levels of STAT6, which is critical for IL-4 signaling and Th2 response, are found in asthmatic patients (Mullings et al., 2001). There is a correlation between the levels of SOCS3 and allergic diseases including dermatitis and asthma associated with the role for SOCS3 in mediating Th2 responses (Seki et al., 2003). Furthermore, constitutively activated STAT3 is found in intestinal cells from patients with Crohn's disease (Lovato et al., 2003). Given these associations of signaling molecules in disease, the measurement of the levels, activation status or subcellular location of signaling molecules is likely to become an important component of assessing the status of immune activation in diseases and likely underlying causes.

PATHOGEN EVASION OF IMMUNE RESPONSE BY TARGETING SIGNALING MOLECULES

Viral evasion of host defense by blocking the immune response is a well established phenomenon. Molecules involved in signaling for responses to TLR and cytokines and IFNs are prime targets of pathogen-encoded inhibitory molecules.

Vaccinia virus (VV) is a pox-virus that encodes several genes that subvert host immune responses. Two of these, A46R and A52R, encode proteins that block TLR-mediated signal transduction. A46R has homology to the TIR family of adaptors and blocks MyD88 dependent signaling (Bowie et al., 2000). A52R blocks IRAK2 and TRAF6 mediated signaling (Harte et al., 2003).

Viral inhibition of cytokine signaling is also very well reported. HPV E7 inhibits IFNα signaling by binding to IRF9 and preventing its translocation to the nucleus and participation in ISGF3 formation (Barnard and McMillan, 1999). The HPV E6 protein interferes with IFNα signaling by interaction with Tyk2 and consequent inhibition of Stat activation (Li et al., 1999b). The adenovirus E1A protein also inhibits IFNα signaling at the level of ISGF3 formation (Gutch and Reich, 1991; Kalvakolunu et al.,1991). Paramyxoviruses target STATs 1, 2 and 3 for degradation thereby inhibiting cytokine signal transduction (Ulane and Horvath, 2002; Ulane et al., 2003). Human cytomegalovirus inhibits IFNγ-induction of class II MHC by targeting JAK1 for degradation (Miller et al., 1998).

SUMMARY AND CONCLUSIONS

The signal transducing molecules are necessary for the immune response; they are often important points of regulation (positive and negative); mutations in their genes can lead to human immunodeficiency disease and they are targeted by infectious agents for the purpose of subverting the host immune response. Determination of the levels of activation or translocation of signal transducing molecules such as STATs can be a valuable indicator of cell/status/function and therefore makes an important contribution to measuring immunity. While this field has come a long way in the past decade, the future promises more riches. Current genome information tells us that there are hundreds of kinases, phosphatases, adaptor protein receptors and secreted proteins in the human genome. Genome-wide analyses of polymorphisms, mutations, expression profiling and proteomic approaches to determine protein interactions and enumerate biomarkers will elaborate the function of more signaling pathways and components and markers of immune responses.

REFERENCES

Adams, T.E., Hansen, J.A., Starr, R., Nicola, N.A., Hilton, D.J. and Billestrup, N. (1998). Growth hormone preferentially induces the rapid, transient expression of SOCS3, a novel inhibitor of cytokine signaling. J Biol Chem 273, 1285–1287.

Adib-Conquy, M. and Cavaillon, J.M. (2002). Gamma interferon and granulocyte/monocyte colony-stimulating factor prevent endotoxin tolerance in human monocytes by promoting interleukin-1 receptor-associated kinase expression and its association to MyD88 and not by modulating TLR4 expression. J Biol Chem 277, 27927–27934.

Akira, S., Takeda, K. and Kaisho, T. (2001). Toll-like receptors: critical proteins linking innate and acquired immunity. Nat Immunol 2, 675–680.

Akira, S., Nishio, Y., Inoue, M. et al. (1994). Molecular cloning of APRF, a novel IFN-stimulated gene factor 3 p91-related transcription factor involved in the gp130-mediated signaling pathway. Cell 77, 63–71.

Alexander, W.S., Starr, R., Fenner, J.E. et al. (1999). SOCS1 is a critical inhibitor of interferon γ signaling and prevents the potentially fatal neonatal actions of this cytokine. Cell 98, 597–608.

Aringer, M., Cheng, A., Nelson, J.W. et al. (1999). Janus kinases and their role in growth and disease. Life Sci 64, 2173–2186.

Azam, M., Erdjument-Bromage, H., Kreider, B.L. et al. (1995). Interleukin-3 signals through multiple isoforms of Stat5. EMBO J 14,1402–1411.

Barahmand-Pour, F., Meinke, A., Groner, B. and Decker, T. (1998). Jak2-Stat5 interactions analyzed in yeast. J Biol Chem 273, 12567–12575.

Barnard, P. and McMillan, N.A. (1999). The human papillomavirus E7 oncoprotein abrogates signaling mediated by interferon-alpha. Virology 259, 305–313.

Boulay, J.L., O'Shea, J.J. and Paul, W.E. (2001). Molecular phylogeny within type I cytokines and their cognate receptors. Immunity 19, 159–163.

Bowie, A., Kiss-Toth, E., Symons, J.A., Smith, G.L., Dower, S.K. and O'Neill, L.A. (2000). A46R and A52R from vaccinia virus are antagonists of host IL-1 and toll-like receptor signaling. Proc Natl Acad Sci USA 97, 10162–10267.

Bromberg, J. and Darnell, J.E. Jr (2000). The role of STATs in transcriptional control and their impact on cellular function. Oncogene 19, 2468–2473.

Byth, K.F., Conroy, L.A., Howlett, S. et al. (1996). CD45-null transgenic mice reveal a positive regulatory role for CD45 in early thymocyte development, in the selection of CD4+CD8+ thymocytes, and B cell maturation. J Exp Med 183, 1707–1718.

Cao, X., Shores, E.W., Hu-Li, J. et al. (1995). Defective lymphoid development in mice lacking expression of the common cytokine receptor gamma chain. Immunity 2, 223–238.

Cao, Z., Xiong, M., Takeuchi, T., Kurama, T. and Goeddel, D.V. (1996). TRAF6 is a signal transducer for interleukin-1. Nature 383, 443–446.

Charbonneau, H., Tonks, N.K., Walsh, K.A. and Fischer, E.H. (1988). The leukocyte common antigen (CD45): a putative receptor-linked protein tyrosine phosphatase. Proc Natl Acad Sci USA 85, 7182–7186.

Chauhan, D., Kharbanda, S.M., Ogata, A. et al. (1995). Oncostatin M induces association of Grb2 with Janus kinase JAK2 in multiple myeloma cells. J Exp Med 182, 1801–1806.

Chen, F.E. and Ghosh, G. (1999). Regulation of DNA binding by Rel/NF-kappa B transcription factors: structural views. Oncogene 18, 6845–6852.

Chen, H.E., Chang, S., Trub, T. and Neel, B.G. (1996). Regulation of colony-stimulating factor 1 receptor signaling by the SH2 domain-containing tyrosine phosphatase SHPTP1. Mol Cell Biol 16, 3685–3697.

Chen, X., Vinkemeier, U., Zhao, Y., Jeruzalmi, D., Darnell, J.E. Jr and Kuriyan, J. (1998). Crystal structure of a tyrosine phosphorylated STAT-1 dimer bound to DNA. Cell 93, 827–829.

Chong, M.M., Cornish, A.L., Darwiche, R. et al. (2003). Suppressor of cytokine signaling-1 is a critical regulator of interleukin-7-dependant CD8+ T cell differentiation. Immunity 18, 475–487.

Chung, C.D., Liao, J., Liu, B. et al. (1997). Specific inhibition of Stat3 signal transduction by PIAS3. Science 278, 1803–1805.

Colamonici, O.R., Poterfield, B., Domanaski, P., Constantinescu, S. and Pfeffer, L.M. (1994). Complementation of the interferon alpha response in resistant cells by expression of the cloned subunit of the interferon alpha receptor. A central role of this subunit in interferon alpha signaling. J Biol Chem 269, 9598–9602.

Copeland, N.G., Gilbert, D.J., Schindler, C. et al. (1995). Distribution of the mammalian Stat gene family in mouse chromosome. Genomics 29, 225–228.

Cornish, A.L, Chong, M.M., Davey, G.M. et al. (2003). Suppressor of cytokine signaling-1 regulates signaling in response to interleukin-2 and other gamma c-dependent cytokines in peripheral T cells. J Biol Chem 278, 22755–22761.

Crespo, A., Filla, M.B., Russell, S.W. and Murphy, W.J. (2000). Indirect induction of suppressor of cytokine signaling-1 in macrophages stimulated with bacterial lipopolysaccharide: partial role of autocrine/paracrine interferon-alpha/beta. Biochem J 349, 99–104.

Croker, B.A., Krebs, D.L., Zhang, J.G. et al. (2003). SOCS3 negatively regulates IL-6 signaling in vivo. Nat Immunol 4, 540–545.

Dalpke, A.H., Opper, S., Zimmermann, S. and Heeg, K. (2001). Suppressors of cytokine signaling (SOCS)-1 and SOCS-3 are induced by CpG-DNA and modulate cytokine responses in APCs. J Immunol 166, 7082–7089.

Darnell, J.E. Jr (1997): STATs and gene regulation. Science 277, 1630–1635.

Darnell, J.E. Jr, Kerr, I.M. and Stark, G.R. (1994). Jak-STAT pathways and transcriptional activation in response to IFNs and other extracellular signaling proteins. Science 264, 1415–1421.

David, M., Chen, H.E., Goelz, S., Larner, A.C. and Neel, B.G. (1995). Differential regulation of the alpha/beta interferon-stimulated Jak/Stat pathway by the SH2 domain-containing tyrosine phosphatase SHPTP1. Mol Cell Biol 15, 7050–7058.

Di Santo, J.P., Kuhn, R. and Muller W. (1995). Common cytokine receptor gamma chain (gamma c)-dependent cytokines: understanding in vivo functions by gene targeting. Immunol Rev 148, 19–34.

Diebold, S.S., Kaisho, T., Hemmi, H., Akira, S., Reis, E. and Sousa, C. (2004). Innate antiviral responses by means of TLR7-mediated recognition of single-stranded RNA. Science 303, 1529–1531.

Driggers, P.H., Ennist, D.L., Gleason, S.L. et al. (1990). An interferon gamma-regulated protein that binds the interferon-inducible enhancer element of major histocompatibility complex class I genes. Proc Nal Acad Sci USA 87, 3743–3747.

Duncan, G.S., Mittrucker, H.W., Kagi, D., Matsuyama, T. and Mak, T.W. (1996). The transcription factor interferon regulatory factor-1 is essential for natural killer cell function in vivo. J Exp Med 184, 2043–2048.

Dupuis, S., Jouanguy, E. Al-Hajjar, S. et al. (2003). Impaired response to interferon-alpha/beta and lethal viral disease in human STAT1 deficiency. Nat Genet 33, 388–391.

Dupuis, S., Dargemont, C., Fieschi, C. et al. (2001). Impairment of mycobacterial but not viral immunity by a germline human STAT1 mutation. Science 29, 3300–3303.

Durbin, J.E., Hackenmiller, R., Simon, M.C. and Levy, D.E. (1996). Targeted disruption of the mouse Stat1 gene results in compromised innate immunity to viral disease. Cell 84, 443–450.

Eisenbeis, C.F., Singh, H. and Storb, U. (1995). Pip, a novel IRF family member, is a lymphoid-specific, PU.1-dependent transcriptional activator. Genes Dev 9,1377–1387.

Endo, T.A., Masuhara, M., Yokouchi, M. et al. (1997). A new protein containing an SH2 domain that inhibits JAK kinases. Nature 387, 921–924.

Eyles, J.L., Metcalf, D., Grusby, M.J., Hilton, D.J. and Starr, R. (2002). Negative regulation of interleukin-12 signaling by suppressor of cytokine signaling 1. J Biol Chem 277, 43735–43740.

Farrar, J.D., Smith, J.D., Murphy, T.L., Leung, S., Stark, G.R. and Murphy, K.M. (2000). Selective loss of type I interferon-induced STAT4 activation caused by a minisatellite insertion in mouse Stat2. Nat Immunol 1, 65–69.

Fenner et al., (2004). Submitted for publication.

Finbloom, D.S. and Winestock, K.D. (1995). IL-10 induces the tyrosine phosphorylation of tyk2 and jak1 and the differential assembly of Stat1a and Stat3 complexes in human T cells and monocytes. J Immunol 155, 1079–1090.

Fitzgerald, K.A., McWhirter, S.M., Faia, K.L. et al. (2003). IKK epsilon and TBK1 are essential components of the IRF3 signaling pathway. Nat Immunol 4, 491–496.

Fitzgerald, K.A., Palsson-McDermott, E.M., Bowie, A.G. et al. (2001). Mal (MyD88-adapter-like) is required for Toll-like receptor-4 signal transduction. Nature 413, 78–83.

Fu, X.Y. and Zhang, J.J. (1993). Transcription factor p91 interacts with the epidermal growth factor receptor and mediates activation of the c-fos gene promoter. Cell 74, 1135–1145.

Fu, X.Y., Schindler, C., Improta, T., Aebersold, R. and Darnell, J.E. Jr (1992). The proteins of isgf-3, the interferon alpha-induced transcriptional activator, define a gene family involved in signal transduction. Proc Natl Acad Sci USA 89, 7840–7843.

Gadina, M., Hilton, D., Johnston, J.A. et al. (2001). Signaling by type I and II cytokine receptors: ten years after. Curr Opin Immunol 13, 363–373.

Gough, N.M., Raker, S., Harpur, A. and Wilks, A.F. (1995). Localisation of genes for two members of the JAK family of protein tyrosine kinases to murine chromosomes 4 and 19. Mamm Genome 6, 247–248.

Ghosh, S. and Baltimore, D. (1990). Activation in vitro of NFκB by phosphorylation of its inhibitor I kappa B. Nature 344, 678–682.

Gupta, S., Yan, H., Wong, L.H., Ralph, S., Krolewski, J. and Schindler, C. (1996). The SH2 domains of Stat1 and Stat2 mediate multiple interactions in the transduction of IFN-α signals. EMBO J 15, 1075–1084.

Gutch, M.J. and Reich, N.C. (1991). Repression of the interferon signal transduction pathway by the adenovirus E1A oncogene. Proc Natl Acad Sci USA 88, 7913–7917.

Hamilton, J.A., Whitty, G.A., Kola, I. and Hertzog, P.J. (1996). Endogenous IFN-alpha beta suppresses colony-stimulating factor (CSF)-1-stimulated macrophage DNA synthesis and mediates inhibitory effects of lipopolysaccharide and TNF-alpha. J Immunol 156, 2553–2557.

Haque, S.J., Harbor, P., Tabrizi, M., Yi, T. and Williams, B.R. (1998). Protein-tyrosine phosphatase Shp-1 is a negative regulator of IL-4- and Il-13-dependent signal transduction. J Biol Chem 273, 33893–33896.

Harpur, A.G., Andres, A.C., Ziemiecki, A., Aston, R.R. and Wilks, A.F. (1992). JAK2 a third member of the JAK family of protein tyrosine kinases. Oncogene 7, 1347–1353.

Harte, M.T., Haga, I.R., Maloney, G. et al. (2003). The poxvirus protein A52R targets Toll-like receptor signaling complexes to suppress host defense. J Exp Med 197, 343–351.

Heil, F., Hemmi, H., Hochrein, H. et al. (2004). Species-specific recognition of single-stranded RNA via toll-like receptor 7 and 8. Science 303, 1526–1529.

Hertzog, P.J., O'Neill, L.A.J. and Hamilton, J.A. (2003). The interferon in TLR signaling: more than just antiviral? Trends Immunol 24, 534–539.

Hida, S., Ogasawara, K., Sato, K. et al. (2000). CD8(+) T cell-mediated skin disease in mice lacking IRF-2, the transcriptional attenuator of interferon-alpha/beta signalling. Immunity 13, 643–655.

Hoebe, K., Du, X., Georgel, P. et al. (2003). Identification of Lps2 as a key regulator of MyD88-independent TIR signaling. Nature 424, 743–748.

Holtschke, T., Lohler, J., Kanno, Y. et al. (1996). Immunodeficiency and chronic myelogenous leukemia-like syndrome in mice with a targeted mutation of the ICSBP gene. Cell 87, 307–317.

Hornig, T., Barton, G.M., Flavell, R.A. and Medzhitov, R. (2002). The adaptor molecule TIRAP provides signalling specificity for Toll-like receptors. Nature 420, 329–333.

Horvath, C.M. (2000). STAT proteins and transcriptional responses to extracellular signals. Trends Biochem Sci 25, 496–502.

Horvath, C.M. and Darnell, J.E. Jr (1996). The antiviral state induced by alpha interferon and gamma interferon requires transcriptionally active Stat 1 protein. J Virol 70, 647–650.

Hou, J., Schindler, U., Henzel, W.J., Ho, T.C., Brasseur, M. and McKnight, S.L. (1994). An interleukin-4-induced transcription factor: IL-4 Stat. Science 265, 1701–1706.

Hou, X.S., Melnick, M.B. and Perrimon, N. (1996). Marelle acts downstream of the Drosophila HOP/JAK kinase and encodes a protein similar to the mammalian STATs. Cell 84, 411–419.

Hu, Y., Baud, V., Delhase, M. et al. (1999). Abnormal morphogenesis but intact IKK activation in mice lacking the IKK alpha subunit if IkappaB kinase. Science 284, 31603–31620.

Hu, J., Jacinto, R., McCall, C. and Li, L. (2002). Regulation of IL-1 receptor-associated kinases by lipopolysaccharide. J Immunol 168, 3910–3914.

Hwang, S.Y., Hertzog, P.J., Holland, K.A. et al. (1995). A null mutation in the gene encoding a type I interferon receptor component eliminates antiproliferative and antiviral responses to interferons α and β and alters macrophage responses. Proc Natl Acad Sci USA 92, 1124–1128.

Ihle, J.N. (1995). Cytokine receptor signaling. Nature 377, 591–594.

Irie-Sasaki, J., Sasaki, T., Matsumoto, W. et al. (2001). CD45 is a JAK phosphatase and negatively regulates cytokine receptor signaling. Nature 409, 349–354.

Jacinto, R., Hartung, T., McCall, C. and Li, L. (2002). Lipopolysaccharide- and lipoteichoic acid-induced tolerance and cross-tolerance: distinct alterations in IL-1 receptor-associated kinase. J Immunol 168, 6136–6141.

Janeway, C.A. Jr and Medzhitov, R. (2002). Innate immune recognition. Ann Rev Immunol 20, 197–216.

Kalvakolanu, D.V.R., Bandyopadhyay, S.K., Harter, M.L. and Sen, G.C. (1991). Inhibition of interferon-inducible gene expression by adenoviral E1A proteins: Block in transcriptional complex formation. Proc Natl Acad Sci USA 88, 7459–7463.

Kanakaraj, P., Ngo, K., Wu, Y. et al. (1999). Defective interleukin (IL)-18-mediated natural killer and T helper cell type 1 responses in IL-1 receptor-associated kinase (IRAK)-deficient mice. J Exp Med 189, 1129–1138.

Kanakaraj, P., Schafer, P.H., Cavender, D.E. et al. (1998). Interleukin (IL)-1 receptor-associated kinase (IRAK) requirement for optimal induction of multiple IL-1 signaling pathways and IL-6 production. J Exp Med 187, 2073–2079.

Kaplan, M.H., Sun, Y.L., Hoey, T. and Grusby, M.J. (1996). Impaired IL12 responses and enhanced development of Th2 cells in Stat4 deficient mice. Nature 382, 174–177.

Karaghiosoff, M., Steinborn, R., Kovarik, O. et al. (2003). Central role for typeI interferons and Tyk2 in lipopolysaccharide-induced endotoxin shock. Nat Immunol 4, 471–477.

Karin, M. (1999). How NF-kappaB is activated: the role of the IkappaB kinase (IKK) complex. Oncogene 18, 6867–6874.

Kawai, T., Takeuchi, O., Fujita, T. et al. (2001). Lipopolysaccharide stimulates the MyD88-independent pathway and results in activation of IFN-regulatory factor3 and the expression of a subset of lipopolysaccharide-inducible genes. J Immunol 167, 5887–5894.

Kawai, T., Adachi, O., Ogawa, T., Takeda, K. and Akira, S. (1999). Unresponsiveness of MyD88-deficient mice to endotoxin. Immunity 11, 115–122.

Kimura, T., Kadokawa, Y., Harada, H. et al. (1996). Essential and non-redundant roles of p48 (ISGF3 gamma) and IRF-1 in both type I and type II interferon responses, as revealed by gene targeting studies. Gene Cells 1, 115–124.

Kinjyo, I., Hanada, T., Inagaki-Ohara, K. et al. (2002). SOCS1/JAB is a negative regulator of LPS-induced macrophage activation. Immunity 17, 583–591.

Kishihara, K., Penninger, J., Wallace, V.A. et al. (1993). Normal B lymphocyte development but impaired T cell maturation in CD45-exon6 protein tyrosine phosphatase-deficient mice. Cell 74, 43–56.

Klingmuller, U., Lorenz, U., Cantley, L.C., Neel, B.G. and Lodish, H.F. (1995). Specific recruitment of SH-PTP1 to the erythropoietin receptor causes inactivation of JAK2 and termination of proliferative signals. Cell 80, 729–738.

Kobayashi, K., Hernandez, L.D., Galan, J.E., Janeway, C.A. Jr, Medzhitov, R. and Flavell, R.A. (2002). IRAK-M is a negative regulator of Toll-like receptor signaling. Cell 110, 191–202.

Kono, D.H., Owens, D.G. and Wechsler, A.R. (1996). Jak3 maps to chromosome 8. Mamm Genome 7, 476–477.

Krolewski, J.J., Lee, R., Eddy, R., Shows, B. and Dalla-Favera, R. (1990). Identification and chromosomal mapping of new human tyrosine kinase genes. Oncogene 5, 277–282.

Larner, A.C., David, M., Feldman, G.M. et al. (1993). Tyrosine phosphorylation of DNA binding proteins by multiple cytokines. Science 261, 1730–1733.

Leonard, W.J. and O'Shea, J.J. (1998). Jaks and STATs: biological implications. Ann Rev Immunol 16, 293–322.

Leung, S., Qureshi, S.A., Kerr, I.M., Darnell, E.J. Jr and Stark, G.R. (1995). Role of stat2 in the alpha interferon signaling pathway. Mol Cell Biol 15, 1312–1317.

Levy, D.E., Lew, D.J., Decker, T., Kessler, D.S. and Darnell, J.E. Jr (1990). Synergistic interaction between interferon-alpha and interferon-gamma through induced synthesis of one subunit of the transcription factor ISGF3. EMBO J 9, 1105–1111.

Li, Q., Mercurio, F., Lee, K.-F. and Verma, I.M. (1999a). Severe liver degeneration in mice lacking the IκB kinase. Science 284, 321–325.

Li, S., Labrecque, S., Gauzzi, M.C. et al. (1999b). The human papilloma virus (HPV)-18 E6 oncoprotein physically associates with Tyk2 and impairs Jak-STAT activation by interferon-alpha. Oncogene 18, 5727–5737.

Lin, J.X., Mietz, J., Modi, W.S., John, S. and Leonard, W.J. (1996). Cloning of human Stat5B. Reconstitution of interleukin-2-induced Stat5A and Stat5B DNA binding activity in COS-7 cells. J Biol Chem 271, 10738–10744.

Lin, J.X., Migone, T.S., Tsang, M. et al. (1995). The role of shared receptor motifs and common Stat proteins in the generation of cytokine pleiotropy and redundancy by IL-2, IL-4, IL-7, IL-13 and IL-15. Immunity 2, 331–339.

Liu, K.D., Gaffen, S.L. and Goldsmith, M.A. (1998). JAK/STAT signaling by cytokine receptors. Curr Opin Immunol 10, 271–278.

Liu, X., Robinson, G.W., Wagner, K., Garret, L., Ulynshaw-Boris, A. and Hennighausen, L. (1997). Stat5a is mandatory for adult mammary gland development and lactogenesis. Genes Dev 11, 179–186.

Lohoff, M., Duncan, G.S., Ferrick, D. et al. (2000). Deficiency in the transcription factor interferon regulatory factor (IRF)-2 leads to severely compromised development of natural killer and T helper type 1 cells. J Exp Med 192, 325–336.

Losman, J.A., Chen, X.P., Hilton, D. and Rothman, P. (1999). Cutting edge: SOCS1 is a potent inhibitor of IL4 signal transduction. J Immunol 162, 3770–3774.

Lovato, P., Brender, C., Agnholt, J. et al. (2003). Constitutive STAT3 activation in intestinal T cells from patients with Crohn's disease. J Biol Chem 278, 16777–16781.

Macchi, P., Villa, A., Giliani, S. et al. (1995). Mutations of Jak-3 gene in patients with autosomal severe combined immune deficiency (SCID). Nature 377, 65–68.

Malakhov, M.P., Kim, K., Malakhova, O.A., Jacobs, B.S., Borden, E.C. and Zhang, D.E. (2003). High-throughput immunoblotting. Ubiquitiin-like protein ISG15 modifies key regulators of signal transduction. J Biol Chem 278, 16608–16613.

Marie, I., Durbin, J.E. and Levy, D.E. (1998). Differential viral induction of distinct interferon-alpha genes by positive feedback through interferon regulatory factor-7. EMBO J 17, 6660–6669.

Marine, J.C., McKay, C., Wang, D. et al. (1999). SOCS3 is essential in the regulation of fetal liver erythropoiesis. Cell 98, 617–627.

Martinez-Moczygemba, M., Gutch, M.J., French, D.L. and Reich, N.C. (1997). Distinct STAT structure promotes interaction of STAT2 with the p48 subunit of the interferon-alpha-stimulated transcription factor ISGF3. J Biol Chem 272, 20070–20076.

Matsuguchi, T., Inhorn, R.C., Carless, N., Xu, G., Druker, B. and Griffin JD. (1995). Tyrosine phosphorylation of p95Vav in myeloid cells is regulated by GM-CSF, IL-3 and steel factor and is constitutively increased by p210BCR/ABL. EMBO J 14, 257–265.

Matsumoto, M., Tanaka, N., Harada, H. et al. (1999). Activation of the transcription factor ISGF3 by interferon-gamma. Biol Chem 380, 699–703.

Matsuyama, T., Grossman, A., Mittrucker, H.W. et al. (1995). Molecular cloning of LSIRF, a lymphoid-specific member of the interferon regulatory factor family that binds the interferon-stimulated response element (ISRE). Nucleic Acids Res 23, 2127–2136.

Matsuyama, T., Kimura, T., Kitagawa, M. et al. (1993). Targeted disruption of IRF1 or IRF2 results in abnormal typeI IFN gene induction and aberrant lymphocyte development. Cell 75, 83–97.

Medzhitov, R., Preston-Hurlburt, P., Kopp, E. et al. (1998). MyD88 is an adaptor protein in the hToll/IL-1 receptor family signalling pathways. Mol Cell 2, 253–258.

Meraz, M.A., White, M., Sheehan, K.C.F. et al. (1996). Targeted disruption of the STAT1 gene in mice reveals unexpected physiologic specificity in the JAK-STAT signalling pathway. Cell 84, 431–442.

Mercurio, F., Zhu, B.W., Murray A. et al. (1997). IKK-1 and IKK-2: cytokine-activated IkappaB kinases essential for NF-kappaB activation. Science 278, 860–866.

Metcalf, D., Greenhalgh, C.J., Viney, E. et al. (2000). Gigantism is mice lacking suppressor of cytokine signaling-2. Nature 405, 1069–1073.

Migone, T.S., Cacalone, N.A., Taylor, N., Yi, T., Waldmann, T.A. and Johnston, J.A. (1998). Recruitment of SH2-containing protein tyrosine phosphatase SHP-1 to the interleukin 2 receptor; loss of SHP-1 expression in human T-lymphotropic virus typ I-transformed T cells. Proc Natl Acad Sci USA 95, 3845–3850.

Miller, D.M., Rahill, B.M., Boss, J.M. et al. (1998). Human cytomegalovirus inhibits major histocompatibility complex class II expression by disruption of the Jak/Stat pathway. J Exp Med 187, 675–683.

Mittrucker, H.W., Matsuyama, T., Grossman, A. et al. (1997). Requirement for the transcription factor LSIRF/IRF4 for mature B and T lymphocyte function. Science 275, 540–543.

Miyata, S., Matsuyama, T., Kodama, T. et al. (1999). STAT6 deficiency in a mouse model of allergen-induced airways inflammation abolishes eosinophilia but induces infiltration of CD8+ T cells. Clin Exp Allergy 29, 114–123.

Mui, A.L., Wakao, H., Harada, N., O'Farrell, A.M. and Miyajima, A. (1995). Interleukin-3 granulocyte-macrophage colony-stimulating factor, and interleukin-5 transduce signals through two forms of STAT5. J Leukoc Biol 57, 799–803.

Müller, M., Laxton, C., Briscoe, J. et al. (1993). Complementation of a mutant cell line: central role of the 91 kDa polypeptide of ISGF3 in the interferon-alpha and -gamma signal transduction pathways. EMBO J 12, 4221–4228.

Mustlin,T. and Tasken, K. (2003). Positive and negative regulation of T-cell activaton through kinases and phosphatases. Biochem J 371, 15–27.

Muzio, M., Ni, J., Feng, P. and Dixit, V.M. (1997). IRAK (Pelle) family member IRAK-2 and MyD88 as proximal mediators of IL-1 signaling. Science 278, 1612–1615.

Naka, T., Narazaki, M., Hirata, M. et al. (1997). Structure and function of a new STAT induced STAT inhibitor. Nature 387, 924–929.

Nelson, N., Marks, M.S., Driggers, P.H. and Ozato, K. (1993). Interferon consensus sequence-binding protein, a member of the interferon regulatory factor family, suppresses interferon-induced gene transcription. Mol Cell Biol 13, 588–599.

Neubauer, H., Cumano, A., Muller, M., Wu, H., Huffstadt, U. and Pfeffer, K. (1998). Jak2 deficiency defines an essential developmental checkpoint in definitive hematopoiesis. Cell 93, 397–409.

Nguyen, H., Hiscott, J. and Pitha, P.M. (1997). The growing family of interferon regulatory factors. Cytokine Growth Factor Rev 8, 293–312.

Nicholson, S.E., Willson, T.A., Farley, A. (1999). Mutational analyses of the SOCS proteins suggest a dual domain requirement but distinct mechanisms for inhibition of LIF and IL6 signal transduction. EMBO J 18, 375–385.

Noah, D.L., Blum, M.A. and Sherry, B. (1999). Interferon regulatory factor 3 is required for viral induction of beta interferon in primary cardiac myocyte cultures. J Virol 73, 10208–10213.

Nosaka, T., van Deursen, J.M., Tripp, R.A. et al. (1995). Defective lymphoid development in mice lacking Jak3. Science 270, 800–802.

Oakes, S.A., Candotti, F., Johnston, J.A. et al. (1996). Signaling via IL12 and IL4 in JAK3 dependent and independent pathways. Immunity 5, 605–615.

O'Neill, L.A.J. (2002). Toll-like receptor signal transduction and the tailoring of innate immunity: a role for Mal? Trends Immunol 23, 96–300.

O'Neill, L.A.J. (2004). Immunology. After the toll rush. Science 303, 1481–1482.

Oshiumi, H., Matsumoto, M., Funami, K., Akazawa, T. and Seya, T. (2003). TICAM1 an adapter molecule that participates in Toll-like receptor 3-mediated interferon-β induction. Nat Immunol 4, 161–167.

Owczarek, C.M., Hwang, S.Y., Holland, K.A. et al. (1997). Cloning and characterization of soluble and transmembrane isoforms of a novel component of the murine type I interferon receptor, IFNAR 2. J Biol Chem 272, 23865–23870.

Parganas, E., Wang, D., Stravopodis, D. et al. (1998). Jak2 is essential for signaling through a variety of cytokine receptors. Cell 93, 385–395.

Park, C., Li, S., Cha, E. and Schindler, C. (2000). Immune response in Stat 2 knockout mice. Immunity 13, 795–804.

Park, S.Y., Saijo, K., Takahashi, T. et al. (1995). Developmental defects of lymphoid cells in Jak3 kinase-deficient mice. Immunity 3, 771–782.

Paulson, R.F., Vesely, S., Siminovitch, K.A. and Bernstein, A. (1996). Signaling by the W/Kit receptor tyrosine kinase is negatively regulated in vivo by the protein tyrosine phosphatase Shp1. Nat Genet 13, 309–315.

Penninger, J.M., Irie-Sasaki, J., Sasaki, T. and Oliveira-dos-Santos, A.J. (2001). CD45: new jobs for an old acquaintance. Nat Immunol 2, 389–396.

Petricoin, E.F., Ito, S., Williams, B. L. et al. (1997). Antiproliferative action of interferon-alpha requires componenets of T-cell-receptor signalling. Nature 390, 677–687.

Pfeffer, L.M., Mullersman, J.E., Pfeffer, S.R., Murti, A., Shi, W. and Yang, C.H. (1997). Stat3 as an adapter to couple phosphatidylinositol 3-kinase to the IFNAR1 chain of the type I interferon receptor. Science 279, 1418–1420.

Platanias, L.C. (2003). The p38 mitogen-activated protein kinase pathway and its role in interferon signaling. Pharmacol Ther 98, 129–142.

Platanias, L.C., Uddin, S., Yeter, A., Sun, X.J. and White, M.F. (1996). The type I interferon receptor mediates tyrosine phosphorylation of insulin receptor substrate-2. J Biol Chem 271, 278–282.

Pritchard, M.A., Baker, E., Callen, D.F., Sutherland, G.R. and Wilks, A.F. (1992). Two members of the JAK family of protein tyrosine kinases map to chromosome 1p31.3 and 9p24. Mamm Genome 3, 36–38.

Qureshi, S.A., Salditt-Georgieff, M. and Darnell, J.E. Jr (1995). Tyrosine-phosphorylated Stat1 and Stat2 plus a 48-kDa protein all contact DNA in forming interferon-stimulated-gene factor 3. Proc Natl Acad Sci USA 92, 3829–3833.

Ramana, C.V., Gil, M.P., Schreiber, R.D. and Stark, G.R. (2002). Stat1-dependent and -independent pathways in IFN-gamma-dependent signaling. Trends Immunol 23, 96–101.

Riedy, M.C., Dutra, A.S., Blake, T.B. et al. (1996). Genomic sequence, organization, and chromosomal localisation of human JAK3. Genomics 37, 57–61.

Rodig, S.J., Meraz, M.A., White, J.M. et al. (1998). Disruption of the Jak1 gene demonstrates obligatory and nonredundant roles of the Jaks in cytokine-induced biologic responses. Cell 93, 373–383.

Russell, S.M., Tayebi, N., Nakajima, H. et al. (1995). Mutation of Jak3 in a patient with SCID: essential role of Jak3 in lymphoid development. Science 270, 797–800.

Sakamoto, H., Yasukawa, H., Masuhara, M. et al. (1998). A Janus kinase inhibitor, JAB, is an interferon gamma inducible gene and confers resistance to interferons. Blood 92, 1668–1676.

Sato, M., Hata, N., Asagiri, M., Nakaya, T., Taniguchi, T. and Tanaka, N. (1998). Positive feedback regulation of type I IFN genes by the IFN-inducible transcription factor IRF-7. FEBS Lett 441, 106–110.

Schindler, C. and Strehlow, I. (2000). Cytokines and STAT signaling. Adv Pharmacol 47, 113–174.

Schmidt, M., Nagel, S., Proba, J. et al. (1998). Lack of interferon consensus sequence binding protein (ICSBP) transcripts in human myeloid leukemias. Blood 91, 22–29.

Schultz, L.D., Rajan, T.V. and Greiner, D.L. (1997). Severe defects in immunity and hematopoiesis caused by SHP-1 protein-tyrosine-phosphatase deficiency. Trends Biotechnol 15, 302–307.

Schultz, L.D., Schweitzer, P.A., Rajan, T.V. et al. (1993). Mutations at the murine motheaten locus are within the hematopoietic cell protein-tyrosine phosphatase (Hcph) gene. Cell 73, 1445–1454.

Seki, Y., Inoue, H., Nagata, N. et al. (2003). SOCS-3 regulates onset and maintenance of T(H)2-mediated allergic responses. Nat Med 9, 1047–1054.

Sharma, S., tenOever, B.R., Grandvaux, N., Zhou, G.P., Lin, R. and Hiscott, J. (2003). Triggering the interferon antiviral response through an IKK-related pathway. Science 300, 1148–1151.

Shimoda, K., Kato, K., Aoki, K. et al. (2000). Tyk2 plays an restricted role in IFN alpha signaling, although it is required for IL-12-mediated T cell function. Immunity 13, 561–571.

Shimoda, K., van Deursen, J., Sangster, M.Y. et al. (1996). Lack of IL4 induced Th2 response and IgE class switching in mice with disrupted Stat6 gene. Nature 380, 630–633.

Shinobu, N., Iwamura, T., Yoneyama, M. et al. (2002). Involvement of TIRAP/MAL in signaling for the activation of interferon regulatory factor 3 by lipopolysaccharide. FEBS Lett 517, 251–256.

Shuai, K. (2000). Modulation of STAT signaling by STAT-interacting proteins. Oncogene 19, 2638–2644.

Shuai, K., Horvath, C.M., Huang, L.H., Qureshi, S.A., Cowburn, D. and Darnell, J.E. Jr (1994). Interferon activation of the transcription factor Stat91 involves dimerization through SH2-phosphotyrosyl peptide interactions. Cell 76, 821–828.

Song, M.M. and Shuai, K. (1998). The suppressor of cytokine signaling (SOCS) 1 and SOCS3 but not SOCS2 proteins inhibit interferon mediated antiviral and antiproliferative activities. J Biol Chem 273, 35056–35062.

Starr, R., Willson, T.A., Viney, E.M. et al. (1997). A family of cytokine inducible inhibitors of signaling. Nature 387, 917–921.

Stoiber, D., Kovarik, P., Cohney, S. et al. (1999). Lipopolysaccharide induces in macrophages the synthesis of the suppressor of cytokine signaling 3 and suppresses signal transduction in response to the activating factor IFN gamma. J Immunol 163, 2640–2647.

Suzuki, N., Suzuki, S. and Yeh, W.C. (2002a). IRAK-4 as the central TIR signaling mediator in innate immunity. Trends Immunol 23, 503–506.

Suzuki, N., Suzuki, S., Duncan, G.S. et al. (2002b). Severe impairment of interleukin-1 and Toll-like receptor signalling in mice lacking IRAK-4. Nature 416, 750–756.

Swantek, J.L., Tsen, M.F., Cobb, M.H. and Thomas, J.A. (2000). IL-1 receptor-associated kinase modulates host responsiveness to endotoxin. J Immunol 164, 4301–4306.

Takeda, K., Takeuchi, O., Tsujimura, T. et al. (1999). Limb and skin abnormalities in mice lacking IKK alpha. Science 284, 313–316.

Takeda, K., Tanaka, T., Shi, W. et al. (1996). Essential role of Stat6 in IL4 signaling. Nature 380, 627–630.

Takeda, K. and Akira, S. (2004). Microbial recognition by Toll-like receptors. J Derm Sci 34, 73–82.

Takeshita, T., Arita, T., Higuchi, M. et al. (1997). STAM, signal transducing adaptor molecule, is associated with Janus kinases and involved in signaling for cell growth and c-myc induction. Immunity 6, 449–457.

Taniguchi, T., Ogasawara, K., Takaoka, A. and Tanaka, N. (2001). IRF family of transcription factors as regulators of host defense. Ann Rev Immunol 19, 623–655.

Thierfelder, W.E., van Deursen, J.M., Yamamoto, K. et al. (1996). Requirement for Stat4 in interleukin 12 mediated responses of natural killer and T cells. Nature 382, 171–174.

Thomas, J.A., Allen, J.L., Tsen, M. et al. (1999). Impaired cytokine signaling in mice lacking the IL-1 receptor-associated kinase. J Immunol 163, 978–984.

Thomis, D.C., Gurniak, C.B., Tivol, E., Sharpe, A.H. and Berg, L.J. (1995). Defects in the B lymphocyte maturation and T lymphocyte activation in mice lacking Jak3. Science 270, 794–797.

Tsui, H.W., Siminovitch, K.A., de Souza, L. and Tsui, F.W. (1993). Motheaten and viable motheaten mice have mutations in the haematopoietic cell phosphatase gene. Nat Genet 4, 124–129.

Uddin, S., Yennush, L., Sun, X.-J., Sweet, M.E., White, M.F. and Platanias, L.C. (1995). Interferon α engages the insulin receptor substrate-1 to associate with the phosphatidylinositol 3'-kinase. J Biol Chem 270, 15938–15941.

Udy, G.B., Towers, R.P., Snell, R.G. et al. (1997). Requirement of STAT5b for sexual dimorphism of body growth rates and liver gene expression. Proc Natl Acad Sci USA 94, 7239–7244.

Ulane, C.M., Rodriguez, J.J., Parisien, J.P. and Horvath, C.M. (2003). STAT3 ubiquitylation and degradation by mumps virus suppress cytokine and oncogene signaling. J Virol 7, 6385–6393.

Ulane, C.M. and Horvath, C.M. (2002). Paramyxoviruses SV5 and HPIV2 assemble STAT protein ubiquitin ligase complexes from cellular components. Virology 304, 160–166.

Uze, G., Lutfalla, G. and Gresser, I. (1990). Genetic transfer of a functional human interferon alpha receptor into mouse cells: cloning and expression of its cDNA. Cell 60, 225–234.

Velazquez, L., Mogensen, K.E., Barbieri, G., Fellous, M., Uze, G. and Pelligrini, S. (1995). Distinct domains of the protein tyrosine kinase tyk2 required for binding of interferon-alpha/beta and for signal transduction. J Biol Chem 270, 3327–3334.

Wakao, H., Gouilleux, F. and Groner, B. (1994). Mammary gland factor (MGF) is a novel member of the cytokine regulated transcription factor gene family and confers the prolactin response. EMBO J 13, 2182–2191.

Wang, C.L., Deng, L., Hong, M., Akkaraju, G.R., Inoue, J. and Chen, Z.J. (2001). TAK1 is a ubiquitin-dependent kinase of MKK and IKK. Nature 412, 346–351.

Watling, D., Guschin, D., Müller, M., et al. (1993). Complementation by the protein tyrosine kinase JAK2 of a mutant cell line defective in the interferon-α gamma; signal transduction pathway. Nature 366, 166–170.

Weiss, A. and Schlessinger, J. (1998). Switching signals on or off by receptor dimerization. Cell 94, 277–280.

Weiz, A., Marx, P., Sharf, R. et al. (1992). Human interferon consensus sequence binding protein is a negative regulator of enhancer elements common to interferon-inducible genes. J Biol Chem 267, 25589–25596.

Wen, Z., Zhong, Z. and Darnell, J.E. Jr (1995). Maximal activation of transcription by STAT1 and STAT3 requires both tyrosine and serine phosphorylation. Cell 82, 241–250.

Wesche, H., Gao, X., Li, X., Kirschning, C.J., Stark, G.R. and Cao, Z. (1999). IRAK-M is a novel member of the Pelle/interleukin-1 receptor-associated kinase (IRAK) family. J Biol Chem 274, 19403–19410.

White, L.C., Wright, K.L., Felix, N.J. et al. (1996). Regulation of LMP2 and TAP1 genes by IRF-1 explains the paucity of CD8+ T cells in IRF-1-/- mice. Immunity 5, 365–376.

Wilks, A.F. (1991). Cloning members of protein-tyrosine kinase family using polymerase chain reaction. Methods Enzymol 200, 533–546.

Yamamoto, H., Lamphier, M.S., Fujita, T., Taniguchi, T. and Harada, H. (1994). The oncogenic transcription factor irf-2 possesses a transcriptional repression and a latent activation domain. Oncogene 9, 1423–1428.

Yamamoto, M., Sato, S., Hemmi, H. et al. (2003a). Role of adaptor TRIF in the MyD88-independent Toll-like receptor signaling pathway. Science 301, 640–643.

Yamamoto, M., Sato, S., Hemmi, H. et al. (2003b). TRAM is specifically involved in the TLR4 mediated MyD88-independent signaling pathway. Nat Immunol 4, 1140–1150.

Yamamoto, M., Sato, S., Hemmi, H. et al. (2002a). Essential role for TIRAP in activation of the signalling cascade shared by TLR2 and TLR4. Nature 420, 324–329.

Yamamoto, M., Sato, S., Mori, K. et al. (2002b). Cutting edge: A novel Toll/Il-1 receptor domain-containing adapter that preferentially activates the IFN-β promoter in the Toll-like receptor signalling. J Immunol 169, 6668–6672.

Yang, C.H., Shi, W., Basu, L. et al. (1996). Direct association of STAT3 with the IFNAR-1 chain of the human type I interferon receptor. J Biol Chem 271, 8057–8061.

Yasukawa, H., Misawa, H., Sakamoto, H. et al. (1999). The JAK binding protein JAB inhibits Janus tyrosine kinase activity through binding in the activation loop. EMBO J 18, 1309–1320.

Yeow, W.S., Au, W.C., Juang, Y.T. et al. (2000). Reconstitution of virus-mediated expression of interferon alpha genes in human fibroblast cells by ectopic interferon regulatory factor-7. J Biol Chem 275, 6313–6320.

Yi, T., Mui, A.L., Krystal, G. and Ihle, J.N. (1993). Hematopoietic cell phosphatase associates with the interleukin-3 (IL-3) receptor beta chain and down-regulates IL-3-induced tyrosine phosphorylation and mitogenesis. Mol Cell Biol 13, 7577–7586.

Yin, T., Shen, R., Feng, G.S. and Yang, Y.C. (1997). Molecular characterization of specific interactions between SHP-2 phosphatase and JAK tyrosine kinases. J Biol Chem 272, 1032–1037.

Yoneyama, M., Suhara, W., Fukuhara, Y., Fukuda, M., Nishida, E. and Fujita, T. (1998). Direct triggering of the type I interferon system by virus infection: activation of a transcription factor complex containing IRF-3 and CBP/p300. EMBO J 17, 1087–1095.

Zhang, D., Zhang, G., Hayden, M.S. et al. (2004). A toll-like receptor that prevents infection by uropathogenic bacteria. Science 303, 1522–1526.

Zhang, L. and Pagano, J.S. (1997). IRF-7, a new interferon regulatory factor associated with Epstein–Barr virus latency. Mol Cell Biol 17, 5748–5757.

Zhong, Z., Wen, Z. and Darnell, J.E. Jr (1994). Stat3 and Stat4 members of the family of signal transducers and activators of transcription. Proc Natl Acad Sci USA 91, 4806–4810.

Toll-like Receptors in Innate Immunity

Chapter 6

Thomas R. Hawn[*,†] and David M. Underhill[†]

[*]Division of Infectious Diseases, University of Washington Medical Center, Seattle, WA, USA; [†]Institute for Systems Biology, Seattle, WA 98103, USA

Toll!

C. Nüsslein-Volhard

INTRODUCTION

When doing a screen in the mid-1980s for mutations that affected embryonic patterning in *Drosophila*, Christiane Nüsslein-Volhard of the Max Planck Institute in Tubingen, Germany, exclaimed, 'Toll!' upon first seeing a mutant with disrupted dorsal-ventral patterning (Anderson, 2000). Toll, a German slang term for 'far out', became the name of the mutated gene which turned out to encode a transmembrane receptor. The receptor consisted of a long extracellular domain with leucine- rich repeats and an intracellular domain that bore curious homology to the mammalian interleukin-1 (IL-1) receptor. Further mutational analyses revealed that Toll activated a signaling pathway in flies, having many components that are similar to signaling proteins utilized by the mammalian IL-1 receptor, including orthologues of NF-κB transcription factor family members. In the mid-1990s, Jules Hoffmann and coworkers made the startling discovery that, in addition to playing a role in fly development, Toll is also important for innate immune responses (Lemaitre et al., 1996). Unlike mammals, flies have no adaptive immunity and rely solely on innate defenses for effective immunity. Adult Toll mutant flies succumb readily to fungal infections due to a failure to induce antimicrobial peptides that are required for antifungal defense.

The role of Toll in innate immunity in flies prompted mammalian immunologists to look for proteins similar to Toll. Due to readily available DNA sequences, 10 mammalian homologues, called Toll-like receptors (TLRs), were identified between 1997 and 2001 (Medzhitov et al., 1997; Rock et al., 1998; Takeuchi et al., 1999; Du et al., 2000; Chuang and Ulevitch, 2000, 2001). The importance of TLRs in mammalian innate immunity first became clear from studies on C3H/HeJ mice that are hyporesponsive to lipopolysaccharide (LPS), the major surface component of gram-negative bacterial cell walls. In Bruce Beutler's laboratory, genetic mapping of the defect identified a mutation in a TLR homologue that is now known as Toll-like receptor 4 (TLR4) (Poltorak et al., 1998). As discussed below, we now understand that the family of mammalian Toll-like receptors plays a key role in innate immune responses to a wide range of bacteria, viruses, fungi and parasites. Further, variations in human susceptibility to infection are linked to polymorphisms in TLRs and components of TLR signaling pathways.

TOLL-LIKE RECEPTORS AND SIGNALING

Mammalian TLRs are type I transmembrane proteins with large extracellular domains consisting of multiple leucine-rich repeat structures that vary substantially between the receptors. The intracellular domains are more highly conserved and consist largely of a well-defined domain called the Toll/IL-1 receptor (TIR) homology domain. TLRs

Measuring Immunity, edited by Michael T. Lotze and Angus W. Thomson
ISBN 0-12-455900-X, London

are expressed widely, but the specific subsets expressed vary considerably between different tissues and cell types. For example, monocytes and macrophages express all of the TLRs except TLRs 3 and 9 (Jarrossay et al., 2001). Myeloid dendritic cells express TLRs 1, 2, 5, 6 and 8 while plasmacytoid dendritic cells express exclusively TLRs 7 and 9 (Kadowaki et al., 2001; Jarrossay et al., 2001). Intestinal epithelial cells express TLR5, express low levels of TLR4 and TLR2 and do not express TLRs 1 and 6 (Steiner et al., 2000; Sierro et al., 2001; Gewirtz et al., 2001; Abreu et al., 2002; Melmed et al., 2003). Similarly, lung epithelial cells can be activated through TLR5, but are poorly stimulated through TLR4 (Standiford et al., 1990; DiMango et al., 1995; Hawn et al., 2003; Liaudet et al., 2003). TLR expression in tissues is dynamically regulated by inflammatory stimuli and can therefore change during infection. While TLR4 is not expressed strongly in intestinal epithelia, its expression is upregulated in patients with inflammatory bowel disease (Cario and Podolsky, 2000). Similarly, viral infection strongly upregulates TLR expression in macrophages (Miettinen et al., 2001). Thus, TLR expression can be quite diverse and the role of any particular TLR in inflammatory responses to a specific pathogen must be carefully analyzed with respect to where the TLR is likely to be able to detect the pathogen, and whether TLR expression is regulated during infection.

TLRs are implicated in inflammatory responses to a wide range of microbial products (Table 6.1). There is increasing evidence that TLRs directly bind the microbial products that they respond to, although this is a contentious area. Genetic evidence strongly suggests that LPS binds to TLR4. Certain minimal LPS structures such as lipid IVa and *Rhodobacter sphaeroides* lipid A are antagonists for human cells, but agonists in mouse cells. Several groups have demonstrated that expression of mouse TLR4 in human cells is sufficient to permit the antagonists to become agonists, strongly suggesting that TLR4 is responsible for the direct discrimination of LPS structures (Poltorak et al., 2000; Lien et al., 2000). Similarly, *Pseudomonas aeruginosa* modifies its LPS during growth in lungs of cystic fibrosis patients to enhance resistance to antimicrobial peptides. This modification results in an LPS that is more strongly recognized by human cells and contributes to the chronic inflammation in lungs of these patients. The modification does not affect recognition by mouse cells and the enhanced recognition is attributable to a region of the extracellular domain of human TLR4 (Hajjar et al., 2002). TLR5 has also been reported to bind directly to its ligand, flagellin. Purified flagellin co-immunoprecipitates with the extracellular leucine-rich domain of TLR5 (Smith et al., 2003; Mizel et al., 2003). However, no TLR extracellular domains have yet been fully purified for characterization of binding affinities and structures.

TLRs have also been implicated in recognition of host molecules (Table 6.1). The reason for recognizing these molecules is not entirely clear, but it appears that they may play a role in recognizing 'danger' as manifested by inappropriate cell death or breakdown of tissue barriers. For example, TLR recognition of host heat shock proteins such as Hsp70 may contribute to recognition of necrotic versus apoptotic cell death. Also, the EDA domain of fibronectin is an alternatively spliced variant of fibronectin that is produced during wound healing and recognition

Table 6.1 Toll-like receptors and their ligands

Receptor complex		Ligand	Source	Typical detection range
TLR2 +	TLR1	Tri-acylated lipoproteins	Bacteria	1–1000 ng/ml
		Di-acylated lipoproteins	Bacteria/mycobacteria	1–1000 ng/ml
		Zymosan	Fungi	1–100 µg/ml
		Peptidoglycan	Gram-positive bacteria	0.1–100 µg/ml
		Glycoinositolphospholipids	Trypanosomes	0.1–10 nM
	TLR6	Atypical LPSs	Some gram-negative bacteria	1–1000 ng/ml
		HSP70	Host	10–1000 ng/ml
TLR3		Double stranded RNA	Viruses	1–100 µg/ml
		LPS	Gram-negative bacteria	0.1–1000 ng/ml
		Envelope fusion (F) protein	Respiratory syncytical virus	0.1–1 µg/ml
TLR4 + MD2		Hyaluronan (small MW)	Host	5–100 µg/ml
		HSP70	Host	10–1000 ng/ml
		Fibronectin EDA domain	Host	10–1000 µg/ml
TLR5		Flagellin	Motile bacteria	0.1–1000 ng/ml
TLR7		Imidazoquinoline	Synthetic (natural ligand unknown)	0.1–100 ng/ml
TLR8		Imidazoquinoline	Synthetic (natural ligand unknown)	1–1000 ng/ml
TLR9		CpG DNA	Bacteria/viruses/fungi	Bacterial DNA: 1–100 µg/ml Synthetic oligos: 0.1–100 µg/ml
TLR10		Unknown	–	

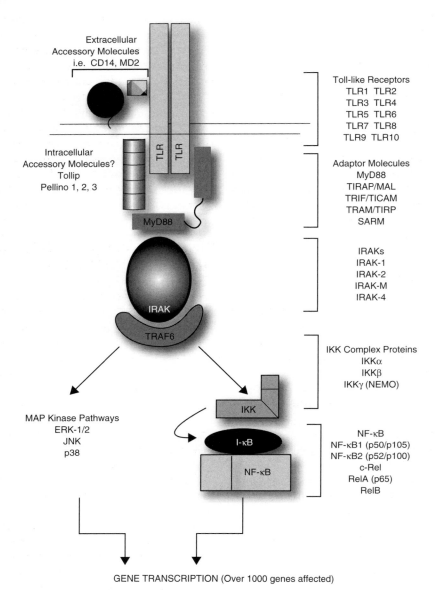

Extracellular
Accessory Molecules
i.e. CD14, MD2

Toll-like Receptors
TLR1 TLR2
TLR3 TLR4
TLR5 TLR6
TLR7 TLR8
TLR9 TLR10

TLR

TLR

Intracellular
Accessory Molecules?
Tollip
Pellino 1, 2, 3

Adaptor Molecules
MyD88
TIRAP/MAL
TRIF/TICAM
TRAM/TIRP
SARM

MyD88

IRAKs
IRAK-1
IRAK-2
IRAK-M
IRAK-4

IRAK

TRAF6

IKK Complex Proteins
IKKα
IKKβ
IKKγ (NEMO)

IKK

MAP Kinase Pathways
ERK-1/2
JNK
p38

I-κB

NF-κB

NF-κB
NF-κB1 (p50/p105)
NF-κB2 (p52/p100)
c-Rel
RelA (p65)
RelB

GENE TRANSCRIPTION (Over 1000 genes affected)

Figure 6.1 TLR signaling pathway. Transmembrane TLRs interact with various extracellular proteins that assist in efficient ligand recognition. Ligand binding triggers signaling though a host of intracellular molecules, and at each step in the pathway multiple related proteins may participate. Mutations in many of these molecules cause specific immunodeficiencies in humans and mice.

of this protein by neighboring or infiltrated cells may contribute to a heightened inflammatory state at these sites (Okamura et al., 2001). Studies showing activation of TLRs by purified host proteins are often met with skepticism due to possible contamination of the preparations with LPS or other microbial products. While these concerns are usually carefully addressed, it is extremely difficult to exclude totally the possibility that the proteins bind and concentrate some small amount of these contaminants.

TLR activation stimulates signal transduction through a complex cascade of molecules that ultimately coordinates transcriptional and translational inflammatory responses (Figure 6.1). In general, TLR activation leads to recruitment of an adaptor molecule called MyD88 through homotypic interactions between the TLR TIR

domain and a TIR domain in MyD88. MyD88 stimulates recruitment and phosphorylation of the kinase IRAK, which in turn recruits TRAF6. Through TRAF6, MAP kinase cascades are stimulated and I-κB kinases (IKKs) are activated. IKKs phosphorylate and trigger degradation of I-κB, releasing NF-κB transcription factors to travel into the nucleus and stimulate transcription of inflammatory genes. The full details of the mechanisms of TLR signal transduction are certainly more complex than this simple model and will take years to work out. As illustrated in Figure 6.1, there are multiple proteins that participate at each stage of signaling, which suggests a relatively deep level of regulation and complexity. Additionally, not all TLRs signal identically. For example, TLR4 triggers production of IFNβ through a mechanism that requires the signaling adaptor molecule TRAM, while TLR2 does not stimulate production of IFNβ and does not signal through TRAM (Yamamoto et al., 2003; Fitzgerald et al., 2003). It has been suggested that such differential signaling by TLRs leads to 'tailoring' of the immune response to be most effective against the specific pathogen detected (Underhill and Ozinsky, 2002). One of the best-characterized examples of tailoring of the immune response is the initiation of Th1 or Th2 type T cell immunity, a polarization that is directed by the innate immune system. Similarly, different local inflammatory responses may lead to extensive cellular infiltration, or to granuloma formation. The specific roles of TLRs in coordinating different types of inflammatory responses and in directing adaptive immunity are still being explored.

DIRECTING ADAPTIVE IMMUNITY

The direct role of TLRs in orchestrating adaptive immune responses is probably best illustrated by the fact that most adjuvants are TLR stimuli. Commonly studied adjuvants such as LPS, CpG DNA and mycobacterial lysates are potent TLR stimuli. The first specific demonstration of the requirement for TLR signaling in directing the adaptive immune response came from studies with MyD88 deficient mice. MyD88 deficient mice immunized with ovalbumin in complete Freund's adjuvant (CFA, a mycobacterial lysate that stimulates through TLR2) fail to develop an efficient T cell response as measured by antigen-induced proliferation or IFN-γ production (Schnare et al., 2001). However, T cells produced IL-4 in response to stimulation with antigen and, although production of antigen specific IgG2a was not detected, antigen specific IgG1 was produced. These characteristics are indicative of Th2 immunity and suggest that MyD88-dependent signaling is required for Th1 immunity that is normally activated by CFA.

Further support for TLR activation in coordinating Th1/Th2 polarization comes from studies directly comparing immune responses when purified TLR2 or TLR4 agonists are used as adjuvants. Pulendran and coworkers demonstrated that mice immunized with ovalbumin together with E. coli LPS (a TLR4 agonist) produce strong Th1 type immune responses to ovalbumin (Pulendran et al., 2001). However, mice immunized with ovalbumin together with P. gingivalis LPS (a TLR2 agonist), fail to produce a strong Th1 response as demonstrated by reduced antigen specific IFN-γ production and increased IL-5 production compared to the TLR4 stimulated mice. Since CFA (discussed above) is a TLR2 activator and induces Th1 responses, while P. gingivalis LPS is not a strong inducer of Th1 responses, there are likely stimulating components in CFA in addition to its TLR2 activity that support the TH1 polarization.

To conclude that TLR4 stimulation assures a Th1 response and that lack of TLR4 activation assures a Th2 response is certainly an oversimplification. First, TLR4

stimulation has been demonstrated to be important in establishing Th2 responses as well. Bottomly and coworkers observed that in a mouse experimental model of allergic asthma (a classic Th2 driven disease) low level exposure to inhaled LPS strongly enhanced Th2 responses to inhaled antigens (Eisenbarth et al., 2002). Second, in addition to TLRs, many receptors including lectins, scavenger receptors and complement receptors participate in orchestrating inflammatory responses to microbes. Many of these receptors have inflammatory activity of their own or modify the effects of TLR stimulation and the complex effects of recognition of microbes through different sets of receptors is only beginning to be understood (Underhill, 2003).

INNATE IMMUNITY AND MURINE MODELS OF INFECTION

Mice with TLR deficiencies have been used to understand the in vivo role of innate immune pathways in regulating the host response to infection (Table 6.2). Several general conclusions can be made from these studies. First, although TLR knockout mice have increased susceptibility to infection with specific pathogens, there are many examples where deletion of a TLR that is known to respond to a pathogen causes no change in susceptibility. These studies demonstrate that the role of any specific TLR in infection varies with the pathogen, probably due to the level of redundancy in the recognition systems (TLRs and other receptors) available for defense to the pathogen. Second, TLRs can play an important role in the development of adaptive immune responses to whole organisms (as well as to pure TLR stimuli as discussed above). Finally, there are some surprising examples where mice deficient in specific TLR pathways are less susceptible to infection. These examples underscore the fact that TLR mediated inflammatory responses are potent and that the innate immune system must carefully balance the overall benefits of these responses with the dangers.

Although not recognizable at the time, the pivotal role of the TLR pathway during in vivo infection was first evident in work performed over 20 years ago showing that the C3H/HeJ mouse is more susceptible to infection with gram-negative bacteria (O'Brien et al., 1980; Hagberg et al., 1984; Woods et al., 1988). This mouse strain has now been demonstrated to carry a mutation in TLR4 that disrupts the receptor's signaling domain (Poltorak et al., 1998). The susceptibility profile of these mice is largely restricted to gram-negative bacteria, which contain LPS. For example, C3H/HeJ mice are not more susceptible to several pathogens, such as Mycobacterium avium and Toxoplasma gondii, that do not contain LPS (Mun et al., 2003; Feng et al., 2003).

The ligand specificity of TLRs (see Table 6.1) predicts that TLR2-/- mice would be more susceptible to a wide variety of pathogens that contain lipopeptides. Consistent with this hypothesis, TLR2-/- mice are more susceptible to infection

Table 6.2 *In vivo* infection murine models with TLR pathway defects

Strain	Strain comparison	Pathogen, route of infection	Susceptibility	Magnitude[a]	Reference
C3H/HeJ	C3H/HeN	*E. coli, S. typhimurium,* urinary tract	↑ cfu by ~150-fold	+2	(Hagberg et al., 1984)
C3H/HeJ	C3H/HeN or C3HeB/FeJ	*N. meningitidis,* i.p.	↑ cfu by ~1000-fold	+3	(Woods et al., 1988)
C3H/HeJ	C3H/HeN	*S. typhimurium*	↑ cfu by ~1000-fold	+3	(O'Brien et al., 1980)
C3H/HeJ	C3H/HeOuJ	*S. pneumoniae* with pneumolysin, nasopharyngeal	↑ mortality 56% vs. 12.5% ($P = 0.02$)	+2	(Malley et al., 2003)
C3H/HeJ	C3H/HeOuJ	Anaerobic bone infection of molar teeth	↓ bone destruction	+1	(Hou et al., 2000)
C3H/HeJ	Several	MTb, Erdman, aerosol 350 cfu	↔ mortality or cfu	0	(Kamath et al., 2003)
C3H/HeJ	C3H/HeN	MTb, H37Rv, aerosol 100 or 2000 cfu	↔ mortality or cfu	0	(Reiling et al., 2002)
C3H/HeJ	C3H/HeN	MTb, H37Rv, aerosol 50–100	↑ mortality, ↑ cfu by ~100-fold	+2	(Abel et al., 2002)
C3H/HeJ	C3H/HeOuJ	BCG, i.v., 2×10^6 cfu	↔ mortality or cfu	0	(Fremond et al., 2003)
C3H/HeJ	C3H/HeN	Sepsis, polymicrobial from colonic puncture	↔ mortality	0	(Weighardt et al., 2002)
C3H/HeJ	C3H/HeN	*Klebsiella pneumoniae,* 10^2–10^3 cfu	↑ cfu by ~1000-fold	+3	(Wang et al., 1999)
C3H/HeJ	C3H/HeN	*Haemophilus influenzae,* 5×10^5 intranasal	↑ cfu by ~10-100-fold	+2	(Wang et al., 2002)
TRL4-/-	C57Bl/6	BCG, i.p., 10^6–10^8 cfu	↔ cfu	0	(Heldwein et al., 2003)
TLR4-/-	C57Bl/6	MTb, H37Rv, aerosol 50–100 cfu	↔ mortality or cfu	0	(Shim et al., 2003)
TRL4-/-	C57Bl/6	*M. avium,* i.v. 10^6 cfu	↔ survival or cfu	0	(Feng et al., 2003)
TLR4-/-	C57Bl/6	*Trichuris muris* (nematode)	↓ worm burden	+2	(Helmby and Grencis, 2003)
TLR4-/-	C57Bl/6	*Toxoplasma gondii,* 50–300 cysts i.p.	↔ mortality	0	(Mun et al., 2003)
TLR2-/-	C57Bl/6	MTb, H37Rv, aerosol 100 or 2000 cfu	↔ mortality or cfu for low dose	0	(Reiling et al., 2002)
			↑ mortality for high dose	+2	
TLR2-/-		MTb	↔ mortality or cfu for low dose	0	(Sugawara et al., 2003a)
TLR2-/-	C57Bl/6	BCG, i.p., 10^6–10^8 cfu	↑ cfu by ~10-fold	+1	(Heldwein et al., 2003)
TLR2-/-	C57Bl/6	*M. avium,* i.v. 10^6 cfu	↑ mortality, ↑ cfu by ~100-fold	+2	(Feng et al., 2003)
TLR2-/-	C57Bl/6	*Listeria monocytogenes,* 5×10^5 cfu i.p.	↔ cfu	0	(Edelson and Unanue, 2002)
TLR2-/-	C57Bl/6	*Staphylococcus aureus,* i.v. 10^6–10^7 cfu i.v.	↑ mortality, ↑ cfu by variable amt	+2	(Takeuchi et al., 2000)
TLR2-/-	C57Bl/6	*S. pneumoniae* meningitis, 10^2–10^3 cfu intracerebral	↑ mortality	+1	(Echchannaoui et al., 2002)
		Listeria monocytogenes, 5×10^2 cfu intracerebral	↑ mortality	+1	
TLR2-/-	C57Bl/6	*Toxoplasma gondii,* 50–300 cysts i.p.	↑ mortality	+3	(Mun et al., 2003)
TLR2-/-	C57Bl/6	Sepsis, polymicrobial from colonic puncture	↔ mortality	0	(Weighardt et al., 2002)

Table 6.2 (Continued)

Strain	Strain comparison	Pathogen, route of infection	Susceptibility	Magnitude[a]	Reference
MyD88-/-	C57Bl/6	*M. avium*, i.v. 10^6 cfu	↑ mortality, ↑ cfu by ~1000-fold	+3	(Feng et al., 2003)
MyD88-/-	C57Bl/6	*Trichuris muris* (nematode)	↓ worm burden	+2	(Helmby and Grencis, 2003)
MyD88-/-	C57Bl/6	*Listeria monocytogenes*, 5×10^5 i.v.	↑ mortality, ↑ cfu by ~1000-fold	+3	(Seki et al., 2002)
MyD88-/-	C57Bl/6	*Listeria monocytogenes*, 5×10^5 i.p.	↑ cfu by ~1000-fold	+3	(Edelson and Unanue, 2002)
MyD88-/-	C57Bl/6	*Staphylococcus aureus*, i.v. 10^6–10^7 cfu	↑ mortality, ↑ cfu by variable amt	+3	(Takeuchi et al., 2000)
MyD88-/-	C57Bl/6	*Toxoplasma gondii*, 50–300 cysts i.p.	↑ mortality	+3	(Mun et al., 2003)
MyD88-/-	C57Bl/6	*Toxoplasma gondii*, 20 cysts i.p.	↑ mortality	+3	(Scanga et al., 2002)
MyD88-/-	C57Bl/6	*Leishmania major*, 5×10^6 footpad	↑ lesion size	+3	(Muraille et al., 2003)
MyD88-/-	C57Bl/6	*Leishmania major*, 1×10^6 intradermal	↑ lesion size	+2	(de Veer et al., 2003)
MyD88-/-	C57Bl/6	MTb, Kurono strain, aerosol 100 cfu	↔ mortality, ↑ lung cfu by ~100-fold	+1	(Sugawara et al., 2003b)
MyD88-/-	C57Bl/6	Sepsis, polymicrobial from colonic puncture	↓ mortality, ↔ cfu	+2	(Weighardt et al., 2002)

[a] Scale: +3 = large effect, +2 = modest, +1 = mild, 0 = no effect. Cfu, colony-forming units, i.p., intraperitoneal, i.v., intravenous. MTb, *Mycobacterium tuberculosis*.

with *S. aureus* and *S. pneumoniae* (Takeuchi et al., 2000; Echchannaoui et al., 2002). In contrast, TLR2-/- mice are not more susceptible to infection with *L. monocytogenes*, another gram-positive organism that signals through TLR2 (Ozinsky et al., 2000). Resistance of TLR2-/- mice to *Listeria* is likely attributable to redundancy of the TLR recognition system, since MyD88-/- mice are highly susceptible to *Listeria* infection (Edelson and Unanue, 2002; Seki et al., 2002). *Listeria* contains flagellin and therefore is recognized by TLR5 as well as TLR2 (Hayashi et al., 2001). For this pathogen, TLR5 recognition may be sufficient to confer resistance (Hayashi et al., 2001; Edelson and Unanue, 2002; Seki et al., 2002). Taken together, the above studies demonstrate the *in vivo* importance of the TLR recognition system in regulating resistance to infection. They also demonstrate that some pathogen susceptibility can be predicted from the types of ligands recognized by each receptor, but that redundancy in the system can often compensate for specific deficiencies.

In vivo studies have illustrated three key features of immune responses regulated by TLRs that contribute to susceptibility in TLR deficient animals. First, cytokine and chemokine release is impaired in knockout mice. Many of the studies in Table 6.2 show that TLR knockout mice have decreased levels of pro-inflammatory cytokines such as TNF-α, IL-6 and IL-12p40. Second, effector mechanisms utilized to kill pathogens are often dysregulated in TLR deficient animals. TLR pathways control production of nitric oxide (NO), an important component of microbicidal activity of phagocytes (Brightbill et al., 1999). MyD88-/- or TLR2-/- mice infected with *Toxoplasma* are more susceptible to infection, carry higher parasite burdens and fail to produce NO as compared to wild type animals (Scanga et al., 2002; Mun et al., 2003). Third, TLR signaling affects the Th1/Th2 balance of the adaptive immune response *in vivo*. C57Bl/6 mice infected with *Leishmania major* normally manifest a strong IL-12 mediated Th1 T cell response and resist the infection. However, MyD88-/- mice (on a C57Bl/6 background) shift their T cell response to a Th2 profile with impaired production of IL-12 and IFN-γ and become susceptible to *Leishmania* infection (de Veer et al., 2003; Muraille et al., 2003). The tendency for MyD88-/- mice to exhibit a Th2 profile has also been observed after infection with *Toxoplasma gondii* (Mun et al., 2003). In contrast to infection with intracellular pathogens such as *Leishmania* and *Toxoplasma*, the host relies on a strong Th2 response to control worm infections. When compared to wild type C57Bl/6 mice, MyD88-/- and TLR4-/- strains are highly resistant to infection with *Trichuris muris*, an intestinal nematode (Helmby and Grencis, 2003). This resistance is associated with enhanced production of Th2 type cytokines, such as IL-4 and IL-13 (Brightbill et al., 1999; Scanga et al., 2002; Mun et al., 2003).

While impairment of the TLR pathway can lead to reduced inflammation and enhanced susceptibility to infection, there are cases where the reduced inflammatory responses are beneficial. For example, MyD88-/- mice are less susceptible than wild type mice to polymicrobial sepsis induced by colon puncture (Weighardt et al., 2002). Similarly, using an anaerobic molar teeth bone infection model, Hou et al. demonstrated that C3H/HeJ mice have less bone destruction than control mice (Hou et al., 2000). These studies illustrate that TLR-mediated inflammation is a two-edged sword: while inflammatory responses are required for effective innate and adaptive immunity, inflammation can also be pathologic.

INNATE IMMUNITY AND SUSCEPTIBILITY TO HUMAN INFECTION

Molecular, cellular and *in vivo* studies have established the importance of TLRs in immunity and suggest that human variation in susceptibility to disease may be in part due to variations in TLR function. Previous studies have shown that genetic factors influence production of TNF-α and other cytokines produced by the innate immune system (Westendorp et al., 1997; Yaqoob et al., 1999). These findings suggest that individuals can be stratified into high and low inflammatory response phenotypes. Furthermore, these inflammatory phenotypes may correlate with clinical outcome as suggested by the association of TNF-α production with fatal meningococcal disease (Westendorp et al., 1997). We will consider two types of clinical syndromes that demonstrate the role of TLR signaling in human susceptibility to disease: congenital immunodeficiency syndromes and common infections in the general population (Table 6.3).

TLR/NF-κB pathway and congenital immunodeficiency syndromes

A series of studies of pediatric immunodeficiency syndromes have convincingly shown that defects in the TLR/NF-κB pathway predispose individuals to serious, recurrent bacterial infections. Mutations in three genes have been identified. Picard et al. demonstrated that a nonsense or deletion mutation in IRAK-4 predisposes children to infection with pyogenic bacteria (predominantly *S. aureus* and *S. pneumoniae*) (Picard et al., 2003; Medvedev et al., 2003). IRAK-4 is a kinase that is recruited to the TLR-MyD88 signaling complex and is essential for signal transduction (see Figure 6.1) (Suzuki et al., 2002). Cells from these individuals are unable to mediate signaling from any of the TLR ligands or IL-1. Interestingly, after several years of debilitating infections, these children improve and have less frequent problems. This observation suggests that the innate immune system defect, while initially severe, can eventually be compensated for by adaptive immune responses.

Several investigators have described mutations in NEMO, one of the regulatory subunits of the IKK family (Zonana et al., 2000; Jain et al., 2001; Doffinger et al., 2001). The IKK proteins phosphorylate IκB and stimulate its degradation, which is necessary to release NF-κB for translocation to the nucleus and activation of NF-κB dependent cytokine gene transcription. NEMO mutations inhibit NF-κB activation and the subsequent cytokine response. Children with NEMO mutations are more susceptible to gram-positive, gram-negative and mycobacterial infections. In addition, they have ectodermal dysplasia as well as elevated IgM levels.

A mutation in IκBα was also recently identified that affects TLR signaling (Courtois et al., 2003). Unlike the IRAK-4 and NEMO mutations, the IκBα defect is a gain-of-function mutation. Mutation of a serine residue prevents phosphorylation, blocks degradation and thus enhances the inhibitory capacity of IαBα by impairing NF-κB translocation. Children with the IκBα mutation are more susceptible to gram-positive and gram-negative infections and also have a T-cell deficiency.

TLR polymorphisms and susceptibility to common infections

While the above studies establish a role for the TLR signaling pathway in congenital immunodeficiency syndromes, recent studies also demonstrate that variations in this pathway also affect susceptibility to common infections in the general population. The most common type of human genetic variation is the single nucleotide polymorphism (SNP), where two alternative bases occur at appreciable frequency (>1%) in the population (Cooke and Hill, 2001; Casanova and Abel, 2002). Two coding region SNPs in TLR4 (D299G and T399I) have been associated with gram-negative bacterial infections in several small studies. One of these SNPs (D299G) is associated with LPS hyporesponsiveness as measured by bronchospasm in response to inhalation of endotoxin (Arbour et al., 2000). Initial *in vitro* studies suggested that this polymorphism was unable to mediate LPS signaling and acted in a dominant fashion with respect to the wild type allele (Arbour et al., 2000). However, separate studies have found no defect in LPS signaling in cells from individuals who are heterozygous for the D299G SNP (Erridge et al., 2003; von Aulock et al., 2003). Several genetic studies have examined whether there is an association of TLR4 D299G with sepsis susceptibility and outcome. Although some of these studies show an association of the 299G allele with increased susceptibility to sepsis, these findings have not been consistently observed (see Table 6.3). One problem may be that that the etiology of sepsis is heterogeneous and that TLR4 SNPs would only be predicted to alter susceptibility to gram-negative infections. To address this point, investigators have examined whether the D299G variant specifically influences susceptibility to gram-negative bacterial infections. While

Table 6.3 Genetic variation in the TLR-NF-κB pathway and susceptibility to infection

Protein	Variation: BP (AA)	Diseases	Variant	Case (frequency)	Control (frequency)	References
3A. Mendelian inheritance						
IRAK-4	(congenital immunodeficiency) C877T (Q293X[a]) 821delT 620delAC Multiple variants	*Case reports* Predominantly gram-positive extracellular pyogenic bacteria (S. pneumoniae, S. aureus). Occasional gram-negative bacteria				(Picard et al., 2003; Medvedev et al., 2003)
NEMO (IKKγ)	including deletions, nonsense and missense mutations	Bacteria including mycobacteria, gram-negative, and gram-positive (many with S.pneumoniae).Elevated IgM levels. Ectodermal dysplasia				(Zonana et al., 2000; Doffinger et al., 2001; Jain et al., 2001)
IκBα	G94T (S32I)	Gram-positive and gram-negative pyogenic bacteria. Also T cell deficiency				(Courtois et al., 2003)
3B. Complex inheritance (common infections in population)						
TLR4	A896G (D299G) C1196T (T399I)	*Case and control cohort definitions* Septic shock (n = 91) vs control (n = 73). No difference in frequency for all subjects with 299G (which includes 399T and 399I). Subgroup with genotype 299G399T was only found in cases (0.055 vs 0 frequency, P = 0.05)	299GD	0.12	0.11	(Lorenz et al., 2002)
		Sepsis (n = 77) vs control (n = 37)	299GD	0.18	0.13	(Agnese et al., 2002)
		SIRS in ICU (n = 94). Dead (n = 21) vs alive (n = 58)	299DG/GG	0.19	0.05, p = 0.076	(Child et al., 2003)
		Sepsis after surgery (n = 153) vs control (n = 154)	299GD	0.065	0.12	(Feterowski et al., 2003)
		Acute infections (n = 53) vs no acute infections (n = 757)	299DG/GG	0.151	0.062, p = 0.013	(Kiechl et al., 2002)
		Meningococcus (n = 1047) vs controls (n = 879)	299G	0.065	0.059	(Read et al., 2001)
		Meningococcus (n = 262) vs controls (n = 262)	299DG/GG	0.213	0.211	(Allen et al., 2003)
TLR4	Multiple rare mutations	Meningococcus (n = 197) vs controls (n = 127)	Multiple	3.42	0.42, p = 0.03	(Smirnova et al., 2001)
TLR5	C1174T (R392X)	Legionnaires' disease (n = 108) vs control (n = 508)	392RX[a]	0.167	0.095, p = 0.03	(Hawn et al., 2003)

[a] X = stop codon; 299G indicates allele frequency; 299GD indicates genotype frequency of heterozygotes; 299GD/GG indicates genotype frequency of heterozygotes and homozygotes; 392RX = genotype frequency of individuals heterozygous for the stop codon.

two studies found an association of the D299G allele with the frequency of gram-negative bacteremia, a third study did not (Lorenz et al., 2002; Agnese et al., 2002; Feterowski et al., 2003). There have also been studies of other types of infections. One study found that D299G predisposed individuals to acute infections such as pyelonephritis and pneumonia (Agnese et al., 2002; Lorenz et al., 2002; Kiechl et al., 2002). Finally, Smirnova et al. found that there was an increased prevalence of multiple rare polymorphisms in TLR4 in meningococcus patients as compared to controls (Smirnova et al., 2003). Taken together, these initial studies suggest a possible association of TLR4 SNPs with susceptibility to gram-negative infections. Studies with larger cohorts are needed to answer this question more definitively.

We recently described four common coding region DNA polymorphisms in TLR5, including a stop codon variant (C1174T, R392STOP) that is unable to mediate flagellin signaling (Hawn et al., 2003). The stop codon (found in the extracellular domain of the protein) is present in ~10 per cent of the population and acts in a dominant fashion with respect to the wild type allele. In a case-control study, we found that two TLR5 polymorphisms, including the stop codon variant, are associated with susceptibility to pneumonia caused by *Legionella pneumophila*, a flagellated bacterium that causes anywhere from 1 to 30 per cent of cases of community-acquired pneumonia (Fraser et al., 1977). The frequency of the stop codon variant was 0.167 in cases and 0.095 in controls (odds ratio 1.90, 95 per cent confidence interval 1.06 to 3.42, $P = 0.03$). We also found that flagellin is a principal activator of pro-inflammatory cytokine production in lung epithelial cells exposed to *Legionella*. Together, these observations implicate genetic variations in TLR5 in susceptibility to human infection and demonstrate an important role for TLR5 in the lung epithelial innate immune response. The data also suggest that expression of TLR4 and TLR5 in different cell types (i.e. TLR4 in macrophages versus TLR5 in epithelial cells) alters the nature of the innate immune response. As a result, the influence of these polymorphisms on disease susceptibility is predicted not only to vary depending on the pathogen, but also on the primary site of infection. The high frequency of the TLR5 stop codon mutation in apparently healthy individuals suggests that there has been some evolutionary advantage to having this genetic variant, although the nature of this benefit is not known.

CONCLUSIONS AND FUTURE PROSPECTS

Since polymorphisms in the TLR signaling pathway can affect susceptibility to common infections, it is possible that in the near future a more complete understanding of this variation will be exploited as a predictive and preventive tool in medicine. Genetic factors may be used to identify patients who are at increased risk for specific infections

or for poor disease progression, leading to more aggressive treatment interventions. Additionally, understanding of the role of TLR signaling in infectious diseases may lead to novel strategies for immune modulation through drugs or vaccines targeting these pathways. Since the first description of a mammalian TLR in 1997, enormous progress has been made in elucidating the role of TLRs in disease through combining *in vitro* cellular/molecular studies, *in vivo* animal studies and human genetic population studies of the innate immune response. Together these approaches will continue to extend our understanding of TLRs in immunity in exciting and unexpected ways.

REFERENCES

Abel, B. et al. (2002). Toll-like receptor 4 expression is required to control chronic Mycobacterium tuberculosis infection in mice. J Immunol *169*, 3155–3162.

Abreu, M.T., Arnold, E.T., Thomas L.S. et al. (2002). TLR4 and MD-2 expression is regulated by immune-mediated signals in human intestinal epithelial cells. J Biol Chem *277*, 20431–20437.

Agnese, D.M., Calvano, J.E., Hahm, S.J. et al. (2002). Human toll-like receptor 4 mutations but not CD14 polymorphisms are associated with an increased risk of gram-negative infections. J Infect Dis *186*, 1522–1525.

Anderson, K.V. (2000). Toll signaling pathways in the innate immune response. Curr Opin Immunol *12*, 13–19.

Arbour, N., Lorenz, E., Schutte, B. et al. (2000). TLR4 mutations are associated with endotoxin hyporesponsiveness in humans. Nat Genet *25*, 187–191.

Brightbill, H.D., Libraty, D.H., Krutzik, S.R. et al. (1999). Host defense mechanisms triggered by microbial lipoproteins through toll-like receptors. Science *285*, 732–736.

Cario, E. and Podolsky, D.K. (2000). Differential alteration in intestinal epithelial cell expression of toll-like receptor 3 (TLR3) and TLR4 in inflammatory bowel disease. Infect Immun *68*, 7010–7017.

Casanova, J.L. and Abel, L. (2002). Genetic dissection of immunity to mycobacteria: the human model. Annu Rev Immunol *20*, 581–620.

Chuang, T. and Ulevitch, R.J. (2001). Identification of hTLR10: a novel human Toll-like receptor preferentially expressed in immune cells. Biochim Biophys Acta *1518*, 157–161.

Chuang, T.H. and Ulevitch, R.J. (2000). Cloning and characterization of a sub-family of human toll-like receptors: hTLR7, hTLR8 and hTLR9. Eur Cytokine Netw *11*, 372–378.

Cooke, G.S. and Hill, A.V. (2001). Genetics of susceptibility to human infectious disease. Nat Rev Genet *2*, 967–977.

Courtois, G., Smahi, A., Reichenbach, J. et al. (2003). A hypermorphic IkappaBalpha mutation is associated with autosomal dominant anhidrotic ectodermal dysplasia and T cell immunodeficiency. J Clin Invest *112*, 1108–1115.

de Veer, M.J., Curtis, J.M., Baldwin, T.M. et al. (2003). MyD88 is essential for clearance of Leishmania major: possible role for lipophosphoglycan and Toll-like receptor 2 signaling. Eur J Immunol *33*, 2822–2831.

DiMango, E., Zar, H.J., Bryan, R. et al. (1995). Diverse Pseudomonas aeruginosa gene products stimulate respiratory epithelial cells to produce interleukin-8. J Clin Invest 96, 2204–2210.

Doffinger, R., Smahi, A., Bessia, C. et al. (2001). X-linked anhidrotic ectodermal dysplasia with immunodeficiency is caused by impaired NF-kappaB signaling. Nat Genet 27, 277–285.

Du, X., Poltorak, A., Wei, Y. et al. (2000). Three novel mammalian toll-like receptors: gene structure, expression, and evolution. Eur Cytokine Netw 11, 362–371.

Echchannaoui, H., Frei, K., Schnell, C., Leib, S.L., Zimmerli, W. and Landmann, R. (2002). Toll-like receptor 2-deficient mice are highly susceptible to Streptococcus pneumoniae meningitis because of reduced bacterial clearing and enhanced inflammation. J Infect Dis 186, 798–806.

Edelson, B.T. and Unanue, E.R. (2002). MyD88-dependent but Toll-like receptor 2-independent innate immunity to Listeria: no role for either in macrophage listericidal activity. J Immunol 169, 3869–3875.

Eisenbarth, S.C., Piggott, D.A., Huleatt, J.W., Visintin, I., Herrick, C.A. and Bottomly, K. (2002). Lipopolysaccharide-enhanced, toll-like receptor 4-dependent T helper cell type 2 responses to inhaled antigen. J Exp Med 196, 1645–1651.

Erridge, C.J., Stewart and Poxton, I.R. (2003). Monocytes heterozygous for the Asp299Gly and Thr399Ile mutations in the Toll-like receptor 4 gene show no deficit in lipopolysaccharide signalling. J Exp Med 197, 1787–1791.

Feng, C.G., Scanga, C.A., Collazo-Custodio, C.M. et al. (2003). Mice lacking myeloid differentiation factor 88 display profound defects in host resistance and immune responses to Mycobacterium avium infection not exhibited by toll-like receptor 2 (TLR2)- and TLR4-deficient animals. J Immunol 171, 4758–4764.

Feterowski, C., Emmanuilidis, K., Miethke, T. et al. (2003). Effects of functional Toll-like receptor-4 mutations on the immune response to human and experimental sepsis. Immunology 109, 426–431.

Fitzgerald, K.A., Rowe, D.C., Barnes, B.J. et al. (2003). LPS-TLR4 signaling to IRF-3/7 and NF-kappaB involves the toll adapters TRAM and TRIF. J Exp Med 198, 1043–1055.

Fraser, D.W., Tsai, T.R., Orenstein, W. et al. (1977). Legionnaires' disease: description of an epidemic of pneumonia. N Engl J Med 297, 1189–1197.

Fremond, C.M. et al. (2003). Control of Mycobacterium bovis BCG infection with increased inflammation in TLR4-deficient mice. Microbes Infect 5, 1070–1081.

Gewirtz, A.T., Navas, T.A., Lyons, S., Godowski, P.J. and Madara, J.L. (2001). Cutting edge: bacterial flagellin activates basolaterally expressed TLR5 to induce epithelial proinflammatory gene expression. J Immunol 167, 1882–1885.

Hagberg, L., Hull, R., Hull, S., McGhee, J.R., Michalek, S.M. and Svanborg Eden, C. (1984). Difference in susceptibility to gram-negative urinary tract infection between C3H/HeJ and C3H/HeN mice. Infect Immun 46, 839–844.

Hajjar, A.M., Ernst, R.K., Tsai, J.H., Wilson, C.B. and Miller, S.I. (2002). Human Toll-like receptor 4 recognizes host-specific LPS modifications. Nat Immunol 3, 354–359.

Hawn, T., Verbon, R.A., Lettinga, K.D. et al. (2003). A common dominant TLR5 stop codon polymorphism abolishes flagellin signaling and is associated with susceptibility to Legionnaires' Disease. J Exp Med 198, 1563–1572.

Hayashi, F., Smith, K.D., Ozinsky, A. et al. (2001). The innate immune response to bacterial flagellin is mediated by Toll-like receptor 5. Nature 410, 1099–1103.

Heldwein, K.A. et al. (2003). TLR2 and TLR4 serve distinct roles in the host immune response against Mycobacterium bovis BCG. J Leukoc Biol 74, 277–286.

Helmby, H. and Grencis, R.K. (2003). Essential role for TLR4 and MyD88 in the development of chronic intestinal nematode infection. Eur J Immunol 33, 2974–2979.

Hou, L., Sasaki, H. and Stashenko, P. (2000). Toll-like receptor 4-deficient mice have reduced bone destruction following mixed anaerobic infection. Infect Immun 68, 4681–4687.

Jain, A., Ma, C.A., Liu, S., Brown, M., Cohen, J. and Strober, W. (2001). Specific missense mutations in NEMO result in hyper-IgM syndrome with hypohydrotic ectodermal dysplasia. Nat Immunol 2, 223–228.

Jarrossay, D., Napolitani, G., Colonna, M., Sallusto, F. and Lanzavecchia, A. (2001). Specialization and complementarity in microbial molecule recognition by human myeloid and plasmacytoid dendritic cells. Eur J Immunol 31, 3388–3393.

Kadowski, N., Ho, S., Antonenko, S. et al. (2001). Subsets of human dendritic cell precursors express different toll-like receptors and respond to different microbial antigens. J Exp Med 194, 863–869.

Kamath, A.B. et al. (2003). Toll-like receptor 4-defective C3H/HeJ mice are not more susceptible than other C3H substrains to infection with Mycobacterium tuberculosis. Infect Immun 71, 4112–4118.

Kiechl, S., Lorenz, E., Reindl, M. et al. (2002). Toll-like receptor 4 polymorphisms and atherogenesis. N Engl J Med 347, 185–192.

Lemaitre, B., Nicolas, E., Michaut, L., Reichhart, J.M. and Hoffmann, J.A. (1996). The dorsoventral regulatory gene cassette spatzle/Toll/cactus controls the potent antifungal response in Drosophila adults. Cell 86, 973–983.

Liaudet, L., Szabo, C., Evgenov, O.V. et al. (2003). Flagellin from gram-negative bacteria is a potent mediator of acute pulmonary inflammation in sepsis. Shock 19, 131–137.

Lien, E., Means, T.K., Heine, H. et al. (2000). Toll-like receptor 4 imparts ligand-specific recognition of bacterial lipopolysaccharide. J Clin Invest 105, 497–504.

Lorenz, E., Mira, J.P., Frees, K.L. and Schwartz, D.A. (2002). Relevance of mutations in the TLR4 receptor in patients with gram-negative septic shock. Arch Intern Med 162, 1028–1032.

Malley, R. et al. (2003). Recognition of pneumolysin by Toll-like receptor 4 confers resistance to pneumococcal infection. Proc Natl Acad Sci USA 100, 1966–1971.

Medvedev, A.E., Lentschat, A., Kuhns, D.B. et al. (2003). Distinct mutations in IRAK-4 confer hyporesponsiveness to lipopolysaccharide and interleukin-1 in a patient with recurrent bacterial infections. J Exp Med 198, 521–531.

Medzhitov, R., Preston-Hurlburt, P. and Janeway, C.A. Jr (1997). A human homologue of the Drosophila Toll protein signals activation of adaptive immunity. Nature 388, 394–397.

Melmed, G., Thomas, L.S., Lee, N. et al. (2003). Human intestinal epithelial cells are broadly unresponsive to Toll-like receptor 2-dependent bacterial ligands: implications for host-microbial interactions in the gut. J Immunol 170, 1406–1415.

Miettinen, M., Sareneva, T., Julkunen, I. and Matikainen, S. (2001). IFNs activate toll-like receptor gene expression in viral infections. Genes Immun 2, 349–355.

Mizel, S.B., West, A.P. and Hantgan, R.R. (2003). Identification of a sequence in human toll-like receptor 5 required for the binding of Gram-negative flagellin. J Biol Chem 278, 23624–23629.

Mun, H.S., Aosai, F., Norose, K. et al. (2003). TLR2 as an essential molecule for protective immunity against Toxoplasma gondii infection. Int Immunol 15, 1081–1087.

Muraille, E., De Trez, C., Brait, M., De Baetselier, P., Leo, O. and Carlier, Y. (2003). Genetically resistant mice lacking MyD88-adapter protein display a high susceptibility to Leishmania major infection associated with a polarized Th2 response. J Immunol 170, 4237–4241.

O'Brien, A.D., Rosenstreich, D.L., Scher, I., Campbell, G.H., MacDermott, R.P. and Formal, S.B. (1980). Genetic control of susceptibility to Salmonella typhimurium in mice: role of the LPS gene. J Immunol 124, 20–24.

Okamura, Y., Watari, M., Jerud, E.S. et al. (2001). The extra domain A of fibronectin activates Toll-like receptor 4. J Biol Chem 276, 10229–10233.

Ozinsky, A., Underhill, D.M., Fontenot, J.D. et al. (2000). The repertoire for pattern recognition of pathogens by the innate immune system is defined by cooperation between toll-like receptors. Proc Natl Acad Sci USA 97, 13766–13771.

Picard, C., Puel, A., Bonnet, M. et al. (2003). Pyogenic bacterial infections in humans with IRAK-4 deficiency. Science 299, 2076–2079.

Poltorak, A., He, X., Smirnova, I. et al. (1998). Defective LPS signaling in C3H/HeJ and C57BL/10ScCr mice: mutations in Tlr4 gene. Science 282, 2085–2088.

Poltorak, A., Ricciardi-Castagnoli, P., Citterio, S. and Beutler, B. (2000). Physical contact between lipopolysaccharide and toll-like receptor 4 revealed by genetic complementation. Proc Natl Acad Sci USA 97, 2163–2167.

Pulendran, B., Kumar, P., Cutler, C.W., Mohamadzadeh, M., Van Dyke, T. and Banchereau, J. (2001). Lipopolysaccharides from distinct pathogens induce different classes of immune responses in vivo. J Immunol 167, 5067–5076.

Reiling, N. et al. (2002). Cutting edge: Toll-like receptor (TLR)2- and TLR4-mediated pathogen recognition in resistance to airborne infection with Mycobacterium tuberculosis. J Immunol 169, 3480–3484.

Rock, F., Hardiman, L.G., Timans, J.C., Kastelein, R.A. and Bazan, J.F. (1998). A family of human receptors structurally related to Drosophila Toll. Proc Natl Acad Sci USA 95, 588–593.

Scanga, C.A., Aliberti, J., Jankovic, D. et al. (2002). Cutting edge: MyD88 is required for resistance to Toxoplasma gondii infection and regulates parasite-induced IL-12 production by dendritic cells. J Immunol 168, 5997–6001.

Schnare, M., Barton, G.M., Holt, A.C., Takeda, K., Akira, S. and Medzhitov, R. (2001). Toll-like receptors control activation of adaptive immune responses. Nat Immunol 2, 947–950.

Seki, E., Tsutsui, H., Tsuji, N.M. et al. (2002). Critical roles of myeloid differentiation factor 88-dependent proinflammatory cytokine release in early phase clearance of Listeria monocytogenes in mice. J Immunol 169, 3863–3868.

Shim, T.S., Turner, O.C. and Orme, I.M. (2003). Toll-like receptor 4 plays no role in susceptibility of mice to Mycobacterium tuberculosis infection. Tuberculosis (Edinb) 83, 367–371.

Sierro, F., Dubois, B., Coste, A., Kaiserlian, D., Kraehenbuhl, J.P. and Sirard, J.C. (2001). Flagellin stimulation of intestinal epithelial cells triggers CCL20- mediated migration of dendritic cells. Proc Natl Acad Sci USA 98, 13722–13727.

Smirnova, I., Mann, N., Dols, A. et al. (2003). Assay of locus-specific genetic load implicates rare Toll-like receptor 4 mutations in meningococcal susceptibility. Proc Natl Acad Sci USA 2, 2.

Smith, K.D., Andersen-Nissen, E., Hayashi, F. et al. (2003). Toll-like receptor 5 recognizes a conserved site on flagellin required for protofilament formation and bacterial motility. Nat Immunol 4, 1247–1253.

Standiford, T.J., Kunkel, S.L., Basha, M.A. et al. (1990). Interleukin-8 gene expression by a pulmonary epithelial cell line. A model for cytokine networks in the lung. J Clin Invest 86, 1945–1953.

Steiner, T.S., Nataro, J.P., Poteet-Smith, C.E., Smith, J.A. and Guerrant, R.L. (2000). Enteroaggregative Escherichia coli expresses a novel flagellin that causes IL-8 release from intestinal epithelial cells. J Clin Invest 105, 1769–1777.

Sugawara, I. et al. (2003a). Mycobacterial infection in TLR2 and TLR6 knockout mice. Microbiol Immunol 47, 327–336.

Sugawara, I. et al. (2003b). Mycobacterial infection in MyD88-deficient mice. Microbiol Immunol 47, 841–847.

Suzuki, N., Suzuki, S., Duncan, G.S. et al. (2002). Severe impairment of interleukin-1 and Toll-like receptor signalling in mice lacking IRAK-4. Nature 416, 750–756.

Takeuchi, O., Hoshino, K. and Akira, S. (2000). Cutting edge: TLR2-deficient and MyD88-deficient mice are highly susceptible to Staphylococcus aureus infection. J Immunol 165, 5392–5396.

Takeuchi, O., Kawai, T., Sanjo, H. et al. (1999). TLR6: A novel member of an expanding toll-like receptor family. Gene 231, 59–65.

Underhill, D.M. (2003). Toll-like receptors: networking for success. Eur J Immunol 33, 1767–1775.

Underhill, D.M. and Ozinsky, A. (2002). Toll-like receptors: key mediators of microbe detection. Curr Opin Immunol 14, 103–110.

von Aulock, S., Schroder, N.W., Gueinzius, K. et al. (2003). Heterozygous toll-like receptor 4 polymorphism does not influence lipopolysaccharide-induced cytokine release in human whole blood. J Infect Dis 188, 938–943.

Wang, M., Jeng, K.C. and Ping, L.I. (1999). Exogenous cytokine modulation or neutralization of interleukin-10 enhance survival in lipopolysaccharide-hyporesponsive C3H/HeJ mice with Klebsiella infection. Immunology 98, 90–97.

Wang, X. et al. (2002). Toll-like receptor 4 mediates innate immune responses to Haemophilus influenzae infection in mouse lung. J Immunol 168, 810–815.

Weighardt, H., Kaiser-Moore, S., Vabulas, R.M., Kirschning, C.J., Wagner, H. and Holzmann, B. (2002). Cutting edge: myeloid differentiation factor 88 deficiency improves resistance against sepsis caused by polymicrobial infection. J Immunol 169, 2823–2827.

Westendorp, R.G., Langermans, J.A., Huizinga, T.W. et al. (1997). Genetic influence on cytokine production and fatal meningococcal disease. Lancet 349, 170–173.

Woods, J.P., Frelinger, J.A., Warrack, G. and Cannon, J.G. et al. (1988). Mouse genetic locus Lps influences susceptibility to Neisseria meningitidis infection. Infect Immun 56, 1950–1955.

Yamamoto, M., Sato, S., Hemmi, H. et al. (2003). TRAM is specifically involved in the Toll-like receptor 4-mediated MyD88-independent signaling pathway. Nat Immunol 4, 1144–1150.

Yaqoob, P., Newsholme, E.A. and Calder, P.C. (1999). Comparison of cytokine production in cultures of whole human blood and purified mononuclear cells. Cytokine 11, 600–605.

Zonana, J., Elder, M.E., Schneider, L.C. et al. (2000). A novel X-linked disorder of immune deficiency and hypohidrotic ectodermal dysplasia is allelic to incontinentia pigmenti and due to mutations in IKK-gamma (NEMO). Am J Hum Genet 67, 1555–1562.

DNA Sequence-Specific Transcription Factors

Chapter 7

Philip E. Auron

University of Pittsburgh School of Medicine, Pittsburgh, PA, USA

There are one-story intellects, two-story intellects and three-story intellects with skylights. All fact collectors with no aim beyond their facts are one-story men. Two-story men compare reason and generalize, using labors of the fact collectors as well as their own. Three-story men idealize, imagine and predict. Their best illuminations come from above through the skylight.

Oliver Wendell Holmes

INTRODUCTION

The role of gene expression in immunity cannot be over emphasized. The development of the immune response depends upon the transcriptional activation of gene collectives that result in the expansion of cell lineages and the expression of gene products that function within, on the surface, and, via secretion, on remote target cells. The activation of transcription depends upon numerous protein factors that target chromatin and DNA. In many cases these are rendered functionally competent as a result of extracellular signaling through surface receptors. This signal-dependent competence can take two major forms. First, the *induction* of *de novo* gene expression generates the presence, or increased concentration, of factors Second, constitutively expressed factors lie dormant in an inactive state awaiting immediate-early activation that can take various molecular forms. These include inherent intramolecular conformational suppression (e.g. C/EBPβ) (Kowenz-Leutz et al., 1994; Williams et al., 1995; Engelman et al., 1998; Baldassare

et al., 1999); intermolecular inhibitory associations (e.g. NF-κB·IκB) (Li and Verma, 2002); and post-DNA binding chemical modification, resulting in association with a cofactor that activates transcription (e.g. CBP/p300 binding to phosphorylated CREB) (De Cesare and Sassone, 2000). Activation then results from chemical modifications directed either toward the transcription factor and the inhibitor or both. In addition to activation, transcription factors can also inhibit transcription, a process essential to generating some cell types, like the effect of the Id factor in favoring NK over T and B cell development (Spits et al., 2000).

The transcription factors involved in messenger RNA synthesis represent a collection of proteins that use diverse mechanisms to regulate gene expression. Factors are grossly categorized as either general or specific. General factors are involved in the expression of most, if not all, RNA polymerase II (Pol II)-dependent protein coding genes. These factors include proteins such as the TFIIA, IIB, TATA binding protein (TBP) and its associated factors (TAFs) that constitute TFIID, the mediator complex that recruits Pol II, and numerous other factors involved in the process of transcription activation, elongation and termination (Naar et al., 2001; Cosma, 2002). Among these, cofactors like SWI/SNF, ISWI, NuRD and CBP/p300 involved in chromatin remodeling and modification as well as enzymes involved in DNA methylation can also be included (Narlikar et al., 2002). Specific factors, by virtue of cognate protein-DNA sequence recognition, target distinct groups of genes. These DNA sequence-specific factors represent the vast repertoire of

Measuring Immunity, edited by Michael T. Lotze and Angus W. Thomson
ISBN 0-12-455900-X, London

proteins that have commonly been associated with specific gene expression and signal transduction responses. It will be these proteins that the remainder of this overview will primarily focus on. General and cofactors will only be briefly discussed for those that possess a developmental- and tissue-specific functional association with a DNA sequence-specific factor.

Although there are approximately 1500 different specific transcription factor genes in humans (alternative splicing may generate as many as 2000 different proteins, as judged from the initial inspection of the genome sequence), there are probably less than 20 specific family types, classified by convention according to the nature of the DNA binding domain (DBD). In fact, four classes (C2H2 Zn Finger, HTH, bHLH and bZIP) collectively constitute between 75 and 96 per cent of the factors and one class, the C2H2 zinc fingers, represents more than half of all factor types (Lander et al., 2001; Venter et al., 2001). In addition to the DBD, general transcription factors contain other types of domains essential to function. These include transcription activation domains (TAD) essential for function, which are involved in protein–protein interactions with various general and specific factors; regulatory domains that control post-translational activity (as described above by either chemical modification or protein–protein interaction); nuclear localization signals (NLS), which facilitate translocation from the cytoplasm to the nucleus and are often integrated into the DBD; and nuclear export signals (NES) that permit recycling of factors whose regulation involves compartmental sequestration away from the DNA into the cytoplasm. Finally, factors can also multimerize via DBD and extra-DBD domains (Figure 7.1). This multimerization serves at least three distinct functions. One is the expansion of target sequence binding specificity due to combinatorial rearrangements. Another is increased binding affinity for the composite target because of an increase in molecular contacts. The third is the recruitment of a secondary TAD,

Sequence-specific transcription factors
interact with DNA and proteins

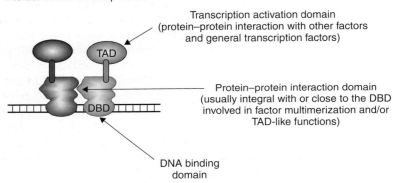

Transcription activation domain
(protein–protein interaction with other factors
and general transcription factors)

Protein–protein interaction domain
(usually integral with or close to the DBD
involved in factor multimerization and/or
TAD-like functions)

DNA binding
domain

Examples of protein-tethered transactivation

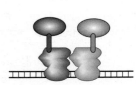

Factors bind at adjacent DNA sites
(HSF-1, homeodomain factors,
Spi-1 with PIP on Ig light chain 3'
enhancer)

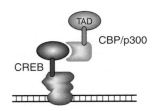

No DBD on co-activator
(CREB with CBP/p300)

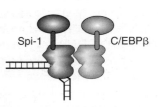

Only one factor binds DNA
(Spi-1 with C/EBP on *IL 1b* promoter,
Ets 1 with USF 1 on HIV-LTR)

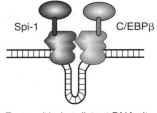

Factors bind at distant DNA sites
(*IL 1b* gene: Spi-1 on promoter with C/EBP
on enhancer)

Figure 7.1 Sequence-specific transcription factors bind DNA and interact with other proteins. The upper panel is a schematic representation of two factors simultaneously binding DNA as dimers. The DNA binding domains (DBD) and transcription activation domains (TAD) are indicated. The lower panel illustrates example configurations as indicated.

provided by a tethered factor, that can serve to facilitate the formation of a productive transcription complex called an enhancesome (Maniatis et al., 1998). This phenomenon, which has been referred to as protein-tethered transactivation (PTT) (Waraswapati et al., 1999), may be especially critical to permit the long-distance interaction between some enhancers and core promoters.

The activation of gene transcription depends upon a hierarchical process. The first step involves the binding of specific factors to exposed DNA target sequences that can initiate chromatin remodeling, thus permitting the exposure of additional sequences that result in a concerted binding of factors that collectively generate an enhancesome. The enhancesome often contains multiple specific factors that cooperatively recruit general factors and Pol II, thus initiating transcription. The specific factors that bind to compacted chromatin, permitting remodeling, may likely be those that possess a structure that is consistent with binding to the single surface of exposed DNA within a nucleosome. For example HTH proteins tangentially bind to one DNA surface (as in the nucleosome), whereas Rel and bZIP proteins wrap completely around the DNA (inconsistent with nucleosome binding). This could explain why some factors bind at early stages, while others do not (Cirillo et al., 2002). Therefore, transcription initiation is a highly regulated and cooperative event involving both sequential and simultaneous binding of numerous proteins. Furthermore, the fact that there are many factors that can bind to the same or very similar sequences (e.g. in humans, there are 140 bHLH proteins that all bind to similar E-box sequences of the type CANNTG), means that more than one factor can bind to a gene and potentially activate transcription. However, the tissue-specific expression, signal-dependent activation and distinct TAD domains, with their specificity for interaction with protein partners, function in concert to limit non-specific activation.

Consequently, the ability of a transcription factor to serve as a marker or surrogate is dependent upon its mode of action and the nature of the chosen assay. For example, a constitutively expressed, dormant, factor may have the potential to be a marker. However, measurement of its abundance either by immunoreactive techniques such as ELISA and Western blot or by measurement of messenger RNA levels, such as by DNA microarray, will not necessarily correlate with functional competence. However, measurement of attributes such as nuclear localization, activating chemical modification (e.g. phosphorylation and acetylation) and DNA binding can (but for some systems like CREB may not) be useful measurable parameters. Also because factors often act on genes in concert with specific partners, the simultaneous expression and/or activation of such cognate pairs can be critical. For this reason, some of the details of specific factor activation, cooperation and expression in light of some key immunological processes will be discussed. Attention will also be paid to the methods of assaying function, critical to the qualification of a valid marker.

CLASSIFICATION OF SPECIFIC FACTOR SUPERFAMILIES

Historically, the easiest and most practical method of identifying novel transcription factor classes has been the direct binding to cognate DNA sequences. This also permitted an immediate correlation with specific target genes via binding specificity. Consequently, the DBD has been the preferred domain by which these proteins have been classified, even if additional regulatory and, especially, TAD sequences may be dispersed among other proteins that do not share a common DBD structure. This convention will be used in this overview and Table 7.1 lists numerous immunologically relevant factors grouped according to the nature of the primary DBD.

Helix-turn-helix (HTH)

Members of the HTH superfamily were the first to be studied in molecular detail and represent numerous important sub-families which include the homeodomain proteins that bind homeo-boxes (Hox); the winged HTH (wHTH) proteins which include the forked-head, ETS and heat shock factor (HSF) proteins; and the POU-domain factors (Garvie and Wolberger, 2001). All of these proteins contain three or four amphipathic α-helices held together by hydrophobic patches that are found consistently on one surface of each helix. Collectively they fold into a tight globular structure with the aliphatic residues clustered into an interior core. One helix usually serves as a primary DNA-binding 'recognition' helix that fits along its length into the major groove of the common B-form of DNA (Figure 7.2A). This interaction usually provides most of the binding specificity, but usually has an insufficient number of molecular contacts to provide stable association. The additional less-specific contacts are provided by accessory interactions mediated by a variety of molecular mechanisms.

For example, some homeodomain proteins have a 'disordered' positively-charged (basic) tail that wraps around the DNA and penetrates the narrow minor groove providing charge-interactions with the negatively-charged (acidic) DNA phosphate backbone (Figure 7.2A). Instead of a tail, other homeodomain proteins interact directly with another binding factor to support binding to two adjacent sites, such as is the case with HoxB1 and Pbx1 (Wilson and Desplan, 1999; LaRonde-LeBlanc and Wolberger, 2003). In addition, other factors like POU-domain and Cut-like factors possess covalently linked multiple HTH domains (Harada et al., 1995). The wHTH proteins have structural extensions such as loops and β-sheets with basic residues that provide additional backbone phosphate contact. The presence of these extra-HTH domain sequences, such as basic tails and wings, results in the ability of HTH proteins to bind DNA as monomers, as well as homotypic dimers and in complexes with other disparate DNA binding proteins. This property manifests upon these factors a tremendous diversity of combinatorial

Table 7.1 Selected transcription factor properties

Factor	Function	Representative target genes	DNA recognition sequence	Representative cofactors
HTH:				
Homeo (Pbx1, HoxB4, A10, Hlx)	Maint. hematopoietic stem cells	Rap1, Irx5	TGAT TNAT	Pbx-Hox heterodimer
Pax5/BSAP/Prd	B cell development, oncogene, suppresses plasma cell development	BLNK, CD19, N-Myc	(G/C)AAAC(A/T)C	Ets 1, Fli 1, GABP, Pax homodimer
Pou(Oct 1)	represses IL8 gene at C/EBP site	IL8	ATNNGCAT	
ETS (Sap, Tel, Spi/PU.1, others)	Hematopoiesis oncogenes, Viral forms	Ig genes, IL 1B, Fms, IL 7RA, E2A, EBF	(G/A)GA(A/T)	bZIP, IRF, Rel, GATA, Pax SRF, Runx, viral proteins
X-box (RFX 5, AP, B)	MHCII, B-Cell, unfolded prot. response	MHCII, UPR genes	GTNRCC(No-3) RGYAAC	CIITA
X-box (XBP1)	Terminal plasma cell development		CRC GTCA	
Y-box (NF-Y/CBF)	Regulation of stem cells	Hox B4, TGFβR	(T/CA/GA/G) CCAATCA	NF-Y(A, B.C)
HSF	Antiinflammatory	IL 1B	GAAATTTC	C/EBPβ
Cut (CDP)	Inhibition of CBF		CCAAT	
IRF 1 to 9	Inflammation, ant-viral, viral forms	IFNB κ & λ Ig, LB 1 B	(A/G)NGAAA	Spi 1, Stat 1, 2
Myb	Monocyte differentiation Inflammation	COX2, PDCD4	YAAC(G/T)G	
Foxp3/Scurfin	Induces CD4+ /CD25+ regulatory T cells			
bZIP:				
Jun, Fos, Fra	Inflammation, myeloid responses	IL 1B, IL2, GMCSF, MMP1	TGAC TCA	Fos, Spi1, NFAT, GR, Maf
C/EBP	Inflammation, myeloid responses	IL 1B, Fms, IL-8, TNFA, IL6	TTRC GYAA	Spi1, CREB, ATF
MafB, c-Maf	Monocyte differentiation	Jun/Fos target genes	tgc TGAC TCAgca	Fos, Jun
NFE2	Megakaryocyte & platelet development		TGAC TCA	
CREB, CREM, ATF	cAMP responses	Fos, ICER, IL1B, NUR77, Nor1	TGAC GTCA	CBP
bHLH:				
Mitf	Osteoclast & mast cell development	TRAP	CAC GTG	Spi1
E2A (E12/E47)	Multiple functions in hematopoiesis	Mb-1	CAC GTG	HEB, SCL, GATA 1, Lmo2
HEB, SCL/Tal1, Id				E2A, HEB, SCL form heterodimers and bind other factors like Lmo2 and GATA 1 to generate complexes
Myc, Max, Mad	Myb granulocyte block, oncogene	B23, PRDX3, JPo1, CD34	CAC GTG	Myc, Max, Mad, Id
Mxi1	Tumor suppressor, Myc repressor		CAC GTG	Myc, Mad
Id1, 2, 3, 4	Selective bHLH repressor, E2A inhibition		CAC GTG	E2A, E47
COE:				
EBF	B-cell development	Mb-1, B29, Pax5	ANNCNCNNGGGAAT	E2A, HEB
C4 Zn Finger:				
Nuclear Receptors	Inflammation, development	Steroid & lipid response genes	RG(G/T)TCA	Dimers bind inverted, everted, Direct DNA repeats
GATA 1, 2, 3	Multiple functions in hematopoiesis	MBP, ε, γ-Hgb, α-1Lb	AGATAAA	Spi1, Fli1, FOG, Sp 1
C2H2 Zn Finger:				
Sp1		CD95, COL2A1	CGGGGGCGG	Spi1, GATA
Egr1/Krox24/ Zif268	Inflammatory response factor	TGFβ, TF, PDGF A&B, COL2A1	GNGNGGGNG	
MZF1	Inhibits CFU-G in myeloid cells		RR(T/G)GGGGA	
WT1	Acute myeloid leukemia marker	TGFβ1, FREAC-4, IGFII	GCGGGGCG	
Ikaros (Ik)	Lymphoid over myeloid development	λ5, TdT, GMCSFR, IL2Rβ, Flk2	(C/T)GGGAA(T/C)	Ik1, 2, Ai, He, Peg, EosNURD

Table 7.1 continued

Factor	Function	Representative target genes	DNA recognition sequence	Representative cofactors
Aiolos (Ai)	B cell development		(C/T)GGGAA(T/C)	Ik1, 2, Ai, He, Peg, EosNURD
Helios (He)	Hematopoietic stem cells & T cells		(C/T)GGGAA(T/C)	Ik1, 2, Ai, He, Peg, EosNURD
Pegasus (Peg)	Lymphoid cells		GNNNGNNG	Ik1, 2, Ai, He, Peg, EosNURD
Eos	Lymphoid cells		GNNNGNNG	Ik1, 2, Ai, He, Peg, EosNURD
Blimp1	Terminal plasma cell development, suppresses B cell Txn			
Bc16	B cell development, suppresses Plasma cell development, oncogene	CyclinD2, MIP1α, MCP1, CD23	TTCCNRGAA (Binding competes with similar Stat6 DNA site)	Stat4-Bc-16-IRF-4 complex, BCoR repressor
C3H Zn β-Hairpin:				
Smad1, 2, 3, 5, 8	Mediators of TGFβ function	PAI-2, IgCα	R(T/G)CT	Dimer-like binding to direct & inverted repeats
Ig-like:				
Runx/CBFα/AML			YGYGGT	CBFα,
NFAT1, 2, 3, 4, 5	Hematopoiesis, activatable response in macrophages, osteoclasts, T, B, & mast cells	IL2, 4, 5, 8, 13, GMCSF, IFNG, HIV-LTR, TRAP, CTR	(T/A) GGAAR	AP-1, NFAT1 & 5 can bind as homodimers
STAT 1, 2, 3, 4 5a, b, 6	Cytokine signaling, hematopoiesis, inflammation, oncogene	Cytokine target genes	TT(C/A)(N$_{2-4}$) (G/T)AA	Various homotypic dimers, Spi 1
T-box (TBX, Tbet, Eomesodermin/ Eomes)	Effectors of helper T cell development	IFNG, GranzymeB, IL12Rβ2	TTTNNCACCT AGGTGNNAA	
p53			RRRC(A/TT/A)GYYY	
NF-κB1, 2, RelA, B, c-Rel	Activatable response in many cell types, represses erythropoiesis, innate & adaptive immunity	IL2, 6, 8, TNFA, IL12p40, COX2, IFN-γ, HIV-LTR, yCAM, ICAM1	gGGRr(N$_{1-2}$)YYCC	C/EBPβ, Stat3, 6, Spi 1, IκBα,β,γ,ζ, Bcl3 Various homotypic dimers
CSL/CBF 1	Activated via intracellular Notch domain		GTGGGAA	Active ternary complex is CSL/ICN/MAML 1
MADS:				
SRF, Mef	Activation of immediate-early genes	Fos, Egr 1, Pip92, Nur77	CC(A/T)5 GG	TCF ETS factors (e.g. Eik1, Sap 1, Net), SRF homodimer
AT-hook:				
MLL	Induces Hox proteins and hematopoietic stem cells	Hox3.1, Foxc2, Gremlin, DCom, Col6A3	AAAATA	
Tcf1, Lef1	Lymphofietic developmental factors Mediators of Wnt function	TCRα	GGAAACTT	Lef1 complexes with ATF, CREB, Po, PEBP2, & Ets 1 on the T cell receptor α chain gene.

interactions, as exemplified by the ETS group of wHTH proteins (Sharrocks et al., 1997; Verger and Duterque, 2002).

Basic leucine zipper (bZIP) and basic helix-loop-helix (bHLH)

The bZIP and bHLH proteins bind DNA as obligate dimers. The basic region of each monomer forms a helix that contacts DNA in a manner somewhat similar to that of the HTH recognition helix. Unlike the HTH helix, the basic region does not benefit from the stabilization of amphipathic-driven intramolecular association and is disordered until stabilized by direct interaction with DNA (Weiss et al., 1990; Anthony-Cahill et al., 1992). In addition, rather than taking advantage of additional tails and

wings to provide binding stability, the formation of a homotypic dimer results in simultaneous binding of two geometrically linked basic regions to opposite sides of the B-DNA helix (Figure 7.2B). This dimeric binding results in a palindromic recognition sequence. However, the presence of two associated proteins can mean that strong binding to a 'perfect' half binding site can be supported by 'imperfect' binding to the second half-site. This hypothesis is supported by reports of bZIP monomer interactions with DNA (Stanojevic and Verdine, 1995; Carroll et al., 1997; Wu et al., 1998; Hollenbeck and Oakley, 2000). Consequently, half-site recognition may be an important mode of DNA binding for these factors.

The mode of dimerization is somewhat different between the bZIP and bHLH proteins. The former dimerizes via

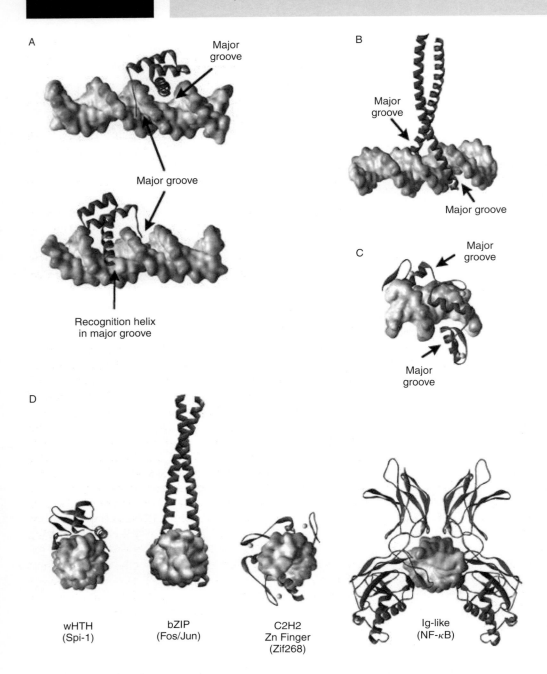

Figure 7.2 Examples of transcription factor-DNA interaction geometries. A. Interaction of the HTH protein engrailed (1HDD) with the major and minor grooves of DNA. B. Binding of the Fos-Jun bZIP dimer (1FOS) to two adjacent major grooves. C. The Zif268 protein (1ZAA) positions three C2H2 Zn fingers continuously along the major groove. D. Axial DNA views of Spi-1/PU.1 (1PUE), Fos/Jun dimer, Zif268 and NF-κB p50 homodimer (1SVC) revealing distinct geometries.

hydrophobic interactions (usually leucines, hence leucine zipper) along the surfaces of two mutually interacting helices that generate a coiled-coil structure that continues into the basic region, following DNA binding. The latter dimerizes via a shared α-helical 4-coil bundle, generating 2-loops that each contain a single basic residue that binds to 2-DNA backbone phosphates, thus providing additional stabilization (Ellenberger et al., 1994; Ma et al., 1994). A variation on the bHLH is the bHLH ZIP in which a leucine zipper coiled-coil extends beyond the HLH module (Ferre-D'Amare et al., 1993). The differences between the bZIP and bHLH dimerization structures results in two distinct DNA binding geometries for the basic regions and a less stable dimerization interaction

for bZIP proteins. The greater propensity for exchange among dimerization partners for the bZIP means that following initial post-translational association, bZIPs can be more effectively regulated by dimer exchange. This has manifested itself in some exotic regulatory mechanisms (Tsukada et al., 1994; Newman and Keating, 2003).

COE helix-loop-helix

An important factor for B cell development, named early B cell factor (EBF), is a member of a novel family of DNA binding proteins designated as COE for the founding members Collier (Col), Olfactory factor1 (Olf-1) and EBF (Dubois and Vincent, 2001). These proteins possess an

HTH motif that neither contains nor is immediately adjacent to a basic region. The recognition sequence for the dimer (ATTCCCNNGGGAAT) does not conform to that of the classic CANNTG E-box.

C4, C2H2, and C3H zinc fingers

This classification is really a consolidation of several different families of DBD possessing at least one Zn atom-containing DNA-binding module. Subclassification depends upon the nature of the amino acids involved in direct zinc coordination (Laity et al., 2001). Domains containing four cysteine residues are referred to as C4, those with two cysteines and two histidines are C2H2. Another family representing the DNA-binding MH1 domain of SMAD proteins contains three cysteines and one histidine (Chai et al., 2003). Other C3H types exist, but they have not been associated with DNA binding and are found in some protein–protein interaction modules. The C4 fingers have also been associated with protein–protein interaction and provide both functionalities in some transcription factors. For example, the nuclear and cytoplasmic steroid/hormone receptors possess monomers that contain two sets of C4 Zn finger modules. In some cases, dimerization is mediated by one set of fingers, while DNA binding with another (Mangelsdorf and Evans, 1995; Chawla et al., 2001; Laity et al., 2001).

The C4 and C2H2 DNA binding finger modules possess distinct structural architectures and DNA binding modes. C4 modules structurally resemble HTH domains, except that the α-helices are not amphipathic and the globular helical structure is held together by Zn coordination, rather than a hydrophobic core. Consequently, the mode of DNA binding is similar to that of HTH in that there is extensive contact with the B-DNA major groove along the length of the helix. This results, like HTH, in a tangential contact between a recognition helix and the DNA helix. In contrast, the C2H2 Zn finger (also called ββα Zn fingers) consists of a single α-helix connected to a 2-stranded anti-parallel β-hairpin, which is stabilized by coordination to a single Zn atom. Rather than extensive contact with the B-DNA major groove via most of the length of the recognition helix, only amino acid residues in the helix near the loop are involved in DNA binding. Instead of tangential contact with the DNA helix, as is the case for HTH, the end of the helix (and its attached loop) points perpendicularly into the major groove much like the finger for which the module is named. As a consequence, the C2H2 Zn finger can closely pack many modules into the major groove along a considerable length of DNA. For this reason, many of these proteins possess numerous and varied arrangements of finger modules that are often rearranged by alternative mRNA splicing. One such protein, CTCF (CCCTC binding factor) possesses 11 finger modules that contact 60 continuous base pairs of DNA major groove (Ladomery and Dellaire, 2002).

Both of these varieties of Zn finger have variants that contain a single finger plus a basic tail, similar to some HTH proteins. Examples include the C4 GATA (Omichinski et al., 1993) and the C2H2 GAGA proteins (Omichinski et al., 1997). Thus, like the HTH proteins, these factors have the potential to bind DNA as monomers.

The R-SMAD proteins that are activated via TGF-β signaling, possess a unique MH1 domain in which a DNA-binding β-hairpin physically extends out of a globular domain. This domain consists of 4 α-helices and 2 antiparallel β-strands stabilized by the coordination of three cysteines and one histidine with Zn. This C3H Zn β-hairpin interacts with a short 4 bp SMAD binding half-site. However, unlike other palindromic sites suggestive of obligatory dimer binding, R-SMADs seem to be capable of binding to isolated half-sites (Chai et al., 2003; Derynck and Zhang, 2003).

Immunoglobulin (Ig)-like

At least 30 human genes code for transcription factors that contain Ig-like DBDs. These are a diverse group of structurally-related proteins that are divided into five different subtypes (Rudolph and Gergen, 2001). Three of these types, the Rel, STAT and T-domain families represent some of the most important molecules in immunology. The Rel family can be subdivided into two related subdivisions, the NF-κB and NFAT factors. Rounding out this grouping are the Runx factors, p53 and the CSL factor (Nam et al., 2003) that is activated by association of the proteolytically-released intracellular portion of notch (ICN). The ICN resembles and acts much like activating forms (Martinez Arias et al., 2002) of IκB (e.g. Bcl-3 and IMAP). All of these factors have structural similarity to the multi-anti-parallel β-stranded Ig-fold and interact with DNA either as homotypic dimers or as partners with disparate partners. Consequently, Ig-like proteins appear to be incapable of binding to DNA as monomers.

MADS

The MADS domain (term taken from the names of the first four members, MCM1, Agamous, Deficiens and Serum response factor) is a DBD that binds as a dimer and strikingly bends DNA. The structure contains a coiled-coil that binds two adjacent DNA grooves along a majority of its length forcing a severe curvature in the DNA molecule (Pellegrini et al., 1995). The coiled-coil is part of a three-tiered sandwich structure that extends away from the DNA. The additional components include another, smaller, coiled coil and an interpositioned β-sheet. This additional structure serves both to hold together the two component monomers as well as provide for additional protein interaction (Garvie and Wolberger, 2001), such as that which has been observed (Hassler and Richmond, 2001) for the interactions between the ETS factor Sap1 (a wHTH protein) and serum response factor (SRF).

AT-hook

A number of important proteins do not favor binding to any specific target via a single DBD, but rather contain multiple DBD domains of low specificity that cooperate to provide specific targeting. One such class of proteins consists of the AT-hook proteins like HMGI(Y), Tcf1 and Lef1, which contain a short disordered peptide having the sequence Arg-Gly-Arg-Pro that binds with low selectivity to the minor groove of A-rich DNA sequences. Additionally, hydrophobic α-helices bind to and expand a minor groove surface, resulting in extensive DNA bending (Aravind and Landsman, 1998). The developmental factor MLL is an AT-hook protein that also contains an MT domain that recognizes unmethylated CpG sequences which are found near the upstream ends of many protein-coding genes (Love et al., 1995; Birke et al., 2002).

SAND

A small number of proteins possess a novel DNA binding motif that is named SAND for the first four identified proteins (human *Sp100*, *Aire1*, *NUDR*, and *Drosophila DEAF1*). Proteins containing this domain often bind DNA as a dimer (Bottomley et al., 2001; Surdo et al., 2003). This domain possesses a 5-stranded anti-parallel β-sheet which stabilizes a multi-α-helical bundle that mediates binding to DNA via a conserved Lys-Asn-Trp-Lys peptide. The SAND domain is usually found in association with a protein–protein interaction module, which appears to be responsible for dimerization.

MODULATION OF FACTOR ACTIVITY

Protein–protein interactions in transcription factors

As described above, strong binding and high target site selectivity between transcription factors and DNA often depends upon direct protein–protein interactions among factors. Although many of these interactions are homotypic between two either identical or similar factors targeting symmetrical palindromic sequences, many others are heterotypic on asymmetric sites that cooperatively bind two or more proteins. For these types of sites, activity is dependent upon the simultaneous presence of all components. The protein–protein interactions can be mediated by DBDs and/or by other domains (see Figure 7.1). For example, the interaction between the bZIP Jun-Fos dimer and NFAT2 involves three DBDs (Chen et al., 1998); the interaction between SRF and Sap1 is between the DBD of one protein and an extra-DBD sequence of another (Hassler and Richmond, 2001); and IRF-2/PIP (IRF-2) and Spi-1/PU.1 (Spi-1) associate by both mutual DBD and extra-DBD interactions (Escalante et al., 2002).

Transcription factor activation pathways

As described above in the Introduction, pre-expressed factors like C/EBPβ, NF-κB, and CREB are not generally constitutively active and must be activated. Additional examples include Notch activation of CSL via a proteolytic pathway (Martinez Arias et al., 2002; Nam et al., 2003); TGF-β activation of SMADs via phosphorylation (Derynck and Zhang, 2003); Wnt signaling through Frizzled resulting in phosphorylation of the β-catenin cofactor, thus leading to activation of LEF/TCF (Moon et al., 2002); and NFAT factors activated by calcium-induced calcinuerin-mediated dephosphorylation (Hogan et al., 2003).

Modulation mechanisms also exist for constitutively active factors and previously activated factors to be rendered more active. The obligatory tyrosine phosphorylation of Stat1 (which is required for dimerization, nuclear localization and transactivation), can be increased by secondary serine phosphorylation within the TAD (Zhang et al., 1998; Nair et al., 2002). Following primary activation via release from the IκB inhibitor (Ghosh and Karin, 2002), the p65 form of NF-κB can be independently positively modulated by serine phosphorylation within both the DBD and the TAD (Madrid et al., 2001; Zhong et al., 2002). Such super-activation beyond the primary signal are likely ways in which responses can be fine-tuned.

THE ROLE OF SPECIFIC FACTORS IN IMMUNITY

Factor balance and combinatorial associations drive hematopoiesis

The development of blood cells lies at the very heart of immunity. Students of immunology have been exposed to hematopoietic tree schemes providing a road-map for describing the developmental pathways that lead to the production of essential immune cell-types. The arrows in these trees have been historically populated with extracellular factors that target specific cell type progenitors that either accelerate or impede progression down a specific pathway. More recently, some of these schemes have added intracellular components that are essential to the process (Cantor and Orkin, 2002; Warren and Rothenberg, 2002; Zhu and Emerson, 2002). Many of these intracellular molecules are the specific transcription factors that target key genes required for a differentiation event. Figure 7.3 presents such a scheme, focusing on transcription factors that either characterize a particular cell type or are required for the differentiation process. The role for these factors has been determined by various methods using animals and *in vitro* differentiation systems. Techniques include the suppression of gene expression either by ablation or other methods of inhibition, ectopic expression and characterization of requirements for expression of target genes by transfection and co-transfection. Additionally, the expression and/or activity of many have been correlated

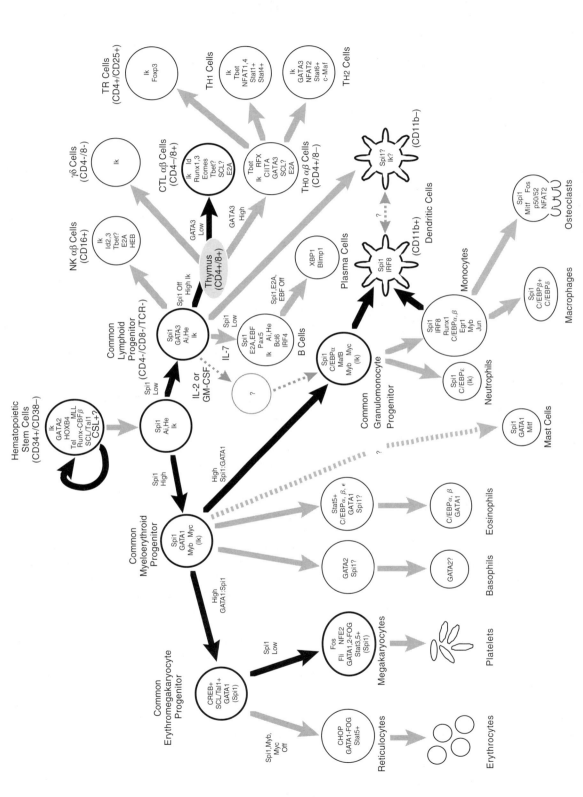

Figure 7.3 Specific transcription factors involved in hematopoiesis. The scheme shows various lineages of cells connected by arrows. Cell types are represented as circles and other closed figures containing designations for critical transcription factors. Factor designations blue followed by a plus sign (+) are pre-existing factors that are activated by an exogenous signal; red represents factors that are key for specific developmental stages; black represents other lineage-specific and critical factors. Black arrows represent stages that are dependent upon engagement of Notch receptors on the cell surface that may activate the CSL factor that binds the intracellular Notch peptide, ICN. Gray arrows are Notch-independent stages. Dotted lines indicate possible, unsubstantiated alternative pathways. Red labels over the arrows note important details regarding expression of selected key factors. **See colour plate 7.3.**

with specific pathologies. Consequently, these important molecules are prime marker and surrogate candidates. Many have been used, similar to extracellular CD molecular markers, as a means of characterizing developmental and disease stages. The use of such factors for these purposes offers advantages and difficulties that must be well understood prior to embarking on their use for practical purposes.

Hematopoietic stem cells

Hematopoiesis is a developmental program that depends upon differential expansion of clonal cells from precursors. An important element of the hematopoietic developmental scheme is that it is regulated by a collection of transcription factors that not only coordinately activate the expression of key genes, but also interact with each other to repress alternate lineages. This paradigm reflects the decision-point nature of hematopoiesis, where a collection of precursor cell types form a nexus where a choice is made regarding upon which developmental path to proceed. At the top of this developmental scheme is the CD34 pluripotent hematopoietic stem cell (HSC). The HSC is a self-renewing stem cell and this function depends upon the activity of a collection of genes. An essential component of this gene activation program is the supportive function of stromal cells which activate via Notch signaling. This dependence on Notch permeates throughout the hematopoietic lineage at several key decision points (Krause, 2002) and these are indicated in Figure 7.3 as dark arrows. The ultimate target of Notch must necessarily be one or more transcription factors. However, the exact nature of such factors has not yet been determined. In particular it is not yet clear whether Notch plays its role via direct activation of a downstream target like the factor CSL (Martinez Arias et al., 2002) or via some indirect role that affects the function of a secondary factor like GATA2 (Kumano et al., 2001), which has also been argued to be important for maintaining HSC immaturity (Minegishi et al., 2003).

In addition to the involvement of Notch and GATA2, other factors have been reported to be essential for HSC (see Figure 7.3). In mice, HoxB3 and B4 have been reported to be important for HSC maintenance and HoxB4 overexpression stimulates HSC regeneration (Bjornsson et al., 2003). Also, Ikaros null mutations have revealed that this factor is important for maximal HSC repopulation, as well as playing a prominent role in lymphopoiesis (Nichogiannopoulou et al., 1999). The wHTH factor Tel also appears to be important for establishment of hematopoiesis of all lineages in the bone marrow (Wang et al., 1998b). The fusion of the TEL and AML1/Runx1 protein derived from the t(12;21) translocation associated with ALL, results in inhibition of AML1/Runx target genes (Scandura et al., 2002), consistent with the important role for the AML1/Runx protein (Lacaud et al., 2002) in early hematopoietic development. Recently, a factor named

early hematopoietic zinc finger (EHZF) which contains 30 C2H2 fingers was reported to be a specific marker of CD34 HSC that is lost upon subsequent differentiation. This factor complexes SMAD factors and inhibits the important B cell factor EBF (Bond et al., 2002).

Post-HSC hematopoietic decisions

The developmental pathway proceeds from the HSC to a decision point for either a common lymphoid or common myeloerythroid progenitor. The molecular nature of the decision process is unclear. However, an important component appears to be the relative expression levels of several key transcription factors. One factor that appears critical at this stage is the wHTH ETS-like factor Spi-1, which is expressed early in hematopoiesis. However, its levels decrease as cells progress toward lymphocytes and increase in the common myeloerythroid progenitors. This variation in expression levels for the two different lineages may be critical, in part, because of a physical interaction that occurs between Spi-1 and GATA proteins, which are another class of factors key to differential development (Zhang et al., 1999; Nerlov et al., 2000). This interaction inhibits Spi-1 from associating with various other cooperative transcription factors like c-Jun and C/EBP via the Spi-1 DNA binding domain, thus decreasing Spi-1-dependent transactivation. Symmetrically, the interaction also inhibits GATA function, possibly by competing for the interaction of GATA with cooperative factors like the C2H2 Zn finger protein Sp1 and the non-DNA binding ubiquitous transactivator CBP/P300 (Cantor and Orkin, 2002). Therefore, the relative abundance of Spi-1 and mutually competing forms of GATA may facilitate the decision process. Consistent with this hypothesis, early lymphopoiesis depends upon GATA3 expression and a decrease in Spi-1. An increase in Spi-1 is consistent with progression toward myeloerythropoiesis, with a maintanance of high Spi-1 driving subsequent myelopoiesis and a decrease in Spi-1 accompanying an increase in GATA1, driving erythromegakaryocyte development. Consequently, the relative expression of mutually inhibitory factors may be an important component of hematopoietic lineage commitment.

Lymphopoietic precursor

Although a decrease in Spi-1 may be critical for lymphopoiesis, the progression toward the B cell lineage nonetheless requires Spi-1 activity. The gene for IL7Rα is dependent upon Spi-1 (DeKoter et al., 2002). Mice, in particular, require IL-7 for early B cell commitment and the efficient development of T cells (Purohit et al., 2003). However, the expression of IL7Rα in T cells, in contrast to B cells, appears to be independent of Spi-1 (DeKoter et al., 2002). The critical Ig heavy chain gene enhancer requires Spi-1 binding (McCarthy et al., 2003), as do the 3′ enhancers from κ and λ light chain genes (Pongubala et al., 1992; Eisenbeis et al., 1993). Also, the PEST domain of Spi-1 recruits the critical B cell factor IRF4, which in turn can associate with E2A, another critical B cell factor that cooperates with Pax5 /BSAP (Pax5), and EBF to set B cell lineage commitment and directly support RAG1 and RAG2 V(D)J gene rearrangements (see Schebesta et al., 2002 for a review). These three factors appear to be capable of generating a stable quaternary complex with the DNA of the Ig light chain 3′ enhancer (Nagulapalli and Atchison, 1998). It should also be noted that a collection of studies argue that Pax5 plays an important role in limiting stem-cell-like self renewal and may be the most important factor for B cell lineage commitment (Schebesta et al., 2002). In addition, Spi-1 cooperates with Stat6 on the Ig ϵ gene (Pesu et al., 2003) and is essential for expression of IL7Rα (reviewed in Schebesta et al., 2002). Ultimately, the differentiation of B cells into antibody secreting plasma cells appears to require a complete loss of Spi-1 expression (Pettersson et al., 1995; Ying et al., 1998; Nagy et al., 2002). In addition to a loss of Spi-1, the HTH protein XBP1 and the C2H2 Zn finger protein Blimp1 are required for terminal B cell differentiation (Mock et al., 1996).

Notch signaling also plays a role in the B versus T cell fate decision. The activation of Notch-1 by cell-surface ligands in the thymus has been shown to induce the expression of the bHLH inhibitor Hes1, which homotypically dimerizes with and inhibits E2A, thus blocking B cell development. Consequently, T cell development is supported by Notch signaling, while B cells are inhibited (reviewed in Schebesta et al., 2002). Another example of inhibition by bHLH homotypic dimerization occurs when expression of the NK cell-specific Id2 inhibitor specifically commits cells to that lineage by blocking the expression of essential bHLH-dependent genes (Ikawa et al., 2001).

An important factor in lymphopoiesis is the C2H2 zinc finger protein Ikaros. This protein is essential for maximal hematopoietic stem cell activity and is absolutely required for all T and B cell downstream progeny during embryogenesis. The genetic loss severely affects lymphopoiesis in adults (Georgopoulos, 2002). Ikaros gene ablation in mice appears to have little effect on myeloid cell development, although it is expressed in that lineage. However, it should be noted that a mutation of the Ikaros DNA binding domain results in developmental effects on myeloid and erythroid lineage cells (Papathanasiou et al., 2003). Additional Ikaros-related factors Helios and Aiolos partially overlap Ikaros function and appear to subdivide along the two major lymphoid branches (Rebollo and Schmitt, 2003). Specifically, Helios (Kelley et al., 1998) appears to be more important for B cell development, while Aiolos (Wang et al., 1998a) plays an Ikaros-like role in T cells. Two additional Ikaros-like factors Eos, which is closely related to Helios, and Pegasus, which is more unique, may also play a role in lymphoid cells (Perdomo et al., 2000).

Thymopoiesis

The maturation of most T cells requires antigenic selection in the thymus. This process results in both the elimination of most self-directed cells and the generation of distinct subtypes and it is dependent upon specific gene expression in both lymphoid and stromal cells (Starr et al., 2003). The subtypes include CD4 and CD8 single positive $\alpha\beta$ T cell receptor-harboring cytotoxic (CTL) and helper (T$_H$) cells and CD4/CD8 double negative $\gamma\delta$ T cell receptor cells. The T$_H$ cells include types 1, 2 and regulatory R cells. In addition there is a CD4/CD8 double negative ab T cell receptor natural killer (NK) cell that is thymus-independent, deriving directly from the bone marrow common lymphoid progenitor. The transcription factors involved in this process are presently under detailed scrutiny. One such factor is the HTH protein FoxN1, a key element in stromal cell function that is the altered gene in the thymic-deficient nude mouse. The gene for FoxN1 is induced via a Wnt-Frizzled pathway (Balciunaite et al., 2002) that likely functions through the β-catenin-activated LEF/TCF AT-hook trascription factors. Similarly, stromal cell-dependent differentiation of NK cells has been reported to be dependent upon a signaling pathway that activates the RelB form of NF-κB (Elewaut et al., 2003). Rel B deficient mice are also deficient in thymic and myeloid-derived dendritic cells (see Gerondakis et al., 1999 for a review of Rel knockouts). The activation of NF-κB family transcription factors is of central importance to many immunological processes, including lymphocyte responses to antigen mediated by membrane Ig on B cells and the T cell receptor. The signal transduction pathway for activation of NF-κB that is essential for T cell maturation and survival is distinct from the more common activation pathways that have been studied for innate immunity (Schmitz et al., 2003).

Transcription factors have also been characterized for T cells. It has been reported that Runx3 and 1 are repressors of CD4 expression in CD8 cells (Woolf et al., 2003). Strikingly, Runx3 protein is only expressed in CD8 single positive cells, while the mRNA is present in both CD4 and CD8 cells (Ehlers et al., 2003). This suggests that the regulation of Runx3 activity is post-transcriptional. The transcription factor Aire is mutated in autoimmune polyendocrinopathy syndrome type 1, a disorder characterized by a spectrum of organ-specific autoimmune diseases. Aire deficiency results in a deficiency in the ability of the thymus to delete self-directed cells (Liston et al., 2003; Pitkanen and Peterson, 2003). This factor likely binds DNA via a SAND domain that is immediately adjacent to an essential zinc-containing RING finger-like PHD domain that usually mediates protein–protein interactions and may be responsible for dimerization.

Although the C4 Zn finger factor GATA3 is important for all lymphopoiesis, it is especially critical in T$_{H2}$ cell maturation (reviewed in Grogan and Locksley, 2002; Ho and Glimcher, 2002; Holloway et al., 2002), where it is initially induced via Stat6 activation by IL-4 (although it ultimately appears to be capable of autoinduction) and leads to the induction of c-Maf expression that cooperates with NFAT2 to induce the IL-4 gene, a hallmark of T_{H2} cells. GATA-3 is expressed throughout the T cell lineage. However, its expression is higher in CD4 than in CD8 single positive cells and acts by inhibiting CD8 single positive cell development (Hernandez et al., 2003). In contrast to GATA3, the T-box binding factor T-bet activates T_{H1} genes and represses T_{H2} gene expression. The expression of GATA3 has also been reported to be dependent upon the expression of the p50 form of NF-κB. The T-bet gene is induced via Stat1 which is activated by IFN-γ. The gene for IL12Rβ2 and the T_{H1} hallmark IFN-γ gene are T-bet targets. Like GATA3, T-bet is capable of autoinduction, although it may be indirectly induced via induction of the homeodomain HTH protein Hlx (Mullen et al., 2002). Expression of IL12Rβ2 is essential for IL-12-dependent activation of Stat4, which cooperates with T-bet to activate the IFN-γ gene. The NFAT class of Ig-like Rel proteins also appears to play a role in T_{H1} versus T_{H2} cell development. Specifically, NFAT2 is important for T_{H2} responses, whereas NFAT1 and NFAT4 repress the T_{H2} response. A proposed mechanism involves blockage of GATA3 access to the IL-4 gene by competitive gene binding. Consequently, the development of specific helper T cell responses seems to depend upon mutual inhibition of GATA3 and T-bet, a process modulated by the action of additional cell-specific transcription factors. Regulatory T cells are another type of CD4 cell that also expresses CD25. These cells are derived from T_{H0} cells and depend upon the expression of the HTH transcription factor Foxp3 (Fontenot et al., 2003; Sakaguchi, 2003; Walker et al., 2003). Overall, helper T cell subset differentiation, like other developmental choice decisions in hematopoiesis, appears to depend upon a complex interplay and balance among cell type-specific factors which cooperate and/or inhibit gene expression. An additional layer of regulation also may depend upon chromatin accessibility and the coordinate regulation of locus-clustered genes by a unifying regulator (Grogan and Locksley, 2002; Lee et al., 2003; Smale, 2003).

As mentioned above, GATA3 inhibits CD8 cells and T-bet represses T_{H2} cells. However, Eomesodermin, a distinct T-bet-like T-box protein, appears to cooperate with T-bet to play an important role in the development of the cytotoxic CD8 response and may be able to mediate CD8 effector cell development in the absence of T-bet (Hatton and Weaver, 2003; Pearce et al., 2003). Therefore, although T-bet may be relevant for CD8 cells, Eomesodermin is presently considered to be the key factor in the development of this cell type.

B cell lymphopoiesis

Like thymopoiesis, early B cell development appears to depend upon Ikaros expression. In contrast to T cells where Spi-1 expression is shut off, B cells require low levels of Spi-1 for expression of numerous essential genes. High levels of Spi-1 inhibit B cells and activate myeloid development (DeKoter and Singh, 2000). The Spi-1 B cell target genes include IgH and IgL genes, IL-7Rα, Rag-1 and 2, mb-1 and, in cooperation with E2A, the COE factor EBF (O'Riordan and Grosschedl, 2000; DeKoter et al., 2002). The EBF factor in turn activates Pax5, which cooperates with EBF and E2A and, in some cases, Spi-1, to activate a vast array of B cell genes. Expression of E2A and EBF is critical for B cell development (see Schebesta et al., 2002 for a review). The activation of the gene for IL-7Rα by Spi-1 is also noteworthy because pro-B cells depend upon IL-7 for survival (see Schebesta et al., 2002). The Wnt/κ-catenin pathway-activated factor LEF1 is also important for pro-B cells. Its presence is mitogenic and maintains adequate numbers of pro-B cells (Reya et al., 2000). TGF-β signaling activates SMAD factors which target the inhibitory bHLH factor Id (Miyazawa et al., 2002). Specifically, TGF-β induction of Id3 blocks B cell development, likely via the direct inhibition of the critical bHLH factor E2A by heterodimer formation (Kee et al., 2001).

Strikingly, EBF expression is lost with plasma cell maturation and EBF-deficient mice have an early block in B cell development (Lin and Grosschedl, 1995). Unlike EBF, Pax5 appears to be important for downstream B cell differentiation and not only activates B cell-specific genes, but actively inhibits non-B cell lineage gene expression (O'Riordan and Grosschedl, 2000). Pax5, along with another B cell factor, Bcl6, suppresses progression toward mature plasma cells by inhibiting, respectively, the master plasma cell regulators Blimp1 and XBP1 (Schebesta et al., 2002). Expression of Bcl6 appears to be dependent upon exposure of B cells to T cell-dependent antigen and is followed by somatic hypermutation and class-switching. In the absence of Bcl6 upregulation, Blimp1 is expressed which in turn inhibits E2A, EBF, Pax5, Ikaros, Spi-1 and Spi-B, and in a permanent step toward plasma cell commitment, also inhibits Bcl6. Although Bcl6 is the switch, plasma cell differentiation is absolutely dependent upon XBP1 and RAG2 complemented mice lacking this gene are incapable of secreting any immunoglobulin (Reimold et al., 2001).

Myeloerythropoiesis

The transcription factor Spi-1 plays an essential regulatory role in non-lymphoid hematopoietic development. Although this transcription factor has been directly implicated in myelopoiesis, its presence also affects erythroid development (Scott et al., 1994; Nerlov and Graf, 1998; Cantor and Orkin, 2001, 2002). In fact, the ratio of Spi-1 to the erythroid-dependent GATA-1 factor dictates the developmental path (see above, under *Post-HSC Hematopoietic Decisions*). Consequently, Spi-1 plays important roles at several hematopoietic decision points, including lymphoid versus myeloerythroid; T cell versus B cell; and erythromegakaryoid versus myeloid. This suggests that along with Notch downstream signaling, Spi-1 serves as a master control for hematopoietic development.

Granulomonopoiesis

Myeloid development is absolutely dependent upon the presence of the Spi-1 transcription factor (Scott et al., 1994; McKercher et al., 1999; Friedman, 2002). Numerous myeloid genes depend upon cognate binding of this protein as recently reviewed by Friedman (Friedman, 2002). The Friedman review comprehensively covers much of the current knowledge regarding transcription factors in myeloid development. This includes the critical role played by Spi-1 which cooperates with C/EBP bZIP factors. In particular C/EBPα is essential for neutrophil and eosinophil development and its absence results in a loss of G-CSF receptor gene expression (Zhang et al., 1997b). Two retinoic acid receptors, RARα1 and RARγ, in concert are also important for neutrophil maturation (Labrecque et al., 1998) as is the C/EBPε isoform (Yamanaka et al., 1997). The C2H2 Zn finger proteins Egr-1 and MZF-1 may not only be important for monocyte differentiation, but their expression may also inhibit granulocytes (see Friedman, 2002). Other factors such as IRF-8, Runx-1, c-Myb, Maf, HoxA10, CDP, p53, E2f and Stat3 may all play varied roles in this developmental pathway.

Macrophages are derived from monocytes following various sorts of extracellular challenges and stress. One of the most important modes of activation is via the Toll-like receptor (TLR) family which responds to many types of direct foreign stimuli (Medzhitov, 2001) as well as endogenous agents (Asea et al., 2002). The TLR signaling pathway activates molecules like TRAF6 which results in the activation of MAP kinase and IκB kinase pathways which in turn activate pre-existing transcription factors like C/EBPβ and NF-κB, respectively. Target genes like IL1B and TNFA depend upon these factors and other factors like IRF-8 for expression (Tsukada et al., 1994; Marecki et al., 2001). Myeloid-derived dendritic cells may require similar sorts of factors for function and may depend upon Stat6 (IL-4) and Stat5 (GM-CSF) for development (Cella et al., 1999; Shortman and Liu, 2002). Osteoclasts are another myeloid-derived cell type which are dependent upon Spi-1, Mitf and c-Fos for development (Grigoriadis et al., 1994; Fleischmann et al., 2000; Luchin et al., 2001) and NFAT2 plus NF-κB activation for bone resorption (Anusaksathien et al., 2001; Gravallese et al., 2001; Takayanagi et al., 2002).

Erythromegakaryopoiesis

The common myeloerythroid progenitor acts as the decision point between myelo- and erythromegakaryopoiesis. When the Spi-1 to GATA-1 ratio is high, cells progress down the myeloid lineage. However, when the ratio tends toward the other direction, erythromegakaryopoiesis results. This decision appears to be dependent upon the mutual antagonism observed between Spi-1 and GATA-1

described above and functions in concert with the GATA cofactor FOG-1. In addition Stat5 activation via the erythropoietin receptor is important for early erythroblast survival (Socolovsky et al., 2001). Another factor that appears to play a role in erythropoiesis is CHOP (Gadd153), an inhibitory C/EBP isoform (Coutts et al., 1999). This may relate to the observation that FOG is not only important for erythroid development in concert with GATA-1, but is also inhibitory for eosinophil development, a phenomenon which is counteracted by C/EBPβ inhibition of FOG gene expression (Querfurth et al., 2000). Therefore, FOG and C/EBP are antagonistic and the expression of a C/EBP inhibitor in erythroid cells may enhance FOG function.

The FOG cofactor is also important for megakaryocyte development (Cantor and Orkin, 2001, 2002; Cantor et al., 2002). Furthermore, PDGF induces other key factors such as c-Fos, GATA-1, NF-E2 and Spi-1 (Lecine et al., 1998; Orkin et al., 1998; Chui et al., 2003). The expression of low levels of Spi-1 has been reported to be important for the expression of platelet-specific proteins (Zhang et al., 1997a). There is also a prominent role for Stat5 and Stat3 activation via the thrombopoietin and G-CSF receptors, respectively (Yang et al., 1999).

Basophils, mast cells and eosinophils

Mast cells appear to be derived from a myeloerythroid progenitor and their development is dependent upon Spi-1, GATA-1, GATA-2 and the activation of Stat6 by IL-4 (Henkel and Brown, 1994) as well as the bHLH factor Mitf (Kataoka et al., 2002). Expression of the eosinophil and basophil granule major basic protein gene is dependent upon GATA-1, but not GATA-2 (Yamaguchi et al., 1998).

Transcription factors and immune disease

Specific transcription factors have been implicated in various diseases. Chromosomal translocations and point mutations have been associated with, and in some cases have been shown to be the cause of, pathologies. This has been especially true for malignancies of the hematopoietic system. Chromosomal fusions involving transcription factors are well known and examples of factors involved in fusions include AML1/Runx1, Tel, MLL and RARα.

These have been recently reviewed regarding their relevance to acute myelogenous leukemia (Scandura et al., 2002). Isoforms of Myc are almost universally disregulated in tumor cells; these include translocations in Burkitt's lymphoma and amplification in neuroblastoma (Hermeking, 2003). Transcription factor mutations have also been reported in specific diseases. GATA-1 mutation is associated with leukemogenesis in Down syndrome (Gurbuxani et al., 2003) and with disregulation of its target gene WT1 gene in myelodysplastic syndrome and acute myeloid leukemia (Patmasiriwat et al., 1999). It is also known that p53 and Bcl-6 mutations can provide additional growth stimulation and apoptosis protection for tumors (Lindstrom and Wiman, 2002). Mutations in FoxP3 and Aire factor genes have been associated with severe autoimmune disease in humans (Ramsdell and Ziegler, 2003). Disregulation of c-Myb plays an important role in cancer progression and metastasis (Ramsay et al., 2003). The IRF factors have been associated with general pathogenic and viral responses (Mamane et al., 1999). Recently, IRF-1 expression has been associated with natural resistance to tuberculosis (Pine, 2002). BSAP and Oct-2 have been reported to be useful in the differential diagnosis of classic Hodgkin's lymphoma (Browne et al., 2003). Members of the ETS group of wHTH proteins have been implicated in many different diseases, including rheumatoid arthritis, systemic lupus erythematosus, breast cancer and leukemia (Dittmer and Nordheim, 1998). Various forms of NF-κB are critical for hematopoietic development and in the processes of innate immunity. In particular, c-Rel appears to be important for IFN-γ expression by T_{H1} cells and IL-12 expression by dendritic cells (Liou and Hsia, 2003). Numerous tumor cells including Hodgkin's disease cells exhibit constitutively active NF-κB, suggesting a possible relevance (Younes et al., 2003). The STAT transcription factors are similarly disregulated in diseases like primary acute myelogenous leukemia (Spiekermann et al., 2001). Truncated dominant-negative forms of Ikaros and Helios have been reported in patients with adult T-cell leukemia/lymphoma (Fujii et al., 2003).

METHODOLOGIES FOR MEASURING TRANSCRIPTION FACTORS

As stated in the Introduction, the measurement of mRNA levels can be a valid approach to determining the importance of a transcription factor. As detailed above, it should be remembered that the presence of mRNA is a necessary prerequisite for factor function, but may not be sufficient because of the potential for ribosome-mediated translational and signal-dependent post-translational regulation. Presently, gene expression profiling is a powerful method for simultaneously analyzing many mRNA types (Ricciardi and Granucci, 2002). However, it should be noted that the dynamic range and precision of microarray technology is not necessarily as broad as that offered by more conventional techniques such as Northern blots and quantitative PCR. Nonetheless, important observations can be made and these can be subsequently verified via traditional approaches. Some recent examples of this approach include profiling for several autoimmune diseases (Aune et al., 2003); diagnosis of lymphoblastic leukemia (Staal et al., 2003); the expression of genes in germinal center B cells and its relationship to B cell lymphoma (Shaffer et al., 2001); the responses of dendritic cells (Huang et al., 2001) and macrophages (Nau et al., 2002) to pathogens; and the effects of tamoxifen on breast cancer (Hodges et al., 2003).

Another approach to analyzing specific transcription factor function is the use of electrophoretic mobility shift assay (EMSA), which directly measures mobility changes on a native polyacrylamide gel, resulting from the in vitro DNA binding activity of cell extracts to radiolabeled DNA (Carey and Smale, 2000). The technique can be extended to include tests for specificity by the use of unlabeled competitor DNA and specific antibodies which can either abrogate binding or, for some antibodies, result in slower-migrating antibody-factor complexes. The advantage of this technique is that the use of an in vitro DNA binding probe results in a precise identification of binding to a specific target sequence with a resolution that is measurable to within one base-pair. Disadvantages relate to the in vitro approach which relies on experimental conditions such as ionic strength, counter-ion charge and cell disruption, which may affect the outcome. Another disadvantage of this technique is that only a small number of factors can be assayed at one time. However, a recent solution-based method employs biotinylated probes that are mixed with cell extracts and then depleted of unbound probe. The protein-bound probes are then dissasociated and analyzed by hybridization to a DNA array, thus providing a high-throughput approach to conventional EMSA (Zeng et al., 2003). The in vitro limitation of EMSA has also been recently addressed by the use of chromatin immunoprecipitation (ChIP) in which the binding of factors to specific DNA regions of chromatin is determined in vivo by a technique that uses immunoprecipitation in association with genomic PCR (Shang and Brown, 2002; Weinmann and Farnham, 2002; Wells and Farnham, 2002). This technique provides an in vivo examination of factor binding to specific genome regions, as determined by the use of selective PCR primers. However, it suffers from a resolution limitation imposed by the size of the fragmented DNA derived, usually by sonication, during the procedure. Interesting variations on this technique can include the ability to execute a whole genome scan of transcription factor binding by combining ChIP with microarray analysis, the so-called 'ChIP on a Chip' technique (Lee et al., 2002).

PRECIS

Transcription factors, especially those that bind to specific DNA sequences, are rapidly becoming an important source of markers for immunologic processes. Although studies of hematopoiesis have traditionally focused on the differential expression and activities of these proteins, other aspects of immunology are benefiting and will benefit from measurements of these molecules. Specifically, the importance of these proteins and the general transcription factors that they physically engage, are key to the understanding of both normal biological processes and to the pharmacogenomic changes that occur as the result of disease and therapeutic intervention. However, it must be emphasized that a simplistic approach to the measurement of these factors may not be appropriate, since many are regulated at various levels beyond that of simple gene induction.

REFERENCES

Anthony-Cahill, S., Benfield, P.A., Fairman, R. et al. (1992). Molecular characterization of helix-loop-helix peptides. Science *255*, 979–983.

Anusaksathien, O., Laplace, C., Li, X. et al. (2001). Tissue-specific and ubiquitous promoters direct the expression of alternatively spliced transcripts from the calcitonin receptor gene. J Biol Chem *276*, 22663–22674.

Aravind, L. and Landsman, D. (1998). AT-hook motifs identified in a wide variety of DNA-binding proteins. Nucleic Acids Res *26*, 4413–4421.

Asea, A., Rehli, M., Kabingu, E. et al. (2002). Novel signal transduction pathway utilized by extracellular HSP70: role of toll-like receptor (TLR) 2 and TLR4. J Biol Chem *277*, 15028–15034.

Aune, T.M., Maas, K., Moore, J.H. and Olsen, N.J. (2003). Gene expression profiles in human autoimmune disease. Curr Pharm Des *9*, 1905–1917.

Balciunaite, G., Keller, M., Balciunaite, P.E. et al. (2002). Wnt glycoproteins regulate the expression of FoxN1, the gene defective in nude mice. Nat Immunol *3*, 1102–1108.

Baldassare, J.J., Bi, Y. and Bellone, C.J. (1999). The role of p38 mitogen-activated protein kinase in IL-1 beta transcription. J Immunol *162*, 5367–5373.

Birke, M., Schreiner, S., Garcia, C.M., Mahr, K., Titgemeyer, F. and Slany, R.K. (2002). The MT domain of the proto-oncoprotein MLL binds to CpG-containing DNA and discriminates against methylation. Nucleic Acids Res *30*, 958–965.

Bjornsson, J.M., Larsson, N., Brun, A.C. et al. (2003). Reduced proliferative capacity of hematopoietic stem cells deficient in Hoxb3 and Hoxb4. Mol Cell Biol *23*, 3872–3883.

Bond, H.M., Mesuraca, M., Carbone, E. et al. (2002). Early hematopoietic zinc finger protein (EHZF), the human homologue to mouse Evi3, is highly expressed in primitive human hematopoietic cells. Blood.

Bottomley, M.J., Collard, M.W., Huggenvik, J.I., Liu, Z., Gibson, T.J. and Sattler, M. (2001). The SAND domain structure defines a novel DNA-binding fold in transcriptional regulation. Nat Struct Biol *8*, 626–633.

Browne, P., Petrosyan, K., Hernandez, A. and Chan, J.A. (2003). The B-cell transcription factors BSAP, Oct-2, and BOB.1 and the pan-B-cell markers CD20, CD22, and CD79a are useful in the differential diagnosis of classic Hodgkin lymphoma. Am J Clin Pathol *120*, 767–777.

Cantor, A.B., Katz, S.G. and Orkin, S.H. et al. (2002). Distinct domains of the GATA-1 cofactor FOG-1 differentially influence erythroid versus megakaryocytic maturation. Mol Cell Biol *22*, 4268–4279.

Cantor, A.B. and Orkin, S.H. (2001). Hematopoietic development: a balancing act. Curr Opin Genet Dev *11*, 513–519.

Cantor, A.B. and Orkin, S.H. (2002). Transcriptional regulation of erythropoiesis: an affair involving multiple partners. Oncogene *21*, 3368–3376.

Carey, M. and Smale, S.T. (2000). Transcriptional Regulation in Eukaryotes. Cold Spring Harbor, NY: Cold Spring Harbor Laboratory Press.

Carroll, A.S., Gilbert, D.E., Liu, X. et .al. (1997). SKN-1 domain folding and basic region monomer stabilization upon DNA binding. Genes Dev *11*, 2227–2238.

Cella, M., Salio, M., Sakakibara, Y., Langen, H., Julkunen, I. and Lanzavecchia, A. (1999). Maturation, activation, and protection of dendritic cells induced by double-stranded RNA. J Exp Med *189*, 821–829.

Chai, J., Wu, J.W., Yan, N., Massague, J., Pavletich, N.P. and Shi, Y. (2003). Features of a Smad3 MH1-DNA complex. Roles of water and zinc in DNA binding. J Biol Chem *278*, 20327–20331.

Chawla, A., Repa, J.J., Evans, R.M. and Mangelsdorf, D.J. (2001). Nuclear receptors and lipid physiology: opening the X-files. Science *294*, 1866–1870.

Chen, L., Glover, J.N., Hogan, P.G., Rao, A. and Harrison, S.C. (1998). Structure of the DNA-binding domains from NFAT, Fos and Jun bound specifically to DNA. Nature *392*, 42–48.

Chui, C.M., Li, K., Yang, M. et al. (2003). Platelet-derived growth factor up-regulates the expression of transcription factors NF-E2, GATA-1 and c-Fos in megakaryocytic cell lines. Cytokine *21*, 51–64.

Cirillo, L.A., Lin, F.R., Cuesta, I., Friedman, D., Jarnik, M. and Zaret, K.S. (2002). Opening of compacted chromatin by early developmental transcription factors HNF3 (FoxA) and GATA-4. Mol Cell *9*, 279–289.

Cosma, M.P. (2002). Ordered recruitment: gene-specific mechanism of transcription activation. Mol Cell *10*, 227–236.

Coutts, M., Cui, K. et al. (1999). Regulated expression and functional role of the transcription factor CHOP (GADD153) in erythroid growth and differentiation. Blood *93*, 3369–3378.

De Cesare, D. and Sassone, C.P. (2000). Transcriptional regulation by cyclic AMP-responsive factors. Prog Nucleic Acid Res Mol Biol *64*, 343–369.

DeKoter, R.P., Lee, H.J. and Singh, H. (2002). PU.1 regulates expression of the interleukin-7 receptor in lymphoid progenitors. Immunity *16*, 297–309.

DeKoter, R.P. and Singh, H. (2000). Regulation of B lymphocyte and macrophage development by graded expression of PU.1. Science *288*, 1439–1441.

Derynck, R. and Zhang, Y.E. (2003). Smad-dependent and Smad-independent pathways in TGF-beta family signalling. Nature *425*, 577–584.

Dittmer, J. and Nordheim, A. (1998). Ets transcription factors and human disease. Biochim Biophys Acta *1377*, F1–11.

Dubois, L. and Vincent, A. (2001). The COE – Collier/Olf1/ EBF – transcription factors: structural conservation and diversity of developmental functions. Mech Dev *108*, 3–12.

Ehlers, M., Laule, K.K., Petter, M. et al. (2003). Morpholino antisense oligonucleotide-mediated gene knockdown during thymocyte development reveals role for Runx3 transcription factor in CD4 silencing during development of CD4−/ CD8+ thymocytes. J Immunol *171*, 3594–3604.

Eisenbeis, C.F., Singh, H. and Storb, U. et al. (1993). PU.1 is a component of a multiprotein complex which binds an essential site in the murine immunoglobulin lambda 2-4 enhancer. Mol Cell Biol *13*, 6452–6461.

Elewaut, D., Shaikh, R.B., Hammond, K.J. et al. (2003). NIK-dependent RelB activation defines a unique signaling pathway for the development of V alpha 14i NKT cells. J Exp Med *197*, 1623–1633.

Ellenberger, T., Fass, D., Arnaud, M. and Harrison, S.C. (1994). Crystal structure of transcription factor E47: E-box recognition by a basic region helix-loop-helix dimer. Genes Dev *8*, 970–980.

Engelman, J.A., Lisanti, M.P. and Scherer, P.E. (1998). Specific inhibitors of p38 mitogen-activated protein kinase block 3T3-L1 adipogenesis. J Biol Chem *273*, 32111–32120.

Escalante, C.R., Brass, A.L., Pongubala, J.M. et al. (2002). Crystal structure of PU.1/IRF-4/DNA ternary complex. Mol Cell *10*, 1097–1105.

Ferre-D'Amare, A.R., Prendergast, G.C., Ziff, E.B. and Burley, S.K. (1993). Recognition by Max of its cognate DNA through a dimeric b/HLH/Z domain. Nature *363*, 38–45.

Fleischmann, A., Hafezi, F., Elliott, C., Reme, C.E., Ruther, U. and Wagner, E.F. (2000). Fra-1 replaces c-Fos-dependent functions in mice. Genes Dev *14*, 2695–2700.

Fontenot, J.D., Gavin, M.A. and Rudensky, A.Y. (2003). Foxp3 programs the development and function of CD4+CD25+ regulatory T cells. Nat Immunol *4*, 330–336.

Friedman, A.D. (2002). Transcriptional regulation of granulocyte and monocyte development. Oncogene *21*, 3377–3390.

Fujii, K., Ishimaru, F., Nakase, K. et al. (2003). Over-expression of short isoforms of Helios in patients with adult T-cell leukaemia/lymphoma. Br J Haematol *120*, 986–989.

Garvie, C.W. and Wolberger, C. (2001). Recognition of specific DNA sequences. Mol Cell *8*, 937–946.

Georgopoulos, K. (2002). Haematopoietic cell-fate decisions, chromatin regulation and ikaros. Nat Rev Immunol *2*, 162–174.

Gerondakis, S., Grossmann, M., Nakamura, Y., Pohl, T. and Grumont, R. (1999). Genetic approaches in mice to understand Rel/NF-kappaB and IkappaB function: transgenics and knock-outs. Oncogene *18*, 6888–6895.

Ghosh, S. and Karin, M. (2002). Missing pieces in the NF-kappaB puzzle. Cell S81–96.

Gravallese, E.M., Galson, D.L., Goldring, S.R. and Auron, P.E. (2001). The role of TNF-receptor family members and other TRAF-dependent receptors in bone resorption. Arthritis Res *3*, 6–12.

Grigoriadis, A.E., Wang, Z.Q., Cecchini, M.G. et al. (1994). c-Fos: a key regulator of osteoclast-macrophage lineage determination and bone remodeling. Science *266*, 443–448.

Grogan, J.L. and Locksley, R.M. (2002). T helper cell differentiation: on again, off again. Curr Opin Immunol *14*, 366–372.

Gurbuxani, S., Vyas, P. and Crispino, J.D. (2003). Recent insights into the mechanisms of myeloid leukemogenesis in Down syndrome. Blood.

Harada, R., Berube, G., Tamplin, O.J., Denis, L.C. and Nepveu, A. (1995). DNA-binding specificity of the cut repeats from the human cut-like protein. Mol Cell Biol *15*, 129–140.

Hassler, M. and Richmond, T.J. (2001). The B-box dominates SAP-1-SRF interactions in the structure of the ternary complex. EMBO J *20*, 3018–3028.

Hatton, R.D. and Weaver, C.T. (2003). Immunology. T-bet or not T-bet. Science *302*, 993–994.

Henkel, G. and Brown, M.A. (1994). PU.1 and GATA: components of a mast cell-specific interleukin 4 intronic enhancer. Proc Natl Acad Sci USA *91*, 7737–7741.

Hermeking, H. (2003). The MYC oncogene as a cancer drug target. Curr Cancer Drug Targets *3*, 163–175.

Hernandez, H.G., Anderson, M.K., Wang, C., Rothenberg, E.V. and Alberola, I.J. (2003). GATA-3 expression is controlled by TCR signals and regulates CD4/CD8 differentiation. Immunity *19*, 83–94.

Ho, I.C. and Glimcher, L.H. (2002). Transcription: tantalizing times for T cells. Cell S109–120.

Hodges, L.C., Cook, J.D., Lobenhofer, E.K. et al. (2003). Tamoxifen functions as a molecular agonist inducing cell cycle-associated genes in breast cancer cells. Mol Cancer Res *1*, 300–311.

Hogan, P.G., Chen, L., Nardone, J. and Rao, A. (2003). Transcriptional regulation by calcium, calcineurin, and NFAT. Genes Dev *17*, 2205–2232.

Hollenbeck, J.J. and Oakley, M.G. (2000). GCN4 binds with high affinity to DNA sequences containing a single consensus half-site. Biochemistry *39*, 6380–6389.

Holloway, A.F., Rao, S. and Shannon, M.F. (2002). Regulation of cytokine gene transcription in the immune system. Mol Immunol *38*, 567–580.

Huang, Q., Liu, D., Majewski, P. et al. (2001). The plasticity of dendritic cell responses to pathogens and their components. Science *294*, 870–875.

Ikawa, T., Fujimoto, S., Kawamoto, H., Katsura, Y. and Yokota, Y. (2001). Commitment to natural killer cells requires the helix-loop-helix inhibitor Id2. Proc Natl Acad Sci USA *98*, 5164–5169.

Kataoka, T.R., Morii, E., Oboki, K., Jippo, T., Maeyama, K. and Kitamura, Y. (2002). Dual abnormal effects of mutant MITF encoded by Mi(wh) allele on mouse mast cells: decreased but recognizable transactivation and inhibition of transactivation. Biochem Biophys Res Commun *297*, 111–115.

Kee, B.L., Rivera, R.R. and Murre, C. (2001). Id3 inhibits B lymphocyte progenitor growth and survival in response to TGF-beta. Nat Immunol *2*, 242–247.

Kelley, C.M., Ikeda, T., Koipally, J. et al. (1998). Helios, a novel dimerization partner of Ikaros expressed in the earliest hematopoietic progenitors. Curr Biol *8*, 508–515.

Kowenz-Leutz, E., Twamley, G., Ansieau, S. and Leutz, A. (1994). Novel mechanism of C/EBP beta (NF-M) transcriptional control: activation through derepression. Genes Dev *8*, 2781–2791.

Krause, D.S. (2002). Regulation of hematopoietic stem cell fate. Oncogene *21*, 3262–3269.

Kumano, K., Chiba, S., Shimizu, K. et al. (2001). Notch1 inhibits differentiation of hematopoietic cells by sustaining GATA-2 expression. Blood *98*, 3283–3289.

Labrecque, J., Allan, D., Chambon, P., Iscove, N.N., Lohnes, D. and Hoang, T. (1998). Impaired granulocytic differentiation in vitro in hematopoietic cells lacking retinoic acid receptors alpha1 and gamma. Blood *92*, 607–615.

Lacaud, G., Gore, L., Kennedy, M. et al. (2002). Runx1 is essential for hematopoietic commitment at the hemangioblast stage of development in vitro. Blood *100*, 458–466.

Ladomery, M. and Dellaire, G. (2002). Multifunctional zinc finger proteins in development and disease. Ann Hum Genet *331*, 342.

Laity, J.H., Lee, B.M. and Wright, P.E. (2001). Zinc finger proteins: new insights into structural and functional diversity. Curr Opin Struct Biol *11*, 39–46.

Lander, E.S., Linton, L.M., Birren, B. et al. (2001). Initial sequencing and analysis of the human genome. Nature *409*, 860–921.

LaRonde-LeBlanc, N.A. and Wolberger, C. (2003). Structure of HoxA9 and Pbx1 bound to DNA: Hox hexapeptide and DNA recognition anterior to posterior. Genes Dev *17*, 2060–2072.

Lecine, P., Villeval, J.L., Vyas, P., Swencki, B., Xu, Y. and Shivdasani, R.A. (1998). Mice lacking transcription factor NF-E2 provide in vivo validation of the proplatelet model of thrombocytopoiesis and show a platelet production defect that is intrinsic to megakaryocytes. Blood *92*, 1608–1616.

Lee, G.R., Fields, P.E., Griffin, T.J. and Flavell, R.A. (2003). Regulation of the Th2 cytokine locus by a locus control region. Immunity 19, 145–153.

Lee, T.I., Rinaldi, N.J., Robert, F. et al. (2002). Transcriptional regulatory networks in Saccharomyces cerevisiae. Science 298, 799–804.

Li, Q. and Verma, I.M. (2002). NF-kappaB regulation in the immune system. Nat Rev Immunol 2, 725–734.

Lin, H. and Grosschedl, R. (1995). Failure of B-cell differentiation in mice lacking the transcription factor EBF. Nature 376, 263–267.

Lindstrom, M.S. and Wiman, K.G. (2002). Role of genetic and epigenetic changes in Burkitt lymphoma. Semin Cancer Biol 12, 381–387.

Liou, H.C. and Hsia, C.Y. (2003). Distinctions between c-Rel and other NF-kappaB proteins in immunity and disease. Bioessays 25, 767–780.

Liston, A., Lesage, S., Wilson, J., Peltonen, L. and Goodnow, C.C. (2003). Aire regulates negative selection of organ-specific T cells. Nat Immunol 4, 350–354.

Love, J.J., Li, X., Case, D.A., Giese, K., Grosschedl, R. and Wright, P.E. (1995). Structural basis for DNA bending by the architectural transcription factor LEF-1. Nature 376, 791–795.

Luchin, A., Suchting, S., Merson, T. et al. (2001). Genetic and physical interactions between Microphthalmia transcription factor and PU.1 are necessary for osteoclast gene expression and differentiation. J Biol Chem 276, 36703–36710.

Ma, P.C., Rould, M.A., Weintraub, H. and Pabo, C.O. (1994). Crystal structure of MyoD bHLH domain-DNA complex: perspectives on DNA recognition and implications for transcriptional activation. Cell 77, 451–459.

Madrid, L.V., Mayo, M.W., Reuther, J.Y. and Baldwin, A.J. (2001). Akt stimulates the transactivation potential of the RelA/p65 Subunit of NF-kappa B through utilization of the Ikappa B kinase and activation of the mitogen-activated protein kinase p38. J Biol Chem 276, 18934–18940.

Mamane, Y., Heylbroeck, C., Genin, P. et al. (1999). Interferon regulatory factors: the next generation. Gene 237, 1–14.

Mangelsdorf, D.J. and Evans, R.M. (1995). The RXR heterodimers and orphan receptors. Cell 83, 841–850.

Maniatis, T., Falvo, J.V., Kim, T.H. et al. (1998). Structure and function of the interferon-beta enhanceosome. Cold Spring Harb Symp Quant Biol 63, 609–620.

Marecki, S., Riendeau, C.J., Liang, M.D. and Fenton, M.J. (2001). PU.1 and multiple IFN regulatory factor proteins synergize to mediate transcriptional activation of the human IL-1 beta gene. J Immunol 166, 6829–6838.

Martinez Arias, A., Zecchini, V. and Brennan, K. (2002). CSL-independent Notch signalling: a checkpoint in cell fate decisions during development? Curr Opin Genet Dev 12, 524–533.

McCarthy, K.M., McDevit, D., Andreucci, A., Reeves, R. and Nikolajczyk, B.S. (2003). HMGA1 co-activates transcription in B cells through indirect association with DNA. J Biol Chem 278, 42106–42114.

McKercher, S.R., Henkel, G.W. and Maki, R.A. (1999). The transcription factor PU.1 does not regulate lineage commitment but has lineage-specific effects. J Leukoc Biol 66, 727–732.

Medzhitov, R. (2001). Toll-like receptors and innate immunity. Nat Rev Immunol 1, 135–145.

Minegishi, N., Suzuki, N., Yokomizo, T. et al. (2003). Expression and domain-specific function of GATA-2 during differentiation of the hematopoietic precursor cells in midgestation mouse embryos. Blood 102, 896–905.

Miyazawa, K., Shinozaki, M., Hara, T., Furuya, T. and Miyazono, K. (2002). Two major Smad pathways in TGF-beta superfamily signalling. Genes Cells 7, 1191–1204.

Mock, B.A., Liu, L., LePaslier, D. and Huang, S. (1996). The B-lymphocyte maturation promoting transcription factor BLIMP1/PRDI-BF1 maps to D6S447 on human chromosome 6q21-q22.1 and the syntenic region of mouse chromosome 10. Genomics 37, 24–28.

Moon, R.T., Bowerman, B., Boutros, M. and Perrimon, N. et al. (2002). The promise and perils of Wnt signaling through beta-catenin. Science 296, 1644–1646.

Mullen, A.C., Hutchins, A.S., High, F.A. et al. (2002). Hlx is induced by and genetically interacts with T-bet to promote heritable T(H)1 gene induction. Nat Immunol 3, 652–658.

Naar, A.M., Lemon, B.D. and Tjian, R. et al. (2001). Transcriptional coactivator complexes. Annu Rev Biochem 70, 475–501.

Nagulapalli, S. and Atchison, M.L. (1998). Transcription factor Pip can enhance DNA binding by E47, leading to transcriptional synergy involving multiple protein domains. Mol Cell Biol 18, 4639–4650.

Nagy, M., Chapuis, B. and Matthes, T. (2002). Expression of transcription factors Pu.1, Spi-B, Blimp-1, BSAP and oct-2 in normal human plasma cells and in multiple myeloma cells. Br J Haematol 116, 429–435.

Nair, J.S., DaFonseca, C.J., Tjernberg, A. et al. (2002). Requirement of Ca2+ and CaMKII for Stat1 Ser-727 phosphorylation in response to IFN-gamma. Proc Natl Acad Sci USA 99, 5971–5976.

Nam, Y., Weng, A.P., Aster, J.C. and Blacklow, S.C. (2003). Structural requirements for assembly of the CSL.intracellular Notch1.Mastermind-like 1 transcriptional activation complex. J Biol Chem 278, 21232–21239.

Narlikar, G.J., Fan, H.Y. and Kingston, R.E. (2002). Cooperation between complexes that regulate chromatin structure and transcription. Cell 108, 475–487.

Nau, G.J., Richmond, J.F., Schlesinger, A., Jennings, E.G., Lander, E.S. and Young, R.A. (2002). Human macrophage activation programs induced by bacterial pathogens. Proc Natl Acad Sci USA 99, 1503–1508.

Nerlov, C. and Graf, T. (1998). PU.1 induces myeloid lineage commitment in multipotent hematopoietic progenitors. Genes Dev 12, 2403–2412.

Nerlov, C., Querfurth, E., Kulessa, H. and Graf, T. (2000). GATA-1 interacts with the myeloid PU.1 transcription factor and represses PU.1-dependent transcription. Blood 95, 2543–2551.

Newman, J.R. and Keating, A.E. (2003). Comprehensive identification of human bZIP interactions with coiled-coil arrays. Science 300, 2097–2101.

Nichogiannopoulou, A., Trevisan, M., Neben, S., Friedrich, C. and Georgopoulos, K. (1999). Defects in hemopoietic stem cell activity in Ikaros mutant mice. J Exp Med 190, 1201–1214.

Omichinski, J.G., Clore, G.M., Schaad, O. et al. (1993). NMR structure of a specific DNA complex of Zn-containing DNA binding domain of GATA-1. Science 261, 438–446.

Omichinski, J.G., Pedone, P.V., Felsenfeld, G., Gronenborn, A.M. and Clore, G.M. (1997). The solution structure of a specific GAGA factor-DNA complex reveals a modular binding mode. Nat Struct Biol 4, 122–132.

O'Riordan, M. and Grosschedl, R. (2000). Transcriptional regulation of early B-lymphocyte differentiation. Immunol Rev 175, 94–103.

Orkin, S.H., Shivdasani, R.A., Fujiwara, Y. and McDevitt, M.A. (1998). Transcription factor GATA-1 in megakaryocyte development. Stem Cells 2, 79–83.

Papathanasiou, P., Perkins, A.C., Cobb, B.S. et al. (2003). Widespread failure of hematolymphoid differentiation caused by a recessive niche-filling allele of the Ikaros transcription factor. Immunity 19, 131–144.

Patmasiriwat, P., Fraizer, G., Kantarjian, H. and Saunders, G.F. (1999). WT1 and GATA1 expression in myelodysplastic syndrome and acute leukemia. Leukemia 13, 891–900.

Pearce, E.L., Mullen, A.C., Martins, G.A. et al. (2003). Control of effector CD8+T cell function by the transcription factor Eomesodermin. Science 302, 1041–1043.

Pellegrini, L., Tan, S. and Richmond, T.J. (1995). Structure of serum response factor core bound to DNA. Nature 376, 490–498.

Perdomo, J., Holmes, M., Chong, B. and Crossley, M. (2000). Eos and pegasus, two members of the Ikaros family of proteins with distinct DNA binding activities. J Biol Chem 275, 38347–38354.

Pesu, M., Aittomaki, S., Valineva, T. and Silvennoinen, O. (2003). PU.1 is required for transcriptional activation of the Stat6 response element in the Igepsilon promoter. Eur J Immunol 33, 1727–1735.

Pettersson, M., Sundstrom, C., Nilsson, K. and Larsson, L.G. (1995). The hematopoietic transcription factor PU.1 is down-regulated in human multiple myeloma cell lines. Blood 86, 2747–2753.

Pine, R. (2002). IRF and tuberculosis. J Interferon Cytokine Res 22, 15–25.

Pitkanen, J. and Peterson, P. (2003). Autoimmune regulator: from loss of function to autoimmunity. Genes Immun 4, 12–21.

Pongubala, J.M., Nagulapalli, S., Klemsz, M.J. et al. (1992). PU.1 recruits a second nuclear factor to a site important for immunoglobulin kappa 3' enhancer activity. Mol Cell Biol 12, 368–378.

Purohit, S.J., Stephan, R.P., Kim, H.G., Herrin, B.R., Gartland, L. and Klug, C.A. (2003). Determination of lymphoid cell fate is dependent on the expression status of the IL-7 receptor. EMBO J 22, 5511–5521.

Querfurth, E., Schuster, M., Kulessa, H. et al. (2000). Antagonism between C/EBPbeta and FOG in eosinophil lineage commitment of multipotent hematopoietic progenitors. Genes Dev 14, 2515–2525.

Ramsay, R.G., Barton, A.L. and Gonda, T.J. (2003). Targeting c-Myb expression in human disease. Expert Opin Ther Targets 7, 235–248.

Ramsdell, F. and Ziegler, S.F. (2003). Transcription factors in autoimmunity. Curr Opin Immunol 15, 718–724.

Rebollo, A. and Schmitt, C. (2003). Ikaros, Aiolos and Helios: transcription regulators and lymphoid malignancies. Immunol Cell Biol 81, 171–175.

Reimold, A.M., Iwakoshi, N.N., Manis, J. et al. (2001). Plasma cell differentiation requires the transcription factor XBP-1. Nature 412, 300–307.

Reya, T., O'Riordan, M., Okamura, R. et al. (2000). Wnt signaling regulates B lymphocyte proliferation through a LEF-1 dependent mechanism. Immunity 13, 15–24.

Ricciardi, C.P. and Granucci, F. (2002). Opinion: Interpretation of the complexity of innate immune responses by functional genomics. Nat Rev Immunol 2, 881–889.

Rudolph, M.J. and Gergen, J.P. (2001). DNA-binding by Ig-fold proteins. Nat Struct Biol 8, 384–386.

Sakaguchi, S. (2003). The origin of FOXP3-expressing CD4+ regulatory T cells: thymus or periphery. J Clin Invest 112, 1310–1312.

Scandura, J.M., Boccuni, P., Cammenga, J. and Nimer, S.D. (2002). Transcription factor fusions in acute leukemia: variations on a theme. Oncogene 21, 3422–3444.

Schebesta, M., Heavey, B. and Busslinger, M. (2002). Transcriptional control of B-cell development. Curr Opin Immunol 14, 216–223.

Schmitz, M.L., Bacher, S. and Dienz, O. (2003). NF-kappaB activation pathways induced by T cell costimulation. Faseb J 17, 2187–2193.

Scott, E.W., Simon, M.C., Anastasi, J. and Singh, H. (1994). Requirement of transcription factor PU.1 in the development of multiple hematopoietic lineages. Science 265, 1573–1577.

Shaffer, A.L., Rosenwald, A., Hurt, E.M. et al. (2001). Signatures of the immune response. Immunity 15, 375–385.

Shang, Y. and Brown, M. (2002). Molecular determinants for the tissue specificity of SERMs. Science 295, 2465–2468.

Sharrocks, A.D., Brown, A.L., Ling, Y. and Yates, P.R. (1997). The ETS-domain transcription factor family. Int J Biochem Cell Biol 29, 1371–1387.

Shortman, K. and Liu, Y.J. (2002). Mouse and human dendritic cell subtypes. Nat Rev Immunol 2, 151–161.

Smale, S.T. (2003). A Th2 cytokine LCR. Adding a new piece to the regulatory puzzle. Immunity 19, 1–2.

Socolovsky, M., Nam, H., Fleming, M.D., Haase, V.H., Brugnara, C. and Lodish, H.F. (2001). Ineffective erythropoiesis in Stat5a(-/-)5b(-/-) mice due to decreased survival of early erythroblasts. Blood 98, 3261–3273.

Spiekermann, K., Biethahn, S., Wilde, S., Hiddemann, W. and Alves, F. (2001). Constitutive activation of STAT transcription factors in acute myelogenous leukemia. Eur J Haematol 67, 63–71.

Spits, H., Couwenberg, F., Bakker, A.Q., Weijer, K. and Uittenbogaart, C.H. (2000). Id2 and Id3 inhibit development of CD34 (+) stem cells into predendritic cell (pre-DC)2 but not into pre-DC1. Evidence for a lymphoid origin of pre-DC2. J Exp Med 192, 1775–1784.

Staal, F.J., van der Burg, M., Wessels, L.F. et al. (2003). DNA microarrays for comparison of gene expression profiles between diagnosis and relapse in precursor-B acute lymphoblastic leukemia: choice of technique and purification influence the identification of potential diagnostic markers. Leukemia 17, 1324–1332.

Stanojevic, D. and Verdine, G.L. (1995). Deconstruction of GCN4/GCRE into a monomeric peptide-DNA complex. Nat Struct Biol 2, 450–457.

Starr, T.K., Jameson, S.C. and Hogquist, K.A. (2003). Positive and negative selection of T cells. Annu Rev Immunol 21, 139–176.

Surdo, P.L., Bottomley, M.J., Sattler, M. and Scheffzek, K. (2003). Crystal structure and nuclear magnetic resonance analyses of the SAND domain from glucocorticoid modulatory element binding protein-1 reveals deoxyribonucleic acid and zinc binding regions. Mol Endocrinol 17, 1283–1295.

Takayanagi, H., Kim, S., Koga, T. et al. (2002). Induction and activation of the transcription factor NFATc1 (NFAT2) integrate RANKL signaling in terminal differentiation of osteoclasts. Dev Cell 3, 889–901.

Tsukada, J., Saito, K., Waterman, W.R., Webb, A.C. and Auron, P.E. (1994). Transcription factors NF-IL6 and CREB recognize a common essential site in the human prointerleukin 1 beta gene. Mol Cell Biol *14*, 7285–7297.

Venter, J.C., Adams, M.D., Myers, E.W. et al. (2001). The sequence of the human genome. Science *291*, 1304–1351.

Verger, A. and Duterque, C.M. (2002). When Ets transcription factors meet their partners. Bioessays *24*, 362–370.

Walker, M.R., Kasprowicz, D.J., Gersuk, V.H. et al. (2003). Induction of FoxP3 and acquisition of T regulatory activity by stimulated human CD4+CD25- T cells. J Clin Invest *112*, 1437–1443.

Wang, J.H., Avitahl, N., Cariappa, A. et al. (1998a). Aiolos regulates B cell activation and maturation to effector state. Immunity *9*, 543–553.

Wang, L.C., Swat, W., Cariappa, A. et al. (1998b). The TEL/ETV6 gene is required specifically for hematopoiesis in the bone marrow. Genes Dev *12*, 2392–2402.

Waraswapati, N., Yang, Z., Waterman, W.R. et al. (1999). Cytomegalovirus IE2 protein stimulates interleukin 1beta gene transcription via tethering to Spi-1/PU.1. Mol Cell Biol *19*, 6803–6814.

Warren, L.A. and Rothenberg, E.V. (2002). Regulatory coding of lymphoid lineage choice by hematopoietic transcription factors. Curr Opin Immunol *15*, 166–175.

Weinmann, A.S. and Farnham, P.J. (2002). Identification of unknown target genes of human transcription factors using chromatin immunoprecipitation. Methods *26*, 37–47.

Weiss, M.A., Ellenberger, T., Wobbe, C.R., Lee, J.P., Harrison, S.C. and Struhl, K. (1990). Folding transition in the DNA-binding domain of GCN4 on specific binding to DNA. Nature *347*, 575–578.

Wells, J. and Farnham, P.J. (2002). Characterizing transcription factor binding sites using formaldehyde crosslinking and immunoprecipitation. Methods *26*, 48–56.

Williams, S.C., Baer, M., Dillner, A.J. and Johnson, P.F. (1995). CRP2 (C/EBP beta) contains a bipartite regulatory domain that controls transcriptional activation, DNA binding and cell specificity. EMBO J *14*, 3170–3183.

Wilson, D.S. and Desplan, C. (1999). Structural basis of Hox specificity. Nat Struct Biol *6*, 297–300.

Woolf, E., Xiao, C., Fainaru, O. et al. (2003). Runx3 and Runx1 are required for CD8 T cell development during thymopoiesis. Proc Natl Acad Sci USA *100*, 7731–7736.

Wu, X., Spiro, C., Owen, W.G. and McMurray, C.T. (1998). cAMP response element-binding protein monomers cooperatively assemble to form dimers on DNA. J Biol Chem *273*, 20820–20827.

Yamaguchi, Y., Ackerman, S.J., Minegishi, N., Takiguchi, M., Yamamoto, M. and Suda, T. (1998). Mechanisms of transcription in eosinophils: GATA-1, but not GATA-2, transactivates the promoter of the eosinophil granule major basic protein gene. Blood *91*, 3447–3458.

Yamanaka, R., Barlow, C., Lekstrom, H.J. et al. (1997). Impaired granulopoiesis, myelodysplasia, and early lethality in CCAAT/enhancer binding protein epsilon-deficient mice. Proc Natl Acad Sci USA *94*, 13187–13192.

Yang, F.C., Tsuji, K., Oda, A. et al. (1999). Differential effects of human granulocyte colony-stimulating factor (hG-CSF) and thrombopoietin on megakaryopoiesis and platelet function in hG-CSF receptor-transgenic mice. Blood *94*, 950–958.

Ying, H., Chang, J.F. and Parnes, J.R. (1998). PU.1/Spi-1 is essential for the B cell-specific activity of the mouse CD72 promoter. J Immunol *160*, 2287–2296.

Younes, A., Garg, A. and Aggarwal, B.B. (2003). Nuclear transcription factor-kappaB in Hodgkin's disease. Leuk Lymphoma *44*, 929–935.

Zeng, G., Gao, L., Xia, T., Tencomnao, T. and Yu, R.K. (2003). Characterization of the 5'-flanking fragment of the human GM3-synthase gene. Biochim Biophys Acta *1625*, 30–35.

Zhang, C., Gadue, P., Scott, E., Atchison, M. and Poncz, M. (1997a). Activation of the megakaryocyte-specific gene platelet basic protein (PBP) by the Ets family factor PU.1. J Biol Chem *272*, 26236–26246.

Zhang, D.E., Zhang, P., Wang, D., Hetherington, C.J., Darlington, G.J. and Tenen, D.G. (1997b). Absence of granulocyte colony-stimulating factor signaling and neutrophil development in CCAAT enhancer binding protein alpha-deficient mice. Proc Natl Acad Sci USA *94*, 569–574.

Zhang, J.J., Zhao, Y., Chait, B.T. et al. (1998). Ser727-dependent recruitment of MCM5 by Stat1alpha in IFN-gamma-induced transcriptional activation. Embo J *17*, 6963–6971.

Zhang, P., Behre, G., Pan, J. et al. (1999). Negative cross-talk between hematopoietic regulators: GATA proteins repress PU.1. Proc Natl Acad Sci USA *96*, 8705–8710.

Zhong, H., May, M.J., Jimi, E. and Ghosh, S. et al. (2002). The phosphorylation status of nuclear NF-kappa B determines its association with CBP/p300 or HDAC-1. Mol Cell *9*, 625–636.

Zhu, J. and Emerson, S.G. (2002). Hematopoietic cytokines, transcription factors and lineage commitment. Oncogene *21*, 3295–3313.

Genetic Diversity in NK and NKT Cells

Chapter 8

Rachel Allen and Anne Cooke
University of Cambridge, Cambridge, UK

> Biologists must constantly keep in mind that what they see was not designed, but rather evolved.
>
> Francis Crick

INTRODUCTION

The mammalian immune system has evolved complex strategies to detect and destroy foreign antigens. Its cells and factors can act towards eliminating a pathogen immediately upon encounter, then develop a subsequent response with specificity and memory. Because a successful immune response relies upon a complex web of interactions between many agents, slight alterations in any of these components can exert an influence on multiple immunological pathways. As a result, naturally occurring variations in genes encoding immune factors are often reflected in the susceptibility of an individual to infectious disease or autoimmunity. Natural selection is likely to select a range of genotypes which balance the threat of these extremes.

The most obvious starting point from which to consider the impact of genetic variation upon immune-related disease is to focus upon the genes (or gene families) that are known to exhibit the highest levels of genetic variation. The major histocompatibility complex (MHC) was first identified as the main agent of transplant compatibility and encodes the MHC-1 and MHC-2 proteins required for antigen presentation to the T cell receptor (TCR). It became clear early on that the most outstanding feature of MHC-1 and MHC-2 genes is their polymorphism. In line with their classical antigen presenting role, the majority of MHC variations are found within the peptide binding groove (Parham et al., 1995). Association studies have shown that expression of certain MHC alleles or haplotypes can influence susceptibility to infection or predispose to autoimmune disease. For example, the human MHC-1 allele HLA-B27 shows a strong association with ankylosing spondylitis and related arthritic conditions (Brewerton et al., 1973; Schlosstein et al., 1973). MHC-2 associations include HLA-DR4 with narcolepsy and HLA DR3, 4 and 2 with diabetes. Pathogenic mechanisms to explain the role of MHC in such diseases have yet to be fully determined.

Specific recognition of individual MHC/peptide combinations is mediated by the T cell receptor. However, MHC-1 proteins are now known to act as ligands for a variety of other cell surface immune receptors that are expressed on alternative cell populations. For example, natural killer (NK) cells are large granular lymphocytes capable of lysing targets that have lost surface expression of MHC-1. Because natural killer cells can provide immediate defense against infection (reviewed in Biron, 1999; Cerwenka and Lanier, 2001) they are regarded as agents of the innate immune system. Observations of their MHC-1 dependent but unprimed killing activity, led to the proposal of the 'missing self' theory (Karre et al., 1985, Karre, 2002) and eventual identification of the MHC-1 specific receptors involved. Subsequent analyses indicate that, like their MHC ligands, some of these 'NK receptors' exhibit a high degree of genetic variation and appear to be evolving rapidly (Canavez et al., 2001; reviewed in

Measuring Immunity, edited by Michael T. Lotze and Angus W. Thomson
ISBN 0-12-455900-X, London

Copyright © 2005, Elsevier. All rights reserved.

Trowsdale and Parham, 2004). Here we describe the genetic variations that have been identified in MHC-1 specific NK receptors and their ligands in human and mouse systems. The potential implications of these variations and their relevance to immune mediated disease will also be discussed.

NK RECEPTOR COMPLEXES

While receptor systems vary between mouse and human, MHC-1 receptors fall into two main categories: C–type lectins and members of the Ig superfamily (Figure 8.1). Representatives of each are active in both species and include receptors with a degree of allele specificity, receptors with a broad spectrum of MHC-1 ligands and receptors that recognize non-classical MHC-1. Recognition of allele subsets is performed by Ig-like receptors in humans, whereas in mice this role is filled by a lectin-like receptor family. Similar to their target MHC proteins, NK receptor genes are found in clusters – Ig-like receptors are encoded within the leukocyte receptor complex (LRC) found on human chromosome 19 and mouse chromosome 7. Lectin NK receptor genes are located in the natural killer complex (NKC) on human chromosome 12 and mouse chromosome 6. Like the MHC, these gene complexes each contain several families of closely related genes. The level of conservation observed between human and rodent NK receptor complexes indicates that Ig-like and lectin-like receptor complexes existed before species divergence.

ACTIVATING VERSUS INHIBITORY RECEPTORS

When an NK cell is stimulated by a target, its subsequent response is dependent upon a delicate balance between signals from activating and inhibitory receptors. Residues within the cytoplasmic domain determine the immunomodulatory effects of any given NK receptor. Inhibitory receptors possess a long cytoplasmic tail containing immunoreceptor tyrosine-based motifs (ITIMs), which mediate the binding of SH2 domain tyrosine phosphatase (SHP) to transmit inhibitory signals to the nucleus. In contrast, activating receptors display a short cytoplasmic tail, with no signaling motifs of their own. Activating receptors carry a charged residue in the transmembrane domain, allowing them to associate with adaptor molecules such as DAP12, DAP10 or FcRIγ to convey their activating signals (Lanier et al., 1998; Nakajima et al., 1999; Wu et al., 1999). Following ligand engagement by an activating receptor, immunoreceptor tyrosine-based activation motifs (ITAMs) in the cytoplasmic domain of the adaptor protein become phosphorylated then recruit tyrosine kinases such as Syk and ZAP70 for signal transduction. NK receptors often appear to act in paired inhibitory/activatory receptor combinations. From this, a combined input of activating and inhibitory signals determines whether an NK cell response, occurs although inhibitory receptors appear to have a higher affinity for ligand and act as the dominant force.

LECTIN RECEPTORS

CD94/NKG2 are genetically conserved receptors whose ligands show a high degree of genetic variation.

The human NK complex (NKC) on chromosome 12 encodes C-type lectins including the NKG2 proteins, CD64 and CD69. Lectin-like receptors and their MHC-1 ligands are described in Table 8.1. While some differences are observed between humans and mice, functional forms of the NKG2 lectin-like receptor family are expressed by both species. These type 2 membrane proteins are found as heterodimers in association with CD94 on the surface of NK cells and a subset of CTL (Lopez-Botet et al., 1997). CD94 combines with NKG2A, B and C to form a structure for recognition of the non-classical MHC-1 protein HLA-E (Braud et al., 1998; Lee et al., 1998; Borrego et al., 1998). HLA-E is not generally regarded as an antigen presenting molecule. Structural constraints in the peptide binding groove limit the peptide binding ability of HLA-E, which

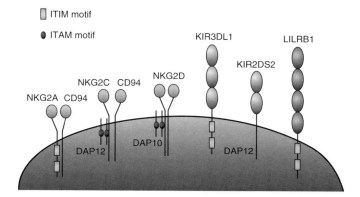

Figure 8.1 'NK' receptors

Table 8.1 Lectin-like receptors and their MHC-1 ligands

Receptor	Activating/inhibitory	Ligand(s)
NKG2A/CD94	Inhibitory	HLA-E (humans) Qa-1b (mice)
NKG2B/CD94	Inhibitory	HLA-E (humans) Qa-1b (mice)
NKG2C/CD94	Activating (associates with DAP12)	HLA-E (humans) Qa-1b (mice)
NKG2D	Activating (associates with DAP10)	MICA (humans) MICB (humans) ULBPs (humans) LETAL (humans) Rae-1 (mice) H60 (mice) MULT1(mice)

binds a short peptide derived from the leader sequence of classical MHC-1 alleles (O'Callaghan et al., 1998; Braud et al., 1997). Recognition of HLA-E by CD94/NKG2 thus provides an indirect means by which to survey expression of other, classical, MHC-1. The murine CD94/NKG2 ligand is Qa-1b. Like HLA-E, this MHC-1-like protein binds leader peptides obtained as a by-product from the expression of classical alleles (Decloux et al., 1997; Cotterill et al., 1997). The CD94/NKG2 family contains both activating and inhibitory receptors; NKG2A and NKG2B carry ITIMs within their cytoplasmic tail and can inhibit the lytic activity of NK and T cells, while CD94/NKG2C associates with the adaptor molecule DAP12 to form an activating receptor complex (Cantoni et al., 1998).

Another activating receptor, NKG2D, is encoded in the NKC nearby the NKG2A, B and C genes. Unlike its relatives, NKG2D does not associate with CD94. Instead, it is found as a homodimer on the surface of NK cells, $\gamma\delta$ T cells and activated $\alpha\beta$ T cells (Bauer et al., 1999, Wu et al., 1999). Signaling through NKG2D leads to NK cell cytotoxicity and co-stimulation of T cell receptor signaling. Alternatively spliced isoforms of NKG2D associate with different adapter proteins – DAP12 and DAP10. Differential expression of these NKG2D/adapter combinations determines whether NKG2D functions as a stimulatory or a co-stimulatory molecule (Diefenbach et al., 2002). One unusual feature of the NKG2D protein is that it recognizes multiple MHC-1-like ligands including membrane-bound and GPI-linked molecules. In humans, NKG2D recognizes two families of stress-inducible ligands, the MICA/MICB proteins and the ULBPs (Bauer et al., 1999; Cosman et al., 2001). ULBPs are upregulated following viral infection (Rolle et al., 2003). NKG2D ligands are known for their polymorphism; MICA and MICB are encoded within the human MHC and unlike other 'non-classical' MHC-1 show a high degree of variation (Perez-Rodriguez et al., 2002; Collins et al., 2002). Association studies for MIC alleles are starting to indicate a potential relevance for these proteins in several disease situations. MICA polymorphisms can affect NKG2D binding and might be expected to exert differential signaling effects (Steinle et al., 2001).

The NKG2D receptor is also found in mice, where again it recognizes multiple ligand families. The three families of ligands recognized by murine NKG2D are H60, retinoic acid early inducible-1 (RAE-1) proteins and the murine ULBP-like transcripts (MULT) (Carayannopoulos et al., 2002). The binding interaction between murine NKG2D and its different ligand families can differ by 25 fold (O'Callaghan et al., 2001). Of these, the RAE-1 proteins are expressed on activated macrophages following toll-like receptor signaling. Recognition of RAE-1 on activated macrophages may provide a means of macrophage/NK cell cross-talk during an innate immune response (Hamerman et al., 2004). Upregulation or ectopic expression of NKG2D ligands leads to MHC unrestricted killing and tumor rejection in mice (Diefenbach et al., 2001; Cerwenka et al., 2001; Verneris et al., 2003).

Table 8.2 The murine Ly49 receptor family and their MHC-1 ligands

Receptor	Activating/inhibitory	Ligand(s)
Ly49A	Inhibitory	H2-Dd, H2-Dk
Ly49C	Inhibitory	H2-Kb, H2-Db, H2-Kd, H2-Dd, H2-Dk
Ly49D	Activating	H2-Dd
Ly49F	Inhibitory	H2^d
Ly49G2	Inhibitory	H2-Dd, H2-Dk, H2-Kd
Ly49I	Inhibitory	H2-Dd, H2-Kb, H2-Kd, H2-Kk
Ly49O	Inhibitory	H2-Ld, H2-Dd, H2-Dk, H2-Db
Ly49P	Activating	H2-Dd
Ly49R	Activating	H2-Dd, H2-Dk
Ly49V	Inhibitory	H2-Ld, H2-Dd, H2-Dk, H2-Db
Ly49W	Activating	H2-Dk, H2-Dd

Activating receptors associate with the DAP12 adaptor protein

THE MURINE LY49 RECEPTOR FAMILY

In addition to NKG2 proteins, the mouse NKC encodes the Ly49 receptors responsible for recognition of MHC-1 allele subsets. Although the mouse NKC encodes several proteins in the Ly49 family, only one Ly49 gene has been identified for humans and appears to be a pseudogene (Westgaard et al., 1998; Barten and Trowsdale, 1999). Murine Ly49 receptor specificities are described in Table 8.2. Ly49 proteins exist as homodimers on the surface of NK cells, T cells and NKT cells where they can influence lytic activity. A high degree of genetic variation is observed between Ly49 receptors in different mouse strains (Wilhelm et al., 2002; Makrigiannis et al., 2002). This is evidenced at the phenotypic level in the enhanced cellular activity of NK cells from C57BL/6 mice compared to BALB/c (Idris et al., 1998). Despite their similarity to C type lectins, binding of MHC by Ly49s does not appear to be carbohydrate dependent.

IG-LIKE RECEPTORS

The KIR family

Genes for the major human family of NK receptors are clustered within the leukocyte receptor complex (LRC) on chromosome 19 (Wilson et al., 1999). The LRC encodes two families of Ig-like receptors that recognize MHC-1: the killer Ig-like receptors (KIR) and the leukocyte immunobulin-like receptors (LILR). Receptor specificities are described in Table 8.3. KIR are expressed on NK cells where they inhibit lytic activity and may influence cytokine secretion and are also observed on subsets of memory T lymphocytes where they exert a similar immunoregulatory effect (Phillips et al., 1995). A systematic nomenclature is used to classify KIR in order to define both the extracellular and intracellular nature of each receptor. Inhibitory receptors have a long cytoplasmic tail carrying ITIM motifs and are given an 'L' suffix. Activating receptors have a short

Table 8.3 Human Ig-like receptors and their MHC-1 ligands

Receptor	Activating/inhibitory	Ligand(s)
KIR2DL1	Inhibitory	HLA-Cw2, Cw4, Cw6 etc (Asn77, Lys80)
KIR2DL2	Inhibitory	HLA-Cw1, Cw3, Cw7 etc (Ser77, Asn80)
KIR2DL3	Inhibitory	HLA-Cw1, Cw3, Cw7 etc (Ser77, Asn80)
KIR2DL4	Inhibitory	HLA-G
KIR2DS1	Activating (associates with DAP12)	HLA-Cw2, Cw4, Cw6 etc (asn77, lys80)
KIR2DS4	Activating (associates with DAP12)	HLA-Cw1, Cw3, Cw7 etc (Ser77, Asn80)
KIR3DL1	Inhibitory	HLA-Bw4 alleles
KIR3DL2	Inhibitory	HLA-A2, A11, HLA B27 free heavy chains
LILRB1	Inhibitory	UL18, HLA-A, B, F, G
LILRB2	Inhibitory	HLA-A, B, F, G
LILRA1	Activating (adaptor unknown)	HLA-B27

cytoplasmic tail and are given an 'S' suffix. Thus, an activating receptor with two extracellular domains would fall into the KIR2DS group, while an inhibitory receptor with three extracellular domains would be classified as KIR3DL.

KIR and genetic variation

KIR exhibit a high degree of genetic variation. For example, KIR haplotypes vary in the number and nature of receptors that they encode. Three 'framework' genes (KIR3DL3, KIR2DL4 and KIR3DL2) are present in all haplotypes (Wilson et al., 2000). Combinations of the remaining receptors vary between haplotypes, with a range of 7–11 different KIR encoded on each (Witt et al., 1999). The 'A' haplotype is the most common and contains only one activating receptor (KIR2DS4). Other haplotypes encode increased numbers of activating KIR. Conventional polymorphism is also observed and multiple alleles of individual KIR receptors continue to be identified. A final level of variation is seen at the cellular level; from the available genetic repertoire, only a subset of receptors will be expressed by a given NK or T cell clone, with no evidence of allelic exclusion. The high level of genetic variation seen for the KIR genes makes them ideal candidates for studies of genetic association in immune-mediated diseases.

The Loukocyte Ig-Like Receptors (LILR)

LILR are the second group of Ig-like receptors encoded within the LRC, but unlike other 'NK receptors' are expressed by cells of the myelomonocytic lineage. Three receptors in this family have been shown to recognize MHC class I as indicated in Table 8.3. LILR signaling can induce a range of effects including alterations in cellular activity and inhibition of other signalling pathways. Expression of LILRA2 and LILRB2 renders dendritic cells tolerogenic

(Chang et al., 2002) and ELILR signaling has been shown to skew the cytokine secretion profile and antimicrobial activity of monocytes (Bleharski et al., 2003). Such functions would indicate that LILR could play a major role in a range of disease situations. Although they do not exhibit the same degree of genetic variation as KIR, ELILR are polymorphic, various alleles are now being identified and disease association studies are beginning to emerge (Torkar et al., 2000; Young et al., 2001).

PIR

The murine leukocyte receptor complex encoding Ig-like NK receptors is located on chromosome 7. Although KIR proteins are absent from this system, homologs of the LILR receptors are found. Like LILR, these receptors, known as paired inhibitory receptors (PIR), are expressed on B cells and myelomonocytic cells where they modulate cellular activity. Activating receptors are termed PIR-A and inhibitory forms PIR-B. PIR are known to affect dendritic cell activity to influence Th1/Th2 phenotype selection (Ujike et al., 2002). The negative influence of PIR-B on B cell activity can be overcome by addition of IL-4, which downregulates the inhibitory isoform, while upregulating activating PIR-A receptor. IL-4 can therefore free B cells from PIR-B inhibitory receptor-mediated suppression to enhance B cell and Th2 responses (Rudge et al., 2002).

NKT CELLS

NK receptors are regarded as agents of innate immunity although they are expressed on both NK cells and T cell subsets. Another unique lymphocyte subset known as NKT cells is also found and bears characteristics of innate and acquired immune systems with an invariant TCR and various NK receptors on their surface. In mice, these cells can also be identified by their expression of the NK1.1 marker (although this is absent from some mouse strains). The invariant T cell receptor (Vα14 in mice, Vα28 in humans) on NKT cells recognizes lipid antigens presented by the MHC-like protein, CD1. Upon stimulation, NKT cells provide a rapid source of IL-4 and IFNγ (Yoshimoto and Paul, 1994), which may allow them to polarize Th1/Th2 differentiation of a subsequent T cell response. Genetic factors can influence the behaviour of NKT cells during infection. In a murine model of malaria, strain specific differences were observed in the regulatory role of NKT cells. These effects mapped to the NKC and could indicate an influence of other NK receptors on NKT cell activity (Hansen et al., 2003). In humans, another potential source of genetic influence could result from polymorphisms in CD1 (Han et al., 1999)

The NKT cell population has been implicated in the maintenance of tolerance and consequently, when this system breaks down, autoimmunity. Several autoimmune diseases highlight the relevance of NKT cells. Reduced numbers of NKT cells are seen in the NOD mouse model of diabetes where they appear to provide a less efficient source of IL-4 than equivalent cells from other mouse strains (Gombert et al., 1996; Baxter et al., 1997; Lehuen et al., 1998; Hammond et al., 2001, Poulton et al., 2001). Genetic factors underlying this deficiency have been mapped to several loci, including two loci that had previously been implicated in diabetes (Esteban et al., 2003; Matsuki et al., 2003; Zhang et al., 2003). In humans, patients with type 1 diabetes may show a similar deficiency of NKT cells with impaired IL-4 production (Wilson et al., 1998). NKT cells have also been implicated in several other autoimmune situations (reviewed in Hammond and Kronenberg, 2003).

NK receptor variation in immune-mediate disease

Viral infection

NK receptors are suitable candidates for involvement in many immune-mediated disease pathologies. Genetic variations would therefore give rise to phenotypic effects in the form of disease susceptibility. This was first observed in the context of viral infection. NK cells are known to be important in the response to CMV infection (Biron and Brossay, 2001). The importance of NKG2D in the response to viral infection is implied by the existence of a viral immune evasion mechanism which has evolved to subvert it. HCMV encodes the UL16 protein which retains ULBPs inside the cell to prevent their recognition by NKG2D (Rolle et al., 2003). KIR and Ly49 receptors are also predicted to play a role in the clearance of viral infection. One particular mouse strain, C57BL/6, was known to be resistant to infection when compared to susceptible BALB/c mice. The gene responsible for this effect was mapped to the Cmv1 locus in the NK complex and subsequently shown to encode an activating Ly49 receptor, Ly49H present in the C57BL/6 Ly49 haplotype (Scalzo et al., 1990; Lee et al., 2001). The Cmv1 locus is also implicated in resistance to other infections (Delona and Brownstein, 1995), although the role of Ly49H has not been formally shown in these cases and another Ly49 receptor may therefore be involved.

In humans, studies are beginning to show the influence of NK receptor polymorphisms on the response to viral infection. Delayed progression to AIDS following HIV infection has been known to be associated with possession of certain HLA alleles such as HLA B27 (Goulder et al., 1997). More recently, an activating KIR allele, KIR3DS1 has been shown in combination with certain HLA B alleles to confer delayed progression in HIV positive individuals (Martin et al., 2002a). This study also demonstrates the combined importance of polymorphisms in both MHC ligand and NK receptor clusters (which are encoded on separate chromosomes) and suggests an epistatic interaction between the two loci. Such effects should be considered in future studies of Ly49 and KIR disease associations.

Autoimmunity

As mentioned above, MHC-1 specific leukocyte receptors are likely to play a role in a range of immune-related diseases. However, as immunomodulators, their greatest clinical relevance is likely to be in diseases involving immune dysregulation. Extensive expression of LILR is seen during early to intermediate stages of rheumatoid arthritis, reflecting the presence of neutrophils and macrophages whose activity they are likely to control. Similarly, there is already evidence of KIR involvement in psoriatic arthritis (PsA). Expression of the activating receptors KIR2DS1 and KIR2DS2 predisposes to disease when MHC ligands for the corresponding inhibitory receptors are absent (Martin et al., 2002b). KIR2DS2 may also play a role in rheumatoid vasculitis, where expansions of CD4(+)CD28(null) T cells expressing this receptor are observed (Yen et al., 2001). It is interesting to note that the receptors identified in the studies described above were all activating isoforms. As described earlier, KIR haplotypes vary in the number of activating receptors they encode with the most common haplotype carrying only one receptor. The implication of activating KIR in arthritis and the observation that the frequency of activating haplotypes is increased in patients with diabetes (van der Slik et al., 2003) could indicate a role for activating receptors in autoimmunity. Activating receptors may favor inflammatory responses and could therefore be useful as a means to combat infection. If, however, they also predispose to autoimmune disease then the continued presence of activating haplotypes within a population may indicate the need to maintain a fine balance between susceptibility to infection and susceptibility to autoimmunity.

Non-obese diabetic (NOD) mice provide an animal model of insulin-dependent diabetes mellitus. These animals show an impairment of NK cell function, directed by upregulation of RAE-1 on activated NK cells and consequent NKG2D modulation (Ogasawara et al., 2003). It is important to note that these findings illustrate how polymorphisms on both receptor and ligand may exert an influence in immune cell activity. In the human system, MICA polymorphisms may be associated with diabetes (Gupta et al., 2003). Studies are now also looking at the influence of MIC polymorphisms in other autoimmune diseases such as psoriatic arthritis (Gonzalez et al., 2002). Thus, differences in induction of NKG2D ligands during inflammation could trigger immune pathology.

Tumors

Ectopic expression of NKG2D ligands on the surface of tumor cells in mice leads to tumor rejection and the development of memory responses (Diefenbach et al., 2001). A similar upregulation of MIC proteins has been observed in human leukemias. This phenomenon is accompanied by the presence of high levels of soluble MIC in serum, which may impair NKG2D mediated control of tumors (Salih et al., 2003). The association of particular MIC alleles with cancers should provide a useful field of study (Chung-Ji et al., 2002).

Transplantation

Having discussed the potential pathologies associated with NK receptor polymorphisms, it is also worth noting that such variabilities may be used to our medical advantage in certain situations. Despite what might be predicted from classical graft versus host disease (GvHD), MHC mismatching for patients with acute myeloid leukemia (AML) appears to improve the rate of survival (Ruggeri et al., 2002). One possible mechanism is that alloreactive NK cells arise from the graft and undergo expansion to kill leukemia cells, yet spare tissues that are targeted by T cells in classical GvHD. KIR and MHC typing to provide mismatch could represent the first clinical application resulting from an increased knowledge of NK receptor diversity.

CONCLUSIONS

As our understanding of the various NK receptor systems grows, we are becoming increasingly aware of their immunological effects and impact upon a disease. Already genetic studies are pointing towards a relevance of NK receptors to infectious and autoimmune disease. In classical genetics, diseases involving mutation and/or loss of function can give clear phenotypic results. Immunological outcomes that result from genetic polymorphism in NK receptors are likely to be subtle in their effects and require detailed association studies. We know already that these receptors and/or their ligands tend to show high levels of genetic variability, probably resulting from their role in combat with rapidly evolving pathogens. A full understanding of the effects of such variations must be accompanied by a clear knowledge of receptor function. As our understanding of NK receptor functions increases we will be able to apply this to our understanding of infectious and autoimmune diseases, throwing new light on pathogenic mechanisms and the influence of genetics.

REFERENCES

Barten, R. and Trowsdale, J. (1999). The human Ly-49L gene. Immunogenetics 49, 731–734.

Bauer, S., Groh, V., Wu, J. et al. (1999). Activation of NK cells and T cells by NKG2D, a receptor for stress-inducible MICA. Science 285, 727–729.

Baxter, A.G., Kinder, S.J., Hammond, K.J.L., Scollay, R. and Godfrey, D.I. (1997). Association between abTCR+CD4-CD8- T-cell deficiency and IDDm in NOD/Lt mice. Diabetes 46, 572–582.

Biron, C.A. (1999). Initial and innate responses to viral infections–pattern setting in immunity or disease. Curr Opin Microbiol 2, 374–381.

Biron, C.A. and Brossay, L. (2001). NK cells and NKT cells in innate defense against viral infections. Curr Opin Immunol 1, 458–464.

Bleharski, J.R., Li, H., Meinken, C. et al. (2003). Use of genetic profiling in leprosy to discriminate clinical forms of the disease. Science 30, 1527–1530.

Borrego, F., Ulbrecht, M., Weiss, E.H., Coligan, J.E. and Brooks, A.G. (1998). Recognition of human histocompatibility leukocyte antigen (HLA)-E complexed with HLA class I signal sequence-derived peptides by CD94/NKG2 confers protection from natural killer cell-mediated lysis. J Exp Med 187, 813–818.

Braud, V., Jones, E.Y. and McMichael, A. (1997). The human major histocompatibility complex class Ib molecule HLA-E binds signal sequence-derived peptides with primary anchor residues at positions 2 and 9. Eur J Immunol 27, 1164–1169.

Braud, V.M., Allan, D.S., O'Callaghan, C.A. et al. (1998). HLA-E binds to natural killer cell receptors CD94/NKG2A, B and C. Nature 391, 795–799.

Brewerton, D.A., Hart, F.D., Nicholls, A., Caffrey, M., James, D.C. and Sturrock, R.D. (1973). Ankylosing spondylitis and HLA-A 27. Lancet 1, 904.

Canavez, F., Young, N.T., Guethlein, L.A. et al. (2001). Comparison of chimpanzee and human leukocyte Ig-like receptor genes reveals framework and rapidly evolving genes. J Immunol 167, 5786–5794.

Cantoni, C., Biassoni, R., Pende, D. et al. (1998). The activating form of CD94 receptor complex: CD94 covalently associates with the Kp39 protein that represents the product of the NKG2-C gene. Eur J Immunol 28, 327–338.

Carayannopoulos, L.N., Naidenko, O.V., Fremont, D.H. and Yokoyama, W.M. (2002). Cutting edge: murine UL16-binding protein-like transcript 1: a newly described transcript encoding a high-affinity ligand for murine NKG2D. J Immunol 169, 4079–4083.

Cerwenka, A., Bakker, A.B., McClanahan, T. et al. (2000). Retinoic acid early inducible genes define a ligand family for the activating NKG2D receptor in mice. Immunity 12, 721–727.

Cerwenka, A. and Lanier, L.L. (2001). Natural killer cells, viruses and cancer. Nat Rev Immunol 1, 41–49.

Chang, C.C., Ciubotariu, R., Manavalan, J.S. et al. (2002). Tolerization of dendritic cells by T(S) cells: the crucial role of inhibitory receptors ILT3 and ILT4. Nat Immunol 3, 237–243.

Chung-Ji, L., Yann-Jinn, L., Hsin-Fu, L. et al. (2002). The increase in the frequency of MICA gene A6 allele in oral squamous cell carcinoma. J Oral Pathol Med 31, 323–328.

Collins, R.W., Stephens, H.A., Clare, M.A. and Vaughan, R.W. (2002). High resolution molecular phototyping of MICA and MICB alleles using sequence specific primers. Hum Immunol 63, 783–794.

Cosman, D., Mullberg, J., Sutherland, C.L. et al. (2001). ULBPs, novel MHC class I-related molecules, bind to CMV glycoprotein UL16 and stimulate NK cytotoxicity through the NKG2D receptor. Immunity 14, 123–133.

Cotterill, L.A., Stauss, H.J., Millrain, M.M. et al. (1997). Qa-1 interaction and T cell recognition of the Qa-1 determinant modifier peptide. Eur J Immunol 27, 2123–2132.

DeCloux, A., Woods, A.S., Cotter, R.J., Soloski, M.J. and Forman, J. (1997). Dominance of a single peptide bound to the class I(B) molecule, Qa-1b. J Immunol 158, 2183–2191.

Delano, M.L. and Brownstein, D.G. (1995). Innate resistance to lethal mousepox is genetically linked to the NK gene complex on chromosome 6 and correlates with early restriction of virus replication by cells with an NK phenotype. J Virol 69, 5875–5877.

Diefenbach, A., Jamieson, A.M., Liu, S.D., Shastri, N. and Raulet, D.H. (2000). Ligands for the murine NKG2D receptor: expression by tumor cells and activation of NK cells and macrophages. Nat Immunol 1, 119–126.

Diefenbach, A., Jensen, E.R., Jamieson, A.M. and Raulet, D.H. (2001). Rae1 and H60 ligands of the NKG2D receptor stimulate tumour immunity. Nature 13, 165–171.

Diefenbach, A., Tomasello, E., Lucas, M. et al. (2002). Selective associations with signaling proteins determine stimulatory versus costimulatory activity of NKG2D. Nat Immunol 3, 1142–1149.

Esteban, L.M., Tsoutsman, T., Jordan, M.A. et al. (2003). Genetic control of NKT cell numbers maps to major diabetes and lupus loci. J Immunol 15, 2873–2878.

Gombert, J.M., Herbelin, A., Tancredeb-bohin, E., Dy, M., Carnaud, C. and Bach, J.F. (1996). Early quantitative and functional deficiency of NK1+-lke thymocytes in the NOD mouse. Eur J Immunol 26, 2989–2998.

Gonzalez, S., Martinez-Borra, J., Lopez-Vazquez, A., Garcia-Fernandez, S., Torre-Alonso, J.C. and Lopez-Larrea, C. (2002). MICA rather than MICB, TNFA, or HLA-DRB1 is associated with susceptibility to psoriatic arthritis. J Rheumatol 29, 973–978.

Goulder, P.J., Phillips, R.E., Colbert, R.A. et al. (1997). Late escape from an immunodominant cytotoxic T-lymphocyte response associated with progression to AIDS. Nat Med 3, 212–217.

Gupta, M., Nikitina-Zake, L., Zarghami, M. et al. (2003). Association between the transmembrane region polymorphism of MHC class I chain related gene-A and type 1 diabetes mellitus in Sweden. Hum Immunol 64, 553–561.

Hamerman, J.A., Ogasawara, K. and Lanier, L.L. (2004). Cutting Edge: Toll-like receptor signalling in macrophages induces ligands for the NKG2D receptor. J Immunol 172, 2001–2005.

Hammond, K.J., Pellicci, D.G., Poulton, L.D. et al. (2001). CD1d-restricted NKT cells: an interstrain comparison. J Immunol 167, 1164–1173.

Hammond, K.J.L. and Kronenberg, M. (2003). Natural killer T cells: natural or unnatural regulators of autoimmunity? Curr Opin Immunol 15, 683–689.

Han, M., Hannick, L.I., DiBrino, M. and Robinson, M.A. (1999). Polymorphism of human CD1 genes. Tissue Antigens 54, 122–127.

Hansen, D.S., Siomos, M.A., Buckingham, L., Scalzo, A.A. and Schofield, L. (2003). Regulation of murine cerebral malaria pathogenesis by CD1d-restricted NKT cells and the natural killer complex. Immunity 18, 391–402.

Idris, A.H., Iizuka, K., Smith, H.R., Scalzo, A.A. and Yokoyama, W.M. (1998). Genetic control of natural killing and in vivo tumor elimination by the Chok locus. J Exp Med 188, 2243–2256.

Karre K, Ljunggren HG, Piontek G, Kiessling R. (1985) Selective rejection of H-2-deficient lymphoma variants suggests alternative immune defence strategy. Nature 319(6055), 675–678.

Karre, K. (2002). NK cells, MHC class I molecules and the missing self. Scand J Immunol 55, 221–228.

Koike, J., Wakao, H., Ishizuka, Y. et al. (2004). Bone marrow allograft rejection mediated by a novel murine NK receptor, NKG2I. J Exp Med 199, 137–144.

Lanier, L.L., Corliss, B., Wu, J. and Phillips, J.H. (1998). Association of DAP12 with activating CD94/NKG2C NK cell receptors. Immunity 8, 693–701.

Lee, N., Llano, M., Carretero, M. et al. (1998). HLA-E is a major ligand for the natural killer inhibitory receptor CD94/NKG2A. Proc Natl Acad Sci USA 28, 5199–5204.

Lee, S.H., Girard, S., Macina, D. et al. (2001). Susceptibility to mouse cytomegalovirus is associated with deletion of an activating natural killer cell receptor of the C-type lectin superfamily. Nat Genet 28, 42–45.

Lehuen, A., Lantz, O., Nbeaudoin, L. et al. (1998). Overexpression of natural killer T cells protects Va14-Ja281 transgenic nonobese diabetic mice against diabetes. J Exp Med 188, 1831–1839.

Lopez-Botet, M., Perez-Villar, J.J., Carretero, M. et al. (1997). Structure and function of the CD94 C-type lectin receptor complex involved in recognition of HLA class I molecules. Immunol Rev 155, 165–174.

Makrigiannis, A.P., Pau, A.T., Schwartzberg, P.L., McVicar, D.W., Beck, T.W. and Anderson, S.K. (2002). A BAC contig map of the Ly49 gene cluster in 129 mice reveals extensive differences in gene content relative to C57BL/6 mice. Genomics 79, 437–444.

Martin, M.P., Gao, X., Lee, J.H. et al. (2002a). Epistatic interaction between KIR3DS1 and HLA-B delays the progression to AIDS. Nat Genet 31, 429–434.

Martin, M.P., Nelson, G., Lee, J.H. et al. (2002b). Cutting edge: susceptibility to psoriatic arthritis: influence of activating killer Ig-like receptor genes in the absence of specific HLA-C alleles. J Immunol 169, 2818–2822.

Matsuki, N., Stanic, A.K., Embers, M.E., Van kaer, L., Morel, L. and Joyce, S. (2003). Genetic dissection of Va14Ja18 natural T cell number and function in autoimmunbe-prone mice J Immunol 170, 5429–5437.

Nakajima, H., Samaridis, J., Angman, L. and Colonna, M. (1999). Human myeloid cells express an activating ILT receptor (ILT1) that associates with Fc receptor gamma-chain. J Immunol 162, 5–8.

O'Callaghan, C.A., Tormo, J., Willcox, B.E. et al. (1998). Structural features impose tight peptide binding specificity in the non-classical MHC molecule HLA-E. Mol Cell 1, 531–541.

O'Callaghan, C.A., Cerwenka, A., Willcox, B.E., Lanier, L.L. and Bjorkman, P.J. (2001). Molecular competition for NKG2D: H60 and RAE1 compete unequally for NKG2D with dominance of H60. Immunity 15, 201–211.

Ogasawara, K., Hamerman, J.A., Hsin, H. et al. (2003). Impairment of NK cell function by NKG2D modulation in NOD mice. Immunity 18, 41–51.

Parham, P., Adams, E.J. and Arnett, K.L. (1995). The origins of HLA-A,B,C polymorphism. Immunol Rev 143, 141–180.

Perez-Rodriguez, M., Arguello, J.R., Fischer, G. et al. (2002). Further polymorphism of the MICA gene. Eur J Immunogenet 29, 35–46.

Phillips, J.H., Gumperz, J.E., Parham, P. and Lanier, L.L. (1995). Superantigen-dependent, cell-mediated cytotoxicity inhibited by MHC class I receptors on T lymphocytes. Science 268, 403–405.

Poulton, L.D., Smyth, M.J., Hawke, C.G. et al. (2001). Cytometric and functional analysis of NK and NKT cell deficiencies in NOD mice. Int Immunol 13, 887–896.

Rolle, A., Mousavi-Jazi, M., Eriksson, M. et al. (2003). Effects of human cytomegalovirus infection on ligands for the activating NKG2D receptor of NK cells: up-regulation of UL16-binding protein (ULBP)1 and ULBP2 is counteracted by the viral UL16 protein. J Immunol 171, 902; Diabetes 52, 2639–2642.

Rudge, E.U., Cutler, A.J., Pritchard, N.R. and Smith, K.G. (2002). Interleukin 4 reduces expression of inhibitory receptors on

B cells and abolishes CD22 and Fc gamma RII-mediated B cell suppression. J Exp Med *195*, 1079–1085.

Ruggeri, L., Capanni, M., Tosti, A. et al. (2002). Innate immunity against hematological malignancies. Cytotherapy *4*, 343–346.

Salih, H.R., Antropius, H., Gieseke, F. et al. (2003). Functional expression and release of ligands for the activating immuno-receptor NKG2D in leukemia. Blood *102*, 1389–1396.

Scalzo, A.A., Fitzgerald, N.A., Simmons, A., La Vista, A.B. and Shellam, G.R. (1990). Cmv-1, a genetic locus that controls murine cytomegalovirus replication in the spleen. J Exp Med *171*, 1469–1483.

Schlosstein, L., Teraskaki, P.I., Bluestone, R. and Pearson, C.M. (1973). High association of an HLA-A antigen, W27, with anky-losing spondylitis. N Engl J Med *288*, 704.

Steinle, A., Li, P., Morris, D.L. et al. (2001). Interactions of human NKG2D with its ligands MICA, MICB, and homologs of the mouse RAE-1 protein family. Immunogenetics *53*, 279–287.

Torkar, M., Haude, A., Milne, S., Beck, S., Trowsdale, J. and Wilson, M.J. (2000). Arrangement of the ILT gene cluster: a common null allele of the ILT6 gene results from a 6.7-kbp deletion. Eur J Immunol *30*, 3655–3662.

Trowsdale, J. and Parham, P. (2004). Mini-review: defense strategies and immunity-related genes. Eur J Immunol *34*, 7–17.

Ujike, A., Takeda, K., Nakamura, A., Ebihara, S., Akiyama, K. and Takai, T. (2002). Impaired dendritic cell maturation and increased T(H)2 responses in PIR-B(-/-) mice. Nat Immunol *3*, 542–548.

van der Slik, A.R., Koeleman, B.P., Verduijn, W. et al. (2003). KIR in type 1 diabetes: disparate distribution of activating and inhibitory natural killer cell receptors in patients versus HLA-matched control subjects.

Verneris, M.R., Karami, M., Baker, J., Jayaswal, A. and Negrin, R.S. (2003). The role of NKG2D signalling in the cytotoxicity of activated and expanded CD8+ T cells. Blood

Westgaard, I.H., Berg, S.F., Orstavik, S., Fossum, S. and Dissen, E. (1998). Identification of a human member of the Ly-49 multi-gene family. Eur J Immunol *28*, 1839–1846.

Wilhelm, B.T., Gagnier, L. and Mager, D.L. (2002). Sequence analysis of the ly49 cluster in C57BL/6 mice: a rapidly evolving multigene family in the immune system. Genomics *80*, 646–661.

Wilson, S.B., Kent, S.C., Patton, K.T. et al. (1998). Extreme Th1 bias of invariant Va24-JaQ T cells in type 1 diabetes. Nature *391*, 177–181.

Wilson, M.J., Torkar, M., Haude, A. et al. (2000). Plasticity in the organization and sequences of human KIR/ILT gene families. Proc Natl Acad Sci USA *97*, 4778–4783.

Witt, C.S., Dewing, C., Sayer, D.C., Uhrberg, M., Parham, P. and Christiansen, F.T. (1999). Population frequencies and putative haplotypes of the killer cell immunoglobulin-like receptor sequences and evidence for recombination. Transplantation *68*, 1784–1789.

Wu, J., Song, Y., Bakker, A.B. et al. (1999). An activating immunore-ceptor complex formed by NKG2D and DAP10. Science *285*, 730–732.

Yen, J.H., Moore, B.E., Nakajima, T. et al. (2001). Major histo-compatibility complex class I-recognizing receptors are dis-ease risk genes in rheumatoid arthritis. J Exp Med *193*, 1159–1167.

Yoshimoto, T. and Paul, W.E. (1994). CD4pos, NK1.1pos T cells promptly produce interleukin 4 in response to in vivo chal-lenge with anti-CD3. J Exp Med *179*, 1285–1295.

Young, N.T., Canavez, F., Uhrberg, M., Shum, B.P. and Parham, P. (2001). Conserved organization of the ILT/LIR gene family within the polymorphic human leukocyte receptor complex. Immunogenetics *53*, 270–278.

Zhang, F., Liang, Z., Matsuki, N. et al. (2003). A murine locus on chromosome 18 controls NKT cell homeostasis and Th cell differentiation. J Immunol *171*, 4613–4620.

Section II

Serologic assays

Handling Sera and Obtaining Fluid from Different Compartments: Practical Considerations

Chapter 9

Dmitriy W. Gutkin[1], Diana Metes[2] and Michael R. Shurin[3]

[1]VA Pittsburgh Healthcare System, Pittsburgh, PA, USA; Departments of [2]Surgery and [3]Pathology, [3]Division of Clinical Immunopathology, University of Pittsburgh Medical Center, Pittsburgh, PA, USA

We hear and apprehend only what we already half know.

Henry David Thoreau

INTRODUCTION

Body fluids are analyzed for a variety of reasons. Some analyses confirm a diagnosis, others identify the cause and nature of an effusion and still others may have more diverse purposes. In addition, body fluids analysis offers a comprehensive view into monitoring disease progression, therapy effectiveness and occurrence of complications. In fact, hematologic, chemical/biochemical, cytologic, microbiologic, serologic, molecular, or genetic techniques are commonly used for evaluation of body fluids. Only biological fluids and procedures related to the immune system or immunological techniques are discussed in this chapter.

Biological fluids include blood, urine, semen (seminal fluid), vaginal secretions, cerebrospinal fluid (CSF), synovial fluid, pleural fluid (pleural lavage), pericardial fluid, peritoneal fluid, amniotic fluid, saliva, nasal fluid, otic fluid, gastric fluid, breast milk, as well as cell culture supernatants. Analysis and characterization of cellular and non-cellular components of the immune system in blood and serum specimens are described and discussed in corresponding chapters. This chapter will explain and illustrate immunological procedures used to characterize other biological fluids. CSF, joint, pleural, pericardial, peritoneal and bronchoalveolar lavage fluids generally require analysis for lymphocyte phenotypes and for involvement in leukemias and lymphomas. Saliva is usually evaluated for the levels of IgA. Clinical immunology tests on urine are usually limited to evaluation of proteinuria aiming to assess renal insufficiency or the presence of a monoclonal gammopathy.

Some procedures to remove body fluids pose serious risks to the patients. This requires obtaining an informed consent. Specimens should be collected in the correct containers, which is usually dictated by the type of anticoagulant needed. All body fluids should be handled as if contaminated with bloodborne pathogens. Researchers, clinical laboratory personnel, students who can reasonably expect to have skin, eye, mucous membrane, or parenteral contact with blood or other potentially infectious specimens must observe these precautions. Examples of potentially infectious or contaminated samples include blood, serum, plasma, CSF, vaginal, pericardial, pleural, amniotic fluids, semen and any non-fixed human tissues and organs. However, standard precautions generally do not apply to the following specimens unless they are visibly contaminated with blood: urine, sputum, sweat, feces, tears, saliva, nasal fluid, vomitus and breast milk.

SERUM HANDLING

Serum samples are widely used in clinical and research laboratories for evaluation of immune responses, state of the immune system, immunomonitoring of clinical trials, generation of antiserum preparations and analysis of

Measuring Immunity, edited by Michael T. Lotze and Angus W. Thomson
ISBN 0-12-455900-X, London

serum proteins and biologically active factors, such as hormones, regulatory peptides, nutritional components, etc. Serum specimens should be clotted prior to centrifugation. Clotting normally takes 30–40 min at room temperature (22°C) and a few hours at 4°C. Clotting can be accelerated to about 15 min by the addition of clotting activators, such as glass beads or silica particles. The time required for clot formation may vary if the patient is on anticoagulant therapy. All tubes after clotting should be centrifuged at 1000–1200 g for 10 min in a swinging-bucket rotor at 22°C and then stored at 2–8°C prior to analysis.

Although sera for most serological tests are safe at room temperature for a short time, perhaps 30–60 min, specimens for some tests must receive special handling. These include blood drawn for complement and cryoglobulins assays. For instance, determination of total hemolytic complement (CH50) requires stat transportation. Serum for complement assays must be frozen at −20°C within 2 h of venepuncture. This is an absolute requirement for the CH50 assay and is strongly recommended for the assay of the C3 and C4 components of complement by nephelometry. Furthermore, for C3 and C4 analyses, the specimen should be refrigerated if delivery will be delayed.

Analysis of cryoglobulins also requires special handling procedures. Cryoglobulins are protein complexes that can precipitate when blood or serum is cooled below 37°C. In cold (4°C), they become reversibly insoluble and either precipitate or gel. Thus, they are referred to as cryoprecipitate or cryogel. The precipitation of cryoglobulins may occur at higher temperatures *in vivo* in blood vessels with very serious consequences. Cryoglobulins are mostly immunoglobulins with small amounts of other plasma proteins. Identification of the immunoglobulin components of cryoglobulins requires isolation of the cryoprecipitate (cryogel), its solubilization and immunofixation with appropriate antisera. Therefore, blood samples for this test must be collected in a warm tube without anticoagulant using a pre-heated needle and syringe and kept at 37°C until clotted. The specimen must be centrifuged at 37°C to maintain solubility of any cryoglobulins before the serum is cooled to 4°C to allow precipitation to occur (up to 7 days). Isolation of precipitated cryoglobulins by centrifugation, as well as washing of the pellet, must be done at 4°C in a pre-cooled centrifuge and with cold PBS or saline. Isolated cryoglobulins should next be dissolved in a buffer at room temperature and used for quantitative analysis of immunoglobulins by nephelometry and qualitative characterization of immunoglobulin subclasses by immunoelectrophoresis and immunofixation.

IMMUNOLOGICAL ANALYSIS OF HUMAN BODY FLUIDS

Urine analysis

Collection and preservation of urine for analytical testing must follow a carefully prescribed procedure to ensure valid results (NCCLC Pub. GP16-T, 1992). Laboratory testing of urine generally falls under three categories – chemical, bacteriologic and microscopic examination. There are also three kinds of urine specimen collection: (i) random, (ii) timed and (iii) 24-h total volume. Random specimens may be obtained any time, but a first morning voided aliquot is optimal for many tests. Although urine specimens are easy to collect, the quality of the results very much depends on the quality of the specimen handling and preservation.

Urine analysis serves for evaluation of kidney function, body homeostasis and general metabolic/autoimmune/neoplastic disorders. Chemical examination of urine consists of pH measurements for acid–base balance, detection of blood as a sign of renal and urinary tract diseases, nitrites as a sign of asymptomatic urinary tract infection and proteins as a sign of (i) increased low-molecular-weight proteins in serum, (ii) glomerular or tubular diseases and (iii) proteins produced in the urinary tract. In addition, other chemical analyses refer to the detection of glucose as a sign of diabetes mellitus, liver, pancreatic and renal tubular diseases; ketones as a sign of type-1 diabetes; bilirubin and urobilinogen as a sign of increased heme degradation and hepatocellular disease. Assessment

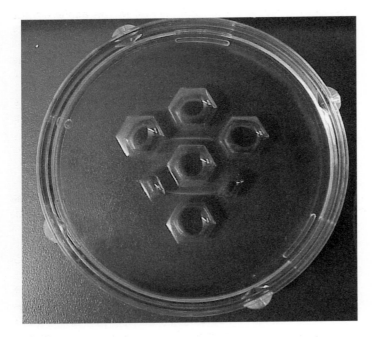

Figure 9.1 Detection of specific antibodies in serum specimens by double diffusion in the gel (Ouchterlony). Double diffusion is the method used to identify anti-Scl-70 antibodies in patient sera. The antigen is prepared by purification and concentration of a rabbit thymus extract. Antibodies to the DNA Topoisomerase Scl-70, are seen almost exclusively in progressive systemic sclerosis (PSS or scleroderma). Results are reported as either positive or negative for anti-Scl-70 antibody. Two precipitin lines demonstrate the presence of anti-Scl-70 antibodies in tested samples. NOVA Gel Scl-70 'T' is commonly used for this assay (INOVA Diagnostics, Inc, San Diego, CA).

of urine sediment, analyses of casts, cellularity and crystals, as well as bacteriologic analysis complete the microscopic examination of urine.

Immunologic analysis of urine specimens consists of identification of immune cells in urine such as PMN, lymphocytes, monocytes and eosinophils that are present in acute or chronic inflammatory tubulo-interstitial nephritis (Nanni-Costa et al., 1992; Yamamoto et al., 2003). Next, urine samples are used for detection of abnormal proteins in urine such as monoclonal immunoglobulin light chains (Bence Jones protein) by immunoelectrophoresis (Graziani et al., 2003) as a sign of multiple myeloma or other lymphoproliferative diseases. Detection of monoclonal κ and λ light chains in urine by nephelometry and total protein electrophoresis methods is the most common urinalysis test in clinical immunology laboratories. Immunoglobulin light chains are produced by plasma cells, slightly in excess of immunoglobulin heavy chains and therefore are present in the serum of healthy adults in free form at low concentrations. Both κ and λ forms of these polyclonal immunoglobulin light chains are mainly metabolized by the kidney and appear under normal conditions only in small amounts in the urine. In patients with a reduced or abolished kidney function, immunoglobulin light chain levels are increased. When overproduced in multiple myeloma and deposited in the kidney, immunoglobulin light chains can be, by themselves, a causative factor of renal diseases and the development of uremia (Cohen, 2003).

Additional immunological tests include examination of anti-DNA antibodies as a sign of lupus (Macanovic et al., 1999) and anti-HIV-1 antibodies to monitor HIV infection in different categories of patients (Gottfried et al 1999; Urnovitz et al., 1999). Finally, evaluation of mRNA specific for activated CD8+ alloreactive T cells in urine may serve as an early indicator for acute cellular rejection in renal transplantation (Dadhania et al., 2003; Ding et al., 2003).

CSF

Cerebrospinal fluid is formed from plasma by ultrafiltration at choroid plexuses. It circulates in the ventricular system and subarachnoid spaces and is resorbed into the blood through villi (Adam et al., 2001). Total CSF volumes are 90 to 150 ml in adults and 10 to 60 ml in neonates. Cerebrospinal fluid may be obtained by an aseptic lumbar puncture. Indications for lumbar puncture include meningeal infection, subarachnoid hemorrhage, CNS malignancy and demyelinating diseases. Up to 20 ml of spinal fluid may normally be removed. Ordinarily, the specimen is divided into three sterile tubes: tube 1 for chemistry and immunology studies, tube 2 for microbiologic examination and tube 3 for cell count and differential.

Cell counts are performed on undiluted CSF in a manual counting chamber. The normal leukocyte cell count in adults is 0 to 5 cells/μl and is higher in neonates, ranging from 0 to 30 cells/μl. The CSF normally contains a small number

of lymphocytes and monocytes in a ratio of approximately 70:30. Increased lymphocytes are seen in various infections (viral meningitis, tuberculous meningitis, fungal meningitis, syphilitic meningoencephalitis, or leptospiral meningitis), in neurodegenerative disorders (multiple sclerosis, subacute sclerosing panencephalitis, Gullain-Barre syndrome, or acute disseminated encephalomyelitis) and in several rheumatic diseases. Plasma cells are not normally present in the CSF but appear in a variety of inflammatory conditions. Increased neutrophil numbers in CSF may occur in bacterial meningitis, viral meningoencephalitis, tuberculous meningitis, mycotic meningitis, or cerebral abscess. Eosinophils may rarely be seen in normal CSF, while increased eosinophil counts are associated with a variety of infectious and non-infectious conditions with parasitic invasions and fungal infections being the most frequent causes.

Immunologic examination of CSF consists of various techniques such as co-agglutination, radioimmunoassay, immune-electrophoresis, enzyme-linked immunosorbent assay (ELISA) and PCR to detect the presence of various antigens, antibodies, abnormal immune proteins and cytokines. Among the diagnostic procedures aimed at defining the etiology and the pathogenesis of inflammatory myelopathies, the examination of the CSF plays a central role. Indeed, for several autoimmune and inflammatory syndromes and diseases involving the spinal cord, in addition to immunological screening of the blood, a detailed analysis of the CSF may allow the achievement of the diagnosis (Perini et al., 2001). Routine CSF analysis might include a detailed cytology, the evaluation of the blood–brain barrier dysfunction, quantitative and qualitative analysis of the intrathecal IgG synthesis and immunological and virological tests based on immunoenzymatic (ELISA, RIA) and molecular biology techniques (PCR). A more advanced step includes fluorescence-activated cell sorting (FACS) analysis of CSF lymphocytes and, when possible, virological and immunological tests on cell culture supernatants.

Most common clinical immunologic tests include evaluation of CSF gamma-globulins by immunochemical methods and CSF protein electrophoresis. Over 80 per cent of CSF protein content is derived from the plasma, in concentrations of less than 1 per cent of the blood level. Mean CSF protein values in adults range from 23 to 38 mg/dl with a generally accepted range of 15 to 45 mg/dl (Roos, 2003). It is clinically important to detect an increase in gamma-globulin synthesis in the cerebrospinal system (intrathecal synthesis) since it is a marker of demyelinating disorders, specifically, multiple sclerosis. Increased intrathecal IgG synthesis is reflected by an elevated CSF/serum IgG ratio. Upregulation of IgG synthesis has a sensitivity of 90 per cent in patients with definite multiple sclerosis, although it is lower in patients with possible multiple sclerosis. In association with the presence of CD8+ T lymphocytes (Skulina et al., 2004), increased levels of TNFα and soluble VCAM-1 (Baraczka et al., 2003) and specific IgG antibodies against myelin-basic protein

(O'Connor et al., 2003) are helpful in a positive diagnosis of multiple sclerosis. Recently, the increased synthesis of IgM and free kappa light chains have been suggested as more specific markers of multiple sclerosis (Rudick et al., 1989; Lolli et al., 1991).

Protein electrophoresis of concentrated CSF is widely used in clinical laboratories for screening of oligoclonal bands, defined as two or more discrete bands in the gamma region that are absent in the concurrently run patient's serum. To enhance the sensitivity of oligoclonal band detection, isoelectrofocusing and immunofixation electrophoresis can be used since these methods provide better resolution and can identify specific light and heavy chains. CSF oligoclonal bands have been demonstrated in 83–94 per cent of patients with definite multiple sclerosis, 40–60 per cent of those with probable disease and 20–30 per cent of possible multiple sclerosis cases. They are also seen in nearly all patients with subacute sclerosing panencephalitis and in 25–50 per cent of patients with various viral, bacterial and fungal CNS infections, as well as in malignant diseases involving the CNS (Brinar, 2002; Brinar and Pozer, 2002; Wolinsky 2003). In summary, elevated IgG indices and the presence of oligoclonal bands are complementary findings useful in the diagnosis of multiple sclerosis, but the positive predictive value of these tests largely depends on the degree of clinical suspicion.

Joint fluid analysis

Joint fluid analysis or synovianalysis is an important asset to the evaluation of different joint diseases, or arthritides. Synovial fluid is a viscous liquid that lubricates the joint spaces and is formed by ultrafiltration of plasma across the synovial membrane and from secretions by synoviocytes. The proteins and immunoglobulin concentrations of the synovial fluid are approximately one fourth those of plasma, while electrolytes, glucose and uric acid concentrations are similar to those of the blood (Kjeldsberg and Knight, 1993).

Specimen collection is performed by aseptic percutaneous aspiration called arthrocentesis and there are no absolute contraindications to joint aspiration. Synovianalysis includes macroscopic (volume, viscosity, color, clarity), microscopic (total white blood cell count, per cent of PMN/mononuclear cells, evaluation for crystals and other materials), chemical (glucose, protein, uric acid), immunologic (immune cells, autoantibodies, cytokines) and bacteriologic (gram stains and cultures) examination. Analysis of synovial fluid plays a major role in the diagnosis of four categories of joint diseases: non-inflammatory (osteoarthritis, Paget's disease, ochronosis, etc), inflammatory (rheumatoid arthritis, lupus erythematosus, sarcoidosis, scleroderma, etc), septic/infectious (viral, bacterial, fungal, etc), and hemorrhagic (traumatic arthritis, hemangioma, thrombocytopenia, etc).

For the chronic inflammatory rheumatic diseases, immunological analyses of synovial liquid are of great relevance in helping to define and classify such clinical entities. For example, for rheumatoid arthritis (RA), a clinical autoimmune syndrome characterized by relapsing-remitting inflammation within the synovial membrane and erosive destruction of adjacent cartilage and bones, the following immune tests of joint fluid may be performed:

1. flow cytometry to detect the frequency and phenotype of immune cells present in synovial fluid (i.e. PMN, monocyte/macrophages, NK cells and CD4/CD8 T cells) (Yavin et al., 2000; Gregory et al., 2003; Pridgeon et al., 2003)
2. serological tests to detect the presence of rheumatoid factor of both IgG and IgM isotypes and other autoantibodies (Hueber et al., 2003)
3. detection of acute-phase proteins (serum amyloid A-SAA) (Yavin et al., 2000)
4. ELISAs to detect proinflammatory cytokine levels in joint fluid (IL-15, IL-18, TNFα, IL-6, IL-8) (McInnes and Liew, 1998; Kaneko et al., 2000; Canetti et al., 2003).

However although analysis of cytokines has considerable research importance, there is no current clinical usefulness in measuring them in joint fluid (Kjeldsberg and Knight, 1993).

Antinuclear antibodies (ANA) are detected in serum in nearly all patients with systemic lupus erythematosus (SLE). Approximately 70 per cent of patients with SLE and about 20 per cent of patients with RA will also have ANA in the synovial fluid (Cracchiolo and Barnett, 1972). Total synovial fluid complement values are normal or slightly elevated in traumatic or degenerative joint disease. However, in addition to RA and SLE, decreased levels of synovial fluid complement are usually seen in septic arthritis (Cracchiolo, 1971).

Pleural, pericardial and peritoneal fluid analysis

Serosal fluids include pleural fluid, pericardial fluid and peritoneal fluid. These fluids are found between potential spaces of pleura, in the pericardial sac, or from the peritoneum. The pleural cavity normally contains a small amount of fluid that facilitates movement of the visceral and parietal pleurae against each other. This fluid is a plasma filtrate derived from capillaries of the parietal pleura. It is produced continuously at a rate that depends on capillary hydrostatic pressure, plasma oncotic pressure and capillary permeability and is reabsorbed through the lymphatics and venules of the visceral pleura (Kjeldsberg and Knight, 1993). The volume of pleural fluid in normal conditions is 4–12 ml on each side (right pleural and left pleural space) (Noppen et al., 2000). Pericardial fluid is present in the pericardial sac in the amount of 10–50 ml and is produced by a transudative process similar to pleural fluid. Peritoneal fluid (up to 50 ml) is normally present in the mesothelium-lined space that represents the peritoneal cavity. Like pleural and pericardial fluid, peritoneal fluid is produced as an ultrafiltrate of plasma that is

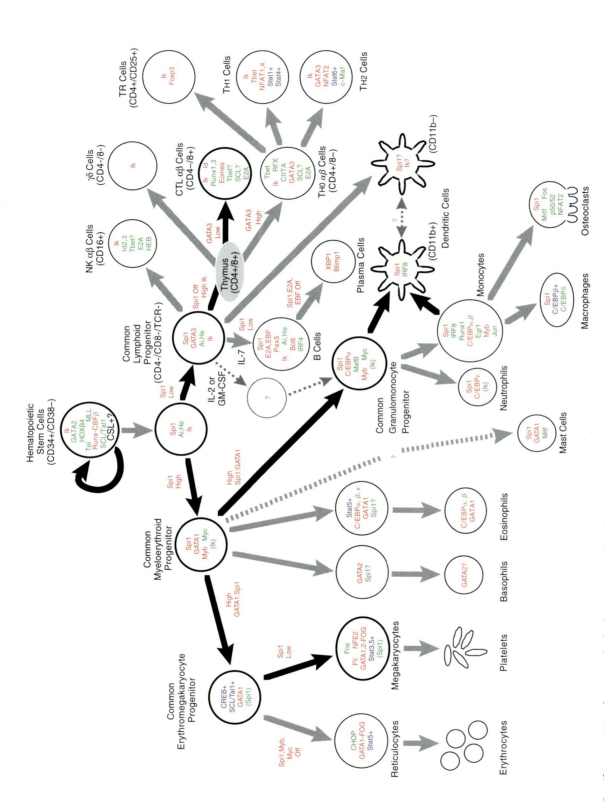

Figure 7.3 Specific transcription factors involved in hematopoiesis. The scheme shows various lineages of cells connected by arrows. Cell types are represented as circles and other closed figures containing designations for critical transcription factors. Factor designations blue followed by a plus sign (+) are pre-existing factors that are activated by an exogenous signal; red represents factors that are key for specific developmental stages; black represents other lineage-specific and critical factors. Black arrows represent stages that are dependent upon engagement of Notch receptors on the cell surface that may activate the CSL factor that binds the intracellular Notch peptide, ICN. Gray arrows are Notch-independent stages. Dotted lines indicate possible, unsubstantiated alternative pathways. Red labels over the arrows note important details regarding expression of selected key factors.

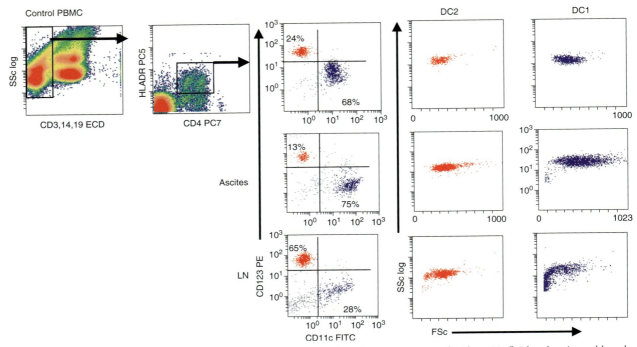

Figure 20.1 Detection of DC1 and DC2. DCs in the peripheral blood of a healthy subject are contrasted with ascitic fluid and peritoneal lymph node (LN) from a patient with newly diagnosed untreated ovarian cancer. Cell suspensions were stained with antibodies CD11c-FITC, CD123-PE, a cocktail of CD3, CD14 and CD19-PE, HLADR-PC5 and CD4-PC7. Cells were acquired on a Beckman-Coulter FC500 cytometer. In this analysis, lymphoid DCs have been color-evented red and myeloid DCs have been colored blue. The differences in scatter properties of these two populations are shown in the last column. In ovarian cancer, myeloid DCs are larger in ascites, compared to control peripheral blood. In LN, where lymphoid DCs predominate, the myeloid DC evidence a population with low forward and side scatter, consistent with apoptosis.

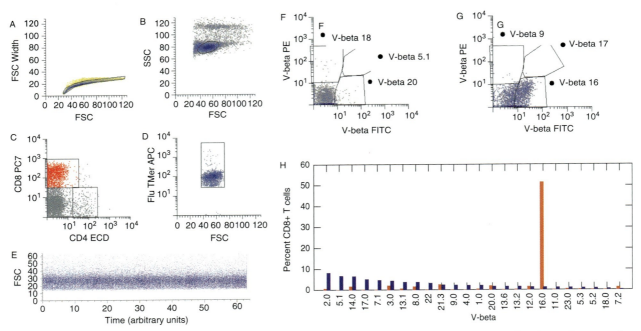

Figure 20.4 Rare event detection of TCR V-beta usage among Flu tetramer+ CD8+ T cells. In panel A, a gate is created on forward scatter pulse height and forward scatter pulse width, excluding doublets (high pulse width for a given pulse height). In panel B the analysis is limited to events displaying lymphoid forward and side light scatter properties. Panel C (*dump gate*) is used both to positively identify CD8+ T cells and to eliminate CD4+ T cells (and anything else appearing positive in the ECD channel). Panel D is the *live gate* on tetramer+ events. Only tetramer+ events falling within this gate were saved in the listmode file, greatly reducing the size of the datafile and increasing the speed of analysis. Forward scatter is shown versus Time (panel E), a calculated parameter that is used to identify and eliminate any spurious event bursts (none were detected here). Finally, panels F and G (from separately stained tubes) show the results of the application of this compound gating strategy. Panel F shows the usage of V-beta 18 (0.04 per cent), 5.1 (0.0 per cent) and 20 (1.9 per cent) among Flu tetramer+/CD8+/CD4− cells. Panel G shows that the majority of Flu tetramer+ T cells (51.4 per cent) are V-beta 16+. Panel H shows the final result, the V-beta repertoire of flu tetramer− and flu tetramer+ CD8+ T cells. Data from tetramer+ events were collected for 24 V-beta specificities. Data were acquired separately for determination of V-beta usage in tetramer negative T cells (without the use of the live gate D). The results are plotted in the order of frequency of V-beta usage in tetramer negative CD8+ T cells (blue bars). Common specificities such as V-beta 2, 5.1, 14 and 17 were very underrepresented in flu tetramer+ T cells (red bars), whereas V-beta 16, which comprised only 1.2 per cent of total CD8+ T cells, accounted for 51.4 per cent of flu tetramer+ T cells. These results are consistent with the clonality (or pauci-clonality) of the majority of influenza matrix peptide specific T cells in this sample.

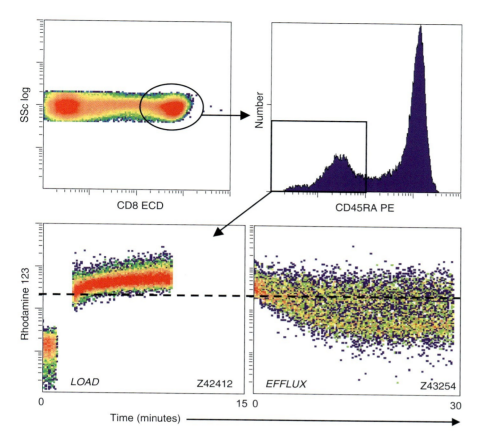

Figure 20.5 R123 load and efflux in CD45RA negative central memory/effector memory peripheral CD8+ T cells. Peripheral blood mononuclear cells were obtained from a normal healthy volunteer. Cells were stained with antibodies CD45RA-PE, CD8-ECD and CD4 plus CD3 PE-Cy5. Cells were acquired on a Beckman-Coulter XL cytometer. Cells were gated on CD3+ events (not shown). Low side scatter CD8+, CD45RA- T cells were identified using a compound gate (top panels). The lower panels show R123 fluorescence as a function of acquisition time. During the first 2 min of acquisition and prior to addition of R123, baseline autofluorescence was determined. R123 LOAD: Acquisition of R123 unstained sample was paused, R123 was added (0.13 μM final concentration) and acquisition was immediately resumed; cells were acquired continuously for an additional 15 min. R123 EFFLUX: Loaded cells were chilled and washed 2 times with 10 ml of ice cold PBS, resuspended in culture medium at 37°C and returned to the cytometer. Cells were maintained at 37°C and data acquired continuously for 30 min. R123 loading and efflux were also determined for CD3+ CD8+ CD45RA+ cells and for the analogous CD4+ T-cell subsets (not shown).

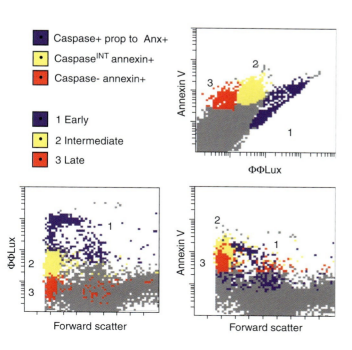

Figure 20.6 Early events in T cell apoptosis. Ficoll/Hypaque separated mononuclear cells recovered from the ascitic fluid of an untreated ovarian cancer patient were stained with antibodies CD45RA-ECD, CD27-PC5 and CD4-PC5. Cells were washed and incubated with Phi Phi Lux-G1D2, washed again, resuspended in high calcium buffer and incubated with Annexin V-PE. Cells were acquired immediately on a Beckman-Coulter FC500 cytometer. CD4+ effector memory cells were identified by gating on CD4+, low and intermediate side scatter, CD27− and CD45RA− events (not shown). Color eventing was used to identify three populations of cells based on caspase 3 activity and annexin V binding. In the first population (blue), caspase activity and annexin V binding increase coordinately, forming a diagonal in the bivariate scatter plot. In the second population (yellow) annexin V binding remains high, but caspase activity, while still present, is reduced. In the third population (red), annexin binding is positive and somewhat decreased, but at this point caspase activity is lost. The temporal sequence of apoptotic events was confirmed by backgating on Phi Phi Lux versus forward light scatter, using color eventing to identify the three populations. Here, it can be seen that the first population (blue) forms an arc as it gains and then loses caspase activity as it collapses in forward scatter. The second population already has low light scatter and further loses caspase activity. The red population, the last in the sequence, consists of small annexin V low, caspase 3 negative cells. Note that a few red colored events have normal forward scatter characteristic. These represent annexin V- cells that were misclassified when the red color event gate was created in the top right panel.

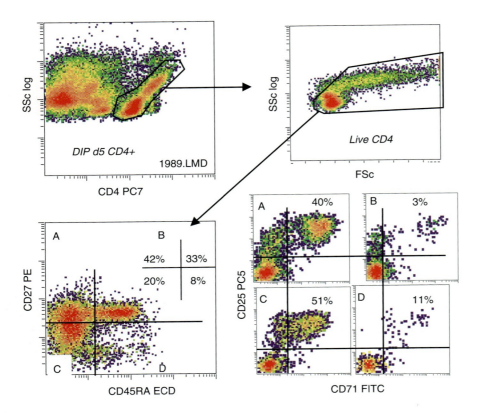

Figure 20.7 Antigen-driven upregulation of CD25 and CD71 in CD4+ T cell subsets. Peripheral blood mononuclear cells were obtained from a healthy subject and cultured for 5 days in the presence of diphtheria toxoid (2 μg/ml). Cultured cells were harvested and stained with antibodies CD71-FITC, CD27-PE, CD45RA-ECD, CD25-PC5 and CD4-PC7. Cells were acquired on a Beckman-Coulter FC500 cytometer. In the top left panel, responding cells can be visualized as CD4+ T cells with high log side scatter. CD4+ cells were filtered through a scatter gate (top right panel) used to eliminate late apoptotic cells, if present and subsetted on the basis of CD45RA and CD27 expression (A, B, C, D). The outcome parameters, CD71 and CD25 were determined in each subset.

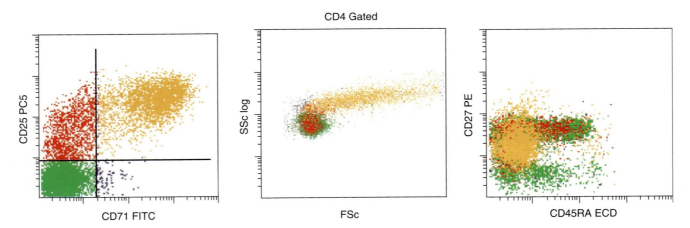

Figure 20.8 The use of color-eventing simultaneously to view outcome and classification parameters. The data are the same as those displayed in Figure 20.7. Here the outcome parameters CD71 and CD25 have been divided into quadrants and each quadrant used as a color-evented gate. For example, CD71/CD25 double positive cells were colored gold. These events are then displayed in bivariate scatter plots of forward by log side scatter and CD45RA by CD71 expression. Proliferating cells (gold) can clearly be visualized as CD45RA negative, CD27 intermediate cells with high forward scatter and high log side scatter.

dependent on vascular permeability and hydrostatic and oncotic forces.

Thoracentesis is a surgical procedure that is performed to drain accumulated fluids (effusions) from the thoracic cavity and is helpful in the diagnosis of inflammation and neoplastic diseases in the lung or pleura. Likewise, pericardiocentesis and peritoneocentesis refer to the collection of fluid from the pericardium and the peritoneal cavities, respectively (Henry, 1996).

Serosal fluids are clinically evaluated if they are accumulated in abnormally high amounts. Such accumulation is called an effusion and results from an imbalance of fluid production and reabsorption. Depending on the mechanism of accumulation, effusions are classified as transudates and exudates. The former result from increased hydrostatic pressure or decreased plasma oncotic pressure, while the latter result from increased vascular permeability or inadequate resorption. Analysis of serosal fluid is usually performed in order to distinguish transudates from exudates, to identify an infectious agent in exudates and to diagnose an involvement of serous membranes by a malignant process (Kjeldsberg and Knight, 1993).

Immunologic studies are performed infrequently and are mainly directed towards diagnosis of serosal involvement by rheumatoid arthritis (RA) and systemic lupus erythematosus (SLE). Pleural effusions can be seen in approximately 5 per cent of patients with RA and 50 per cent of those with SLE (Kjeldsberg and Knight, 1993). Pericardial effusions can also be seen and have a negative impact on prognosis (Hara et al., 1990). Rheumatoid factor (RF) is commonly present in pleural effusions associated with seropositive RA. It is accepted that a pleural fluid titer of 1:320 or greater in a patient with known RA is reasonable evidence of rheumatic pleuritis (Halla et al., 1980). However, elevated RF titers in pleural fluid should be interpreted with caution, since they have been identified in patients with bacterial pneumonia, tuberculosis and malignant effusions (Levine et al., 1968).

Lupus effusion is a common complication in patients with SLE. ANA titers are useful in the diagnosis of lupus pleuritis and pericarditis because they have a sensitivity of about 85 per cent using a cut-off titer of 1:160 (Good et al., 1983). However, this test is not specific because elevated ANA titers also occur in other clinical conditions (Leventhal et al., 1990; Wang et al., 2000).

Decreased complement levels (CH50 below 10 U/ml or C4 levels below 10×10^{-5} U/g protein) are seen in most, but not all, patients with rheumatoid or lupus pleuritis (Hunder et al., 1972; Musher et al., 1972; Halla et al., 1980). However, these tests are not highly specific.

Amniotic fluid analysis

Amniotic fluid is a product of fetal metabolism and continuous exchanges of chemicals and water take place between the fluid, the fetus and the maternal circulation.

The composition of amniotic fluid is similar to maternal plasma. In addition, small numbers of fetal cells can be also detected. After the first trimester, the amniotic fluid contains fetal urine and its constant volume is maintained by fetal swallowing. Amniocentesis is the transabdominal needle aspiration of 10–20 ml of amniotic fluid for laboratory analysis. This test is performed to detect fetal abnormalities (chromosomal and neural tube defects), diagnose metabolic disorders, determine fetal age and maturity, identify fetal gender and access fetal health. Analysis of amniotic fluid may be also helpful for the early diagnosis of hemolytic disease of the newborn (HDN). In HDN, the fetal erythrocytes serve as antigens and, if they access the maternal circulation, may stimulate production of antibodies. Maternal IgG passes through the placenta, and interacts with the fetal red blood cells causing hemolysis and hemolytic disease.

The cytologic analysis of amniotic fluid is of limited clinical value. Biochemical analyses of amniotic fluid to test fetal distress consist of measurement of bilirubin, as a sign of hemolytic disease of the newborn, as well as detection of alpha-fetoprotein as an indicator of fetal neural tube defects. In instances where preterm delivery is indicated, fetal maturity testing of the amniotic fluid is performed. Specifically, maturity of fetal lungs is assessed by biochemical and immunologic measurements of surfactant and its components such as lecithin/sphingomyelin (Poggi et al., 2003), phosphatidyl glycerol (Eisenbrey et al., 1989) and phospholipids (Moore, 2002). Detection of IL-1α and β, IL-6, TNFα and IL-8 in amniotic fluid by ELISA may implicate the inflammatory cytokines in immune-pathogenesis of preterm labor induction (Hillier et al., 1993; Witczak et al., 2003). In fact, alteration of cytokine levels in pregnancy, as well as changes in Th1/Th2 cytokine balance has been documented (Shurin et al., 1999). Elevated second-trimester amniotic fluid IL-6 levels have been associated with preterm delivery, confirming that this indicator of early intrauterine inflammation predicts birth before 34 weeks' gestation (Wenstrom et al., 1998; El-Bastawissi et al., 2000). Furthermore, amniotic fluid C-reactive protein concentrations of >110 ng/ml have a sensitivity of 80.8 per cent and a specificity of 69.5 per cent in the prediction of spontaneous preterm delivery at <34 weeks (Ghezzi et al., 2002). However, since no relationships between amniotic fluid and maternal serum levels of proinflammatory cytokines were observed (Witczak et al., 2003), it is likely that there is a barrier which limits cytokine transfer by the placenta and regulates the separation of these two compartments. These results also confirm the fact that amniotic fluid not only provides a physical barrier to protect the fetus from trauma, but serves as an immunologic barrier against intrauterine infections. Immunoglobulins IgG, IgA, IgM, and IgD, as well as complement factors (C3, C4, C5, factors B, H and I), lactoferrin, lysozyme, β-lysin and IFNα are present in amniotic fluid and are responsible for antibacterial and antiviral activity found therein (Kjeldsberg and

Knight, 1993; Quan et al., 1999). Measurements of antibody levels in amniotic fluid, such as for fetal syphilis, may suggest the severity of fetal disease associated with the risk of treatment failure (Hollier et al., 2001). Importantly, occult infection accounts for up to 12 per cent of pregnancy losses following genetic amniocentesis. Recent studies characterizing the association between amniotic fluid ferritin (acute-phase reactant) levels and post-amniocentesis pregnancy loss documented that ferritin is a suitable marker of inflammation in asymptomatic women destined to have an early pregnancy loss (Ramsey et al., 2002).

Nasal and ear fluid

In the clinical immunology laboratory, nasal and ear fluids are tested for detection of the beta-2 transferrin band by immunofixation electrophoresis (IFE) or Western blot analysis as a diagnostic tool for the presence of CSF or perilymph. This test is helpful in the differential diagnosis for CSF otorrhea or CSF rhinorrhea. The beta-2 transferrin band has not been detected in multiple fluids including serum, ear fluid, nasal secretions, saliva, tears or endolymph, indicating the specificity of the slower beta-2 transferrin isoform for CSF.

Transferrin is a ubiquitous monomeric glycoprotein consisting of 679 amino acids, two iron-binding sites and two N-linked complex glycan chains. Two isoforms of transferrin are present in the cerebrospinal fluid. One band is seen normally in serum and migrates in what has been termed the beta-1 protein fraction. The slower isoform in CSF results from digestion of sialic acid side chains by cerebral neuraminidase and migrates in the beta-2 fraction. Thus, beta-2-transferrin is a protein produced by neuraminidase activity in the brain, and is uniquely found in the CSF and perilymph. Its absence in other body secretions makes its detection invaluable in diagnosing a CSF leak or perilymphatic fistula.

The leakage of CSF into nasal or oral cavities and its subsequent drainage from these cavities may be caused by different reasons. CSF rhinorrhea results from a breakdown of the dura and supporting structures of the skull base. Trauma is responsible for 81–90 per cent of the cases of CSF rhinorrhea and it occurs in approximately 2 per cent of all head injuries. Leakage of CSF may also occur after fracture of the skull base or after surgery on the skull base, nose or paranasal sinuses. Further causes of cerebrospinal fluid leakage are infection, hydrocephalus, congenital malformations and tumors.

Usually 0.5 ml of body fluid (nasal, otic, etc.) is required for the beta-2 transferrin analysis and direct collections may be done with a pipette, syringe, test tube or microcollection device. Although results may be obtainable on smaller specimens (as little as 0.05 ml, depending on the protein concentrations and percentage of spinal fluid in the sample), reliable results are best obtained with an adequate sample volume. If direct collection is not feasible, samples may be collected using cotton swabs, but the fluid must be expressed from the swabs and placed into a microcollection container. All specimens should be kept frozen in a plastic vial on dry ice, unless the analysis will be done immediately.

Seminal fluid analysis

Infertility is a significant medical problem that affects many couples. Evaluation is the starting point for treatment of infertility as it may suggest specific causes and appropriate treatment modalities (Makar and Toth, 2002). Although the history and physical examination provide important information, specific diagnostic tests are required to evaluate infertility. Because the causes of infertility can be multifactorial, a systematic approach typically is used and involves testing for male factor, ovulatory factor, uterotubal factor and peritoneal factor. Many of these diagnostic tests are laboratory based, including semen analysis, serum progesterone level, serum basal follicle-stimulating hormone level and clomiphene citrate challenge (McLachlan et al., 2003).

Sperm-reactive antibodies (SpAb) are found attached to sperm, or present in serum or seminal fluid, in approximately 6 per cent of men presenting with infertility (McLachlan, 2002). A growing body of data supports their pathophysiological role in some cases by the interference with sperm motility and/or sperm–egg interaction. The occurrence of SpAbs may follow disruption of either the cellular barrier separating sperm antigens from the immune system (e.g. testis trauma or obstruction to sperm outflow), or dysregulation of normal immunosuppressive activities within the male reproductive tract. The epididymis is likely to be the key site of antibody generation, especially in the setting of obstruction. Antisperm antibodies may be measured by many methods, including agglutination, immobilization, immunofluorescence assays, etc. (Carson et al., 1988). Detection methods are all based on the assessment of immunoglobulin isotypes rather than specific antibody–antigen interactions, which limits their usefulness (McLachlan, 2002).

Interestingly, allergy or increased adult female sensitivity to human semen has been described, including episodes of severe anaphylaxis (Kooistra et al., 1980; Wasson et al., 1987; Yocum et al., 1996). Increased levels of specific IgE antibodies in serum can be detected in these patients and PSA was considered as a potential major allergen.

Screening for polymorphonuclear neutrophils (PMN) seminal elastase-inhibitor complex (Ela/alpha1-PI) is another example of immunological analysis of seminal fluid, which is easy to perform, reproducible and a reliable quantitative test for diagnosis and prognosis of silent genital tract inflammation of couples (Zorn et al., 2003). Elastase is a protease released by PMN during the inflammatory process. Since 1987, seminal elastase-inhibitor complex has been proposed as a marker of male silent genital tract inflammation. Measured by immunoassay in seminal plasma, Ela/alpha1-PI at a cut-off level of ≥230 μ/l, is useful in the detection of genital tract inflammation. The prevalence of increased seminal Ela/alpha1-PI in infertile men is significantly higher than that observed in fertile men (Zorn et al., 2003). The Ela/alpha1-PI level is positively correlated with other seminal fluid markers of male genital tract inflammation, including reduced semen volume, citric acid and fructose and increased albumin, complement component C3, ceruloplasmin, immunoglobulins IgG and IgA and IL-6 and IL-8. A higher seminal Ela/alpha1-PI is associated with a lower percentage of sperm with single-stranded DNA and better fertilization rate in in vitro fertilization. Besides infertility, the determination of Ela/alpha1-PI is useful to confirm the presence of prostate and other male accessory gland bacterial inflammation (Zorn et al., 2003).

HUMAN BODY FLUIDS PRECAUTIONS AND REGULATIONS

Policy

Each Medical Center/University/Hospital should establish, adopt and enforce a comprehensive set of standards, guidelines and procedures that will minimize the risk to students, faculty and staff of occupational exposure to human body fluids and other materials that may contain agents of human infection. In areas and activities similar to non-campus settings (e.g. clinical and research laboratories, health care facilities, core laboratories, etc.), the policy shall apply regulations, standards and practices that have been developed by relevant governmental or professional agencies (e.g. US Public Health Service, Centers for Disease Control, Occupational Safety and Health Administration, State Department of Public Health, National Collegiate Athletic Association, etc.) insofar as they are not in conflict with laws governing the particular Medical Center/University or the ethical standards of the academic community. In other areas or activities in which risks are identified or suspected and for which legal or professional standards have not been developed and/or published, the particular clinical or research laboratory shall adopt standards, guidelines and practices that are appropriate for the level of risk identified. Included are educational activities to explain risks and to allay unwarranted fears arising from misconceptions of risk.

Implementation

Inherent in this or similar policies is the responsibility of each clinical or research facility to identify risks, to differentiate them according to severity and to maintain adherence to reasonable or established standards, guidelines and practices. Administrative oversight for the risk identification and reduction program is usually the responsibility of

Environmental Health and Safety, in collaboration with all segments of each Medical Center/University/Hospital community. Actual implementation of the policy and adherence to the policy is the responsibility of the department or unit involved. The primary goal of the program is to provide a systematic approach aimed at the primary recognition, evaluation and control of exposures to human blood, body fluids and other potentially infectious materials.

It is the responsibility of the principal investigator, researcher or administrative unit head to be aware of appropriate federal, state or university regulations involving the safe handling of human body fluids, to implement policies and procedures that adequately protect the environment and those working in the environment and to request assistance whenever potential or actual violations of prudent practices occur. Inadequate attention to human body fluid precautions may lead to appropriate sanctions or disciplinary actions within approved health and safety practices of the Medical Center/University/Hospital.

Medical Centers/Universities/Hospitals are responsible for providing all necessary immunizations and the medical treatment of employees and students following occupational contacts with human blood and other potentially infectious materials.

Specific terminology

Infectious body fluids shall include blood, semen, vaginal secretions, cerebrospinal fluid, synovial fluid, pleural fluid, pericardial fluid, peritoneal fluid, amniotic fluid, saliva in dental procedures, any body fluid that is visibly contaminated with blood and all body fluids in situations where it is difficult or impossible to differentiate between body fluids.

Other potentially infectious materials shall include infectious body fluids, any unfixed human tissue or organ, cell or tissue cultures containing human immunodeficiency virus (HIV), hepatitis C virus (HCV), or hepatitis B virus (HBV), organ cultures, culture medium, or blood, organs, or other tissues from experimental animals infected with HIV, HCV, HBV, or other viruses like adenoviruses, vaccinia viruses, HSV and others.

Occupational exposure means reasonably anticipated skin, eye, mucous membrane or parenteral contact with blood or other potentially infectious materials during the performance of an employee's duties or assignments of a student in a class.

HIV infection shall include all stages in the progression of infection, including HIV seropositivity and AIDS.

Levels of exposure. The Medical Center/University/Hospital Human Body Fluids Precaution policy must apply to occupational exposure to human blood or other materials which may be potentially infected with HIV, HBV, HCV or any other bloodborne pathogen or potentially infectious material. Each activity in which students, faculty or staff may participate must be classified as Category I (exposure) or Category II (non-exposure). This is consistent with occupational exposure as established by the US Department of Labor, Occupational Safety and Health Administration standards (OSHA, 1991).

Category I (Exposure): Procedures and activities that involve (known or predictable) contact with human blood, body fluids, or tissues, including spills or splashes. Risks are identifiable, since they are inherent in regular job-related tasks – for instance, clinical and research laboratories, dental offices and other health care settings. Appropriate protective measures should be identified, adopted and required for every person whose work or activity is classified as Category I. Administration is responsible for providing appropriate protective supplies and equipment (e.g. gloves for routine use by anyone drawing human blood samples) and offering immunization to protect against HBV infection and appropriate medical treatment following contact with human blood and other potentially infectious materials for all students and employees whose work involves this level of risk.

Category II (Non-exposure). Procedures and activities that do not involve regular or occasional contact with human blood, body fluids or tissue and in which there is an extremely low risk of transmission of HBV, HCV or HIV. For instance, sharing instruments, hand shaking, use of public or shared toilets or phones. However, this does not suggest or imply that other infectious diseases, i.e. upper respiratory infections, are not transmitted via direct or indirect contact. These diseases are either self-limited or treatable by available therapeutic agents. Furthermore, appropriate educational programs should be introduced to explain lack of risk to persons active in these settings, but suitable medical treatment following contacts with human blood and other potentially infectious materials must be provided if an accidental exposure occurs.

Bloodborne pathogens

Human blood, body fluids and other body tissues are widely recognized as vehicles for the transmission of human disease. Although many of these diseases are readily identified and can be prevented and/or treated successfully, e.g. syphilis and tuberculosis, others are not. At least three common infectious agents transmitted through human blood products and body fluids continue to present a serious health problem, including hepatitis B virus (HBV), hepatitis C virus (HCV) and human immunodeficiency virus (HIV). Because of difficulties in identifying, preventing and treating the diseases they cause, special precautions for minimizing the risk of infection are warranted.

HBV, the more common of the three infectious agents, causes a serious form of hepatitis which can lead to a permanent loss of liver function or even death. When suspected, it can be detected readily in blood or body fluids. Persons exposed can be protected temporarily by the use of hepatitis B immune globulin. An available vaccine provides long-term protection for those whose work or travel entails a high risk of exposure. Its cost is high but readily justifiable in view of the serious consequences of clinical disease.

HCV, once called non-A non-B hepatitis, also causes a serious form of hepatitis which can lead to a permanent loss of liver function and death. There is no vaccine to protect against this type of hepatitis but this disease can be partially treated in some cases with interferon.

HIV may cause acquired immunodeficiency syndrome (AIDS). In addition, once introduced, it may exist in humans for many years before causing symptoms; during this long latent period, it can be transmitted through blood products and other body fluids. Unprotected sexual contact is widely recognized as the most common mode of transmission but transmission is well recognized via transfusion, shared use of intravenous needles and pregnancy. Documented cases have been traced to work related inadvertent contact, such as needle sticks with infected blood. HIV appears to be very fragile, hence unable to survive for substantial periods outside the body of humans. Efforts to develop a useful vaccine have not been successful; researchers generally hold out scant hope for success in the near future. Although there is no cure for HIV disease, it is important to recognize the disease at an early stage so that treatment can be initiated. A particularly disturbing feature of the HIV infection is the long latent period between introduction of the virus into a person's body and clinical symptoms, which may average 5–7 years. There appears to be no bar to transmission during the latent period. This characteristic poses an especially serious threat to human health since there is neither an effective cure nor an agent for prevention, such as a vaccine. Disease control must rest solely, therefore, with behavioral strategies at both the individual and collective levels. Individual protective behaviors can result from programs to provide information and alter attitudes; the adoption of collective measures is an institutional and social responsibility.

Examples of guidelines for management of occupational exposure to human blood or body fluids

Transmission of hepatitis B virus (HBV), human immunodeficiency virus (AIDS virus, HIV) and other pathogenic microorganisms to health care and research workers through human blood, body fluids and other body tissues has been documented. Although all efforts should be made to prevent exposure, employees who are performing known or predictable procedures and activities with human body fluids (see campus policy Human Body Fluids Precautions), may be exposed to infectious agents. If an employee has a parenteral (e.g. needlestick, cut, bite) or mucous membrane (splash to the eye or mouth) exposure to human blood or other body fluids, or has a skin exposure involving large amounts of human blood or prolonged contact with blood especially when the exposed skin is chapped, abraded, or afflicted with dermatitis (eczema):

1 This incident should be reported to the supervisor.
2 The employee should report to Emergency Care immediately to have the exposure evaluated. If necessary, post-exposure treatment should be initiated within 2 h of exposure.
3 The supervisor should report accidents to the Department/Division of Environmental Health and Safety or similar.

REFERENCES

Adam, P., Taborsky, L., Sobek, O. et al. (2001). Cerebrospinal fluid. Adv Clin Chem 36, 1–62.

Baraczka, K., Pozsonyi, T., Szuts, I., Ormos, G. and Nekam, K. (2003). Increased levels of tumor necrosis alpha and soluble vascular endothelial adhesion molecule-1 in the cerebrospinal fluid of patients with connective tissue diseases and multiple sclerosis. Acta Microbiol Immunol Hung 50, 339–348.

Brinar, V.V. (2002). The differential diagnosis of multiple sclerosis. Clin Neurol Neurosurg 104, 211–220.

Brinar, V.V., Pozer, Ch. M. (2002). [The laboratory diagnosis of multiple sclerosis.] Zh Nevrol Psikhiatr Im S S Korsakova Suppl 7–14.

Canetti, C.A., Leung, B.P., Culshaw, S., McInnes, I.B., Cunha, F.Q. and Liew, F.Y. (2003). IL-18 enhances collagen-induced arthritis by recruiting neutrophils via TNF-alpha and leukotriene B4. J Immunol 171, 1009–1015.

Carson, S.A., Reiher, J., Scommegna, A. and Prins, G.S. (1988). Antibody binding patterns in infertile males and females as detected by immunobead test, gel-agglutination test, and sperm immobilization test. Fertil Steril 49, 487–492.

Cohen, G. (2003). Immunoglobulin light chains in uremia. Kidney Int Suppl: S15–18.

Cracchiolo, A. 3rd (1971). Joint fluid analysis. Am Fam Physician 4, 87–94.

Cracchiolo, A. 3rd and Barnett, E.V. (1972). The role of immunological tests in routine synovial fluid analysis. J Bone Joint Surg Am 54, 828–840.

Dadhania, D., Muthukumar, T., Ding, R. et al. (2003). Molecular signatures of urinary cells distinguish acute rejection of renal allografts from urinary tract infection. Transplantation 75, 1752–1754.

Ding, R., Li, B., Muthukumar, T. et al. (2003).103 mRNA levels in urinary cells predict acute rejection of renal allografts. Transplantation 75, 1307–1312.

Eisenbrey, A.B., Epstein, E., Zak, B., McEnroe, R.J., Artiss, J.D. and Kiechle, F.L. (1989). Phosphatidylglycerol in amniotic fluid. Comparison of an 'ultrasensitive' immunologic assay with TLC and enzymatic assay. Am J Clin Pathol 91, 293–297.

El-Bastawissi, A.Y., Williams, M.A., Riley, D.E., Hitti, J. and Krieger, J.N. (2000). Amniotic fluid interleukin-6 and preterm delivery: a review. Obstet Gynecol 95, 1056–1064.

Ghezzi, F., Franchi, M., Raio, L. et al. (2002). Elevated amniotic fluid C-reactive protein at the time of genetic amniocentesis is a marker for preterm delivery. Am J Obstet Gynecol 186, 268–273.

Good, J.T. Jr, King, T.E., Antony, V.B. and Sahn, S.A. (1983). Lupus pleuritis. Clinical features and pleural fluid characteristics with special reference to pleural fluid antinuclear antibodies. Chest 84, 714–718.

Gottfried,T.D., Sturge, J.C. and Urnovitz, H.B. (1999). A urine test system for HIV-1 antibodies. Am Clin Lab 18, 4.

Graziani, M., Merlini, G. and Petrini, C. (2003). Guidelines for the analysis of Bence Jones protein. Clin Chem Lab Med 41, 338–346.

Gregory, B., Kirchem, A., Phipps, S. et al. (2003). Differential regulation of human eosinophil IL-3, IL-5, and GM-CSF receptor alpha-chain expression by cytokines: IL-3, IL-5, and GM-CSF down-regulate IL-5 receptor alpha expression with loss of IL-5 responsiveness, but up-regulate IL-3 receptor alpha expression. J Immunol 170, 5359–5366.

Halla, J.T., Schrohenloher, R.E. and Volanakis, J.E. (1980). Immune complexes and other laboratory features of pleural effusions: a comparison of rheumatoid arthritis, systemic lupus erythematosus, and other diseases. Ann Intern Med 92, 748–752.

Hara, K.S., Ballard, D.J., Ilstrup, D.M., Connolly, D.C. and Vollertsen, R.S. (1990). Rheumatoid pericarditis: clinical features and survival. Medicine (Baltimore) 69, 81–91.

Henry, J.B. (1996). W.B. Saunders Company, Philadelphia, PA.

Hillier, S.L., Witkin, S.S., Krohn, M.A., Watts, D.H., Kiviat, N.B. and Eschenbach, D.A. (1993). The relationship of amniotic fluid cytokines and preterm delivery, amniotic fluid infection, histologic chorioamnionitis, and chorioamnion infection. Obstet Gynecol 81, 941–946.

Hollier, L.M., Harstad, T.W., Sanchez, P.J., Twickler, D.M. and Wendel, G.D. Jr (2001). Fetal syphilis: clinical and laboratory characteristics. Obstet Gynecol 97, 947–953.

Hueber, W., Utz, P.J. and Robinson, W.H. (2003). Autoantibodies in early arthritis: advances in diagnosis and prognostication. Clin Exp Rheumatol 21, S59–64.

Hunder, G.G., McDuffie, F.C. and Hepper, N.G. (1972). Pleural fluid complement in systemic lupus erythematosus and rheumatoid arthritis. Ann Intern Med 76, 357–363.

Kaneko, S., Satoh, T., Chiba, J., Ju, C., Inoue, K. and Kagawa, J. (2000). Interleukin-6 and interleukin-8 levels in serum and synovial fluid of patients with osteoarthritis. Cytokines Cell Mol Ther 6, 71–79.

Kjeldsberg, C. and Knight, J. (1993). Body fluids. ASCP Press, Chicago.

Kooistra, J.B., Yunginger, J.W., Santrach, P.J. and Clark, J.W. (1980). In vitro studies of human seminal plasma allergy. J Allergy Clin Immunol 66, 148–154.

Leventhal, L.J., DeMarco, D.M. and Zurier, R.B. (1990). Antinuclear antibody in pericardial fluid from a patient with primary cardiac lymphoma. Arch Intern Med 150, 1113–1115.

Levine, H., Szanto, M., Grieble, H.G., Bach, G.L. and Anderson, T.O. (1968). Rheumatoid factor in nonrheumatoid pleural effusions. Ann Intern Med 69, 487–492.

Lolli, F., Siracusa, G., Amato, M.P. et al. (1991). Intrathecal synthesis of free immunoglobulin light chains and IgM in initial multiple sclerosis. Acta Neurol Scand 83, 239–243.

Macanovic, M., Hogarth, M.B. and Lachmann, P.J. (1999). Anti-DNA antibodies in the urine of lupus nephritis patients. Nephrol Dial Transplant 14, 1418–1424.

Makar, R.S. and Toth, T.L. (2002). The evaluation of infertility. Am J Clin Pathol 117 Suppl, S95–103.

McInnes, I.B. and Liew, F.Y. (1998). Interleukin 15: a proinflammatory role in rheumatoid arthritis synovitis. Immunol Today 19, 75–79.

McLachlan, R.I. (2002). Basis, diagnosis and treatment of immunological infertility in men. J Reprod Immunol 57, 35–45.

McLachlan, R.I., Baker, H.W., Clarke, G.N. et al. (2003). Semen analysis: its place in modern reproductive medical practice. Pathology 35, 25–33.

Moore, T.R. (2002). A comparison of amniotic fluid fetal pulmonary phospholipids in normal and diabetic pregnancy. Am J Obstet Gynecol 186, 641–650.

Musher, D.R., Hunder, G.G. and McDuffie, F.C. (1972). Pleural fluid complement. Ann Intern Med 77, 482–483.

Nanni-Costa, A., Iannelli, S., Vangelista, A. et al. (1992). Flow cytometry evaluation of urinary sediment in renal transplantation. Transpl Int 5 Suppl 1, S8–12.

Noppen, M., De Waele, M., Li, R. et al. (2000). Volume and cellular content of normal pleural fluid in humans examined by pleural lavage. Am J Respir Crit Care Med 162, 1023–1026.

O'Connor, K.C., Chitnis, T., Griffin, D.E. et al. (2003). Myelin basic protein-reactive autoantibodies in the serum and cerebrospinal fluid of multiple sclerosis patients are characterized by low-affinity interactions. J Neuroimmunol 136, 140–148.

OSHA (1991). Occupational Exposure to Bloodborne Pathogens, 29 CFR 1910, December 6.

Perini, P., Calabrese, M., Ranzato, F., Tiberio, M. and Gallo, P. (2001). Cerebrospinal fluid examination in the differential diagnosis of inflammatory myelopathies. Neurol Sci 22 Suppl 2, S65–68.

Poggi, S.H., Spong, C.Y., Pezzullo, J.C. et al. (2003). Lecithin/sphingomyelin ratio and lamellar body count. What values predict the presence of phosphatidylglycerol? J Reprod Med 48, 330–334.

Pridgeon, C., Lennon, G.P., Pazmany, L., Thompson, R.N., Christmas, S.E. and Moots, R.J. (2003). Natural killer cells in the synovial fluid of rheumatoid arthritis patients exhibit a CD56bright,CD94bright,CD158negative phenotype. Rheumatology (Oxford) 42, 870–878.

Quan, C.P., Forestier, F. and Bouvet, J.P. (1999). Immunoglobulins of the human amniotic fluid. Am J Reprod Immunol 42, 219–225.

Ramsey, P.S., Andrews, W.W., Goldenberg, R.L., Tamura, T., Wenstrom, K.D. and Johnston, K.E. (2002). Elevated amniotic fluid ferritin levels are associated with inflammation-related pregnancy loss following mid-trimester amniocentesis. J Matern Fetal Neonatal Med 11, 302–306.

Roos, K.L. (2003). Lumbar puncture. Semin Neurol 23, 105–114.

Rudick, R.A., French, C.A., Breton, D. and Williams, G.W. (1989). Relative diagnostic value of cerebrospinal fluid kappa chains in MS: comparison with other immunoglobulin tests. Neurology 39, 964–968.

Shurin, M.R., Lu, L., Kalinski, P., Stewart-Akers, A.M. and Lotze, M.T. (1999). Th1/Th2 balance in cancer, transplantation and pregnancy. Springer Semin Immunopathol 21, 339–359.

Skulina, C., Schmidt, S., Dornmair, K. et al. (2004). Multiple sclerosis: brain-infiltrating CD8+ T cells persist as clonal expansions in the cerebrospinal fluid and blood. Proc Natl Acad Sci USA 101, 2428–2433.

Urnovitz, H.B., Sturge, J.C., Gottfried, T.D. and Murphy, W.H. (1999). Urine antibody tests: new insights into the dynamics of HIV-1 infection. Clin Chem 45, 1602–1613.

Wang, D.Y., Yang, P.C., Yu, W.L., Kuo, S.H. and Hsu, N.Y. (2000). Serial antinuclear antibodies titre in pleural and pericardial fluid. Eur Respir J 15, 1106–1110.

Wasson, A.W., Coy, E.A., Kooistra, J.B. and Yunginger, J.W. (1987). Seminal plasma immunosuppressive factors in the spouse of a woman with seminal fluid allergy. Am J Reprod Immunol Microbiol 15, 99–100.

Wenstrom, K.D., Andrews, W.W., Hauth, J.C., Goldenberg, R.L., DuBard, M.B. and Cliver, S.P. (1998). Elevated second-trimester amniotic fluid interleukin-6 levels predict preterm delivery. Am J Obstet Gynecol 178, 546–550.

Witczak, M., Torbe, A. and Czajka, R. (2003). [Maternal serum and amniotic fluid IL-1 alpha, IL-1 beta, IL-6 and IL-8 levels in preterm and term labor complicated by PROM.] Ginekol Pol 74, 1343–1347.

Wolinsky, J.S. (2003). The diagnosis of primary progressive multiple sclerosis. J Neurol Sci 206, 145–152.

Yamamoto, K., Okamura, D., Kurahara, D. et al. (2003). Do urinary mononuclear cells reflect disease activity in lupus nephritis? Cell Mol Biol (Noisy-le-grand) 49, 1333–1337.

Yavin, E.J., Preciado-Patt, L., Rosen, O. et al. (2000). Serum amyloid A-derived peptides, present in human rheumatic synovial fluids, induce the secretion of interferon-gamma by human CD(4)(+) T-lymphocytes. FEBS Lett 472, 259–262.

Yocum, M.W., Jones, R.T. and Yunginger, J.W. (1996). Concurrent sensitization to natural rubber latex and human seminal fluid. J Allergy Clin Immunol 98, 1135–1136.

Zorn, B., Sesek-Briski, A., Osredkar, J. and Meden-Vrtovec, H. (2003). Semen polymorphonuclear neutrophil leukocyte elastase as a diagnostic and prognostic marker of genital tract inflammation – a review. Clin Chem Lab Med 41, 2–12.

Acute-Phase Proteins and Inflammation: Immunological and Clinical Implications

Chapter 10

Chau-Ching Liu and Joseph M. Ahearn

Division of Rheumatology and Clinical Immunology, Department of Medicine, University of Pittsburgh School of Medicine, Lupus Center of Excellence University of Pittsburgh Schools of Health Sciences, Pittsburgh, PA, USA

This operation of the body, termed inflammation, requires our greatest attention, for it is one of the most common and most extensive in its causes, and it becomes itself the cause of many local effects, both salutary and diseased.

> John Hunter, 1794 (from A Treatise on the Blood, Inflammation, and Gun-Shot Wounds. London: G. Nicol; 1794, p. 249 (Reprinted in Birmingham, AL: Classics of Medicine Library; 1982, p. 249)

INTRODUCTION

Host defense against infection or injury is essential for self-preservation. When faced with such challenges, the body quickly mounts a complex series of reactions to eliminate infectious pathogens, prevent ongoing tissue damage and facilitate repair of injured tissues. Initial interest in these reactions was sparked in 1930 when C-reactive protein (CRP; so named because of its ability to bind the C-polysaccharide of *Pneumococcus*) was discovered in the plasma of patients with acute pneumococcal pneumonia (Tillett and Francis, 1930). Investigators soon realized that CRP was involved in the systemic changes that occur during the acute phase of an inflammatory condition (MacLeod and Avery, 1941). These well-orchestrated changes are now collectively known as the 'acute-phase response', a term coined by Avery and colleagues in 1941 (MacLeod and Avery, 1941). Because of its apparent role in host defense against infectious pathogens, the acute-phase response can be viewed as an important manifestation of innate immunity.

Since 1930, numerous studies have been conducted to characterize the acute-phase response in various diseases and experimental systems. An intense interest in this 'ancient' biological phenomenon has recently been rekindled, owing primarily to its newly discovered association with chronic inflammatory disorders such as cardiovascular disease. In this chapter, we will summarize the pathophysiological sequences of the acute-phase response, discuss the biochemical and functional characteristics of two major acute-phase proteins in humans, describe methods commonly used to measure the acute-phase response and review recent data implicating a pivotal role of acute-phase proteins in cardiovascular disease.

ACUTE-PHASE RESPONSE AND ACUTE-PHASE PROTEINS

Acute-phase response

The acute-phase response (APR) refers to a wide range of neuroendocrine, physiological and metabolic changes that are initiated immediately after a tissue is afflicted with an infection or injury (e.g. trauma, burns, surgery, etc.) (Baumann and Gauldie, 1994; Gabay and Kushner, 1999). At times, intense physical exercise or psychological stress can also induce mild to moderate APR-like changes (Strachan et al., 1984). Such changes may take place locally or systemically. While the APR may first be involved in initiating and amplifying tissue inflammation, this complex response can ultimately aid in attenuating and

Measuring Immunity, edited by Michael T. Lotze and Angus W. Thomson
ISBN 0-12-455900-X, London

resolving inflammation. Normally, the APR is elicited within a few hours after the initial insult and the majority of the response subsides over a period of 24–72 h. Consequently, the body is likely to return to homeostasis and normal function within a few days. However, this process can be prolonged and converted into a chronic reaction if the initial stimulus persists or a normal regulatory step is disrupted. As a result, an aberrantly prolonged APR may not only contribute to ongoing tissue damage and metabolic disturbance associated with the disease (e.g. cachexia in patients with acquired immunodeficiency syndrome or cancer), but also lead to further complications (e.g. cardiovascular disease or reactive amyloidosis) (Uhlar and Whitehead, 1999; Gabay and Kushner, 1999).

In humans, the APR is characterized by fever, altered vascular permeability and changes in the biosynthetic and metabolic profiles in different organs (Baumann and Gauldie, 1994). The cascade of APR is initiated and coordinated by a diverse spectrum of cells and inflammatory mediators. Macrophages at sites of infection/injury and monocytes in the blood are primarily responsible for initiating the APR. These cells produce cytokines such as interleukin (IL)-1 and tumor necrosis factor-α (TNF-α), which can then stimulate cells in the surrounding tissue to release additional cytokines (e.g. IL-6) and chemokines (e.g. monocyte chemoattractant protein-1 (MCP-1) and IL-8). These mediators in turn exert chemotactic and other systemic effects, thereby setting off a full-blown APR (Figure 10.1).

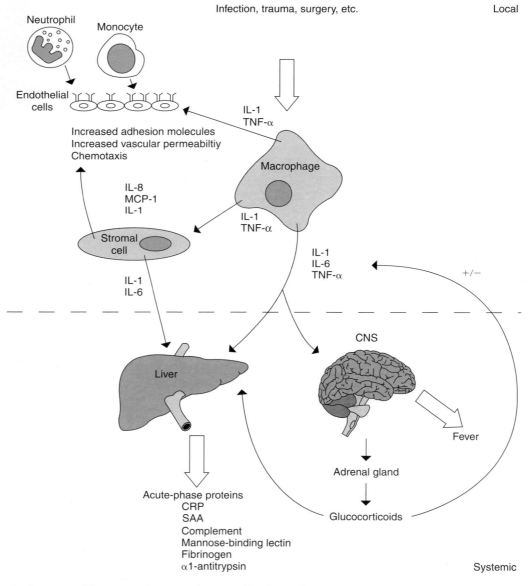

Figure 10.1 Schematic illustration of the major inducers, mediators and local as well as systemic changes during the acute-phase response. Macrophages secrete early cytokines, such as IL-1, IL-6 and TNF-α, at the site of tissue injury. These cytokines stimulate adjacent cells, such as stromal cells and endothelial cells, to release additional cytokines and chemokines and initiate inflammatory cell infiltration. Cytokines released into systemic circulation play important roles in eliciting the hepatic APR (i.e. production of acute-phase proteins) and fever. Cytokines and acute-phase proteins, which have been extensively studied and are the focus of this chapter, are indicated in bold characters.

Locally at the site of inflammation, IL-1, IL-6 and TNF-α produced by macrophages/monocytes can activate endothelial cells, upregulate their expression of adhesion molecules and thus enhance attachment/migration of leukocytes into the inflamed tissue (Baumann and Gauldie, 1994). Inflammatory cytokines, in combination with various molecules (e.g. nitric oxide, reactive oxygen species and prostaglandins) produced by cytokine-stimulated cells, can also influence the vascular tone and permeability (Baumann and Gauldie, 1994). Together, these mediators induce dilatation and leakage of the blood vessels, particularly the post-capillary venules and cause tissue edema and erythema (redness) – hallmark changes of local inflammation.

Systemically, fever and a set of biochemical/metabolic changes occurring in the liver are the two most prominent components of the APR. Fever is thought to be induced by inflammatory cytokines released from the site of inflammation and IL-6 produced in the brain stem (Baumann and Gauldie, 1994; Gabay and Kushner, 1999), probably via the induction of prostaglandin E_2 synthesis (Dinarello et al., 1988). IL-1 and IL-6 also stimulate the hypothalamic– pituitary–adrenal axis to release adrenocorticotropic hormone and subsequently glucocorticoids (Akira et al.,1993; Baumann and Gauldie, 1994), which play important roles in regulating the APR. Moreover, IL-1 and IL-6 trigger a series of changes in the liver that is referred to as the 'hepatic APR'. The hepatic APR includes alterations in the transport of ions and metabolites, changes in the activities of many metabolic pathways and, most importantly, profound modifications in the regulation and production of the 'acute-phase proteins'.

Acute-phase proteins

Although cells and molecules involved in or invoked by the APR can be collectively called the 'acute-phase reactants', the proteinaceous reactants are specifically referred to as 'acute-phase proteins'. There are approximately 30 acute-phase proteins that vary considerably in structure and function. By definition, an acute-phase protein is one whose concentration in the plasma increases (for a 'positive' acute-phase protein) or decreases (for a 'negative' acute-phase protein) by at least 25 per cent during the acute phase (approximately the first 7 days) of inflammatory conditions (Morley and Kushner, 1982; Steel and Whitehead, 1994; Gabay and Kushner, 1999) (Table 10.1). The biological significance of the decrease of certain plasma proteins (e.g. albumin) during the acute inflammatory state is not well understood. However, it is reasonable to postulate that such 'negative' proteins may be non-essential for the protection of the host during inflammatory conditions. Thus, diminished production of these proteins during the acute phase may allow the biosynthetic machinery of the host to concentrate on generating the 'positive' proteins that are crucial for controlling any potentially harmful situations. The following discussion will focus on the positive acute-phase proteins.

Table 10.1 Human acute-phase proteins[a]

'Positive' acute-phase proteins[b]
C-reactive protein[c]
Serum amyloid A
Fibrinogen
von Willebrand factor
Plasminogen
Tissue plasminogen activator
Plasminogen activator inhibitor-1
α_1-Antitrypsin
α_1-Antichymotrypsin
α_2-Antiplasmin
Complement (C3, C4, C9, factor B, C4-binding protein, mannose-binding lectin)
Granulocyte colony-stimulating factor
Ceruloplasmin
Haptoglobin
Ferritin
Fibronectin
Surfactant A
Surfactant D
α_1-Acid glycoprotein
Secreted phospholipase A_2
Lipopolysaccharide-binding protein
Interleukin 1-receptor antagonist

'Negative' acute-phase proteins[d]
Albumin
α-Fetoprotein
Transferrin
Transthyretin
Thyroxine-binding globulin
Insulin-like growth factor I
Fetuin

[a] This table is not meant to be exclusive. Many other 'minor' acute-phase proteins are not listed here.
[b] Proteins whose plasma concentrations increase during the acute phase.
[c] Serum amyloid P component, also a pentraxin, is the counterpart for human CRP in mice.
[d] Proteins whose plasma concentrations decrease during the acute phase.

Most acute-phase proteins are synthesized by hepatocytes in the liver (Steel and Whitehead, 1994). Hepatocytes respond to inflammatory mediators through specific cell surface receptors. Mediators capable of regulating the hepatic APR can be divided into four general categories:

1 IL-6-type cytokines
2 IL-1-type cytokines
3 growth factors
4 glucocorticoids.

Many of these regulators act in a complementary or coordinated fashion and each may influence more than one acute phase protein. Among these regulators, IL-6 is perhaps the most important and most studied. IL-6 binds to IL-6 receptors expressed on hepatocytes and induces the transcription of several genes encoding acute-phase proteins. The IL-6 receptor uses the gp130 glycoprotein as the signaling component. Other cytokines that signal through the gp130, such as oncostatin M, leukemia inhibitory factor, IL-11 and ciliary neurotrophic factor, are also capable of inducing production of acute-phase proteins (Taga and Kishimoto, 1997). The involvement of IL-6 in the hepatic APR has primarily been investigated *in vitro* using cultured hepatocytes (Ganapathi et al., 1991) and *in vivo* with IL-6-knockout mice (Kopf et al., 1994). The IL-6-knockout mice displayed significantly suppressed APR initiated by either injections of turpentine or infections with gram-positive bacteria, but not by lipopolysaccharides (endotoxins derived from gram-negative bacteria) (Kopf et al., 1994). These results establish a critical role of IL-6 in the APR initiated by some, but not all, stimuli. Moreover, these data suggest that different stimuli may preferentially trigger a spectrum of inflammatory cytokines to initiate the APR.

The IL-1-type cytokines, such as IL-1$_\alpha$ and IL-1$_\beta$, have been shown to induce a set of acute-phase proteins that are distinct from those induced by the IL-6-type cytokines. The acute-phase proteins induced by IL-1 are called type 1 acute-phase proteins and by IL-6, type 2 acute-phase proteins (Baumann and Gauldie, 1994). The major type 1 acute-phase proteins are serum amyloid A (SAA), complement proteins and haptoglobin, whereas type 2 acute-phase proteins include fibrinogen, C-reactive protein (CRP) and some anti-proteases. Interestingly, although IL-6 often enhances the inducing effect of IL-1 on type 1 acute-phase proteins, IL-1 does not enhance the inducing effects of IL-6 on type 2 acute-phase proteins (Gauldie et al., 1987). In fact, it may sometimes inhibit these effects. As with IL-6, gene-knockout mice have been used to demonstrate the important role of IL-1$_\beta$ in the induction of acute-phase proteins. As seen in IL-6-knockout mice, IL-1$_\beta$-knockout mice have a diminished APR in response to injections of turpentine (Zheng et al., 1995).

While IL-1 and IL-6 are efficient inducers of acute-phase proteins, growth factors and glucocorticoids function mainly as modulators. Among the growth factors with this capability are insulin, transforming growth factor-β (TGF-β), hepatocyte growth factor and fibroblast growth factor (Baumann and Gauldie, 1994). For example, insulin can attenuate the stimulatory effects of IL-1 and IL-6 on hepatocytes (Campos and Baumann, 1992). The action of TGF-β is more complex. It suppresses the effects of IL-1 on type 1 acute-phase proteins, but enhances the effects of IL-6 on type 2 acute-phase proteins (Mackiewicz et al., 1990). Glucocorticoids have a modest ability to induce directly the expression of some acute-phase proteins (Baumann and Gauldie, 1994). The principal function of glucocorticoids, however, is synergistically to enhance the inducing effects of IL-1 and IL-6 (Besedovsky et al., 1986; Ganapathi et al., 1991). In addition to these direct and indirect stimulatory functions, glucocorticoids may play a negative-feedback role in controlling the propagation/persistence of the APR through inhibiting the production of inflammatory cytokines by macrophages and monocytes.

The primary mechanism by which acute-phase proteins are regulated appears to be through enhanced transcription of their coding genes (Baumann and Gauldie, 1994; Steel and Whitehead, 1994; Uhlar and Whitehead, 1999; Volanakis, 2001); however, additional regulatory mechanisms appear to be involved. For example, increased secretion of acute-phase proteins by hepatocytes has been reported to contribute to the increase in acute-phase proteins in the plasma (Macintyre et al., 1985). In addition, post-translational modifications, such as alterations in glycosylation, may occur to some acute-phase proteins during inflammatory states (Jiang et al., 1995). While the majority of acute-phase proteins eventually increase in the plasma during the APR, they do not all increase at the same time or to the same extent in patients with similar or even the same illness. A unique sequence of acute-phase protein increase has repeatedly been observed in different experimental or clinical situations (Colley et al., 1983; Yamada, 1999). For example, cytokines such as IL-1 and IL-6 increase within 2–3 h after tissue injury, followed by CRP and SAA, which start to increase at 3–6 hours (Colley et al., 1983; Yamada, 1999). Complement components and fibrinogen may increase after 1–2 days. Likewise, the magnitude of changes in plasma concentrations varies considerably among different acute-phase proteins. Whereas complement proteins, ceruloplasmin, fibrinogen and haptoglobin usually increase by 50 per cent to several times their normal concentrations, CRP and SAA may increase up to 1000 times their baseline concentrations (Baumann and Gauldie, 1994; Steel and Whitehead, 1994; Volanakis, 2001). Furthermore, distinct sets of acute-phase proteins may be preferentially induced in patients with different illnesses or even with similar illnesses. These differences may be due to the types of inflammatory cytokines induced in a given stimulatory condition or a variation in the sensitivity of the host to a particular inducer. The great variability in the induction of acute-phase proteins in different pathophysiological conditions suggests that individual acute-phase proteins are independently regulated by a complex network of regulatory mechanisms.

ROLES OF ACUTE-PHASE PROTEINS IN INFLAMMATION, IMMUNE DEFENSE AND DISEASE

Because of the prompt changes in the plasma concentrations of acute-phase proteins after an infection or injury occurs, investigators have speculated that the APR may benefit the host. Acute-phase proteins, which differ considerably in molecular structure and biochemical activity, may serve different purposes in the evolutionary sequences of the APR by participating in the propagation or restriction of acute inflammatory reactions, the adaptation to disturbed homeostasis during acute inflammation, or the repair of injured tissue. For example, elevated concentrations of complement proteins not only may generate increasing amounts of chemotaxins C3a and

C5a that can trigger movement of leukocytes into the inflamed tissue, but also can result in direct damage of infectious microorganisms. Together, these actions facilitate the clearance of debris from injured tissue and prevent the spread of infectious agents. Increased concentrations of anti-proteases (e.g. α_1-antitrypsin) may neutralize the action of lysosomal enzymes released following the infiltration of activated leukocytes, thus preventing tissue damage. In addition, fibrinogen may aid in tissue repair. In humans, CRP and SAA are the two acute-phase proteins that increase most swiftly and abundantly during the APR. Therefore, their biological characteristics and functional roles in inflammatory disease deserve special attention and will be discussed in detail (see Table 10.2).

C-reactive protein (CRP)

Human CRP and its homologue in mouse, serum amyloid P component (SAP), are members of a phylogenetically ancient and highly conserved family of proteins called the 'pentraxins'. The name 'pentraxin' (from the Greek for 'five berries') was derived from the unique structure of

Table 10.2 Functions of C-reactive protein and serum amyloid A

C-reactive protein
Opsonization (binding to phosphorylcholine expressed on pathogens and apoptotic cells; enhancing phagocytosis via Fc receptors expressed on phagocytes)

Activation of the classical pathway of complement (resulting in C3/C4 opsonization of pathogens and apoptotic cells; enhancing phagocytosis via complement receptors expressed on phagocytes)

Immune-modulation
  Proinflammatory
    Inducing tumoricidal activity of monocytes/macrophages
    Inducing production of H_2O_2 and secretion of IL-1 and TNF by monocytes/macrophages

  Anti-inflammatory
    Inducing shedding of L-selectin and IL-6 receptors from neutrophils
    Downregulating activities of neutrophils

Atherogenesis?

Serum amyloid A
Modulation of cholesterol metabolism/transport

Immune-modulation
  Proinflammatory
    Activation of leukocytes
    Chemotaxis of neutrophils, monocytes and T cells
    Induction of proinflammatory cytokines produced by monocytes (e.g. IL-1)
    Upregulation of adhesion molecules expressed by leukocytes
    Enhancement of phagocytic activity of neutrophils
    Induction of extracellular matrix-degrading enzymes (e.g. collagenase, stromelysin and matrix metalloproteinases 2 and 3)

  Anti-inflammatory
    Suppression of antibody production
    Inhibition of reactive oxygen burst response in neutrophils
    Inhibition of platelet aggregation
    Inhibition of T cell–macrophage interaction

these proteins, which consists of five identical subunits non-covalently associated and arranged symmetrically around a central pore (Volanakis, 2001). Phylogenetic studies have shown that the pentraxins have been conserved over 500 million years of evolution, with the most ancient member identified in the hemolymph of the invertebrate *Limulus polyphemus* (horseshoe crab). This evolutionary conservation, in conjunction with the lack of reported CRP-deficient humans and animals, underscores the biological indispensability of CRP for host defense and survival.

Human CRP was discovered in 1930 when Tillett and Francis reported an interesting observation that precipitants formed when the C-polysaccharide of *Pneumococcus pneumoniae* was added to the plasma of patients with pneumonia in the acute stage (Tillett and Francis, 1930). Because of the observed reactivity to C-polysaccharides, they named the then elusive plasma protein 'C-reactive protein'. CRP was later isolated and has since been characterized extensively. CRP is capable of binding in a Ca^{2+}-dependent manner to phosphorylcholine, a component of many bacterial and fungal polysaccharides and of surface membranes of most cells (Volanakis, 2001). Under normal circumstances, the conformation of phosphorylcholine in cellular membranes renders it unavailable to bind CRP. However, during apoptosis and necrosis, membrane lipid constituents are perturbed or oxidized and the conformation of phosphorylcholine in the membrane is altered. As a result, CRP can bind to phosphorylcholine and opsonized damaged host cells in addition, thereby facilitating their removal by phagocytic cells. Recent studies by Du Clos and colleagues have shown that phagocytic cells recognize CRP-opsonized targets through type I and type II_A Fc-gamma receptors (FcγRI and FcγII$_A$) (Marnell et al., 1995; Bharadwaj et al., 1999).

CRP can also opsonize microorganisms and damaged cells in an indirect way. Once CRP is bound to its ligands, it can bind complement component C1q and efficiently activate the classical pathway of the complement cascade (Kaplan and Volanakis, 1974; Volanakis, 1982; Mold et al., 1999). This activation process leads to the formation of C3 convertases but not C5 convertases; the formation of the latter is inhibited by factor H that also binds to CRP (Mold et al., 1984). Thus, when CRP activates the complement cascade, the microorganisms and damaged cells are opsonized by complement ligands but are not lysed (Berman et al., 1986). The CRP-initiated, complement-mediated opsonization of pathogens and cell debris may further facilitate their removal by phagocytic cells that express abundant levels of complement receptors. In addition to enhancing phagocytosis, CRP can also modulate other functional activities of phagocytic cells through engagement of complement receptors and Fcγ receptors. For example, CRP has been shown to enhance the tumoricidal activity of monocytes (Barna et al., 1987), induce the production of proinflammatory cytokines by macrophages (Galve-de Rochemonteix et al., 1993), stimulate the synthesis of tissue factors by monocytes (Nakagomi et al., 2000) and trigger the shedding of IL-6 receptors from neutrophils (Jones et al., 1999). As a result, not only is CRP an important component of innate immunity, but it also serves as a bridge linking the humoral and cellular arms of the immune system.

CRP has also been shown to bind chromatin (Robey et al., 1984) as well as several other nuclear constituents such as histones (Du Clos et al., 1988; Pepys et al., 1994). Therefore, CRP can bind necrotic and apoptotic cells not only through phosphorylcholine in the damaged membranes but also through the nuclear contents exposed on the cell surface. From an immunological point of view, the increased clearance of apoptotic cells and their derived nuclear contents by phagocytic cells via CRP opsonization may prevent the development of potential nuclear antigen-specific autoimmune responses (Andrade et al., 2000; Gershov et al., 2000; Liu et al., 2003).

Serum amyloid A (SAA)

Interest in SAA began 40 years ago when a unique protein was isolated from tissues obtained from patients with amyloidosis secondary to chronic inflammatory diseases (reactive amyloidosis; also known as amyloidosis type A) (Benditt and Eriksen, 1966). SAA was later identified as the precursor protein of amyloid fibrils and is now known as a family of differentially expressed apolipoproteins encoded by multiple genes (Malle et al., 1993; Uhlar and Whitehead, 1999). Similar to CRP, SAA has been evolutionarily conserved for over 400 million years (Uhlar et al., 1994). However, unlike CRP, SAA does not share structural homology with any known proteins. Structurally, SAA is a single polypeptide with a predicted conformation as a globular protein. Two types of SAA exist in humans, one produced constitutively (C-SAA) and one induced during the APR (A-SAA) (Uhlar and Whitehead, 1999). The A-SAA, encoded by the SAA1 and SAA2 genes, is produced primarily in the liver and minimally in several extrahepatic sites (Meek and Benditt, 1986). In response to an infection or tissue injury, A-SAA can quickly be induced by IL-1, IL-6 and TNF-α with an increase approaching 1000-fold (from a baseline concentration of 1 μg/ml to 1 mg/ml) (Uhlar and Whitehead, 1999; Yamada, 1999). As in the case for CRP, the increase of A-SAA during inflammation is mainly due to upregulated gene transcription.

The primary physiological function of A-SAA remains largely unknown, but various activities have been reported (Uhlar and Whitehead, 1999; Yamada, 1999). In vitro studies have shown that SAA can bind rapidly with high-density lipoprotein (HDL) during the APR, thereby displacing or replacing apolipoprotein A1 (apoA1) within the lipoprotein complex (Benditt and Eriksen, 1977; Hoffman and Benditt, 1982; Coetzee et al., 1986). Moreover, A-SAA may enhance the activity of lecithin-cholesterol acyltransferase, a key enzyme mediating

cholesterol esterification (Steinmetz et al., 1989). Based on these findings, it is postulated that A-SAA may play a role in the metabolism and transport of cholesterol by modifying the HDL complexes and redirecting them from hepatocytes to macrophages during the APR (Banka et al., 1995; Uhlar and Whitehead, 1999). This notion is supported by experimental data that demonstrated a preferential binding of SAA-HDL complexes to macrophages rather than hepatocytes (Kisilevsky and Subrahmanyan, 1992). It is possible that macrophages may use this SAA-mediated mechanism effectively to engulf cholesterol and lipid debris at the site of inflammation where cell death occurs profusely. Furthermore, as the APR evolves, excess cholesterol may be redistributed for use in tissue repair.

Besides the potential involvement in cholesterol metabolism, A-SAA may also be involved in immune-related functions. For example, in vitro studies have shown that SAA is capable of inducing adhesion, migration and tissue infiltration of monocytes, neutrophils and lymphocytes (Badolato et al., 1994), increasing production of cytokines by T lymphocytes and monocytes (Patel et al., 1998) and stimulating generation of extracellular matrix-degrading enzymes (Migita et al., 1998). Recently, it has been suggested that the chemotactic activity of SAA is mediated through low-affinity receptors for N-formyl-methionyl-leucyl-phenylalanine, a chemotactic peptide, expressed on phagocytic cells (Su et al., 1999). In contrast, several earlier studies have suggested an anti-inflammatory role for SAA. For instance, SAA has been reported to suppress production of antibodies by lymphocytes (Benson and Aldo-Benson, 1982), to inhibit oxygen burst reaction in neutrophils (Linke et al., 1991), to limit platelet aggregation (Zimlichman et al., 1990) and to interfere with T cell–macrophage interaction (Aldo-Benson and Benson, 1982). These seemingly inconsistent data, collectively, indicate that SAA is a multifunctional protein that may play an important role in preserving tissue homeostasis by transiting between proinflammatory and anti-inflammatory functions according to the stage of the APR. However, it remains to be verified whether SAA indeed executes all or some of these functions in vivo.

MEASUREMENT OF THE ACUTE-PHASE RESPONSE IN DISEASE: ERYTHROCYTE SEDIMENTATION RATE AND PLASMA CRP LEVELS

Despite lack of specificity for a particular disease, the wide-ranging biochemical, physiological, neuroendocrinal and hematological changes occurring during the APR provide physicians with many potential biomarkers to accurately diagnose and monitor the severity of inflammatory disease and to evaluate the efficacy of disease management. For example, since changes in plasma concentrations of acute-phase proteins may reflect the presence or intensity of an inflammatory process, measurements of these proteins can help differentiate inflammatory from non-inflammatory diseases and thus allow for the institution of proper treatment. Currently, the most widely used methods for assessing inflammatory conditions are the erythrocyte sedimentation rate (ESR) and plasma CRP concentration.

Erythrocyte sedimentation rate (ESR)

In 1921, Fahraeus reported that aggregation and sedimentation of erythrocytes may be enhanced by plasma fibrinogen (now known as an acute-phase protein) (Fahraeus, 1921). His observation eventually led to the development of the ESR, which measures the rate of settlement of erythrocytes in a tube of anticoagulated blood within a specific period of time. The ESR measurement is quick, simple and inexpensive and, in many situations, is a useful indicator of inflammation (Sox and Liang, 1986; Saadeh, 1998).

Erythrocytes, the most abundant cells in the blood, normally circulate as single, unaggregated cells. The 'single' status of erythrocytes is maintained primarily by their net negative surface charge, causing them to repel each other. Under pathological conditions, however, erythrocytes may aggregate and form the so-called 'rouleaux' (rolls of stacked coins), which are bigger and heavier than single erythrocytes. Because they are bigger and heavier, aggregated erythrocytes settle more readily under gravity than do single erythrocytes. Therefore, an increase in the ESR *in vitro* may indicate the presence of any factors that may increase erythrocyte aggregation *in vivo*. The ESR is usually measured using either the Westergren method or the Wintrob method. In general, the blood is drawn from a patient into a tube containing anticoagulants and a sample of anticoagulated blood is placed in a calibrated tube of standard dimensions and incubated in a vertical position for exactly one hour. The distance the layer of erythrocytes has fallen from the plasma surface (the zero mark) in that hour is measured and reported in millimeter (mm)/h. In the Westergren method, blood is anticoagulated using sodium citrate (original Westergren method) or EDTA (modified Westergren method), diluted 1:4 and placed in a standard 200-mm glass tube. In the Wintrob method, the anticoagulated blood is not diluted but is placed directly into a graduated 100-mm tube. The Wintrob method is relatively simpler, but may be less sensitive than the Westergren method.

It should be noted that the ESR is not a specific indicator of a particular disease but a non-specific parameter of inflammation. For example, the ESR value may increase in patients with an acute inflammation (e.g. acute infection or injury) or a chronic disease (e.g. rheumatoid arthritis or cancer). Furthermore, there are situations in which an elevated ESR may be unrelated to inflammation. To understand these distinctions, it is necessary to consider the

factors that influence erythrocyte aggregation:

1 plasma proteins
2 sizes of erythrocytes
3 shapes of erythrocytes
4 number of erythrocytes.

The effects of plasma proteins are most profound during the APR. Plasma proteins that are positively charged can neutralize and reduce the negative surface charge on erythrocytes, thereby decreasing the repulsive force and prompting erythrocytes to aggregate. In inflammatory states, acute-phase proteins in the plasma, particularly fibrinogen, may efficiently facilitate aggregation of erythrocytes and hence increase the ESR. Abnormally increased or decreased concentrations of plasma proteins unrelated to inflammation can also affect the ESR. Patients with paraproteinemia in diseases such as multiple myeloma may have an increased ESR. In contrast, patients with hypoalbuminemia, seen in many chronic diseases, may have a decreased ESR. Within the general population, the elderly (possibly secondary to increased fibrinogen or occult disease), women and obese individuals generally have higher ESR values (Sox and Liang, 1986). Pregnant women (possibly due to increased fibrinogen and plasma volume) and patients with diabetes mellitus and renal diseases (probably due to the underlying disease) have also been reported to have an elevated ESR (Sox and Liang, 1986). Since the aggregation of erythrocytes is significantly influenced by the sizes, shapes and numbers of those cells, hematological abnormalities may also alter ESR values. For example, patients with anemia generally have an elevated ESR. These patients have fewer erythrocytes and the resulting reduced friction between those cells can lead to faster sedimentation rates *in vitro*. However, patients with macrocytic (large erythrocyte) anemia usually have a higher ESR than do patients with microcytic (small erythrocyte) anemia, because large cells tend to sediment more rapidly than do small cells. Moreover, because irregularly shaped or rounded erythrocytes do not aggregate as well as normal disc-shaped erythrocytes, patients with diseases such as sickle cell anemia may have low (even zero) ESR values. Normal ESR values and the conditions in which the ESR may be increased or decreased are summarized in Table 10.3.

Plasma CRP levels

Although the ESR is easy to measure, it is essentially an indirect assessment of plasma fibrinogen concentration and can easily be affected by physiological and pathological 'non-inflammatory' factors as discussed above. Measuring plasma concentrations of CRP appears to have several advantages over the ESR. For example, whereas the ESR changes relatively slowly in response to changes in the inflammatory condition of a patient, the

Table 10.3 ESR: Reference values in healthy individuals and changes in disease

Westergren (modified) ESR (mm/h)		Wintrob ESR (mm/h)	
Men <50 years	0–15	Men	0–9
Men >50 years	0–20		
Women <50 years	0–20	Women	0–20
Women >50 years	0–30		

Increased ESR	Decreased ESR
Acute and chronic infections	Sickle cell disease (irregular-shaped erythrocytes)
Rheumatic diseases	Microcytosis (small erythrocytes)
Malignancies	Spherocytosis (round-shaped erythrocytes)
Diabetes	Polycythemia (increased number of erythrocytes)
Anemia	Waldenstrom's syndrome (increased plasma viscosity)
Macrocytosis (large erythrocytes)	
Multiple myeloma	
Obesity	
Pregnancy	
Female gender (slight increase)	
Age (increasing 0.85 mm/h per 5 years of age)	

plasma CRP changes promptly. The broader range of the abnormal values of CRP (1–1000 µg/ml) also provides a more sensitive means to detect inflammatory conditions in which the ESR may only vary by a narrow range. Moreover, the plasma concentrations of CRP do not seem to be affected by age and gender to the same degree as does the ESR.

Plasma concentrations of CRP can be measured by a variety of experimental and commercially available assays such as enzyme-linked immunosorbent assays, radioimmunoassays, immunonephelometric assays and immunoturbidimetric assays (Kapyaho et al., 1989; Ledue et al., 1998). These assays are generally excellent in terms of specificity and have sensitivity limits of 3–5 µg/ml. In the wake of recent appreciation for CRP as an indicator of chronic inflammatory diseases such as atherosclerosis, high-sensitivity CRP assays have been developed for quantifying plasma CRP concentrations in the low physiological range (0.1–2 µg/ml) more precisely (Wilkins et al., 1998; Rifai and Ridker, 2001) (see next section for further discussion). CRP assays are now routinely performed in many commercial laboratories, but the technical details will not be elaborated here due to space constraint. Instead, the clinical implications of CRP will be discussed.

Plasma levels of CRP in most healthy individuals are about or less than 2 µg/ml, but some individuals may have CRP as high as 10 µg/ml. This rather wide 'normal' range of plasma CRP levels may be due to the presence of clinically insignificant injury or infections in some 'healthy' individuals. However, increasing evidence

suggests that slightly elevated, but still physiological, CRP levels may predict the development of cardiovascular disease in apparently healthy individuals. Numerous clinical studies suggest that significant changes in plasma CRP levels have a quantitative correlation with inflammatory states. For example, markedly elevated CRP levels are often found in patients with severe bacterial infections (e.g. bacterial meningitis, septic arthritis, bacterial pneumonia, etc.) (Morley and Kushner, 1982) and hence CRP levels may be of value in distinguishing serious infections from less serious infections (e.g. acute pyelonephritis versus acute cystitis, acute bacterial pneumonia versus acute bronchitis, bacterial meningitis versus aseptic meningitis, etc.). A number of retrospective and prospective studies have recently demonstrated that plasma CRP levels may be used as a systemic marker of focal inflammation and infection such as acute appendicitis (Gronroos and Gronroos, 1999; Zimmerman et al., 2003). In postoperative patients, increased CRP levels were shown to predict septic complications before their clinical manifestation (Mustard et al., 1987). Serial measurements of CRP levels in patients with serious trauma appeared to help differentiate complications of bacterial sepsis from non-infectious systemic inflammatory responses (Miller et al., 1999). Elevated CRP is also frequently detected in patients with malignancies or in patients with rheumatic diseases (e.g. rheumatoid arthritis) (Kushner, 1991). Interestingly, most patients with systemic lupus erythematosus do not have high plasma CRP levels during the active disease (flare) state (Pepys et al., 1982). However, the CRP levels do rise significantly in these patients when they suffer from a concurrent bacterial infection (Pepys et al., 1982).

CRP AND CHRONIC INFLAMMATORY DISEASE: CARDIOVASCULAR DISEASE AS A MODEL

Accumulating evidence suggests that atherosclerosis is a chronic inflammatory disease (Ross, 1999; Libby, 2002). It is believed that vascular wall injury associated with hyperlipidemia, hypertension, physical stress or infections (e.g. *Chlamydia pneumoniae*) may lead to endothelial cell dysfunction, adhesion molecule expression, cytokine and inflammatory mediator production, inflammatory cell infiltration and vascular smooth muscle cell proliferation. This sequence of changes is probably provoked and exacerbated by immune reactions against infectious antigens, altered lipids such as oxidized low-density lipoprotein (LDL), or yet-unidentified autoantigens within the vessel wall. These 'smoldering' immune-inflammatory responses not only can drive the development of atherosclerotic plaques, but also, upon acute exacerbation, may cause plaque instability and the ensuing acute ischemic events (Ross, 1999; Libby, 2002). Therefore, it is intuitively attractive to investigate the correlation between inflammatory markers and the natural course of atherosclerotic cardiovascular disease. It has previously been shown that the serum levels of IL-6, a major inducer of acute-phase proteins, are elevated in patients with acute coronary syndromes (unstable angina or acute myocardial infarction (MI)) (Biasucci et al., 1996). This finding suggests that serum levels of acute-phase proteins (e.g. CRP and SAA), conventional markers of systemic inflammation, may provide clues to the development and/or progression of focal inflammation such as that occurring within the atherosclerotic vessel wall. The urgency to identify novel, reliable biomarkers (or, ideally, bio-predictors) of atherosclerotic cardiovascular disease is further prompted by the fact that half of all MI occur in patients who have normal plasma lipid levels, a traditional risk factor for coronary artery disease (Ridker, 1999).

CRP as a biomarker of cardiovascular disease

Recently, an enormous effort has been initiated to elucidate the associations between CRP levels and cardiovascular disease. Several epidemiological and laboratory-based studies have demonstrated a remarkable correlation between plasma CRP levels and the size of acute MI (de Beer et al., 1982), post-infarction adverse events (including mortality) (Haverkate et al., 1997; Toss et al., 1997; Morrow et al., 1998; Lindahl et al., 2000), as well as the risk of future acute coronary events (Ferreiros et al., 1999). Moreover, plasma CRP levels have also been found to be significantly higher in patients with unstable angina than in patients with stable angina or non-angina disease, and patients with unstable angina and high CRP appeared to have worse outcomes (Berk et al., 1990). For example, the European Concerted Action on Thrombosis and Disabilities Angina Pectoris Study showed that patients with a CRP level greater than 3.6 μg/ml (a level traditionally considered within the 'normal' range) have a twofold increased risk of MI and sudden cardiac death (Toss et al., 1997). Collectively, these studies demonstrate clearly that plasma CRP levels can serve as an indicator of the severity of cardiovascular disease and/or a predictor for prognosis.

CRP as a predictor of cardiovascular disease

Much enthusiasm has recently been elicited by several studies showing that CRP levels may also aid in predicting cardiovascular risk in individuals who are apparently healthy. Kuller et al. reported a positive correlation between CRP and coronary artery disease in healthy, but high-risk, men (e.g. smokers) (Kuller et al., 1996). In this prospective study, the risk of subsequent cardiovascular death was 4.3-fold higher in asymptomatic smokers whose CRP levels were in the highest quartile than in those in the lowest quartile. Similarly, Ridker et al. showed that healthy asymptomatic men who had higher baseline CRP levels were more prone to develop MI, stroke or peripheral vascular disease (Ridker et al., 1997, 1998a), and the risk of developing MI was nearly three times higher for men whose CRP levels were in the highest quartile than for those

in the lowest quartile (Ridker et al., 1997). Furthermore, it was shown that preventive use of aspirin significantly reduced the risk of MI only in men in the highest CRP quartile, implicating a pathogenic role for CRP in coronary artery disease (Ridker et al., 1997). Interestingly, the increased risk of coronary artery disease for individuals with high CRP levels does not appear to correlate with their plasma lipid levels, a traditional risk factor (Ridker et al., 1998b). Although individuals with high levels of both CRP and cholesterol were clearly at the highest risk to develop future MI, healthy individuals with high levels of cholesterol alone or individuals with high levels of CRP alone still had a significantly higher risk than those with low levels of both CRP and cholesterol (Ridker et al., 1998b, 2000). The notion that CRP may be more important than lipid levels is supported by a recent study in which CRP levels were shown to predict cardiovascular events more accurately than did LDL-cholesterol levels (Ridker et al., 2002). In that study, more than 75 per cent of patients with elevated CRP levels experienced a major cardiovascular event despite low LDL-cholesterol levels. Although many studies investigating the associations between CRP and cardiovascular disease have been performed in middle-aged men (Kuller et al., 1996; Ridker et al., 1997; Koenig et al., 1999), similar results have recently been obtained in women (Ridker et al., 1998c, 2000) and the elderly (Tracy et al., 1997; Harris et al., 1999). Taken together, these studies provide convincing evidence that CRP levels can potentially be used to predict risks of atherosclerotic cardiovascular disease and to monitor its progression. It should be pointed out, however, that in all studies, the 'high' CRP levels (2–4 μg/ml) detected in the healthy individuals who were predicted to be at higher risks were still well within the 'physiological' range (1–10 μg/ml). Therefore, in order to use CRP levels properly as a predictor or biomarker of atherosclerotic cardiovascular disease, it will be necessary to use the recently developed high-sensitivity CRP assays, instead of conventional assays (Wilkins et al., 1998; Rifai and Ridker, 2001).

CRP as a pathogenic factor of cardiovascular disease

The mechanisms underlying the correlation between CRP and atherosclerotic cardiovascular disease are still being investigated. At first glance, elevated CRP levels may simply reflect inflammation and tissue injury within the established atherosclerotic lesions, with more advanced disease giving rise to higher levels of CRP. However, several lines of evidence have suggested that CRP may be directly involved in the pathogenesis of atherosclerosis. First, CRP has been shown to bind selectively to LDL, particularly the partially degraded LDL found within atherosclerotic plaques (Torzewski et al., 1998, 2000). The presence of CRP within plaques not only may lead to activation of the complement system within plaques and promote tissue damage (Torzewski et al., 1998), but also may enhance recruitment of monocytes into atherosclerotic lesions (Torzewski et al., 2000). Second, it has been reported that CRP can stimulate endothelial cells to express adhesion molecules and monocyte chemoattractant protein-1 (Pasceri et al., 2001), thereby enhancing inflammatory cell infiltration into the atherosclerotic plaques. Third, it has been shown that CRP-bound LDL was efficiently taken up by macrophages (Zwaka et al., 2001; Fu and Borensztajn, 2002) and may thus contribute to the formation of foam cells within atherosclerotic plaques. Fourth, CRP present in the arterial wall lesions may stimulate macrophages to produce tissue factor, an important initiator of coagulation (Nakagomi et al., 2000). As a result, CRP may both aggravate the atherosclerotic process and increase the propensity of occlusive thrombosis. Lastly, it has recently been shown that injection of human CRP into rats could provoke complement-mediated tissue damage and increase the size of myocardial infarct induced by experimental coronary artery ligation (Griselli et al., 1999). It is possible that similar CRP-triggered, complement-dependent tissue damage mechanisms may actually mediate ischemic myocardial injury in patients with MI (Lagrand et al., 1997).

FUTURE PROSPECTS

Although solitary measurements of acute-phase proteins clearly do not have diagnostic specificity for a particular disease, serial measurements can be helpful in monitoring the progress of diseases and improving clinical management. The studies summarized in this chapter strongly suggest that CRP and probably other acute-phase proteins do not merely reflect the inflammatory process of atherosclerosis, but may be directly involved in the pathogenesis of atherosclerosis. Although not discussed in this chapter, recent studies have also shown that SAA, like CRP, may serve as a predictor/indicator of cardiovascular disease (Liuzzo et al., 1994; Urieli-Shoval et al., 2000). Moreover, the expression of SAA by several cell types within atherosclerotic lesions and the binding of SAA to HDL raise the possibility that it is involved in the pathogenesis of atherosclerosis (Benditt and Eriksen, 1977; Hoffman and Benditt, 1982; Meek et al., 1994). Together, this mounting evidence supports a renascent role for acute-phase proteins, particularly CRP and SAA, as promising predictors and indicators of chronic inflammatory diseases such as atherosclerotic cardiovascular disease. Future studies deciphering the pathogenic mechanisms of CRP and SAA are warranted for developing sensitive assays for early detection and implementing novel preventive/therapeutic interventions of cardiovascular and, perhaps, other yet-to-be-defined, diseases of inflammation and immunity.

ACKNOWLEDGEMENTS

We thank Dr Janice M. Sabatine for expert editorial assistance and Jason Brickner for skilled graphic assistance.

REFERENCES

Akira, S., Taga, T. and Kishimoto, T. (1993). Interleukin-6 in biology and medicine. Adv Immunol 54, 1–78.

Aldo-Benson, M.A. and Benson, M.D. (1982). SAA suppression of immune response in vitro: evidence for an effect on T cell-macrophage interaction. J Immunol 128, 2390–2392.

Andrade, F., Casciola-Rosen, L. and Rosen, A. (2000). Apoptosis in systemic lupus erythematosus. Clinical implications. Rheum Dis Clin North Am 26, 215–217.

Badolato, R., Wang, J.M., Murphy, W.J. et al. (1994). Serum amyloid A is a chemoattractant: induction of migration, adhesion, and tissue infiltration of monocytes and polymorphonuclear leukocytes. J Exp Med 180, 203–209.

Banka, C.L., Yuan, T., de Beer, M.C., Kindy, M., Curtiss, L.K. and de Beer, F.C. (1995). Serum amyloid A (SAA): influence on HDL-mediated cellular cholesterol efflux. J Lipid Res 36, 1058–1065.

Barna, B.P., James, K. and Deodhar, S.D. (1987). Activation of human monocyte tumoricidal activity by C-reactive protein. Cancer Res 47, 3959–3963.

Baumann, H. and Gauldie, J. (1994). The acute phase response. Immunol Today 15, 74–80.

Benditt, E.P. and Eriksen, N. (1966). Amyloid. 3. A protein related to the subunit structure of human amyloid fibrils. Proc Natl Acad Sci USA 55, 308–316.

Benditt, E.P. and Eriksen, N. (1977). Amyloid protein SAA is associated with high density lipoprotein from human serum. Proc Natl Acad Sci USA 74, 4025–4028.

Benson, M.D. and Aldo-Benson, M.A. (1982). SAA suppression of in vitro antibody response. Ann NY Acad Sci 389, 121–125.

Berk, B.C., Weintraub, W.S. and Alexander, R.W. (1990). Elevation of C-reactive protein in 'active' coronary artery disease. Am J Cardiol 65, 168–172.

Berman, S., Gewurz, H. and Mold, C. (1986). Binding of C-reactive protein to nucleated cells leads to complement activation without cytolysis. J Immunol 136, 1354–1359.

Besedovsky, H., del Rey, A., Sorkin, E. and Dinarello, C.A. (1986). Immunoregulatory feedback between interleukin-1 and glucocorticoid hormones. Science 233, 652–654.

Bharadwaj, D., Stein, M.P., Volzer, M., Mold, C. and Du Clos, T.W. (1999). The major receptor for C-reactive protein on leukocytes is fcgamma receptor II. J Exp Med 190, 585–590.

Biasucci, L.M., Vitelli, A., Liuzzo, G. et al. (1996). Elevated levels of interleukin-6 in unstable angina. Circulation 94, 874–877.

Campos, S.P. and Baumann, H. (1992). Insulin is a prominent modulator of the cytokine-stimulated expression of acute-phase plasma protein genes. Mol Cell Biol 12, 1789–1797.

Coetzee, G.A., Strachan, A.F., van der Westhuyzen, D.R., Hoppe, H.C., Jeenah, M.S. and de Beer, F.C. (1986). Serum amyloid A-containing human high density lipoprotein 3. Density, size, and apolipoprotein composition. J Biol Chem 261, 9644–9651.

Colley, C.M., Fleck, A., Goode, A.W., Muller, B.R. and Myers, M.A. (1983). Early time course of the acute phase protein response in man. J Clin Pathol 36, 203–207.

de Beer, F.C., Hind, C.R., Fox, K.M., Allan, R.M., Maseri, A. and Pepys, M.B. (1982). Measurement of serum C-reactive protein concentration in myocardial ischaemia and infarction. Br Heart J 47, 239–243.

Dinarello, C.A., Cannon, J.G. and Wolff, S.M. (1988). New concepts on the pathogenesis of fever. Rev Infect Dis 10, 168–189.

Du Clos, T.W., Zlock, L.T. and Rubin, R.L. (1988). Analysis of the binding of C-reactive protein to histones and chromatin. J Immunol 141, 4266–4270.

Fahraeus, R. (1921). The suspension-stability of the blood. Acta Med Scand 55, 1–288.

Ferreiros, E.R., Boissonnet, C.P., Pizarro, R. et al. (1999). Independent prognostic value of elevated C-reactive protein in unstable angina. Circulation 100, 1958–1963.

Fu, T. and Borensztajn, J. (2002). Macrophage uptake of low-density lipoprotein bound to aggregated C-reactive protein: possible mechanism of foam-cell formation in atherosclerotic lesions. Biochem J 366, 195–201.

Gabay, C. and Kushner, I. (1999). Acute-phase proteins and other systemic responses to inflammation. N Engl J Med 340, 448–454.

Galve-de Rochemonteix, B., Wiktorowicz, K., Kushner, I. and Dayer, J.M. (1993). C-reactive protein increases production of IL-1 alpha, IL-1 beta, and TNF-alpha, and expression of mRNA by human alveolar macrophages. J Leukoc Biol 53, 439–445.

Ganapathi, M.K., Rzewnicki, D., Samols, D., Jiang, S.L. and Kushner, I. (1991). Effect of combinations of cytokines and hormones on synthesis of serum amyloid A and C-reactive protein in Hep 3B cells. J Immunol 147, 1261–1265.

Gauldie, J., Richards, C., Harnish, D., Lansdorp, P. and Baumann, H. (1987). Interferon beta 2/B-cell stimulatory factor type 2 shares identity with monocyte-derived hepatocyte-stimulating factor and regulates the major acute phase protein response in liver cells. Proc Natl Acad Sci USA 84, 7251–7255.

Gershov, D., Kim, S., Brot, N. and Elkon, K.B. (2000). C-Reactive protein binds to apoptotic cells, protects the cells from assembly of the terminal complement components, and sustains an antiinflammatory innate immune response: implications for systemic autoimmunity. J Exp Med 192, 1353–1364.

Griselli, M., Herbert, J., Hutchinson, W.L. et al. (1999). C-reactive protein and complement are important mediators of tissue damage in acute myocardial infarction. J Exp Med 190, 1733–1740.

Gronroos, J.M. and Gronroos, P. (1999). Leucocyte count and C-reactive protein in the diagnosis of acute appendicitis. Br J Surg 86, 501–504.

Harris, T.B., Ferrucci, L., Tracy, R.P. et al. (1999). Associations of elevated interleukin-6 and C-reactive protein levels with mortality in the elderly. Am J Med 106, 506–512.

Haverkate, F., Thompson, S.G., Pyke, S.D., Gallimore, J.R. and Pepys, M.B. (1997). Production of C-reactive protein and risk of coronary events in stable and unstable angina. European Concerted Action on Thrombosis and Disabilities Angina Pectoris Study Group. Lancet 349, 462–466.

Hoffman, J.S. and Benditt, E.P. (1982). Secretion of serum amyloid protein and assembly of serum amyloid protein-rich high density lipoprotein in primary mouse hepatocyte culture. J Biol Chem 257, 10518–10522.

Jiang, S.L., Lozanski, G., Samols, D. and Kushner, I. (1995). Induction of human serum amyloid A in Hep 3B cells by IL-6 and IL-1 beta involves both transcriptional and post-transcriptional mechanisms. J Immunol 154, 825–831.

Jones, S.A., Novick, D., Horiuchi, S., Yamamoto, N., Szalai, A.J. and Fuller, G.M. (1999). C-reactive protein: a physiological activator of interleukin 6 receptor shedding. J Exp Med 189, 599–604.

Kaplan, M.H. and Volanakis, J.E. (1974). Interaction of C-reactive protein complexes with the complement system. I. Consumption of human complement associated with the reaction of C-reactive protein with pneumococcal C-polysaccharide and with the choline phosphatides, lecithin and sphingomyelin. J Immunol 112, 2135–2147.

Kapyaho, K., Welin, M.G., Tanner, P., Karkkainen, T. and Weber, T. (1989). Rapid determination of C-reactive protein by enzyme immunoassay using two monoclonal antibodies. Scand J Clin Lab Invest 49, 389–393.

Kisilevsky, R. and Subrahmanyan, L. (1992). Serum amyloid A changes high density lipoprotein's cellular affinity. A clue to serum amyloid A's principal function. Lab Invest 66, 778–785.

Koenig, W., Sund, M., Frohlich, M. et al. (1999). C-Reactive protein, a sensitive marker of inflammation, predicts future risk of coronary heart disease in initially healthy middle-aged men: results from the MONICA (Monitoring Trends and Determinants in Cardiovascular Disease) Augsburg Cohort Study, 1984 to 1992. Circulation 99, 237–242.

Kopf, M., Baumann, H., Freer, G. et al. (1994). Impaired immune and acute-phase responses in interleukin-6-deficient mice. Nature 368, 339–342.

Kuller, L.H., Tracy, R.P., Shaten, J. and Meilahn, E.N. (1996). Relation of C-reactive protein and coronary heart disease in the MRFIT nested case-control study. Multiple Risk Factor Intervention Trial. Am J Epidemiol 144, 537–547.

Kushner, I. (1991). C-reactive protein in rheumatology. Arthritis Rheum 34, 1065–1068.

Lagrand, W.K., Niessen, H.W., Wolbink, G.J. et al. (1997). C-reactive protein colocalizes with complement in human hearts during acute myocardial infarction. Circulation 95, 97–103.

Ledue, T.B., Weiner, D.L., Sipe, J.D., Poulin, S.E., Collins, M.F., and Rifai, N. (1998). Analytical evaluation of particle-enhanced immunonephelometric assays for C-reactive protein, serum amyloid A and mannose-binding protein in human serum. Ann Clin Biochem 35 (Pt 6), 745–753.

Libby, P. (2002). Inflammation in atherosclerosis. Nature 420, 868–874.

Lindahl, B., Toss, H., Siegbahn, A., Venge, P. and Wallentin, L. (2000). Markers of myocardial damage and inflammation in relation to long-term mortality in unstable coronary artery disease. FRISC Study Group. Fragmin during Instability in Coronary Artery Disease. N Engl J Med 343, 1139–1147.

Linke, R.P., Bock, V., Valet, G. and Rothe, G. (1991). Inhibition of the oxidative burst response of N-formyl peptide-stimulated neutrophils by serum amyloid-A protein. Biochem Biophys Res Commun 176, 1100–1105.

Liu, C.-C., Navratil, J.S., Sabatine, J.M. and Ahearn, J.M. (2003). Apoptosis, Complement, and SLE: A mechanistic view. Curr Dir of Autoimmun. In press. 7, 49–86.

Liuzzo, G., Biasucci, L.M., Gallimore, J.R. et al. (1994). The prognostic value of C-reactive protein and serum amyloid, a protein in severe unstable angina. N Engl J Med 331, 417–424.

Macintyre, S.S., Kushner, I. and Samols, D. (1985). Secretion of C-reactive protein becomes more efficient during the course of the acute phase response. J Biol Chem 260, 4169–4173.

Mackiewicz, A., Ganapathi, M.K., Schultz, D. et al. (1990). Transforming growth factor beta 1 regulates production of acute-phase proteins. Proc Natl Acad Sci USA 87, 1491–1495.

MacLeod, C.M. and Avery, O.T. (1941). The occurrence during acute infections of a protein not normally present in the blood. III. Immunological propertities of the C-reacitve protein and its differentiation from normal blood proteins. J Exp Med 85, 491–498.

Malle, E., Steinmetz, A. and Raynes, J.G. (1993). Serum amyloid A (SAA): an acute phase protein and apolipoprotein. Atherosclerosis 102, 131–146.

Marnell, L.L., Mold, C., Volzer, M.A., Burlingame, R.W. and Du Clos, T.W. (1995). C-reactive protein binds to Fc gamma RI in transfected COS cells. J Immunol 155, 2185–2193.

Meek, R.L. and Benditt, E.P. (1986). Amyloid A gene family expression in different mouse tissues. J Exp Med 164, 2006–2017.

Meek, R.L., Urieli-Shoval, S. and Benditt, E.P. (1994). Expression of apolipoprotein serum amyloid A mRNA in human atherosclerotic lesions and cultured vascular cells: implications for serum amyloid A function. Proc Natl Acad Sci USA 91, 3186–3190.

Migita, K., Kawabe, Y., Tominaga, M., Origuchi, T., Aoyagi, T. and Eguchi, K. (1998). Serum amyloid A protein induces production of matrix metalloproteinases by human synovial fibroblasts. Lab Invest 78, 535–539.

Miller, P.R., Munn, D.D., Meredith, J.W. and Chang, M.C. (1999). Systemic inflammatory response syndrome in the trauma intensive care unit: who is infected? J Trauma 47, 1004–1008.

Mold, C., Gewurz, H. and Du Clos, T.W. (1999). Regulation of complement activation by C-reactive protein. Immunopharmacology 42, 23–30.

Mold, C., Kingzette, M. and Gewurz, H. (1984). C-reactive protein inhibits pneumococcal activation of the alternative pathway by increasing the interaction between factor H and C3b. J Immunol 133, 882–885.

Morley, J.J. and Kushner, I. (1982). Serum C-reactive protein levels in disease. Ann NY Acad Sci 389, 406–418.

Morrow, D.A., Rifai, N., Antman, E.M. et al. (1998). C-reactive protein is a potent predictor of mortality independently of and in combination with troponin T in acute coronary syndromes: a TIMI 11A substudy. Thrombolysis in Myocardial Infarction. J Am Coll Cardiol 31, 1460–1465.

Mustard, R.A. Jr, Bohnen, .M., Haseeb, S. and Kasina, R. (1987). C-reactive protein levels predict postoperative septic complications. Arch Surg 122, 69–73.

Nakagomi, A., Freedman, S.B. and Geczy, C.L. (2000). Interferon-gamma and lipopolysaccharide potentiate monocyte tissue factor induction by C-reactive protein: relationship with age, sex, and hormone replacement treatment. Circulation 101, 1785–1791.

Pasceri, V., Cheng, J.S., Willerson, J.T., Yeh, E.T. and Chang, J. (2001). Modulation of C-reactive protein-mediated monocyte chemoattractant protein-1 induction in human endothelial cells by anti-atherosclerosis drugs. Circulation 103, 2531–2534.

Patel, H., Fellowes, R., Coade, S. and Woo, P. (1998). Human serum amyloid A has cytokine-like properties. Scand J Immunol 48, 410–418.

Pepys, M.B., Booth, S.E., Tennent, G.A., Butler, P.J. and Williams, D.G. (1994). Binding of pentraxins to different nuclear structures: C-reactive protein binds to small nuclear ribonucleoprotein particles, serum amyloid P component binds to chromatin and nucleoli. Clin Exp Immunol 97, 152–157.

Pepys, M.B., Lanham, J.G. and de Beer, F.C. (1982). C-reactive protein in SLE. Clin Rheum Dis 8, 91–103.

Ridker, P.M. (1999). Evaluating novel cardiovascular risk factors: can we better predict heart attacks? Ann Intern Med 130, 933–937.

Ridker, P.M., Buring, J.E., Shih, J., Matias, M. and Hennekens, C.H. (1998c). Prospective study of C-reactive protein and the risk of future cardiovascular events among apparently healthy women. Circulation 98, 731–733.

Ridker, P.M., Cushman, M., Stampfer, M.J., Tracy, R.P. and Hennekens, C.H. (1997). Inflammation, aspirin, and the risk of cardiovascular disease in apparently healthy men. N Engl J Med 336, 973–979.

Ridker, P.M., Cushman, M., Stampfer, M.J., Tracy, R.P. and Hennekens, C.H. (1998a). Plasma concentration of C-reactive protein and risk of developing peripheral vascular disease. Circulation 97, 425–428.

Ridker, P.M., Glynn, R.J. and Hennekens, C.H. (1998b). C-reactive protein adds to the predictive value of total and HDL cholesterol in determining risk of first myocardial infarction. Circulation 97, 2007–2011.

Ridker, P.M., Hennekens, C.H., Buring, J.E. and Rifai, N. (2000). C-reactive protein and other markers of inflammation in the prediction of cardiovascular disease in women. N Engl J Med 342, 836–843.

Ridker, P.M., Rifai, N., Rose, L., Buring, J.E. and Cook, N.R. (2002). Comparison of C-reactive protein and low-density lipoprotein cholesterol levels in the prediction of first cardiovascular events. N Engl J Med 347, 1557–1565.

Rifai, N. and Ridker, P.M. (2001). High-sensitivity C-reactive protein: a novel and promising marker of coronary heart disease. Clin Chem 47, 403–411.

Robey, F.A., Jones, K.D., Tanaka, T. and Liu, T.Y. (1984). Binding of C-reactive protein to chromatin and nucleosome core particles. A possible physiological role of C-reactive protein. J Biol Chem 259, 7311–7316.

Ross, R. (1999). Atherosclerosis – an inflammatory disease. N Engl J Med 340, 115–126.

Saadeh, C. (1998). The erythrocyte sedimentation rate: old and new clinical applications. South Med J 91, 220–225.

Sox, H.C. Jr. and Liang, M.H. (1986). The erythrocyte sedimentation rate. Guidelines for rational use. Ann Intern Med 104, 515–523.

Steel, D.M. and Whitehead, A.S. (1994). The major acute phase reactants: C-reactive protein, serum amyloid P component and serum amyloid A protein. Immunol Today 15, 81–88.

Steinmetz, A., Hocke, G., Saile, R., Puchois, P. and Fruchart, J.C. (1989). Influence of serum amyloid A on cholesterol esterification in human plasma. Biochim Biophys Acta 1006, 173–178.

Strachan, A.F., Noakes, T.D., Kotzenberg, G., Nel, A.E. and de Beer, F.C. (1984). C reactive protein concentrations during long distance running. Br Med J (Clin Res Ed) 289, 1249–1251.

Su, S.B., Gong, W., Gao, J.L. et al. (1999). A seven-transmembrane, G protein-coupled receptor, FPRL1, mediates the chemotactic activity of serum amyloid A for human phagocytic cells. J Exp Med 189, 395–402.

Taga, T. and Kishimoto, T. (1997). Gp130 and the interleukin-6 family of cytokines. Annu Rev Immunol 15, 797–819.

Tillett, W. S. and Francis, T. Jr (1930). Serological reactions in pneumonia with non-protein somatic fraction of pneumococcus. J Exp Med 52, 561–571.

Torzewski, J., Torzewski, M., Bowyer, D.E. et al. (1998). C-reactive protein frequently colocalizes with the terminal complement complex in the intima of early atherosclerotic lesions of human coronary arteries. Arterioscler Thromb Vasc Biol 18, 1386–1392.

Torzewski, M., Rist, C., Mortensen, R.F. et al. (2000). C-reactive protein in the arterial intima: role of C-reactive protein receptor-dependent monocyte recruitment in atherogenesis. Arterioscler Thromb Vasc Biol 20, 2094–2099.

Toss, H., Lindahl, B., Siegbahn, A. and Wallentin, L. (1997). Prognostic influence of increased fibrinogen and C-reactive protein levels in unstable coronary artery disease. FRISC Study Group. Fragmin during Instability in Coronary Artery Disease. Circulation 96, 4204–4210.

Tracy, R.P., Lemaitre, R.N., Psaty, B.M. et al. (1997). Relationship of C-reactive protein to risk of cardiovascular disease in the elderly. Results from the Cardiovascular Health Study and the Rural Health Promotion Project. Arterioscler Thromb Vasc Biol 17, 1121–1127.

Uhlar, C.M., Burgess, C.J., Sharp, P.M. and Whitehead, A.S. (1994). Evolution of the serum amyloid A (SAA) protein super-family. Genomics 19, 228–235.

Uhlar, C.M. and Whitehead, A.S. (1999). Serum amyloid A, the major vertebrate acute-phase reactant. Eur J Biochem 265, 501–523.

Urieli-Shoval, S., Linke, R.P. and Matzner, Y. (2000). Expression and function of serum amyloid A, a major acute-phase protein, in normal and disease states. Curr Opin Hematol 7, 64–69.

Volanakis, J.E. (1982). Complement activation by C-reactive protein complexes. Ann NY Acad Sci 389, 235–250.

Volanakis, J.E. (2001). Human C-reactive protein: expression, structure, and function. Mol Immunol 38, 189–197.

Wilkins, J., Gallimore, J.R., Moore, E.G. and Pepys, M.B. (1998). Rapid automated high sensitivity enzyme immunoassay of C-reactive protein. Clin Chem 44, 1358–1361.

Yamada, T. (1999). Serum amyloid A (SAA): a concise review of biology, assay methods and clinical usefulness. Clin Chem Lab Med 37, 381–388.

Zheng, H., Fletcher, D., Kozak, W. et al. (1995). Resistance to fever induction and impaired acute-phase response in inter-leukin-1 beta-deficient mice. Immunity 3, 9–19.

Zimlichman, S., Danon, A., Nathan, I., Mozes, G. and Shainkin-Kestenbaum, R. (1990). Serum amyloid A, an acute phase pro-tein, inhibits platelet activation. J Lab Clin Med 116, 180–186.

Zimmerman, M.A., Selzman, C.H., Cothren, C., Sorensen, A.C., Raeburn, C.D. and Harken, A.H. (2003). Diagnostic implica-tions of C-reactive protein. Arch Surg 138, 220–224.

Zwaka, T.P., Hombach, V. and Torzewski, J. (2001). C-reactive protein-mediated low density lipoprotein uptake by macrophages: implications for atherosclerosis. Circulation 103, 1194–1197.

Complement in Health and Disease

Chapter 11

Chau-Ching Liu and Joseph M. Ahearn

*Division of Rheumatology and Clinical Immunology, Department of Medicine,
University of Pittsburgh School of Medicine, Lupus Center of Excellence
University of Pittsburgh Schools of Health Sciences, Pittsburgh, PA, USA*

Discovery consists in seeing what everyone else has seen
and in thinking what no one else has thought.

Albert Szent-Györgi, 1937 Nobel Prize in Physiology or
Medicine

HISTORICAL OVERVIEW

Although its name may imply an ancillary role in immunity,
the complement system is indeed a vital component of
host defense. Incidentally, the discovery and research of
such an important system intertwine with the development of modern immunology and coincide with the revolution in biochemical as well as molecular biological
technology (Ross, 1986; Frank, 1998).

Investigation of complement originated during the
nascence of microbiology in the second half of the nineteenth century. In the 1870s, investigators first observed
that bacteria injected into the circulation were rapidly
destroyed and cleared from the bloodstream. Nuttall,
Buchner, Bordet, and others later discovered that cell-
free serum was capable of killing bacteria (Nuttall, 1888;
Buchner, 1889; Bordet, 1909). The bactericidal activity was
found to be mediated by a heat-labile fraction with non-
specific activity (now known to be complement) and a
heat-stable component with antigen specificity (now
known to be antibodies). Buchner named the heat-labile
bactericidal factors 'alexins' (*alexis* – Greek word meaning
'to ward off or protect') and proposed an enzymatic
action for them. Subsequently, Bordet made several

important observations, which later won him a Nobel
Prize, demonstrating that lysis of erythrocytes sensitized by immune sera was similarly mediated by those
heat-labile and heat-stable factors (Bordet, 1909).

In 1899, the term 'complement', which soon replaced
alexins, was introduced by Ehrlich as a part of his 'side-
chain' theory to emphasize the fact that the heat-labile
factors present in fresh serum 'complemented' the heat-
stable specific factors in mediating immune bacteriolysis
and hemolysis (Ehrlich, 1899). At that time, there was substantial debate over whether complement was a group of
factors or a uniform substance. Protein biochemistry studies conducted in the early 1900s soon began to provide
some answers. Since then, laborious studies by many
investigators have established that complement is not a
single substance but consists of multiple proteins. By the
1920s, it was thought that complement consisted of at
least three factors, which were later identified as C1, C2 and
C4. However, the currently accepted order of complement
components in the classical pathway was not established
until 1938 when Ueno described a cellular intermediate
consisting of erythrocytes, antibody, C1, C4 and a certain
'endpiece' (Frank, 1998). The then-elusive endpiece was
still thought to be a single factor. By the late 1950s, Mayer
and colleagues proposed a mathematical model of complement action that suggested the final component,
termed C3, might actually be a multi-factor component
(Levine et al., 1954; Rapp, 1958). During the 1960s and
1970s, investigators in the laboratories of Nelson (Nelson
et al., 1966), Muller-Eberhard (Muller-Eberhard, 1975),

*Measuring Immunity, edited by Michael T. Lotze and Angus W. Thomson
ISBN 0-12-455900-X, London*

and others (Klein and Wellensieck, 1965) separated and characterized these components that are now known as C3, C5, C6, C7, C8 and C9.

In parallel with the much-noticed studies on antibody-dependent activation of complement, Pillemer and colleagues made a series of observations in the 1940s and 1950s that eventually led to the discovery of the alternative pathway of complement activation. While studying the ability of zymosan, an insoluble glycoprotein of baker's yeast, to interact with serum factors, they observed that the zymosan particles could bind the 'classical C3' (now understood to be the late complement components) but spared the early components (i.e. C1, C2 and C4) (Pillemer et al., 1953). In 1954, Pillemer hypothesized that zymosan interacts with a previously unknown serum protein named 'properdin' (Latin for 'destruction-bringing') and mediates activation of C3 in an antibody-independent fashion (Pillemer et al., 1954). Pillemer further proposed that several co-factors, which he named properdin factor A and properdin factor B, are needed for this mode of complement activation. Although criticized and neglected at the time, this hypothetical model was later corroborated by other investigators and proven to be a second complement activation pathway that does not depend on antibodies.

Mayer and colleagues originally hypothesized a 'one-hit' theory to explain complement-mediated cell lysis (Mayer, 1961a). This model proposed that one 'donut' lesion consisting of all complement components present in the surface membrane of an erythrocyte can destabilize the osmotic equilibrium and cause cell lysis. This hypothetical model was validated in the 1960s when Dourmashkin and Humphrey used electron microscopy to identify complement 'donut' (or 'pore') lesions on erythrocytes (Borsos et al., 1964; Humphry and Dourmashkin, 1969). Subsequent biochemical studies, conducted primarily by the Muller-Eberhard group (Muller-Eberhard, 1986) and the Bhakdi group (Bhakdi and Tranum-Jensen, 1983), demonstrated that such pore structures, now known as 'membrane attack complexes', consist of one molecule each of C5, C6, C7, C8 and multiple (from 1 up to 16) C9 molecules. By the late 1960s and throughout the1970s and 1980s, the biochemical nature of complement was nearly resolved and research in complement genes was rapidly progressing. Consequently, significant investigative efforts were geared toward delineating the biological functions and regulatory mechanisms of complement. As a result, an unexpectedly large number of regulatory proteins and receptors have been identified and characterized (reviewed by Ross and Atkinson, 1985; Carroll, 1998). These studies have laid a solid foundation for our understanding of complement in health and disease.

The complement system is far more complex than one would have imagined for an 'ancillary' component of immunity. A third activation pathway, the lectin pathway, was discovered in the 1990s and has not yet been fully characterized (reviewed by Wallis, 2002; Turner, 2004).

Undoubtedly, many previously unrecognized functions of complement are yet to be discovered. Despite considerable advances in complement research since its discovery more than 100 years ago, we are only in the early stages of investigating the involvement of complement in clinical diseases as diverse as systemic lupus erythematosus, atherosclerosis and Alzheimer's disease. Important insights into the roles of complement in disease may be obtained from patients deficient in any of the complement components. However, such cases are rare. Since the 1990s, advances in gene knock-out techniques have created an unprecedented opportunity to evaluate the pathophysiologic relevance of complement using highly sophisticated animal models (Holers, 2000; Linton, 2001).

Equipped with a wealth of information accumulated over the past one and half centuries and an armory of sophisticated techniques, investigators are now poised to elucidate the role of complement in numerous diseases, to evaluate its utility as biomarkers of disease and to explore the potential of novel therapeutic approaches targeting the complement system. In this chapter, we will review briefly the biology and roles of complement in health and disease, describe traditional methods for complement measurement and discuss recent advances for measuring the state of complement activation in vivo. We will conclude this chapter by discussing, in perspective, the great potential of the complement system to provide valuable biomarkers for inflammatory diseases. For information pertaining specifically to systemic lupus erythematosus (SLE), the prototypic complement-involving autoimmune disorder, readers are encouraged to consult the Chapter 44 on SLE associated tests later in this book.

BIOLOGY OF THE COMPLEMENT SYSTEM

The complement system comprises more than 30 plasma and membrane-bound proteins that form three distinct pathways (classical, alternative and lectin) designed to protect against invading pathogens (Figure 11.1). Many of the complement proteins exist in plasma as functionally inactive pro-proteins until appropriate events trigger their activation. Once activated, the proteins within each pathway undergo a cascade of sequential serine protease-mediated cleavage events, release biologically active fragments and self-assemble into multi-molecular complexes. This activation process is a series of enzymatic reactions in which each enzyme (complement) molecule generated at one step can generate multiple enzyme (complement) molecules at the next step, thus allowing for tremendous amplification of activated molecules. In general, the activation of the complement system can be viewed as a two-stage process. The first stage, unique to each of the three activation pathways, involves the 'early' complement components that lead to the formation of the so-called 'C3 convertases'. The second stage, common to all three pathways once they

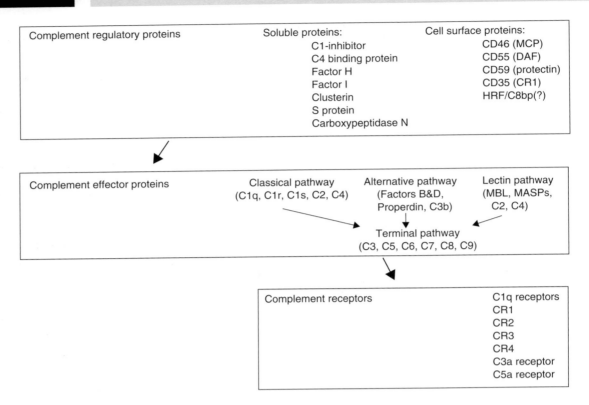

Figure 11.1 The complement system.

converge, results in the formation of a lytic complex consisting of the 'terminal' complement components. In humans and other mammals, the complement system is controlled by many regulatory proteins to ensure that this effective machinery does not become overactive and inflict undesirable inflammatory reactions on the host (Table 11.1).

Complement activation pathways

The classical pathway of complement activation is responsible for executing a major effector mechanism of antibody-mediated immune responses. There are five proteins specific to activation of the classical pathway: C1q, C1r, C1s, C4 and C2 (see Figure 11.1). Activation of this pathway begins when C1q binds to the Fc portion of IgG (particularly IgG1 and IgG3) or IgM molecules that are bound to an antigen. The binding of C1q to an antigen–antibody complex (immune complex) leads to activation of C1r (a serine protease) which, in turn, leads to activation of C1s (also a serine protease). C1s enzymatically cleaves the other two classical pathway proteins, C4 and C2, generating and releasing two small soluble polypeptides, C4a and C2b. At the same time, this proteolytic cleavage leads to the formation of a surface-bound bimolecular complex, C4b2a, which functions as an enzyme and is referred to as the classical pathway C3 convertase. It should be noted that in addition to the conventionally accepted mode of activation triggered by antigen–antibody complexes, the classical pathway can

also be activated in an antibody-independent manner. Recent studies have shown that C1q is capable of interacting with a variety of non-immune substances such as C-reactive protein (Jiang et al., 1991), fibronectin, amyloid P component (Ying et al., 1993), β-amyloid protein (Rogers et al., 1992; Velazquez et al., 1997), neurofibrillary tangles (Shen et al., 2001) and molecules that have anionic charges such as DNA and lipopolysaccharides (Jiang et al., 1992). Most recently, C1q has also been shown to bind directly to surfaces of apoptotic cells (Korb and Ahearn, 1997; Navratil et al., 2001). As a result, these interactions can also initiate the complement activation cascade.

Unlike activation of the classical pathway, activation of the alternative pathway is not dependent on antibodies. Three plasma proteins are unique to the alternative pathway: factor B, factor D and properdin (see Figure 11.1). Normally, complement C3 undergoes a so-called 'C3 tick-over' process, a continuous, low-rate hydrolysis that generates C3b (Pangburn and Muller-Eberhard, 1983). A fraction of these spontaneously generated C3b molecules may covalently attach to the surface of microbial pathogens and host cells via thioester bonds. The bound C3b molecules are capable of binding factor B. Once bound, factor B is cleaved into Ba and Bb fragments by factor D (a serine protease). While the small, soluble Ba fragment diffuses away from the activation site, the Bb fragment remains associated with C3b. Similar to the C4b2a complex in the classical pathway, the surface-bound C3bBb complex serves as the alternative pathway

Table 11.1 Effector components and regulatory proteins of the human complement system

Effector proteins	Function /pathway involved	M_r (kD)
C1q	Recognition, binding/Classical	450 (a six-subunit bundle)
C1r	Serine protease/Classical	85
C1s	Serine protease/Classical	85
C4[a]	Serine protease (C4b); anaphylatoxin (C4a)/Classical	205 (a 3-chain, $\alpha\beta\gamma$, complex)
C2	Serine protease (C2a); small fragment with kinin-activity (C2b)/Classical	102
C3[b]	Membrane binding, opsonization (C3b); anaphylatoxin (C3a)/Terminal	190 (a 2-chain, $\alpha\beta$, complex)
C5	MAC component (C5b), anaphylatoxin (C5a)/Terminal	190 (a 2-chain, $\alpha\beta$, complex)
C6	MAC component/Terminal	110
C7	MAC component/Terminal	100
C8	MAC component/Terminal	150 (a 3-chain, $\alpha\beta\gamma$, complex)
C9	MAC component/Terminal	70
Factor B	Serine protease/Alternative	90
Factor D	Serine protease/Alternative	24
Properdin	Stabilizing C3bBb complexes/Alternative	55 (monomers) 110, 165, 220, or higher (oligomers)
MBL	Recognition, binding/Lectin	200–400 (2–4 subunits with three 32 kD chains each)
MASP-1	Serine protease/Lectin	100
MASP-2	Serine protease/Lectin	76

Regulatory protein	Function	M_r (kD)
C1-inhibitor (C1-INH)	Removing activated C1r and C1s from the C1 complex	105
C4-binding protein (C4bp)	Displacing C2b in the C4bC2b complex; cofactor for factor I	570 (a 7-subunit complex)
Factor H	Displacing Bb in the C3bBb complex; cofactor for factor I	160
Factor I	Serine protease cleaving C3b and C4b	88
Clusterin	Preventing insertion of soluble C5b–7 complexes into cell membranes	70
S protein (Vitronectin)	Preventing insertion of soluble C5b–7 complexes into cell membranes	84
Carboxypeptidase N	Inactivating anaphylatoxins	280 (a multi-subunit complex)
CD35 (CR1[c])	Binding C3b and C4b; cofactor for factor I	160–250 (4 isoforms)
CD46 (MCP[d])	Promoting C3b and C4b inactivation by factor I	45–70 (different glycosylation forms)
CD55 (DAF[e])	Accelerating decay of the C3bBb and C4b2a complexes	70
CD59 (Protectin; H19)	Preventing C9 incorporation into the MAC in a homologous restriction manner	18–20

[a] serum concentration range considered normal: 20–50 mg/dl.
[b] serum concentration range considered normal: 55–120 mg/dl.
[c] Complement receptor 1.
[d] Membrane cofactor protein.
[e] Decay accelerating factor.

C3 convertase. The C3bBb complexes, if bound to mammalian cells, will be rapidly degraded by several regulatory proteins, thereby preventing self-damage of the host cells and tissue. However, the C3bBb complexes associated with microbial pathogens, which do not express these regulatory proteins, will remain intact and can be further stabilized by the binding of properdin. Traditionally, the alternative pathway is studied *in vitro* using a variety of activators including zymosan, cobra venom factor, endotoxin and rabbit erythrocytes.

The lectin pathway shares several components with the classical pathway (see Figure 11.1). Initiation of the lectin pathway is mediated through the binding of mannose-binding lectin (MBL; also known as mannose-binding protein (MBP)) to a variety of repetitive carbohydrate moieties such as mannose, N-acetyl-D-glucosamine and N-acetyl-mannosamine, which are abundantly present on a variety of microorganisms (Wallis, 2002). MBL, a plasma protein composed of a collagen-like region and a carbohydrate-binding domain, is structurally similar to C1q. As in the case of the C1qC1rC1s complex, MBL forms complexes in the plasma with other proteins such as mannose-binding protein-associated serine proteases (MASPs, such as MASP-1, MASP-2 and MASP-3) and Map19 (Thiel et al., 1997; Gal and Ambrus, 2001; Dahl et al., 2001). Under physiological conditions, MBL does not bind to mammalian cells, probably because these cells lack mannose residues on their surface. Once bound to microbial pathogens, MASPs, particularly MASP-2 within the MBL complex, can cleave C4 and initiate the complement cascade. Alternatively, MBL, in place of C1q, may trigger the activation cascade by activating C1r and C1s. At this point, the lectin pathway intersects with the classical pathway and a C3 convertase, i.e. the C4b2a complex, is eventually generated.

C3 convertases, generated during the first stage of complement activation, cleave C3, the central and most abundant component of the complement system. This proteolytic cleavage gives rise to a smaller C3a fragment and a larger C3b fragment. Similar to C4a, C3a is a soluble polypeptide that diffuses away. C3b molecules, if not hydrolyzed and inactivated in the fluid phase, can bind covalently to the surface of microbial pathogens or to immune complexes initially responsible for activating the system. The C3b molecules associate with C4bC2a or C3bBb complexes to form the C5 convertase. The C5 convertase cleaves C5 and initiates activation and assembly of the terminal components, C5, C6, C7, C8 and C9, into the membrane attack complex (MAC) (C_{5b-9}; also called 'terminal complement complex (TCC)') on the surface of foreign pathogens.

Effector functions of complement

The complement system is traditionally thought to have four biological functions (Walport, 2001):

1 opsonization
2 activation of inflammation
3 clearance of immune complexes
4 osmotic lysis of invading microorganisms.

These functions are mediated by the soluble or surface-bound fragments of activated complement proteins (generally referred to as 'complement split products'), which in turn interact with specific membrane receptors expressed on various cell types.

The soluble proteolytic fragments, C3a, C4a and C5a, are small polypeptides (approximately 9–10 kD) and are highly potent proinflammatory molecules. They attract and activate leukocytes, by binding to specific receptors expressed on those cells. The larger fragments, C3b, C4b and their derivatives (e.g. iC3b and iC4b), can remain bound to the surface of microbial pathogens (opsonization) and facilitate recognition and uptake of the opsonized pathogens by phagocytic cells. This function is mediated through the binding of these complement-derived fragments to complement receptor (CR) 1 (for C3b and C4b), CR3 (for iC3b), and perhaps CR4 (for iC3b) expressed on phagocytes.

The binding of C4b and C3b to immune complexes prevents their aggregation into insoluble complexes and enhances their clearance. The clearance of C3b/C4b-opsonized immune complexes is believed to be mediated by erythrocytes that express CR1 and are capable of transporting immune complexes to macrophages of the reticuloendothelial system in the spleen and liver (Schifferli, 1986). Finally, the C_{5b-9} MACs may perturb the osmotic equilibrium and/or disrupt the integrity of the surface membrane of target cells, thereby causing lysis of these cells. Interestingly, on nucleated cells, sublytic levels of MACs can instead stimulate cellular activities including Ca^{2+} influx, activation of phospholipases and protein kinases and production of proinflammatory cytokines and arachidonic acid-derived mediators (Imagawa et al., 1983; Wiedmer et al., 1987; Morgan, 1989).

For several decades, the role of the complement system was thought to be limited to these four effector functions. However, there has been a recent explosion in discovery of additional roles for complement, particularly in linking the innate and acquired immune responses. For example, we (Korb and Ahearn, 1997; Navratil et al., 2001) and others (Mevorach et al., 1998; Nauta et al., 2002) have recently shown that C1q can bind directly to keratinocytes, endothelial cells and monocytes that are undergoing apoptosis and this binding can subsequently trigger activation and deposition of C4 and C3 on these apoptotic cells. Thus, apoptotic cells and blebs become opsonized and can be effectively taken up by phagocytic cells via a complement receptor-mediated mechanism (Mevorach et al., 1998; Nauta et al., 2002). Accumulation of apoptotic bodies in the kidneys and delayed removal of apoptotic cells from the peritoneal cavity of C1q-knockout mice have been reported. Moreover, mice deficient in C1q or C4 have been shown to develop autoimmune responses to nuclear autoantigens. Taken together, these studies strongly suggest that complement is involved in facilitating the clearance of autoantigen-containing apoptotic bodies and therefore plays a pivotal role in maintaining immune tolerance (Pickering et al., 2000; Liu et al., 2004a).

Complement – an important bridge between innate immunity and adaptive immunity

An increasing number of studies have shown that innate immunity and adaptive immunity, the two arms of the immune system, collaborate in an intricate way to elicit efficient immune responses against infectious agents (Fearon and Locksley, 1996; Carroll, 1998). The complement system, particularly C3, its derivative fragments and their cognate receptors, plays an important role in this collaboration. Most effector cell types crucial for mounting effective immune responses are known to express receptors specific for complement components and derivatives. For example, phagocytic cells (e.g. neutrophils and macrophages) and antigen-presenting cells (e.g. dendritic cells and macrophages) express CR3 and CR4 on their surface. These receptors bind iC3b and possibly iC4b. B cells and follicular dendritic cells express CR2, the major receptor for C3d (Fang et al., 1998; Carroll, 2000). There are several ways whereby complement serves as a bridge between innate immunity and adaptive immunity. First, antigens (and immune complexes) decorated with C3d, the end cleavage product of C3 and a major ligand for CR2, are capable of cross-linking the B cell receptors to the CR2/CD19/TAPA-1 co-receptor complexes and thus facilitating B cell activation and enhancing humoral immune responses (Fearon and Carter, 1995). Second, antigens (and immune complexes) opsonized by C3 can be retained in the germinal centers of secondary lymphoid follicles via binding to CR2-expressing follicular dendritic cells (Fang et al., 1998); the retained antigens provide essential signals for survival and affinity maturation of B cells as well as for generation of memory B cells (Fischer et al., 1998). Third, opsonization of pathogens by complement components facilitates their uptake by phagocytes and antigen-presenting cells and thus may enhance presentation of antigens and initiation of specific immune responses. Fourth, complement activation products generated at sites of infection can recruit inflammatory cells and immune effector cells to help eliminate pathogenic antigens.

COMPLEMENT AND DISEASE

The versatile function and ubiquitous presence of complement in immune/inflammatory responses dictate its double-edged nature. Complement is important for host defense against infectious pathogens and invading foreign cells. At times, however, over-zealous activation of the complement system can cause tissue damage associated with many clinical situations. Furthermore, deficiencies of complement components are associated with a number of clinical disorders.

Complement and inflammatory diseases

Complement is involved in virtually all clinical conditions associated with inflammation. Prominent among these conditions are acute infections, sepsis and immune complex disorders. Other clinical conditions with well-established complement-mediated pathogenesis include

Table 11.2 Clinical conditions in which complement-mediated injury is implicated*

Autoimmune disease	Systemic lupus erythematosus
	Rheumatoid arthritis
	Dermatomyositis
	Sjogren's syndrome
	Scleroderma
	Autoimmune hemolytic anemia
	Idiopathic thrombocytopenic purpura
	Multiple sclerosis
	Myasthenia gravis
	Autoimmune myocarditis
	Anti-phospholipid syndrome
	Vasculitis
Neurological disease	Alzheimer's disease
	Parkinson's disease
	Guillain-Barre syndrome
	Prion disease
Ischemia/reperfusion injury	Myocardial infarction
	Stroke
	Shock
Cardiovascular disease	Atherosclerosis
Miscellaneous	Paroxysmal nocturnal hematuria
	Serum sickness
	Transplant hyperacute rejection
	Acute respiratory distress syndrome
	Pre-eclampsia

* This table is not meant to be exclusive. Listed are representative examples.

ischemia/reperfusion injury during myocardial infarction, stroke and shock. Most recently, complement has been shown to play important roles in atherosclerotic cardiovascular disease and neurodegenerative diseases. Table 11.2 summarizes the broadening spectrum of clinical conditions involving complement-mediated tissue damage. We will briefly discuss a few representative clinical conditions.

Because the primary function of complement is to eliminate invading microorganisms and probably cell debris, tissue damage mediated by complement almost always occurs when the complement system is faithfully executing its physiologic function. Neutrophils, macrophages and other inflammatory cells recruited to the infected site may release large bursts of inflammatory mediators that can inadvertently damage surrounding cells and tissue. For example, during reperfusion of ischemic tissue, complement may be activated by ischemia-injured cells and inflict significant damage on surrounding cells and tissue. Profound activation of the complement system during bacterial sepsis undoubtedly also enhances secretion of cytokines and inflammatory mediators that in turn intensify local and systemic tissue damage.

Another major function of complement is to facilitate removal of antigen–antibody complexes. Immune complexes, if not solubilized and cleared properly, can form insoluble aggregates that deposit in various tissues. Activation of the complement system may ensue and cause damage to surrounding tissue. The kidneys, skin and vessels appear to be most susceptible to such pathogenesis. The resulting glomerulonephritis, rashes and vasculitis commonly occur in patients with immune complex diseases such as SLE.

Increasingly, it is thought that neurodegenerative disorders such as Alzheimer's disease (AD) are inflammatory in nature (Akiyama et al., 2000) and that complement mediates, at least in part, brain tissue damage characteristic of these diseases (McGeer and McGeer, 2002; Van Beek et al., 2003). This is suggested by the following observations:

1 epidemiological studies have shown that the use of anti-inflammatory agents, particularly certain non-steroidal anti-inflammatory drugs, significantly reduces the risk of developing AD and/or retards AD progression (McGeer et al., 1996)
2 histopathological studies have demonstrated that various complement components and split products localize in β-amyloid plaques and neurofibrillary tangles, hallmark lesions of AD and that MACs are associated with dystrophic neurites (Eikelenboom and Stam, 1982; Yasojima et al., 1999)
3 in vitro studies have shown that C1q can bind to β-amyloid and neurofibrillary tangles, activating the classical pathway in an antibody-independent manner (Rogers et al., 1992; Velazquez et al., 1997).

Collectively, these findings suggest complete activation of the complement cascade within the brains of AD patients. Together with other pathogenic factors, the complement system may exert detrimental effects and contribute to the inflammatory damage in the brain tissue of AD patients (McGeer and McGeer, 2002; Van Beek et al., 2003).

The involvement of complement in a wide variety of inflammatory diseases not only supports its pathogenic role, but also suggests that complement proteins in the circulation and in other body fluids (e.g. cerebrospinal fluid) may serve as a source of biological markers to guide disease management (Jongen et al., 2000). Moreover, the realization of the role of complement in inflammatory diseases has fostered a new research effort to modulate and/or prevent complement-mediated pathogenic mechanisms in conditions such as myocardial infarction and Alzheimer's disease.

Complement deficiency and disease

Complement deficiency in humans has been reported for almost every component of the complement system (Morgan and Walport, 1991; Barilla-LaBarca and Atkinson, 2003). Although the overall incidence of hereditary complement deficiency is low in the general population, a deficiency of any complement component is significantly associated with specific human diseases (Table 11.3). The clinical manifestations associated with the hereditary deficiency of individual complement components vary widely. Because complement deficiencies are inherited in an autosomal recessive fashion (except for C1-inhibitor deficiency) and may involve different mutations within a given

Table 11.3 Complement deficiencies and associated diseases

Deficient component	Associated diseases
C1	SLE[a,b]; bacterial infections
C2	SLE[a,b]; bacterial infections
C4	SLE[a,b]; bacterial infections
C3	Bacterial infections[c]
C5	Bacterial infections[c]
C6	Bacterial infections[c]
C7	Bacterial infections[c]
C8	Bacterial infections[c]
C9	Bacterial infections[c]
Properdin	Bacterial infections[c]
C1-inhibitor	Hereditary angioedema
MBL	Bacterial and viral infections

[a] predominant phenotype.
[b] risk hierarchy for developing SLE : C1 deficiency (~90%) > C4 deficiency (~75%) > C2 deficiency (~40%).
[c] most frequently infections with encapsulated bacteria, especially *Neisseria meningitidis*.

complement component gene, the severity of clinical manifestation in patients deficient in the same component may range from none to partial (heterozygous gene defects) to complete (homozygous gene defects).

Given the crucial role for complement in host defense, it is not surprising that complement deficiency predisposes an individual to infections. Most patients deficient in complement, particularly C3 and the terminal components, are susceptible to certain bacterial and viral agents, especially encapsulated bacteria such as *Neisseria meningitidis*. Interestingly, patients deficient in the early components of the classical pathway, C1, C4 and C2, are prone to develop autoimmune diseases such as SLE and Sjogren's syndrome (Ratnoff, 1996; Barilla-LaBarca and Atkinson, 2003). It has been postulated that this intriguing clinical association is due to impaired clearance of immune complexes and apoptotic cells in the absence of these early complement components. Increased susceptibility to infections and SLE has also been reported in patients with MBL deficiency (Turner, 2004).

Complement deficiencies may also be acquired. When complement is increasingly consumed during heightened active states of an underlying disease, acquired deficiencies can occur and usually involve multiple components simultaneously.

MEASUREMENT OF COMPLEMENT

During clinical inflammatory states in which complement activation occurs, complement proteins would presumably be consumed at a rate proportional to activity of the disease. Thus, measuring complement activation may be useful for diagnosing disease, assessing disease status and determining response to therapy. Measuring complement activity and individual component levels is also essential for detecting and diagnosing complement deficiency. Conventionally, the complement system is measured by one of two types of assays. Functional assays measure complement-mediated hemolytic activity: CH50 (indicative of the activity of the classical pathway) and APH50 (indicative of the activity of the alternative pathway). Immunochemical assays measure serum concentrations of individual complement components and their split products. A synopsis of commonly performed complement measurement assays, with special emphasis on the underlying principles and noteworthy precautions, will be provided in this section. For detailed protocols, readers are recommended to consult several recently published laboratory manuals (Shevach, 1994; Wurzner et al., 1997; Morgan, 2000).

Measurement of complement functional activity

Assays that measure complement-mediated hemolysis, such as the CH50 and APH50 assays, are simple quantitative tests for functional complement components in serum or other fluid samples. These assays depend on sequential activation of the classical pathway components (C1, C4 and C2) or alternative pathway components (properdin, factor B and factor D) followed by the terminal components (C3, C5, C6, C7, C8 and C9). Target erythrocytes are lysed when the resultant MACs are assembled and inserted into their plasma membranes (Mayer, 1961a, 1972). Complement activity is quantitated by determining the dilution of a serum (or other fluid sample) required to lyse 50 per cent of sheep erythrocytes sensitized with anti-sheep IgM (for CH50 assays) or unsensitized rabbit erythrocytes (for APH50 assays) under standard conditions. Hemolysis assays are often the first line of tests used to determine whether a patient is deficient in complement. However, since these assays measure the functional integrity of the complement system as a whole, abnormal results may reflect either the absence of any complement protein or the presence of a non-functional component. Additional tests are required to identify the missing or functionally abnormal component.

Functional hemolytic assay for total complement activity: CH50 and APH50

Because complement components are heat-labile, samples for complement assays should be handled with proper precautions. The functional hemolytic assays are routinely performed using serum. To prepare serum samples, blood should be drawn into a plain tube (avoiding tubes with 'serum separators' or 'clot activators'), allowed to clot at room temperature or 37°C for 30–60 min and separated by centrifugation. If not used immediately, serum samples should be stored at −70°C to optimize the preservation of complement proteins in functionally active forms.

Traditionally, limiting dilution assays are used to assess CH50 and APH50. A typical protocol for determining CH50 entails the following steps. A series of twofold dilutions of each serum sample should be prepared in ice-cold gelatin-veronal (barbitone) buffer containing Ca^{2+} and Mg^{2+} (GVB^{2+}). To prepare antibody-sensitized sheep erythrocytes (EA), sheep erythrocytes are washed sequentially with GVB containing EDTA (GVBE) and GVB^{2+}, resuspended in GVB^{2+}, mixed with rabbit antiserum containing anti-sheep erythrocyte IgM/G (commercially available), incubated for 15 min at 37°C, washed to remove unbound antibodies and resuspended in GVB^{2+}. The EA suspension is added to the diluted serum samples in equal volumes, mixed, incubated for 60 min at 37°C and the reaction mixtures are subsequently centrifuged. Hemoglobin released from the erythrocytes lysed during the incubation remains in the supernatant. Hemolysis is quantitated by measuring the optical density of hemoglobin in the supernatants by spectrophotometry. The dilution of serum capable of lysing 50 per cent of erythrocytes can be calculated using a probability plot, Kabat and Mayer plot, or other chosen method (Mayer, 1961b; Shevach, 1994; Wurzner et al., 1997; Morgan, 2000). The reciprocal of this dilution represents complement activity in Units/ml of serum. For example, if a 1:160 dilution of a serum sample lyses 50 per cent of erythrocytes, complement activity in that sample is reported as 160 CH50 U/ml.

To obtain reliable results, the proper controls should be included in each CH50 assay. A negative control containing erythrocytes in buffer alone will control for spontaneous lysis of erythrocytes, a positive control sample should contain fresh calibrated human serum and a total lysis control should be prepared using water to induce 100 per cent hemolysis. Although the CH50 assay is often performed in test tubes with analysis using spectrophotometry, alternative techniques have been used in various laboratories. These include blood agarose assays resembling the radial immunodiffusion (RID) assay, EIA (enzymatic immunoassays), ELISA (enzyme-linked immunosorbent assays) or microtiter plate-adapted spectrophotometric assays (Liu and Young, 1988; Shevach, 1994). The microtiter method is convenient when testing a large number of samples.

The APH50 assay is similar to the CH50 assay, with two modifications. First, because sheep erythrocytes are inefficient in activating the alternative pathway, unsensitized rabbit erythrocytes are used in this assay (Platts-Mills and Ishizaka, 1974). Second, since the classical pathway requires both Ca^{2+} and Mg^{2+} for activation but the alternative pathway requires only Mg^{2+}, EGTA (ethyleneglycol bis(β-aminoethyl ether)-N,N-tetraacetic acid), a chelator of Ca^{2+} but not of Mg^{2+}, is included in the assay buffer to permit activation of the alternative pathway but prevent concomitant activation of the classical pathway.

Functional hemolytic assay for individual complement components

The presence and functional activity of individual complement proteins can easily be examined using a modified

CH50 or APH50 assay. The modified limiting dilution assay is performed using a control serum containing an excess of all complement components except the one being tested for, a serially diluted test sample and EA (for C1–C9) or rabbit erythrocytes (for factor B and factor D). Human sera that are deficient in individual complement components can be obtained from commercial sources. Because erythrocytes are lysed only when the test sample contains the complement component missing from the control serum (i.e. the component being tested for), negative hemolysis indicates a deficiency of the tested-for component in the test sample. Positive hemolysis should be proportional to the amount and functional activity of the tested-for component present in the test sample. These assays, although not particularly sensitive or quantitative, are useful for further work-up of patients whose CH50 and/or APH50 are abnormally low or absent.

Measurement of concentrations of complement components

Measurement of serum levels of complement components is commonly used to diagnose and assess disease activity in chronic rheumatic diseases such as SLE. These tests also help to identify deficiencies of individual complement components.

Traditionally, serum is used for complement measurements. As cautioned above for the functional hemolysis assays, serum samples should be handled promptly and carefully to minimize possible degradation of complement proteins. A number of immunochemical methods, which are generally based on the antigen–antibody reactivity between complement components in the test sample and added anti-complement antibodies, are available for such measurement. The selection of a proper method depends on several factors such as the level of sensitivity required, the availability of specific antibody, the number of samples and the types of samples. In most clinical immunology laboratories, nephelometry is routinely used to measure complement components that are present at relatively high concentrations in the serum (e.g. C3 and C4). Other components that are usually at low concentrations (e.g. C1, C2, C5 through C9, factor B, factor D, properdin, etc.) can be measured using RID or ELISA, with the latter being more sensitive and robust in terms of quantitation. Similarly, concentrations of soluble regulatory proteins of the complement system (e.g. C4 binding protein, C1-inhibitor, factor H, etc.) can be measured by RID or ELISA. When C3 and C4 concentrations are too low to be measured accurately by nephelometry, i.e. <20 mg/dl and <10 mg/dl, respectively, RID is the alternative method of choice. For other body fluids or cell culture supernatants, in which the levels of complement components may be very low, ELISA is the most practical method to use. With regard to the test reagents, some antibodies, which are usually polyclonal in nature, may react with both native molecules and their respective split products. Such cross-reactivity

may result in overestimation of the concentrations of the tested-for components and hence should be taken into consideration when interpreting the results.

Measurement of complement split products

Measurement of serum concentrations of complement components is essentially a static appraisal of an extremely dynamic process that includes activation, consumption, catabolism and synthesis of these components. Unlike their parental molecules, which are also acute-phase proteins (Sturfelt and Sjoholm, 1984; Gabay and Kushner, 1999), complement split products are generated only when complement activation occurs and thus acute-phase responses do not increase their concentrations. Therefore, direct determination of complement split products is thought to reflect more precisely the activation process of complement *in vivo* and may even allow investigators to differentiate the activation mechanisms (e.g. classical versus alternative). Measures of complement split products, yielded from activation of the classical pathway (C1rs-C1 inhibitor complex, C4a and C4d), alternative pathway (Bb and C3bBbP), lectin pathway (C4a and C4d) and terminal pathway (C3a, iC3b, C3d, C5a and sC_{5b-9}), are currently performed in many clinical immunology laboratories.

When measuring complement split products, plasma, instead of serum, should be used. Plasma is used to avoid generating complement split products *in vitro* during the coagulation process of serum derivation. Typically, blood is drawn into tubes containing EDTA (a Ca^{2+}/Mg^{2+} chelator serving as both an anticoagulant and an inhibitor of complement activation) and centrifuged to separate plasma from cells. Plasma should be promptly collected, aliquoted and stored at $-70°C$ until use.

Tests to detect complement split products have been made possible with the development of monoclonal antibodies specific for 'neoepitopes' generated following proteolytic cleavage of complement molecules during activation. Since only low levels of complement split products may be present in the circulation, even after significantly increased complement activation, ELISA and EIA are the most practical methods for their measurement. The complement split products have different, but commonly short, half-lives in the plasma. Some split products, such as C3a, C4a and C5a, are quickly converted to more stable, less active forms, such as C3a-desArg, C4a-desArg and C5a-desArg. In comparison, complement products that form multi-molecular complexes usually have a relatively long half-life in the circulation. Examples of the latter include C1rs-C1 inhibitor complexes (products of classical pathway activation), C3bBbP complexes (products of alternative pathway activation) and sC_{5b-9} (the ultimate product of complement activation). sC_{5b-9} is the soluble form of MAC that consists of C5b, C6, C7, C8, poly-C9 and the solubilizing protein, S, protein, Reagent kits for detecting and quantitating C3a-desArg,

C4a-desArg, C4d, iC3b, C3d, C5a-desArg and sC$_{5b-9}$ are now readily available from commercial sources.

Drawbacks and potential problems associated with complement measurement

Potential problems of functional hemolytic assays

The CH50 and APH50 assays are probably the simplest and fastest tests for assessing complement function of an individual and a convenient assay for screening hereditary as well as acquired complement deficiencies. However, they are biological assays and are inevitably influenced by many factors ranging from stability of complement in test samples to quality of experimental reagents to conditions of laboratory environment. Laboratory factors that may affect the results of functional hemolysis assays include: fragility and concentration of erythrocytes, quantity and quality of the antibody used to sensitize sheep erythrocytes, pH and concentrations of Ca^{2+} and Mg^{2+} of buffer solutions and temperature and reaction time of the assays. The test samples should always be properly handled and stored, avoiding repeated freezing/thawing or delays between the times of dilution, preparation and testing. If all laboratory factors are carefully controlled and standardized, however, the results are usually highly reproducible from assay to assay. With respect to sensitivity and specificity, these assays effectively reflect the function of the complement system as a whole entity, but they are relatively insensitive for detecting decreases in specific components. Nevertheless, functional hemolysis assays represent first-line screening tests for complement function that combine simplicity and efficiency with reproducibility. Definite and accurate diagnosis of deficiency of individual complement components may be achieved by combining the functional assays with immunochemical tests that measure serum concentrations of individual complement components.

Potential problems associated with measurement of complement proteins

The discrepant reports regarding the value of measuring serum C4 and C3 to monitor disease activity of chronic inflammatory diseases such as SLE may originate from several factors that particularly confound measurement of C3 and C4 in disease. First, there is a wide range of variation in serum C3 and C4 levels among healthy individuals and this range overlaps with that observed in patients with different diseases. Second, traditional concentration measurements reflect the presence of C3 and C4 protein entities irrespective of their functional integrity. Third, acute-phase responses during inflammation may lead to an increase in C4 and C3 synthesis (Sturfelt and Sjoholm, 1984; Gabay and Kushner, 1999), which can counterbalance the consumption of these proteins during activation. Fourth, genetic variations, such as partial deficiency of

C4, which is commonly present in the general population and in patients with autoimmune diseases (Ratnoff, 1996; Barilla-LaBarca and Atkinson, 2003), may result in lower than normal serum C4 levels in some patients because of decreased synthesis rather than increased complement consumption during disease flares. Fifth, tissue deposition of immune complexes may result in complement activation at local sites in patients with certain diseases; such activity may not be faithfully reflected by the levels of complement products in the systemic circulation. Additional concerns should be raised regarding the measurements of complement split products. As mentioned above, many of the split products have an undefined, most likely short, half-life both *in vivo* and *in vitro*. Moreover, complement activation can easily occur *in vitro* after blood sampling. In combination, these factors may hamper accurate measures of activation products that are derived solely from complement activation occurring in patients. However, the recent development of a broad range serine protease inhibitor, FUT-175, may minimize this concern (Inagi et al., 1991; Pfeifer et al., 1999). When added to plasma samples at the time of collection, this inhibitor prevents *in vitro* complement activation and thus ensures more accurate measurements of complement split products circulating at the time of sample collection.

COMPLEMENT AS A SOURCE OF BIOMARKERS FOR DISEASE DIAGNOSIS AND MONITORING

Hereditary complement deficiency should be considered in any individuals experiencing recurrent infections for which other possible causes have been excluded. Acquired complement deficiency should be suspected if patients have low serum complement levels and exhibit immune complex disease-like symptoms. In the latter case, an autoimmune disorder, in which complement activation occurs during active states, is likely the primary disease. Complement measurements can be helpful in the diagnosis and monitoring of such primary diseases.

For the purpose of diagnosing or differentiating hereditary complement deficiency and underlying diseases, an algorithm for complement analysis can be formulated (Figure 11.2). Any patients suspected to be complement deficient should first be tested using the CH50 and APH50 assays. Normal results of these assays almost always allow physicians to exclude the possibility of complement deficiency. Complete lack of CH50 and/or APH50 activity is a strong indication of complement deficiency and should be followed with further tests to determine which component is missing. Functional hemolysis assays and/or concentration measurements for selected complement components can be performed according to the following rationales:

1 if both CH50 and APH50 are absent or extremely low, the defect is most likely C3 or one of the terminal components (C5 through C9)

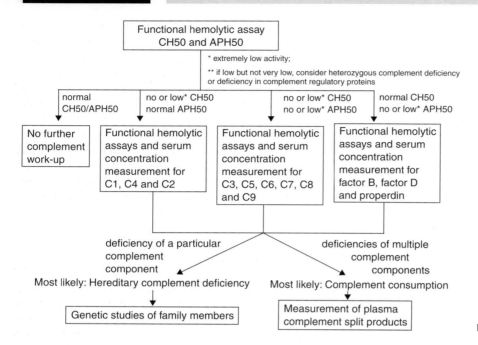

Figure 11.2 Algorithm for complement analysis.

2 if CH50 is absent or very low but APH50 is normal, the defect is in one of the early components of the classical pathway (C1q, C1r, C1s, C4, C2)

3 if CH50 is normal but APH50 is absent or very low, the defect is one of the alternative pathway components (factor B, factor D, properdin)

4 if both CH50 and APH50 are moderately but not dramatically low, the defect is most likely an acquired phenomenon due to *in vivo* complement activation caused by an underlying disease.

As a general rule, the absence or decrease of multiple components also point toward an acquired complement deficiency due to consumption. It should be kept in mind, however, that patients with a partial complement deficiency due to heterozygous genetic defects may also exhibit lower than normal (but not extremely low) CH50 and APH50 activities. Additionally, deficiencies of complement regulatory proteins (C1-inhibitor, factor I and factor H) may cause uncontrolled activation of complement that consumes C3. Such a 'secondary' C3 deficiency may also lead to absent or extremely low CH50 and APH50 and should be differentiated from 'primary' (hereditary) deficiency of C3 or terminal components.

Measuring levels of complement proteins and their split products may be useful in monitoring disease activity of certain chronic inflammatory conditions. This utility is probably best exemplified in patients with SLE (Walport, 2002; Liu et al., 2004b) (see Chapter 44 on SLE related tests). Interestingly, while some studies have supported the usefulness of CH50, serum C3 and C4 concentrations, or plasma levels of complement split products as markers or predictors of SLE disease activity (Falk et al., 1985; Valentijn et al., 1985; Esdaile et al., 1996a), other studies have found these tests to be minimally useful (Abrass et al., 1980;

Walz LeBlanc et al., 1994; Esdaile et al., 1996b). Some investigators have suggested that complement measurement may be more informative when it is performed chronologically in the same patient and the interpretation is based on the specific genetic and clinical characteristics of the patient. Detailed discussion on those studies, however, is beyond the scope of this chapter. Such diversified data may reflect limitations of current standard complement assays in monitoring patients with chronic diseases like SLE who have variable clinical manifestations and unpredictable courses. Few studies have been conducted to evaluate rigorously the potential for complement as a source of biomarkers for disease activity/progression in other chronic inflammatory diseases such as atherosclerosis, an area that undoubtedly warrants further investigation.

FUTURE PROSPECTS: MEASUREMENT OF CELL-SURFACE COMPLEMENT SPLIT PRODUCTS AND RECEPTORS

Given the ubiquitous participation of the complement system in the pathogenesis of inflammatory- and immune-mediated disorders, remarkably little attention has been paid to developing complement-based biomarkers. Measurement of serum C3 and C4 has been the gold standard in the field for several decades, despite the extremely limited utility of this approach as described above. Assays for soluble complement split products such as C3d and C4d, although theoretically advantageous to measurements of the parent molecules, have not been embraced as generally more useful. These observations have led to more recent consideration of measurement of the products of complement activation on surfaces of circulating hematopoietic cells.

Complement proteins are abundant in the circulation and thus can readily interact with circulating blood cells. Complement split products that have the capacity to attach covalently to cell-surface components are likely to persist longer than soluble split products in plasma and hence may be detected more readily and reliably. Because erythrocytes and platelets are, respectively, the two most abundant cells in the circulation, they are potentially abundant 'magnets' for products of complement activation generated either locally or systemically. Based on this rationale, erythrocytes and platelets may serve as circulating 'biological beacons' of the inflammatory condition *in vivo*.

This hypothesis was recently tested with flow cytometric assays to measure rigorously the levels of C4d on surfaces of erythrocytes and platelets. For erythrocytes, complement receptor 1 (CR1) and C4d levels were analyzed simultaneously. Initial studies focused on SLE because the pathogenesis of SLE is characterized, in part, by defects in clearance of complement-bearing immune complexes via erythrocytes expressing CR1. We aimed to determine whether these SLE-specific defects might be reflected by abnormal and diagnostic patterns of complement ligand and receptor expression on erythrocytes of patients with SLE (Ross et al., 1985; Wilson et al., 1987). Although numerous previous studies have demonstrated reduced levels of erythrocyte CR1 in patients with SLE, concurrent analysis of CR1 and complement ligand C4d has not been previously reported. Using these assays, we conducted a cross-sectional study that included patients with SLE, patients with other inflammatory- and immune-mediated diseases and healthy control subjects (King et al., 2002).

The data from this pilot study support several conclusions. First, erythrocyte-bound C4d (E-C4d) and erythrocyte-expressed CR1 (E-CR1) are present on surfaces of all normal erythrocytes. Second, E-C4d and E-CR1 levels demonstrate minimal fluctuation in normal individuals over time. Third, abnormally high E-C4d and abnormally low E-CR1 is a pattern with high diagnostic sensitivity and specificity for SLE. Fourth, E-C4d and E-CR1 levels in a given patient with SLE fluctuate over time and correlate with disease activity. Fifth, measurement of C4d on reticulocytes (R-C4d) may serve as an 'instant messenger' of disease activity in SLE because R-C4d fluctuates with disease activity and the life span of a reticulocyte is approximately 24–48 h. This study demonstrates for the first time, in a systematic fashion, that considerable levels of a complement split product are present and readily detected on surfaces of erythrocytes in patients with an inflammatory disease.

Measurement of C4d on platelets (P-C4d) has also been explored as a potential source of complement-based biomarkers (Johnson et al., 2003). Comparisons of a single determination of P-C4d in SLE patients, patients with other inflammatory diseases and healthy control subjects have demonstrated that detection of C4d on platelet surfaces is 100 per cent specific in distinguishing SLE patients from healthy controls and 98 per cent specific in distinguishing SLE patients from patients with other diseases. Together, these recent investigations suggest that measurement of complement ligands and receptors on cell surfaces, such as E-C4d, E-CR1, R-C4d, and P-C4d are simple, rapid and inexpensive methods that may identify a new approach to mining the complement system for biomarkers. Such biomarkers may serve a number of needs such as diagnosis, assessment of disease activity, identification of subsets of disease, prediction of disease course, demonstration of response to therapy and prediction of response to therapy.

ACKNOWLEDGEMENTS

We thank Dr Janice M. Sabatine for expert editorial assistance. We also thank our colleagues in the Lupus Center of Excellence and Division of Rheumatology and Clinical Immunology for providing clinical samples, helpful discussion and skilled technical as well as administrative support. Investigations in the authors' laboratory are supported by grants from the National Institutes of Health (RO1 AR-4676402, RO1 HL074335, RO1 AR-46588, NCRR/GCRC MO1-RR-00056, K24 AR02213 and P30 AR47372), the Lupus Foundation of Pennsylvania, the Alliance for Lupus Research, the Lupus Foundation of America, Southeastern Pennsylvania Chapter and the Arthritis Foundation.

REFERENCES

Abrass, C.K., Nies, K.M., Louie, J.S., Border, W.A. and Glassock, R.J. (1980). Correlation and predictive accuracy of circulating immune complexes with disease activity in patients with systemic lupus erythematosus. Arthrit Rheum 23, 273–282.

Akiyama, H., Barger, S., Barnum, S. et al. (2000). Inflammation and Alzheimer's disease. Neurobiol Aging 21, 383–421.

Barilla-LaBarca, M.L. and Atkinson, J.P. (2003). Rheumatic syndromes associated with complement deficiency. Curr Opin Rheumatol 15, 55–60.

Bhakdi, S. and Tranum-Jensen, J. (1983). Membrane damage by complement. Biochem Biophys Acta 737, 343–372.

Bordet, J. (1909). Resume of Immunology. In Studies in Immunology. New York: Wiley and Sons.

Borsos, T., Dourmashkin, R. R. and Humphry, J. H. (1964). Lesions in erythrocyte membranes caused by immune hemolysis. Nature 202, 251–252.

Buchner, H. (1889). Uber die baterientodtende Wirkung des zellfreien Blutserums. Zbl Bakt 5, 817.

Carroll, M.C. (1998). The role of complement and complement receptors in induction and regulation of immunity. Annu Rev Immunol 16, 545–568.

Carroll, M.C. (2000). The role of complement in B cell activation and tolerance. Adv Immunol 74, 61–88.

Dahl, M.R., Thiel, S., Matsushita, M.C. et al. (2001). A new mannan-binding lectin associated serine protease, MASP-3, and its association with distinct complexes of the MBL complement activation pathway. Immunity 15, 1–10.

Ehrlich, P. (1899). Uber Hamolysine. Berl Klin Wochenschr 36, 481–486.

Eikelenboom, P. and Stam, F.C. (1982). Immunoglobulins and complement factors in senile plaques. An immunoperoxidase study. Acta Neruopathol 57, 239–242.

Esdaile, J.M., Joseph, L., Abrahamowicz, M., Danoff, D. and Clarke, A.E. (1996a). Routine immunologic tests in systemic lupus erythematosus: Is there a need for more studies? J Rheumatol 23, 1891–1896.

Esdaile, J.M., Abrahamowicz, M., Joseph, L., MacKenzie, T., Li, Y. and Danoff, D. (1996b). Laboratory tests as predictors of disease exacerbations in systemic lupus erythematosus: why some tests fail. Arthrit Rheum 39, 370–378.

Falk, R.J., Agustin, M.D., Dalmasso, P., Kim, Y., Lam, S. and Michael, A. (1985). Radioimmunoassay of the attack complex of complement in serum from patients with systemic lupus erythematosus. N Engl J Med 312, 1594–1599.

Fang,Y., Xu, C., Fu, Y.X., Holers, V.M. and Molina, H. (1998). Expression of complement receptors 1 and 2 on follicular dendritic cells is necessary for the generation of a strong antigen-specific IgG response. J Immunol 160, 5273–5279.

Fearon, D.T. and Carter, R.H. (1995). The CD19/CR2/TAPA-1 complex of B lymphocytes: linking natural to acquired immunity. Annu Rev Immunol 13, 127–149.

Fearon, D.T. and Locksley, R.M. (1996). The instructive role of innate immunity in the acquired immune response. Science 272, 50–53.

Fischer, M.B., Goerg, S., Shen, L. et al. (1998). Dependence of germinal center B cells on expression of CD21/CD35 for survival. Science 280, 582–585.

Frank, M.M. (1998). Introduction and Historical Notes. In The Human Complement System in Health and Disease, J.E. Volanakis and M.E. Frank, eds. New York: Marcel Dekker, Inc., pp. 1–8.

Gabay, C. and Kushner, I. (1999). Acute-phase proteins and other systemic responses to inflammation. N Engl J Med 340, 448–454.

Gal, P. and Ambrus, G. (2001). Structure and function of complement activating complexes: C1 and MBL-MASPs. Curr Prot Pept Sci 2, 43–59.

Holers, V.M. (2000). Phenotypes of complement knockouts. Immunopharmacology 49, 125–131.

Humphry, J.H. and Dourmashkin, R.R. (1969). The lesions in cell membranes caused by complement. Adv Immunol 11, 75–115.

Imagawa, D.K., Osifchin, N.E., Paznekas, W.A. et al. (1983). Consequences of cell membrane attack by complement: release of arachidonate and formation of inflammatory derivatives. Proc Natl Acad Sci USA 80, 6647–6651.

Inagi, R., Miyata, T., Madea, K., Sugiyama, S., Miyama, A. and Nakashima, I. (1991). Fut-175 as a potent inhibitor of C5/C3 convertase activity for production of C5a and C3a. Immunol Lett 27, 49.

Jiang, H., Cooper, B., Robey, F.A. and Gewurz, H. (1992). DNA binds and activates complement via residues 14–26 of the human C1q A chain. J Biol Chem 267, 25597–25601.

Jiang, H.X., Siegel, J.N. and Gewurz, H. (1991). Binding and complement activation by C-reactive protein via the collagen-like region of C1q and inhibition of these reactions by monoclonal antibodies to C-reactive protein and C1q. J Immunol 146, 2324–2330.

Johnson, J. J., Manzi, S., Navratil, J. S., Kao, A., Nilson, S.E., and Ahearn, J. M. (2003). Platelets are decorated by complement ligands in patients with systemic lupus erythematosus (SLE): An etiologic clue and biomarker for cardiovascular disease. Arthrit Rheum 48, S656.

Jongen, P.J.H., Doesburg, W.H., Ibrahim-Stappers, J.L.M., Lemmens, W.A.J.G., Hommes, O.R. and Lamers, K.J.B. (2000). Cerebrospinal fluid C3 and C4 indexes in immunological disorders of the central nervous system. Acta Neurol Scand 101, 116–121.

King, D.E., Navratila, J.S., Liu, C.-C. et al. (2002). A new assay for SLE diagnosis and assessment of disease activity. Arthrit Rheum 46, S294.

Klein, P.G. and Wellensieck, H.J. (1965). Multiple nature of the third component of guinea pig complement. I. Separation and characterization of three factors a, b, and c, essential for hemolysis. Immunology 8, 590–603.

Korb, L.C. and Ahearn, J.M. (1997). C1q binds directly and specifically to surface blebs of apoptotic human keratinocytes. Complement deficiency and systemic lupus erythematosus revisited. J Immunol 158, 4525–4528.

Levine, L., Mayer, M.M. and Rapp, H.J. (1954). Kinetic studies on immune hemolysis. VI. Resolution of the C'y reaction step into two successive processes involving C'2 and C'3. J Immunol 73, 435–442.

Linton, S. (2001). Animal models of inherited complement deficiency. Mol Biotechnol 18, 135–148.

Liu, C.-C., Navratil, J.S., Sabatine, J.M. and Ahearn, J.M. (2004a). Apoptosis, Complement, and SLE: A mechanistic view. Curr Direct Autoimmun 7, 49–86.

Liu, C.-C., Ahearn, J.M. and Manzi, S. (2004b). Complement as a source of biomarkers in systemic lupus erythematosus: past, present, and future. Curr Rheumatol Reports 6, 85–88.

Liu, C.-C. and Young, J.D.E. (1988). A semi-automated microassay for complement activity. J Immunol Methods 113, 33–39.

Mayer, M.M. (1961a). Development of a one-hit theory of immune hemolysis. In Immunochemical approaches to problems in microbiology, M. Heidelberger and D.J. Plescia, eds. New Brunswick: Rutgers, pp. 268–279.

Mayer, M.M. (1961b). Complement v. complement fixation. In Experimental Immunochemistry, E.A. Kabat and M.M. Mayer, eds. Springfield, IL: Charles C. Thomas Publisher, pp. 133–239.

Mayer, M.M. (1972). Mechanism of cytolysis by complement. Proc Natl Acad Sci USA 69, 2954–2958.

McGeer, P.L. and McGeer, E.G. (2002). The possible role of complement activation in Alzheimer's disease. Trends Mol Med 8, 519–523.

McGeer, P.L., Schulzer, M. and McGeer, E.G. (1996). Arthritis and anti-inflammatory agents as possible protective factors for Alzheimer's disease: a review of 17 epidemiological studies. Neurology 47, 425–432.

Mevorach, D., Mascarenhas, J.O., Gershov, D. and Elkon, K.B. (1998). Complement-dependent clearance of apoptotic cells by human macrophages. J Exp Med 188, 2313–2320.

Morgan, B.P. (1989). Complement membrane attack on nucleated cells: resistance, recovery and non-lethal effects. Biochem J 264, 1–14.

Morgan, B.P. (2000). Complement methods and protocols. Methods Mol Biol 150, 1–268.

Morgan, B.P. and Walport, M.J. (1991). Complement deficiency and disease. Immunol Today 12, 301–306.

Muller-Eberhard, H.J. (1975). Complement. Annu Rev Biochem 44, 697–724.

Muller-Eberhard, H.J. (1986). The membrane attack complex of complement. Annu Rev Immunol 4, 503–528.

Nauta, A.J., Trouw, L.A., Daha, M.R. et al. (2002). Direct binding of C1q to apoptotic cells and cell blebs induces complement activation. Eur J Immunol 32, 1726–1736.

Navratil, J.S., Watkins, S.C., Wisnieski, J.J. and Ahearn, J.M. (2001). The globular heads of C1q specifically recognize surface blebs of apoptotic vascular endothelial cells. J Immunol 166, 3231–3239.

Nelson, R.A., Jensin, J., Gigli, I. and Tamura, N. (1966). Methods for the separation, purification and measurement of nine components of hemolytic complement in guinea pig serum. Immunochemistry 3, 111–135.

Nuttall, G. (1888). Experimente uber die bacterienfeindlichen Einfluesse des thierischen Korpers. Z Hyg Infekrionskr 4, 353.

Pangburn, M.K. and Muller-Eberhard, H.J. (1983). Initiation of the alternative complement pathway due to spontaneous hydrolysis of the thioester of C3. Ann NY Acad Sci 421, 291–298.

Pfeifer, P.H., Kawahara, M.S. and Hugli, T.E. (1999). Possible mechanism for in vitro complement activation in blood and plasma samples: Futhan/EDTA controls in vitro complement activation. Clin Chem 45, 1190–1199.

Pickering, M.C., Botto, M., Taylor, P.R., Lachmann, P.J. and Walport, M.J. (2000). Systemic lupus erythematosus, complement deficiency, and apoptosis. Adv Immunol 76, 227–324.

Pillemer, L., Blum, L., Lepow, I.H., Ross, O.A., Todd, E.W. and Wardlaw, A.C. (1954). The properdin system and immunity. I. Demonstration and isolation of a new serum protein, properdin, and its role in immune phenomena. Science 120, 279–285.

Pillemer, L., Lepow, I.H. and Blum, L. (1953). The requirement for a hydrozine-sensitive serum factor and heat-labile serum factors in the inactivation of human C'3 by zymosan. J Immunol 71, 339–345.

Platts-Mills, T.A.E. and Ishizaka, K. (1974). Activation of the alternative pathway of human complement by rabbit cells. J Immunol 113, 348–358.

Rapp, H.J. (1958). Mechanism of immune hemolysis: recognition of two steps in the conversion of EAC' 1,4,2 to E. Science 127, 234–236.

Ratnoff, W.D. (1996). Inherited deficiencies of complement in rheumatic diseases. Rheum Dis Clin North Am 22, 75–94.

Rogers, J., Cooper, N.R., Webster, S. et al. (1992). Complement activation by beta-amyloid in Alzheimer disease. Proc Natl Acad Sci USA 89, 10016–10020.

Ross, G.D. (1986). Introduction and history of complement research. In Immunobiology of the Complement System, G.D. Ross, ed. New York: Academic Press, pp. 1–19.

Ross, G.D. and Atkinson, J.P. (1985). Complement receptor structure and function. Immunol Today 6, 115–119.

Ross, G.D., Yount, W.J., Walport, M.J. et al. (1985). Disease-associated loss of erythrocyte complement receptors (CR1, C3b receptors) in patients with systemic lupus erythematosus and other diseases involving autoantibodies and/or complement activation. J Immunol 135, 2005–2014.

Schifferli, J.A. (1986). The role of complement and its receptor in the elimination of immune complexes. N Engl J Med 315, 488–495.

Shen, Y., Lue, L., Yang, L. et al. (2001). Complement activation by neurofibrillary tangles in Alzheimer's disease. Neurosci Lett 305, 165–168.

Shevach, E.M. (1994). Complement. In Current Protocols in Immunology, J.E. Coligan, A.M. Kruisbeek, D.H. Margulies, E.M. Shevach, and W. Strober, eds. New York: John Wiley & Sons, Inc., pp. 13.0.1–13.2.9.

Sturfelt, G. and Sjoholm, A.G. (1984). Complement components, complement activation, and acute phase response in systemic lupus erythematosus. Int Arch Allerg Appl Immunol 75, 75–83.

Thiel, S., Vorup-Jensen, T., Stover, C.M. et al. (1997). A second serine protease associated with mannan-binding lectin that activates complement. Nature 386, 506–510.

Turner, M.W. (2004). The role of mannose-binding lectin in health and disease. Mol Immunol 40, 423–429.

Valentijn, R.M., van Overhagen, H., Hazevoet, H.M. et al. (1985). The value of complement and immune complex determinations in monitoring disease activity in patients with systemic lupus erythematosus. Arthrit Rheum 28, 904–913.

Van Beek, J., Elward, K. and Gasque, P. (2003). Activation of complement in the central nervous system: roles in neurodegenration and neuroprotectin. Ann NY Acad Sci 992, 56–71.

Velazquez, P., Cribbs, D.H., Poulos, T.L. and Tenner, A.J. (1997). Aspartate residue 7 in amyloid beta-protein is critical for classical complement pathway activation: implications for Alzheimer's disease pathogenesis. Nat Med 3, 77–79.

Wallis, R. (2002). Structural and functional aspects of complement activation by mannose-binding protein. Immunobiology 205, 433–445.

Walport, M.J. (2001). Complement. First of two parts. N Engl J Med 344, 1058–1066.

Walport, M.J. (2002). Complement and systemic lupus erythematosus. Arthritis Res 4 (suppl. 3), S279–S293.

Walz LeBlanc, B.A., Gladman, D.D. and Urowitz, M.B. (1994). Serologically active clinically quiescent systemic lupus erythematosus-predictors of clinical flares. J Rheumatol 21, 2239–2241.

Wiedmer, T., Ando, B. and Sims, P.J. (1987). Complement C5b-9-stimulated platelet secretion is associated with a Ca2+-initiated activation of cellular protein kinases. J Biol Chem 262, 13674–13681.

Wilson, J.G., Wong, W.W., Murphy, E.E.I., Schur, P.H. and Fearon, D.T. (1987). Deficiency of the C3b/C4b receptor (CR1) of erythrocytes in systemic lupus erythematosus: Analysis of the stability of the defect and of a restriction fragment length polymorphism of the CR1 gene. J Immunol 138, 2706–2710.

Wurzner, R., Mollnes, T.E. and Morgan, B.P. (1997). Immunochemical assays for complement components. In Immunochemistry 2: a practical approach, A.P. Johnstone and M.W. Turner, eds. Oxford: Oxford University Press, pp. 197–223.

Yasojima, K., Schwab, E.G., McGeer, E.G., and McGeer, P.L. (1999). Up-regulated production and activation of the complement system in Alzheimer's disease brain. Am J Pathol 154, 927–936.

Ying, S.C., Gewurz, A.T., Jiang, H. and Gewurz, H. (1993). Human serum amyloid P component oligomers bind and activate the classical complement pathway via residues 14–26 and 76–92 of the A chain collagen-like region of C1q. J Immunol 150, 169–176.

Immunoglobulin Titers and Immunoglobulin Subtypes

Popovic Petar[1], Diane Dubois[2], Bruce S. Rabin[2] and Michael R. Shurin[2,3]

*Departments of Surgery[1], Pathology[2] and Immunology[3]
Division of Clinical Immunopathology[2], University of Pittsburgh Medical Center,
Pittsburgh, PA, USA*

Thinking is more interesting then knowing, but less interesting than looking.

Johann Wolfgang von Goethe

IMMUNOGLOBULINS

Immunoglobulins (antibodies) are a group of heterogeneous proteins that exhibit the unique property of being able to bind to proteins or polysaccharides that stimulated the production of the antibody. Antibodies are one of two important antigen recognition components of the immune system. Antibodies recognize antigen directly in a three-dimensional conformation while the other antigen recognition system, the T lymphocytes, recognizes antigen in conjunction with MHC molecules. Antibodies are expressed on the membrane of developing and mature B cells where they function as B-cell receptors for antigens. The interaction of antigen with membrane bound immunoglobulins initiates activation of the B cell and, with proper stimulation, there is synthesis and secretion of the specific antibody into the circulation.

Immunoglobulins specifically recognize a particular antigenic determinant on a larger molecule. The site recognized by a specific antibody is called an 'epitope'. Antigen binding is the primary function of antibodies. Physiologic benefits provided by antibodies include helping to rid the body of disease-causing bacteria, protection from viral infection and neutralizing bacterial toxins. The significant biological effects of antibody are mediated by a variety of secondary 'effector functions' including activation of the complement cascade or attachment of antibody-covered bacterial antigens to phagocytic cells through the specific receptors on the phagocytic cell for the portion of the antibody molecule that does not directly bind to the antigen.

In addition to their unique and central role in host protection, antibody contributes to the pathogenesis of a variety of reactions that are called hypersensitivity reactions. Hypersensitivity implies that the individual has been exposed to the antigen in the past and when exposed for a second time, there is a rapid onset of an immune reaction. Allergies are an example of a hypersensitivity reaction.

There are three other types of hypersensitivity reaction in addition to the allergic type, which is called Type 1. Type 2 hypersensitivity reactions occur when antibodies specifically recognize and bind to receptors on cell membranes. If the receptor is involved with altering cell function there may be increased (for example, Graves' disease) or decreased (for example, myasthenia gravis) cell activity. Finally, antibodies binding to circulating cells could induce cell removal or lysis and cause severe clinical conditions like anemia and thrombocytopenia.

Type 3 hypersensitivity reactions occur when circulating antibody binds to the specific antigen and form immune complexes. The phagocytic cells of the spleen, liver and lung normally remove immune complexes from the circulation. If there are more complexes formed than can be removed by mononuclear phagocytes, the complexes

*Measuring Immunity, edited by Michael T. Lotze and Angus W. Thomson
ISBN 0-12-455900-X, London*

will become deposited in tissue. In tissue the complexes will activate the complement system. This will induce an inflammatory response and damage to the tissue that is caused by enzymes released from the inflammatory cells and anoxia (the lack of oxygen) caused by occlusion of small blood vessels.

Type 4 hypersensitivity is mediated by T lymphocytes and does not involve antibody.

All immunoglobulins consist of two identical low molecular weight polypeptide light chains (23 kD) and two identical polypeptide heavy chains (50–70 kD). The chains are held together by inter-chain disulfide bonds and by non-covalent interactions. While all immunoglobulin molecules share the same basic structural characteristics, the amino terminal end displays remarkable variability that accounts for the capability of antibodies of different specificities to bind to an almost infinite number of antigens.

Based on the variability in the amino acid sequences, both the heavy and light chain can be divided into variable (V) and constant (C) regions. The antigen binding site involves the variable region. Structural differences outside their antigen binding sites, i.e. in the constant region, correlate with the different effector function mediated by antibodies, such as complement activation or binding to specific receptors expressed on different cell types. For example, mast cells have a receptor for the constant region of the IgE class of antibody and polymorphonuclear leukocytes have a receptor for the constant region of IgG.

Based on the total number of different variable regions or antigen binding sites, it can be estimated that an individual can produce antibodies with more than 10 million different specificities.

Analysis of immunoglobulin fragments produced by proteolytic digestion has been useful in elucidating structural and functional relationships of immunoglobulins. Digestion with papain breaks the immunoglobulin molecule into two identical fragments that contain the whole light chain and the V_H and C_{H1} domains of the heavy chain. They are called Fab fragments because they contain the antigen binding sites of the antibody. Each Fab fragment is monovalent whereas the original molecule is divalent. Digestion with papain also produces a fragment that contains the remainder of the two heavy chains each containing a C_{H2} and C_{H3} domain. This fragment was called Fc fragment because it was easily crystallized. The effector functions of immunoglobulins are mediated by the Fc part of the molecule, while other domains in this fragment intercede in different functions. In contrast to the papain-mediated digestion, treatment of immunoglobulins with pepsin results in cleavage of the heavy chain in a fragment that contains both antigen-binding sites. This fragment was called $F(ab')_2$ because it was divalent. The $F(ab')_2$ strongly binds antigen but it does not mediate the effector functions of antibodies, since it misses the Fc part of the whole molecule.

IMMUNOGLOBULIN CLASSES

The immunoglobulin classes are IgG, IgA, IgM, IgD and IgE. The constant region is the same for all immunoglobulins within a given class, indeed it is the constant region that provides a means of differentiating one class of immunoglobulin from another. Thus, all immunoglobulin molecules that are of the IgG class have identical aspects to their constant regions that allow them to be identified as IgG. Similarly IgA, IgM, IgD and IgE have identical characteristics to their constant regions.

Not every part of the variable region is as variable as every other part of the variable region. The variable end of the H and L chains begins at the amino terminal end of the chain. The first 110 amino acids are involved in the variable portion of the H and L chains. The amino acids at positions 30–34, 48–56 and 94–99 are much more variable than the amino acids at the other positions. The highly variable regions are termed the hypervariable regions and the amino acids between the hypervariable regions are termed the framework regions. The intrachain disulfide bonds bring the hypervariable regions together to form the actual site that combines with the antigen.

Another aspect of the immunoglobulin molecule is termed the hinge region. The hinge region is located between the first (CH1) and second (CH2) constant regions of the H chain. This region allows the two Fab portions to have mobility so that the two portions that combine with antigen can move. The primary shape of the immunoglobulin molecule is that of a 'Y' with flexibility of the two arms given by the hinge region.

The heavy chain is assigned a specific designation for each isotype.

Isotype	Heavy chain
IgG	Gamma
IgA	Alpha
IgM	Mu
IgD	Delta
IgE	Epsilon

The molecular weight of the light chain is approximately 22 000 daltons. There are only two classes of L chains and they are termed kappa and lambda. The two L chains which comprise a single basic immunoglobulin unit are both kappa or both lambda. Thus each immunoglobulin class (IgG, IgA, IgM, IgD, IgE) is composed of kappa containing molecules and lambda containing molecules. The difference between kappa and lambda is due to different amino acid sequences.

IgG

Immunoglobulin G (IgG) is a major class of immunoglobulins found in the blood comprising 75 per cent of total serum immunoglobulins (Table 12.1). IgG is also the major immunoglobulin in the extravascular spaces and the only type of immunoglobulin that binds to receptors on placental trophoblasts and crosses the placenta. Transferred maternal IgG provides immunity for the fetus and newborn. The IgG is capable of carrying out all of the functions of immunoglobulin molecules. In general, IgG is strong at activating complement and is the best antibody for phagocytosis of opsonized microorganisms through the Fcγ receptors on phagocytes. IgG also plays an important role in neutralizing bacterial toxins in the blood and tissues. Antibodies of the IgG class express their predominant activity during a secondary immune response. Thus, the appearance of specific IgG antibodies normally reflects the 'maturation' of the immune response, which is switched on upon repeated contact with a specific antigen. The subclasses of IgG are produced depending on the cytokine present (especially IL-4 and IL-2) and each subclass has its own specific activity (Table 12.2) (Schur, 1987). For instance, IgG2 does not cross the placenta, IgG4 does not fix complement and IgG2 and IgG4 do not bind to Fc receptors with a high affinity (Meulenbroek and Zeijlemaker, 1996). IgG2 levels are also slowly increased during childhood and reach adult levels only by 6–8 years of age. IgG2 antibodies are usually induced by some carbohydrate antigens, such as pneumococcal polysaccharide, whereas protein antigens induce predominantly IgG1 and/or IgG3 responses. However, *Haemophilus influenzae* type b polyribose phosphate (*H. influenzae* vaccine) and *Neisseria meningitidis* capsular polysaccharide induce IgG1 and IgG2 antibodies.

IgA

Immunoglobulin A (IgA) can be detected in the circulation in low levels and in the monomeric form. IgA is the second most common immunoglobulin in human serum after IgG (see Table 12.1). IgA is widespread, does not fix complement and is most active at mucosal surfaces such as bronchioles, nasal mucosa, prostate, vagina and intestine, where it presents as a dimeric protein (Fagarasan and Honjo, 2003). IgA is also common in saliva, tears and breast milk, especially colostrums (Van de Perre, 2003). Secretory IgA is found in association with another protein, the so-called secretory piece or T piece. Unlike the IgA that is produced by plasma cells, the secretory piece is expressed in epithelial cells and added to the IgA molecules as they pass into the secretions. The secretory piece mediates IgA transport across the mucosa and protects IgA from degradation. Secretory IgA can neutralize toxins, bind viruses, agglutinate bacteria, prevent bacteria from binding to mucosal epithelial cells and bind to various food antigens, thus preventing their entry into the general circulation. The role of serum IgA is less unclear. IgA subclasses differ in distribution and function. IgA1 is present mainly in the serum (it accounts for 85 per cent of serum IgA) and predominates in secretion in the upper intestine and in the various mucosal glands. IgA2 predominates in secretion in the large intestine and in the female genital tract.

IgM

Immunoglobulin M (IgM) is the third most common serum immunoglobulin accounting for 5–10 per cent of total levels. It is also a component of secretory immunoglobulins at the mucosal surfaces and in breast milk. Secreted IgM normally exists as a pentamer but it can be also detected as a monomer. As a consequence of its pentameric structure,

Table 12.1 Estimated ranges for normal levels of serum immunoglobulins*

	IgG (mg/dl)	IgA (mg/dl)	IgM (mg/dl)	IgE (IU/ml)
3 months	140–650	1–45	20–120	<15.0
1 year	250–1100	10–100	25–160	<60.0
5 years	515–1450	25–200	40–200	<90.0
10 years	770–1650	40–360	40–250	<200.0
Adult	560–1770	40–390	60–360	<100.0

* Normal ranges of serum immunoglobulins vary between laboratories, since the estimation of immunoglobulin concentration in serum specimens strongly depends on analytical methods, calibration curves, specificity and type of antiglobulin antibodies, provided standards.

Table 12.2 Properties of immunoglobulin G subclasses*

	IgG$_1$	IgG$_2$	IgG$_3$	IgG$_4$
Serum concentration (adult ranges) (mg/dl)	420–1100	150–600	20–140	1–180
Proportion of total Ig (%)	40–80	15–50	1.5–10	0.5–15
Serum half-life (days)	21	21	7	21
Complement activation	++	+	+++	−
Response to protein antigens	++	+/−	++	+/−
Response to polysaccharide antigens	+	++	−	−
Placental cross-transfer	+	+	+	+

* Normal ranges of serum immunoglobulins vary between laboratories, since the estimation of immunoglobulin concentration in serum specimens strongly depends on analytical methods, calibration curves, specificity and type of antiglobulin antibodies, provided standards.

IgM is a powerful agglutinating and precipitating antibody, a strong complement fixing immunoglobulin and thus is efficient in leading to the lysis of microorganisms. It is also involved in neutralization of toxins (Stahl and Sibrowski, 2003). Biological significance of this immunoglobulin is based on the facts that IgM is the first immunoglobulin to be made by the fetus and the first antibody to be produced by virgin B cells after the primary antigen stimulation. IgM is the first antibody to be produced in response to infection since it does not require 'class switch' to another antibody class. However, it is only synthesized as long as antigen remains present because there are no memory cells for IgM. As a B-cell surface immunoglobulin, IgM exists as a monomer and functions as a receptor for antigens. The surface IgM is structurally different in the Fc region from the secreted form since it must bind through the membrane. Surface IgM binds directly as an integral membrane protein; it does not bind to an IgM Fc receptor like IgE does. A deficiency of IgM makes the host extremely susceptible to septicemia or other forms of sepsis. Being a large molecule (900 kD), the majority (80 per cent) of IgM exists within the vascular space.

IgD

Immunoglobulin D (IgD) is primarily found on the surface of B lymphocytes where it functions as a receptor for antigen. IgD does not bind complement or cells through the Fc receptor. A small amount of IgD is secreted accounting for about 0.25 per cent of the total serum immunoglobulins (Vladutiu, 2000). With use of sensitive assays, IgD has been found in all of the mammalian and avian species tested and is conserved across species, which suggests an evolutionary advantage (Blattner and Tucker, 1984). However, the physiologic function of serum IgD is not clear; it has even been thought that IgD might have no function (Blattner and Tucker, 1984). This was investigated in animals treated with anti-IgD and, more recently, in IgD-deficient mice. In one model of IgD knockout mice, there was only a slight decrease in the number of B cells in the periphery and immunoglobulin isotypes were almost normal (Nitschke et al., 1993). In another model, there was a delayed affinity maturation during T-cell-dependent antigen response (Roes and Rajewsky, 1993). IgD may also have a regulatory role by enhancing a protective antibody response of the IgM, IgG or IgA isotype, or by interfering with viral replication (Moskophidis et al., 1997). IgD can also participate in the generation and maintenance of B-cell memory and might have an important role in the transition from a stage of susceptibility to induction of B-cell tolerance to one of responsiveness (Vladutiu, 2000). In mice, IgD may substitute for some functions of IgM when IgM is absent. Studies in IgM-deficient IgM-/- mice reveal that B cells with surface expression of IgM were replaced by B cells with surface expression of IgD.

Immunization of IgM-/- mice revealed an IgD immune response in place of the now absent IgM response, although with a delayed increase in antibody concentration as compared to normal (Orinska et al., 2002). Finally, IgD is a potent inducer of TNF-α, IL-1β and IL-1 receptor antagonist (Drenth et al., 1996). IgD also induces release of IL-6, IL-10 and leukemia inhibitory factor from peripheral blood mononuclear cells.

IgE

Immunoglobulin E (IgE) exists as a monomer and has an extra domain in the constant region. IgE does not fix complement and is the least common serum immunoglobulin since it binds with a high affinity to the specific Fc receptors on basophils and mast cells even before interacting with antigen (Gould et al., 2003). Binding of the antigen to IgE on the cells results in immediate release of various mediators, including histamine, serotonin, leukotrienes and others. This class of antibody is responsible for Type I hypersensitivity reactions or immediate hypersensitivity reactions such as hay fever, asthma, hives and anaphylaxis. Although IgE is commonly involved in allergic reactions, the main function of IgE seems to be to protect the host against invading parasites (Gould et al., 2003). Eosinophils have Fc receptors for IgE and binding of eosinophils to IgE-coated helminths results in killing of the parasite. Since serum IgE levels rise in parasitic diseases, measuring IgE levels is helpful in diagnosing parasitic infections. IgE is distributed throughout the body, although cells synthesizing IgE are found predominantly in association with mucosal tissues and, like IgA, this class of antibody is particularly effective at mucosal surfaces. However, IgE is not found in breast milk, and only in very low amounts in other secretions such as saliva. IgE is found to increase significantly in response to parasitic infection.

Of the five classes of immunoglobulins, IgG, IgA and IgM are the main components found in serum. Measurement of serum levels of these immunoglobulins is essential for the diagnosis and monitoring of primary and secondary immunodeficiencies and lymphoid malignancies. In addition, elevated levels of polyclonal immunoglobulins may occur in autoimmune diseases, liver diseases and chronic infections. Since total serum IgE is significantly raised in only 50–75 per cent of patients with asthma, the routine use of serum IgE analysis is limited.

IMMUNOGLOBULIN DEFICIENCIES

Immunodeficiencies affecting either antibody production or cell-mediated immunity are commonly subdivided in two groups – primary and secondary. The primary immunodeficiency diseases are the naturally occurring defects that increase susceptibility to infections. The disorders constitute a spectrum of more than 80 different innate defects in the immune system (Cooper et al., 2003). The overall incidence of these immunodeficiency diseases is estimated at approximately 1 in 10 000, excluding selective immunoglobulin A deficiency. There may be as many as 500 000 cases in the USA, of which about 50 000 cases are diagnosed each year. Common primary immunodeficiencies include disorders of antibody immunity, affecting B-cell differentiation and/or antibody production, isolated T-cell abnormalities, combined B- and T-cell defects, phagocytic disorders and complement deficiencies (Cooper et al., 2003). The majority of immune defects involve antibody production; these immune deficiencies are found more often in adults than infants and children (Ballow, 2002).

The immune system can also be adversely affected secondarily by a variety of conditions, such as malnutrition, malignancy, metabolic diseases, infections, as well as immunosuppressive drugs or radiation. Antibody deficiencies need to be excluded in patients who have recurrent, severe or unusual pyogenic infections. The commonest sites of infection are the upper and lower respiratory tracts and the infections caused by capsulated bacterial pathogens like *Streptococcus pneumoniae* and *Haemophilus influenzae*. Some patients also develop diarrhea and malabsorption due to bacterial overgrowth in the small intestine or chronic infection with *Giardia*, *Campylobacter* or *Cryptosporidium* (Puck, 1997; IUIS Scientific Committee, 1999).

Immunoglobulin A deficiency

IgA deficiency is the most frequent primary immunodeficiency, with an average prevalence of 1:400–1:700. IgA deficiency is defined as a serum IgA concentration of less than 7 mg/dl with normal serum IgM and IgG levels (Table 12.3). Both IgA subclasses, IgA1 and IgA2, are usually markedly reduced or absent, although isolated deficiencies of each subclass have been described. In general, an IgA2 deficiency would be expected to lead to more serious infections than an IgA1 deficiency, due to the stronger protease susceptibility of the IgA1 molecule.

Approximately 50 per cent of individuals with selective IgA deficiency are clinically asymptomatic. IgA deficient patients usually have sino-pulmonary infections, involvement of the gastrointestinal tract with giardiasis and nodular lymphoid hyperplasia. An increased frequency of autoimmune disorders has also been associated with IgA deficiency, including arthritis, a lupus-like illness, autoimmune endocrinopathies, chronic active hepatitis, ulcerative colitis, Crohn's disease, a sprue-like disease and autoimmune hematologic disorders (Ballow, 2002). Selective IgA deficiency is also strongly associated with atopy. IgA deficiencies are often found in association with other immune abnormalities, including ataxia-telangiectasia and IgG subclass deficiencies. The occurrence of IgA

Table 12.3 Common levels of immunoglobulins in immunodeficiency diseases*

Diseases	IgG	IgA	IgM	IgE	IgD
Selective IgA deficiency	n	↓↓	n	n	
Selective IgG deficiency	↓↓	n/↓	n	n	
Selective Ig class deficiency	n/↓	n/↓	n/↓	n/↓	n/↓
X-linked agammaglobulinemia	↓↓	↓↓	↓↓	n/↑	
Hyper-IgM syndrome	↓	↓	↑	↓	
Common variable immunodeficiency	↓↓	↓↓	n/↓	↓	
Ataxia telangiectasia	↓	↓↓	n	↓	
Wiskott-Aldrich syndrome	n/↑	n/↑	↓	n/↑	
'Bare-lymphocyte syndrome' (MHC deficiencies)	n/↓	↓↓	↓↓	n/↓	
SCID	↓↓	↓↓	↓↓	↓↓	

* n, normal levels; ↓, decreased levels; ↑, increased levels.

deficiency in both male and female patients and its clustering in families suggest an autosomal inheritance.

The pathogenesis of IgA deficiency is still unknown, although abnormalities in immunoglobulin class switching and the cytokines involved in isotype switching have been implicated. The pathogenesis of IgA deficiency may share a common cause with common variable immunodeficiency because these two disorders share many immunological aspects.

Immunoglobulin G deficiency

A deficiency of total IgG will generally result in serious infectious problems. IgG subclass deficiency also occurs and is a common feature in a number of primary as well as secondary immunodeficiency syndromes (Ballow, 2002). Since a decreased level of one IgG subclass may be accompanied by increased levels of one or more of the other subclasses, the total IgG level may be within the normal range. Therefore, evaluation of IgG subclass levels is important, even when the total IgG level is within or only slightly below the reference range of healthy individuals (Meulenbroek and Zeijlemaker, 1996). As IgG1 comprises up to 70 per cent of the total IgG serum concentration, patients with IgG1 deficiency usually have reduction in total IgG. Interest in IgG subclass deficiencies arose from a report of a family with recurrent sinopulmonary infections who had normal serum IgG, IgA and IgM concentration but reduced IgG2 and IgG4 levels. These patients were shown to be unable to produce antibodies to polysaccharide antigens but have normal antibody responses to the protein antigens.

Deficiencies can occur in single or multiple IgG subclasses (Morell, 1994). Deficiencies of IgG subclasses can be subdivided in different groups. A complete deficiency of one or more subclasses, caused by deletions in chromosome 14 loci, is rare (Bottaro et al., 1989). Most abnormalities are based upon regulatory defects resulting in decreased levels rather than a total lack of one or more immunoglobulin subclasses. IgG2 deficiency may occur either as an isolated finding or in association with IgA or IgG4 deficiency. Among the combined IgG subclass deficiencies, an IgG2/IgG4 deficiency predominates (Jefferis and Kumararatne, 1990). The relevance of selective IgG4 deficiency is uncertain, as approximately up to 15 per cent of the general population have IgG4 concentrations in serum below the limit of detection. Interestingly, the genes encoding IgG2, IgG4 and IgA are closely linked and this combined deficiency is due to a regulation defect of the 'downstream switch' in the heavy chain loci (Meulenbroek and Zeijlemaker, 1996). It seems that the expression of the immunoglobulins whose genes are located downstream in the C(H) region, such as IgG4 and IgE, requires more help from Th2 cells compared to the upstream isotypes, IgG1 and IgG3 (Mayumi et al., 1983; Bich-Thuy and Revillard, 1984). IgG4 and IgG2 deficiencies are often found to be associated with a predominant T-cell defect, such as in ataxia telangiectasia, AIDS and immune reconstitution after bone marrow transplantation. It has been noticed that patients with IgG1 and/or IgG3 deficiency are more likely to have more chronic and recurrent infections of the lower respiratory tract, whereas patients with IgG2 and/or IgG4 deficiency are more likely to have sinusitis and otitis (Herrod, 1993a,b).

Immunoglobulin M deficiency

Selective IgM deficiency implies correct gene rearrangements in B cells and might be caused by the failure of polysaccharide recognition systems. In this case, a certain decrease in the IgG2 and IgG4 subclasses would be also anticipated, because of their specificity for bacterial polysaccharide antigens.

Patients with a combined X-linked Wiskott-Aldrich deficiency syndrome display low or absent serum IgM levels, while IgG, IgA and IgE levels may be normal or elevated (Thrasher, 2002). WASP patients are unable to respond to polysaccharide antigens and thus isoagglutinins are absent.

Immunoglobulin D deficiency

IgD deficiency is a defect of humoral immunity that is characterized by abnormally low serum levels of this immunoglobulin (Alper et al., 2003). It has been reported that approximately 11 per cent of 371 American Red Cross blood donors and 6 per cent of 1529 study subjects had low or undetectable IgD levels (<0.002 mg/ml). In the study group, a number of the individuals with low IgD had rheumatologic disease (e.g. juvenile rheumatoid arthritis, lupus, psoriatic arthritis, vasculitis), but the frequency of low IgD within groups of patients with each disease did not differ from the normal controls using chi-square analysis. In another study, using a cutoff of 2.15 IU/ml, assays of 245 healthy adults and 301 healthy children revealed that approximately 13 per cent of each group had low levels of IgD. Unfortunately, little is known

about the normal function of IgD and few clinical signs or symptoms are associated with its absence. Individuals with low or absent levels of IgD do not appear unusually predisposed to infections.

Other immunodeficiencies associated with hypogammaglobulinemia

Common variable immunodeficiency (CVID)

Common variable immunodeficiency, also known as adult-onset hypogammaglobulinemia, acquired hypogammaglobulinemia or dysgammaglobulinemia, is a heterogeneous group of disorders involving both B-cell and T-cell immune function (Ballow, 2002). The average age of onset of symptoms is 25 years and the average age at diagnosis is 28 years. CVID is characterized by recurrent bacterial infections (recurrent otitis, chronic sinusitis and recurrent pneumonia), decreased serum immunoglobulin levels, especially IgG and IgA and abnormal antibody responses to specific immunization (Fischer, 2004). Most individuals with CVID are panhypogammaglobulinemic, but some produce substantial amounts of IgM. Although markedly diminished, the serum Ig levels are usually higher than those found in patients with X-linked agammaglobulinemia. Autoimmune disorders occur frequently in patients with CVID (approximately 22 per cent of patients) and include rheumatoid arthritis, autoimmune hematologic disorders, such as hemolytic anemia, idiopathic thrombocytopenic purpura and pernicious anemia, autoimmune neurologic diseases, such as Guillain-Barré syndrome, chronic active hepatitis often related to hepatitis C virus and autoimmune endocrinopathies, particularly involving the thyroid gland (Etzioni, 2003).

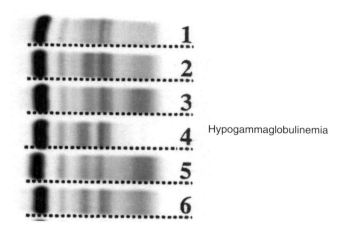

Hypogammaglobulinemia

Figure 12.1 Evaluation of gammaglobulins by total protein electrophoresis in serum specimens. Normal range of immunoglobulins is shown in samples 1, 2 and 6. Samples 3 and 5 demonstrate a polyclonal increase in immunoglobulin levels, which might be associated with infections, autoimmune diseases or certain liver abnormalities. Sample 4 is an example of hypogammaglobulinemia, which may be a sign of primary or secondary immunodeficiency or light chain myeloma. The automated SPIFE 3000 electrophoresis system was used for serum protein separation and staining (Helena Laboratories, Beaumont, TX).

Immunodeficiency with hyper-IgM

During the last few years, a series of primary immune deficiencies characterized by a defect of class switch recombination and the inability to produce immunoglobulins other than IgM or IgD have been described. Some of these defects are collectively referred to as hyper-IgM immunodeficiency (HIGM) syndrome. This syndrome mainly affects males (55–65 per cent) and is characterized by decreased serum levels of IgG, IgA and IgE, but elevated IgM and accompanied with severe recurrent bacterial infections. Patients with HIGM syndrome can also develop autoimmune disorders (Etzioni, 2003). Coombs positive hemolytic anemia, inflammatory bowel disease, hepatitis, seronegative arthritis, hypothyroidism and discoid lupus erythematosus have all been reported in HIGM patients. A variety of serum autoantibodies have been detected as well, including anti-erythrocyte, anti-erythropoietin, anti-platelet, anti-smooth muscle, anti-cardiolipin, anti-Ro, anti-RNP, antinuclear and anti-thyroid antibodies.

HIGM type 1 (HIGM1) is inherited as an X-linked trait (Gaspar et al., 2002). The disease is caused by defective expression of CD40 ligand (CD40L, CD154), a molecule predominantly expressed by activated CD4+ T cells. CD40–CD40L interaction is essential for final maturation of B cells after their activation by antigen and supports class switch recombination. Immunological features include very low serum levels of IgG and IgA, with normal to increased IgM. The number and distribution of T-cell subsets are normal, as are proliferative responses to mitogens. Patients with HIGM1 syndrome are clinically and immunologically indistinguishable from subjects carrying genetic defects of CD40 (a molecule constitutively expressed by B lymphocytes, monocytes, dendritic cells and by endothelial and some epithelial cells) that results in an autosomal recessive form of HIGM, which has been recently described and termed HIGM type 3 (Puck, 1994).

In contrast, patients with HIGM type 2 (HIGM2) present with a distinct clinical phenotype characterized by enlargement of tonsils and lymph nodes and recurrent bacterial sino-pulmonary infections, without increased susceptibility to opportunistic pathogens. Pathologic examination of lymph nodes reveals aberrantly large germinal centers, a finding that clearly distinguishes HIGM2 from HIGM1 and HIGM3. In addition to the characteristic immunoglobulin profile similar to HIGM1 and HIGM3, patients with HIGM2 show a lack of switched IgD-negative B cells and a profound defect of somatic hypermutation. The association of both somatic hypermutation and class switch recombination deficiency is explained by mutations in the recently cloned activation-induced cytidine deaminase (AID) gene that plays a critical role in both processes.

A fourth form of HIGM affects males and is characterized by the association of hypogammaglobulinemia with hypohydrotic ectodermal dysplasia (HIGM-ED). Similarly to other forms of HIGM, HIGM-ED is not a pure humoral deficiency since defects of T and natural killer (NK) cells have been also reported (Imai et al., 2003).

X-linked aggammaglobulinemia (XLA)

X-linked aggammaglobulinemia, also called Bruton's agammaglobulinemia, or congenital agammaglobulinemia, occurs with a frequency of about 1 per 3–6 million. Total absence or marked deficiency of serum immunoglobulins, extremely low percentages (<2 per cent) or absent B cells, but normal or even increased numbers of pro-B cell in the bone marrow due to the block of their maturation, are typical findings in XLA (Fischer, 2004). The upper respiratory tract is the most common site of infection. Other types of infection include pyoderma, chronic conjunctivitis, gastroenteritis, arthritis and meningitis-encephalitis. Capsulated bacteria, particularly *H. influenzae* and *S. pneumoniae*, are commonly associated with these infections. Arthritis and a dermatomyositis-like syndrome can also occur in patients with XLA, although autoimmune disorders do not seem to be a frequent problem in patients with XLA (Ballow, 2002).

HYPERIMMUNOGLOBULINEMIA

Increased levels of serum immunoglobulin may be a consequence of upregulated synthesis or lowered catabolism. Distinctively, hypergammaglobulinemia may arise from monoclonal, polyclonal or oligoclonal pathological or physiological processes. For instance, monoclonal increase of immunoglobulins commonly results from a malignant or premalignant clonal B or plasma cell proliferation, while a polyclonal increase in serum antibodies could be the consequence of autoimmune or inflammatory reactions. Increase of total IgG, IgA and IgM can be detected in patients with hepatitis or cirrhosis, rheumatoid arthritis and systemic lupus erythematosus. In most infections the first antibodies to appear will be of the IgM class, while those of the IgG class will be produced later. In general, microbial protein antigens will mainly evoke antibody responses of the IgG1 and IgG3 subclasses, with a minor contribution of IgG2 and IgG4. On the other hand, polysaccharide antigens will predominantly induce IgG2 antibodies.

Monoclonal gammopathy

Numerous terms such as monoclonal gammopathy (MG), paraprotein, M-component or M-protein are applied to describe the immunoglobulins overproduced by a single clone of B cells. The term M-protein is generally preferred, because it does not imply structural characteristics of the molecule other than its homogeneous nature and does mean that the patient exhibits a pathological condition. M-protein corresponds to the observation of an electrophoretically restricted migration pattern at serum protein electrophoresis, but does not reflect a particular cellular mechanism involved in the clonal production of the immunoglobulin. In an attempt to unify the various names mentioned above, the general term 'immunoglobulinopathy' has been proposed for clonal overproduction of immunoglobulins. The search for an M-component may be of relevance in patients presenting unexplained peripheral neuropathy, carpal tunnel syndrome, nephrotic syndrome, renal insufficiency, cardiomyopathy, refractory heart failure, orthostatic hypotension, acquired von Willebrand's disease, or malabsorption, because all these abnormalities have been associated with MG.

The detection of a single overproduced immunoglobulin is classically associated with B-cell lymphoproliferative disorders, like multiple myeloma, Waldenstrom's macroglobulinemia, non-Hodgkin's lymphoma, chronic lymphocytic leukemia and amyloidosis, but it can also be observed in the absence of a malignant disease (Chaibi et al., 2002). The latter situation is known as monoclonal gammopathy of undetermined significance (MGUS). B-cell lymphoproliferative disorders should be suspected instead of MGUS in patients with M-protein associated with unexplained anemia, back pain, weakness or fatigue, osteolytic lesions, fractures, osteopenia, hypercalcemia, renal insufficiency, proteinuria, diffuse failure of reabsorption in the proximal renal tubule resulting in glycosuria, generalized aminoaciduria and hypophosphatemia (acquired Fanconi's syndrome), or with the history of recurrent bacterial infections.

Plasma cell neoplasms usually manifest as disseminated bone marrow lesions (multiple myeloma) and infrequently as solitary extramedullary tumors classified as plasmacytomas. Malignant plasma cells usually secrete monoclonal IgG (60 per cent) or IgA (20 per cent) and rarely IgD (1–2 per cent) (Ho et al., 2002). There is a quantitative increase in the immunoglobulin concentration in the blood of multiple myeloma patients, but all of the immunoglobulins have identical specificity and therefore do not contribute to immune defense. The concentration of normal immunoglobulins is usually decreased due to dysregulation of lymphopoiesis and B-cell differentiation.

The term 'monoclonal gammopathy of undetermined significance' denotes the presence of a monoclonal protein in patients without evidence of plasma or B-cell proliferative disorders (Kyle and Rajkumar, 2003). This type of gammopathy is relatively common, with a prevalence of about 0.15 per cent of the general population. However, occurrences rise with age as MGUS has been found in approximately 1 per cent of persons older than 50 years, 3 per cent of persons older than 70 years and 4 per cent of individuals over 80 years old (Chaibi et al., 2002). Monoclonal gammopathy of undetermined significance may be associated with various disorders, including non-B-cell hematological malignancies, autoimmune diseases, secondary immunodeficiency states, von Willebrand disease, connective tissue diseases and neurologic disorders. A significant proportion of patients with MGUS will develop multiple myeloma or related disorders during a long-term follow-up. In addition, there are a number of unusual clinical findings that are due to the specific binding properties of the MG. These particular antibodies can lead to severe clinical problems in the absence of signs of malignancy and were named 'perverse' MG.

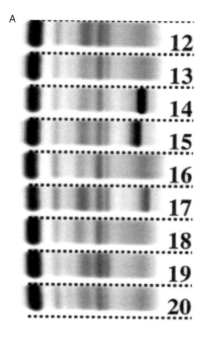

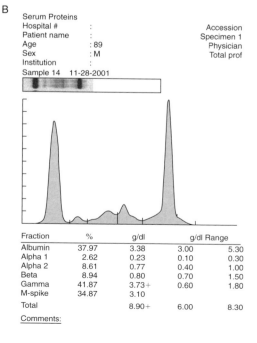

Figure 12.2 Detection of monoclonal gammopathies in serum specimens by total protein electrophoresis. A. Samples 14, 15 and 17 are examples of monoclonal gammopathy visible as the presence of significant band (M-protein) in gamma region. B. Densitometric analysis of sample 14 reveals the concentration of monoclonal protein in serum specimen. Windows-based QuickScan 2000 flat-bed densitometry (Helena Laboratories, Beaumont, TX) was used to image visible electrophoretic analytes on the agarose gel.

Biclonal, triclonal and oligoclonal gammopathies

Biclonal gammapathies occur in more than 5 per cent of patients with MG and are characterized by the presence of two homogeneous plasma immunoglobulins. The biclonal gammopathy may result from proliferation of two clones of plasma cells, each producing an unrelated mono-clonal protein or from the production of two M-proteins by one clone of plasma cells (Ho et al., 2002). Triclonal gammopathies or oligoclonal gammopathies have been also reported. The identification of multiple clonal immunoglobulins largely depends on the sensitivity of the technique utilized. Although it has been proposed that oligoclonal gammopathies should be considered to form a separate category of immunoglobulinopathies, studies in healthy volunteers, patients and animal models confirm that oligoclonal gammopathies and MG usually result from different pathophysiolological processes. MG is most frequently observed in patients with a malignant disease involving a single B-cell clone (Ho et al., 2002), whereas oligoclonal gammopathies are often detected in patients without overt B-cell malignancies. Immunoglobulin oligo-clonality may reflect a T-cell/B-cell imbalance, a selective antigenic pressure, or both. In all cases, however, identification of an immunoglobulinopathy may have important clinical implications.

Immunoglobulin M paraproteins

IgM paraproteins are IgM antibodies derived from the same B-cell clone and hence have identical immuno-chemical properties and functional activity (Roberts-Thomson et al., 2002). They are identified as monoclonal γ or β bands on serum protein electrophoresis with immunofixation having μ heavy chain and κ or λ light chain antigenicity. Circulating IgM paraprotein in large quantities is an essential feature of Waldenstrom's macroglobulinemia (Ghobrial et al., 2003) but may also occur in other B-cell lymphoproliferative disorders or as a 'benign' finding, particularly in the elderly. It is important that the clinical distinction is made between these possi-bilities, as Waldenstrom's macroglobulinemia and similar lymphoproliferative disorders with IgM paraproteinemia are potentially life-threatening disorders with unique clinico-pathological features.

IgM paraproteins accounted for ~20 per cent of all new paraproteins detected. IgM paraproteinemia occurs more commonly in males and its frequency increases with age (Roberts-Thomson et al., 2002). Approximately 30 per cent of IgM paraproteins are associated with B-cell lympho-proliferative disorders with the remainder being identi-fied as monoclonal IgM gammopathies of uncertain significance. IgM paraproteins frequently exist in multiple molecular forms, the pentamer being the dominant species in all patients but decamers also being observed in most patients, particularly those with high levels of IgM (Ghobrial et al., 2003). Monomeric and oligomeric IgM

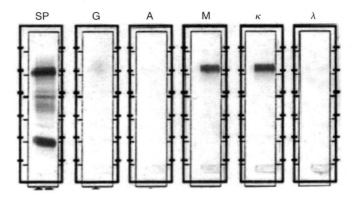

Figure 12.3 Analysis of monoclonal immunoglobulins in serum specimens by serum electrophoresis with immunofixation. Using specific antibodies against heavy and light chains of immunoglobulins allows detection of the nature of monoclonal immunoglobulins after electrophoretic separation of serum proteins on agarose gels. Immunofixation analysis of sample 14 (see Figure 9.2) revealed the presence of monoclonal IgM/k. The automated SPIFE 3000 electrophoresis system was used for serum protein separation, staining and development (Helena Laboratories, Beaumont, TX).

were also evident, notably in those patients having a malignant form of lymphoproliferative disorder.

Monoclonal heavy chain disease

Heavy chain disease (HCD) is a rare disorder characterized by the secretion of monoclonal proteins consisting of incomplete heavy chains of the immunoglobulins. Gamma-HCD is associated with the increased synthesis and release of monoclonal γ chains of IgG and accompa-nied by lymphoadenopathy and osteolysis. Alpha-HCD, or Mediterranean lymphoma, is characterized by the secretion of α chains of IgA by mucosal plasma cells in the intestines. This results in the development of progressive malabsorption syndrome, diarrhea and abdominal pain. Mu-HCD occurs in conjunction with lymphoproliferative diseases, particularly B-CLL.

Light chain disorders

Bence Jones plasmacytomas are characterized by the exclusive secretion of light chains, which can be detected in serum and urine (Bence Jones proteins) in different concentrations depending on the stage of disease pro-gression (Stone, 2002). Protein electrophoresis of serum obtained from these patients often demonstrates marked decrease of total immunoglobulins (secondary antibody deficiency) due to replacement of hematopoietic precur-sors in the bone marrow with myeloma cells and thus deficient lymphopoiesis.

Production of light chains is also associated with primary, non-hereditary light chain (AL) amyloidosis, which is characterized by the deposition of fibrils from fragments of immunoglobulin light chains (Buxbaum, 2004). AL occurs in plasma cell disorders, especially multiple myeloma or Waldenstrom's macroglobulinemia. Amyloidosis most commonly induces renal symptoms, although cardiac and gastrointestinal involvement is also typically observed.

Hyper-IgD syndrome

A definite increase in serum IgD was found in patients with Hodgkin's disease several months after splenectomy (Corte et al., 1978). A correlation with the histologic type was observed; e.g. patients in the lymphocyte-depleted group had extremely high levels of IgD. Increased concentrations of serum IgD were found in other diseases and conditions, e.g. in children with kwashiorkor (Rowe et al., 1968) and after allogeneic bone marrow transplantation (Mizuma et al., 1987). High values of serum IgD were also reported in children following chemotherapy for malignancies (Azuma et al., 1991), in some patients with hyperparathyroidism (Papadopoulos and Frieri, 1984) and in cigarette smokers (Bahna et al., 1983). IgD was also increased (>100 U/ml) in many children with periodic fever, aphthous stomatitis, pharyngitis and adenopathy syndrome (Padeh et al, 1999).

The new syndrome – hyperimmunoglobulinemia D syndrome (HIDS) – was described in 1984 by Van der Meer et al. and seems to have boosted the measurement of serum IgD in various patients in the hope of detecting more patients with HIDS and also of finding increased IgD in other conditions (Vladutiu, 2000). HIDS is the only entity for which the measurement of polyclonal IgD is necessary for diagnosis. This syndrome is characterized by recurrent febrile attacks accompanied by abdominal pain, arthralgia, headache and skin lesions. HIDS is probably inherited as an autosomal recessive trait and mutations in the mevalonate kinase gene were shown to cause HIDS (Houten et al., 1999). It has been proposed that patients exhibit an uncontrolled type 3 hypersensitivity reaction, possibly with involvement of IgD-containing complexes (Boom et al., 1990).

ANALYSIS OF SPECIFIC ANTIBODIES IN SERUM

Evaluation of the serum levels of specific antibodies is essential for diagnosis of certain immunodeficiency diseases, many autoimmune disorders, allergies and a number of infectious diseases.

Specific antibodies in immunodeficiencies

The ability to produce specific antibodies against defined antigens is the most sensitive method of detecting certain malfunctions of antibody production. The incidence of specific antibody defects in patients with normal immunoglobulins is unknown (Bird, 1991). However, in the presence of history suggestive of immunodeficiency without gross deficiency of total serum immunoglobulins,

detection of specific antibodies before and after immunization should be assessed. The levels of specific antibodies are usually determined using a panel of protein and carbohydrate antigens. This includes (i) thymus-dependent antigens tetanus toxoid, diphtheria toxoid, influenza vaccine and Salk vaccine (inactivated polio) and (ii) thymus-independent antigens, such as E. coli LPS, pneumococcal polysaccharide, H. influenzae type b polyribose phosphate and meningococcal polysaccharide type A and C (Bird, 1991). If initial levels of specific antibodies are low, the patient should be immunized with the appropriate antigen and the antibody response should be reassessed in 3–4 weeks. However, immunization with live vaccines is contraindicated in patients with suspected immunodeficiency.

Specific antibodies in autoimmune diseases

Autoimmune diseases are conditions in which structural or functional damage to organs and tissues results from immunological mechanisms mediated by autoantibodies or autoreactive cells. The autoantibody in organ-specific autoimmune diseases is directed predominantly at particular target organs or tissues, which are also the site of immunopathology. This includes autoimmune thyroiditis (Hashimoto's thyroiditis and Graves' disease), autoimmune gastritis, autoimmune hepatitis (chronic active hepatitis and primary biliary cirrhosis) and other autoimmune diseases of skin (bullous pemphigoid), GI tract (celiac disease), CNS (multiple sclerosis), muscles (myasthenia gravis), kidney (Goodpasture's syndrome), pancreas (insulin-dependent diabetes mellitus) and erythrocytes (autoimmune hemolytic anemia). In non-organ specific autoimmune diseases, which include systemic lupus erythematosus, rheumatoid arthritis and the vasculitides, the autoantibodies are not organ restricted and present in many different tissues. Autoantibodies can be grouped into primary antibodies, which are directly pathogenic, and secondary antibodies, which recognize intracellular antigens. Secondary antibodies are usually not involved in the pathogenesis of many conditions, but can serve as useful diagnostic markers of different autoimmune diseases (Bird, 1991).

The ease of detection of antibodies recognizing a variety of tissue and intracellular antigens has led to the description of a wide range of autoantibody specificities. The list of autoantibodies and corresponding antigens is constantly growing. For instance, rheumatoid factor (RF) for many years served as the only serological factor associated with rheumatoid arthritis (RA). RF consists naturally occurring autoantibodies with specificity for the Fc region of IgG (Moore and Dorner, 1993). A number of other autoantibodies associated with RA have been described, most of which remain largely experimental tools. Furthermore, no single antibody marker is sufficiently sensitive to be used solely in the diagnosis of RA as was concluded on the basis of their sensitivity range (Marcelletti and Nakamura, 2003). However, a few markers are highly specific for RA suggesting that a diagnostic panel consisting of two or three markers may achieve sufficient sensitivity. Of particular interest are those autoantibodies that recognize citrullinated forms of native proteins. Antikeratin and antiperinuclear factor antibodies have been tested for several years and were found to be highly specific for RA (van Boekel et al., 2002). New studies indicate that these antibodies recognize an epitope that includes the deimidated form of arginine called citrulline (Schellekens et al., 1998). Cyclic peptides containing citrulline (CCP) have been used to develop a highly sensitive and specific assay for the differential diagnosis of RA. Subsequent clinical studies demonstrated predictive value of the anti-CCP plus RF combination suggesting that the disease could potentially be identified solely on the basis of serology (Marcelletti and Nakamura, 2003).

Determination of tissue-specific autoantibodies is of great value for disease diagnosis, monitoring of therapy and prediction of the disease progression. For instance, Hashimoto's thyroiditis involves antibodies to various intracellular antigens, including thyroglobulin and thyroid peroxidase. Hyperthyroidism in Graves' disease is due to antibodies to the thyrotropin receptor that cause overstimulation of the gland (Reiterer and Borkenstein, 2003). Autoimmune liver diseases are associated with an autoimmune attack on hepatocytes and bile duct epithelial cells mediated by antibodies recognizing a sialoglycoprotein receptor and 2-oxo acid dehydrogenase enzyme complexes on mitochondrial membranes. Autoantibodies to myelin basic protein and myelin-associated glucoprotein are found in multiple sclerosis and polyneuropathy, respectively (Lutton et al., 2004). Goodpasture's syndrome is characterized by the presence of autoantibody to glomerular, renal tubular and alveolar basement membranes, resulting primarily in injury to the glomerulus that can rapidly progress to renal failure (Jara et al., 2003). Autoantibody-mediated damage to the acetylcholine receptors in skeletal muscles leads to the progressive muscle weakness and is the pathogenetic basis of myasthenia gravis (Vincent et al., 2003).

A diagnosis of autoimmune disease implies that the autoimmune response is a significant component of the disease process. In most instances the initiating events of autoimmune disease are not understood and autoantibodies are an effect of disease, not a cause. Even though the cause may not be known, the presence of autoantibodies can be clinically useful and their titers may have prognostic value.

Specific antibodies in infectious diseases

Medical importance of serological, i.e. antibody-based test in the diagnosis of infectious diseases is evident when

1 the microorganism cannot be cultured, e.g. syphilis and hepatitis A, B and C

2 the microorganism is too dangerous to culture, e.g. rickettsial diseases
3 culture techniques are not readily available, e.g. HIV and EBV
4 the microorganism takes too long to grow, e.g. *Mycoplasma* (Gaur et al., 1994).

For instance, infection with *Treponema pallidum* provokes a complex antibody response and serological tests for syphilis are based on the detection of one or more of these antibodies. No 'perfect' single test is available at present and although more than 200 methods have been reported, only a few are routinely used. Detection of antibodies of two types are currently used for screening and diagnostic purposes: (i) non-treponemal antibodies, or regain, which react with lipid antigens and (ii) treponemal antibodies, which react with *T. pallidum* and closely related strains (Young, 1998).

Infection with hepatitis B virus (HBV) stimulates strong immunological responses to a number of HBV antigens. Acute and chronic phases of the disease are discernible based on specific serologic profile. In acute HBV hepatitis, HBsAg, HBeAg and HBcAb (antibody to the core protein) may be detected in the blood during viral replication. In chronic hepatitis, the development of HBeAb (antibody to the e antigen) indicates that the disease is no longer infectious. During a 'window' period, IgM HBcAb may be the only detectable serologic marker.

Serology tests are commonly used in both the diagnosis of different infections and in screening for specific immunity (Gaur et al., 1994). For instance, primary infection is indicated by the presence of specific IgM antibodies or by a fourfold rise in specific IgG antibody titers between acute- and convalescent-phase samples.

QUANTITATIVE IMMUNOGLOBULINS

Quantitative measurement of serum, urine or CSF immunoglobulins is used in the workup of both immunodeficiency states and some lymphoproliferative disorders. If an abnormality in humoral immunity is suspected, initial evaluation should include determination of IgG, IgA and IgM levels. The IgA level is especially helpful in that IgA concentrations in serum are low in almost all permanent types of agammaglobulinemia and in selective IgA deficiency. IgA measurement yields information about the body's resistance to mucosal infection as well as information related to specific diseases, such as myeloma and infection. Decreased levels are associated with immune deficiencies, protein losing conditions, non-IgA myelomas, mucosal infection and otitis media. Increased levels are associated with IgA myelomas, alcohol-related cirrhosis, chronic infection, active rheumatic disease and malabsorption syndrome. IgA deficiency may be associated with an anaphylactic reaction to blood products containing IgA and with development of antibodies to animal proteins.

IgE level assessment would be appropriate in patients with suspected atopy, Wiskott-Aldrich syndrome or suspected hyperimmunoglobulin E syndrome (Emanuel, 2003). Serum IgE concentrations are also increased in parasitic infestations and bronchopulmonary aspergillosis. Since total serum IgE is markedly elevated in about one half of patients with asthma, measurement of total IgE is not essential in any allergic conditions (Haeney, 1991). However, total serum IgE levels can be of value in infants with a positive family history of atopic disease and troublesome symptoms of suspected allergic origin, since levels are normally very low under the age of 2 years (Haeney, 1991). On the contrary, detection of antigen-specific IgE antibodies is of a great importance for patients with asthma. There are several available techniques to detect antigen-specific IgE in serum. These are radioallergosorbent test (RAST), radioimmunoassay (RIA) and enzyme-linked immunosorbent assay (ELISA) (Dolen, 2003).

IgG subclass testing should not be used for screening patients for suspected immunodeficiency, but should be reserved for patients who lack specific antibody responses to antigenic challenge yet have slightly low or normal immunoglobulin serum concentrations. Occasionally serum and urine protein electrophoresis may be helpful in evaluating patients with polyclonal or oligoclonal gammapathies and immunodeficiencies (Keren et al., 1999). Serum protein electrophoresis (SPE) is a technique in which molecules are separated on the basis of their size and electrical charge. SPE profile is traditionally divided into five regions: albumin, α-1, α-2, β and γ regions. IgG, IgM, IgD and IgE migrate in the γ-globulin region, while IgA migrates as a broad band in the β and γ regions. Additional evaluation of serum immunoglobulins is conducted if the SPE results reveal a monoclonal component, or if there is a significant quantitative abnormality of serum immunoglobulins. Another method of evaluating immunoglobulins in serum is immunofixation electrophoresis (IFE). In IFE, serum specimens are electrophoresed first and then specific antibodies recognizing γ, α, μ, δ and ϵ heavy chains and κ and λ light chains are applied directly to the gel. The antibody–antigen complexes are formed and can be visualized by staining. Polyclonal immunoglobulins are pointed out by diffuse staining, whereas monoclonal bands are reflected by narrow and intensely stained bands. Lack of staining indicates immunodeficiencies of one or more immunoglobulin classes (Keren, 1999).

Multiple immunological methods are also available for the quantitation of immunoglobulin levels. These methods can be classified into two general classes. The first group involves evaluation of physical properties from immune complexes generated by serum immunoglobulins and specific antibodies, such as light scattering, precipitation in gels, or agglutination of different particles. The second group involves assessment of serum immunoglobulins using specifically labeled antibodies. Three commonly used procedures include rate nephelometry, radial immunodiffusion (RID) in the first group and ELISA in the second group.

In the RID procedure, an antigen solution is placed in a well cut in the agarose gel containing specific antibodies. As the antigen diffuses into the gel, it reacts with the antibody forming a precipitin ring and its diameter is proportional to the antigen concentration. Nephelometry is based on the detection of light scattered from antigen–antibody complexes formed in a cuvette where serum samples are mixed with a specific antibody solution. Nephelometry is automated, fast and accurate.

Detection of autoantibodies is usually done by ELISA for known specific antigens or by immunofluorescence for initial screening of different groups of autoantibodies. For instance, known antigen is attached to a slide in form of cell lines or tissue with a known pattern of antigen distribution. The patient's serum is added and if it contains antibody against the antigen, it will remain fixed to it on the slide and can be detected on addition of a fluorescent-dye-labeled antibody to human IgG and examination by fluorescent microscopy. This method is commonly used to detect nuclear, gastric parietal cell, mitochondrial, smooth muscle and reticulin autoantibodies when frozen sections from a composite block of several tissues, rat kidney, liver, and stomach served as a substrate. Antinuclear antibodies (ANA) can be detected by the same technique using human epithelial cell line HEp-2 as a substrate.

CONCLUSIONS

Immunoglobulins play a key role in host defense against infections. Thus evaluation of the titers of each immunoglobulin subclasses as well as the levels of specific antibodies is essential for diagnosis of many immunological diseases. Similarly analysis of the presence and titer of a number of specific antibodies is widely used for prognosis and diagnosis of a variety of autoimmune diseases and allergies. However, immunoglobulins serve not only as a diagnostic tool, but could be also used for different therapeutic modalities. For instance, replacement therapy with γ-globulin in patients with immunodeficiencies, passive immunization for prophylaxis of some infectious diseases or neutralization of toxins or poisons and antibody-based immunotherapeutic approaches for cancer patients.

REFERENCES

Alper, C.A., Xu, J., Cosmopoulos, K. et al. (2003). Immunoglobulin deficiencies and susceptibility to infection among homozygotes and heterozygotes for C2 deficiency. J Clin Immunol 23, 297–305.

Azuma, E., Masuda, S., Hanada, M. et al. (1991). Hyperimmunoglobulinemia D following cancer chemotherapy. Oncology 48, 387–391.

170   Immunoglobulin Titers and Immunoglobulin Subtypes

Bahna, S.L., Heiner, D.C. and Myhre, B.A. (1983). Changes in serum IgD in cigarette smokers. Clin Exp Immunol 51, 624–630.

Ballow, M. (2002). Primary immunodeficiency disorders: antibody deficiency. J Allergy Clin Immunol 109, 581–591.

Bich-Thuy, L.T. and Revillard, J.P. (1984). Modulation of polyclonally activated human peripheral B cells by aggregated IgG and by IgG-binding factors: differential effect on IgG subclass synthesis. J Immunol 133, 544–549.

Bird, A.G. (1991). Organ-specific autoantibodies. In Clinical immunology. A practical Approach, H.G. Gooi and H. Chapel, eds. New York: Oxford University Press, pp. 175–194.

Blattner, F.R. and Tucker, P.W. (1984). The molecular biology of immunoglobulin D. Nature 307, 417–422.

Boom, B.W., Daha, M.R., Vermeer, B.-J. and van der Meer, J.W.M. (1990). Immune complex vasculitis in a patient with hyperimmunoglobulinemia D and periodic fever. Arch Dermatol 126, 1621–1624.

Bottaro, A., DeMarchi, M., DeLange, G.G. et al. (1989). Human IGHC locus restriction fragment length polymorphisms in IgG4 deficiency: evidence for a structural IGHC defect. Eur J Immunol 19, 2159–2162.

Buxbaum, J.N. (2004). The systemic amyloidoses. Curr Opin Rheumatol 16, 67–75.

Chaibi, .P, Merlin, L., Thomas, C. and Piette, F. (2002). Monoclonal gammapathy of undetermined significance. Ann Med Intern 153, 459–466.

Cooper, M.A., Pommering, T.L. and Koranyi, K. (2003). Primary immunodeficiencies. Am Fam Physician 68, 2001–2008.

Corte, G., Ferraris, A.M., Rees, J.K., Bargellesi, A. and Hayhoe, F.G. (1978). Correlation of serum IgD level with clinical and histologic parameters in Hodgkin disease. Blood 52, 905–910.

Dolen, W.K. (2003). IgE antibody in the serum – detection and diagnostic significance. Allergy 58, 717–723.

Drenth, J.P., Goertz, J., Daha, M.R. and van der Meer, J.W. (1996). Immunoglobulin D enhances the release of tumor necrosis factor-alpha, and interleukin-1 beta as well as interleukin-1 receptor antagonist from human mononuclear cells. Immunology 88, 355–362.

Emanuel, I.A. (2003). In vitro testing for allergy diagnosis. Otolaryngol Clin North Am 36, 879–893.

Etzioni, A. (2003). Immune deficiency and autoimmunity. Autoimmun Rev 2, 364–369.

Fagarasan, S. and Honjo, T. (2003). Intestinal IgA synthesis: regulation of front-line body defences. Nat Rev Immunol 3, 63–72.

Fischer, A. (2004). Human primary immunodeficiency diseases: a perspective. Nat Immunol 5, 23–30.

Gaspar, H.B., Sharifi, R., Gilmour, K.C. and Thrasher, A.J. (2002). X-linked lymphoproliferative disease: clinical, diagnostic and molecular perspective. Br J Haematol 119, 585–595.

Gaur, S., Kesarwala, H., Gavai, M., Gupta, M., Whitley-Williams, P. and Frenkel, L.D. (1994). Clinical immunology and infectious diseases. Pediatr Clin North Am 41, 745–782.

Ghobrial, I.M., Gertz, M.A. and Fonseca, R. (2003). Waldenstrom macroglobulinaemia. Lancet Oncol 4, 679–685.

Gould, H.J., Sutton, B.J., Beavil, A.J. et al. (2003). The biology of IgE and basis of allergic disease. Annu Rev Immunol 21, 579–628.

Haeney, M. (1991). Allergy. In Clinical immunology. A practical Approach, H.G. Gooi and H. Chapel, eds. New York: Oxford University Press, pp. 221–250.

Herrod, H.G. (1993a). Clinical significance of IgG subclasses. Curr Opin Pediatr 5, 696–699.

Herrod, H.G. (1993b). Management of the patient with IgG subclass deficiency and/or selective antibody deficiency. Ann Allergy 70, 3–8.

Ho, P.J., Campbell, L.J., Gibson, J., Brown, R. and Joshua, D. (2002).The biology and cytogenetics of multiple myeloma. Rev Clin Exp Hematol 6, 276–300.

Houten, S.M., Kuis, W., Duran, M. et al. (1999). Mutations in MVK, encoding mevalonate kinase, cause hyperimmunoglobulinaemia D and periodic fever syndrome. Nat Genet 22, 175–177.

Imai, K., Catalan, N., Plebani, A. et al. (2003). Hyper-IgM syndrome type 4 with a B lymphocyte-intrinsic selective deficiency in Ig class-switch recombination. J Clin Invest. 112, 136–142.

IUIS Scientific Committee. (1999). Report. Primary immunodeficiency diseases. Clin Exp Immunol 118 (Suppl 1), 1–28.

Jara, L.J., Vera-Lastra, O. and Calleja, M.C. (2003). Pulmonary-renal vasculitic disorders: differential diagnosis and management. Curr Rheumatol Rep 5, 107–115.

Jefferis, R. and Kumararatne, D.S. (1990). Selective IgG subclass deficiency: quantification and clinical relevance. Clin Exp Immunol 81, 357–367.

Keren, D.F. (1999). Procedures for the evaluation of monoclonal immunoglobulins. Arch Pathol Lab Med 123, 126–132.

Keren, D.F., Alexanian, R., Goeken, J.A., Gorevic, P.D., Kyle, R.A. and Tomar, R.H. (1999). Guidelines for clinical and laboratory evaluation patients with monoclonal gammopathies. Arch Pathol Lab Med 123, 106–107.

Kyle, R.A. and Rajkumar, S.V. (2003). Monoclonal gammopathies of undetermined significance: a review. Immunol Rev 194, 112–139.

Lutton, J.D., Winston, R. and Rodman, T.C. (2004). Multiple sclerosis: etiological mechanisms and future directions. Exp Biol Med (Maywood) 229, 12–20.

Marcelletti, J.F. and Nakamura, R.M. (2003). Assessment of serological markers associated with rheumatoid arthritis. Diagnostic autoantibodies and conventional disease activity markers. Clin Applied Immunol Rev 4, 109–123.

Mayumi, M., Kuritani, T., Kubagawa, H. and Cooper, M.D. (1983). IgG subclass expression by human B lymphocytes and plasma cells: B lymphocytes precommitted to IgG subclass can be preferentially induced by polyclonal mitogens with T cell help. J Immunol 130, 671–677.

Meulenbroek, A.J. and Zeijlemaker, W.P. (1996). Human IgG Subclasses: Useful diagnostic markers for immunocompetence. Amsterdam: CLB.

Mizuma, H., Zolla-Pazner, S., Litwin, S. et al. (1987). Serum IgD elevation is an early marker of B cell activation during infection with the human immunodeficiency viruses. Clin Exp Immunol 68, 5–14.

Moore, T.L. and Dorner, R.W. (1993). Rheumatoid factors. Clin Biochem 26, 75–84.

Morell, A. (1994). Clinical relevance of IgG subclass deficiencies. Ann Biol Clin (Paris) 52, 49–52.

Moskophidis, D., Moskophidis, M. and Lohler, J. (1997). Virus-specific IgD in acute viral infection of mice. J Immunol 158, 1254–1261.

Nitschke, L., Kosco, M.H., Kohler, G. and Lamers, M.C. (1993). Immunoglobulin D-deficient mice can mount normal immune responses to thymus-independent and -dependent antigens. Proc Natl Acad Sci USA 90, 1887–1891.

Orinska, Z., Osiak, A., Lohler, J. et al. (2002). Novel B cell population producing functional IgG in the absence of membrane IgM expression. Eur J Immunol 32, 3472–3480.

Padeh, S., Brezniak, N., Zemer, D. et al. (1999). Periodic fever, aphthous stomatitis, pharyngitis, and adenopathy syndrome: clinical characteristics and outcome. J Pediatr 135, 98–101.

Papadopoulos, N.M. and Frieri, M. (1984). The presence of immunoglobulin D in endocrine disorders and diseases of immunoregulation, including the acquired immunodeficiency syndrome. Clin Immunol Immunopathol 32, 248–252.

Puck, J.M. (1994). Molecular basis for three X-linked immune disorders. Hum Mol Genet 3, 1457–1461.

Puck, J.M. (1997). Primary immunodeficiency diseases. J Am Med Assoc 278, 1835–1841.

Reiterer, E. and Borkenstein, M.H. (2003). [Disorders of the thyroid gland in neonates and youth: latent hypothyroidism and hyperthyroidism.] Acta Med Austr 30, 107–109.

Roberts-Thomson, P.J., Nikoloutsopoulos, T. and Smith, A.J. (2002). IgM paraproteinaemia: disease associations and laboratory features. Pathology 34, 356–361.

Roes, J. and Rajewsky, K. (1993). Immunoglobulin D (IgD)-deficient mice reveal an auxiliary receptor function for IgD in antigen-mediated recruitment of B cells. J Exp Med 177, 45–55.

Rowe, D.S., Crabbe, P.A. and Turner, M.W. (1968). Immunoglobulin D in serum, body fluids and lymphoid tissues. Clin Exp Immunol 3, 477–490.

Rupolo, B.S., Mira, J.G. Kantor Junior, O. (1998). [IgA deficiency.] J Pediatr (Rio J) 74, 433–440.

Schellekens, G.A., de Jong, B.A., van den Hoogen, F.H.J., Van de Putte, L.B. and van Venrooij, W.J. (1998). Citrulline is an essential constituent of antigenic determinants recognized by rheumatoid arthritis-specific autoantibodies. J Clin Invest 101, 273–281.

Schur, P.H. (1987). IgG subclasses – a review. Ann Allergy 58, 89–96, 99.

Stahl, D. and Sibrowski, W. (2003). Regulation of the immune response by natural IgM: lessons from warm autoimmune hemolytic anemia. Curr Pharm Des 9, 1871–1880.

Stone, M.J. (2002). Myeloma and macroglobulinemia: what are the criteria for diagnosis? Clin Lymphoma 3, 23–25.

Thrasher, A.J. (2002). WASp in immune-system organization and function. Nat Rev Immunol 2, 635–646.

van Boekel, M.A.M., Vossenaar, E.R., van den Hoogen, F.H.J. and van Venrooij, W.J. (2002). Autoantibody systems in rheumatoid arthritis: specificity, sensitivity and diagnostic value. Arthrit Res 4, 87–93.

Van de Perre, P. (2003). Transfer of antibody via mother's milk. Vaccine 21, 3374–3376.

Vincent, A., McConville, J., Farrugia, M.E. et al. (2003). Antibodies in myasthenia gravis and related disorders. Ann NY Acad Sci 998, 324–335.

Vladutiu, A.O. (2000). Immunoglobulin D: properties, measurement, and clinical relevance. Clin Diagn Lab Immunol 7, 131–140.

Young, H. (1998). Syphilis. Serology. Dermatol Clin 16, 691–698.

Human Antiglobulin Responses

Chapter 13

Lorin K. Roskos[1], Sirid-Aimée Kellermann[1] and Kenneth A. Foon[2]

[1]Abgenix, Inc., [2]Division of Hematology-Oncology, University of Pittsburgh Cancer Institute, Pittsburgh, PA, USA

Without tolerance, our world turns into hell.

> Friedrich Dürrenmatt (1921–1990),
> Swiss dramatist, novelist, essayist.
> Trans. by Gerhard P. Knapp (1995).
> *About Tolerance* (1977)

Ha has are nothing to laugh about.

> Anonymous

INTRODUCTION

Although the ability to generate monoclonal antibodies was pioneered nearly three decades ago (Kohler and Milstein, 1975), only three murine monoclonal antibodies (mAbs) have been approved in the USA for therapeutic use. OKT®3 was approved in 1986; but over 16 years elapsed before the approvals of Zevalin™ and Bexxar® in 2002 and 2003, respectively. In contrast, twelve therapeutic mAbs with reduced murine protein content have been approved in the last decade. The recent resurgence in therapeutic mAb development and approval is attributable to the development of chimeric, humanized and fully-human mAb technology. These technologies have limited the magnitude and clinical relevance of antiglobulin responses directed against murine protein in the constant and variable regions of mAbs.

The clinical impact of immunogenicity was recognized soon after murine mAbs entered clinical trials (Cosimi et al., 1981; Sears et al., 1982; Miller et al., 1983; Dillman

et al., 1984). Antiglobulin responses negatively impact pharmacokinetics, efficacy and safety (Dillman, 1990; Isaacs, 1990). As an example (see Figure 13.1), a human anti-mouse antibody (HAMA) response against the murine anti-CD5 mAb, T101, resulted in accelerated clearance and neutralization of T101 and blocked the depletion of circulating target cells (Dillman et al., 1984). Similarly, neutralizing HAMA responses developed against OKT®3 despite intense immunosuppression; in some patients these HAMA responses were associated with accelerated clearance and loss of efficacy (Cosimi et al., 1981; Chatenoud et al., 1986a; Jaffers et al., 1986; Hooks et al., 1991). The HAMA responses against OKT®3 have been well characterized and consist of anti-isotypic and anti-idiotypic oligoclonal IgM and IgG antibodies against the murine constant and variable regions of OKT®3 (Chatenoud et al., 1986a,b; Jaffers et al., 1986). The immunogenicity of murine mAbs led to a general recognition that the therapeutic success of mAbs would be severely restricted until technologies were developed to limit or eliminate xenogeneic elements (Dillman, 1990; Isaacs, 1990; Kuus-Reichel et al., 1994).

The development of chimeric, humanized and fully-human mAb technology has decreased the immunogenicity of therapeutic mAbs. The immunogenicity profiles of the 15 therapeutic mAbs currently approved in the USA (as of November 2003) are listed in Table 13.1. For each mAb the technology platform, isotype, dosing route, patient immunocompetence (as determined by mAb target and comedications) and immunogenicity incidence are indicated. Because the patient population, assay sensitivity,

Measuring Immunity, edited by Michael T. Lotze and Angus W. Thomson
ISBN 0-12-455900-X, London

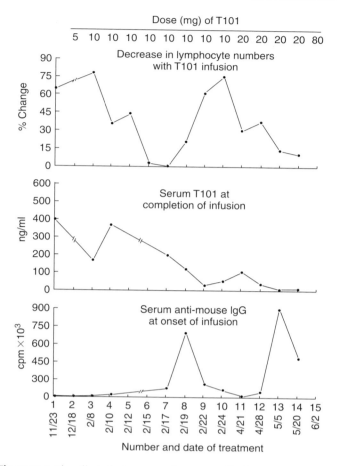

Figure 13.1 The effect of a human anti-mouse antibody response (HAMA) on the pharmacokinetics and activity of the murine anti-CD5 monoclonal antibody, T101. Appearance of HAMA was associated with accelerated clearance and decreased serum levels of T101 and loss of target cell depletion despite continued therapy at higher dose levels (from Dillman et al., 1984).

ANTIGENIC DETERMINANTS

Antibody structure and engineering

Monoclonal antibodies present several main antigenic determinants that can potentially elicit an antiglobulin response. A schematic illustration of mAb structure and potential antigenic determinants is given in Figure 13.2. MAbs consist of two identical Fabs and an Fc. Each Fab contains an antigen-binding site. The Fc determines the ability of the mAb to bind complement and interact with immune effector cells and governs the antibody half-life. The antibody half-life, the ability to recruit complement and the ability to interact with Fc receptors on immune effector cells may be important contributors to the risk of mAb immunogenicity (Fearon, 1998a,b; Kuus-Reichel et al., 1994; Reitan and Hannestad, 2002).

Each mAb molecule contains two identical heavy chains and two identical light chains. The heavy chain has one variable domain (VH) and three constant domains (CH1, CH2 and CH3). Each light chain has one variable domain (VL) and one constant domain (CL). The VH and VL domains contain unique amino acid sequences in the complementarity determining regions (CDR) and the framework regions that determine specificity and affinity for antigen binding. The uniqueness of the antibody variable region contributes to the potential immunogenicity of mAb products (Stein, 2002). Additionally, each heavy chain contains an N-linked carbohydrate moiety in CH2. The specific composition of the carbohydrate moiety can be critical to the antibody's effector function and may directly impact immunogenicity (Jefferis and Lund, 1997; Jefferis et al., 1998; Davies et al., 2001; Shields et al., 2002). The human IgG class is subdivided into four isotypes: IgG1, IgG2, IgG3 and IgG4. Antibodies of the IgG1 isotype have a greater capacity for effector function (Gessner et al., 1998) than the IgG2 and IgG4 isotypes, which are comparatively inactive regarding effector function.

The predominant determinant of mAb immunogenicity is the extent of xenogeneic protein content. Recombinant DNA techniques have enabled replacement of progressively larger portions of mouse mAbs with human sequences. Chimeric mAbs have the constant domains of both heavy and light chains replaced with human immunoglobulin sequences. Retention of murine V regions results in about one-third of the antibody being of xenogeneic origin (Morrison et al., 1984). Humanized mAbs have the framework of the V regions replaced with human sequences, but the CDRs (about 5–10 per cent of the total mAb) are retained as murine (Riechmann et al., 1988). Fully-human mAbs can now be generated from bacteriophage (Huse et al., 1989; McCafferty et al., 1990) or ribosome (Hanes and Pluckthun, 1997) display libraries or using transgenic mice that have been genetically engineered to produce human antibodies (Lonberg et al., 1994; Mendez et al., 1997; Kuroiwa et al., 2000).

Development of an antibody fragment is sometimes desired to decrease mAb half-life, eliminate effector

sample timing and sample handling can impact the reported incidence of immunogenicity, quantitative comparisons of incidence should not be made between similar products. However, general trends across mAb technology platforms can be observed. When dosing route, duration of treatment and immune status are considered, it is evident that humanization and fully-human antibody technology have allowed extended mAb therapy in immunocompetent patients and have permitted mAbs to be administered subcutaneously, a dosing route commonly considered to be more immunogenic than the intravenous route.

All the approved mAbs to date have exhibited some level of immunogenicity, regardless of the technology platform, antigen target or patient population. For those involved in the development and clinical use of mAbs, a general understanding of the clinical aspects of antiglobulin responses is essential. This chapter provides an overview of antibody structure, antigenic determinants, the clinical impact of immunogenicity and methods to detect, predict or prevent human antiglobulin responses.

Table 13.1 Immunogenicity of approved therapeutic monoclonal antibodies

mAB	Technology	Isotype	Dosing route	Immunosuppression?		Immunogenicity Incidence	Reference
				Antigen	Comedication		
OKT®3	Mu	IgG2a	IV	Yes	Yes	80%	Hooks et al. (1991)
Zevalin™	MuRc	IgG1	IV	Yes	Yes	3.8%	PI
Bexxar®	MuRc	IgG2a	IV	Yes	Yes	10–70%	PI
Reopro®	Ch	Fab	IV	No	No	5.8% (1 dose) 25% (2+ doses)	PI, Tcheng et al. (2001)
Rituxan®	Ch	IgG1	IV	Yes	No	1.1%	PI
Simulect®	Ch	IgG1	IV	Yes	Yes	1.2–3.5% (2 doses)	PI
Remicade®	Ch	IgG1	IV	Yes	Yes	10–61%	PI, Baert et al. (2003)
Zenapax®	Hz	IgG1	IV	Yes	Yes	8.4%	PI
Synagis®	Hz	IgG1	IM	No	No	0.7–1.8%	PI
Herceptin®	Hz	IgG1	IV	No	Yes	0.1%	PI
Mylotarg™	HzADC	IgG4	IV	Yes	Yes	0% HAHA 2 pts. HADA	PI
Campath®	Hz	IgG1	IV	Yes	No	1.9% CLL patients 63% RA patients	PI, Weinblatt et al. (1995)
Xolair®	Hz	IgG1	SC	No	No	<0.1%	PI
Raptiva™	Hz	IgG1	SC	Yes	No	6.3%	PI
Humira™	HuPD	IgG1	SC	Yes	Yes	1% with MTX 12% monotherapy	PI

Data are from the product prescribing information (PI) or other sources as indicated. Mu: murine; MuRC: murine radioconjugate; Ch: chimeric; Hz: humanized; HzADC: humanized antibody-drug conjugate; HuPD: human phage-display derived; MTX: methotrexate; IV: intravenous; IM: intramuscular; SC: subcutaneous. PI The immunosuppression columns designate whether the antibody–antigen interaction is immunosuppressive and if immunosuppressive therapies are usually given concurrently with the antibody.

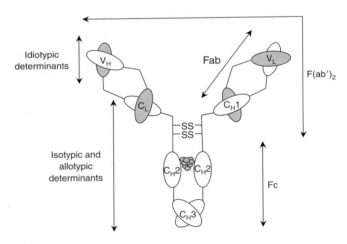

Figure 13.2 A schematic of the structure of IgG and its major antigenic determinants.

function or enhance tissue penetration (see Figure 13.2). A Fab fragment eliminates the Fc domain and retains the VH, VL, CH1 and CL domains. If divalent binding or a longer half-life is desired, F(ab')₂ fragments may be developed. F(ab')₂ fragments consist of two Fab fragments linked at their carboxyterminal ends by disulfide bonds. An alternative to the Fab or F(ab')₂ format is the single-chain

Fv, which consists of the VH and VL domains joined in tandem by a linker peptide. Diabodies and triabodies are alternative, multivalent structures based on the scFv format (Weiner and Adams, 2000; Hudson and Souriau, 2003). Following a single dose, murine antibody fragments are generally less immunogenic than intact murine mAbs (Kuus-Reichel et al., 1994). The decreased, single-dose immunogenicity of mAb fragments may be related to the short duration of exposure relative to intact mAbs and to the absence of the complement and effector cell binding properties imparted by the Fc domain.

Antiglobulin nomenclature

A human antiglobulin antibody (HAGA) response is designated according to the construct of the mAb immunogen: human anti-mouse antibody (HAMA); human anti-chimeric antibody (HACA); and human anti-humanized or anti-human antibody (HAHA). A HACA response against the variable region of a chimeric antibody may be referred to as a HAMA response to provide more information about the antigenic determinant. However, an antibody response against the murine, complementarity determining regions of humanized antibodies has been traditionally designated as a HAHA response. An antibody that develops against the toxin moiety of an immunoconjugate, e.g. anti-*Pseudomonas* exotoxin, is designated as a human anti-toxin antibody (HATA). An antibody response against the small molecule moiety of an antibody-drug conjugate (ADC) is designated as a human anti-drug antibody (HADA) response. HAGA responses may be anti-isotypic, anti-idiotypic or anti-allotypic. An anti-isotypic response is directed against the constant regions of the heavy or light chains. Anti-idiotypic antibodies develop against unique idiotopes of the antibody variable region. Anti-allotypic responses may potentially develop against polymorphic regions of the constant domains.

Idiotypic determinants

The adaptive immune system is able to recognize virtually any antigen by virtue of a highly diverse repertoire of antigen receptors on circulating B cells and T cells. Antibody diversity is achieved at several levels. During B cell maturation in the bone marrow, a wide array of antibody specificities is created when each B cell recombines one of over 50 VH genes with one of several DH and JH genes (to create the antibody heavy chain variable region) and one of approximately 40 Vκ genes with one of several Jκ genes (or, alternatively one of approximately 30 Vλ genes with one of several Jλ genes) to create the light chain variable region. During this recombination process, nucleotides are added or deleted at the junctions of V, D and J genes, leading to the introduction or deletion of a novel sequence; the combination of heavy and light chains introduces additional diversity.

When the immunoglobulin expressed on the cell membrane of a naïve B cell recognizes a specific antigen, the B cell becomes activated and begins to proliferate. A process known as somatic hypermutation is triggered, whereby mutations are introduced in the heavy and light chain variable regions. B cells expressing somatically hypermutated antibodies with enhanced binding to the particular antigen are positively selected to survive and proliferate and may undergo further rounds of somatic hypermutation (referred to as 'affinity maturation'), resulting in a population of B cells with progressively refined affinity and specificity.

The antigen recognition site of an antibody is formed by three hypervariable loops, or CDRs, within the heavy and light chain variable regions. The combined processes of junctional diversity during recombination, somatic hypermutation/affinity maturation results in antibodies with mutations concentrated within the CDRs. Mutations in the surrounding framework regions are less frequent, as these may impact an antibody's basic secondary structure and are therefore selected against during the affinity maturation process. The hypervariable loops combine to create the antibody's unique antigen recognition site known as its *idiotypic determinant* and each loop is an individual *idiotope*.

While junctional diversity and somatic hypermutation are beneficial for creating a diverse array of antibodies

with unique idiotypes able to recognize foreign proteins, on the other hand the same idiotypic determinants may be perceived as immunogenic in patients receiving an antibody drug. Anti-idiotypic antibodies generated in patients can block the antibody drug from binding to its antigen and therefore have a neutralizing effect. Since anti-idiotypic responses are directed against mutations that can be found in murine, chimeric, humanized and even human antibodies, all of these can be potentially immunogenic. Indeed, anti-idiotypic responses to antibody drugs have been described (Schroeder et al., 1993; Weinblatt et al., 1995; Regan et al., 1997; Baudouin et al., 2003).

Isotypic and allotypic determinants

Antibodies also possess isotypic and allotypic determinants. Anti-isotypic responses in patients are usually a consideration for antibodies with non-human constant regions; lack of tolerance to human antibody isotypes is rare. However, patients with rheumatoid factor (RF) may be HAHA positive prior to receiving monoclonal antibody therapy. Rheumatoid factor is typically comprised of low affinity IgM antibodies against the constant regions of human IgG; most frequently RF is directed against the CH2-CH3 domain interface (Sasso et al., 1988; Jefferis and Mageed, 1989; Mageed et al., 1997).

Allotypes, in contrast, are allelic polymorphisms within the constant domain of antibody heavy chain and kappa light chains. Because the polymorphisms segregate with particular ethnic groups (Pandey, 2000) and can be found on the antibody surface (Hougs et al., 2003), the patient allotype may be a contributing factor to immunogenicity. In principle, a patient who is homozygous for an allotypic variant may have an increased risk for development of an anti-allotypic HAHA response; however, little to no information is available regarding the contribution of anti-allotypic responses to mAb immunogenicity.

Post-translational modifications

Antibodies can undergo a number of post-translational modifications and these modifications are affected to a greater or lesser degree by the technology platform and expression system used to create and produce the antibody.

Mammalian antibodies possess a complex biantennary oligosaccharide on heavy chain residue Asn297 (Chadd and Chamow, 2001). Expression of human antibodies in non-human systems – most commonly hamster CHO cells and mouse NS0 cells and hybridomas – results in distinct glycosylation patterns (Chadd and Chamow, 2001). The particular glycosylation pattern may lead to complement activation or antibody binding to mannose-binding lectin. Increased binding to the mannose receptor on dendritic cells may enhance antibody uptake and processing by these antigen presenting cells, thereby increasing the potential for triggering anti-idiotypic antibody responses (Dong et al., 1999).

Other expression systems, such as yeast or transgenic livestock, also exhibit differences in glycosylation. Antibodies made in plants and *E.coli* lack oligosaccharides altogether. The glycosylation pattern may directly contribute to immunogenicity or may alter antibody structure (Krapp et al., 2003), thus creating potentially immunogenic conformers. However, to date there is little information regarding immunogenicity of non-human glycosylation patterns in antibody drugs in the clinic and the more important repercussions are likely to be on the antibody's effector capabilities.

CLINICAL RELEVANCE OF ANTIGLOBULIN RESPONSES

Impact on pharmacokinetics

Antiglobulin responses against mAb products usually alter pharmacokinetics and biodistribution. Immune complex formation accelerates mAb clearance, reduces serum levels and impairs targeting of therapeutic mAbs (Dillman, 1990; Weiner, 1999a,b). These pharmacokinetic effects have been commonly observed following repeated administration of murine mAbs. For example, the formation of large immune complexes in serum, altered biodistribution and increased deposition of the murine mAb 791T/36 in liver and spleen have been demonstrated in clinical studies (Pimm et al., 1985; Perkins et al., 1988) and animal models (Pimm et al., 1988, 1989) following development of an antiglobulin response. The observations were consistent with rapid elimination of the immune complexes by the reticuloendothelial system. A polyclonal response is not required to promote immune complexation and accelerated clearance. In a mouse model, an anti-idiotypic mAb αTS1 against the radiolabeled mAb TS1 produced dose-dependent increases in TS1 clearance as the ratio of TS1:αTS1 was varied from 1:0.3 to 1:1.2 (Johansson et al., 2002). Immune complexes in serum were observed, most commonly as tetrameric and hexameric rings and rings containing more than eight mAbs. Relative to TS1 alone, a substantial amount of radioactivity was relocated from blood to liver 1 h after concurrent dosing of TS1 and αTS1.

Altered pharmacokinetics and biodistribution are also seen following HAGA responses to chimeric, humanized and human mAbs. In rheumatoid arthritis patients receiving retreatment with infliximab between 1 and 6 months following their initial therapy, the mean area under the curve in HACA-positive patients was approximately one-fourth that of HACA-negative patients; the terminal half-life in HACA-positive patients was 48 h compared to 190 h in HACA-negative patients (Wagner et al., 2003). Following the development of a HAHA response to the humanized mAb sibrotuzumab in ovarian cancer patients,

accelerated clearance of the mAb, increased deposition in liver and decreased tumor targeting was observed (Scott et al., 2003). Accelerated clearance of the human mAb adalimumab also occurs upon development of HAHA responses (Abbott Laboratories, 2002).

Impact on efficacy

Accelerated clearance of therapeutic mAbs or neutralization of the antigen-binding domain can result in loss of product efficacy, impaired antigen targeting or interference with antibody-based diagnostic tests (Dillman, 1990; Kuus-Reichel et al., 1994; Klee, 2000; Stein, 2002). Loss of efficacy of OKT®3 has been observed when HAMA titers exceeded 1:1000 (Stein, 2002). The development of HACA responses to infliximab in patients with Crohn's disease was associated with a decreased duration of response to treatment (Baert et al., 2003). ACR20 response to adalimumab at the proposed dosage of 40 mg was reduced from 50 per cent in HAHA-negative rheumatoid arthritis patients to 30 per cent in HAHA-positive patients (Kress, 2002). In colon cancer patients receiving the humanized antibody A33, initial declines in CEA levels were observed only in the absence of HAHA-positive responses (Welt et al., 2003a,b).

Impact on safety

Serious safety risks may be associated with immunogenicity. Adverse reactions may be local or systemic and may vary from mild injection site reactions to life-threatening anaphylaxis (Dillman, 1990; Stein 2002). Acute hypersensitivity reactions to xenogeneic protein may occur on administration of the first dose and delayed hypersensitivity may be associated with the development of HAGA responses (Dillman, 1990). Patients developing HACA responses to infliximab (Baert et al., 2003) and HAHA responses to sibrotuzumab (Scott et al., 2003) and A33 (Ritter et al., 2001; Welt et al., 2003a,b) have shown an increased risk of hypersensitivity reactions relative to HAGA-negative patients. Anaphylactic shock caused by IgE sensitization has been described in a patient receiving retreatment with the chimeric mAb, basiliximab (Baudouin et al., 2003).

Infusion reactions to mAbs are reported frequently, but hypersensitivity reactions may be difficult to distinguish from target-mediated cytokine release (Koren et al., 2002). Mild to moderate infusion reactions are commonly observed following administration of the humanized mAb, trastuzumab. Serious and fatal infusion reactions have been rare; in post-marketing surveillance until March 2000, 74 worldwide cases, including nine fatal cases, occurred in 25 000 patients treated with trastuzumab (Cook-Bruns, 2001). Most of the serious reactions occurred within 2 h after starting the first infusion. Infusion and anaphylactoid reactions have been seen following infusion with the chimeric anti-EGFr antibody cetuximab, but not the fully human anti-EGFr antibody ABX-EGF

(Figlin et al., 2002; Needle, 2002; Schwartz et al., 2002), suggesting the reactions may be against the murine protein in cetuximab. An association of elevated lymphocyte counts with severity of infusion reactions has been reported following rituximab treatment, suggesting that the toxicity may be directly related to antibody binding to CD20 on circulating B lymphocytes (Winkler et al., 1999). Cytokine release after treatment with murine OKT®3 is believed to be caused by T-cell opsonization and subsequent lympholysis (Gaston et al., 1991). Cross-linking of effector cells may be a contributing factor, as bispecific antibodies targeting FcγRI and FcγRIII have been commonly associated with infusion reactions (Curnow, 1997; McCall et al., 2001).

Immunogenicity may precipitate or exacerbate target-mediated toxicity. In patients receiving re-administration of abciximab, 5.6 per cent of HACA-positive patients developed severe thrombocytopenia (platelets <20 000/μl) compared to 1.7 per cent of HACA-negative patients (Tcheng et al., 2001; Wagner et al., 2003). Consistent with these trends, severe thrombocytopenia after a second exposure to abciximab has been traced to antibodies specific to murine sequences in abciximab that recognize abciximab-coated platelets (Curtis et al., 2002).

Idiotype vaccines

Certain cancer therapeutics are actually designed to elicit anti-idiotypic antibodies (Bhattacharya-Chatterjee et al., 2002). Immunotherapy is very effective in certain animal model systems and it has been used to treat human cancers for several decades. Numerous investigators have studied active immunotherapy of cancer patients with tumor-derived material, with positive clinical responses reported. The major problem in using human material for immunization is that tumor-associated antigens (TAAs) are typically weak immunogens. A common explanation for the absence of anti-tumor immunity is that the immune system has become tolerant to tumor antigens. The large majority of TAAs in humans are non-mutated self-antigens. They are likely to be expressed at a higher level by malignant cells than by normal cells because of systemic gene deregulation associated with the cell transformation process. Therefore, the development strategies effective in inducing a strong immune response against self-TAAs represents one of the major challenges for the active immunotherapy of cancer. Among the many immunization strategies utilized to break unresponsiveness of self-TAAs, one effective method is to present the critical epitope to the now tolerant host in a different molecular environment. While this can be done with well-defined antigens such as haptens, it is impossible with most tumor antigens because they are chemically ill defined and difficult to purify. Carbohydrate antigens are even more problematic because they cannot be produced by recombinant techniques.

The immune network hypothesis offers a unique approach to transforming epitope structures into idiotypic determinants expressed on the surface of antibodies. Jan Lindemann (Lindenmann, 1973) and Niels Jerne (Jerne, 1974) proposed theories that described the immune system as a network of interacting antibodies and lymphocytes. According to the original network hypothesis, the Id-anti-Id interactions regulate the immune response of a host to a given antigen. Both Id and anti-Id have been used to manipulate cellular and humoral immunity.

The network hypothesis predicts that, within the immune network, the universe of external antigen (Ag) is mimicked by Ids expressed by antibodies and T-cell receptors. According to the network concept, immunization with a given Ag will generate the production of antibodies against this Ag, termed Ab1. This Ab1 can generate a series of anti-Id antibodies against Ab1, termed Ab2. Some of these Ab2 molecules can effectively mimic the three-dimensional structure of external Ag. These particular anti-Id, called Ab2β, which fit into the paratopes of Ab1, can induce specific immune responses similar to the responses induced by nominal Ag. Anti-Id antibodies of the β type express the internal image of the Ag recognized by the Ab1 antibody and can be used as surrogate Ag. Immunization with Ab2β can lead to the generation of anti-anti-Id antibodies (Ab3) that recognize the corresponding original Ag identified by the Ab1. Because of this Ab1-like reactivity, the Ab3 is also called Ab1' to indicate that it might differ in its other idiotopes from Ab1. Several such Ab2β have been used in animal models to trigger the immune system to induce specific and protective immunity against bacterial, viral (including HIV) and parasitic infections (Bhattacharya-Chatterjee, 1990). Similarly, a number of human trials have demonstrated that anti-idiotypic antibodies can break immune tolerance to a number of TAAs (Mellstedt et al., 1991; Mittelman et al., 1992; Denton et al., 1994; Herlyn et al., 1994; Durrant et al., 1995; Fagerberg et al., 1995; Foon et al., 1995, 1997, 1999).

DETECTING ANTIGLOBULIN RESPONSES

Because of the clinical relevance of immunogenicity, numerous analytical methods have been developed to assess antigenic responses to biological products (Mire-Sluis, 2002; Wadhwa et al., 2003). Each of the analytical methods has advantages and important limitations. Most notably, the sensitivity of all methods for detection of HAGA responses will be reduced by the presence of mAb in serum, as mAb will complex HAGA in serum and compete with assay capture and detection reagents. Choice of analytical methodology should be made based on considerations of sensitivity, specificity and efficiency.

Positive and negative controls

Positive and negative controls should be incorporated into all HAGA assays. The negative control may be pooled normal human serum. A similar reactivity of the negative control relative to naïve patient serum samples should be established. The positive control may be an anti-idiotypic neutralizing monoclonal antibody with a determined affinity to the therapeutic mAb. Inclusion of a high-affinity and a low-affinity control should be considered. Since the sensitivity of the assay will depend on the affinity of the positive control, a well-characterized monoclonal antibody standard is preferable to a polyclonal antibody preparation, where a quantitative assessment of affinity is not feasible. While 'authentic' positive controls have been proposed using HAGA positive samples from animals or patients, the availability of a well-characterized monoclonal anti-idiotypic antibody with long-term stability data is preferable to provide consistency over long periods of sample analysis. If an anti-idiotypic mAb is not available as a standard, a monoclonal or polyclonal antibody against the mAb constant regions may be used. However, if the therapeutic mAb contains human constant regions, this positive control will be cross-reactive with endogenous human IgG; therefore, the positive control must be added to buffer or animal serum rather than a human serum matrix.

Double-antigen bridging immunoassay

The assay most commonly used to detect HAGA responses uses the therapeutic mAb as the capture and detection reagent and is referred to as the 'double-antigen method' or the 'antigen bridging immunoassay'. This assay may be established using an immunoradiometric assay (IRMA) (Khazaeli et al., 1988) or an enzyme-linked immunosorbent assay (ELISA) (Buist et al., 1995; Ritter et al., 2001). Since the ELISA method does not involve the use of radioisotopes, the ELISA is usually the preferred format for routine application. The ELISA format is illustrated in Figure 13.3 (upper panel). The method incorporates the analyte and three sandwich reagents. First, the therapeutic mAb is coated on the ELISA plate. Following a wash step, the serum samples to be analyzed are diluted in blocking buffer and are added to the plate, allowing HAGA, if present, to bind to the plated mAb. After another wash step, biotinylated therapeutic mAb is added, which binds to the divalent HAGA. Finally, streptavidin-conjugated horseradish peroxidase (HRP) is added, which binds to the biotinylated mAb; after another wash a colorimetric substrate of HRP, such as TMB, is added and developed and the optical density (OD) of the sample is determined. As the only requirement for reagent bridging is that the HAGA is multivalent, this assay format will detect anti-idiotypic and anti-isotypic HAGA responses of any class or isotype.

Assay validation should be conducted to establish assay specificity, sensitivity, the threshold value associated with a seropositive sample and the appropriate concentration of the positive control. An example of assay validation for a fully-human mAb to interleukin-8,

ABX-IL8, is shown in Figure 13.3 (lower panel). Specificity is established by determining the OD of replicate serum samples from several individual normal serum donors and a pooled normal human serum source. The mean and standard deviation of replicates across sources are determined to factor in intra-assay, inter-assay and inter-subject variability. The OD threshold for a seropositive sample is generally set three standard deviations above the mean OD of the negative control samples. This threshold value should be calculated as a multiple of the negative control OD; each assay plate containing unknowns will include negative control samples and use of the OD multiple rather than the absolute OD value will more readily accommodate inter-assay variability. The positive control is evaluated over a range of concentrations to find a level that consistently yields OD values just above the OD threshold.

Use of patient samples during initial assay validation may not be practible or feasible due to availability of patient samples or because of informed consent limitations. Thus, use of healthy volunteer samples and commercial pooled serum during the initial validation is reasonable. However, naïve patient samples may yield a different range of negative OD values. For example, rheumatoid arthritis patients may show a wide range of OD values due to the presence of rheumatoid factor. In other cases, particularly for studies of mAbs containing xenogeneic protein, pre-existing anti-animal antibodies or heterophile antibodies may be present in serum prior to treatment (Kaplan and Levinson, 1999; Kricka, 1999). In all clinical studies, a pre-study baseline sample should be collected from patients to establish the individual patient's baseline reactivity and the range of OD values at baseline in the study patient population. If baseline positive samples are observed, then outlier tests should be used to exclude these positive values from the mean and standard deviation calculations used to establish the seropositive threshold. Thus, 'in process' validation should be conducted on an ongoing basis to confirm that the threshold established in the initial assay validation study is valid for the intended patient population.

If a HAGA sample is collected while the therapeutic mAb is still in the serum, then the assay sensitivity will be reduced. This is illustrated in Figure 13.3 (lower panel) where the therapeutic mAb was spiked at a level equal to the limit of quantification of the pharmacokinetic assay into serum containing the anti-idiotypic positive control. In this case, the sensitivity was reduced by approximately two orders of magnitude. Because of competition between the therapeutic mAb in serum and therapeutic mAb used as capture reagent, detection of the positive control required that the anti-idiotypic concentration exceed the therapeutic mAb concentration in serum before detection was feasible. This example illustrates the importance of assessing pharmacokinetics and collecting HAGA samples following washout of the therapeutic mAb.

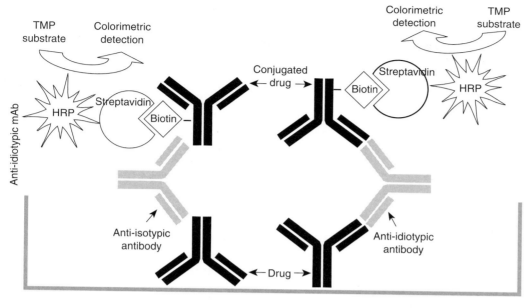

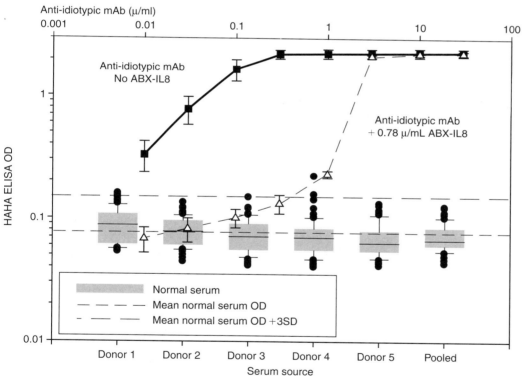

Figure 13.3 Configuration of a double-antigen, bridging ELISA for immunogenicity screening (upper panel) and assay validation results for a similarly configured, HAHA screening ELISA developed for the fully-human antibody, ABX-IL8 (lower panel, data on file at Abgenix, Inc).

The double-antigen method is typically very sensitive, fast and inexpensive to conduct. Thus, the double-antigen method often provides the best balance between efficiency and practicality. However, the primary limitation of this method is in the detection of low affinity antibodies. Because of the wash steps that are conducted after addition of the serum sample, low affinity antibodies may be washed off of the capture reagent, reducing assay sensitivity. Single-step methods, such as biosensor immunoassays, are useful alternatives for detection of low affinity HAGA responses such as an early IgM response.

Biosensor immunoassays

The biosensor immunoassay is based on detection by surface plasmon resonance (Swanson et al., 2002). The BIACORE 3000 (BIACORE Inc., Uppsala, Sweden) is an example of an instrument that utilizes this technology.

In this method, the therapeutic mAb is immobilized covalently on a biosensor surface in a flow cell. Diluted serum is then injected through the flow cell, allowing binding of HAGA to the immobilized mAb on the biosensor surface. The instrument detects binding to the immobilized mAb; the response unit (RU) signal is proportional to the added mass on the biosensor surface. The surface can then be regenerated by injection of acidic or basic solutions, allowing the analysis of multiple samples.

The application of a biosensor immunoassay for the detection of HAHA responses to the humanized mAb, A33, is illustrated in Figure 13.4 (Ritter et al., 2001). The relative magnitude of the RU is affected by the serum HAHA concentration and affinity. The dissociation phase from the immobilized mAb provides an indication of the dissociation constant and thus a rough indication of the relative HAHA affinity. The biosensor method has been able to detect positive HAHA responses earlier than an ELISA bridging assay (Ritter et al., 2001). Since the biosensor assay does not involve a wash step that could dissociate HAGA bound to immobilized mAb prior to detection, this method has enhanced sensitivity to detect low affinity HAGA responses, such as early IgM or IgG responses that occur prior to affinity maturation. The biosensor assay can be readily adapted to further characterization of a HAGA response, including determination of HAGA class and isotype, relative affinity and binding specificity (Ritter et al., 2001; Swanson et al., 2002).

The biosensor immunoassay is one of the most robust and sensitive methods available for the detection of HAGA responses. However, the primary limitations of this method are cost and efficiency. Instrument costs may be prohibitive for some organizations. Also, sample throughput per instrument is low relative to the ELISA method.

Confirmatory assay

Upon detection of a seropositive sample in a HAGA screening assay, a confirmatory assay should be conducted to verify the presence of a HAGA response. Frequently the confirmatory assay is conducted by titrating the therapeutic mAb into the HAGA serum sample (Swanson, 2002). A concentration-dependent decrease in assay signal should be observed as the spiked mAb complexes HAGA in serum. To avoid a sample retest bias (a seropositive sample that is retested may randomly yield a false negative retest result), a seronegative patient sample should be evaluated in parallel with each seropositive sample that is retested. Further characterization of the HAGA response may include quantitation, determination of class and isotype, neutralizing capacity and epitope mapping (Mire-Sluis, 2001, 2002).

Neutralization assay

An antibody response to a biotherapeutic product can affect the drug's biological activity in several ways. For example, antibodies may enhance the clearance of the drug from the circulation (Maini et al., 1998), or specifically inhibit the drug's ability to interact with other proteins necessary to exert its desired biological effect. Neutralizing assays can be used to determine whether patient antiglobulin antibodies fall in the latter category (Mire-Sluis, 2001). In competition assays, the ability of the antibody drug to

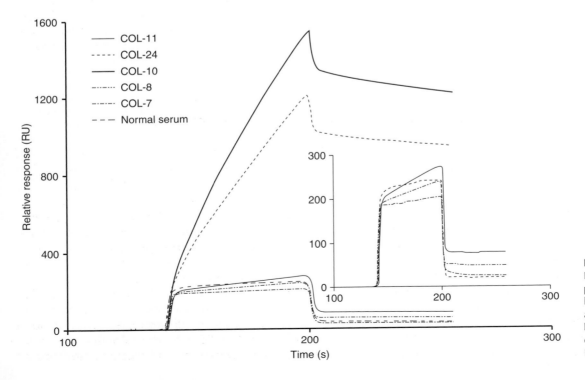

Figure 13.4 Detection of HAHA responses in cancer patients directed against the humanized monoclonal antibody, A33, using a biosensor assay developed on a Biacore 2000 (from Ritter, 2002).

bind to its target in the presence of patient serum is assessed. More sophisticated approaches can investigate the effect of antiglobulin antibodies on an antibody drug's effects on live cells using readouts such as cell proliferation or cytokine release.

Pharmacokinetic assay

Because of pharmacokinetic sensitivity to the development of HAGA responses, pharmacokinetics should be evaluated in parallel with immunogenicity assays where feasible. Collection of 'trough' samples just prior to the next administered dose is often sufficient to detect a change in the pharmacokinetic profile as a HAGA response develops. Trough levels are usually the most sensitive to the development of a HAGA response as the ratio of HAGA levels to drug levels will be highest at trough. Ideally, the pharmacokinetic assay should be established using the antigen as the capture reagent. Such a format may detect neutralizing HAGAs that block binding to antigen as well as HAGAs that accelerate clearance of the mAb. Because of decreased HAGA assay sensitivity that occurs when the therapeutic mAb is present in serum, the pharmacokinetic assay may be more sensitive than the HAGA assay during the dosing period. However, a change in the pharmacokinetic profile in absence of supportive HAGA assay data should be interpreted cautiously. If the mAb is subject to antigen-mediated clearance ('antigen sink'), then a time-dependent change in the pharmacokinetic profile may reflect altered antigen expression rather than development of a HAGA response.

Other assay formats

Other technologies can be applied to detect immunogenicity in animal models or in patients. A radioimmunoassay (RIA) approach uses radiolabeled drug that is mixed with the patient sample, whereupon antibody drug complexes are precipitated, for example with *Staphylococcus* Protein A. Radioactivity measured in the complex is a function of the amount of anti-drug antibodies present in the patient sample. When the drug is an IgG antibody, this approach must be adjusted in order to avoid Protein A-mediated precipitation of the drug in the absence of patient antiglobulin antibodies. The RIA approach for immunogenicity testing is further complicated by the difficulty in automating it for high-throughput applications.

An electrochemiluminescent-based strategy, such as the Origen® technology (Igen, Inc.), is an extremely sensitive format (Grimshaw et al., 1997) that may be used as a pharmacokinetic or HAGA assay. To detect the therapeutic mAb, the antibody drug is captured via an anti-idiotypic antibody or the antigen coupled to paramagnetic beads. A reporter anti-idiotypic antibody or the antigen labeled with a ruthenium chelate is added; the ternary complex emits a chemiluminescent signal in the presence of an electrical potential. In the HAGA assay format, the therapeutic mAb is used as the capture reagent and ruthenium-conjugated therapeutic mAb is used to detect. An advantage of this format, besides sensitivity, is that the method does not involve a wash step that could remove low-affinity HAGAs from the capture reagent. However, the assay may be subject to a prozone effect, thus routine analysis at more than one dilution factor may be necessary. Instrumentation and assay reagents are generally more expensive than for the bridging ELISA method.

Finally, the Luminex multiple analyte profiling system offers a multiplexed immunofluorescent approach for immunogenicity testing and quantitation (Seideman and Peritt, 2002; Opalka et al., 2003). This may be a means, for example, to determine the isotype(s) of the antiglobulin antibodies in patient serum (Gordon and McDade, 1997); another application may be basic epitope mapping based on binding of patient antiglobulin antibodies to Fab, Fc, or smaller fragments of the antibody drug, or competition with a panel of mAbs whose epitope specificity has been previously defined.

Collection of serum samples for immunogenicity assessment

Serum samples for use in HAGA assays should be collected pretreatment, during mAb treatment and in a follow-up after therapy has been discontinued and the mAb has been eliminated from serum. Samples collected during treatment should be collected just prior to the next dose, when mAb levels are lowest and will provide the least interference with the HAGA assay. For chronic therapy, collection of HAGA samples every 1–2 months or after each cycle of chemotherapy may be appropriate. Pharmacokinetic samples should be collected simultaneously with the HAGA sample to determine the effect of HAGA on pharmacokinetics and provide additional assurance against false-negative HAGA determinations while mAb is present in serum.

PREDICTING AND AVOIDING ANTIGLOBULIN RESPONSES

Ideally, the process of therapeutic antibody discovery and development should avoid immunogenicity altogether. Biophysical properties of the mAb and clinical factors are significant contributors to the risk of immunogenicity (Table 13.2). The choice of technology platform for generating monoclonal antibody drugs is a key factor in mitigating immunogenicity. Thus, phage display and human immunoglobulin-transgenic mice can deliver fully human antibodies that avoid the immunogenic xenogeneic elements of murine, chimeric and humanized antibodies. Nevertheless, decreasing muricinity does not necessarily eliminate immunogenicity. For example, adalimumab, a fully human anti-TNF antibody, is immunogenic in approximately 12 per cent of patients as a monotherapy (Abbott

Table 13.2 Factors potentially modulating the immunogenicity of monoclonal antibodies

Risk factor	Relative risk
Xenogeneic protein content	murine ≫ chimeric > humanized > fully-human
Antibody construct	intact > fragment
Antibody class	IgM, monomeric IgA > IgG, polymeric IgA
Antibody isotype	IgG1, IgG3 > IgG2, IgG4
Antigen localization	cell membrane antigen > secreted antigen
Immunosuppression	immunocompetent > immunosuppressed
Dose level	low dose > high dose
Dosing frequency	infrequent > frequent
Dosing route	subcutaneous > intramuscular ≥ intravenous

Laboratories, 2002; Kress, 2002). The observations with adalimumab further raise the interesting possibility that phage display technology may result in antibodies with unnatural structural features, due to *in vitro* pairing of heavy and light chain variable regions that have not affinity matured in tandem as would be found in antibodies generated *in vivo*. Clinical data on additional phage-display derived antibodies will be needed to address this hypothesis.

Regardless of the technology employed, mutations introduced into the heavy chain and light chain variable regions during the V(D)J recombination and somatic hypermutation processes may generate novel immunogenic sequences. The heavy and light chain CDRs (particularly the CDR3) are, by definition, hypervariable and can contain a number of mutations. Mutations in the framework region can be found in chimeric antibodies and ones generated in transgenic mice, while humanization and phage display approaches are able to engineer the CDR sequences of a desired antibody into selected recombinant antibody templates that *a priori* lack framework mutations. Molecular biological techniques can be used to revert framework or even CDR mutations in cloned recombinant antibodies back to the germline sequence, although this can potentially impact on potency and affinity. Currently, the success of reverse engineering to reduce antibody immunogenicity while retaining specificity and potency can only be tested empirically.

Besides immunogenicity conferred by unusual conformers or sequence mutations, antibodies whose variable regions are encoded by certain V genes may be immunogenic in patients who themselves do not express these V gene products. While the human genome can contain numerous functional VH, Vκ and Vλ genes, polymorphisms exist in individual genomic and expressed repertoires (Huang et al., 1996; Ignatovich et al., 1997; Wang and Stollar, 1999; Li et al., 2002). In addition, a number of V genes have several alleles (Tomlinson et al., 1995; Li et al., 2002) and, similar to what has been reported for antibody constant region allotypes, in the case of some V genes, certain alleles are common in some ethnic groups and rare in others (Atkinson et al., 1996; Juul et al., 1997).

In order to avoid immunogenicity, we must be able to predict it; this has taken on increasing importance as antibody drugs are entering the clinic in increasing numbers. Clearly it would be desirable to recognize immunogenic 'risk factors' prior to initiating costly clinical trials in patients and either reject antibodies that are suspect or modify them to reduce their immunogenic potential. For example, a systematic assessment of all VH, Vκ and Vλ genes present and expressed in a large number of subjects representing a variety of ethnic backgrounds may be a valuable resource in immunogenicity prediction. With increased clinical experience as well as insight from progressively more sophisticated *in vitro* and *in vivo* preclinical models, diverse approaches are being used to address the challenge.

The immunogenicity of a biologic can be predicted by assaying for the presence of B- and T-cell epitopes using, for example, PEPSCAN or peptide scanning. In this approach, an array of overlapping peptides is generated that represents the sequence of the biologic and this array is then queried (scanned) with anti-biologic antibodies to identify epitopes (i.e. immunogenic sites). This approach is either retrospective (human patients must be exposed to the biologic and develop an immune response so that their sera can then tested for epitope reactivity) or, alternatively, it extrapolates from antibody responses elicited in animals. Testing human patient serum may reveal reactivity to one or more sequences in the biologic, but it will not be possible to dissect which of the epitopes triggers antibodies with clinical sequelae. The situation is further complicated by the fact that antibodies' specificity may be for a linear sequence, but may also be directed against discontinuous sequences and conformational epitopes (including, for example, antibody drug idiotypic determinants). Peptide scanning techniques can identify immunogenicity directed against conformational or discontinuous epitopes by a process of elimination (the patient antibodies bind to the native molecule but not to any of the peptides), but it is difficult at best to pinpoint the location of the epitope in hope of engineering the biologic to have a less immunogenic sequence or structure.

Another tactic is to use *ex vivo* prediction methods, in which lymphocytes isolated from human peripheral blood are stimulated with the biologic and the ensuing response is assessed. This can be used to predict the presence of T-cell epitopes (which are a necessary precursor for the induction of antigen-specific IgG antibodies) in a drug (Stickler et al., 2003). Assaying lymphocytes from a large panel of donors identifies immunodominant epitopes recognized by a diverse population. Such an approach can also compare the original biologic and variants thereof (such as a reverse-engineered antibody drug). While *ex vivo* immunogenicity prediction is attractive because it uses human lymphocytes, it cannot reproduce the complexity of an *in vivo* immune response and cannot answer questions about the effects of the immune response on pharmacokinetic parameters.

Animal models have predicted immunogenicity of biologics in humans with variable success (Wierda et al., 2001; Bussiere, 2003). Generally, animal models are poor predictors of immunogenicity, in part due to a lack of tolerance of the animal to the human protein (i.e. the biologic is inherently immunogenic in non-human species). Certain biomolecules may be accurately tested in non-human primates where there is a high degree of homology to the animal ortholog (Zwickl et al., 1991). This problem has been addressed in some cases by creating transgenic mice expressing human proteins such as tissue plasminogen activator, insulin and interferon-$\alpha2$; these mice, being tolerant, are useful tools for testing immunogenicity of recombinant biologics based on the human protein (Stewart et al., 1989; Ottesen et al., 1994; Palleroni et al., 1997).

In our own experience, all fully-human antibodies are immunogenic in non-human primates and other animal species (unpublished observations). However, the same human immunoglobulin-transgenic mouse strains that are used to generate fully human therapeutic antibodies may also serve as valuable tools to test immunogenicity of human or humanized antibodies. Since these mice are de facto tolerant to human antibodies, they should not mount spurious immune responses to innocuous antibody sequences. XenoMouse® transgenic mice are ideally suited for this purpose, as they possess approximately 80 per cent of the functional human VH genes and about half of all functional Vκ genes and certain strains also contain all Vλ genes (Mendez et al., 1997; Kellermann and Green, 2002). Thus, these mice are theoretically tolerant to many, if not most, variable region germline sequences. This model furthermore can immortalize an antiglobulin response in the XenoMouse® mice by fusing B cells with myelomas to create hybridomas, which can then be used to dissect the immune response into individual antiglobulin antibody components and analyze their affinity, epitope specificity and effects on the antibody drug's bioactivity and pharmacokinetics.

CONCLUSIONS

The evolution of monoclonal antibody technology over the last three decades has been driven primarily by the clinical need to mitigate antiglobulin responses against therapeutic mAbs. Antiglobulin responses may negatively impact pharmacokinetics, efficacy and safety. Thus, monitoring and assessment of antiglobulin responses remain an essential part of clinical studies of antibody products. The development of fully-human antibody technology that eliminates xenogeneic protein and new methods to help predict immunogenicity may further support the development of mAbs with decreased immunogenicity, enhanced efficacy and improved safety profiles.

ACKNOWLEDGEMENTS

The authors gratefully acknowledge Hong Lu, MS (Abgenix, Inc), for the development and validation of the ABX-IL8 HAHA screening ELISA; and Pat Torello and Juan Li for their assistance in preparation of this manuscript.

REFERENCES

Abbott Laboratories. (2002). Adalimumab prescribing information. North Chicago, IL.: Abbot Laboratories.
Atkinson, M.J., Cowan, M.J. and Feeney, A.J. (1996). New alleles of IGKV genes A2 and A18 suggest significant human IGKV locus polymorphism. Immunogenetics 44, 115–120.
Baert, F., Noman, M., Vermeire, S. et al. (2003). Influence of immunogenicity on the long-term efficacy of infliximab in Crohn's disease. N Engl J Med 348, 601–608.
Baudouin, V., Crusiaux, A., Haddad, E. et al. (2003). Anaphylactic shock caused by immunoglobulin E sensitization after retreatment with the chimeric anti-interleukin-2 receptor monoclonal antibody basiliximab. Transplantation 76, 459–463.
Bhattacharya-Chatterjee, M., Chatterjee, S.K. and Foon, K.A. (2002). Anti-idiotype antibody vaccine therapy for cancer. Expert Opin Biol Ther 2, 869–881.
Buist, M.R., Kenemans, P., van Kamp, G.J. and Haisma, H.J. (1995). Minor human antibody response to a mouse and chimeric monoclonal antibody after a single i.v. infusion in ovarian carcinoma patients: a comparison of five assays. Cancer Immunol Immunother 40, 24–30.
Bussiere, J.L. (2003). Animal models as indicators of immunogenicity of therapeutic proteins in humans. Dev Biol (Basel) 112, 135–139.
Chadd, H.E. and Chamow, S.M. (2001). Therapeutic antibody expression technology. Curr Opin Biotechnol 12, 188–194.
Chatenoud, L., Baudrihaye, M.F., Chkoff, N., Kreis, H., Goldstein, G. and Bach, J.F. (1986a). Restriction of the human in vivo immune response against the mouse monoclonal antibody OKT3. J Immunol 137, 830–838.
Chatenoud, L., Jonker, M., Villemain, F., Goldstein, G. and Bach, J.F. (1986b). The human immune response to the OKT3 monoclonal antibody is oligoclonal. Science 232, 1406–1408.
Cook-Bruns, N. (2001). Retrospective analysis of the safety of Herceptin immunotherapy in metastatic breast cancer. Oncology 61 Suppl 2, 58–66.
Cosimi, A.B., Burton, R.C., Colvin, R.B. et al. (1981). Treatment of acute renal allograft rejection with OKT3 monoclonal antibody. Transplantation 32, 535–539.
Curnow, R.T. (1997). Clinical experience with CD64-directed immunotherapy. An overview. Cancer Immunol Immunother 45, 210–215.
Curtis, B.R., Swyers, J., Divgi, A., McFarland, J.G. and Aster, R.H. (2002). Thrombocytopenia after second exposure to abciximab is caused by antibodies that recognize abciximab-coated platelets. Blood 99, 2054–2059.
Davies, J., Jiang, L., Pan, L.Z., LaBarre, M.J., Anderson, D. and Reff, M. (2001). Expression of GnTIII in a recombinant anti-CD20 CHO production cell line: Expression of antibodies with altered glycoforms leads to an increase in ADCC through higher affinity for FC gamma RIII. Biotechnol Bioeng 74, 288–294.

Denton, G.W., Durrant, L.G., Hardcastle, J.D., Austin, E.B., Sewell, H.F. and Robins, R.A. (1994). Clinical outcome of colo-rectal cancer patients treated with human monoclonal anti-idiotypic antibody. Int J Cancer 57, 10–14.

Dillman, R.O. (1990). Human antimouse and antiglobulin responses to monoclonal antibodies. Antibody Immunocon Radiopharm 3, 1–15.

Dillman, R.O., Shawler, D.L., Dillman, J.B. and Royston, I. (1984). Therapy of chronic lymphocytic leukemia and cutaneous T-cell lymphoma with T101 monoclonal antibody. J Clin Oncol 2, 881–891.

Dong, X., Storkus, W.J. and Salter, R.D. (1999). Binding and uptake of agalactosyl IgG by mannose receptor on macrophages and dendritic cells. J Immunol 163, 5427–5434.

Durrant, L.G., Doran, M., Austin, E.B. and Robins, R.A. (1995). Induction of cellular immune responses by a murine mono-clonal anti-idiotypic antibody recognizing the 791Tgp72 anti-gen expressed on colorectal, gastric and ovarian human tumours. Int J Cancer 61, 62–66.

Fagerberg, J., Steinitz, M., Wigzell, H., Askelof, P. and Mellstedt, H. (1995). Human anti-idiotypic antibodies induced a humoral and cellular immune response against a colorectal carcinoma-associated antigen in patients. Proc Natl Acad Sci USA 92, 4773–4777.

Fearon, D.T. (1998a). Non-structural determinants of immuno-genicity and the B cell co-receptors, CD19, CD21, and CD22. Adv Exp Med Biol 452, 181–184.

Fearon, D.T. (1998b). The complement system and adaptive immunity. Semin Immunol 10, 355–361.

Figlin, R.A., Belldegrun, A.S., Crawford, J. et al. (2002). ABX-EGF, a fully human anti-epidermal growth factor receptor (EGFR) monoclonal antibody (mAb) in patients with advanced cancer: phase 1 clinical results. Proc Am Soc Clin Oncol 21, 10a.

Foon, K.A., Chakraborty, M., John, W.J., Sherratt, A., Kohler, H. and Bhattacharya-Chatterjee, M. (1995). Immune response to the carcinoembryonic antigen in patients treated with an anti-idiotype antibody vaccine. J Clin Invest 96, 334–342.

Foon, K.A., John, W.J., Chakraborty, M. et al. (1999). Clinical and immune responses in resected colon cancer patients treated with anti-idiotype monoclonal antibody vaccine that mimics the carcinoembryonic antigen. J Clin Onco 17, 2889–2895.

Foon, K.A., John, W.J., Chakraborty, M. et al. (1997). Clinical and immune responses in advanced colorectal cancer patients treated with anti-idiotype monoclonal antibody vaccine that mimics the carcinoembryonic antigen. Clin Cancer Res 3, 1267–1276.

Gaston, R.S., Deierhoi, M.H., Patterson, T. et al. (1991). OKT3 first-dose reaction: association with T cell subsets and cytokine release. Kidney Int 39, 141–148.

Gessner, J.E., Heiken, H., Tamm, A. and Schmidt, R.E. (1998). The IgG Fc receptor family. Ann Hematol 76, 231–248.

Gordon, R.F. and McDade, R.L. (1997). Multiplexed quantifica-tion of human IgG, IgA, and IgM with the FlowMetrix system. Clin Chem 43, 1799–1801.

Grimshaw, C., Gleason, C., Chojnicki, E. and Young, J. (1997). Development of an equilibrium immunoassay using electro-chemiluminescent detection for a novel recombinant protein product and its application to pre-clinical product develop-ment. J Pharm Biomed Anal 16, 605–612.

Hanes, J. and Pluckthun, A. (1997). In vitro selection and evolu-tion of functional proteins by using ribosome display. Proc Natl Acad Sci USA 94, 4937–4942.

Herlyn, D., Harris, D., Zaloudik, J. et al. (1994). Immunomodulatory activity of monoclonal anti-idiotypic antibody to anti-colorectal carcinoma antibody CO17-1A in animals and patients. J Immunother Emphasis Tumor Immunol 15, 303–311.

Hooks, M.A., Wade, C.S. and Millikan, W.J. Jr (1991). Muromonab CD-3: a review of its pharmacology, pharmaco-kinetics, and clinical use in transplantation. Pharmacotherapy 11, 26–37.

Hougs, L., Garred, P., Kawasaki, T., Kawasaki, N., Svejgaard, A. and Barington, T. (2003). Three new alleles of IGHG2 and their prevalence in Danish Caucasians, Mozambican Blacks and Japanese. Tissue Antigens 61, 231–239.

Huang, S.C., Jiang, R., Glas, A.M. and Milner, E.C. (1996). Non-stochastic utilization of Ig V region genes in unselected human peripheral B cells. Mol Immunol 33, 553–560.

Hudson, P.J. and Souriau, C. (2003). Engineered antibodies. Nat Med 9, 129–134.

Huse, W.D., Sastry, L., Iverson, S.A. et al. (1989). Generation of a large combinatorial library of the immunoglobulin repertoire in phage lambda. Science 246, 1275–1281.

Ignatovich, O., Tomlinson, I.M., Jones, P.T. and Winter, G. (1997). The creation of diversity in the human immunoglobulin V(lambda) repertoire. J Mol Biol 268, 69–77.

Isaacs, J.D. (1990). The antiglobulin response to therapeutic antibodies. Semin Immunol 2, 449–456.

Jaffers, G.J., Fuller, T.C., Cosimi, A.B., Russell, P.S., Winn, H.J. and Colvin, R.B. (1986). Monoclonal antibody therapy. Anti-idiotypic and non-anti-idiotypic antibodies to OKT3 arising despite intense immunosuppression. Transplantation 41, 572–578.

Jefferis, R. and Lund, J. (1997). Glycosylation of antibody mol-ecules: structural and functional significance. Chem Immunol 65, 111–128.

Jefferis, R., Lund, J. and Pound, J.D. (1998). IgG-Fc-mediated effector functions: molecular definition of interaction sites for effector ligands and the role of glycosylation. Immunol Rev 163, 59–76.

Jefferis, R. and Mageed, R.A. (1989). The specificity and reactiv-ity of rheumatoid factors with human IgG. Monogr Allergy 26, 45–60.

Jerne, N.K. (1974). Towards a network theory of the immune system. Ann Immunol (Paris) 125C, 373–389.

Johansson, A., Erlandsson, A., Eriksson, D. et al. (2002). Idiotypic-anti-idiotypic complexes and their in vivo metabo-lism. Cancer 94 (4 Suppl), 1306–1313.

Juul, L., Hougs, L., Andersen, V., Garred, P. et al. (1997). Population studies of the human V kappa A18 gene polymor-phism in Caucasians, blacks and Eskimos. New functional alleles and evidence for evolutionary selection of a more restricted antibody repertoire. Tissue Antigens 49, 595–604.

Kaplan, I.V. and Levinson, S.S. (1999). When is a heterophile anti-body not a heterophile antibody? When it is an antibody against a specific immunogen. Clin Chem 45, 616–618.

Kellermann, S.A. and Green, L.L. (2002). Antibody discovery: the use of transgenic mice to generate human monoclonal anti-bodies for therapeutics. Curr Opin Biotechnol 13, 593–597.

Khazaeli, M.B., Saleh, M.N., Wheeler, R.H. et al. (1988). Phase I trial of multiple large doses of murine monoclonal antibody CO17-1A. II. Pharmacokinetics and immune response. J Natl Cancer Inst 80, 937–942.

Klee, G.G. (2000). Human anti-mouse antibodies. Arch Pathol Lab Med 124, 921–923.

Kohler, G. and Milstein, C. (1975). Continuous cultures of fused cells secreting antibody of predefined specificity. Nature 256, 495–497.

Koren, E., Zuckerman, L.A. and Mire-Sluis, A.R. (2002). Immune responses to therapeutic proteins in humans – clinical significance, assessment and prediction. Curr Pharm Biotechnol 3, 349–360.

Krapp, S., Mimura, Y., Jefferis, R., Huber, R. and Sondermann, P. (2003). Structural analysis of human IgG-Fc glycoforms reveals a correlation between glycosylation and structural integrity. J Mol Biol 325, 979–989.

Kress, S. (2002). Clinical review, Abbott, biologic licensing application, adalimumab – for use in the treatment of rheumatoid arthritis. STN 125057.

Kricka, L.J. (1999). Human anti-animal antibody interferences in immunological assays. Clin Chem 45, 942–956.

Kuroiwa, Y., Tomizuka, K., Shinohara, T. et al. (2000). Manipulation of human minichromosomes to carry greater than megabase-sized chromosome inserts. Nat Biotechnol 18, 1086–1090.

Kuus-Reichel, K., Grauer, L.S., Karavodin, L.M., Knott, C., Krusemeier, M. and Kay, N.E. (1994). Will immunogenicity limit the use, efficacy, and future development of therapeutic monoclonal antibodies? Clin Diagn Lab Immunol 1, 365–372.

Li, H., Cui, X., Pramanik, S. and Chimge, N.O. (2002). Genetic diversity of the human immunoglobulin heavy chain VH region. Immunol Rev 190, 53–68.

Lindenmann, J. (1973). Speculations on idiotypes and homobodies. Ann Immunol (Paris) 124, 171–184.

Lonberg, N., Taylor, L.D., Harding, F.A. et al. (1994). Antigen-specific human antibodies from mice comprising four distinct genetic modifications. Nature 368, 856–859.

Mageed, R.A., Borretzen, M., Moyes, S.P., Thompson, K.M. and Natvig, J.B. (1997). Rheumatoid factor autoantibodies in health and disease. Ann NY Acad Sci 815, 296–311.

Maini, R.N., Breedveld, F.C., Kalden, J.R. et al. (1998). Therapeutic efficacy of multiple intravenous infusions of anti-tumor necrosis factor alpha monoclonal antibody combined with low-dose weekly methotrexate in rheumatoid arthritis. Arthritis Rheum 41, 1552–1563.

McCafferty, J., Griffiths, A.D., Winter, G. and Chiswell, D.J. (1990). Phage antibodies: filamentous phage displaying antibody variable domains. Nature 348, 552–554.

McCall, A.M., Shahied, L., Amoroso, A.R. et al. (2001). Increasing the affinity for tumor antigen enhances bispecific antibody cytotoxicity. J Immunol 16, 6112–6117.

Mellstedt, H., Frodin, J.E., Biberfeld, P. et al. (1991). Patients treated with a monoclonal antibody (ab1) to the colorectal carcinoma antigen 17-1A develop a cellular response (DTH) to the 'internal image of the antigen' (ab2). Int J Cancer 48, 344–349.

Mendez, M.J., Green, L.L., Corvalan, J.R. et al. (1997). Functional transplant of megabase human immunoglobulin loci recapitulates human antibody response in mice. Nat Genet 15, 146–156.

Miller, R.A., Oseroff, A.R., Stratte, P.T. and Levy, R. (1983). Monoclonal antibody therapeutic trials in seven patients with T-cell lymphoma. Blood 62, 988–995.

Mire-Sluis, A.R. (2001). Progress in the use of biological assays during the development of biotechnology products. Pharm Res 18, 1239–1246.

Mire-Sluis, A.R. (2002). Challenges with current technology for the detection, measurement and characterization of antibodies against biological therapeutics. Dev Biol (Basel) 10, 59–69.

Mittelman, A., Chen, Z.J., Yang, H., Wong, G.Y. and Ferrone, S. (1992). Human high molecular weight melanoma-associated antigen (HMW-MAA) mimicry by mouse anti-idiotypic monoclonal antibody MK2-23: induction of humoral anti-HMW-MAA immunity and prolongation of survival in patients with stage IV melanoma. Proc Natl Acad Sci USA 89, 466–470.

Morrison, S.L., Johnson, M.J., Herzenberg, L.A. and Oi, V.T. (1984). Chimeric human antibody molecules: mouse antigen-binding domains with human constant region domains. Proc Natl Acad Sci USA 81, 6851–6855.

Needle, M.N. (2002). Safety experience with IMC-C225, an anti-epidermal growth factor receptor antibody. Semin Oncol 29 (Suppl 14), 55–60.

Opalka, D., Lachman, C.E., MacMullen, S.A. et al. (2003). Simultaneous quantitation of antibodies to neutralizing epitopes on virus-like particles for human papillomavirus types 6, 11, 16, and 18 by a multiplexed luminex assay. Clin Diagn Lab Immunol 10, 108–115.

Ottesen, J.L., Nilsson, P., Jami, J. et al. (1994). The potential immunogenicity of human insulin and insulin analogues evaluated in a transgenic mouse model. Diabetologia 37, 1178–1185.

Palleroni, A.V., Aglione, A., Labow, M. et al. (1997). Interferon immunogenicity: preclinical evaluation of interferon-alpha 2a. J Interferon Cytokine Res 17 Suppl 1, S23–S27.

Pandey, J.P. (2000). Immunoglobulin GM and KM allotypes and vaccine immunity. Vaccine 19, 613–617.

Perkins, A.C., Pimm, M.V. and Powell, M.C. (1988). The implications of patient antibody response for the clinical usefulness of immunoscintigraphy. Nucl Med Commun 9, 273–282.

Pimm, M.V., Durrant, L.G. and Baldwin, R.W. (1989). The influence of syngeneic anti-idiotypic antibody on the biodistribution of an anti-tumour monoclonal antibody in BALB/c mice. Int J Cancer 43, 147–151.

Pimm, M.V., Perkins, A.C., Armitage, N.C. and Baldwin, R.W. (1985). The characteristics of blood-borne radiolabels and the effect of anti-mouse IgG antibodies on localization of radiolabeled monoclonal antibody in cancer patients. J Nucl Me. 26, 1011–1023.

Pimm, M.V., Perkins, A.C., Durrant, L.G. and Baldwin, R.W. (1988). A rat model for imaging the effect of anti mouse antibody responses on the biodistribution of radiolabelled mouse monoclonal antibodies. Eur J Nucl Med 14, 507–511.

Regan, J., Campbell, K., van Smith, L. et al. (1997). Characterization of anti-thymoglobulin, anti-Atgam and anti-OKT3 IgG antibodies in human serum with an 11-min ELISA. Transpl Immunol 5, 49–56.

Reitan, S.K. and Hannestad, K. (2002). Immunoglobulin heavy chain constant regions regulate immunity and tolerance to idiotypes of antibody variable regions. Proc Natl Acad Sci USA 99, 7588–7593.

Riechmann, L., Clark, M., Waldmann, H. and Winter, G. (1988). Reshaping human antibodies for therapy. Nature 332, 323–327.

Ritter, G., Cohen, L.S., Williams, C. Jr et al. (2001). Serological analysis of human anti-human antibody responses in colon cancer patients treated with repeated doses of humanized monoclonal antibody A33. Cancer Res 61, 6851–6859.

Sasso, E.H., Barber, C.V., Nardella, F.A., Yount, W.J. and Mannik, M. (1988). Antigenic specificities of human monoclonal and polyclonal IgM rheumatoid factors. The C gamma 2-C gamma 3 interface region contains the major determinants. J Immunol 140, 3098–3107.

Schroeder, T.J., First, M.R., Pouletty, C., Hariharan, S. and Pouletty, P. (1993). Rapid detection of anti-OKT3 antibodies with the Transtat assay. Transplantation 55, 297–299.

Schwartz, G., Dutcher, J., Vogelzang, N. et al. (2002). Phase 2 clinical trial evaluating the safety and effectiveness of ABX-EGF in renal cell cancer (RCC). Proc Am Soc Clin Oncol 21, 24a.

Scott, A.M., Wiseman, G., Welt, S. et al. (2003). A Phase I Dose-Escalation Study of Sibrotuzumab in Patients with Advanced or Metastatic Fibroblast Activation Protein-positive Cancer. Clin Cancer Res 9, 1639–1647.

Sears, H.F., Atkinson, B., Mattis, J. et al. (1982). Phase-I clinical trial of monoclonal antibody in treatment of gastrointestinal tumours. Lancet 1, 762–765.

Seideman, J. and Peritt, D. (2002). A novel monoclonal antibody screening method using the Luminex-100 microsphere system. J Immunol Methods 267, 165–171.

Shields, R.L., Lai, J., Keck, R. et al. (2002). Lack of fucose on human IgG1 N-linked oligosaccharide improves binding to human Fcgamma RIII and antibody-dependent cellular toxicity. J Biol Chem 277, 26733–26740.

Stein, K.E. (2002). Immunogenicity: concepts/issues/concerns. In Biologics 2000 – comparability of biotechnology products. Basel: S. Karger, pp. 15–23.

Stewart, T.A., Hollingshead, P.G., Pitts, S.L., Chang, R., Martin, L.E. and Oakley, H. (1989). Transgenic mice as a model to test the immunogenicity of proteins altered by site-specific mutagenesis. Mol Biol Med 6, 275–281.

Stickler, M., Mucha, J., Estell, D., Power, S. and Harding, F. (2003). A human dendritic cell-based method to identify CD4+ T-cell epitopes in potential protein allergens. Environ Health Perspect 111, 251–254.

Swanson, S.J., Mytych, D. and Ferbas, J. (2002). Use of biosensors to monitor the immune response. Dev Biol (Basel) 109, 71–78.

Tcheng, J.E., Kereiakes, D.J., Lincoff, A.M. et al. (2001). Abciximab readministration: results of the ReoPro Readministration Registry. Circulation 104, 870–875.

Tomlinson, I.M., Cox, J.P., Gherardi, E., Lesk, A.M. and Chothia, C. (1995). The structural repertoire of the human V kappa domain. EMBO J 14, 4628–4638.

Wadhwa, M., Bird, C., Dilger, P., Gaines-Das, R. and Thorpe, R. (2003). Strategies for detection, measurement and characterization of unwanted antibodies induced by therapeutic biologicals. J Immunol Methods 278, 1–17.

Wagner, C.L., Schantz, A., Barnathan, E. et al. (2003). Consequences of immunogenicity to the therapeutic monoclonal antibodies ReoPro and Remicade. Dev Biol (Basel) 112, 37–53.

Wang, X. and Stollar, B.D. (1999). Immunoglobulin VH gene expression in human aging. Clin Immunol 93, 132–142.

Weinblatt, M.E., Maddison, P.J., Bulpitt, K.J. et al. (1995). CAMPATH-1H, a humanized monoclonal antibody, in refractory rheumatoid arthritis. An intravenous dose-escalation study. Arthritis Rheum 38, 1589–1594.

Weiner, L.M. (1999a). An overview of monoclonal antibody therapy of cancer. Semin Oncol 26 (Suppl 12), 41–50.

Weiner, L.M. (1999b). Monoclonal antibody therapy of cancer. Semin Oncol 26 (Suppl 14), 43–51.

Weiner, L.M. and Adams, G.P. (2000). New approaches to antibody therapy. Oncogene 19, 6144–6151.

Welt, S., Ritter, G., Williams, C., Jr et al. (2003a). Phase I study of anticolon cancer humanized antibody a33. Clin Cancer Res 9, 1338–1346.

Welt, S., Ritter, G., Williams, C., Jr et al. (2003b). Preliminary report of a phase I study of combination chemotherapy and humanized A33 antibody immunotherapy in patients with advanced colorectal cancer. Clin Cancer Res 9, 1347–1353.

Wierda, D., Smith, H.W. and Zwickl, C.M. (2001). Immunogenicity of biopharmaceuticals in laboratory animals. Toxicology 158, 71–74.

Winkler, U., Jensen, M., Manzke, O., Schulz, H., Diehl, V. and Engert, A. (1999). Cytokine-release syndrome in patients with B-cell chronic lymphocytic leukemia and high lymphocyte counts after treatment with an anti-CD20 monoclonal antibody (rituximab, IDEC-C2B8). Blood 94, 2217–2224.

Zwickl, C.M., Cocke, K.S., Tamura, R.N. et al. (1991). Comparison of the immunogenicity of recombinant and pituitary human growth hormone in rhesus monkeys. Fundam Appl Toxicol 16, 275–287.

Rheumatoid Factors

Martin A.F.J. van de Laar

Department for Rheumatology, Medisch Spectrum Twente & University Twente, Enschede, the Netherlands

What I am going to tell you about is what we teach our physics students in the third or fourth year of graduate school… It is my task to convince you not to turn away because you don't understand it. You see my physics students don't understand it… That is because I don't understand it. Nobody does.

Richard P. Feynman, QED, The Strange Theory of Light and Matter, Penguin Books, London, 1990, p 9. (1)

INTRODUCTION

Waaler and Rose were the first to demonstrate the presences of a serum factor in patients suffering from rheumatoid arthritis (Waaler, 1940; Rose et al., 1948). They used sheep red blood cells coated with IgG from sensitized rabbits or humans. Incubating these coated cells with serum of patients suffering from rheumatoid arthritis resulted in an agglutination reaction. This phenomenon, not present in the serum of healthy individuals, was named the rheumatoid factor. For many years it was believed that rheumatoid arthritis was caused by the rheumatoid factor, or at least rheumatoid factor played a major role in the pathogenesis of the disease. As a result the rheumatoid factor was studied extensively in many laboratories and by many clinicians. Despite all this, currently, the exact role of rheumatoid factor in rheumatoid arthritis and other immunological conditions remains unclear.

THE STRUCTURE OF RHEUMATOID FACTORS

Rheumatoid factors are defined as autoantibodies reactive with the Fc part of IgG antibodies. Although the classical Waaler-Rose assay depends mainly on IgM antibodies, RF activity can be found in virtually any class of immunoglobulins. The occurrence of IgA-, IgG- as well as IgM-rheumatoid factors is widely established (Kunkel et al., 1966; Dunne et al., 1979). The IgM-rheumatoid factor consists of five subunits of approximately 185 000 Daltons joined by a disulfide, forming a pentamer (Figure 14.1). In addition, IgA-rheumatoid factor consists of two identical subunits, forming a polymeric structure varying between 160 000 and 1 000 000 Daltons (Schrohenloher et al., 1986). IgG-rheumatoid factor is in fact monomeric, however, complex formations with other IgG-rheumatoid factor molecules as well as with other IgG antibodies are found (Pope et al., 1975). Rheumatoid factors of patients suffering from rheumatoid arthritis react with IgG of various species (Butler and Vaughan, 1964). Rheumatoid factors react with various epitopes as represented in the different allotypic subgroups and can be found in some animals also. Moreover, variable degrees of cross-reactivity with other non-immunoglobulin antigens including $\beta2$-microglobulin and DNA histone nucleoprotein have been demonstrated (Aitcheson et al., 1980; Williams et al., 1992).

Measuring Immunity, edited by Michael T. Lotze and Angus W. Thomson
ISBN 0-12-455900-X, London

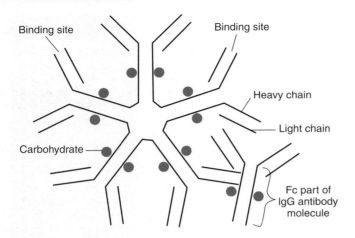

Figure 14.1 Usual rheumatoid factor.

PRODUCTION OF RHEUMATOID FACTORS

As addressed earlier rheumatoid factors (RF) are heterogeneous autoantibodies reactive with multiple determinants mainly localized to the Fc-portion of IgG (Youngblood et al., 1994). Clinical relevance of rheumatoid factors occurring in the spectrum of related diseases differs. These observations suggest that induction of synthesis of rheumatoid factors might involve different pathophysiological mechanisms. Antibodies with rheumatoid factor properties can be induced by immunization of animals and humans, however, rheumatoid arthritis disease is not induced by this process (Nemazee, 1985; Nemazee and Sato, 1983; Tarkowski et al., 1985).

Whether B cells are stimulated to produce rheumatoid factors by either non-specific polyclonal activation or are antigen driven is a matter still under debate. Polyclonal activators are effective inducers of rheumatoid factor *in vivo* as well as *in vitro* (Koopman and Schrohenloher, 1980a; Dalal et al., 1990). This suggests that rheumatoid factor producing B cells constitute the normal B cell repertoire. Obviously, modulating influences regulate rheumatoid factor expression. However, there is also evidence for antigen selection in the expression of autoantibodies in human systemic diseases like rheumatoid arthritis (Shlomchik et al., 1987). Recently, it was demonstrated that a mutation of the *ZAP-70* gene is responsible for autoimmune arthritis in mice which resembles rheumatoid arthritis including the production of rheumatoid factor (Norika et al., 2003).

The production of rheumatoid factor might be induced by abnormal IgG structures. IgG is a glycoprotein with N-linked oligosaccharides, invariably located in the Fc portion at asparagine 297. In rheumatoid arthritis, as well as in aging, an altered glycosylation of IgG is found. An increase in galactose-deficient oligosaccharide terminating in N-acetylglycosamine located at position 297 is demonstrated (Parekh et al., 1988; Tomana et al., 1988). Alterations on the oligosaccharide moiety in the Fc portion

of the IgG can lead to exposure of different epitopes. However, this mechanism is also present in inflammatory diseases in which RF is usually absent like ulcerative colitis and Crohn's disease (Go et al, 1994). Possibly, other mechanisms for alteration of IgG are irradiation or neutrophil driven free-oxygen radicals.

Besides B cells and T cells, monocytes (CD14+) and cytokines (IL-10) also likely stimulate the production of rheumatoid factors (Hirohata et al., 1995; Perez et al., 1995). The B cells bearing the T-cell marker CD5 are increased in the circulation of patients suffering from rheumatoid arthritis of Sjögren's syndrome. These CD5+ B cells seem to elaborate autoantibodies including rheumatoid factors (Casali et al., 1987).

Selection of rheumatoid factor from the host's natural repertoire not only occurs in rheumatoid arthritis but is also found in inflammatory diseases characterized by chronic antigen exposure. The presence of rheumatoid factors in subacute bacterial endocarditis is well known. Moreover, mice immunized with vesicular stomatitis virus respond with production of rheumatoid factors (Fehr et al., 1997). This suggests that rheumatoid factors represent a response to antibodies rather than a disease specific reaction.

B cells can function as antigen-presenting cells. In particular, antigen-specific B cells can bind their specific antigen and function efficiently as antigen-presenting cells (Rock et al., 1984). Thus rheumatoid factor-producing B cells might present antigen contained in immune complexes to antigen-specific T-helper cells. Rheumatoid factor B cells which have migrated to the synovium of patients suffering from rheumatoid arthritis might present a variety of antigens to relevant T cells, thus serving the local immune response (Tighe et al., 1993).

PATHOPHYSIOLOGY OF RHEUMATOID FACTORS

Currently, although frequently investigated, the origin of rheumatoid factors is incompletely understood (Sutton et al., 2000). It is likely that an abnormal immune response appears to select, possibly by antigen stimulation, rheumatoid factor from the natural antibody repertoire (Carayannopulos et al., 2000). IgM-rheumatoid factors can bind to monomeric IgG in serum as well as in synovial fluid to form a soluble complex, which sediments at 22 S. Thus rheumatoid factors are constituents of soluble and precipitated immune complexes in rheumatoid arthritis (Franklin et al., 1957). Remarkably, the complex consists of five IgG molecules for every one IgM-rheumatoid factor molecule. As mentioned earlier IgG-rheumatoid factors can react with themselves as well as with other IgG molecules, forming a wide spectrum of complexes (Nardella et al., 1981).

In patients suffering from rheumatoid arthritis who are negative for rheumatoid factor, B cells capable of producing rheumatoid factor are increased in number compared with normal individuals, however, the number of cells is considerably lower than in patients positive for rheumatoid factor (He et al., 1996).

The presence of rheumatoid factors is associated with the genetic disposition for rheumatoid arthritis of HLA DRB1*0401 as well as with the environmental factor of cigarette smoking (Mattey et al., 2002; Stolt et al., 2003). In twins suffering from rheumatoid arthritis the concentration of rheumatoid factors is related, emphasizing the relation between genetic factors and rheumatoid arthritis (MacGregor et al., 1995).

Currently, the role of rheumatoid factors in the pathogenesis of RA or other rheumatic diseases is unknown. However, local production of rheumatoid factor in synovium is well documented (Wernick et al., 1985). Moreover, rheumatoid factors are constituents of immune complexes in sera and synovial fluid of patients suffering from rheumatoid arthritis (Winchester et al., 1970). Both IgM- and IgG-rheumatoid factors can enhance complement activation (Sabharwal et al., 1982). IgM-rheumatoid factors modify the handling of immune complexes. Although it was postulated that rheumatoid factors stimulate pinocytosis, the opposite effect is demonstrated in some studies. This might be explained by differences in rheumatoid factor concentrations. By cross-linking with their Fcγ receptors rheumatoid factors directly activate natural killer cells (Hendrich et al., 1991). It has been shown that this stimulation induces secretion of interferon-γ and tumor necrosis factor-α (Saxne et al., 1988).

Rheumatoid factors are involved in many physiologic functions. In addition to their possible role in rheumatoid arthritis their frequent association with infections and following immunization argues for rheumatoid factors to be a part of the host response to infectious agents.

CLINICAL UTILITY OF RHEUMATOID FACTORS

Rheumatoid factors can be found in many rheumatic and non-rheumatic disorders. In rheumatoid arthritis, between 30 and 90 per cent of patients have circulating rheumatoid factors. Sensitivity of the rheumatoid factor tests is up to 90 per cent in clinically established disease. In contrast, in epidemiologically defined populations, including limited disease, sensitivity drops to 30 per cent. Since up to 5 per cent of healthy individuals have circulating rheumatoid factors as well, the value of the rheumatoid factor test for screening purposes is limited. Rheumatoid factors are found in other rheumatic diseases in both rheumatoid arthritis patients and in healthy individuals (Table 14.1). Therefore, the diagnostic value of a positive rheumatoid factor test in patients suspected to have rheumatoid arthritis is limited depending on the pre-test probability. In a study that addressed the positive predictive value (the likelihood of having the disease in the presence of one positive rheumatoid factor test),

a predictive value of only 24 per cent for rheumatoid arthritis and 34 per cent for any rheumatic condition was found (Shmerling and Delbanco, 1992). In patients with a chronic symmetrical distal polyarthritis, the presence of rheumatoid factors merely underscores the diagnosis and helps to determine the prognosis (Shmerling and Delbanco, 1991; Green et al., 1995; Hulseman and Zeidler, 1995). In contrast, the absence of rheumatoid factors is reassuring. In a study, the negative predictive value of the rheumatoid factor test for rheumatoid arthritis and any rheumatic disease was 89 and 85 per cent, respectively (Shmerling and Delbanco, 1992). The higher the concentration of rheumatoid factor the greater the likelihood that the patient has a rheumatic disease. However, in these circumstances the differential diagnosis with chronic inflammatory diseases remains relevant (Table 14.2). Increasing specificity by a higher cut off titer for rheumatoid factor reduces sensitivity (Shmerling and Delbanco 1992).

The presence of rheumatoid factors may precede the development of rheumatoid arthritis by many years (Halldorsdottir et al., 2000; Jansen et al., 2003). The Amsterdam study revealed that not only rheumatoid

Table 14.1 Rheumatic disorders and prevalence of rheumatoid factors

Disorder	%
Rheumatoid arthritis	30–90
Sjögren's syndrome	75–95
Mixed connective tissue disease	50–60
Mixed cryoglobulinemia	40–100
Systemic lupus erythematosus	15–35
Polymyositis/dermatomyositis	5–10

From: Shmerling, R.H. and Delbanco, T.L. 1991.

Table 14.2 Other conditions associated with a positive rheumatoid factor test

Condition	% rheumatoid factors
Bacterial endocarditis	25–50
Non-A hepatitis	20–75
Tuberculosis	8
Leprosy	5–58
Syphilis	≤13
Parasitic infection	20v90
(e.g. Chagas disease, leishmaniasis, onchocerciasis, schistosomiasis)	15–65
Viral infection	
(e.g. rubella, CMV, EBV, mumps, influenza, HIV)	3–33
Sarcoidosis	10–50
Interstitial lung fibrosis	30–50
Silicosis	30
Asbestosis	45–70
Primary biliary cirrhosis	5–25
Malignancy (e.g. leukemia, colon carcinoma)	10–15
Post multiple immunization	

From: Shmerling, R.H. and Delbanco, T.L. 1991.

factor but also anticyclic citrullated peptide and C-reactive protein can precede the disease by many years. This suggests that rheumatoid factor is not an initial feature of the disease but that subclinical disease may precede rheumatoid arthritis. Since it is hypothesized that treating early disease might be able to induce stable complete remission, this observation revitalizes the discussion on the window of opportunity to treat early disease.

Patients suffering rheumatoid factor-positive rheumatoid arthritis experience a more aggressive course of the disease. They will develop more erosions and extra-articular manifestations. Moreover, their disease is more destructive and they are more likely to become functionally impaired (Van der Heijde et al., 1988; Knijff-Dutmer et al., 2002). Although recognized by clinical experience, the fluctuation of rheumatoid factors titer with disease activity was formally studied only recently. It was demonstrated that accurately measured concentrations of IgA- as well as IgM-rheumatoid factors are well correlated with other process variables. Moreover, it was demonstrated that the cumulative exposure over time to rheumatoid factors, as representative of disease activity, is related to disease outcome as measured by the erosion score (Knijff-Dutmer et al., 2002). It was demonstrated that each individual patient has a fairly constant relation between exposure to disease activity and progression of joint damage. Determination of this relation, reflecting the ability of the disease to cause serious damage is not currently possible. However, using genetic markers and clinical predictors it might be possible to establish this ratio and guide initial treatment decisions in rheumatoid arthritis (Scott, 2003).

Occasionally, IgA- and or IgG-rheumatoid factors are found in patients in the absence of IgM rheumatoid factor. The value of this finding is suggested by the observation that the prognosis of rheumatoid arthritis is associated with the presence of IgA- and IgG-rheumatoid factor (Van Leeuwen et al., 1995).

In conclusion, the rheumatoid factor tests are probably not very useful for the screening for rheumatoid arthritis or for diagnosing rheumatoid arthritis or any other systemic autoimmune diseases in the general population. However, in the context of a rheumatology practice its value has been proven in confirming the clinical diagnosis, appraising the prognosis, establishing complications and monitoring disease activity.

DETECTION OF RHEUMATOID FACTORS

In the past, rheumatoid factor activity in clinical specimens was based on agglutination tests. Red blood cells or latex particles coated with IgG detect primarily IgM-rheumatoid factors through their ability to augment the agglutination of the IgG coated particles. At present, these agglutination tests are widely replaced by automated tests. Frequently used is nephelometry. It monitors the formation of immune complexes by spectrometry.

Scattering of an incident light is used to detect complexes in dilute solutions of serum either with or without rheumatoid factor with an aggregated IgG reagent. In more concentrated mixtures the formed complexes turn the solution cloudy, which can be measured by light absorption or turbidimetry. Mixing of serum and reagent is performed in a cuvette within a light beam. Measuring is done in a photoelectric cell for optical density. Samples with high concentration of rheumatoid factors may require dilution for accurate measurement. Results are quantified in international units, following calibration with an appropriate reference (Finley et al., 1979; Lowell, 2001). Interesting improvements resulting in increased sensitivity and quantitative accuracy are presently available. The non-competitive solid-phase 'sandwich type' assay is capable of measuring accurately nanograms of rheumatoid factor (Koopman and Schrohenloher, 1980b). In our institute a time-resolved fluoroimmunoassay of the IgM rheumatoid factor was developed. Aggregated rabbit IgG was coated to microtiter plates. Rabbit anti-human IgM were labelled with Eu3+ to mark IgM-rheumatoid factors. The lower detection limit of the assay is 1.3×10^3 IU/l. The range for measuring IgM rheumatoid factor in one dilution is $5–1200 \times 10^3$ IU/l (Van der Sluijs Veer and Soons, 1992).

The occurrence of rheumatoid factors is a bizarre biological phenomenon of autoantibodies directed against the Fc fragment of IgG antibodies. Rheumatoid factors are found in virtually all classes of immunoglobulins. Moreover, rheumatoid factors are found in a spectrum of infectious and autoimmune diseases. Despite extensive insight in the biochemical, biological and clinical aspects of rheumatoid factors, the mystery remains.

REFERENCES

Aitcheson, C.T., Peebles, C., Joslin, F. and Tan, E.M. (1980). Characteristic of antinuclear antibodies in rheumatoid arthritis: reactivity of rheumatoid factor with histone-dependent nuclear antigen. Arthrit Rheum 23, 528–538.

Butler, V.P. and Vaughan, J.H. (1964). Hemagglutination by rheumatoid factor of cells coated with animal gamma globulins. Proc Soc Exp Biol Med 116, 585–593.

Carayannopulos, M.O., Potter, K.N., Li, Y., Natvig, J.B. and Capra, J.D. (2000). Evidence that human immunoglobulin M rheumatoid factors can be derived from the natural autoantibody pool and undergo an antigen driven immune response in which somatically mutated rheumatoid factors have lower affinities for immunoglobulin G Fc than their germline counterparts. Scand J Immunol 51, 327–336.

Casali, P., Burastero, S.E., Nakamura, M., Inghirami, G. and Notkins, A.L. (1987). Human lymphocytes making rheumatoid factor and antibody to ssDNA belong to Leu-1+ B-cell subset. Science 236, 77–81.

Dalal, N., Roman, S. and Levinson, A.I. (1990). In vitro secretion of human IgM Rheumatoid factor: evidence of distinct rheumatoid factor populations in health and disease. Arthrit Rheum 33, 1340–1346.

Dunne, J.V., Carson, D.A., Spiegeleberg, H.L., Alspaugh, M.A. and Vaughan, J.A. (1979). IgA rheumatoid factor in the sera and saliva of patients with rheumatoid arthritis and Sjögren's syndrome. Ann Rheum Dis 38, 161–165.

Fehr, T., Bachmann, M.F., Bucher, E. et al. (1997). Role of repetitive antigen patterns for induction of antibodies against antibodies. J Exp Med 185, 1785–1792.

Finley, P.R., Hicks, M.J., Williams, R.J., Hinlicky, J. and Lichti, D.A. (1979). Rate nephelometric measurement of rheumatoid factor in serum. Clin Chem 25, 1909–1914.

Franklin, E.C., Holman, H.R., Kuller-Eberhard, H.J. and Kunkel, H.G. (1957). An unusual protein component of high molecular weight in the serum of certain patients with rheumatoid arthritis. J Exp Med 105, 425–438.

Go, M.F., Schrohenloher, R.E. and Tomana, M. (1994). Deficient galactosylation of serum IgG in inflammatory bowel disease: correlation with disease activity. J Clin Gastroenterol 18, 86–87.

Green, M., Marzo-Ortega, H., McGonagle, D. et al. (1995). Persistence of mild, early inflammatory arthritis: the importance of disease duration, rheumatoid factor and the shared epitope. Arthrit Rheum 42, 2184–2188.

Halldorsdottir, H.D., Jonsson, T., Thorsteinsson, J. and Valdimarsson, H. (2000). A prospective study on the incidence of rheumatoid arthritis among people with persistent increase of rheumatoid factor. Ann Rheum Dis 59, 149–151.

He, X., Zhong, W., McCarthy, T.G., Weyand, C.M. and Coronzy, J.J. (1996). Increased responsiveness of rheumatoid factor producing B cells in seronegative and seropositive rheumatoid arthritis. Arthrit Rheum 39, 1499–1506.

Hendrich, C., Kuipers, J.G., Kolanus, W., Hammer, M. and Schmidt, R.E. (1991). Activation of CD16+ effector cells by rheumatoid factor complex. Arthrit Rheum 34, 423–431.

Hirohata, S., Yanagida, T., Koda, M., Koiwa, M., Yoshina, S. and Ochi, T. (1995). Selective induction of IgM rheumatoid factors by CD14+ monocyte-lining cells generated from bone marrow of patients with rheumatoid arthritis. Arthrit Rheum 38, 384–388.

Hulsemann, J.L. and Zeidler, H. (1995). Undifferentiated arthritis in an early synovitis out-patient clinic. Clin Exp Rheumatol 13, 37–43.

Jansen, L.M., van Schaardenburg, D., van der Horst-Bruinsma, I., van der Stadt, R.J., de Koning, M.H. and Dijkmans, B.A. (2003). The predictive value of anti cyclic citrullinated peptide antibodies in early arthritis. J Rheumatol 30, 1691–1695.

Knijff-Dutmer, E.A.J., Drossaers-bakker, W.K., Verhoeven, A. et al. (2002). Rheumatoid factor measured by fluoroimmuno assay: a responsive measure of rheumatoid arthritis disease activity that is associated with joint damage. Ann Rheum Dis 61, 603–607.

Koopman, W.J. and Schrohenloher, R.E. (1980a). In vitro synthesis of IgM rheumatoid factor by lymphocytes from healthy adults. J Immunol 125, 934–939.

Koopman, W.J. and Schrohenloher, R.E. (1980b). A sensitive radioimmunoassay for quantitation of IgM rheumatoid factor. Arthrit Rheum 23, 302–308.

Kunkel, H.G., Muller-Eberhard, H.J., Fudenberg, H.H. and Tomasis, T.B. (1966). Gamma globulin complexes in rheumatoid arthritis and certain other conditions. J Clin Invest 40, 117–129.

Lowell, C. (2001). Clinical laboratory methods for detection of antigens and antibodies. In Medical Immunology 10th edn, Parslow, T.G. et al. eds. New York: Lange Medical Books.

MacGregor, A.J., Bamber, S., Carth,y D. et al. (1995). Heterogeneity of disease phenotype in monozygotic twins concordant for rheumatoid arthritis. Br J Rheumatol 34, 215–220.

Mattey, D.L., Dawes, P.T., Clarke, S. et al. (2002). Relationship among HLA-DRB1 shared epitope, smoking and rheumatoid factor production in rheumatoid arthritis. Arthrit Rheum 47, 403–407.

Nardella, F.A., Teller, D.C. and Mannik, M. (1981). Studies on the antigenic determinants in the self association of IgG rheumatoid factor. J Exp Med 154, 112–125.

Nemazee, D.A. and Sato, V.L. (1983). Induction of rheumatoid antibodies in the mouse: regulated production of auto antibodies in the secondary humoral response. J Exp Med 158, 29–545.

Nemazee, D.A. (1985). Immune complexes can trigger specific T-cell dependent auto anti-IgG antibody production in mice. J Exp Med 161, 242–256.

Norika, S., Takeshi, T., Hiroshi, H. et al. (2003). Altered thymic T-cell selection due to a mutation of the ZAP-70 gene causes autoimmune arthritis in ice. Nature 426, 454–460.

Parekh, R., Roitt, I., Isenberg, D., Dwek, R. and Rademacher, T. (1988). Age related galactosylation of the N-linked oligosaccharides of human serum IgG. J Exp Med 167, 1731–1736.

Perez, L., Orte, J. and Brieva, J.A. (1995). Terminal differentiation of spontaneous rheumatoid factor secreting B cells from rheumatoid arthritis patients depends upon endogenous interleukine 10. Arthrit Rheum 38, 1771–1776.

Pope, R.M., Teller, D.C. and Mannik, M. (1975). (1975). The molecular basis of self-association of IgG rheumatoid factors. J Immunol 115, 365–373.

Rock, K.L., Benacerraf, B. and Abbas, A.K. (1984). Antigen presentation by hapten-specific B lymphocytes. I. Role of surface immunoglobulin receptors. J Exp Med 16, 1102–1113.

Rose, H.M., Ragan, C., Pearce, E. and Lipman, M.O. (1948). Differential agglutination of normal and sensitized erythrocytes by sera of patients with rheumatoid arthritis. Proc Soc Exp Biol Med 68, 1–6.

Sabharwal, U.K., Vaughan, J.H., Fong, S., Bennet, P.H., Carson, D.A. and Curd, J.G. (1982). Activation of the classical pathway of complement by rheumatoid factors: assessment by radioimmunoassay for C4. Arthrit Rheum 25, 162–167.

Saxne, T., Palladino, M.A., Heinegard, D., Talal, N. and Wolheim, F.A. (1988). Detection of tumor necrosis factor α but not tumor necrosis factor β in rheumatoid arthritis synovial fluid and serum. Arthrit Rheum 31, 1041–1045.

Schrohenloher, R.E., Koopman, W.J. and Alarcon, G.S. (1986). Molecular forms of IgA rheumatoid factor in serum and synovial fluid of patients with rheumatoid arthritis. Arthrit Rheum 29, 1194–1202.

Scott, D.L. (2003). Genotype and phenotype: should genetic markers and clinical predictors drive initial treatment decisions in rheumatic diseases? Curr Opin Rheumatol 15, 213–218.

Shlomchik, M.J., Marshak-Rothstein, A., Wolfowicz, C.B., Rothsein, T.L. and Weigert, M.G. (1987). The role of clonal selection and somatic mutation in autoimmunity. Nature 328, 805–811.

Shmerling, R.H. and Delbanco, T.L. (1991). The rheumatoid factor: an analysis of clinical utility. Am J Med 91, 528–534.

Shmerling, R.H. and Delbanco, T.L. (1992). How useful is the rheumatoid factor? An analysis of sensitivity, specificity and predictive value. Arch Intern Med 152, 2417–2420.

Stolt, P., Bengtsson, C., Nordmark, B. et al. (2003). Quantification of the influence of cigarette smoking on rheumatoid arthritis:

results from a population based case-control study, using incident cases. Ann Rheum Dis 62, 835–841.

Sutton, B., Corper, A., Bonagura, V. and Taussing, M. (2000). The structure and origin of rheumatoid factors. Immunol Today 21, 177.

Tarkowski, A., Czerkinsky, C. and Nilsson, L.-A. (1985). Simultaneous induction of rheumatoid factor and antigen-specific antibody-secreting cells during the secondary immune response in man. Clin Exp Immunol 51, 299–304.

Tighe, H., Chen, P.P., Tucker, R. et al. (1993). Function of B cells expressing a human immunoglobulin rheumatoid factor autoantibody in transgenic mice. J Exp Med 177, 109–118.

Tomana, M., Schrohenloher, R.E., Koopman, W.J., Alarcon, G.S. and Paul, W.A. (1988). Abnormal glycosylation of serum IgG from patients with chronic inflammatory diseases Arthrit Rheum 31, 333–338.

Van der Heijde, D.M., van Riel, P.L., van Rijswijk, M.H. and van de Putte, L.B. (1988). Influence of prognostic features on the final outcome in rheumatoid arthritis: A review of the literature. Semin Arthrit Rheum 17, 284–292.

Van der Sluijs Veer, G. and Soons, J.W. (1992). A time-resolved fluoroimmuno assay of the IgM-rheumatoid factor. Eur J Clin Chem Clin Biochem 30, 301–305.

Van Leeuwen, M.A., Westra, J., van Riel, P.L., Limburg, P.C. and van Rijswijk, M.H. (1995). IgM, IgA and IgG rheumatoid factors in early rheumatoid arthritis: predictive of radiological progression? Scand J Rheumatol 24, 146–153.

Waaler, E. (1940). On the occurrence of a factor in human serum activating the specific agglutination of sheep blood corpuscles. Acta Pathol Microbiol Scand 17, 172–188.

Wernick, R.M., Lipsky, P.E., Marban-Arcos, E., Maliakkal, J.J., Edelbaum, D. and Ziff, M. (1985). IgG and IgM rheumatoid factor synthesis in rheumatoid synovoid membrane cell cultures. Arthrit Rheum 28, 742–752.

Williams, R.C., Malone, C.C. and Tsuchiya, N. (1992). Rheumatoid factors from patients with rheumatoid arthritis react with β2-microglobulin. J Immunol 149, 1104–1113.

Winchester, R.J., Agnello, V. and Klungel, H.G. (1970). Gamma globulin complexes in synovial fluid of patients with rheumatoid arthritis: partial characterization and relationship to lowered complement levels. Clin Exp Immunol 6, 689–706.

Youngblood, K., Fruchter, L., Ding, G., Lopez, J., Bonagura, V. and Davidson, A. (1994). Rheumatoid factors from the peripheral blood of two patients are genetically heterogeneous and somatically mutated. J Clin Invest 93, 852–861.

Autoantibodies

Ezio Bonifacio and Vito Lampasona

Immunology of Diabetes Unit, and Diagnostica e Ricerca San Raffaele, San Raffaele Scientific Institute, Milan, Italy

A bird in the hand is worth two in the bush.

Anonymous

INTRODUCTION

The quote is meant to bring attention to what is likely to be the greatest asset of autoantibodies, i.e. they are accessible. The humoral autoimmune response is often shunned as being a bystander and irrelevant to the disease process and having no mechanistic value. For type 1 diabetes it was recently described to me as the crumbs that remain after the important cell-mediated events. This may be so, but similar to forensic evidence that remains after the crime has taken place, these crumbs can be very informative if examined wisely. Autoantibodies can change in response to specific disease-related events and not to non-specific inflammation, stay around long enough to tell the story and can be reproducibly measured. Without wanting to dampen the enthusiasm for many of the novel cell-based markers proposed in this book, few of the other markers of immunity can be reproducibly detected without sample manipulation and few remain unaffected by things such as diurnal variation and non-specific infections or inflammation. In autoimmune disease, autoantibodies are *the* specific soluble circulating effectors of the disease process.

Autoantibodies were first identified in 1954 (Adams, 1958; Campbell et al., 1956). Measurement was by a functional assay in which immunoglobulin from a patient with

Graves' disease was found to stimulate thyroid cells (Adams, 1958) and by a crude immunoprecipitation assay in which a thyroid extract overlaid with patient's serum gave a precipitate of immune complexes at the interface (Campbell et al., 1956). These were pivotal findings from opposite sides of the globe that confirmed the existence of autoantibodies and autoimmune disease. The experiments also told us that autoantibodies could cause disease and provided us with a general rule that disease-relevant autoantibodies can (and probably should) bind to native antigen.

After these first findings, autoantibodies to almost every organ or tissue in the body have been described. A minority of these are directly responsible for disease pathology, others contribute indirectly to the disease and the majority are simply markers of the disease or non-specifically associated with disease. This chapter will address how autoantibodies may be useful in clinical practice. Type 1 diabetes will be used as a model disease and examples cited from other diseases or autoantibodies where relevant.

Antibodies are produced by B lymphocytes in response to antigen encounter and in most cases, specific help from T lymphocytes. In a typical antibody response, exposure to antigen in the presence of B cell growth factors results in B lymphocyte expansion and IgM antibody production. Sustained or repeated antigen exposure results in switch from IgM to IgG production and selection of clones that produce antibodies of high affinity to the antigen (Burnet, 1961; Wabl et al., 1999). Autoantibodies are

Measuring Immunity, edited by Michael T. Lotze and Angus W. Thomson
ISBN 0-12-455900-X, London

usually of IgG isotype and therefore are likely to have similar requirements for their production, i.e. a source of antigen and specific T cell help. Changes in the amount of antigen exposure or in T cell help should therefore result in changes in the amount or qualities of autoantibody that is produced and found in the circulation. In view of the fact that many therapies aim to modulate these two parameters in order to prevent or ameliorate autoimmune disease, autoantibodies should be useful indirect markers to monitor the efficacy of intervention. Autoantibodies are also considered aberrant in the concept of tolerance to self-proteins and therefore should be useful markers for disease diagnosis, pathogenesis or prediction.

AUTOANTIBODIES IN DISEASE DIAGNOSIS OR PREDICTION

One of the problems we have as clinical interpreters of tests is to decipher and translate much of what is published into what is practical for the clinical setting. In the case of the diagnostic utility of autoantibodies, like all tests, we need to know three fundamental parameters of the test that is being applied. These are the sensitivity for predicting disease, the specificity in health or confounding disease and the *a priori* probability of disease in the subject being tested. The relationship between these three parameters is described within Bayes theory and forms the basis of clinical diagnosis. In situations where the *a priori* probability of disease is low (e.g. <1%), the specificity of the test has a profound effect on the diagnostic utility. Indeed, one of the limitations of autoantibodies with respect to disease diagnosis or prediction is that the majority of individuals with autoantibodies do not have autoimmune disease (Bingley et al., 1993, 1997; Hagopian et al., 1995). The detection of autoantibodies, therefore, can rarely diagnose disease in the absence of corroborating clinical or laboratory evidence.

What assays should be used for measurement?

Much of the autoantibody detection in health is probably due to inadequacies of the tests that are used for measurement. It is often just as important to know the limitations of the test as it is to know its merits. It should be remembered that measures of autoantibodies rely on *in vitro* binding of immunoglobulin to the antigen(s) of interest and that forces that lead to binding in a test tube can be different to those present *in vivo*. Moreover, unlike the measurement of analytes such as minerals or proteins that are identical or very similar between subjects, autoantibodies to the same protein are heterogeneous and their target epitopes can differ substantially even within the same individual. Two general questions that should be considered when determining the disease

relevance of an autoantibody are:

1 whether the antibodies bind to antigen that is found *in vivo* and
2 whether this binding is of sufficient strength to bind *in vivo*.

Specific examples where these conditions may not be met include the use of peptides or denatured antigen as in Western blot methods. Placing large amounts of altered protein on solid phase matrices is a good way to obtain binding, but much of the binding has not proven to have disease relevance. In type 1 diabetes, for example, autoantibodies binding a protein termed ICA69 were specifically identified by Western blot assay in the majority of patients at disease onset (Pietropaolo et al., 1993). These were of potential etiological relevance since the ICA69 protein had a homology to a cows' milk protein also reported to be immunogenic in patients with type 1 diabetes (Karjalainen et al., 1992). Subsequent studies showed that binding was only found in Western blot and not in assays using antigen sources that were conformationally similar to native antigen and that the binding in Western blot was also frequent in sera from patients with other autoimmune diseases and indeed in healthy controls (Lampasona et al., 1994; Martin et al., 1995, 1996). A similar story occurred in multiple sclerosis for antibodies to myelin basic protein and to MOG (Reindl et al., 1999; Genain et al., 1999; O'Connor et al., 2003; Lampasona et al., 2004). In MS, however, both antigens are still considered of clinical relevance and binding in Western blot was reported to predict clinical outcome in intervention trials (Berger et al., 2003), but the verdict is still out as to whether this truly is the case.

Standardization of autoantibody measurements

The inadequacies of certain tests for autoantibody measurement and the need to provide answers to the specificity and sensitivity of autoantibody tests has led to repeated attempts to validate and standardize autoantibody measurement. For some autoantibodies, e.g. anti-DNA, we are still debating which method should be used (Emlen and O'Neill, 1997), whereas for others such as those relevant to type 1 diabetes, the most sensitive and specific methodology has been established and standardization is aimed at quantitative measurement (Bingley et al., 2003).

The type 1 diabetes autoantibody standardization efforts are indeed, exemplary in their achievements (Table 15.1). What commenced in the mid-80s as a comparison of immunofluorescence assays (Gleichmann and Bottazzo, 1987) has developed WHO standards and units (Mire-Sluis et al., 2000) and brought worldwide consensus to the measurement of autoantibodies to specific target antigens such as GAD and IA-2. The standardization program took two important steps in achieving this. The

Table 15.1 Objectives of an autoantibody standardization program

- Validate disease relevance of autoantibody markers
- Identify methods which achieve sensitive and specific measurement
- Assess and improve assay sensitivity and specificity
- Assess and improve concordance between laboratories

Achievements of the islet autoantibody workshop program
- Blinded assessment of assay performance

  o sensitivity
  o specificity
  o reproducibility
  o limit of detection
  o quantification of antibody levels

- Development of evaluation methods

  o Adjusted sensitivity
  o ROC curve analysis

- Reference reagents and common units

  o identification of suitable sera
  o validation of reference standards and units
  o recommendations for general implementation

- Identification of systematic differences

  o assay format-related
  o antigen-related

- Evaluation of implementation of novel assays
- Training

  o Identification of training labs

- Identification and surveillance of reference laboratories

  o training
  o multicenter studies

first was to establish, validate and make official a WHO reference standard. The second was to collect and distribute a large number of samples from control subjects ($n = 100$) and representative patients at disease onset ($n = 50$) in a relatively large operation that was done in collaboration with the CDC. The large numbers that were distributed allowed meaningful calculations of sensitivity and specificity for each of the participating assays that could (and were expected) to be reported in subsequent publications. It was quickly determined that some assays and laboratories were sensitive and specific and others were not. Laboratories that wanted to set up assays had a reference point as to which assays performed best and had an address for training. Moreover, new methods or commercial kits had target sensitivities and specificity to achieve in order to be competitive and new antibodies could be quickly validated using the blinded samples from health and disease (Bingley et al., 2003).

Predicting future autoimmune disease

Autoantibodies can often be detected prior to disease onset (Gorsuch et al., 1981). In theory, therefore, one could potentially screen for autoantibodies in order to prevent disease (assuming an effective and acceptable prevention therapy was available). As such, they would be

excellent surrogate markers for future disease. As discussed, however, their utility as predictive disease markers is dependent upon the specificity of the test and the *a priori* probability of the disease in the subject being assessed. For example, finding an individual positive for autoantibodies to GAD or to IA-2 will not be a specific finding for type 1 diabetes simply because the prevalence of the disease (around 0.3 per cent) is much too low. Most GAD or IA-2 autoantibody positive subjects found in such a screening will never develop type 1 diabetes. An effective way to increase the predictive value of the test is by increasing the *a priori* risk for type 1 diabetes. The *a priori* risk increases by more than 10-fold to around 5 per cent in first degree relatives of patients with type 1 diabetes (Atkinson and Eisenbarth, 2001). Other ways to increase the *a priori* risk is to identify subjects who have one or more of the symptoms of the disease as is done in connective tissue diseases (Emlen and O'Neill, 1997).

Autoantibody screening in subjects with an *a priori* disease susceptibility starts to have a potential clinical value and at this point the characteristics of the autoantibodies detected markedly influence the likelihood that the subject will progress to disease. In type 1 diabetes, disease development is associated with persistent, high titer, high affinity autoantibodies to more than one antigen (Achenbach et al., 2004). Each of these qualities increases the likelihood that the detection of autoantibodies in a subject has identified pre-clinical disease. Transient autoantibody positivity is rarely associated with the development of type 1 diabetes, and repeat positivity in a second sample is an essential part of risk assessment. Since we have already stated that sustained antibody responses usually require repeated exposure to antigen it makes sense that autoimmune disease that occurs through cell death will be associated with persistent autoantibodies, regardless of whether the autoimmunity is responsible for, or a result of, cell death.

The magnitude of the autoimmune response is also likely to be an indicator of the severity of cell destruction. Although claims of inverse relationships between cellular and humoral autoimmune responses exist (Harrison et al., 1993), such a counter-regulation of the two arms of our adaptive immune system is unlikely to be an effective way to defend against infections. Moreover, although the Th1/Th2 paradigm might predict more antibodies in a Th2 than Th1 biased immune response, the paradigm does not predict that antibodies will be dispensed with when an interferon-gamma cell-mediated response is promoted. In our experience the magnitude of the humoral autoimmune response is indeed directly related to the likelihood of developing autoimmune disease, even in a presumed cell-mediated autoimmune disease such as type 1 diabetes (Bonifacio et al., 1990; Achenbach et al., 2004). Magnitude can be measured by titer and by the breadth or range of autoantigen targets. With respect to titer, several reports have shown that the higher the autoantibody titer the more likely it is diagnostic or predictive of disease (Strieder et al., 2003; Hu et al., 2003; Vencovsky et al., 2003). As the titer of the antibody detected increases, much of the weaker binding found in health is lost and the odds shift in favor of disease. Moreover, in antibody mediated autoimmune diseases, the higher the titer the more likely that the antibodies will have clinical consequences (Garlepp et al., 1982).

High titer responses are often associated with reactivity against more than one epitope or antigen. In diseases that are not directly mediated by autoantibodies, the likelihood that a single autoantibody is associated with disease is less than if autoantibodies to more than one target antigen are detected. In type 1 diabetes, the likelihood of developing disease is directly related to the number of autoantigen targets autoantibodies are found against (Kulmala et al., 1998; Achenbach et al., 2004). The antigens also have their own hierarchy so that autoantibodies to IA-2 are far more specific for disease than autoantibodies to GAD (Decochez et al., 2002; Achenbach et al., 2004). This general rule will apply to autoimmune diseases in which there is cell death. Where there is functional impairment without cell death then it is sufficient to have autoantibodies against the functional target (Flier et al., 1976). Such autoimmune diseases are, however, rare. The breadth of the autoantibody response can also be measured by the number of autoantibody epitopes it is directed against and probably by the subclass usage. Broad, multiple subclass autoantibodies are usually synonymous with high titer, but these features can be separate indicators of disease risk also in low titer autoantibody positive subjects (Achenbach et al., 2004). It makes sense, therefore, to be able to quantify not only titer and affinity, but also the number of epitope targets. This concept was recently used very effectively in multiple sclerosis where an array of antigens and peptides were screened with patient sera to show disease relevance and changes post treatment (Robinson et al., 2003). Although the disease relevance of the target antigens may be questioned in such an approach, it is a promising example of how autoantibody reactivity can be exploited using proteomic technology.

Finally, affinity of autoantibodies can be useful in determining the likelihood of disease. Autoantibody affinity is only sporadically reported. For IgG autoantibodies, it is assumed that they are usually of high affinity. There are, however, IgG that weakly bind to the autoantigen in the detection assay, but of sufficient strength to cause a signal. This is especially true for solid phase assays such as ELISA and Western blots. Once binding has occurred, the antibody assays do not distinguish high and low affinity IgG. Lower affinity IgG may not be specifically directed against the target autoantigen and therefore have little if any clinical consequence. This was well demonstrated for insulin autoantibodies, where high capacity very low affinity antibodies were readily detected by ELISA and not RBA and where such antibodies were not disease relevant (Sodoyez-Goffaux et al., 1988). More recently, differences

in insulin autoantibody affinity at the top end of antibody affinity were also found to have clinical consequence. Insulin autoantibodies (IAA) are the first to appear in childhood (Hummel et al., 2004). Some, but not all children who develop IAA also develop autoantibodies to GAD and/or IA-2 and subsequently progress to diabetes. The development of multiple autoantibodies and disease was strongly associated with an early development of very high affinity IAA (unpublished observations). This points to a mechanism in which the early exposure to autoantigen that evokes an immune response is of sufficient magnitude to effect a high titer antibody response. This principle appears to apply when autoantibodies are markers of a disease process but, in rare cases, the lower affinity antibodies can directly cause disease. Again, the case is insulin autoantibodies, where very high titer lower affinity autoantibodies can bind insulin *in vivo* and through slow dissociation release insulin with profound hypoglycemia (Meschi et al., 1992).

Autoantibodies for tracking preclinical disease

An ability to identify subjects with autoimmunity prior to clinical disease allows us to track the natural history of autoimmune disease. Thus far, autoantibodies have been the most informative markers that have mapped the natural history of autoimmune diabetes. Some of the more informative studies on the natural history have been in type 1 diabetes where children have been prospectively followed from birth through to the development of autoantibodies and eventually diabetes (Ziegler et al., 1999; Nejentsev et al., 1999; Colman et al., 2000; Carmichael et al., 2003; Stanley et al., 2004). Relatively frequent measurement of autoantibodies from birth has shown that the natural history starts with development of autoantibodies to insulin within the first 1–2 years of life in genetically susceptible subjects, that autoantibodies to GAD and/or IA-2 may follow soon after and that clinical diabetes only occurs in children who have at least two of these antibodies. As discussed, progression from insulin autoantibodies to multiple autoantibodies and disease is strongly associated with the affinity of the insulin autoantibody response suggesting that the magnitude of the initial insult leading to autoantibodies is a major determinant of disease risk. The course to disease varies with respect to time from months to many years and autoantibodies may follow a uniform rise toward disease or may wax and wane with several rises before disease onset. Impressive have been the changes in titer and epitope targets of the different autoantibodies in the pre-clinical period potentially heralding pathogenic events relevant to the disease process (Naserke et al., 1998; Bonifacio et al., 1999, 2000). The prospective follow-up of children has also allowed the identification of some of the environmental factors that influence the development of diabetes-associated autoimmunity (Honeyman et al., 2000; Ziegler et al., 2003; Norris et al., 2003; Sadeharju et al., 2003).

Autoantibodies for monitoring disease or treatment efficacy

An important difference in monitoring a disease process as compared to predicting disease is that the autoantibody measurements do not necessarily need to be specific for disease as long as the changes in reactivity associate with changes in the disease process within an individual. In theory, autoantibody production requires the presence of antigen and T cell help and therapies that change these should also alter magnitude of the autoantibody response. Unfortunately, however, changes are generally non-specific and whereas we have a range of autoantibody characteristics that help us predict, diagnose or track disease, it is unlikely that specific changes in autoantibody epitope, affinity or target antigens will provide more information than just titer. Specific examples of therapies that change antibody titer are those that are based on immunosuppression (Weetman et al., 1983; Mandrup-Poulsen et al., 1985) or removal of immunoglobulin (Hummel et al., 1998). Effective treatment usually results in a reduction of autoantibodies (as well as other antibodies) and a reduced ability to mount an immune response to antigen challenge (Boitard et al., 1987; Fuchtenbusch et al., 2000). Measuring autoantibody titer is, therefore, an essential monitor in such therapies, but the reduction in titer of an existing autoantibody response

is marginal as compared to the immunosuppression of immune responses to antigen challenge and autoantibody titer has been stable in immunosuppressive treatments that have had clinically detectable outcomes (Petersen et al., 1994). An unusual finding is a rise in autoantibodies following immunosuppression. Such an unexpected response is likely to identify an adverse event. One of the more intriguing settings where this has been described is in allo-transplantation in autoimmune disease (Braghi et al., 2000; Bosi et al., 2001). Our experience in pancreas and islet transplantation in patients with type 1 diabetes has found a few subjects who, despite being profoundly immunosuppressed to prevent allo-rejection, produced marked rises in their autoantibody titers (Figure 15.1). In the case of pancreas transplantation, these occurred several years after transplant, without concomitant evidence of allo-rejection and were followed by loss of the pancreas graft function (Braghi et al., 2000). In islet transplantation, we observed marked rises in autoantibodies to GAD within 1 week post-transplant in a minority of patients, despite lymphodepletion and immunosuppression. The rises were a clear sign of inadequate immunosuppression in some cases, whereas in others they were probably a response to the transplantation of damaged islets (Bosi et al., 2001).

One of the more classical changes with respect to reduction of antigen exposure is celiac disease. Here, IgA

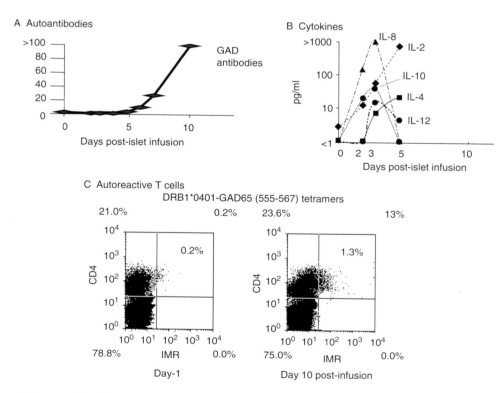

Figure 15.1 Frequent follow-up of circulating surrogate markers of immune activation following the infusion of allogeneic human islets into a patient with autoimmune type 1 diabetes. Despite the administration of immunosuppressive therapy, autoantibody titer to GAD rose sharply within 6 days post-transplant (A). This observation prompted investigation of other circulating markers which found substantial increases in circulating cytokine concentrations (B), including IL-2 and the appearance of autoreactive CD4 positive T cells against the GAD65 555-567 peptide (C).

and/or IgG autoantibodies to tissue transglutaminase C are found in the circulation and can be used to diagnose clinically silent disease (Dieterich et al., 1997). The titer of these autoantibodies is controlled by exposure of the gut to wheat gluten and treatment is by removal of wheat gluten from the diet (Maki et al., 1998). Monitoring of compliance to the dietary treatment can be done by measuring transglutaminase autoantibody titers. The titer falls quickly when gluten is removed and rises quickly when it is reintroduced in the diet (Sategna-Guidetti et al.,1993). In theory, any disease in which exposure to environmental antigen exacerbates autoantibody production can be monitored by measuring autoantibody titer, but unfortunately, the environmental antigen equivalents of gluten in celiac disease are unknown for most autoimmune diseases.

FUTURE PROSPECTS

Standardized quantitative measurement of disease-associated autoantibodies to autoantigen and discrete autoantigen epitopes is currently one of the few surrogate markers that can reliably detect changes in autoimmune disease pathogenesis. These should, therefore, be included in studies that aim to track pathogenic events leading to autoimmune disease or changes that follow immune intervention. These changes may only be suggestive and not conclusive of specific autoimmune events in individual patients but, importantly, they can pin-point changes that can be used to validate assays of cell-mediated autoreactivity, that until now have proven unreliable markers of autoimmune disease (Roep et al., 1999; Peakman et al., 2001). Like all tests, the usefulness of autoantibody measurements largely depends upon the availability of quantitative, sensitive and specific assays and this should be in the forefront of prerequisites when deciding whether the test can be used as a surrogate marker and collaborative initiatives to validate tests should be a continuing international priority.

REFERENCES

Achenbach, P., Warncke, K., Reiter, J. et al. (2004) Stratification of type 1 diabetes risk on the basis of islet autoantibody characteristics. Diabetes 53, 384–392.

Adams, D.D. (1958). The presence of an abnormal thyroid-stimulating hormone in the serum of some thyrotoxic patients. J Clin Endocrinol Metab 8, 699–712.

Atkinson, M.A. and Eisenbarth, G.S. (2001). Type 1 diabetes: new perspectives on disease pathogenesis and treatment. Lancet 358, 221–229.

Berger, T., Rubner, P., Schautzer, F. et al. (2003). Antimyelin antibodies as a predictor of clinically definite multiple sclerosis after a first demyelinating event. N Engl J Med 349, 139–145.

Bingley, P.J., Bonifacio, E. and Gale, E.A. (1993). Can we really predict IDDM? Diabetes 42, 213–220.

Bingley, P.J., Bonifacio, E., Williams, A.J., Genovese, S., Bottazzo, G.F. and Gale, E.A. (1997). Prediction of IDDM in the general population: strategies based on combinations of autoantibody markers. Diabetes 46, 1701–1710.

Bingley, P.J., Bonifacio, E. and Mueller, P.W. (2003). Diabetes Antibody Standardization Program: first assay proficiency evaluation. Diabetes 52, 1128–1136.

Boitard, C., Feutren, G., Castano, L. et al. (1987). Effect of cyclosporin A treatment on the production of antibody in insulin-dependent (type I) diabetic patients. J Clin Invest 80, 1607–1612.

Bonifacio, E., Bingley, P.J., Shattock, M. et al. (1990). Quantification of islet-cell antibodies and prediction of insulin-dependent diabetes. Lancet 335, 147–149.

Bonifacio, E., Scirpoli, M., Kredel, K., Fuchtenbusch, M. and Ziegler, A.G. (1999). Early autoantibody responses in prediabetes are IgG1 dominated and suggest antigen-specific regulation. J Immunol 163, 525–532.

Bonifacio, E., Lampasona, V., Bernasconi, L. and Ziegler, A.G. (2000). Maturation of the humoral autoimmune response to epitopes of GAD in preclinical childhood type 1 diabetes. Diabetes 49, 202–208.

Bosi, E., Braghi, S., Maffi, P. et al. (2001). Autoantibody response to islet transplantation in type 1 diabetes. Diabetes 50, 2464–2471.

Braghi, S., Bonifacio, E., Secchi, A., Di Carlo, V., Pozza, G. and Bosi, E. (2000). Modulation of humoral islet autoimmunity by pancreas allotransplantation influences allograft outcome in patients with type 1 diabetes. Diabetes 49, 218–224.

Burnet, F.M. (1961). The new approach to immunology. N Engl J Med 264, 24–34.

Campbell P.N., Doniach, D., Hudson, R.V. and Roitt, I.M. (1956). Auto-antibodies in Hashimoto's disease (lymphadenoid goitre). Lancet 271, 820–821.

Carmichael, S.K., Johnson, S.B., Baughcum, A. et al. (2003). Prospective assessment in newborns of diabetes autoimmunity (PANDA): maternal understanding of infant diabetes risk. Genet Med 5, 77–83.

Colman, P.G., Steele, C., Couper, J.J. et al. (2000). Islet autoimmunity in infants with a Type I diabetic relative is common but is frequently restricted to one autoantibody. Diabetologia 43, 203–209.

Decochez, K., De Leeuw, I.H., Keymeulen, B et al. (2002). IA-2 autoantibodies predict impending type I diabetes in siblings of patients. Diabetologia 45, 1658–1666.

Dieterich, W., Ehnis, T., Bauer, M. et al. (1997). Identification of tissue transglutaminase as the autoantigen of celiac disease. Nat Med 3, 797–801.

Emlen, W. and O'Neill, L. (1997). Clinical significance of antinuclear antibodies: comparison of detection with immunofluorescence and enzyme-linked immunosorbent assays. Arthritis Rheum 40, 1612–1618.

Flier, J.S., Kahn, C.R., Jarrett, D.B. and Roth, J. (1976). The immunology of the insulin receptor. Immunol Commun 5, 361–373.

Fuchtenbusch, M., Kredel, K., Bonifacio, E., Schnell, O. and Ziegler, A.G. (2000). Exposure to exogenous insulin promotes IgG1 and the T-helper 2-associated IgG4 responses to insulin but not to other islet autoantigens. Diabetes 49, 918–925.

Garlepp, M.J., Kay, P.H. and Dawkins, R.L. (1982). The diagnostic significance of autoantibodies to the acetylcholine receptor. J Neuroimmunol 3, 337–350.

Genain, C.P., Cannella, B., Hauser, S.L. and Raine, C.S. (1999). Identification of autoantibodies associated with myelin damage in multiple sclerosis. Nature Med 5, 170–175.

Gleichmann, H. and Bottazzo, G.F. (1987). Progress toward standardization of cytoplasmic islet cell-antibody assay. Diabetes 36, 578–584.

Gorsuch, A.N., Spencer, K.M., Lister, J. et al. (1981). Evidence for a long prediabetic period in type I (insulin-dependent) diabetes mellitus. Lancet 2, 1363–1365.

Hagopian, W.A., Sanjeevi, C.B., Kockum, I. et al. (1995). Glutamate decarboxylase-, insulin-, and islet cell-antibodies and HLA typing to detect diabetes in a general population-based study of Swedish children. J Clin Invest 95, 1505–1511.

Harrison, L.C., Honeyman, M.C., DeAizpurua H.J. et al. (1993). Inverse relation between humoral and cellular immunity to glutamic acid decarboxylase in subjects at risk of insulin-dependent diabetes. Lancet 341, 1365–1369.

Honeyman, M.C., Coulson, B.S., Stone, N.L. et al. (2000). Association between rotavirus infection and pancreatic islet autoimmunity in children at risk of developing type 1 diabetes. Diabetes 49, 1319–1324.

Hu, P.Q., Fertig, N., Medsger, T.A. Jr and Wright, T.M. (2003). Correlation of serum anti-DNA topoisomerase I antibody levels with disease severity and activity in systemic sclerosis. Arthritis Rheum 48, 1363–1373.

Hummel, M., Durinovic-Bello, I., Bonifacio, E. et al. (1998). Humoral and cellular immune parameters before and during immunosuppressive therapy of a patient with stiff-man syndrome and insulin dependent diabetes mellitus. J Neurol Neurosurg Psychiatry 65, 204–208.

Hummel, M., Bonifacio, E., Schmid, S., Walter, M., Knopff, A. and Ziegler, A.G. (2004). Islet autoantibody development and risk for childhood type 1 diabetes in offspring of affected parents. Ann Intern Med in press.

Karjalainen, J., Martin, J.M., Knip, M. et al. (1992). A bovine albumin peptide as a possible trigger of insulin-dependent diabetes mellitus. N Engl J Med 327, 302–307.

Kulmala, P., Savola, K., Petersen, J.S. et al. (1998). Prediction of insulin-dependent diabetes mellitus in siblings of children with diabetes. A population-based study. The Childhood Diabetes in Finland Study Group. J Clin Invest 101, 327–336.

Lampasona, V., Ferrari, M., Bosi, E., Pastore, M.R., Bingley, P.J. and Bonifacio, E. (1994). Sera from patients with IDDM and healthy individuals have antibodies to ICA69 on western blots but do not immunoprecipitate liquid phase antigen. J Autoimmun 7, 665–674.

Lampasona, V., Franciotta, D., Furlan, R. et al. (2004). Similar low frequency of anti-MOG IgG and IgM in MS patients and healthy subjects. Neurology 62, 2092–2094.

Maki, M., Sulkanen, S. and Collin, P. (1998). Antibodies in relation to gluten intake. Dig Dis 16, 330–332.

Mandrup-Poulsen, T., Nerup, J., Stiller, C.R. et al. (1985). Disappearance and reappearance of islet cell cytoplasmic antibodies in cyclosporin-treated insulin-dependent diabetics. Lancet 1, 599–602.

Martin, S., Kardorf, J., Schulte, B. et al. (1995). Autoantibodies to the islet antigen ICA69 occur in IDDM and in rheumatoid arthritis. Diabetologia 38, 351–355.

Martin, S., Lampasona, V., Dosch, M. and Pietropaolo, M. (1996). Islet cell autoantigen 69 antibodies in IDDM. Diabetologia 39, 747.

Meschi, F., Dozio, N., Bagnetti, E., Carra, M., Cofano, D. and Chiumello, G. (1992). An unusual case of recurrent hypoglycaemia: 10-year follow up of a child with insulin auto-immunity. Eur J Pediatr 151, 32–34.

Mire-Sluis, A.R., Gaines Das, R. and Lernmark, A. (2000). World Health Organization International Collaborative Study for islet cell antibodies. Diabetologia 43, 1282–1292.

Naserke, H.E., Ziegler, A.G., Lampasona, V. and Bonifacio, E. (1998). Early development and spreading of autoantibodies to epitopes of IA-2 and their association with progression to type 1 diabetes. J Immunol 161, 6963–6969.

Nejentsev, S., Sjoroos, M., Soukka, T. et al. (1999). Population-based genetic screening for the estimation of Type 1 diabetes mellitus risk in Finland: selective genotyping of markers in the HLA-DQB1, HLA-DQA1 and HLA-DRB1 loci. Diabet Med 16, 985–992.

Norris, J.M., Barriga, K., Klingensmith, G. et al. (2003). Timing of initial cereal exposure in infancy and risk of islet autoimmunity. J Am Med Assoc 290, 1713–1720.

O'Connor, K.C., Chitnis, T., Griffin, D.E. et al. (2003). Myelin basic protein-reactive autoantibodies in the serum and cerebrospinal fluid of multiple sclerosis patients are characterized by low-affinity interactions. J Neuroimmunol 136, 140–148.

Peakman, M., Tree, T.I., Endl, J. et al. (2001). Characterization of preparation of GAD65, proinsulina, and the islet tyrosine phosphatase 1A-2 for use in detection of autoreactive T-cells in type 1 diabetes: report phase II of the second International Immunology of Diabetes Society Workshop for Standardization of T-cell assays in type 1 diabetes. Diabetes 50, 1749–1754.

Petersen, J.S., Dyrberg, T., Karlsen, A.E. et al. (1994). Glutamic acid decarboxylase (GAD65) autoantibodies in prediction of beta-cell function and remission in recent-onset IDDM after cyclosporin treatment. The Canadian-European Randomized Control Trial Group. Diabetes 43, 1291–1296.

Pietropaolo, M., Castano, L., Babu, S. et al. (1993). Islet cell autoantigen 69 kD (ICA69). Molecular cloning and characterization of a novel diabetes-associated autoantigen. J Clin Invest 92, 359–371.

Reindl, M., Linington, C., Brehm, U. et al. (1999). Antibodies against the myelin oligodendrocyte glycoprotein and the myelin basic protein in multiple sclerosis and other neurological diseases: a comparative study. Brain 122, 2047–2056.

Robinson, W.H., Fontoura, P., Lee, B.J. et al. (2003) Protein microarrays guide tolerizing DNA vaccine treatment of autoimmune encephalomyelitis. Nat Biotechnol 21, 1033–1039.

Roep, B.O., Atkinson, M.A., van Endert, P.M., Gottlieb, P.A., Wilson, S.B. and Sachs, J.A. (1999) Autoreactive T cell responses in insulin-dependent (Type 1) diabetes mellitus, Report of the first international workshop for standardization of T cell assays. J. Autoimmmun. 13, 267–282.

Sadeharju, K., Hamalainen, A.M., Knip, M. et al. (2003). Enterovirus infections as a risk factor for type I diabetes: virus analyses in a dietary intervention trial. Clin Exp Immunol 132, 271–277.

Sategna-Guidetti, C., Pulitano, R., Grosso, S. and Ferfoglia, G. (1993). Serum IgA antiendomysium antibody titers as a marker of intestinal involvement and diet compliance in adult celiac sprue. J Clin Gastroenterol 17, 123–127.

Sodoyez-Goffaux, F., Koch, M., Dozio, N., Brandenburg, D. and Sodoyez, J.C. (1988). Advantages and pitfalls of radioimmune and enzyme linked immunosorbent assays of insulin antibodies. Diabetologia 31, 694–702.

Stanley, H.M., Norris, J.M., Barriga, K. et al. (2004). Is presence of islet autoantibodies at birth associated with development of persistent islet autoimmunity? The Diabetes Autoimmunity Study in the Young (DAISY). Diabetes Care 27, 497–502.

Strieder, T.G., Prummel, M.F., Tijssen, J.G., Endert, E. and Wiersinga, W.M. (2003). Risk factors for and prevalence of thyroid disorders in a cross-sectional study among healthy female relatives of patients with autoimmune thyroid disease. Clin Endocrinol 59, 396–401.

Vencovsky, J., Machacek, S., Sedova, L. et al. (2003). Autoantibodies can be prognostic markers of an erosive disease in early rheumatoid arthritis. Ann Rheum Dis 62, 427–430.

Wabl, M., Cascalho, M. and Steinberg, C. (1999). Hypermutation in antibody affinity maturation. Curr Opin Immunol 11, 186–189.

Weetman, A.P., McGregor, A.M., Ludgate, M. et al. (1983). Cyclosporin improves Graves' ophthalmopathy. Lancet 2, 486–489.

Ziegler, A.G., Hummel, M., Schenker, M. and Bonifacio, E. (1999). Autoantibody appearance and risk for development of childhood diabetes in offspring of parents with type 1 diabetes: the 2-year analysis of the German BABYDIAB Study. Diabetes 48, 460–468.

Ziegler, A.G., Schmid, S., Huber, D., Hummel, M. and Bonifacio, E. (2003). Early infant feeding and risk of developing type 1 diabetes-associated autoantibodies. J Am Med Assoc 290, 1721–1728.

Antibody Affinity Using Fluorescence

Chapter 16

Sergey Y. Tetin[1] and Theodore L. Hazlett[2]

[1]*Core R&D Biotechnology, Abbott Diagnostics Division, Abbott Laboratories, Abbott Park, IL, USA*
[2]*Laboratory for Fluorescence Dynamics, University of Illinois at Urbana-Champaign, Urbana, IL, USA*
TLH supported by NIM Grant PHS 5 P41-RR03155

Nature is not on the surface; it is in the depths. Colors are the surface expression of this depth …

Paul Cezanne

INTRODUCTION

Affinity determination is a central event in the characterization and evaluation of antibodies. Selection of an antibody for a desired application is primarily based on this information. Accurate measurement of an equilibrium binding constant entails measuring the fraction of antibody and ligand bound under a given set of experimental conditions. The chosen method should measure this fraction in the most accurate way without perturbing the system's equilibrium.

It is often possible to determine the concentration of the antibody–hapten complex by tracking binding-induced changes in physical characteristics of either component such as light absorption, fluorescence, diffusion rate, etc. In these cases there is no necessity to separate free and bound components and the measurements can be performed in a solution phase at equilibrium. The level of sensitivity of the binding assay will depend on the specific reporter group and the physical parameters being monitored.

In this chapter we will discuss practical aspects of measuring antibody affinity in solutions and focus on basic fluorescence techniques. The general benefit of using fluorescence-based methods relates to their high sensitivity that extends limits of accurately measurable dissociation constants into the subnanomolar range. Additionally, the fluorescence emission of most fluorophores is sensitive to the probe's microenvironment and may contain valuable information on the structure and dynamics of the molecules under study. However, in ligand binding studies, the nature of the fluorescence changes is less important than the correlation of these changes with the fraction of complex.

Antibody molecules contain many tryptophan residues including several tryptophans in or nearby the antibody binding site. It is possible to use intrinsic antibody fluorescence originating from tryptophan side chains for monitoring. More often researchers must use extrinsic fluorescent labels that are chemically attached to the antigen or antibody in order to register binding events. However, inclusion of extrinsic labels may affect the binding equilibrium and generally requires additional characterizations.

Basic principles of fluorescence and descriptions of experimental arrangements for proper fluorescence measurements have been described elsewhere (Lakowicz, 1999). There are numerous other excellent publications (Jameson and Sawyer, 1995; Brand and Johnson, 1997; Valeur, 2002) dedicated to principles and applications of fluorescence in protein biochemistry and biophysics. We have recently reviewed applications of fluorescence spectroscopy to antibody binding studies (Tetin and Hazlett, 2000).

THE BINDING MODEL

Through all further discussions we shall use terms *site* or *binding site* as equivalents to the term *antibody binding*

Measuring Immunity, edited by Michael T. Lotze and Angus W. Thomson
ISBN 0-12-455900-X, London

site. Under the term *ligand*, we shall recognize any molecule that binds to this site, which would include relatively small organic molecules, also known in the immunology literature as *haptens*, as well as larger biomolecules, such as proteins, that have *independent antigenic epitopes*.

A simple binding model (one ligand per site, independent non-interacting sites) is suitable for describing most solution antibody–ligand interactions:

$$S + L \leftrightarrow SL \tag{1}$$

where S is the concentration of free antibody binding sites, L is the concentration of unbound ligand and SL is the concentration of the complex.

The equilibrium binding constants, the association constant K_a and the dissociation constant K_d for this reaction can be expressed simply in the following equations:

$$K_d = \frac{1}{K_a} = \frac{S \times L}{SL} \tag{2}$$

Association between ligand and site is energetically favored with a negative change in free energy, ΔG. The free energy and the binding constant are related according to the formula:

$$\Delta G = -RT \ln K_a \tag{3}$$

where R is the gas constant and T is the temperature in Kelvin. Additional thermodynamic details can be extracted using the basic expression of the second law of thermodynamics:

$$\Delta G = \Delta H - T\Delta S \tag{4}$$

where ΔH is the enthalpy change and ΔS is the change in entropy. Measuring binding constants at different temperatures, ionic strength, pH, etc., can provide a researcher with information about forces involved in the reaction underlying potential mechanisms (see, for example, Weber, 1992).

There are two simple equations that connect readily measurable initial or *total* concentrations (S_t and L_t) of the reagents and their concentrations after reaching the reaction equilibrium:

$$S_t = S + SL \tag{5}$$
$$L_t = L + SL \tag{6}$$

Using these two equations with equation (1), one can calculate the fraction of the bound sites or, alternatively, the fraction of the bound ligand:

$$F_b^{sites} = \frac{SL}{S_t} = \frac{SL}{S + SL} \tag{7}$$
$$F_b^{ligand} = \frac{SL}{L_t} = \frac{SL}{L + SL} \tag{8}$$

Finally, equations (7) or (8) can be combined with equation (2) and fraction bound (sites or ligand) can then be expressed in terms of the initial (total) reagent concentrations and Kd. For example, the fraction of the bound sites can be calculated from the equation:

$$F_b^{sites} = \frac{L_t + S_t + K_t - \sqrt{L_t^2 + S_t^2 + K_d^2 - 2S_tL_t + 2L_tK_d + 2S_tK_d}}{2S_t} \tag{9}$$

The fraction of the bound ligand can be calculated in the same manner if the denominator in equation (9) is replaced with the term $2L_t$. Equation (9) is helpful for designing binding experiments. It can be used to calculate the fraction of sites bound for an expected K_d with a given total concentrations of ligand and sites and therefore, it is handy for optimization of the initial reagent concentrations.

It can be difficult to chemically determine the component concentrations (S, L, SL) of a sample at equilibrium. There are several experimental techniques, which we will discuss later, that relate a fluorescence signal to the fraction of ligand or sites bound. With a linear relationship between fraction bound and the measured signal, the fluorescence data can be directly fitted to the binding model (equation (10), below). Equation (10) is derived using a simplification of the classic Adair's equation (Adair, 1925) for the simple binding model (non-interacting sites, one ligand per site) and its adaptation for IgG containing two non-interacting binding sites:

$$F_b = \frac{m \times L}{K_d + L} + c \tag{10}$$

where m is a scaling factor and c is a constant for adjustment of the ligand related signal in absence of the antibody for a non-zero value.

DETERMINATION OF THE BINDING STOICHIOMETRY

It is generally accepted that the typical stoichiometry for most antibody reactions is one ligand molecule per one antibody binding site. Nevertheless, it is critical, especially when working with small haptens, to verify this ratio experimentally for every new antibody tested. Several potential experimental artifacts include ligand aggregation, non-specific binding outside of the antibody binding site and more than one ligand per one site ratios.

Maintaining high fractions of the bound reagents is essential for stoichiometry experiments. If we titrate ligand into a solution of an antibody at constant concentration (ten or more times higher than the K_d), the plotted fraction of antibody sites bound rises linearly until sites are filled and then the plot will show saturation.

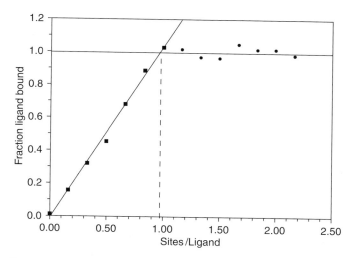

Figure 16.1 Stoichiometric binding plot for an anti-digitoxin mouse monoclonal antibody that binds fluorescein-labeled digitoxin with $K_d = 0.13$ nM. Concentration of the hapten was 10 nM at each point of the titration. The antibody was purified from the serum-free media using a Protein-A column (Amersham Biosciences, NJ). The abscissa on the plot is expressed in terms of the antibody binding sites to hapten molar ratio.

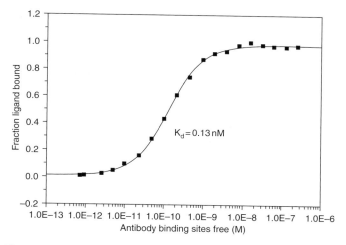

Figure 16.2 Determination of the dissociation constant of an anti-digitoxin mouse monoclonal antibody (the same mAb as shown in Figure 16.1) using fluorescence anisotropy. Concentration of the fluorescein-labeled digitoxin was held constant at 0.1 nM. Free hapten demonstrates the anisotropy value of 0.12. Anisotropy at saturation was 0.246. Binding results in the 45 per cent quenching of the hapten fluorescence. Fraction of hapten bound was calculated with equation (**19**) and the binding plot was fitted with equation (**10**).

The transition should occur at the ratio of two ligand molecules per one IgG. A typical stoichiometric titration is shown in Figure 16.1.

Similar experiments are also useful for measuring the concentrations of active antibody in polyclonal antisera, ascites fluids, tissue culture media or after chemical coupling of antibodies with other molecules. Our experience with polyclonal hyperimmune sera suggests that the amount of high affinity antibodies may vary from 5 to 50 per cent of the entire IgG fraction.

In practice, determination of stoichiometry can be performed by any of the techniques that are used in affinity measurements. It is also a good idea to perform stoichiometric titrations at several fixed concentrations of one of the reagents. Correct experiments should produce identical stoichiometic numbers independent of reagent concentrations.

AFFINITY MEASUREMENTS

General considerations

Affinity determinations are commonly performed by titrations of one of the binding components into another, which is held at a constant concentration, keeping total volume of the reaction mixture unchanged (Figure 16.2). In a typical titration, concentration of one of the components should vary in a broad range, while concentration of the second component is expected to be kept close to the K_d. Experimental conditions including concentrations of the reagents should be thoroughly optimized in order to measure accurately the signal related to the bound antibody or antigen. It can be shown theoretically (Weber,

1965) that the precision in K_d determinations varies across the fraction bound and is highest when the $F_b = 0.5$. Analyzing all titration data together in a single matrix minimizes effects of the random errors at each point of the titration and assures a reliable K_d value.

The reader should note that the random errors in fraction bound result in a systematic error in K_d: binding curves are not symmetric and an error in fraction bound pushes the apparent K_d to higher values (Tetin and Hazlett, 2000). Finding a right balance in sensitivity and versatility of the detection method and optimization of reagent concentration requires preliminary experiments.

Affinity determination using fluorescence quenching

Binding of an antigen to the antibody may result in changes of the antibody (or antigen) intrinsic fluorescence. Frequently, binding leads to fluorescence quenching, though a binding-induced enhancement in the observed fluorescence signal is also possible.

Fluorescence quenching is calculated by the equation:

$$Q = \left(1 - \frac{I_{sample}}{I_{free}}\right) \times 100 \qquad (11)$$

where I_{free} is the emission of the fluorescent species in absence of the second binding component and I_{sample} is the fluorescence intensity of the mixed antibody and antigen (hapten) at any point in the titration. Binding induced fluorescence enhancement results in the opposite sign in the equation. Fraction bound can be calculated by dividing the fluorescence quenching (enhancement) value at each point in the titration series by the corresponding value at saturation. If, for any practical reason, complete saturation cannot be reached, a step-by-step iterative fitting procedure to approximate K_d using equations (10) and (9) is recommended (Tetin et al., 1993).

Tryptophan is the primary intrinsic fluorophore found in proteins; it can be excited by ultraviolet light. The only other measurable protein fluorophore, tyrosine, has a much lower extinction coefficient and a poor quantum yield that diminishes its practical use in binding measurements. In proteins, fluorescence of tryptophan is highly sensitive to the microenvironment, an aspect that has been extensively researched (reviewed by Callis, 1997). Binding-induced wavelength shifts and amplitude changes in the tryptophan emission spectra have been observed for many antibody systems (as examples, see Tetin et al., 1993; Viswanathan et al., 1996). Velik et al. (1960) published the first application of hapten-dependent quenching of antibody intrinsic fluorescence for affinity determinations. The same approach was applied to the study an anti-single strand DNA autoantibody (Tetin et al., 1993) and to affinity measurements of antibodies toward trisubstituted sweeteners (Viswanathan et al., 1996).

It is important to emphasize that affinity determinations using intrinsic protein fluorescence, in principle, are not limited by the size of studied molecules and can be based on changes in the fluorescence of either component including protein antigens. However, quenching of antibody fluorescence is more common, since antibodies typically contain several tryptophan residues in, or in close proximity to the binding site. In many cases, the tryptophan side chain intimately contacts the antigen.

The sensitivity of affinity measurements based on quenching of intrinsic protein fluorescence depends on the number and initial brightness of tryptophans that are affected by the binding and the change in the fluorescence signal. Commonly, one should be able to readily measure affinities at the submicromolar level and, perhaps, to extend this range to a low nanomolar limit when the experimental setup is thoroughly optimized.

Introduction of fluorescent labels (probes) that can be tightly, or covalently, bound to proteins and other molecules expanded use of fluorescence methods for measuring binding events and processes. The idea of using fluorescent labels for protein studies and synthesis of the first probe, dansyl or DNS, belongs to Gregorio Weber (1952b). Currently, researchers have access to numerous labeling chemistries and a wide variety of fluorescent probes produced by Molecular Probes (Eugene, OR), Amersham Biosciences (Piscataway, NJ), Atto-Tec (Siegen, Germany) and other manufacturers, that can satisfy most of our needs in labeling of antibodies and antigens (haptens).

Labeling of relatively small organic molecules (haptens) requires synthetic incorporation of a reactive chemical group into the hapten molecule that will make a covalent bond(s) with the chemically activated label. It is good practice to use well-characterized chemical linkers or spacers to tether the hapten and the probe to prevent direct interactions of a fluorescent label with the antibody. The labeled molecules can then be used in binding studies performed by several fluorescence techniques that are described further in this chapter. However, if binding of a labeled ligand results in a measurable quenching of its fluorescence, the abovementioned quenching-based method can be chosen as possibly the simplest way to evaluate the K_d. As a rule, fluorescent labels are designed to exhibit high extinction coefficients and high quantum efficiencies; they are very bright and easy detectable in subnanomolar concentrations.

Affinity determinations using fluorescence anisotropy

Fluorescence anisotropy is sensitive to changes in rotational motions of fluorophores. Binding of a relatively small fluorescent hapten to a large antibody restricts motions of the hapten molecule as well as reducing the rotational diffusion of its fluorescent moiety leading to an increase in the observed fluorescence anisotropy. The same effect can also be observed with significantly larger antigens where binding of an antibody affects the probe's local rotational freedom and results in a pronounced change in the measured fluorescence anisotropy. Equally, bound antigen may affect local motions of antibody chromophores and change the anisotropy of the antibody fluorescence. The former is far more common and will be the focus of this section. Nevertheless, the following considerations are also appropriate when a ligand-induced increase in the anisotropy of antibody intrinsic fluorescence is employed to monitor binding.

Haptens labeled with fluorescent reporter groups are extensively utilized in various areas of immunology, especially in antibody structure–function studies and immunoassays. Often, the binding of such ligands does not affect the emission intensity and an increase in fluorescence anisotropy may be the only detectable spectroscopic parameter available for monitoring binding.

At first, we should identify the very similar terms anisotropy and polarization. By common agreement, the plane of the tabletop is defined as the horizontal plane, while the vector normal to this plane is the vertical axis. When taking a standard anisotropy measurement, the excitation light is polarized along the *vertical axis* and the emission is collected in both the horizontal and vertical planes. The polarized emission intensities are then used to calculate the polarization (P) and anisotropy (r) using the following equations:

$$P = \frac{I_v - I_h}{I_v + I_h} \qquad (12)$$

and

$$r = \frac{I_v - I_h}{I_v + 2I_h} \qquad (13)$$

where I_v is the emission intensity polarized along the vertical axis and I_h is the component of the emitted light polarized along the horizontal axis. As a rule, optical parts (monochromators, lenses, filters) of fluorometers possess unequal transmission or varying sensitivities (photo detectors) for vertically or horizontally polarized light. Corrections for such instrumental artifacts are made through the use of a correction factor known as the G-factor. The G-factor is calculated with the vertical and horizontal emission intensities measured with the *excitation polarizer set at the horizontal position* according to equation (14):

$$G = \frac{I_{hv}}{I_{hh}} \tag{14}$$

At this condition, excitation with horizontally polarized light will set off equal vertical horizontal emission intensities (G = 1.0). If the instrument has a polarization bias, G will not equal 1.0. Incorporating G-factor will modify equation (13):

$$r = \frac{I_v - G \times I_h}{I_v + 2G \times I_h} \tag{15}$$

Most of the commercially available instruments have the option for correcting the single-point polarization measurements with the G-factor and it is very important to perform such corrections carefully.

More than 50 years ago Weber (1952a) published general principles for application of the fluorescence polarization approach in studying macromolecules and formulated the addition law that relates polarization of a mixture of fluorophores to the individual components present in solution. Later, the same addition law was expressed in terms of anisotropy (Jablonski, 1960):

$$r = \sum_i f_i r_i \tag{16}$$

where r is the anisotropy of the mixture; r_i is anisotropy of the i'th fluorophore and f_i is the associated fractional fluorescence intensities. Thus, in antibody–hapten binding, anisotropy r at any point in the titration is the sum of the products between the individual anisotropies of the free r_{free} and bound r_{bound} species and their respective fractional intensities (f_{free} and f_{bound}; note that $f_{free}+f_{bound} = 1$) as given in equation (17),

$$r = f_{free}r_{free} + f_{bound}r_{bound} \tag{17}$$

If emission of the hapten is not affected by binding to the antibody, the respective fractional contributions of the free and bound hapten will be equivalent to their fractional concentrations. Equation (17) can be rewritten in a form to solve for fraction bound (F_b):

$$F_b = \frac{r - r_{free}}{r_{bound} - r_{free}} \tag{18}$$

In the case where binding changes the hapten emission, the fractional intensities of free and bound hapten will show unequal weighting and will not be equivalent to respective molar fractions. To correct for the brightness differences a ratio of fluorescence intensities of the bound to free hapten measured under the same experimental conditions ($q = \frac{I_{bound}}{I_{free}}$) can be used and equation (18) must be adjusted to:

$$F_b = \frac{r - r_{free}}{(r_{bound} - r) \times q + r - r_{free}} \tag{19}$$

Since free and bound hapten possess different fluorescence intensities, anisotropy data cannot be directly fitted with equation (10). It is necessary first to calculate the fraction of the bound ligand with equation (19) and then use equation (10) for fitting. An example is given in Figure 16.2, where fluorescein-labeled digitoxin was titrated with the anti-digitoxin antibody and binding data were fitted with equation (10).

As was already mentioned in the beginning of this section, fluorescence polarization (or anisotropy) depends on rotational diffusion of a fluorophore and, thus, is sensitive to the dynamics of macromolecules. The steady-state fluorescence anisotropy discussed here gives a weighted average of the rotational modes in the studying system. The more sophisticated measurement of time-resolved anisotropy can extract the individual rotational rates present in the antibody–hapten complex. Since this technique is less likely to be used for evaluation of the binding constants, we will just note that time-resolved anisotropy measurements provide information about local motion of the bound hapten and rigidity of the antibody binding site. It is also possible to determine the motions of protein subunits and protein domains in such experiments. In fact, independent movements of the Fab portions in the IgG molecule and the segmental flexibility of antibody in solution were discovered by means of fluorescence polarization (Zagyansky et al., 1969; Yquerabide et al., 1970).

FLUORESCENCE CORRELATION SPECTROSCOPY

Fluorescence correlation spectroscopy (FCS) is a powerful technique for looking at molecular interactions, organization and dynamics. The first application of this technique toward biochemical problems was published in the early 1970s on the association of a nucleic acid synthesis inhibitor and its DNA counterpart (Magde et al., 1972, 1974). The theory of the method was discussed in detail and the potentials of the technique for cellular and biochemical studies were well recognized in these early publications. Unfortunately, at that time the technology was inadequate for adaptation of FCS to the common experimental problems being addressed. The development of confocal microscopy, advances in detector technology, dramatic enhancement of computational speeds and the arrival of fast, femtosecond pulse-lasers in the 1990s ushered in a revival in the use of FCS toward biochemical and biological questions (for reviews see Thompson, 1991; Eigen and Rigler, 1994; Rigler and Elson, 2000; Hess et al., 2002; Thompson et al., 2002). Since that time, technical understanding has greatly advanced and the practical application of FCS, in turn, has become more focused. In this section of the chapter, we will examine the fundamentals of FCS and its application in determining antibody–antigen binding strength.

The basic data collected in FCS is a time-series of fluorescence intensity fluctuations. These fluctuations can derive from a variety of sources, such as translational diffusion of fluorescent species in and out of an observation volume, dynamic macromolecular conformational shifts and fluorophore photophysics, to name a few. A typical FCS instrument is based on a confocal fluorescence microscope design containing a high numerical aperture objective to tightly focus the excitation beam to a diffraction-limited beam width (beam waist). A pinhole rejects out of plane emission rendering an observation volume limited along the x-, y- and z-axes. A small volume can also be achieved in the absence of a pinhole using a high peak power mode-locked laser as an excitation source and taking advantage of the two-photon effect (Berland et al., 1995, 1996; Yu et al., 1996; Xu et al., 1996). In either case, a three dimensional Gaussian volume of one femtoliter is approximated (Berland et al., 1995; Hess and Webb, 2002).

FCS has the capacity to distinguish between fast and slow moving species that we use to determine the concentrations of free and bound ligand when examining antibody and hapten interactions. The FCS fluorescence time traces contain the intensity peaks due to molecules diffusing in and out of the beam (our defined volume). The number of peaks we observe over time relates to the concentration of molecules and the widths of these peaks reflect the diffusion time of our (fluorescent) species through the volume.

Data can be analyzed for the inherent intensity fluctuations, PCH (Müller et al., 2000, 2001) and FIDA (Kask et al., 1999) or more commonly with the autocorrelation function given in equation:

$$G(\tau) = \frac{\langle \delta F(t) \cdot \delta F(t + \tau) \rangle}{\langle F(t) \rangle^2} \quad (20)$$

where the $\langle \; \rangle$ symbols indicate the time average of the enclosed value(s), F is the fluorescence, δF is the difference between the fluorescence at a given time, t, and the average fluorescence, and τ is the time shift variable. The autocorrelation points generated from the time trace can then be fitted to the diffusion and fractional intensities of 'i' species present using equation (21) (for

one-photon excitation):

$$G(\tau)_{sample} = \sum_{i=1}^{M} f_i^2 \cdot G_i(0) \cdot \left(1 + \frac{\tau}{\tau_{Di}}\right)^{-1} \left(1 + \frac{\tau}{\left(\frac{w}{z}\right)^2 \cdot \left(\frac{\tau}{\tau_{Di}}\right)}\right)^{-1/2} \quad (21)$$

where $G(0)_i$ is the time-zero autocorrelation limit, f_i is the fractional intensity, τ_{Di} is the average diffusion time through the volume, w is the $1/e^2$ radius of the Gaussian volume and z is the axial $1/e^2$ radius. The $G(0)$ values are related to the particle numbers of the individual species.

Using autocorrelation analysis, our ability to distinguish between two fluorescent species is based on the differences in their respective diffusion times. When detecting antibody, hapten and antibody–hapten complex, the hapten demonstrates the largest change in the diffusion rate upon its binding to the antibody and therefore it is best if we design our assay with a fluorescent hapten in mind. The binding constant of fluorescein-labeled digoxin (digoxin tracer, MW = 732) to the rabbit anti-digoxin antibody (MW~150 000) was measured using FCS on a ConfoCor (Carl Zeiss, Germany) microscope in a serial titration experiment. The diffusion times for free ($\tau_d = 330$ μs) and bound ($\tau_d = 73$ μs) tracer were determined from samples of digitoxin tracer without antibody and with a saturating concentration of antibody. These two diffusion times were held constant in a two-component analysis using equation (21). Analysis was performed at each point in the titration series and the fractions of the free and bound tracer were resolved. As is shown in Figure 16.3, the results fit well to the simple binding model (equation (10)) with the K_d value

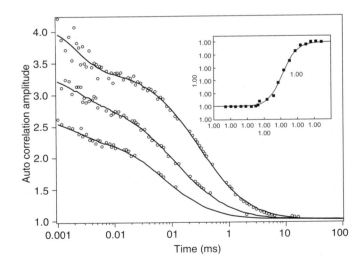

Figure 16.3 Binding of digoxin tracer with anti-digoxin antibody measured by FCS (Tetin et al., 2002). Autocorrelation data points and fits for samples (from bottom to top) with free tracer (no antibody), partially bound tracer and fully bound tracer (saturating antibody). Upper panel: determination of the dissociation constant for anti-digoxin antibody from the FCS experiment. Points correspond to tracer fraction bound as a function of free antibody binding sites. Solid line is the fit to the data to the simple binding model (equation (10)).

of 12 nM. A dissociation constant using fluorescence anisotropy, 11 nM, demonstrated good agreement between the two methods in quantitative determination of antibody affinity (Tetin et al., 2002).

The application of FCS to a competitive immunoassay format was evaluated in the same study. In this assay the analyte, vancomycin, competitively displaces tracer, fluorescein-labeled vancomycin, bound to the antibody. Displacement of the antibody-bound tracer with unlabeled vancomycin resulted in a strong decline of the fraction of the long diffusion time component. Also, the average number of fluorescent molecules in the reaction increased monotonically from 1.2 in the beginning to 2.2 at the end of the titration, when tracer molecules became essentially free. Such a trend is consistent with the bivalent nature of antibody that initially had two bound tracer molecules per molecule diffusing as a single entity, followed by release of two independently diffusing tracer molecules in the presence of competitor.

In both aforementioned antibody systems, the fluorescence intensity of the tracer did not change upon binding. When there is a brightness change between free and bound hapten, photon counting histogram (PCH) analysis, or the similar fluorescence intensity distribution analysis (FIDA) can be applied to the data. These analytical tools work on a principle different from autocorrelation analysis. With PCH we look at the distribution of particles, or molecules, as observed through the photon counts, during our collection time. The random distribution of particles in a volume is a Poisson distribution and thus our photon distribution will be Poissonian with a three dimensional Gaussian excitation volume imposed. Analysis of the resulting broadened Poisson photon distribution will resolve the average particle number and the average molecular brightness (Müller et al., 2000, 2001). Multiple diffusing species can also be analyzed and will result in a distribution that is a convolution of the individual distributions. PCH analysis was fruitfully used to study another anti-digoxin antibody, a mouse monoclonal antibody that quenches about one-half of the digoxin-fluorescein tracer fluorescence upon binding. The analysis resolved free and bound species of the digoxin tracer enabling calculation of the dissociation constant of approximately 0.3 nM (Chen et al., 2000).

Clearly, FCS is well suited for antibody binding studies whether based on differences in the translational diffusion rate of an antibody and the immune complex. There are, however, certain limits in the technique. Resolution of two fluorescent species in the intensity autocorrelation function analysis is only possible if they exhibit at least a 50 per cent difference in the diffusion rates and the experimental conditions are thoroughly optimized (Meseth et al., 1999). In the PCH analysis the resolution of two fluorescent species is achievable if their relative intensities differ by twofold or more (Chen et al., 1999, 2000; Kask et al., 1999). It must be noted that these limits were established for rather perfectly selected systems. More often researchers face various obstacles including high fluorescent background and instability of biological samples, unleashing of labels, photo-bleaching, high level of the triplet state component, low fluorescence signals and other experimental hurdles that complicate broad application of the technique.

Implementation of dual fluorophore labeling and cross-correlation FCS strategies promises additional advantages by making assays more sensitive and resistant to background interferences. The method was successfully used in several biological systems. Foldes-Papp et al. (2001) obtained a measurable cross-correlation signal from the immune complex that included the rhodamine green-labeled protein autoantigen, the autoantibody from a patient serum and the murine anti-human IgG monoclonal antibody labeled with Cy5 fluorescent dye (Amersham Bioscience, New Jersey).

In our laboratory we were able to register a measurable cross-correlation signal when the digitoxin hapten was coupled with the Alexa-488 dye (Molecular Probes, Oregon) and the anti-digitoxin monoclonal mouse antibody was labeled with TexasRed (Molecular Probes, Oregon) (Tetin and Stroupe, 2004). Further development of the labeling chemistry, experimental technique and the data analysis will enable measurements of the binding constants, which will be greatly appreciated by many experimentalists in the field.

CONCLUSIONS AND FUTURE PROSPECTS

Fluorescence-based methods are well suited for affinity determinations. Protocols involving fluorescence quenching or changes in fluorescence anisotropy have become standard experimental approaches in antibody binding characterizations. As a rule, these techniques require introduction of fluorescent labels into the binding system under study. However, in some cases binding studies can be based on measuring intrinsic fluorescence of antibodies or antigens. Sensitivity of the fluorescence based methods permits determination of the equilibrium binding constants in the subnanomolar range.

Revival and fast progress of the FCS methodology has brought a new possibility in studying antibody-binding processes at the single molecule level. This area is undergoing a speedy development in both technique and instrumentation, as well as a continued refinement of theory. Possibly, FCS will grow into a standard quantitative method for antibody characterization and assay development.

In this current review we focused on describing principles and advantages of the fluorescence-based methods in application to antibody affinity determinations. Usually, such measurements do not require a high degree of automation. It is important to indicate that all the aforementioned techniques have been also realized in commercially available highly automated analyzers. The automated systems are widely used for diagnostics immunoassays, or for high throughput assays developed for potential drugs and therapeutic targets in the pharmaceutical industry.

Among other fluorescence-based technologies showing a strong promise for antibody affinity measurements we should name two novel biosensor platforms. One method is based on using total internal reflection fluorescence (Asanov et al., 1998) and the second on directional surface-plasmon-coupled emission as detection technologies (Lakowicz, 2004). These methods combine enhancements in the detection capabilities with a high level of potential automation and possibilities for high throughput antibody screening. However, both methods require measuring antibody–antigen binding interactions on a planar surface where one component is immobilized and, therefore, they may show aberrant binding profiles (Svitel et al., 2003). Solution phase studies will always remain preferable for quantitative binding characterizations.

REFERENCES

Adair, G.S. (1925). The hemoglobin system. VI. The oxygen dissociation curve of hemoglobin. J Biol Chem 63, 529–545.

Asanov, A.N., Wilson, W.W. and Oldham, P.B. (1998). Regenerable biosensor platform:a total internal reflection fluorescence cell with electrochemical control. Anal Chem 70, 1156–1163.

Berland, K.M., So, P.T.C., Chen, Y., Mantulin, W.W. and Gratton, E. (1996). Scanning two-photon fluctuation correlation spectroscopy particle counting measurements for detection of molecular aggregation. Biophys J 71, 410–420.

Berland, K.M., So, P.T.C. and Gratton, E. (1995). Two-photon fluorescence correlation spectroscopy: method and application to the intracellular environment. Biophys J 68, 694–701.

Brand, L. and Johnson, M.L. eds, (1997). Fluorescence spectroscopy. Meth Enzymol 278, 628.

Callis, P.R. (1997). 1La and 1Lb transitions of tryptophan: applications of theory and experimental observations to fluorescence of proteins. Meth Enzymol 278, 113–150.

Chen, Y., Müller, J.D., So, P.T. and Gratton, E. (1999). The photon counting histogram in fluorescence fluctuation spectroscopy. Biophys. J., 77, 553–567

Chen, Y., Müller, J.D., Tetin, S.Y., Tyner, J.D. and Gratton, E. (2000). Probing ligand protein binding equilibria with fluorescence fluctuation spectroscopy. Biophys J 79, 1074–1084.

Eigen, M. and Rigler, R. (1994). Sorting single molecules: application to diagnostics and evolutionary biotechnology. Proc Natl Acad Sci USA 91, 5740–5747.

Foldes-Papp, Z., Demel, U. and Tilz, G.P. (2001). Ultrasensitive detection and identification of fluorescent molecules by fcs: impact for immunobiology. Proc Natl Acad Sci USA 98, 11509–11514.

Hess, S.T., Huang, S., Heikal, A.A. and Webb, W.W. (2002). Biological and chemical applications of fluorescence correlation spectroscopy: a review. Biochemistry 41, 697–705.

Hess, S.T. and Webb, W.W. (2002). Focal volume optics and experimental artifacts in confocal fluorescence correlation spectroscopy. Biophys J 83, 2300–2317.

Jablonski, A. (1960). On the notion of emission anisotropy. Bull Acad Pol Sci 8, 259–264.

Jameson, D.M. and Sawyer, W.H. (1995). In Biochemical Spectroscopy, Vol. 246, K. Sauer, ed. San Diego pp. 283–299.

Kask, P., Palo, K., Ullmann, D. and Gall, K. (1999). Fluorescence-intensity distribution analysis and its application in biomolecular detection technology. Proc Natl Acad Sci USA 96, 1379–1376.

Lakowicz, J.R. (1999). Principles of Fluorescence Spectroscopy, 2nd edn. New York: Kluwer Academic/Plenum Publishers.

Lakowicz, J.R. (2004). Radiative decay engineering 3: surface plasmon coupled directional emission. Anal Biochem 324, 153–169.

Magde, D., Elson, E.L. and Webb, W.W. (1972). Thermodynamic fluctuations in a reacting system – measurement by fluorescence correlation spectroscopy. Phys Rev Lett 29, 705–708.

Magde, D., Elson, E.L. and Webb, W.W. (1974). Fluorescence correlation spectroscopy. II. An experimental realization. Biopolymers 13, 20–61.

Meseth, U., Wohland, T., Rigler, R. and Vogel, H. (1999). Resolution of fluorescence correlation measurements. Biophys J 76, 1619–1631.

Müller, J.D., Chen, Y. and Gratton, E. (2000). Resolving heterogeneity on the single molecular level with the photon counting histogram. Biophys J 76, 474–486.

Müller, J.D., Chen, Y. and Gratton, E. (2001). In Fluorescence Correlation Spectroscopy. Theory and Applications, R. Rigler, and E.L., Elson, eds. Berlin: Springer-Verlag, pp. 410–437.

Rigler, R. and Elson, E. L. (2000). Fluorescence Correlation Spectroscopy. Berlin: Springer-Verlag.

Svitel, J., Balbo, A., Mariuzza, R.A., Gonzales, N.R. and Schuck, P. (2003). Combined affinity and rate constant distributions of ligand populations from experimental surface binding kinetics and equilibria. Biophys J 84, 4062–4077.

Tetin, S.Y. and Hazlett, T.L. (2000). Optical spectroscopy in studies of antibody-hapten interactions. METHODS 20, 341–361.

Tetin, S.Y., Rumbley, C.A., Hazlett, T.L. and Voss, E.W. Jr (1993). Elucidation of anti-ssDNA autoantibody BV 04–01 binding interactions with homooligonucleotides. Biochemistry 32, 9011–9017.

Tetin, S.Y. and Stroupe, S.D. (2004). Antibodies in diagnostic applications. Curr Pharm Biotechnol 5, 9–16.

Tetin, S.Y., Swift, K.M. and Matayoshi, E.D. (2002). Measuring antibody affinity and performing immunoassay at the single molecule level. Anal Biochem 307, 84–91.

Thompson, N.L. (1991). Fluorescence correlation spectroscopy. In Topics in Fluorescence Spectroscopy, Volume 1, J.R., Lakowicz, ed. New York: Plenum Press, pp. 337–378.

Thompson, N.L., Lieto, A.M. and Allen, N.W. (2002) Recent advances in fluorescence correlation spectroscopy. Curr Opin Struct Biol 12, 634–641.

Valeur, B. (2002). Molecular Fluorescence. Principles and Applications. Weinheim: Wiley-VCH.

Velick, S.F., Parker, C.W. and Eisen, H.N. (1960). Excitation energy transfer and the quantitative study of the antibody hapten reaction. Proc Natl Acad Sci USA 46, 1470–1482.

Viswanathan, M., Subramaniam, S., Pledger, D.W., Tetin, S.Y. and Linthicum, D.S. (1996). Modeling the structure of the combining site of an antisweet taste ligand monoclonal antibody NC10.14. Biopolymers 39, 395–406.

Weber, G. (1952a). Polarization of the fluorescence of macromolecules. 1. Theory and experimental method. Biochem J 51, 145–155.

Weber, G. (1952b). Polarization of the fluorescence of macromolecules 2. Fluorescent conjugates of ovalbumin and bovine serum albumin. Biochem J 51, 155–167.

Weber, G. (1965). The binding of small molecules to proteins. In Molecular Biophysics, B. Pulman, and M., WeissBluth, eds. New York: Academic Press, pp. 369–397.

Weber, G. (1992). Protein Interactions. New York: Routledge, Chapman & Hall.

Xu, C., Zipfel, W., Shear, J.B., Williams, R.M. and Webb, W.W. (1996). Multiphoton fluorescence excitation: new spectra windows for biological nonlinear microscopy. Proc Natl Acad Sci USA 93, 10763–10768.

Yguerabide, J., Epstein, H.F. and Stryer, L. (1970). Segmental flexibility in an antibody molecule. J Mol Biol 51, 573–590.

Yu, W., So, P.T.C., French, T. and Gratton, E. (1996). Fluorescence generalized polarization of cell membranes: a two-photon scanning microscopy approach. Biophys J 70, 626–636.

Zagyansky, Y.A., Nezlin, R.S. and Tumerman, L.A. (1969). Flexibility of immunoglobulin G molecules as established by fluorescent polarization measurements. Immunochemistry 6, 787–800.

SLE-Associated Tests

Chapter 17

Maureen McMahon[1] and Kenneth Kalunian[2]
[1]UCLA School of Medicine, Los Angeles, CA, USA
[2]UCSD School of Medicine, La Jolla, CA, USA

Then everything includes itself in power; Power into will, will into appetite; And appetite, a universal wolf, so doubly seconded with will and power, must make perforce a universal prey, and last eat up himself.
The Phoenix and the Turtle,

William Shakespeare (1601)

INTRODUCTION

Systemic lupus erythematosus (SLE) is an autoimmune disease characterized by a diverse array of clinical manifestations and by the production of autoantibodies to components of the cell nucleus. A diagnosis of SLE is likely if four of eleven of the American College of Rheumatology criteria for SLE are met (Table 17.1). The detection of autoantibodies in patients is not only useful in establishing a diagnosis of SLE, but may also reflect disease activity, correlate with organ involvement and predict relapse. It is important to recognize, however, that no one test or test panel can perform all of these activities, as increases in the specificity of a test usually correspond to decreases in sensitivity. Additionally, not all of the clinical features of SLE are mediated by antibodies.

ANTINUCLEAR ANTIBODIES

Antinuclear antibodies (ANA) are autoantibodies that react with a variety of nuclear antigens, including nucleic acids, histones and components of the centromere. Although ANA are very sensitive for SLE, they are common in unwell elderly individuals (Tan et al., 1997) and in patients with Sjogren's syndrome, scleroderma, polymyositis, juvenile rheumatoid arthritis, chronic active hepatitis, infectious mononucleosis, leprosy, vasculitis and endocarditis (Wallace et al., 2001).

The most common screening test is immunoflourescence on rodent liver or human epithelial (Hep-2) tissue, although enzyme-linked immunosorbent assays (ELISA) are available. With rodent tissue substrates, 5–10 per cent of normal subjects will have a positive test at the screening dilution of 1:20, but only approximately 1 per cent will have a positive test at 1:160. With Hep-2 tissue culture cells, 10–15 per cent of normal subjects will have a positive test at the screening dilution of 1:40, but only 1 per cent will have a positive test at 1:320 (Wallace et al., 2001). Thus, ANAs have low positive predictive value when used in unselected populations or at low titers (Shiel and Jason, 1989; Tan et al., 1997). In selected populations, however, ANA are a highly sensitive test for SLE, and when Hep-2 cells are used, over 98 per cent of patients who fulfill the American College of Rheumatology criteria for lupus have a positive test (Wallace et al., 2001). ANA found in healthy people do tend to be polyreactive, low affinity antibodies which are usually of the IgM subclass and are usually present in low titers. In contrast, patients with SLE and Sjogren's syndrome usually have high titers of high-affinity IgG ANA against specific disease associated nuclear antigens (Ulvestad et al., 2000).

Measuring Immunity, edited by Michael T. Lotze and Angus W. Thomson
ISBN 0-12-455900-X, London

Table 17.1 The American College of Rheumatology classification criteria for SLE

Criteria	Detail
Photosensitivity	Photosensitive skin rash
Malar rash	Flat or raised with fixed erythema
Discoid rash	Raised with plugging/scaling/scarring
Oral ulcers	Usually painless
Arthritis	Non-erosive, 2 or more peripheral joints
Serositis	Pleural or cardiac
Renal disorder	Proteinuria or cellular casts
Neurological disorder	Seizures or psychosis without other cause
Hematological disorder	Hemolysis, cytopenia
Immunological disorder	Anti-dsDNA, anti-Smith, antiphospholipid antibodies (anticardiolipin, lupus anticoagulant, or false positive VDRL)
Antinuclear antibody	Abnormal titer ANA at any time point

ANTIBODIES TO DNA

The first reports of antibodies to DNA in the serum of patients with SLE appeared in 1957 (Ceppellini et al., 1957; Holborow et al., 1957; Robbins et al., 1957). Antibodies to DNA have been found even in healthy humans as part of the normal 'natural immune repertoire' (Ebling and Hahn, 1989; Pisetsky et al., 1990). Antibodies to bacteria and to DNA can share similar sequences; therefore, it is likely that the natural antibody repertoire exists to provide quick antibody protection against attack from pathogenic invaders (Wallace et al., 2001). In normal humans, these DNA antibodies are usually of the IgM class, react primarily to single stranded DNA and have low avidity for DNA (Wallace et al., 2001). Some subsets of these DNA antibodies, however, are pathogenic. There is evidence that the anti-double stranded DNA (dsDNA) antibodies found in SLE patients play a direct role in the pathogenesis of the disease. When dsDNA antibodies are introduced into healthy mice, they induce proteinuria and azotemia (Madaio et al., 1987; Tsao et al., 1990). Anti-dsDNA antibodies in both humans and mice have been associated with active disease and with nephritis, especially IgG antibodies (Rothfield and Stollar, 1967; Schur and Sandson 1968). The mechanism of the pathogenic effect of dsDNA antibodies is likely related to their charge; dsDNA antibodies are cationic, while the glomerular basement membrane is poly-anionic. Therefore, the cationic anti-DNA can bind and be trapped by the basement membrane (Ebling and Hahn, 1980). The dsDNA antibodies can then bind to available DNA, form immune complexes and activate complement, thereby causing damage (Gauthier and Mannik, 1990).

High titers of antibodies to dsDNA have a specificity of more than 90 per cent for SLE (Wallace et al., 2001). Low titers, however, are less specific, as they can be detecting ssDNA and can be found in several other disease entities,

such as drug-induced SLE, rheumatoid arthritis, Sjogren's syndrome, chronic infections, chronic liver disease and aging. Several studies have found a close correlation between SLE disease activity and high dsDNA antibody titers (Schur and Sandson, 1968; Gershwin and Steinberg, 1974; Emlen et al., 1986). Weaker correlations with disease activity are found, however, when more sensitive assays such as ELISA are used (Isenberg et al., 1984). In most patients, however, increases in anti-dsDNA titers likely herald a flare of disease and an increased risk of nephritis (Ward et al., 1991). Anti-dsDNA antibodies may also be present in patients prior to the onset of SLE; one recent study found anti-dsDNA antibodies in 55 per cent of patients at a mean of 2.2 years prior to the diagnosis of the disease (Arbuckle et al., 2003). IgM antibodies to dsDNA may be less specific for SLE than IgG antibodies (Ehrenstein et al., 1993; Avina-Zubieta et al., 1995).

There are several laboratory methods for detecting anti-DNA antibodies, with varying sensitivities and specificities. Specific assays should be used for diagnosis, while sensitive assays might be more useful for monitoring (Emlen and O'Neill, 1997). In the Farr assay, radiolabeled DNA is added to diluted serum or plasma. Immunoglobulin is then precipitated by ammonium sulfate; unbound DNA is not precipitated. Radioactivity in the precipitate indicates binding of DNA by anti-DNA. The Farr assay detects only antibodies with high avidity; high avidity antibodies might be more relevant to SLE pathogenesis, especially in nephritis (Leon et al., 1977; Egner, 2000). It is the least sensitive assay and is positive in only 50–60 per cent of patients with SLE. Antibody titers, however, correlate well with disease activity and flare (Wallace et al., 2001).

In the ELISA assay, DNA is bound to wells in microtiter plates (often coated with negatively charged molecules such as methylated bovine serum albumin or protamine sulfate). Diluted patient plasma samples are incubated with DNA in the wells; after several hours, the wells are washed and bound immunoglobulin is incubated with enzyme labeled anti-human IgG or IgM. The binding of the second antibody is detected by color change, read with a spectrophotometer. Both low and high avidity enzymes are detected with this assay. The ELISA assay is very sensitive, being positive in 70–85 per cent of SLE patients, but it is less specific than the Farr assay (Wallace et al., 2001). The best clinical correlations can be made with high titers.

A third method of detecting anti-DNA antibodies uses a kinetoplast containing circular dsDNA from the flagella of the *Crithidia luciliae* organism. Test serum is incubated with *Crithidia* organisms on a slide. After washing, fluorescent anti-human IgG, Ig or IgM are added. Immunoglobulin bound to the DNA structure is then detected using an ultraviolet microscope. This test is most specific for anti-dsDNA and highly specific for SLE. Both low avidity and high avidity antibodies are measured, however, and the sensitivity is generally not as good as with the ELISA assay. Titers of anti-DNA measured by this method have little correlation with disease activity.

ANTIBODIES TO RO AND LA

Human Ro antibodies associate with a common type of human RNA in a complex known as hYRNA (Wallace et al., 2001). Ro exists in two forms: Ro52 and Ro60. In SLE, anti-Ro60 antibodies predominate; both forms are present in Sjogren's syndrome (Slobbe et al., 1991).

Antibodies to Ro and La are associated with a variety of clinical features. Traditionally, anti-Ro and anti-La antibodies are associated with Sjogren's syndrome and are also called anti-SSA and anti-SSB respectively. Anti-Ro antibodies are found in 40–80 per cent of Sjogren's patients and 50 per cent of SLE patients, while anti-La antibodies are found in 15–40 per cent of Sjogren's patients and 10–20 per cent of SLE patients (Harley et al., 1989). These antibodies are associated with a variety of clinical manifestations in SLE patients. For example, anti-Ro antibody positivity has been associated with a variety of dermatologic conditions. Correlations with anti-Ro antibodies and SLE have been found with photosensitive skin rash (Maddison et al., 1978) and 75 per cent of patients with subacute cutaneous lupus erythematosus are anti-Ro positive (Sontheimer et al., 1982). In fact, antibodies to Ro are deposited directly into skin (Lee and Norris, 1989). Associations have also been found between anti-Ro antibodies and hematologic abnormalities, including thrombocytopenia (Morley et al., 1981; Anderson et al., 1985), lymphopenia (Harley et al., 1989) and anemia (Alexander et al., 1983). Additionally, many SLE patients who are ANA negative have anti-Ro antibodies (Alexander et al., 1983). Anti-Ro antibodies have also been associated with interstitial pneumonitis in SLE patients (Hedgpeth and Boulware, 1988). Anti-Ro and anti-La antibodies are also passed across the placenta to the fetus (Buyon and Winchester, 1990) and both antibodies are associated with congenital heart block and neonatal dermatitis (Scott et al., 1983). Interestingly, the presence of anti-La antibodies when present alone without the presence of anti-Ro antibodies has a negative correlation with renal disease in SLE patients (Harley et al., 1989). Although the serum levels of anti-Ro and anti-La vary over time by as much as 10- to 20-fold, the relevance of this to disease activity is not known (Scofield et al., 1996).

The traditional assay performed to detect the Ro antibody is the Ouchterlony double immunodiffusion assay. Although this assay is very specific, it is slow and subject to frequent false negative results (Wallace et al., 2001). More recently, ELISA assays for anti-Ro and anti-La antibodies have been developed. These assays have 10- to 100-fold increases in sensitivity over the traditional immunodiffusion assays (Sanchez-Guerrero et al., 1996). The specificity of these assays, however, is decreased due to increases in artifacts that cause false positive results

(Egner, 2000). Newer enzyme immunoassays and Western blotting techniques are able to discriminate between antibodies to Ro52 and Ro60, although it is still unclear how clinically useful these assays will be (Egner, 2000).

ANTI-snRNP ANTIBODIES

Patients with SLE frequently have antibodies to the U series of small nuclear ribonucleoproteins, the U snRNPs. U1 RNP is a component of the spliceosome complex, whose function is to assist in splicing premessenger RNA to mature RNA (Hoffman and Greidinger, 2000). The most commonly measured of these antibodies are the anti-RNP and the anti-Smith (anti-Sm). When examined under indirect immunofluorescence, anti-Sm and anti-U1 RNP antibodies stain the nucleus of cells in a speckled pattern with sparing of the nucleoli (Wallace et al., 2001).

The antibody to RNP was first identified in sera of patients with SLE in 1971 (Mattioli and Reichlin, 1971). Shortly thereafter, Sharp et al. (1971) described a group of patients characterized by features of SLE, inflammatory muscle disease, scleroderma and the absence of renal disease. They also noted that this group of patients, with what they called mixed connective tissue disease (MCTD), contained high titers of antibodies to extractable nuclear antigens. Subsequent studies revealed that the sera from the MCTD patients was reacting to the RNP antigen (Sharp et al., 1972).

Anti-U1 RNP antibodies are found in approximately 30–40 per cent of patients with SLE (Wallace et al., 2001). The major clinical association of RNP antibodies is with MCTD; indeed, this illness is defined by the presence of the antibody (Sharp et al., 1972). Anti-RNP antibodies can also be found in a small percentage of patients with Sjogren's syndrome, rheumatoid arthritis, scleroderma and polymyositis (Norman, 1975; Sharp et al., 1976; Reeves et al., 1985). They are more common in African-American patients than in those of European descent (Arnett et al., 1988). Anti-RNP antibody titers may correlate with disease activity (Hoet et al., 1992).

Anti-Sm antibodies were first identified in the sera of SLE patients in 1966. These antibodies are found in approximately 25 per cent of all patients with SLE, although they are more common in blacks and Asians as compared to those of European descent. Overall, the anti-Sm antibodies are found in 10–20 per cent of white patients with SLE as opposed to 30–40 per cent of Asian and African-American patients (Homma et al., 1987; Abuaf et al., 1990).

The presence of anti-Sm antibodies is a helpful tool in the diagnosis of SLE and has been included in the American College of Rheumatology classification criteria (Tan et al., 1982). The association of anti-Sm antibodies with specific disease manifestations is less clear. Early studies using immunodiffusion assays suggested that patients with anti-Sm antibodies may have milder renal disease and less central nervous system involvement than patients with anti-DNA antibodies (Winn et al., 1979). Other studies have shown that rising anti-Sm antibody titers may correlate with more active disease (Boey et al., 1988) and may predict disease flare (Barada et al., 1981). One study using the ELISA assay, however, found that the presence of anti-Sm antibodies did not correlate with any particular disease manifestation (Field et al., 1988). In contrast, a large study of over 100 Japanese patients found that anti-Sm antibodies detected by ELISA correlated with a low frequency of progression to end stage renal disease. The anti-Sm positive patients did, however, have both a poorer overall prognosis and a higher prevalence of late onset proteinuria (Takeda et al., 1989) than patients without anti-Sm antibodies.

In the past, laboratories have relied on immunodiffusion for the routine detection of anti-Sm and anti-U1 RNP antibodies. The sensitivity of immunodiffusion can be increased with the use of counterimmunoelectrophoresis (Wallace et al., 2001). In immunodiffusion, a prototype anti-Sm or anti-U1 RNP antibody is placed into a well in an agarose gel. The soluble fraction of a tissue extract such as rabbit or calf thymus is prepared by sonication in a saline buffer and is placed into an adjacent well. During a 24–48-h incubation period, diffusion brings the antibodies into contact with the antigens. As they bind, a lattice structure develops that is visible as a precipitin band. Antibodies in a particular serum can be identified through comparison with a serum of known specificity. More recently, ELISAs for the detection of anti-Sm and anti-U1 RNP antibodies have been utilized. ELISA methods have the advantage of speed, as results are available within hours as opposed to 1–2 days. They have sensitivity that approaches that of the immunodiffusion assay and are easier and safer to perform. As with other antibody testing, however, the ELISA has a somewhat higher rate of false positive results (Wallace et al., 2001).

HISTONE ANTIBODIES

Histones are basic proteins that bind the DNA helical structure to contribute to the supercoil formation in the nucleosome (Rubin and Waga, 1987). They were first detected in the sera of a group of SLE patients in 1960 (Kunkel and Deicher, 1960). Further investigation revealed an incidence of anti-histone antibodies in 93 per cent of patients with drug-induced SLE (Fritzler and Tan, 1978). Around 30–80 per cent of patients with SLE have IgG and IgM anti-histone antibodies detectable by immunoblotting or ELISA (Egner, 2000). Most patients who are treated with procainamide eventually develop anti-histone antibodies, but only 10–20 per cent of patients display evidence of active disease (Totoritis et al., 1988). Most asymptomatic patients have antibodies of the IgM isotype (Hobbs et al., 1987). Symptomatic patients with procainamide-induced SLE have predominantly IgG anti-histone antibodies that react

with the H2A-H2B histone complex (Rubin et al., 1982, 1992, 1995). Antibodies to the H2A-H2B complex have greater than 90 per cent sensitivity for procainamide-induced lupus compared to asymptomatic patients (Rubin et al., 1992, 1995). Titers of anti-histone antibody may correlate with disease activity (Gioud et al., 1982). The antibodies are not specific for SLE, however, and cannot distinguish drug-induced SLE from idiopathic SLE (Rubin and Waga, 1987; Massa et al., 1994).

LUPUS ANTICOAGULANT AND ANTIPHOSPHOLIPID ANTIBODIES

Antiphospholipid (APL) antibody syndrome (APS) refers to the syndrome of antibody-mediated thrombosis. The name is somewhat of a misnomer, as it is now recognized that these antibodies are directed against plasma proteins that may or may not be associated with a phospholipid. The Sapporo classification criteria for the syndrome require either a thrombotic manifestation (venous, arterial or vasculopathy) or pregnancy morbidity in addition to a positive titer for anticardiolipin antibody (aCL) or lupus anticoagulant (LA) (Wilson et al., 1999). More recently, antibodies to B$_2$-glycoprotein I (B$_2$-GPI), a plasma protein that was found to act as a cofactor in the aCL antibody assays, have also been associated with the antiphospholipid antibody syndrome (McNeil et al., 1990; Matsuura et al., 1990). Primary APS may occur in the absence of any rheumatologic condition; in one study of non-SLE patients with verified venous thrombosis, 15 per cent had APL antibodies (Eschwege et al., 1988). The frequency of APL in unselected patients with thrombotic stroke has ranged from 5 to 29 per cent, while in younger patients it ranged from 18 to 46 per cent (Wallace et al., 2001). APS can also occur in conjunction with SLE. Hughes has estimated APS in SLE patients at a frequency of 35 per cent (Hughes, 1993).

The first APL to be recognized was the false-positive test for syphilis. Patients with a false positive test were found to be at risk for the development of SLE (Moore and Mohr, 1952); there have been no consistent data, however, that demonstrate that a false positive VDRL is associated with thrombosis.

APL antibodies are also found commonly in patients with infections (including HIV, bacterial, protozoan and viral illnesses) (Hassell et al., 1994) and other autoimmune diseases (including rheumatoid arthritis (Wolf et al., 1994), Sjogren's syndrome (Rosler et al., 1995), scleroderma (Herrick et al., 1994) and vasculitides such as microscopic polyangiitis and Wegener's granulomatosis (Hergesell et al., 1993) and Takayasu's arteritis (Misra et al., 1994)). They have also been found in patients with malignancies (Malnick et al., 1993; Papagiannis et al., 1994) and sickle cell anemia (Kucuk et al., 1993).

The frequencies of LA, aCL antibody and anti-B$_2$GPI in SLE has varied widely among studies. Some of this variation likely results from differing sensitivities of the assays and differing patient selection criteria and study designs. In addition, levels of the antibody in individual patients may fluctuate over time. Both aCL and LA can fluctuate with disease activity (Cooper et al., 1989) and levels of both can be suppressed with treatment of the disease (Derksen et al., 1986; Alarcon-Segovia et al., 1989).

Lupus anticoagulant

The lupus anticoagulants are IgG or IgM immunoglobulins that can inhibit any of four procoagulant phospholipid complexes or two anticoagulant phospholipid-dependent reactions. In vitro, LAs appear to inhibit the prothrombinase reaction. They were first identified in a group of patients with SLE in 1948 (Conley et al., 1948) and, although as many as 50 per cent of patients with LA do not have SLE, the name has persisted.

Two groups of LA have been found; in the first group, LA activity could be separated from aCL activity and was dependent on human prothrombin (Bevers et al., 1991). In the second group, LA was dependent on the plasma protein B_2-glycoprotein I (B_2-GPI) (Galli et al., 1992).

The LA assay is a functional assay and does not measure antibody titer; because LAs are heterogeneous, however, no one assay is able to detect 100 per cent. Individual assays for LA include the following:

1 Activated partial thromboplastin time (aPTT). It is important to use aPTT reagents that are sensitive to the lupus anticoagulant (Adcock and Marlar, 1992). A sensitive aPTT using a sensitive reagent is an excellent screening test (Triplett, 1992), but may not be an appropriate screening test in pregnancy because it is affected by rising factor VIII.
2 Modified dilute Russell viper venom time (dRVVT). The dRVVT can be used as an initial sensitive screening test for LA or as a confirmatory test (Thiagarajan et al., 1986). Its sensitivity has surpassed the kaolin clotting time (KCT) and the tissue-thromboplastin inhibition tests in two studies (Thiagarajan et al., 1986; Forastiero et al., 1990), but other studies have shown that it is not as sensitive as aPTT (Triplett, 1992). The dRVVT is relatively resistant to clotting factor deficiencies when compared to other tests for LA. However, factor V or X levels below 0.4 U/ml do prolong the dRVVT (Thiagarajan et al., 1986). Both the source of the phospholipid (Brandt and Triplett, 1989) and the source of the venom can lead to variability in the results of the dRVVT (Exner and McRea, 1990).
3 Kaolin clotting time. The KCT is an aPTT without added platelet substitute, with kaolin acting as an activator and phospholipid surface (Margolis, 1958). The KCT is affected by residual platelets and, therefore, requires a filtration step to remove the platelets (Exner, 1985). In some studies, the KCT has not been as sensitive as a sensitive aPTT (Triplett, 1992).
4 Platelet neutralization procedures (PNP). One method of determining that an inhibitor is phospholipid dependent is by increasing the amount of phospholipid in an assay, as in the platelet neutralization procedure (PNP). Another is to accentuate the prolonged coagulation time by reducing the phospholipid (the tissue thromboplastin inhibition time) (Wallace et al., 2001). The tissue thromboplastin inhibition time is not widely used, as most studies show it is both less sensitive and less specific than PNP (Brandt et al., 1987). The PNP can be combined with the aPTT or dRVVT by using freeze-thawed platelets to correct or shorten the abnormal clotting time (Kornberg et al., 1989).

Because of the heterogeneity of LA, it is unlikely that any one assay will be accepted as the preferred standard. A combination of the most sensitive tests, such as the aPTT and the dRVVT, is the best approach to screening.

Laboratory criteria for lupus anticoagulant were established by the Scientific and Standardization Committee Subcommittee for the Standardization of LAs in 1995 (Brandt et al., 1987). These criteria include the following:

1 Prolongation of phospholipid dependent clotting tests (e.g. KCT, dilute Russell viper venom test (dRVVT), tissue thromboplastin inhibition time, plasma-recalcification clotting time, or sensitive partial thromboplastin time (PTT)).
2 The clotting time of a mixture of test and normal plasma should be significantly longer than that of the normal mixed with various plasmas from patients without LA.
3 There should be a relative correction of the defect by the addition of lysed washed platelets or phospholipid liposomes containing phosphatydylserine or hexagonal phase phospholipids.
4 It should be non-specific for any individual clotting factor and should rapidly lose apparent activity on dilution of test plasmas with saline.

It is important to use platelet-poor plasma to maximize the sensitivity of most assays (Arvieux et al., 1994). It is also important to note that no LA screening test is valid in the presence of heparin.

Anticardiolipin antibody

Cardiolipin is a normal plasma component, with more than 94 per cent found as part of very low density lipoprotein, low density lipoprotein and high density lipoprotein fractions (Deguchi et al., 2000). Cardiolipin is the major antigenic component of the false positive test for syphilis (Harris et al., 1983). Because APL antibodies cross-react with other negatively charged phospholipids, such as phosphatidylserine, cardiolipin can serve as a representative antigen in the solid-phase system (Inoue et al., 1986). Several studies have demonstrated that aCL IgG isotypes are a major predictor of thrombosis and pregnancy loss (Harris et al., 1986; Loizou et al., 1988), although there have been reports of similar associations with IgM aCL as well (Cronin et al., 1988; Cervera et al., 1993). IgM aCL has been associated with hemolytic anemia (Deleze et al., 1988). Although the APS classification criteria do not include IgA aCL, some have associated IgA with APS syndrome (Greco et al., 2000), vasculitis (Tajima et al., 1998) and recurrent abortions (Kalunian et al., 1988).

The anticardiolipin antibody (aCL) assay is an ELISA assay, performed as described above, after ELISA plates are coated with negatively charged phospholipid (usually cardiolipin) (Harris, 1990).

Anti-B$_2$-glycoprotein

B$_2$-glycoprotein I (B$_2$‴GPI), also called apolipoprotein H, is a plasma protein that was found to act as a cofactor in the aCL antibody assays, improving the binding of aCL (McNeil et al., 1990; Matsuura et al., 1990). In vivo, anti-B$_2$-GPI has several roles, including the inhibition of ADP-induced platelet aggregation, activation of the intrinsic coagulation pathway and activation of platelet pro-thrombinase activity (Nimpf et al., 1985; Schousboe, 1985). It is now widely accepted that most aCL antibodies are directed against a complex of negatively charged phospholipids with B$_2$-GPI (Shoenfeld and Meroni, 1992). The binding of aCL antibodies made in autoimmune diseases is enhanced by the presence of B$_2$-GPI, as opposed to those made in response to infections (Matsuura et al., 1990). Even though B$_2$-GPI is the target of aCL antibodies, patients can be positive for anti-B$_2$-GPI but negative for aCL; in one study, 11 per cent of SLE patients made antibodies to B$_2$-GPI alone (Day et al., 1998).

As with aCL antibodies, the strongest association of anti-B$_2$-glycoprotein I antibodies with thrombotic events has been demonstrated with the IgG and IgM isotypes (Roubey, 2000). Also similar to aCL antibodies, however, is the accumulating body of evidence that suggests that IgA anti-B$_2$-glycoprotein I antibodies may also be associated with the clinical manifestations of the antiphospholipid syndrome, including recurrent spontaneous abortions (Lakos et al., 1999; Lee et al., 2001). Anti-B$_2$-glycoprotein I may be a more specific marker for thrombotic events than aCL (Viard et al., 1992); however, since it is unusual for a patient with APS to be negative for both aCL and LA, anti-B$_2$-glycoprotein is not yet part of the routine work-up for patients with hypercoagulability.

ANTI-RIBOSOMAL P ANTIBODIES

Antibodies specific for ribosomal P proteins have been reported in SLE patients in frequencies ranging from 5 to 42 per cent (Bonfa and Elkon, 1986; Schneebaum et al., 1991). Correlations between anti-ribosomal P antibodies

and neuropsychological involvement have been described (Bonfa et al., 1987; Nojima et al., 1994), but their predictive value is controversial (Iverson, 1996; Press et al., 1996). Various reports have also described correlations with lupus nephritis (Hulsey et al., 1995; Reichlin and Wolfson-Reichlin, 2003), hepatic involvement (Koren et al., 1993; Arnett and Reichlin, 1995) and disease activity (Sato et al., 1991). Anti-ribosomal P antibodies can be detected by ELISA or immunoblotting.

COMPLEMENT

The complement system comprises at least 30 interacting, circulating blood proteins that serve as mediators and amplifiers of inflammatory responses. Two pathways in this system, the classic (C1, C4, C2) and alternative (factors B, D and properdin) lead to cleavage of the third component of complement (C3). In turn, C3 activates the membrane attack complex (C5–C9). The complement system induces lysis of antibody coated cells, promotes chemotaxis and increases vascular permeability. It also participates in the clearance of immune complexes (Ratnoff, 1996).

The CH50 assay, or total hemolytic complement assay, evaluates the functional integrity of the classical complement pathway by determining the dilution of serum required to lyse 50 per cent of antibody coated red blood cells. Persistently low or absent CH50 suggests an inherited deficiency of a complement component (Frank, 1992). Deficiencies of C1, C2, C3 or C4 increase susceptibility to SLE (Ratnoff, 1996). For example C2 deficiency is one of the most common genetic complement deficiencies in whites; approximately 1 per cent of the population are heterozygous (Schur and Sandson, 1968; Wallace et al., 2001). Among individuals homozygous for C2 deficiency, about 30 per cent have SLE (Schur and Sandson, 1968; Wallace et al., 2001). Most patients with C2 deficiency and SLE have a relatively mild form of the disease with mostly skin and joint manifestations and mild to no renal disease (Ruddy, 1996). C4 deficiency is also associated with SLE, although complete complement deficiency is rare because four alleles (two at C4A and two at C4B) contribute to the production of the protein (Wallace et al., 2001). Nevertheless, C4 null alleles predispose to SLE in multiple ethnic groups (Howard et al., 1986; Kemp et al., 1987; Wilson and Perez, 1988; Sturfelt et al., 1990), even though C4 levels may be normal in these patients.

Decreased levels of serum complement often reflect increased utilization of the system during active periods of immune complex mediated diseases such as SLE (Vaughan and Boling, 1961). Similar changes may occur in non-rheumatic diseases such as subacute bacterial endocarditis and post-streptococcal glomerulonephritis (Bush et al., 1993; Fleisher and Tomar, 1997). Serum levels of C3 and C4 are frequently decreased during and prior to active disease in SLE (Swaak et al., 1979; Clough and Chang, 1990; Egner, 2000). Persistently low C3 has also been associated with lupus nephritis (Sullivan et al., 1996) and hematologic activity (Ho et al., 2001). C3 levels have been reported to be normal, however, in up to 50 per cent of patients with clinically active disease (Valentijn et al., 1985). The measurement of complement as a marker of disease activity is complicated by the fact that complement levels can be elevated in inflammatory states as an acute phase reactant. Also, inherited complement deficiencies can result in chronically low levels. Several studies have therefore suggested that the measurement of complement split products such as C3d, C4d and Bb may be more sensitive predictors of disease flare, as levels are elevated only during complement activation (Buyon et al., 1992; Manzi et al., 1996).

REFERENCES

Abuaf, N., Johanet, C., Chretien, P. et al. (1990). Detection of autoantibodies to Sm antigen in systemic lupus erythematosus by immunodiffusion, ELISA and immunoblotting: variability of incidence related to assays and ethnic origin of patients. Eur J Clin Invest 20, 354–359.

Adcock, D.M. and Marlar, R.A. (1992). Activated partial thromboplastin time reagent sensitivity to the presence of the lupus anticoagulant. Arch Pathol Lab Med 116, 837–840.

Alarcon-Segovia, D., Deleze, M., Oria, C.V. et al. (1989). Antiphospholipid antibodies and the antiphospholipid syndrome in systemic lupus erythematosus. A prospective analysis of 500 consecutive patients. Medicine (Baltimore) 68, 353–365.

Alexander, E.L., Arnett, F.C., Provost, T.T. et al. (1983). Sjogren's syndrome: association of anti-Ro(SS-A) antibodies with vasculitis, hematologic abnormalities, and serologic hyperreactivity. Ann Intern Med 98, 155–159.

Anderson, M.J., Peebles, C.L., McMillan, R. et al. (1985). Fluorescent antinuclear antibodies and anti-SS-A/Ro in patients with immune thrombocytopenia subsequently developing systemic lupus erythematosus. Ann Intern Med 103, 548–550.

Arbuckle, M.R., McClain, M.T., Rubertone, M.V. et al. (2003). Development of autoantibodies before the clinical onset of systemic lupus erythematosus. N Engl J Med 349, 1526–1533.

Arnett, F.C., Hamilton, R.G., Roebber, M.G. et al. (1988). Increased frequencies of Sm and nRNP autoantibodies in American blacks compared to whites with systemic lupus erythematosus. J Rheumatol 15, 1773–1776.

Arnett, F.C. and Reichlin, M. (1995). Lupus hepatitis: an underrecognized disease feature associated with autoantibodies to ribosomal P. Am J Med 99, 465–472.

Arvieux, J., Roussel, B. and Colomb, M.G. (1994). [Antiphospholipid and anti beta 2-glycoprotein I antibodies.] Ann Biol Clin (Paris) 52, 381–385.

Avina-Zubieta, J.A., Galindo-Rodriguez, G., Kwan-Yeung, L. et al. (1995). Clinical evaluation of various selected ELISA kits for the detection of anti-DNA antibodies. Lupus 4, 370–374.

Barada, F.A. Jr, Andrews, B.S., Davis, J.S. 4th et al. (1981). Antibodies to Sm in patients with systemic lupus erythematosus. Correlation of Sm antibody titers with disease activity and other laboratory parameters. Arthrit Rheum 24, 1236–1244.

Bevers, E.M., Galli, M., Barbui, T. et al. (1991). Lupus anticoagulant IgGs (LA) are not directed to phospholipids only, but to a complex of lipid-bound human prothrombin. Thromb Haemost 66, 629–632.

Boey, M.L., Peebles, C.L., Tsay, G. et al. (1988). Clinical and autoantibody correlations in Orientals with systemic lupus erythematosus. Ann Rheum Dis 47, 918–923.

Bonfa, E. and Elkon, K.B. (1986). Clinical and serologic associations of the antiribosomal P protein antibody. Arthrit Rheum 29, 981–985.

Bonfa, E., Chu, J.L., Brot, N. et al. (1987). Lupus anti-ribosomal P peptide antibodies show limited heterogeneity and are predominantly of the IgG1 and IgG2 subclasses. Clin Immunol Immunopathol 45, 129–138.

Brandt, J.T. and Triplett, D.A. (1989). The effect of phospholipid on the detection of lupus anticoagulants by the dilute Russell viper venom time. Arch Pathol Lab Med 113, 1376–1378.

Brandt, J.T., Triplett, D.A., Musgrave, K. et al. (1987). The sensitivity of different coagulation reagents to the presence of lupus anticoagulants. Arch Pathol Lab Med 111, 120–124.

Bush, T.M., Shlotzhauer, T.L. and Grove, W. (1993). Serum complements. Inappropriate use in patients with suspected rheumatic disease. Arch Intern Med 153, 2363–2366.

Buyon, J.P. and Winchester, R. (1990). Congenital complete heart block. A human model of passively acquired autoimmune injury. Arthrit Rheum 33, 609–614.

Buyon, J.P., Tamerius, J., Belmont, H.M. et al. (1992). Assessment of disease activity and impending flare in patients with systemic lupus erythematosus. Comparison of the use of complement split products and conventional measurements of complement. Arthrit Rheum 35, 1028–1037.

Ceppellini, R., Polli, E. and Celada, F. (1957). A DNA-reacting factor in serum of a patient with lupus erythematosus diffusus. Proc Soc Exp Biol Med 96, 572–574.

Cervera, R., Khamashta, M.A., Font, J. et al. (1993). Systemic lupus erythematosus: clinical and immunologic patterns of disease expression in a cohort of 1,000 patients. The European Working Party on Systemic Lupus Erythematosus. Medicine (Baltimore) 72, 113–124.

Clough, J.D. and Chang, R.K. (1990). Effectiveness of testing for anti-DNA and the complement components iC3b, Bb, and C4 in the assessment of activity of systemic lupus erythematosus. J Clin Lab Anal 4, 268–273.

Conley, C.L., Morse, R.H., II, W.I. et al. (1948). Circulating anticoagulant as a cause of hemorrhagic diathesis in man. Bull Johns Hopkins Hosp 83, 288–296.

Cooper, R.C., Klemp, P., Stipp, C.J. et al. (1989). The relationship of anticardiolipin antibodies to disease activity in systemic lupus erythematosus. Br J Rheumatol 28, 379–382.

Cronin, M.E., Biswas, R.M., Van der Straeton, C. et al. (1988). IgG and IgM anticardiolipin antibodies in patients with lupus with anticardiolipin antibody associated clinical syndromes. J Rheumatol 15, 795–798.

Day, H.M., Thiagarajan, P., Ahn, C. et al. (1998). Autoantibodies to beta2-glycoprotein I in systemic lupus erythematosus and primary antiphospholipid antibody syndrome: clinical correlations in comparison with other antiphospholipid antibody tests. J Rheumatol 25, 667–674.

Deguchi, H., Fernandez, J.A., Hackeng, T.M. et al. (2000). Cardiolipin is a normal component of human plasma lipoproteins. Proc Natl Acad Sci USA 97, 1743–1748.

Deleze, M., Oria, C.V. and Alarcon-Segovia, D. (1988). Occurrence of both hemolytic anemia and thrombocytopenic purpura (Evans' syndrome) in systemic lupus erythematosus.

Relationship to antiphospholipid antibodies. J Rheumatol 15, 611–615.

Derksen, R.H., Biesma, D., Bouma, B.N. et al. (1986). Discordant effects of prednisone on anticardiolipin antibodies and the lupus anticoagulant. Arthrit Rheum 29, 1295–1296.

Ebling, F. and Hahn, B.H. (1980). Restricted subpopulations of DNA antibodies in kidneys of mice with systemic lupus. Comparison of antibodies in serum and renal eluates. Arthrit Rheum 23, 392–403.

Ebling, F.M. and Hahn, B.H. (1989). Pathogenic subsets of antibodies to DNA. Int Rev Immunol 5, 79–95.

Egner, W. (2000). The use of laboratory tests in the diagnosis of SLE. J Clin Pathol 53, 424–432.

Ehrenstein, M., Longhurst, C. and Isenberg, D.A. (1993). Production and analysis of IgG monoclonal anti-DNA antibodies from systemic lupus erythematosus (SLE) patients. Clin Exp Immunol 92, 39–45.

Emlen, W. and O'Neill, L. (1997). Clinical significance of antinuclear antibodies: comparison of detection with immunofluorescence and enzyme-linked immunosorbent assays. Arthrit Rheum 40, 1612–1618.

Emlen, W., Pisetsky, D.S. and Taylor, R.P. (1986). Antibodies to DNA. A perspective. Arthrit Rheum 29, 1417–1426.

Eschwege, F., Sancho-Garnier, H., Gerard, J.P. et al. (1988). Ten-year results of randomized trial comparing radiotherapy and concomitant bleomycin to radiotherapy alone in epidermoid carcinomas of the oropharynx: experience of the European Organization for Research and Treatment of Cancer. NCI Monogr 6, 275–278.

Exner, T. (1985). Comparison of two simple tests for the lupus anticoagulant. Am J Clin Pathol 83, 215–218.

Exner, T. and McRea, J. (1990). Studies on the relationship between 'antiphospholipid' antibodies and the lupus anticoagulant. Blood Coagul Fibrinolysis 1, 17–21.

Field, M., Williams, D.G., Charles, P. et al. (1988). Specificity of anti-Sm antibodies by ELISA for systemic lupus erythematosus: increased sensitivity of detection using purified peptide antigens. Ann Rheum Dis 47, 820–825.

Fleisher, T.A. and Tomar, R.H. (1997). Introduction to diagnostic laboratory immunology. J Am Med Assoc 278, 1823–1834.

Forastiero, R.R., Falcon, C.R. and Carreras, L.O. (1990). Comparison of various screening and confirmatory tests for the detection of the lupus anticoagulant. Haemostasis 20, 208–214.

Frank, M.M. (1992). Detection of complement in relation to disease. J Allergy Clin Immunol 89, 641–648.

Fritzler, M.J. and Tan, E.M. (1978). Antibodies to histones in drug-induced and idiopathic lupus erythematosus. J Clin Invest 62, 560–567.

Galli, M., Cortelazzo, S., Daldossi, M. et al. (1992). Increased levels of beta 2-glycoprotein I (aca-Cofactor) in patients with lupus anticoagulant. Thromb Haemost 67, 386.

Gauthier, V.J. and Mannik, M. (1990). A small proportion of cationic antibodies in immune complexes is sufficient to mediate their deposition in glomeruli. J Immunol 145, 3348–3352.

Gershwin, M.E. and Steinberg, A.D. (1974). Qualitative characteristics of anti-DNA antibodies in lupus nephritis. Arthrit Rheum 17, 947–954.

Gioud, M., Kaci, M.A. and Monier, J.C. (1982). Histone antibodies in systemic lupus erythematosus. A possible diagnostic tool. Arthrit Rheum 25, 407–413.

Greco, T.P., Amos, M.D., Conti-Kelly, A.M. et al. (2000). Testing for the antiphospholipid syndrome: importance of IgA anti-beta 2-glycoprotein I. Lupus 9, 33–41.

Harley, J.B., Sestak, A.L., Willis, L.G. et al. (1989). A model for disease heterogeneity in systemic lupus erythematosus. Relationships between histocompatibility antigens, autoantibodies, and lymphopenia or renal disease. Arthrit Rheum 32, 826–836.

Harris, E.N. (1990). Special report. The Second International Anti-cardiolipin Standardization Workshop/the Kingston Anti-Phospholipid Antibody Study (KAPS) group. Am J Clin Pathol 94, 476–484.

Harris, E.N., Chan, J.K., Asherson, R.A. et al. (1986). Thrombosis, recurrent fetal loss, and thrombocytopenia. Predictive value of the anticardiolipin antibody test. Arch Intern Med 146, 2153–2156.

Harris, E.N., Gharavi, A.E., Boey, M.L. et al. (1983). Anticardiolipin antibodies: detection by radioimmunoassay and association with thrombosis in systemic lupus erythematosus. Lancet 2, 1211–1214.

Hassell, K.L., Kressin, D.C., Neumann, et al. (1994). Correlation of antiphospholipid antibodies and protein S deficiency with thrombosis in HIV-infected men. Blood Coagul Fibrinolysis 5, 455–462.

Hedgpeth, M.T. and Boulware, D.W. (1988). Interstitial pneumonitis in antinuclear antibody-negative systemic lupus erythematosus: a new clinical manifestation and possible association with anti-Ro (SS-A) antibodies. Arthrit Rheum 31, 545–548.

Hergesell, O., Egbring, R. and Andrassy, K. (1993). Presence of anticardiolipin antibodies discriminates between Wegener's granulomatosis and microscopic polyarteritis. Adv Exp Med Biol 336, 393–396.

Herrick, A.L., Heaney, M., Hollis, S. et al. (1994). Anticardiolipin, anticentromere and anti-Scl-70 antibodies in patients with systemic sclerosis and severe digital ischaemia. Ann Rheum Dis 53, 540–542.

Ho, A., Barr, S.G., Magder, L.S. et al. (2001). A decrease in complement is associated with increased renal and hematologic activity in patients with systemic lupus erythematosus. Arthrit Rheum 44, 2350–2357.

Hobbs, R.N., Clayton, A.L. and Bernstein, R.M. (1987). Antibodies to the five histones and poly(adenosine diphosphate-ribose) in drug induced lupus: implications for pathogenesis. Ann Rheum Dis 46, 408–416.

Hoet, R.M., Koornneef, I., de Rooij, D.J. et al. (1992). Changes in anti-U1 RNA antibody levels correlate with disease activity in patients with systemic lupus erythematosus overlap syndrome. Arthrit Rheum 35, 1202–1210.

Hoffman, R.W. and Greidinger, E.L. (2000). Mixed connective tissue disease. Curr Opin Rheumatol 12, 386–390.

Homma, M., Mimori, T., Takeda, Y. et al. (1987). Autoantibodies to the Sm antigen: immunological approach to clinical aspects of systemic lupus erythematosus. J Rheumatol 14 Suppl 13, 188–193.

Holborow, E.J., Weir, D.M. and Johnson, G.D. (1957). A serum factor in lupus erythematosus with affinity for tissue nuclei. Br Med J 13, 732–734.

Howard, P.F., Hochberg, M.C., Bias, W.B. et al. (1986). Relationship between C4 null genes, HLA-D region antigens, and genetic susceptibility to systemic lupus erythematosus in Caucasian and black Americans. Am J Med 81, 187–193.

Hughes, G.R. (1993). The antiphospholipid syndrome: ten years on. Lancet *342*, 341–344.

Hulsey, M., Goldstein, R., Scully, L. et al. (1995). Anti-ribosomal P antibodies in systemic lupus erythematosus: a case-control study correlating hepatic and renal disease. Clin Immunol Immunopathol *74*, 252–256.

Inoue, T., Miyakawa, K. and Shimozawa, R. (1986). Interaction of surfactants with vesicle membrane of dipalmitoylphosphatidylcholine. Effect on gel-to-liquid-crystalline phase transition of lipid bilayer. Chem Phys Lipids *42*, 261–270.

Isenberg, D.A., Shoenfeld, Y. and Schwartz, R.S. (1984). Multiple serologic reactions and their relationship to clinical activity in systemic lupus erythematosus. Arthrit Rheum *27*, 132–138.

Iverson, G.L. (1996). Are antibodies to ribosomal P proteins a clinically useful predictor of neuropsychiatric manifestations in patients with systemic lupus erythematosus? Lupus *5*, 634–635.

Kalunian, K.C., Peter, J.B., Middlekauff, H.R. et al. (1988). Clinical significance of a single test for anti-cardiolipin antibodies in patients with systemic lupus erythematosus. Am J Med *85*, 602–608.

Kemp, M.E., Atkinson, J.P., Skanes, V.M. et al. (1987). Deletion of C4A genes in patients with systemic lupus erythematosus. Arthrit Rheum *30*, 1015–1022.

Koren, E., Schnitz, W. and Reichlin, M. (1993). Concomitant development of chronic active hepatitis and antibodies to ribosomal P proteins in a patient with systemic lupus erythematosus. Arthrit Rheum *36*, 1325–1328.

Kornberg, A., Silber, L., Yona, R. et al. (1989). Clinical manifestations and laboratory findings in patients with lupus anticoagulants. Eur J Haematol *42*, 90–95.

Kucuk, O., Gilman-Sachs, A., Beaman, K. et al. (1993). Antiphospholipid antibodies in sickle cell disease. Am J Hematol *42*, 380–383.

Kunkel HG, H.H., Deicher HR. (1960). Multiple autoanitbodies to cell constituents in systemic lupus erythematosus. Ciba Foundation Symposium Cellular Aspects of Immunology, London. Boston: Little, Brown, pp. 429–437.

Lakos, G., Kiss, E., Regeczy, N. et al. (1999). Isotype distribution and clinical relevance of anti-beta2-glycoprotein I (beta2-GPI) antibodies: importance of IgA isotype. Clin Exp Immunol *117*, 574–579.

Lee, L.A. and Norris, D.A. (1989). Mechanisms of cutaneous tissue damage in lupus erythematosus. Immunol Ser *46*, 359–386.

Lee, R.M., Branch, D.W. and Silver, R.M. (2001). Immunoglobulin A anti-beta2-glycoprotein antibodies in women who experience unexplained recurrent spontaneous abortion and unexplained fetal death. Am J Obstet Gynecol *185*, 748–753.

Leon, S.A., Green, A., Ehrlich, G.E. et al. (1997). Avidity of antibodies in SLE: relation to severity of renal involvement. Arthrit Rheum *20*, 23–29.

Loizou, S., Byron, M.A., Englert, H.J. et al. (1988). Association of quantitative anticardiolipin antibody levels with fetal loss and time of loss in systemic lupus erythematosus. Q J Med *68*, 525–531.

Madaio, M.P., Carlson, J., Cataldo, J. et al. (1987). Murine monoclonal anti-DNA antibodies bind directly to glomerular antigens and form immune deposits. J Immunol *138*, 2883–2889.

Maddison, P.J., Mogavero, H. and Reichlin, M. (1978). Patterns of clinical disease associated with antibodies to nuclear ribonucleoprotein. J Rheumatol *5*, 407–411.

Malnick, S., Sthoeger, Z., Attali, M. et al. (1993). Anticardiolipin antibodies associated with hypernephroma. Eur J Med *2*, 308–309.

Manzi, S., Rairie, J.E., Carpenter, A.B. et al. (1996). Sensitivity and specificity of plasma and urine complement split products as indicators of lupus disease activity. Arthrit Rheum *39*, 1178–1188.

Margolis, J. (1958). The kaolin clotting time; a rapid one-stage method for diagnosis of coagulation defects. J Clin Pathol *11*, 406–409.

Massa, M., De Benedetti, F., Pignatti, P. et al. (1994). Anti-double stranded DNA, anti-histone, and anti-nucleosome IgG reactivities in children with systemic lupus erythematosus. Clin Exp Rheumatol *12*, 219–225.

Matsuura, E., Igarashi, Y., Fujimoto, M. et al. (1990). Anticardiolipin cofactor(s) and differential diagnosis of autoimmune disease. Lancet *336*, 177–178.

Mattioli, M. and Reichlin, M. (1971). Characterization of a soluble nuclear ribonucleoprotein antigen reactive with SLE sera. J Immunol *107*, 1281–1290.

McNeil, H.P., Simpson, R.J., Chesterman, C.N. et al. (1990). Antiphospholipid antibodies are directed against a complex antigen that includes a lipid-binding inhibitor of coagulation: beta 2-glycoprotein I (apolipoprotein H). Proc Natl Acad Sci USA *87*, 4120–4124.

Misra, R., Aggarwal, A., Chag, M. et al. (1994). Raised anticardiolipin antibodies in Takayasu's arteritis. Lancet *343*, 1644–1645.

Moore, J.E. and Mohr, C.F. (1952). The incidence and etiologic background of chronic biologic false-positive reactions in serologic tests for syphilis. Ann Intern Med *37*, 1156–1161.

Morley, K.D., Bernstein, R.M., Bunn, C.C. et al. (1981). Thrombocytopenia and anti-Ro. Lancet *2*, 940.

Nimpf, J., Wurm, H. and Kostner, G.M. (1985). Interaction of beta 2-glycoprotein-I with human blood platelets: influence upon the ADP-induced aggregation. Thromb Haemost *54*, 397–401.

Nojima, T., Kamata, M., Matsunobu, T. et al. (1994). [Detection of autoantibodies in sera from patients with rheumatoid arthritis.] Ryumachi *34*, 871–878.

Norman, P.S. (1975). Immunotherapy (desensitization) in allergic disease. Annu Rev Med *26*, 337–344.

Papagiannis, A., Cooper, A. and Banks, J. (1994). Pulmonary embolism and lupus anticoagulant in a woman with renal cell carcinoma. J Urol *152*, 941–942.

Pisetsky, D.S., Jelinek, D.F., McAnally, L.M. et al. (1990). In vitro autoantibody production by normal adult and cord blood B cells. J Clin Invest *85*, 899–903.

Press, J., Palayew, K., Laxer, R.M. et al. (1996). Antiribosomal P antibodies in pediatric patients with systemic lupus erythematosus and psychosis. Arthrit Rheum *39*, 671–676.

Ratnoff, W.D. (1996). Inherited deficiencies of complement in rheumatic diseases. Rheum Dis Clin North Am *22*, 75–94.

Reeves, W.H., Fisher, D.E., Lahita, R.G. et al. (1985). Autoimmune sera reactive with Sm antigen contain high levels of RNP-like antibodies. J Clin Invest *75*, 580–587.

Reichlin, M. and Wolfson-Reichlin, M. (2003). Correlations of anti-dsDNA and anti-ribosomal P autoantibodies with lupus nephritis. Clin Immunol *108*, 69–72.

Robbins, W.C., Holman, H.R., Deicher, H. et al. (1957). Complement fixation with cell nuclei and DNA in lupus erythematosus. Proc Soc Exp Biol Med *96*, 575–579.

Rosler, D.H., Conway, M.D., Anaya, J.M. et al. (1995). Ischemic optic neuropathy and high-level anticardiolipin antibodies in primary Sjogren's syndrome. Lupus 4, 155–157.

Rothfield, N.F. and Stollar, B.D. (1967). The relation of immunoglobulin class, pattern of anti-nuclear antibody, and complement-fixing antibodies to DNA in sera from patients with systemic lupus erythematosus. J Clin Invest 46, 1785–1794.

Roubey, R.A. (2000). Update on antiphospholipid antibodies. Curr Opin Rheumatol 12, 374–378.

Rubin, R.L., Bell, S.A. and Burlingame, R.W. (1992). Autoantibodies associated with lupus induced by diverse drugs target a similar epitope in the (H2A-H2B)-DNA complex. J Clin Invest 90, 165–173.

Rubin, R.L., Burlingame, R.W., Arnott, J.E. et al. (1995). IgG but not other classes of anti-[(H2A-H2B)-DNA] is an early sign of procainamide-induced lupus. J Immunol 154, 2483–2493.

Rubin, R.L., Joslin, F.G. and Tan, E.M. (1982). A solid-phase radioimmunoassay for anti-histone antibodies in human sera: comparison with an immunofluorescence assay. Scand J Immunol 15, 63–70.

Rubin, R.L. and Waga, S. (1987). Antihistone antibodies in systemic lupus erythematosus. J Rheumatol 14 (Suppl 13), 118–126.

Ruddy, S. (1996). Rheumatic diseases and inherited complement deficiencies. Bull Rheum Dis 45, 6–8.

Sanchez-Guerrero, J., Lew, R.A., Fossel, A.H. et al. (1996). Utility of anti-Sm, anti-RNP, anti-Ro/SS-A, and anti-La/SS-B (extractable nuclear antigens) detected by enzyme-linked immunosorbent assay for the diagnosis of systemic lupus erythematosus. Arthrit Rheum 39, 1055–1061.

Sato, T., Uchiumi, T., Ozawa, T. et al. (1991). Autoantibodies against ribosomal proteins found with high frequency in patients with systemic lupus erythematosus with active disease. J Rheumatol 18, 1681–1684.

Schneebaum, A.B., Singleton, J.D., West, S.G. et al. (1991). Association of psychiatric manifestations with antibodies to ribosomal P proteins in systemic lupus erythematosus. Am J Med 90, 54–62.

Schousboe, I. (1985). beta 2-Glycoprotein I: a plasma inhibitor of the contact activation of the intrinsic blood coagulation pathway. Blood 66, 1086–1091.

Schur, P.H. and Sandson, J. (1968). Immunologic factors and clinical activity in systemic lupus erythematosus. N Engl J Med 278, 533–538.

Scofield, R.H., Zhang, F., Kurien, B.T. et al. (1996). Development of the anti-Ro autoantibody response in a patient with systemic lupus erythematosus. Arthrit Rheum 39, 1664–1668.

Scott, J.S., Maddison, P.J., Taylor, P.V. et al. (1983). Connective-tissue disease, antibodies to ribonucleoprotein, and congenital heart block. N Engl J Med 309, 209–212.

Sharp, G.C., Irvin, W.S., LaRoque, R.L. et al. (1971). Association of autoantibodies to different nuclear antigens with clinical patterns of rheumatic disease and responsiveness to therapy. J Clin Invest 50, 350–359.

Sharp, G.C., Irvin, W.S., May, C.M. et al. (1976). Association of antibodies to ribonucleoprotein and Sm antigens with mixed connective-tissue disease, systemic lupus erythematosus and other rheumatic diseases. N Engl J Med 295, 1149–1154.

Sharp, G.C., Irvin, W.S., Tan, E.M. et al. (1972). Mixed connective tissue disease – an apparently distinct rheumatic disease syndrome associated with a specific antibody to an extractable nuclear antigen (ENA). Am J Med 52, 148–159.

Shiel, W.C. Jr and Jason, M. (1989). The diagnostic associations of patients with antinuclear antibodies referred to a community rheumatologist. J Rheumatol 16, 782–785.

Shoenfeld, Y. and Meroni, P.L. (1992). The beta-2-glycoprotein I and antiphospholipid antibodies. Clin Exp Rheumatol 10, 205–209.

Slobbe, R.L., Pruijn, G.J., Damen, W.G. et al. (1991). Detection and occurrence of the 60- and 52-kD Ro (SS-A) antigens and of autoantibodies against these proteins. Clin Exp Immunol 86, 99–105.

Sontheimer, R.D., Maddison, P.J., Reichlin, M. et al. (1982). Serologic and HLA associations in subacute cutaneous lupus erythematosus, a clinical subset of lupus erythematosus. Ann Intern Med 97, 664–671.

Sturfelt, G., Truedsson, L., Johansen, P. et al. (1990). Homozygous C4A deficiency in systemic lupus erythematosus: analysis of patients from a defined population. Clin Genet 38, 427–433.

Sullivan, K.E., Wisnieski, J.J., Winkelstein, J.A. et al. (1996). Serum complement determinations in patients with quiescent systemic lupus erythematosus. J Rheumatol 23, 2063–2067.

Swaak, A.J., Aarden, L.A., Statius van Eps, L.W. et al. (1979). Anti-dsDNA and complement profiles as prognostic guides in systemic lupus erythematosus. Arthrit Rheum 22, 226–235.

Tajima, C., Suzuki, Y., Mizushima, Y. et al. (1998). Clinical significance of immunoglobulin A antiphospholipid antibodies: possible association with skin manifestations and small vessel vasculitis. J Rheumatol 25, 1730–1736.

Takeda, Y., Wang, G.S., Wang, R.J. et al. (1989). Enzyme-linked immunosorbent assay using isolated (U) small nuclear ribonucleoprotein polypeptides as antigens to investigate the clinical significance of autoantibodies to these polypeptides. Clin Immunol Immunopathol 50, 213–230.

Tan, E.M., Cohen, A.S., Fries, J.F. et al. (1982). The 1982 revised criteria for the classification of systemic lupus erythematosus. Arthrit Rheum 25, 1271–1277.

Tan, E.M., Feltkamp, T.E., Smolen, J.S. et al. (1997). Range of antinuclear antibodies in 'healthy' individuals. Arthritis Rheum 40, 1601–1611.

Thiagarajan, P., Pengo, V. and Shapiro, S.S. (1986). The use of the dilute Russell viper venom time for the diagnosis of lupus anticoagulants. Blood 68, 869–874.

Totoritis, M.C., Tan, E.M., McNally, E.M. et al. (1988). Association of antibody to histone complex H2A-H2B with symptomatic procainamide-induced lupus. N Engl J Med 318, 1431–1436.

Triplett, D.A. (1992). Coagulation assays for the lupus anticoagulant: review and critique of current methodology. Stroke 23 (Suppl 2), I11–14.

Tsao, B.P., Ebling, F.M., Roman, C. et al. (1990). Structural characteristics of the variable regions of immunoglobulin genes encoding a pathogenic autoantibody in murine lupus. J Clin Invest 85, 530–540.

Ulvestad, E., Kanestrom, A., Madland, T.M., et al. (2000). Evaluation of diagnostic tests for antinuclear antibodies in rheumatological practice. Scand J Immunol 52, 309–315.

Valentijn, R.M., van Overhagen, H., Hazevoet, H.M. et al. (1985). The value of complement and immune complex determinations in monitoring disease activity in patients with systemic lupus erythematosus. Arthrit Rheum 28, 904–913.

Vaughan, B.E. and Boling, E.A. (1961). Rapid assay procedures for tritium-labeled water in body fluids. J Lab Clin Med *57*, 159–164.

Viard, J.P., Amoura, Z. and Bach, J.F. (1992). Association of anti-beta 2 glycoprotein I antibodies with lupus-type circulating anticoagulant and thrombosis in systemic lupus erythematosus. Am J Med *93*, 181–186.

Wallace, D.J., Hahn, B. and Dubois, E.L. (2001). Dubois' Lupus Erythematosus, 6th edn. Philadelphia: Lippincott Williams & Wilkins. xiii, 1348.

Ward, M.M., Dawson, D.V. and Pisetsky, D.S. (1991). Serum immunoglobulin levels in systemic lupus erythematosus: the effects of age, sex, race and disease duration. J Rheumatol *18*, 540–544.

Wilson, W.A., Gharavi, A.E., Koike, T. et al. (1999). International consensus statement on preliminary classification criteria for definite antiphospholipid syndrome: report of an international workshop. Arthrit Rheum *42*, 1309–1311.

Wilson, W.A. and Perez, M.C. (1988). Complete C4B deficiency in black Americans with systemic lupus erythematosus. J Rheumatol *15*, 1855–1858.

Winn, D.M., Wolfe, J.F., Lindberg, D.A. et al. (1979). Identification of a clinical subset of systemic lupus erythematosus by antibodies to the SM antigen. Arthrit Rheum *22*, 1334–1337.

Wolf, P., Gretler, J., Aglas, F. et al. (1994). Anticardiolipin antibodies in rheumatoid arthritis: their relation to rheumatoid nodules and cutaneous vascular manifestations. Br J Dermatol *131*, 48–51.

Multiplexed Serum Assays

Anna Lokshin

Department of Obstetrics/Gynecology and Reproductive Sciences, University of Pittsburgh, Pittsburgh, PA, USA

Nothing is as simple as we hope it will be.

Jim Horning

INTRODUCTION

Several hundred cytokines, chemokines and growth factors interact as part of a peptide/protein regulatory network that controls many important physiologic processes including immunity, hematopoiesis, angiogenesis, stromagenesis and wound healing and repair. Such factors can be secreted by immune, as well as non-hematopoietic cells and can alter the behavior and properties of immune as well as many other cell types. Cytokines in particular display complex interactions among themselves, including synergy, antagonism, pleiotropy (many activities by one cytokine) and redundancy (many distinct cytokines displaying the same function). Therefore, analysis of the complex interacting set of cytokines expressed within the tissue microenvironments is often of more value than analysis of a single isolated cytokine. Cytokine profiles can be critical indicators distinguishing normal and pathologic states, particularly when expressed at detectable levels within the serum. However, the large number of cytokines expressed in physiologic and pathologic states often make determination of function of each cytokine an elaborate task (Tilg et al., 1992, Tracey and Cerami, 1993). Cytokines can be quantitated using a variety of methods. mRNA can be detected by real-time PCR; intracellular proteins can be measured by flow cytometry following staining of permeabilized cells and secreted cytokines can be quantified with bioassays, such as enzyme-linked immunosorbent assays (ELISAs), radioactive immunosorbent assays and microarrays. The ELISA is the most common method for quantitating secreted cytokines due to its high specificity and sensitivity (Mosmann and Fong, 1989, Hsieh et al., 1992). A typical ELISA involves sandwiching a cytokine between two specific antibodies that bind to individually distinct sites on the cytokine. The first 'capture' antibody tethers the cytokine to a solid support, i.e. the bottom of a 96-well plate. The second 'detection' antibody is usually modified by biotinylation or coupling to horseradish peroxidase in order to link the captured cytokine to a common detection system. ELISAs provide sensitive, specific and precise quantitation of cytokines. When applied to the large number of cytokines that are involved in defining a particular system, they are expensive and time-consuming to perform. Recently, a new technology, allowing the simultaneous measurement of multiple cytokines in one sample, was introduced that can complement the traditional ELISA, particularly when there is small sample size and multiple cytokines are to be measured.

PRINCIPLES BEHIND THE MULTIPLEX PLATFORM

Multiplexed microsphere-based technology (FlowMetrix™) developed by the Luminex Corporation (Austin, TX), is a

Measuring Immunity, edited by Michael T. Lotze and Angus W. Thomson
ISBN 0-12-455900-X, London

highly sensitive, multiplexed assay platform that provides a means to determine qualitative and quantitative measurements of multiple analytes simultaneously in one sample. The assay systems employ small polystyrene/latex microspheres or beads (~3–5 μm in diameter) as solid support for the capture molecules instead of a planar substrate, which is conventionally used for ELISA assays (Figure 18.1) (5–7). The individual microspheres are color-coded by a distinct mixture of red and orange fluorescent dyes resulting in an array of 100 individually addressable populations of microspheres (Figure 18.1) (Fulton et al., 1997). In each individual immunoassay, the capture molecule, i.e. capture antibody, is coupled to a distinct type of bead. The different color-coded bead sets can be pooled and the immunoassay is performed in a single reaction well of a filter-bottom 96-well plate. Individual analyte molecules, e.g. specific cytokines, are allowed to bind to appropriate capture antibodies. The reaction is followed by addition of a mixture of specific biotinylated detection antibodies. The bead mixture is then incubated with PE or ALEXA 488-conjugated Streptavidin. The microspheres provide a high signal-to-noise ratio for detection of low-level fluorescence with PE/ALEXA 488 as the reporter (Fulton et al., 1997). Washing steps are typically performed after each reaction using a vacuum manifold, however they may be omitted. Reactions are then analyzed using a Luminex cytometer, which quantitates the green, orange and red fluorescence of each microsphere using the FL1, Fl2 and FL3 detectors, respectively (see Figure 18.1). Each bead type is identified by its individual spectral address and the concentration of each analyte (cytokine) is measured based on the intensity of second green fluorescence signal associated with a specific color-coded bead (see Figure 18.1). Finally, the concentrations of the analytes in the sample are determined by extrapolation from an internal standard. As the individual bead sets can be discriminated in the flow cytometer, many assays can be performed simultaneously in a single small (50 μl) sample, thus allowing for multiplexed quantitation.

Such strategies can be used for virtually any bioassay that is based on the specific binding of one molecule to another, such as immunoassays (e.g. ELISA); protein–protein interaction assays (e.g. interaction mapping); enzyme assays (e.g. kinase, phosphatase and protease assays); receptor-ligand assays and protein-nucleic acid assays.

HISTORY AND APPLICATIONS OF BEAD-BASED ASSAYS

The first reports used microspheres composed of a variety of materials including latex, polystyrene, polyacrylamide, or glass as solid support for immunoassays and appeared as early as 1982 (Lisi et al., 1982; Renner, 1994; Iannelli et al., 1997, 1998; Kempfer et al., 1999). Capture molecules, e.g. antibodies and antigens, have been adsorbed or directly or indirectly coupled to the microspheres. Early microsphere-based immunoassays included ones for β2-microglobulin (Bishop and Davis, 1997), Clostridium difficile toxin (Renner, 1994), and α-fetoprotein (Frengen et al., 1993). Human IgG (Lisi et al., 1982) and IgE (Kwittken et al., 1994) have been measured with antibodies chemically coupled to microspheres. Bead-based multiplexed assays have been used for bacterial serotyping of multiple strains of Streptococcus pneumoniae (Park et al., 2000; Pickering et al., 2002). Alternatively, antigens have been adsorbed to microspheres to detect antibodies specific for Helicobacter pylori (Best et al., 1992), human IgA (Syrjala et al., 1991), κ-light chains (Wilson and Wotherspoon, 1988) and phospholipids (Obringer et al., 1995; Eschwege et al., 1996; Drouvalakis et al., 1999) or covalently attached to detect antibodies to α-gliadin (Presani et al., 1989). Microspheres coated with human C1q were used to detect circulating immune complexes containing elusive HIV antigens (McHugh et al., 1986, 1988) and collagen has been used to capture von Willebrand factor (Kempfer et al., 1999). In some instances, these assays were more sensitive than the

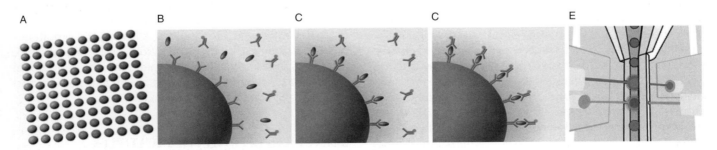

Figure 18.1 Basics of FlowMetrix™ technology. A. The technology uses 5.6 μm polystyrene particles, called microspheres that are internally labeled with two fluorescent dyes. B. Each bead set can be coated with a reagent specific to a particular bioassay (e.g. capture antibody). Coated beads are suspended in a test sample to collect analyte molecules. C. Detection molecules, e.g. detection antibody, coupled with Biotin, are allowed to bind to analyte molecules on the beads. D. Fluorescently labeled reporter tags, e.g. Streptavidin-PE, bind to Biotin on detection molecule. E. Within the Luminex 100 compact analyzer, precision fluidics lines up suspended microspheres in a single file prior to passing through the detection chamber to allow discrete measurement of single beads. As a microsphere passes through the detection chamber, a red laser excites both the internal red and infrared dyes, allowing the proper classification of the microspheres to one of 100 sets. A green laser excites orange fluorescence associated with the binding of a specific analyte. Many readings are made on each bead set, further validating the results.

conventional ELISA and could resolve indeterminate clinical samples (McHugh et al., 1997). Likewise, such assays have also been established to measure RNA for a number of viral antigens (Mehrpouyan et al., 1997; Smith et al., 1998; Van Cleve et al., 1998). Microspheres coated with HLA class I and class II antigens have been used for HLA typing (Moses et al., 2000; Bray, 2001). This technology has recently been implemented on the Luminex platform for DNA-based HLA typing (Fulton et al., 1997), as well as testing for antibodies to specific HLA antigens (Bray, 2001). In addition, a microsphere technique was utilized for analysis of phosphorylation of the signaling protein, ERK-2 (Lund-Johansen et al., 2000).

MEASURING OF CYTOKINE RESPONSES: xMAP VERSUS ELISA

There are several advantages of these bead-based measures when compared with conventional ELISA. The most important advantage is that many assays can be performed simultaneously, thus allowing for the multiplexed quantitation of up to 100 analytes in a single sample. Microsphere-based arrays are more rapid, less expensive and require only 50 μl of sample for analyzing all cytokines as compared with at least 100 μl for each cytokine measured by ELISAs (Oliver et al., 1998; Carson and Vignali, 1999; Vignali, 2000; Cook et al., 2001; Kellar et al., 2001; Camilla et al., 2001). In the near-liquid phase of the microsphere-based assay, equilibrium is reached sooner so incubation times are reduced significantly and analysis can be completed in 30–60 min, particularly if wash steps are eliminated (Millan et al., 1985). Furthermore, the inclusion of new cytokines to this panel only requires the addition of new bead sets. Finally, the near-liquid phase homogeneous assay format confers high sensitivity. The average conventional ELISA assay can detect cytokines at levels as low as 50 pg/ml. Sensitivity in multiplexed assays can be as good as 1 pg/ml (Wilson and Wotherspoon, 1988; Oliver et al., 1998; Carson and Vignali, 1999; Vignali, 2000; Camilla et al., 2001; Cook et al., 2001; Mahanty et al., 2001; Kellar et al., 2001; Hildesheim et al., 2002; de Jager et al., 2003).

The performance of the multiplexed formats for human cytokines has been validated by comparisons with ELISAs (Oliver et al., 1998; Chen et al., 1999; Cook et al., 2001; Kellar et al., 2001; Camilla et al., 2001; Mahanty et al., 2001). Such comparisons have demonstrated that the detection limits were the same or better for the multiplexed assays (Oliver et al., 1998; Chen et al., 1999; Cook et al., 2001; Kellar et al., 2001; Camilla et al., 2001; Mahanty et al., 2001). Sample data from the two methods were highly comparable (correlation coefficients = 0.86–1.0) (Chen et al., 1999; Cook et al., 2001; Kellar et al., 2001; Camilla et al., 2001; Mahanty et al., 2001). Reproducibility was excellent for the multiplexed format: intra-assay CVs were less than 10 per cent (Oliver et al., 1998; Cook et al.,

2001) and inter-assay CVs were less than 5 per cent (Camilla et al., 2001). Recoveries of eight cytokines spiked into a buffer or normal serum matrix averaged 102.5 ± 5 per cent (Kellar et al., 2001).

Multiplexed assays for up to 15 human cytokines have been described (Oliver et al., 1998; Chen et al., 1999; Cook et al., 2001; Kellar et al., 2001; Camilla et al., 2001; Mahanty et al., 2001; Hildesheim et al., 2002). Different combinations of interleukins (IL)-1β, -2, -4, -5, -6, -8, -10, -12, TNFα, IFNγ, GM-CSF, IFN-inducible protein (IP)-10 and RANTES were measured in whole blood, cell-culture supernatants, tears and serum. Secretion of TH1 versus TH2 cytokines from stimulated mouse CD4+ T cells (Carson and Vignali, 1999) or from Staphylococcus aureus-stimulated peripheral blood mononuclear cells obtained from patients with hyperimmunoglobulinemia E syndrome (Martins et al., 2002) was studied with multiplexed bead-based assays. A different group of 15 human cytokines (IL-1α, IL-1β, IL-2, IL-4, IL-5, IL-6, IL-8, IL-10, IL-12p70, IL-13, IL-15, IL-17, IL-18, IFNγ and TNFα) were validated in a study of healthy individuals, rheumatoid arthritis patients and juvenile idiopathic arthritis patients (de Jager et al., 2003). In another study, the multiplex assay was applied to the determination of cytokine profiles in whole blood from atopic and non-atopic asthmatic patients (Camilla et al., 2001). The results showed that atopic subjects' blood has higher levels of IL-4 and less IFNγ than the blood of non-atopic subjects. However, atopic asthmatic subjects' blood has significantly higher concentrations of IFNγ than that of atopic non-asthmatic subjects (Camilla et al., 2001). Finally, this technique allowed determination of six human cytokine (IFNγ, TNFα, IL-2, IL-4, IL-5, IL-10) concentrations simultaneously in a single tear sample. The small volume required (5–10 μl/test) by the bead array decreased collection time, minimizing the confounding effect of stimulation on cytokine concentration in tears, as well as allowing calculation of cytokine ratios (Cook et al., 2001). Together, the results obtained indicate that the multiplexed technology constitutes a powerful system for the quantitative, simultaneous determination of secreted cytokines in pathological conditions.

CYTOKINES IN CANCER

An increasing volume of data suggests a relationship between cytokine levels in human body fluids and disease pathogenesis. Cytokines are implicated in many aspects of tumor growth (Leek et al., 1994; Hotfilder et al., 1997; Tartour and Fridman, 1998; Schneider et al., 2001; Liekens, 2002; Opdenakker and Van Damme, 2002; Arya et al., 2003; Salcedo and Oppenheim, 2003; Rubin, 2003; Miller, 2003). It is widely accepted that cytokines are involved in the anorexia–cachexia syndrome (56). The relationships between cytokines and tumor are multiple and bidirectional. Cytokines play a role by stimulating the host immune system to generate anti-tumor specific responses. Conversely, tumor development may lead to a state of immunosuppression reflected by low cytokine expression in tumor stroma (reviewed in Muller et al., 2002, Muller and Pawelec, 2003). In addition, cancer cells are capable of directly producing cytokines. These cytokines may act on the cancer cells in an autocrine manner or, in a paracrine manner, on the supporting tissues such as fibroblasts and blood vessels to produce an environment conducive to cancer growth and metastasis (Negus and Balkwill, 1996). Cancer cells express growth factors and their cognate receptors, such as EGF, EGFR and Her2/neu, render them independent of exogenous growth stimuli (Powers et al., 2000; Zwick et al., 2001; Normanno et al., 2001; Kopp et al., 2003). Tumor cells also express and produce angiogenic factors, such as VEGF, FGF, PDGFA and B, IL-6 and IL-8 (Lichtenstein et al., 1990; Takeyama et al., 1991; Pisa et al., 1992; Di Blasio et al., 1995; Negus et al., 1995, 1998; Gleich et al., 1996; Huleihel et al., 1997; Wu et al., 1997; Glezerman et al., 1998; Asschert et al., 1999; Keshava et al., 1999; Xu and Fidler, 2000; Berger et al., 2001; Ripley et al., 2001; Savarese et al., 2001; Schwartz et al., 2001; Scotton et al., 2001), that are capable of stimulating migration, proliferation and survival of vascular cells in the established tumor blood vessels (Angiolillo et al., 1995; Voest et al., 1995; Volpert et al., 1998). Tumor cells can produce other cytokines and chemokines, such as MCP-1, G-CSF, GM-CSF, CSF-1, TNFα, IL-1α and IL-1β (Lichtenstein et al., 1990; Takeyama et al., 1991; Pisa et al., 1992; Di Blasio et al., 1995; Negus et al., 1995, 1998; Gleich et al., 1996; Huleihel et al., 1997; Wu et al., 1994, 1997; Glezerman et al., 1998; Asschert et al., 1999; Keshava et al., 1999; Xu and Fidler, 2000; Berger et al., 2001; Ripley et al., 2001; Savarese et al., 2001; Schwartz et al., 2001; Scotton et al., 2001). MCP-1, for example, can cause accumulation of tumor-associated macrophages (TAM) (Negus et al., 1995) which, in turn, can stimulate cancer growth by producing IL-1, IL-6, TNF, TGFβ, EGF, and PDGF (Mantovani, 1994).

These multiple cytokines form a complicated network in blood creating cancer-specific cytokine profiles. Elevated levels of various cytokines have been analyzed using ELISA in blood, ascites, pleural effusions and urine of patients with different types of cancer (reviewed in Dunlop and Campbell, 2000). Individual cytokine combinations were examined in various studies. For example, IL-1, IL-6, IL-7, IL-2, IL-8, IL-10, FGF, TNF, TGF angiogenin, GM-CSF and TNFβ were analyzed in patients with squamous cell carcinoma of the vulva as compared with normal controls (Dunlop and Campbell, 2000). It was concluded that levels of IL-2, IL-10 and IL-8 were elevated in these patients. Furthermore, FGF, TNF and TGF were elevated in patients with early stage cancer, whereas patients with progressive disease had increased levels of angiogenin, GM-CSF and TNFβ. In endometrial cancer, IL-2, IL-7, IL-8, IL-10, FGF, TNF, GM-CSF, angiogenin and

TGFβ were significantly elevated in patients with early stage carcinoma (Chopra et al., 1996, 1997, 1998). Penson et al. (2000) reported the levels of various cytokines (IL-1β, IL-2, IL-6, IL-8, MCP-1, GM-CSF and TNFα) in the serum and ascites of ovarian cancer patients. Increased concentration of only IL-6 and IL-8 were found and the levels of these cytokines correlated with a poor initial response to chemotherapy (Penson et al., 2000). These studies demonstrated that a great diversity in the cytokine profiles is associated with individual tumor types with no single cytokine being present in all patients with cancer (Kerbel and Folkman, 2002). However, different sets of cytokines were evaluated in each study and no systematic evaluation of complete cytokine profiles in each cancer type has been undertaken. Analyzing expanded cytokine panels using fluorescent bead-based immunoassays can further contribute to an understanding of the role of cytokines in cancer. In addition, cancer type-specific cytokine combinations could potentially serve as serum biomarkers for cancer early detection, diagnosis and prognosis.

To verify the hypothesis that identification of cancer-specific cytokine panels may allow for early cancer diagnosis, we have analyzed a panel of 33 cytokines, IL-1β, IL-2, IL-4, IL-5, IL-6, IL-8, IL-10, IL-12p40, IL-13, IL-15, IL-17, IL-18, TNFα, IFNγ, GM-CSF, EGF, VEGF, G-CSF, bFGF, HGF, RANTES, MIP-1α, MIP-1β, MCP-1, EGFR, TGFβ, FasL, MMP 2, MMP 9, TIMP 1, TIMP 2, survivin and CA 125, using multiplexed bead assays in patients with ovarian cancer as compared to healthy control women. Serum samples were obtained from 55 patients diagnosed with early stages (I-II) ovarian cancer and 55 healthy age-matched controls. Serum levels of IL-2, IL-4, IL-5, IL-10, IL-13, IL-15, IL-17, IL-18, TNFα, IFNγ, RANTES, GM-CSF, bFGF and survivin were undetectable in either the control or patient groups. IL-1β, MIP-1α, MIP-1β, HGF, TGFβ, EGFR, MMP 2, MMP 9, TIMP 1, TIMP 2 and FasL, demonstrated measurable serum concentrations, which did not significantly differ between the control and patient groups (data not shown). Serum concentrations of IL-6, IL-8, G-CSF, VEGF, and CA 125, were significantly higher ($P < 0.01$) in ovarian cancer patients as compared to controls. Surprisingly, women with ovarian cancer demonstrated significantly lower blood levels of EGF, IL-12p40 and MCP-1 ($P < 0.001$). The results are presented in Figure 18.2. Statistical analysis was then performed to evaluate usefulness of these data for early detection of ovarian cancer. Classification trees algorithm (Brieman et al., 1984) resulted in selection of a combination of five serum markers CA 125, EGF, VEGF, IL-6, and IL-8 that allowed distinguishing early stage ovarian cancer cases from normal controls with high power, i.e. 91 per cent specificity and 96 per cent sensitivity.

To ascertain whether the cytokine combination described above is specific for ovarian cancer, we have evaluated the same extended cytokine panel in three other cancers, namely, breast, pancreatic and melanoma.

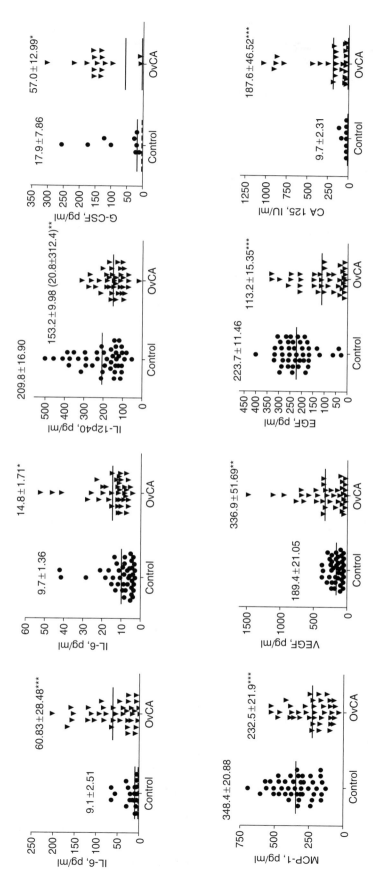

Figure 18.2 Serum levels of cytokines and growth factors in early stage ovarian cancer patients and healthy controls. Blood sera were collected from 55 patients with early stage (I–II) ovarian cancer and from 55 age and sex-matched healthy controls. Sera were analyzed using FlowMetrix technology. Horizontal lines indicate mean values. * denotes statistical significance between controls and cancer patients of $P < 0.05$; ** $P < 0.01$; *** $P < 0.001$. Presented Mean $\pm$ SE.

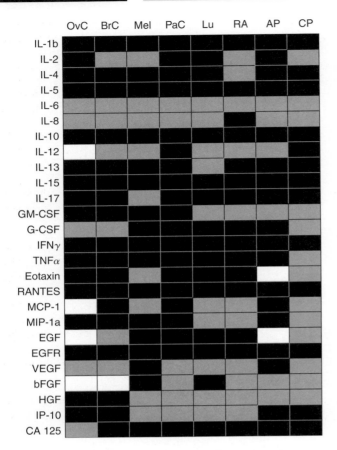

Figure 18.3 Cytokine profiles are cancer-specific. OvC: ovarian cancer, BrC: breast cancer, Mel: melanoma, PaC: pancreatic cancer, Lu: lupus (SLE), RA: rheumatoid arthritis, AP: acute pancreatitis, CP: chronic pancreatitis. Gray bars: marker is elevated in cancer cases as compared to control; white bars: marker is lower in cancer cases; black: no difference.

In addition, two autoimmune diseases, rheumatoid arthritis and lupus, were evaluated. Figure 18.3 clearly demonstrates that cytokine profiles are unique for each disease type. While all cancers have elevated levels of IL-6 and IL-8, other markers differ, thus creating the basis for development of organ site-specific serum cytokine diagnostic cancer assays.

CONCLUSIONS

Multiplexed immunoassay systems possess substantial sensitivity and reproducibility. Multiplexed immunoassays improve the throughput by greatly increasing the amount of information obtained from a single experiment. In addition, they lower the cost of analysis by reducing the amount of material and reagents needed. The reduction of sample volume is of great importance for all those applications where only minimal amounts of samples are available (e.g. analysis of multiple tumor markers from a minimum amount of biopsy material). Simultaneous analysis of multiple cytokines will provide a deeper insight into the immunological mechanisms of normal

and pathological physiological processes. In addition, multiplexed immunoassays will be used in disease screening and elucidating people's predisposition to get a certain disease. Furthermore, multiplexed immunoassays will open up new possibilities with regard to the monitoring of patients during disease treatment and therapy.

REFERENCES

Angiolillo, A.L., Sgadari, C., Taub, D.D. et al. (1995). Human interferon-inducible protein 10 is a potent inhibitor of angiogenesis in vivo. J Exp Med 182, 155–162.

Arya, M., Patel, H.R. and Williamson, M. (2003). Chemokines: key players in cancer. Curr Med Res Opin 19, 557–564.

Asschert, J.G., Vellenga, E., Ruiters, M.H. and de Vries, E.G. (1999). Regulation of spontaneous and TNF/IFN-induced IL-6 expression in two human ovarian-carcinoma cell lines. Int J Cancer 82, 244–249.

Berger, S., Siegert, A., Denkert, C., Kobel, M. and Hauptmann, S. (2001). Interleukin-10 in serous ovarian carcinoma cell lines. Cancer Immunol Immunother 50, 328–333.

Best, L.M., Veldhuyzen van Zanten, S.J., Bezanson, G.S., Haldane, D.J. and Malatjalian, D.A. (1992). Serological detection of Helicobacter pylori by a flow microsphere immunofluorescence assay. J Clin Microbiol 30, 2311–2317.

Bishop, J.E. and Davis, K.A. (1997). A flow cytometric immunoassay for beta2-microglobulin in whole blood. J Immunol Methods 210, 79–87.

Bray, R.A. (2001). Flow cytometry in human leukocyte antigen testing. Semin Hematol 38, 194–200.

Brieman, L.F.J., Olshen, R.A. and Stone, C.J. (1984). Classification and Regression Trees. Monterey: Wadsworth and Brooks/Cole.

Camilla, C., Mely, L., Magnan, A. et al. (2001). Flow cytometric microsphere-based immunoassay: analysis of secreted cytokines in whole-blood samples from asthmatics. Clin Diagn Lab Immunol 8, 776–784.

Carson, R.T. and Vignali, D.A. (1999). Simultaneous quantitation of 15 cytokines using a multiplexed flow cytometric assay. J Immunol Methods 227, 41–52.

Chen, R., Lowe, L., Wilson, J.D. et al. (1999). Simultaneous quantification of six human cytokines in a single sample using microparticle-based flow cytometric technology. Clin Chem 45, 1693–1694.

Chopra, V.V., Dinh, T.V. and Hannigan, E.V. (1996). Serum levels of interleukins, growth factors and angiogenin in patients with endometrial cancer. Cancer J Sci Am 2, 279.

Chopra, V., Dinh, T.V. and Hannigan, E.V. (1997). Circulating serum levels of cytokines and angiogenic factors in patients with cervical cancer. J Cancer Res Clin Oncol 123, 167–172.

Chopra, V., Dinh, T.V. and Hannigan, E.V. (1998). Angiogenin, interleukins, and growth-factor levels in serum of patients with ovarian cancer: correlation with angiogenesis. Cancer Invest 16, 152–159.

Cook, E.B., Stahl, J.L., Lowe, L. et al. (2001). Simultaneous measurement of six cytokines in a single sample of human tears using microparticle-based flow cytometry: allergics vs. nonallergics. J Immunol Methods 254, 109–118.

de Jager, W., te Velthuis, H., Prakken, B.J., Kuis, W. and Rijkers, G.T. (2003). Simultaneous detection of 15 human cytokines in a single sample of stimulated peripheral blood mononuclear cells. Clin Diagn Lab Immunol 10, 133–139.

Di Blasio, A.M., Carniti, C., Vigano, P. and Vignali, M. (1995). Basic fibroblast growth factor and ovarian cancer. J Steroid Biochem Mol Biol 53, 375–379.

Drouvalakis, K.A., Neeson, P.J. and Buchanan, R.R. (1999). Detection of anti-phosphatidylethanolamine antibodies using flow cytometry. Cytometry 36, 46–51.

Dunlop, R.J. and Campbell, C.W. (2000). Cytokines and advanced cancer. J Pain Symptom Manage 20, 214–232.

Eschwege, V., Laude, I., Toti, F., Pasquali, J.L. and Freyssinet, J.M. (1996). Detection of bilayer phospholipid-binding antibodies using flow cytometry. Clin Exp Immunol 103, 171–175.

Frengen, J., Schmid, R., Kierulf, B. et al. (1993). Homogeneous immunofluorometric assays of alpha-fetoprotein with macroporous, monosized particles and flow cytometry. Clin Chem 39, 2174–2181.

Fulton, R.J., McDade, R.L., Smith, P.L., Kienker, L.J. and Kettman, J.R., Jr (1997). Advanced multiplexed analysis with the FlowMetrix system. Clin Chem 43, 1749–1756.

Gleich, L.L., Srivastava, L. and Gluckman, J.L. (1996). Plasma platelet-derived growth factor: preliminary study of a potential marker in head and neck cancer. Ann Otol Rhinol Laryngol 105, 710–712.

Glezerman, M., Mazot, M., Maymon, E. et al. (1998). Tumor necrosis factor-alpha and interleukin-6 are differently expressed by fresh human cancerous ovarian tissue and primary cell lines. Eur Cytokine Netw 9, 171–179.

Hildesheim, A., Ryan, R.L., Rinehart, E. et al. (2002). Simultaneous measurement of several cytokines using small volumes of biospecimens. Cancer Epidemiol Biomarkers Prev 11, 1477–1484.

Hotfilder, M., Nowak-Gottl, U. and Wolff, J.E. (1997). Tumorangiogenesis: a network of cytokines. Klin Padiatr 209, 265–270.

Hsieh, C.S., Heimberger, A.B., Gold, J.S., O'Garra, A. and Murphy, K.M. (1992). Differential regulation of T helper phenotype development by interleukins 4 and 10 in an alpha beta T-cell-receptor transgenic system. Proc Natl Acad Sci USA 89, 6065–6069.

Huleihel, M., Maymon, E., Piura, B. et al. (1997). Distinct patterns of expression of interleukin-1 alpha and beta by normal and cancerous human ovarian tissues. Eur Cytokine Netw 8, 179–187.

Iannelli, D., D'Apice, L., Cottone, C. et al. (1997). Simultaneous detection of cucumber mosaic virus, tomato mosaic virus and potato virus Y by flow cytometry. J Virol Methods 69, 137–145.

Iannelli, D., D'Apice, L., Fenizia, D. et al. (1998). Simultaneous identification of antibodies to Brucella abortus and Staphylococcus aureus in milk samples by flow cytometry. J Clin Microbiol 36, 802–806.

Kellar, K.L., Kalwar, R.R., Dubois, K.A., Crouse, D., Chafin, W.D. and Kane, B.E. (2001). Multiplexed fluorescent bead-based immunoassays for quantitation of human cytokines in serum and culture supernatants. Cytometry 45, 27–36.

Kempfer, A.C., Silaf, M.R., Farias, C.E., Carballo, G.A., Woods, A.I. and Lazzari, M.A. (1999). Binding of von Willebrand factor to collagen by flow cytometry. Am J Clin Pathol 111, 418–423.

Kerbel, R. and Folkman, J. (2002). Clinical translation of angiogenesis inhibitors. Nat Rev Cancer 2, 727–739.

Keshava, N., Gubba, S. and Tekmal, R.R. (1999). Overexpression of macrophage colony-stimulating factor (CSF-1) and its

receptor, c-fms, in normal ovarian granulosa cells leads to cell proliferation and tumorigenesis. J Soc Gynecol Investig·6, 41–49.

Kopp, R., Rothbauer, E., Ruge, M. et al. (2003). Clinical implications of the EGF receptor/ligand system for tumor progression and survival in gastrointestinal carcinomas: evidence for new therapeutic options. Recent Results Cancer Res 162, 115–132.

Kwittken, P.L., Pawlowski, N.A., Sweinberg, S.K., Douglas, S.D. and Campbell, D.E. (1994). Flow cytometric measurement of immunoglobulin E to natural latex proteins. Clin Diagn Lab Immunol 1, 197–201.

Leek, R.D., Harris, A.L. and Lewis, C.E. (1994). Cytokine networks in solid human tumors: regulation of angiogenesis. J Leukoc Biol 56, 423–435.

Lichtenstein, A., Berenson, J., Gera, J.F., Waldburger, K., Martinez-Maza, O. and Berek, J.S. (1990). Resistance of human ovarian cancer cells to tumor necrosis factor and lymphokine-activated killer cells: correlation with expression of HER2/neu oncogenes. Cancer Res 50, 7364–7370.

Liekens, S. (2002). The role of growth factors, angiogenic enzymes and apoptosis in neovascularization and tumor growth-collected publications. Verh K Acad Geneeskd Belg 64, 197–224.

Lisi, P.J., Huang, C.W., Hoffman, R.A. and Teipel, J.W. (1982). A fluorescence immunoassay for soluble antigens employing flow cytometric detection. Clin Chim Acta 120, 171–179.

Lund-Johansen, F., Davis, K., Bishop, J. and de Waal Malefyt, R. (2000). Flow cytometric analysis of immunoprecipitates: high-throughput analysis of protein phosphorylation and protein-protein interactions. Cytometry 39, 250–259.

Mahanty, S., Bausch, D.G., Thomas, R.L. et al. (2001). Low levels of interleukin-8 and interferon-inducible protein-10 in serum are associated with fatal infections in acute Lassa fever. J Infect Dis 183, 1713–1721.

Mantovani, A. (1994). Tumor-associated macrophages in neoplastic progression: a paradigm for the in vivo function of chemokines. Lab Invest 71, 5–16.

Martins, T.B., Pasi, B.M., Pickering, J.W., Jaskowski, T.D., Litwin, C.M. and Hill, H.R. (2002). Determination of cytokine responses using a multiplexed fluorescent microsphere immunoassay. Am J Clin Pathol 118, 346–353.

McHugh, T.M., Stites, D.P., Busch, M.P., Krowka, J.F., Stricker, R.B. and Hollander, H. (1988). Relation of circulating levels of human immunodeficiency virus (HIV) antigen, antibody to p24, and HIV-containing immune complexes in HIV-infected patients. J Infect Dis 158, 1088–1091.

McHugh, T.M., Stites, D.P., Casavant, C.H. and Fulwyler, M.J. (1986). Flow cytometric detection and quantitation of immune complexes using human C1q-coated microspheres. J Immunol Methods 95, 57–61.

McHugh, T.M., Viele, M.K., Chase, E.S. and Recktenwald, D.J. (1997). The sensitive detection and quantitation of antibody to HCV by using a microsphere-based immunoassay and flow cytometry. Cytometry 29, 106–112.

Mehrpouyan, M., Bishop, J.E., Ostrerova, N., Van Cleve, M. and Lohman, K.L. (1997). A rapid and sensitive method for non-isotopic quantitation of HIV-1 RNA using thermophilic SDA and flow cytometry. Mol Cell Probes 11, 337–347.

Millan, J.L., Nustad, K. and Norgaard-Pedersen, B. (1985). Highly sensitive solid-phase immunoenzymometric assay for placental and placental-like alkaline phosphatases with a monoclonal antibody and monodisperse polymer particles. Clin Chem *31*, 54–59.

Miller, A.H. (2003). Cytokines and sickness behavior: implications for cancer care and control. Brain Behav Immun *17* Suppl 1, S132–134.

Moses, L.A., Stroncek, D.F., Cipolone, K.M. and Marincola, F.M. (2000). Detection of HLA antibodies by using flow cytometry and latex beads coated with HLA antigens. Transfusion *40*, 861–866.

Mosmann, T.R. and Fong, T.A. (1989). Specific assays for cytokine production by T cells. J Immunol Methods *116*, 151–158.

Muller, L., Kiessling, R., Rees, R.C. and Pawelec, G. (2002). Escape mechanisms in tumor immunity: an update. J Environ Pathol Toxicol Oncol *21*, 277–330.

Muller, L. and Pawelec, G. (2003). Cytokines and antitumor immunity. Technol Cancer Res Treat *2*, 183–194.

Negus, R.P. and Balkwill, F.R. (1996). Cytokines in tumour growth, migration and metastasis. World J Urol *14*, 157–165.

Negus, R.P., Stamp, G.W., Relf, M.G. et al. (1995). The detection and localization of monocyte chemoattractant protein-1 (MCP-1) in human ovarian cancer. J Clin Invest *95*, 2391–2396.

Negus, R.P., Turner, L., Burke, F. and Balkwill, F.R. (1998). Hypoxia down-regulates MCP-1 expression: implications for macrophage distribution in tumors. J Leukoc Biol *63*, 758–765.

Normanno, N., Bianco, C., De Luca, A. and Salomon, D.S. (2001). The role of EGF-related peptides in tumor growth. Front Biosci *6*, D685–707.

Obringer, A.R., Rote, N.S. and Walter, A. (1995). Antiphospholipid antibody binding to bilayer-coated glass microspheres. J Immunol Methods *185*, 81–93.

Oliver, K.G., Kettman, J.R. and Fulton, R.J. (1998). Multiplexed analysis of human cytokines by use of the FlowMetrix system. Clin Chem *44*, 2057–2060.

Opdenakker, G. and Van Damme, J. (2002). Chemokines and proteinases in autoimmune diseases and cancer. Verh K Acad Geneeskd Belg *64*, 105–136.

Park, M.K., Briles, D.E. and Nahm, M.H. (2000). A latex bead-based flow cytometric immunoassay capable of simultaneous typing of multiple pneumococcal serotypes (Multibead assay). Clin Diagn Lab Immunol *7*, 486–489.

Penson, R.T., Kronish, K., Duan, Z. et al. (2000). Cytokines IL-1beta, IL-2, IL-6, IL-8, MCP-1, GM-CSF and TNFalpha in patients with epithelial ovarian cancer and their relationship to treatment with paclitaxel. Int J Gynecol Cancer *10*, 33–41.

Pickering, J.W., Martins, T.B., Schroder, M.C. and Hill, H.R. (2002). Comparison of a multiplex flow cytometric assay with enzyme-linked immunosorbent assay for auantitation of antibodies to tetanus, diphtheria, and Haemophilus influenzae Type b. Clin Diagn Lab Immunol *9*, 872–876.

Pisa, P., Halapi, E., Pisa, E.K. et al. (1992). Selective expression of interleukin 10, interferon gamma, and granulocyte-macrophage colony-stimulating factor in ovarian cancer biopsies. Proc Natl Acad Sci USA *89*, 7708–7712.

Powers, C.J., McLeskey, S.W. and Wellstein, A. (2000). Fibroblast growth factors, their receptors and signaling. Endocr Relat Cancer *7*, 165–197.

Presani, G., Perticarari, S. and Mangiarotti, M.A. (1989). Flow cytometric detection of anti-gliadin antibodies. J Immunol Methods *119*, 197–202.

Renner, E.D. (1994). Development and clinical evaluation of an amplified flow cytometric fluoroimmunoassay for Clostridium difficile toxin A. Cytometry *18*, 103–108.

Ripley, D., Tang, X.M., Ma, C. and Chegini, N. (2001). The expression and action of granulocyte macrophage-colony stimulating factor and its interaction with TGF-beta in endometrial carcinoma. Gynecol Oncol *81*, 301–309.

Rubin, H. (2003). Cancer cachexia: its correlations and causes. Proc Natl Acad Sci USA *100*, 5384–539.

Salcedo, R. and Oppenheim, J.J. (2003). Role of chemokines in angiogenesis: CXCL12/SDF-1 and CXCR4 interaction, a key regulator of endothelial cell responses. Microcirculation *10*, 359–370.

Savarese, T.M., Mitchell, K., McQuain, C et al. (2001). Coexpression of granulocyte colony stimulating factor and its receptor in primary ovarian carcinomas. Cancer Lett *162*, 105–115.

Schneider, G.P., Salcedo, R., Welniak, L.A., Howard, O.M. and Murphy, W.J. (2001). The diverse role of chemokines in tumor progression: prospects for intervention (Review). Int J Mol Med *8*, 235–244.

Schwartz, B.M., Hong, G., Morrison, B.H. et al. (2001). Lysophospholipids increase interleukin-8 expression in ovarian cancer cells. Gynecol Oncol *81*, 291–300.

Scotton, C., Milliken, D., Wilson, J., Raju, S. and Balkwill, F. (2001). Analysis of CC chemokine and chemokine receptor expression in solid ovarian tumours. Br J Cancer *85*, 891–897.

Smith, P.L., WalkerPeach, C.R., Fulton, R.J. and DuBois, D.B. (1998). A rapid, sensitive, multiplexed assay for detection of viral nucleic acids using the FlowMetrix system. Clin Chem *44*, 2054–2056.

Syrjala, M.T., Tolo, H., Koistinen, J. and Krusius, T. (1991). Determination of anti-IgA antibodies with a flow cytometer-based microbead immunoassay (MIA). J Immunol Methods *139*, 265–270.

Takeyama, H., Wakamiya, N., O'Hara, C. et al. (1991). Tumor necrosis factor expression by human ovarian carcinoma in vivo. Cancer Res *51*, 4476–4480.

Tartour, E. and Fridman, W.H. (1998). Cytokines and cancer. Int Rev Immunol *16*, 683–704.

Tilg, H., Wilmer, A., Vogel, W. et al. (1992). Serum levels of cytokines in chronic liver diseases. Gastroenterology *103*, 264–274.

Tracey, K.J. and Cerami, A. (1993). Tumor necrosis factor, other cytokines and disease. Annu Rev Cell Biol *9*, 317–343.

Van Cleve, M., Ostrerova, N., Tietgen, K. et al. (1998). Direct quantitation of HIV by flow cytometry using branched DNA signal amplification. Mol Cell Probes *12*, 243–247.

Vignali, D.A. (2000). Multiplexed particle-based flow cytometric assays. J Immunol Methods *243*, 243–255.

Voest, E.E., Kenyon, B.M., O'Reilly, M.S., Truitt, G., D'Amato, R.J. and Folkman, J. (1995). Inhibition of angiogenesis in vivo by interleukin 12 (see comments). J Natl Cancer Inst *87*, 581–586.

Volpert, O.V., Fong, T., Koch, A.E. et al. (1998). Inhibition of angiogenesis by interleukin 4. J Exp Med *188*, 1039–1046.

Wilson, M.R. and Wotherspoon, J.S. (1988). A new microsphere-based immunofluorescence assay using flow cytometry. J Immunol Methods *107*, 225–230.

Wu, J., Payson, R.A., Lang, J.C. and Chiu, I.M. (1997). Activation of fibroblast growth factor 8 gene expression in human embryonal carcinoma cells. J Steroid Biochem Mol Biol *62*, 1–10.

Wu, S., Meeker, W.A., Wiener, J.R., Berchuck, A., Bast, R.C., Jr and Boyer, C.M. (1994). Transfection of ovarian cancer cells with tumor necrosis factor-alpha (TNF-alpha) antisense mRNA abolishes the proliferative response to interleukin-1 (IL-1) but not TNF-alpha. Gynecol Oncol 53, 59–63.

Xu, L. and Fidler, I.J. (2000). Interleukin 8: an autocrine growth factor for human ovarian cancer. Oncol Res 12, 97–106.

Zwick, E., Bange, J. and Ullrich, A. (2001). Receptor tyrosine kinase signalling as a target for cancer intervention strategies. Endocr Relat Cancer 8, 161–173.

Section III

Cellular enumeration and phenotyping

Handling and Storage of Cells and Sera: Practical Considerations

Chapter
19

Stephen E. Winikoff, Herbert J. Zeh, Richard DeMarco
and Michael T. Lotze
University of Pittsburgh School of Medicine, Pittsburgh, PA, USA

Get your facts first, and then you can distort them as much
as you please.

Mark Twain

INTRODUCTION

An essential component to many ongoing research
projects is the availability of high quality, appropriately
selected tissue and biological materials. With the explosion of technology development and research interest in
the fields of genomics and proteomics, in addition to
the ongoing advances in immunologic research and
immunotherapy, the importance of appropriately collected and annotated tissue specimens has heightened.
The specimens serve as the starting point for many
types of clinical research and the coordination, collection, handling, storage, transport and retrieval of specimens is a prerequisite for the acquisition of high-quality
data. The procedures and protocols should be validated
and standardized and tailored to the specific nature of
the investigations for which they will be used.

EARLY IDENTIFICATION OF POTENTIAL BIOMARKERS AND CONDITIONS FOR STORAGE

Whenever feasible, the potential biomarkers of interest
should be identified prior to data collection so that
protocols can be appropriately designed and assays can
be validated. A variety of factors may affect the sample
quality and preliminary pilot tests to assess the optimal
collection conditions as well as factors affecting the stability of a particular biomarker should be performed.
These tests should ideally be carried out prior to sample
collection. In a study of the ovarian cancer biomarker,
OVXI, for example, a number of factors were found to
affect the levels of the biomarker, including immediate
separation of the serum, the temperature and length of
storage prior to processing and the transit time of shipping. The authors concluded that for their analysis, samples should be collected in plain EDTA tubes and not in
heparin-containing tubes and that serum should be separated immediately or stored at 4°C (Hogdall et al., 1999).
The relationship between various types of systems biology
gene expression, protein expression and cellular phenotypes is an important aspect of modern immunobiology
(Heath et al., 2003; Pennisi, 2003; Levesque and Benfey,
2004; McDonald et al., 2004; You, 2004). Appropriate
collection and analysis of clinical tissues for such cellular
molecular profiling is dictated by the manner of specimen
handling. Developing 'best practice' methods of tissue
fixation and embedding (Gillespie et al., 2001), serum and
cellular storage, labeling and annotation are important if
the data can be made rapidly available to clinicians and
the research community. Protocols and discussion regarding some of these issues from the perspective of the
National Cancer Institute (NCI) are available on the website, http://cgap-mf.nih.gov.

Measuring Immunity, edited by Michael T. Lotze and Angus W. Thomson
ISBN 0-12-455900-X, London

CONFIDENTIALITY AND OWNERSHIP ISSUES

Public concern about the ethical use of biological samples has led to strict guidelines concerning the acquisition of informed consent for the usage of these materials as well as the protection of confidentiality of the study participants. Study scientists must inform participants not only of any immediate potential risks involved in the study, but also of the current, future and, sometimes, unforeseen uses of the samples. They must understand that the samples may be collected and stored for future use. Written consent should be obtained prior to collection, with the document including a description of the kind of samples to be collected, the means of sample collection and the short- and long-term intended use of the samples. The document should discuss issues of confidentiality and whether communication of interim findings of subsequent studies will be conveyed to subjects (OHSR Information Sheet). More information is available at the following website: http://ohsr.od.nih.gov.

Clear communication is necessary between scientists, staff and study subjects. When possible, collection of blood should be concurrent with phlebotomy or insertion of lines required for clinical evaluation or procedures to minimize inconvenience or discomfort to the study subject. Instructions to staff, including the timing of collection, volumes required and collection containers should be clearly delineated and reinforced by written protocols and frequent communication. The staff of the processing laboratory, especially when in a separate location from that of the sample collection, needs to be aware of the protocol for handling the specimens, in order to avoid unsuccessful delivery attempts, prolonged transport or damage to the tissue.

STABILITY OF BIOLOGICAL SAMPLES

Several factors affect the stability of biological samples (Oldham et al., 1976; Riisbro et al., 2001; Ellis et al., 2004; Perez-Pujol et al., 2004). For blood collection, specific anticoagulants may be required for individual analytical purposes. Citrate-stabilized blood may offer better quality of RNA and DNA and produces a higher yield of lymphocytes for culture. Heparin-stabilized blood, on the other hand, affects T cell proliferation. In addition, heparin has been found to bind to many proteins. EDTA is appropriate for DNA-based assays, but may pose problems for cytogenetic analysis. Collection of whole blood in any type of anticoagulant-containing tubes may induce cytokine production *in vitro*. Many potential biomarkers are labile and the stability of a particular biomarker ought to be explored prior to large-scale collection.

The time interval prior to processing of biological samples may affect their stability. For example, cell viability may decrease with time. For many biomarkers as well, the time between collection and processing affects the stability.

For cytokine analysis, cells should be separated from serum immediately after blood collection, because delays will affect results (Blatt et al., 1965; Kerkay et al., 1977). If the physical distance between collection and processing results in transportation delays, unstable biomarkers should be excluded from analysis.

TEMPERATURE OF STORAGE: PREVENTION OF DEGRADATION

Temperature may affect sample stability during sample collection and processing as well as during storage (Cao et al., 2003; Celluzzi and Welbon, 2003; Dikicioglu et al., 2003; Greco et al., 2003; Itoh et al., 2003; Nederhand et al., 2003; Raabe et al., 2003; Thach et al., 2003; Rentas et al., 2004). The sample is ideally separated into different components and stored at the appropriate temperature. DNA may be stored at 4°C for several weeks, at −20°C for several months and at −80°C for several years. Isolated RNA must be stored at −80°C. Live cells are stable at room temperature for up to 48 h, but must be cultured or cryopreserved in liquid nitrogen at −150°C in order to remain alive. Serum and plasma require temperatures of −80°C to preserve a large number of soluble components. Immunoglobulins in plasma, on the other hand, are stable at room temperature for several days. Many immunologic studies can benefit from the storage of viable cells for future use. Whole blood may be cryopreserved in 10 per cent DMSO. Typically, cells are separated prior to storage and cryopreserved in FBS/DMSO for future use. Lymphocytes can be isolated from whole blood by density centrifugation through gradients such as Ficoll. While separation can be performed with a simple centrifugation step, Ficoll isolation is more complete and allows separation of lymphocytes from granulocytes. Cells may be stored in the vapor phase of liquid nitrogen (−150°C) or the liquid phase (−196°C). Vials stored in the liquid phase may be subject to damage, however, so storage in the vapor phase has become common. Cryopreservation may affect quality of cells, so pilot studies should be performed to determine the extent of cell loss or cell characteristics after freezing. Loss of cell viability has been observed when cells are warmed to −132°C or higher, a situation which occurs each time a rack of boxes is taken out for removal or addition of sample (Lopaczynski et al., 2001).

Samples obtained from surgical specimens can be banked under the supervision of surgical pathologists. The sampling and freezing of the tissue may occur during evaluation of the fresh specimen immediately after receipt in the pathology laboratory. For protein or nucleic acid extraction, viable tissue should be handled with instruments that have not touched other tissue. Uniform containers can facilitate storage and tissue specimens may be stored in screw-cap cryogenic 2 ml vials. The tissue should be placed in a cryogenic vial and held in liquid nitrogen for at least 1 min. The vial should be transported thereafter on dry ice or held temporarily in a −70°C freezer until transfer to a liquid nitrogen freezer for storage. For histologic staining, the tissue is placed in OCT in a cryogenic vial and the vial is similarly immersed in liquid nitrogen. When needed for sectioning, the frozen OCT block can be removed by warming the vial briefly and inverting and tapping the vial. After use, the exposed tissue surface should be covered with a layer of OCT and the block returned to the vial for storage.

Frozen tissues may be held at −70°C for up to 1 week prior to transfer to the liquid nitrogen freezer, where they are stored permanently in the vapor phase (−140−−150°C).

Protection from enzymatic degradation (Bode and Norris, 1992; Noonan et al., 1996; Martin-Valmaseda et al., 1997; Tencer et al., 1997; Roberts et al., 1998; Lakey et al., 2001; Stroh et al., 2002; Waheed and Van Etten, 2002) may be accomplished by the addition of protease inhibitors or RNAase inhibitors. Protease inhibitors are toxic to live cells and must not be added to whole blood if cells are to be protected. DNA, on the other hand, is stable at 37°C for several days.

UNIVERSAL PRECAUTIONS

Universal precautions must be strictly followed at all stages of work with human tissues. All human tissues are considered to be potentially infectious and tests of pathogenicity are generally not done prior to study use. Personnel must be adequately trained to protect themselves and others. Safety regulations and guidelines are available through OSHA (http://www.osha.gov), the NIH (http://www.niehs.nih.gov/odhsb/manual/home.htm) or safety offices established at most large research institutions.

Specific regulations are in place regarding the transport of potentially infectious or hazardous materials. Study participants involved in the shipping of biological materials are required to receive specific training concerning these regulations and training should be repeated every 2 years.

REGULATIONS CONCERN PACKAGING AND LABELING OF GOODS

Training is available through most large research institutions and through Saf-T-Pak (http://www.saftpak.com). The effect of irradiation on biological specimens should be considered, as security measures may involve the irradiation of mail packages.

INVENTORY AND TRACKING SYSTEMS

The importance of a tracking system for tissue specimens cannot be overemphasized. This includes details such as collection date, sample number, volumes and types of samples. The system should track locations and specific

Table 19.1 Factors important for procurement and storage of specimens

Informed consent
Record keeping
  Sample labels
  Custody of samples
  Laboratory log
  Database
  Resolution of problems
Sample integrity
  Identification of analytes
  Protocol development
  Procurement
  Storage conditions
    Temperature during transport and storage
    Preservation conditions (sterility, solutions, inhibitors of degradation)
  Pilot analysis
Education and training
  Communication to participants
  Universal precautions
  Shipping and transport protocols
Quality control and oversight

usage of specimens. Personal information must be encoded in compliance with privacy protection regulations. Electronic database systems, particularly those that use barcodes, are increasingly employed. The CDC, for example, has a capacity of 6 million banked specimens. A sophisticated physical and electronic structure is necessary to support such large repositories. Commercially available software programs can handle smaller numbers of samples (http://www.freezerworks.com/).

The spectrum of technological applications employing biological specimens ranges from substance detection to immunological methods (ELISA, flow cytometry, to advanced genetic analysis or microarray technologies). Large institutions have therefore developed laboratory core facilities responsible for large research programs and epidemiological projects. Responsibilities of these core facilities include development of sample collection, processing protocols and quality assurance procedures, as well as coordination of sample handling, processing and banking.

The validity of the development of new biomarkers, proteomic and genomic analyses, depends on adherence to strict standards and guidelines. These standards begin with ensuring the stability of the sample, analyte, or antigen during collection, processing, storage and analysis. Collection and processing must be standardized and carefully monitored for quality control. Only in this way will clinical investigations be successfully undertaken with reliable and reproducible results.

REFERENCES

Blatt, W.F., Kerkay, J. and Mager, M. (1965). Effect of serum handling on electrophoretic patterns: paper strip and moving boundary analysis. Am J Med Technol 31, 349–354.

Bode, A.P. and Norris, H.T. (1992). The use of inhibitors of platelet activation or protease activity in platelet concentrates stored for transfusion. Blood Cells *18*, 361–380; discussion 381–382.

Cao, E., Chen, Y., Cui, Z. and Foster, P.R. (2003). Effect of freezing and thawing rates on denaturation of proteins in aqueous solutions. Biotechnol Bioeng *82*, 684–690.

Celluzzi, C.M. and Welbon, C. (2003). A simple cryopreservation method for dendritic cells and cells used in their derivation and functional assessment. Transfusion *43*, 488–494.

Chan, B.Y., Buckley, K.A., Durham, B.H., Gallagher, J.A. and Fraser, W.D. (2003). Effect of anticoagulants and storage temperature on the stability of receptor activator for nuclear factor-kappa B ligand and osteoprotegerin in plasma and serum. Clin Chem *49*, 2083–2085.

Dikicioglu, E., Meteoglu, I., Okyay, P., Culhaci, N. and Kacar, F. (2003). The reliability of long-term storage of direct immunofluorescent staining slides at room temperature. J Cutan Pathol *30*, 430–436.

Ellis, V., Charlett, A. and Bendall, R. (2004). A comparison of IgG anti-rubella activity in frozen serum stored in primary gel separation tubes or secondary tubes. J Clin Pathol *57*, 104–106.

Gillespie, J.W., Ahram, M., Best, C.J. et al. (2001). The role of tissue microdissection in cancer research. Cancer J *7*, 32–39.

Greco, N.J., Lee, W.R. and Moroff, G. (2003). Increased transmigration of G-CSF-mobilized peripheral blood CD34+ cells after overnight storage at 37 degrees C. Transfusion *43*, 1575–1586.

Heath, J.R., Phelps, M.E. and Hood, L. (2003). NanoSystems biology. Mol Imaging Biol *5*, 312–325.

Hogdall, E.V., Hogdall, C.K., Kjaer, S.K. et al. (1999). OVX1 radioimmunoassay results are dependent on the method of sample collection and storage. Clin Chem *45*, 692–694.

Itoh, T., Minegishi, M., Fushimi, J. et al. (2003). A simple controlled-rate freezing method without a rate-controlled programmed freezer provides optimal conditions for both large-scale and small-scale cryopreservation of umbilical cord blood cells. Transfusion *43*, 1303–1308.

Kerkay, J., Coburn, C.M. and McEvoy, D. (1977). Effect of sodium ascorbate concentration on the stability of samples for determination of serum folate levels. Am J Clin Pathol *68*, 481–484.

Lakey, J.R., Helms, L.M., Kin, T. et al. (2001). Serine-protease inhibition during islet isolation increases islet yield from human pancreases with prolonged ischemia. Transplantation *72*, 565–570.

Levesque, M.P. and Benfey, P.N. (2004). Systems biology. Curr Biol *14*, R179–180.

Lopaczynski, W., Hruszkewycz, A.M. and Lieberman, R. (2001). Preprostatectomy: A clinical model to study stromal-epithelial interactions. Urology *57*, 194–199.

Martin-Valmaseda, E.M., Sanchez-Yague, J., Marcos, R. and Llanillo, M. (1997). Decrease in platelet, erythrocyte and lymphocyte acetylcholinesterase activities due to the presence of protease inhibitors in the storage buffer. Biochem Mol Biol Int *41*, 83–91.

McDonald, D.M., Teicher, B.A., Stetler-Stevenson, W. et al. (2004). Report from the society for biological therapy and vascular biology faculty of the NCI workshop on angiogenesis monitoring. J Immunother *27*,161–175.

Nederhand, R.J., Droog, S., Kluft, C., Simoons, M.L. and de Maat, M.P. (2003). Logistics and quality control for DNA sampling in large multicenter studies. J Thromb Haemost *1*, 987–991.

Noonan, K., Kalu, M.E., Holownia, P. and Burrin, J.M. (1996). Effect of different storage temperatures, sample collection procedures and immunoassay methods on osteocalcin measurement. Eur J Clin Chem Clin Biochem *34*, 841–844.

Oldham, R.K., Dean, J.H., Cannon, G.B. et al. (1976). Cryopreservation of human lymphocyte function as measured by in vitro assays. Int J Cancer *18*, 45–55.

Pennisi, E. (2003).Systems biology. Tracing life's circuitry. Science *302*, 1646–1649.

Perez-Pujol, S., Lozano, M., Perea, D., Mazzara, R., Ordinas, A. and Escolar, G. (2004). Effect of holding buffy coats 4 or 18 hours before preparing pooled filtered PLT concentrates in plasma. Transfusion *44*, 202–209.

Raabe, A., Kopetsch, O., Gross, U., Zimmermann, M. and Gebhart, P. (2003). Measurements of serum S-100B protein: effects of storage time and temperature on pre-analytical stability. Clin Chem Lab Med *41*, 700–703.

Rentas, F.J., Macdonald, V.W., Houchens, D.M., Hmel, P.J. and Reid, T.J. (2004). New insulation technology provides next-generation containers for 'iceless' and lightweight transport of RBCs at 1 to 10 degrees C in extreme temperatures for over 78 hours. Transfusion *44*, 210–216.

Riisbro, R., Christensen, I.J., Hogdall, C., Brunner, N. and Hogdall, E. (2001). Soluble urokinase plasminogen activator receptor measurements: influence of sample handling. Int J Biol Markers *16*, 233–239.

Roberts, R.F., Nishanian, G.P., Carey, J.N. et al. (1998). Addition of aprotinin to organ preservation solutions decreases lung reperfusion injury. Ann Thorac Surg *66*, 225–230.

Stroh, C., Cassens, U., Samraj, A.K., Sibrowski, W., Schulze-Osthoff, K. and Los, M. (2002). The role of caspases in cryo-injury: caspase inhibition strongly improves the recovery of cryopreserved hematopoietic and other cells. Faseb J *16*, 1651–1653.

Tencer, J., Thysell, H., Andersson, K. and Grubb, A. (1997).Long-term stability of albumin, protein HC, immunoglobulin G, kappa- and lambda-chain-immunoreactivity, orosomucoid and alpha 1-antitrypsin in urine stored at −20 degrees C. Scand J Urol Nephrol *31*, 67–71.

Thach, D.C., Lin, B., Walter, E. et al. (2003). Assessment of two methods for handling blood in collection tubes with RNA stabilizing agent for surveillance of gene expression profiles with high density microarrays. J Immunol Methods *283*, 269–279.

Waheed, A. and Van Etten, R.L. (2002). Protection of prostatic acid phosphatase activity in human serum samples by plasmin inhibitors. Clin Chim Acta *320*, 127–131.

You, L. (2004). Toward computational systems biology. Cell Biochem Biophys *40*, 167–184.

Phenotypic and Functional Measurements on Circulating Immune Cells and their Subsets

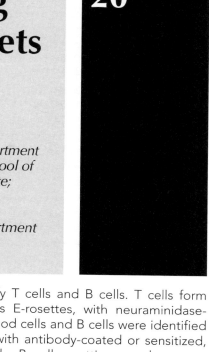

Chapter 20

Albert D. Donnenberg[1] and Vera S. Donnenberg[2]

[1]*Departments of Medicine, University of Pittsburgh School of Medicine; Department of Infectious Disease and Microbiology, University of Pittsburgh Graduate School of Public Health; Flow Cytometry Facility, University of Pittsburgh Cancer Institute; Hematopoietic Stem Cell Laboratory, University of Pittsburgh Medical Center, Pittsburgh, PA, USA*
[2]*Department of Surgery, University of Pittsburgh School of Medicine; Department of Pharmaceutical Sciences, University of Pittsburgh School of Pharmacy, Pittsburgh, PA, USA*

... Whatever you think
It's more than that, more than that ...

Robin Williamson, *Job's Tears*, 1967

INTRODUCTION

Current flow cytometry as applied to the detection of biomarkers is defined by several attributes: application of quality control measures, use of multiple-color measurements, use of the quantitative capacities of flow cytometry (inferring number of molecules from fluorescence, measuring the absolute number of events of interest) and most importantly, measuring function on defined subpopulations of cells within a heterogeneous mixture. The purpose of this chapter is to trace the development of these advances and provide examples and, hopefully, practical suggestions for their implementation in basic and translational research.

IMMUNE BIOMARKERS BEFORE FLOW CYTOMETRY

By the early 1970s it was well appreciated that the morphologically homogeneous peripheral blood lymphocytes could be divided into several subpopulations on the basis of differing surface structures that serve as population markers (Winchester and Ross, 1976). In mice, lymphocyte subpopulations were divided into functionally distinct subsets by alloantisera. In humans, rosetting techniques were used to quantify T cells and B cells. T cells form complexes, known as E-rosettes, with neuraminidase-treated sheep red blood cells and B cells were identified by forming rosettes with antibody-coated or sensitized, sheep red blood cells. B cell rosetting was known to occur because of the presence of Fc receptors on B cells. Although the mechanism for T cell rosetting was obscure at the time that this assay was developed, it is now appreciated that they form because red cells bind avidly to CD2, a signaling molecule that induces costimulation when bound to its natural ligand, the adhesion molecule CD58 (LFA-1) on antigen presenting cells (Arulanandam et al., 1994). Although rosette assays were technically challenging, they became widely adopted by clinical immunology laboratories and were used for diagnosis of lymphoid malignancies, congenital immune deficiency states and studies on the pathogenesis of autoimmunity. An early but classic example of immune monitoring is the study of Noel et al., in which the kinetics of peripheral T and B cell reconstitution was followed in allogeneic bone marrow transplant patients with and without acute graft versus host disease (Noel et al., 1978). The data and normal ranges are still valid today.

FLOW CYTOMETRY AND THE FIRST MONOCLONAL ANTIBODIES

Characterization of lymphocyte subsets was one of the earliest applications of flow cytometry. In the mid-1970s the Herzenberg laboratory combined standard immunofluorescence staining techniques with their newly developed single color 2-parameter fluorescence activated cell sorter and identified and separated murine B cells (Loken and Herzenberg, 1975) and T cells (Cantor et al., 1975). These studies used polyclonal alloantisera, which were well developed in the murine system because of strain-specific polymorphisms. The description of two-color analysis by the same group followed, using fluorescein and rhodamine tagged polyclonal antibodies (Loken et al., 1977). Despite the rapid progress of flow cytometry, its application to human immunology and medicine appeared to be at an impasse. Unlike the murine and rat systems, where strain specific genetic differences could be exploited, surface molecule specific anti-human antisera were difficult to produce. As late as 1984, Kamentsky, a pioneer of analytical cytology, lamented, 'Although there are now flow cytometers in clinical laboratories, their applications remain limited by a lack of specific markers' (Kamentsky, 2003). The creation of monoclonal antibodies by Milstein and colleagues in 1977 (Pearson et al., 1977) gradually changed the field of flow cytometry, providing an inexhaustible supply of reagents of exquisite specificity. Within a year after Milstein's invention, monoclonal antibody specific for rat (White et al., 1978) and murine (Trowbridge, 1978) helper T cells and murine MHC antigens (Hammerling et al., 1978) were described. Shortly thereafter, the description of three murine monoclonal antibodies specific for human T cell surface determinants, designated OKT1, OKT3 and OKT4 (Kung et al., 1979) paved the way for human studies. Today these hybridomas are recognized as producing antibodies against the CD5, CD3 and CD4 determinants, respectively. In 1982 the first Human Leukocyte Differentiation Antigen (HLDA) Workshop was held in Paris, France and the principle of classifying monoclonal antibodies by clusters of differentiation (CDs) was formulated and a total of 15 CDs were defined. To date, 247 CDs have been identified. The eighth HLDA workshop, initiated in 2000 and scheduled for completion in 2004, is an international effort involving several hundred laboratories.

BENCHTOP ANALYTICAL FLOW CYTOMETERS

Advances in instrumentation also played a large role in bringing flow cytometry into routine use in clinical and less specialized research laboratories. The first flow cytometers were designed as cell sorters, with data analysis being a secondary consideration. On some models, data were recorded by taking Polaroid photographs of events plotted on an oscilloscope screen. By the late 1970s small, expensive computers produced by Tektronix, Hewlett-Packard and Digital Equipment Corporation permitted rudimentary computer-assisted data analysis. In these early days, internal random access memory was often limited to 64 kb and low capacity magnetic tapes and giant 256 kb 8-inch floppy disks were the only devices available

for data storage. By 1984, desktop computers and data storage on hard-drives had advanced to the stage that a Flow Cytometry Standard (FCS) for data storage was proposed (Murphy and Chused, 1984), allowing offline reanalysis of 'listmode' data for the first time. At about the same time, affordable benchtop cytometers became available. These instruments had air-cooled argon lasers and fixed optics, eliminating water cooling systems, special power requirements and daily optical alignment. Analytical software also progressed rapidly and analytical tools geared toward offline data exploration, such as Becton-Dickinson's revolutionary Paint-A-Gate (capable of *color-eventing*, which will be discussed later) and Verity's WinList and ModFit became available. In the mid-1990s, Coulter introduced the Elite XL 4-color analytical cytometer with digital electronics. After analog pulse-processing, signals were digitized at high-resolution, eliminating non-linear log amplifiers and paving the way for correct multi-color compensation. The newest generation of Beckman-Coulter, Becton-Dickinson and Dako-Cytomation cytometers all have provisions for listmode storage of uncompensated high-resolution data, extending to offline analysis the ability to recalculate color compensation.

THE HIV EPIDEMIC AND THE RISE OF FLOW CYTOMETRY IN CLINICAL IMMUNOLOGY

The history of the CD4 T-cell assay and its role in the fight against AIDS has been ably recounted by Mandy (Mandy et al., 2002). The finding that CD4 loss was associated with immunodeficiency in this newly described syndrome (Reinherz et al., 1981) led to the adoption of CD4 count as a biomarker of disease progression, standardization of CD4 analysis (Centers for Disease Control, 1992) and, most recently, the development of a bead-calibrated single-platform absolute count assay (Mandy et al., 2003) (discussed below). In the early days of AIDS clinical trials, the AIDS Clinical Trial Group (ACTG) and the National Institutes of Allergy and Infectious Disease Division of AIDS confronted the need for inter-laboratory standardization, ultimately developing protocols incorporating sample send-outs and other measures of quality assessment now widely accepted by the flow community (Paxton et al., 1989; Gelman et al., 1993; Bergeron et al., 1998).

The multi-center AIDS cohort study (MACS), a prospective study of almost 5000 gay men, proved to be an early triumph of standardization (Giorgi et al., 1998). The study, launched in 1984, followed the entire MACS cohort on a twice-yearly basis collecting clinical data, biological specimens and, of course, measuring CD4+ T cells. When inconsistencies were noted in the results from the first two visits, MACS investigators recognized the need for standardization and greatly improved assay agreement across centers during subsequent visits. An important aspect of the MACS study is that gay men were recruited without prior knowledge of their HIV status. More than 600 MACS participants converted from HIV negative to HIV positive while on study, allowing the precise relationship between CD4 count and HIV infection to be defined (Margolick et al., 1993). Follow-up studies demonstrated that total T cell numbers (CD4 plus CD8) are conserved until the onset of clinical AIDS, providing evidence for the homeostatic regulation of T cell generation (Margolick et al., 1995; Margolick and Donnenberg, 1997). Another early MACS innovation was the discovery that assessing activation markers in combination with T cell subset markers could yield additional prognostic information (Giorgi et al., 1993). The MACS, which is still active 20 years since its inception, still relies heavily on flow cytometry for its studies on the immunologic monitoring of HIV+ cohort members who are now on anti-retroviral therapy. In retrospect, the HIV epidemic was a major driving force for the transition of flow cytometers from temperamental research instruments into ubiquitous clinical tools.

CONTEMPORARY FLOW CYTOMETRY

Quality control

Perhaps the least glamorous, but most important aspect of modern flow cytometry is the emphasis on quality control (QC). Like those pesky experimental controls, essential quality control measures are necessary for the valid interpretation of flow cytometric data. The instrument-related elements of a quality control program are shown in Table 20.1. The College of American Pathologists (CAP), which administers a quality assurance program for clinical flow cytometry laboratories, states that quality assurance measures must cover specimen and result integrity throughout pre-analytical, analytical and post-analytical processes (D'hautcourt, 1996; Gratama et al., 1999). CAP provides a helpful checklist covering the areas that must be addressed by a quality assurance program. As a part of their accreditation process, laboratories also participate in surveys conducted twice or three times per year, in which blood samples are aliquoted and sent by express mail to participating laboratories. The results are tabulated and compared to the results of other laboratories using similar instrumentation and methods.

Although the level of quality control required in clinical laboratories may be overkill in the research setting, the careful investigator would do well to review the CAP checklist and decide which standards should be adopted.

The items listed in Table 20.1 are suggested for laboratories involved in human investigation to confirm consistent operation of the cytometer and performance of the reagents. Other QC issues such as sample integrity and consistency of data analysis are beyond the scope of this discussion, but should be considered as well. The first two steps of QC, optics and PMT setting verification, are performed with standard beads such as Beckman-Coulter FlowCheck and FlowSet, respectively. Fluidics/optics verification is performed on a linear scale and the objective is to ensure that the beads give a coefficient of variation (CV, standard deviation divided by the mean) below a predetermined value. Tight CVs indicate proper laser alignment and good hydrodynamic focusing in the flow cell.

Table 20.1 Recommended elements of flow cytometry quality control

Element	Procedure	Frequency	Comments
Fluidics/optics	Check CV of all parameters with standard beads	Daily	Poor CV can result from partial obstruction, drifting optical alignment, failing laser
Electronics	Set gain for all PMTs to place standard beads in target channels	Daily	Assures day-to-day consistency in flourescence measurement. Assures that a balance between PMTs is maintained (important for compensation)
Color compensation	Stain single color control samples	Variable	Stained controls may be cells or beads and may be reagent-specific or fluorochrome-specific
Internal process/reagents	Concurrent staining of normal or preserved standard cells	Daily	For standard cells, mean per cent positive and absolute count with upper and lower limits are published by the vendor
Linearity/sensitivity	Check fluorescence intensity of multi-peak beads	Yearly. More often if quantitative fluorescence measurements are made	Beads of graded fluorescence intensity are run and the expected and observed fluorescence are compared

When a partial obstruction occurs, the most sensitive parameter is forward light scatter and this parameter will fall out of tolerance. Daily assessment of PMT gain is also important and easy to do. During the assay development phase, PMT settings (voltage and gain) will have been chosen appropriate to the test. For each fluorochrome, settings will have been chosen such that cell populations known to be negative are usually placed within the first decade and the brightest positive populations are on scale. At that time, calibration beads, such as Beckman-Coulter FlowSet would have been run and the target channel (channel of bead mean fluorescence intensity) would have been noted for each PMT. During daily calibration, the same calibration beads are run again and PMT gain is adjusted, if necessary, to place the beads at their target channel. This helps ensure that quantitative determination of fluorescence is consistent from day to day. The other ingredients necessary for quantitative fluorescence measurement are linearity of detection and calibration relative to a known standard. Linearity can be measured with multi-peak beads and antibody binding can be calibrated to molecules of equivalent soluble fluorochrome (MESF) using beads of known antibody binding capacity.

The topic of color compensation and how often and by what method it should be confirmed, is controversial. In the two-color world, where fluorescein isothiocyanate (FITC) and phycoerythrin (PE) were the only fluorochromes used, the required amount of color compensation did not vary from day to day, providing that the instrument had been calibrated as described above. Correct two-color compensation can be verified daily, weekly, or even less often, using beads dyed with the fluorochromes of interest, such as Becton-Dickinson CaliBRITE beads. The introduction of tandem dyes such as PE-Texas Red (also known as ECD), PE-Cyanine5 (PC5), PE-Cyanine7 (PC7), Allophycocyanine-Cyanine5 (APC-Cy5) and Allophycocyanine-Cyanine7 (APC-Cy7), opened up the world of polychromatic flow cytometry, but also introduced a twist to compensation. The emissions spectra of single fluorochrome dyes are always the same, regardless of the antibody to which it is conjugated, given that other relevant parameters (such as pH for FITC) are constant. This is not always the case for the tandem dyes, which can vary from manufacturer to manufacturer, lot to lot and, over time, within the same vial. Most of this variability is explained by the amount of free PE, PE that behaves as if it were not part of a tandem dye. Tandem dyes are especially light sensitive and the amount of apparent free PE can increase upon exposure to ambient light. Thus, the simple approach used for two-color cytometry, arriving at a single compensation solution to be used for all cells stained with the same fluorochromes, is not optimal in every setting. A method, advocated by some vendors, is to stain preserved or freshly isolated cells singly, with brightly staining antibodies representing each fluorochrome to be used in the multi-color combination. CD8 or CD45 are frequently used for this purpose.

However, the assumption that the compensation required for the CD8-PC7 in your single stained standard is identical to that required by the CD4-PC7 in your multicolor stained sample may not always be correct. The alterative, to stain cells singly with each antibody used in your panel, is not ideal either, since some of the markers will stain dimly and therefore will yield imprecise compensation settings. A solution advocated by some laboratories is the use of anti-Ig capture beads, which bind all murine monoclonal antibodies equally well, regardless of their specificity or fluorochrome. Such standards could be run with each assay, or even acquired after the fact to confirm that correct compensation settings were used. As mentioned above, many new cytometers have the ability to save uncompensated high-resolution listmode data (16 or 20 bits), allowing compensation to be performed or corrected after acquisition.

Identifying T cell subsets

Lymphocyte subsetting, the idea that immune cells at different stages of development or with distinct functions can be identified and quantified on the basis of expression of cell surface markers, has been one of the major applications to drive the development of current multiparameter flow cytometry. The other major application, the classification and detection of leukemias and lymphomas, is beyond the scope of this article. In Western medicine, the notion of immunologic naiveté and memory can be traced to Jennerian vaccination in the late eighteenth century and the observation that exposure to a pathogen can lead to subsequent resistance to reinfection. Although this insight has led to the eradication of smallpox and the control of polio and many other infectious diseases of major public health significance, the molecular events and changes in lymphocyte populations responsible for the phenomenon of immune memory are still incompletely understood and controversial (Ahmed and Gray, 1996). The first inkling that immune memory was mediated by lymphocytes came from Landsteiner and Chase in 1942, when they showed that transfer of delayed-type hypersensitivity (DTH) from an immune to a naive guinea pig required leukocytes. I was fortunate to hear Dr Merrill Chase, who died at the age of 98 in January of 2004, recount the tale of this discovery and it is worthy of a short digression.

Dr Chase was a young assistant working on this problem at the Rockefeller University in the laboratory of the Nobel Laureate Karl Landsteiner. Since it was well appreciated that immunity to a variety of agents could be transferred from immune to non-immune animals by passive transfer of antibodies, their goal was to identify the humoral factor responsible for DTH. Guinea pigs were immunized with guinea pig stromal cells that had been haptenated with picryl chloride. This is a powerful DTH antigen and upon intradermal challenge, immunized animals developed characteristic erythematous reactions. In an attempt to transfer this response, peritoneal exudates were induced and harvested from immune animals, clarified by centrifugation and injected into naive animals. It was the winter holiday season and the experiments thus far had been entirely negative. Rushing to get out of the laboratory, Dr Chase elected to save a few minutes by skipping the centrifugation step. The naive animals inoculated with cloudy cellular peritoneal exudate fluid responded vigorously to antigen challenge. The good news was that Dr Chase had opened a new field of enquiry. The bad news was that he had to admit to the demanding Dr Landsteiner precisely what he had done. The experiment was repeated with appropriate negative controls and the rest is history.

Decades later, the existence of memory T cells participating in B-cell mediated antibody responses (Mitchell et al., 1972) and in the generation of cytotoxic effector functions (Kedar and Bonavida, 1975) were also demonstrated in adoptive transfer models. The next advance awaited the development of several anti-human monoclonal antibodies that could be used to separate T cells into recall antigen responsive and unresponsive populations. These antibodies included 4B4 (CD29, the adhesion molecule beta-1 integrin) (Morimoto et al., 1985a), HB-11 (CD38, an ectoenzyme ADP-ribosyl cyclase) (Tedder et al., 1985), 2H4 (CD45RA, a high molecular weight isoform of the leukocyte tyrosine phosphatase) (Morimoto et al., 1985b) and UCHL1 (CD45RO, the low molecular weight isoform of the leukocyte tyrosine phosphatase) (Smith et al., 1986). The Shaw laboratory was the first to frame this problem in terms of a dichotomy between naive and memory T cells (Sanders et al., 1988), demonstrating that umbilical cord blood T cells (prototypically naive) expressed low levels of LFA-1 (CD11a/CD18, adhesion and signaling), LFA-3 (CD58, adhesion and costimulation), CD29 and UCHL1 (CD45RO) and high levels of CD45RA, compared to adult peripheral T cells. They also showed that mitogen stimulation of cord blood resulted in upregulation of CD45RO, CD58 and CD29. CD45, the leukocyte common plasma membrane-associated tyrosine phosphatase, has proved to a particularly useful marker of T cell differentiation and activation (Trowbridge and Thomas, 1994). CD45 contains three exons (A, B and C), which can be differentially spliced to produce isoforms of distinct molecular weight. Isoform switching takes place during T cell maturation and activation and multiple isoforms can be expressed in the same cell. As mentioned above, recall-antigen reactive memory T cells were found within the population expressing the lowest molecular weight isoform (CD45RO) in which all three exons have been spliced out. Naive cells, again defined by their predominance in umbilical cord blood, were found within the population retaining the A exon (CD45RA) (Sanders et al., 1988; Bradley et al., 1989). However, the advent of multiparameter cytometry revealed both phenotypic and functional heterogeneity within T cell populations, whether defined on the basis of CD45 isoform expression, or expression of any other single marker. Using four-color

cytometry, then a great novelty, Picker and colleagues integrated the findings of Shaw and definitively mapped the phenotypic changes accompanying the transition from naive to memory T cell (Picker et al., 1993). Among the many important findings in this report was that CD45RA+/CD45RO− naive cells proceed through a CD45RA+/CD45RO+ intermediate on the way to becoming CD45RA−/CD45RO+ and expressing high levels of CD58, CD11a and CD54 (ICAM-1). They also demonstrated that CD62L (L-selectin) was critically involved in T cell homing, being high in peripheral lymph nodes, even during activation, but downregulated in the tonsils and appendix during activation or in vitro after stimulation. This study also set a benchmark for the analysis of multiparameter data, making excellent use of color-eventing (demonstrated later in this chapter) to reveal the relationship of four parameters in a single bi-variate plot.

Chemokine receptor 7 (CCR7) is also important in lymphocyte trafficking. Once CD62L has allowed the lymphocyte to dock on the high endothelial venule, engagement of CCR7 with its endothelial cell ligand SLC, allows lymphocyte to transmigrate into the lymph node (Campbell et al., 2001). Sallusto et al. (1999) looked at the functional properties of CD4+ and CD8+ T cells sorted on the basis of CCR7 and CD45RA expression. Among CD4+ T cells, sort purified CD45RA−/CCR7− cells secreted the highest levels of interferon-gamma, IL-4 and IL-5 upon subsequent polyclonal stimulation. In contrast, all CD4 populations secreted IL-2. For CD8+ T cells, the double negative population and the CD45RA+/CCR7− populations were strong interferon-gamma producers, whereas CD45RA+/CCR7+/CD62L+ cells produced the highest levels of IL-2. They theorized a T cell maturational pathway in which CD45RA+/CCR7− naive T cells (capable of lymph node homing) give rise to CD45RA−/CCR7+ central memory cells (also capable of lymph node homing). These in turn give rise to CD45RA−/CCR7− effector memory cells. The CD45RA+/CCR7− population was too rare to study in CD4+ T cells, but comprised the most powerful effector population, as measured by cytokine secretion and granzyme and perforin expression among CD8+ T-cells.

Appay and colleagues (2002) used MHC-class I tetramer technology to examine the differentiation of antigen specific CD8+ T cells obtained during acute and chronic infections with Epstein Barr virus, hepatitis C virus, human immunodeficiency virus and cytomegalovirus. Defining effector cells as activated, virus specific cells found during acute infection and memory cells as resting virus specific cells found during periods of low viral load (chronic infection), they disputed the hypothesis that antigen specific CD8+ T cells transition from naive cells, to memory cells and then to effector cells. Instead, they proposed that antigen-primed T cells could be divided into three subsets according to CD28 and CD27 expression, evolving unidirectionally with time after antigen exposure from CD28/CD27 double positive, to CD28−/CD27+ and finally to CD28−/CD27−. The early cells in this continuum have greater proliferative potential and later cells greater cytotoxic potential. Depending on the specific virus, memory cells (antigen experienced resting cells) could 'accumulate' at any stage of this continuum.

Approaching the problem of T cell subsetting with the current state of the art in cytometry, DeRosa and colleagues (2001) used 11-color cytometry to define unambiguously the phenotype of naive T cells. In their example, they used a highly modified hybrid cytometer (Becton-Dickinson and Cytomation) fitted with violet, blue and red lasers, succeeding in detecting five colors off the blue laser, four colors off the red laser and two colors off the violet laser. Examining CD4+ and CD8+ T cells simultaneously, they concluded that naive T cells, defined as incapable of producing interferon-gamma, were CD45RA+/CD62L+/CD11a dim/CD27+. Minor cell populations discordant for expression of these markers secreted interferon-gamma and therefore were interpreted as being contaminating memory T cells.

PRACTICAL CONSIDERATIONS AND EXAMPLES

Rare event problems and multiparameter flow cytometry

Discriminating individual cell populations in a heterogeneous mixture always comes down to a signal to noise problem: how to separate the populations of interest from other populations in multiparameter space. Autofluorescence, non-specific antibody binding, multimodal distribution of specific antibody binding and shared antibody specificities (e.g. CD5 is present on T cells, but also a population of B cells, CD8 is present on subsets of T and NK cells), all contribute to this problem. By careful choice of antibodies and fluorochromes, populations of interest can be pulled into unique locations in multiparameter space. This is especially important for populations that are present at low frequency. The advent of polychromatic flow cytometry has given us the unprecedented ability to identify subsets on the basis of multiple parameters and perform functional measurements simultaneously in well-defined cell subsets. Such functional determinations include cytokine secretion (Brosterhus et al., 1999), T-cell receptor specificity (Altman et al., 1996), cytotoxicity (Liu et al., 2002), proliferation (Drach et al., 1989; Li et al., 1995; Nordon et al., 1997; Shapiro, 2003), apoptosis (Guedez et al., 1998), calcium flux (June et al., 1986), viability (Darzynkiewicz et al., 1982), multiple drug resistance pump activity (Donnenberg et al., 2004), mitochondrial membrane potential (Cossarizza et al., 1993), kinase activity (Perez and Nolan, 2002), telomere length (Baerlocher and Lansdorp, 2003) and many others. In this section, we will provide several practical examples from our laboratory of flow cytometry techniques, many of which exemplify the synthesis of phenotypic and functional determinations.

The challenge of rare event problems: dendritic cells in the peripheral circulation

The detection of circulating monocytoid and lymphoid dendritic cells (DC1 and DC2, respectively) requires strategies that are common to all 'rare event' problems in flow cytometry. Technical aspects of rare-event detection have been reviewed by several authors (van den Engh, 1993; Rosenblatt et al., 1997; Donnenberg and Meyer, 1999; Baumgarth and Roederer, 2000; Donnenberg et al., 2003). What follows is a practical discussion of rare event detection strategies as applied to the DC problem, which we have previously discussed in some detail (Donnenberg and Donnenberg, 2003).

Sample concentration and flow rate

Although event frequency is an intrinsic property of the sample, the proportion of events of interest can be greatly increased in the analytical window. For example, knowing that DC1 and DC2 do not express lineage markers present on most peripheral mononuclear cells, it becomes possible to increase greatly the proportion of DCs in the analysis by eliminating irrelevant or interfering cell populations. In the measurement of DC, this virtual depletion is accomplished by staining T cells, monocytes and B cells with a cocktail of lineage markers (CD3, CD14, CD19), all labeled with the same fluorochrome. Cells expressing any of these markers are logically removed from the analysis using what has been called a *dump gate* (Donnenberg et al., 2001). Through judicious use of the threshold parameter or live gating, irrelevant events can be made invisible to the cytometer or eliminated from the list-mode file (an example of the latter will be provided in Figure 20.4). However, it is the absolute frequency of the event of interest which dictates how many total cells must be processed. Obviously the lower the frequency of the events of interest, the more events it will be necessary to acquire. Although the rate of sample acquisition on the flow cytometer can be manipulated by increasing the sample flow rate, best results are obtained when the flow rate is not unduly rapid and the cell concentration of the sample is optimized for the particular instrument.

Signal to noise

Successful detection of rare events depends on maximizing the signal to noise ratio. Noise comes from many sources including the non-specific binding of a fluorochrome of interest, cellular autofluorescence, disruptions in fluidics and other electrical or mechanical problems. One very important aspect of rare event analysis is to characterize the total noise using an appropriate negative control. Sometimes, it is possible to devise a control sample that is identical to the experimental sample in all respects, except that it does not contain the rare event of interest (Barratt-Boyes et al., 2000) or, it may be necessary to use control reagents such as isotype-matched fluorochrome-conjugated antibodies (Donnenberg et al., 2001). In the latter case, a few caveats apply: in addition to being matched for isotype, the control reagent must be similar to the experimental reagent with respect to the ratio of fluorescent dye to protein and it must be used at the same concentration. Additionally, staining must be designed so that the same gating strategy used to detect the rare event can be applied to the negative control sample. Mario Roederer has termed this strategy FMO, or fluorescence minus one (Roederer, 2001), although when we have two outcome parameters (see Figure 20.7) FMT may be more appropriate. It is also important to point out that an identical number of events must be acquired for the negative control sample as for the experimental sample, because it is the frequency of false positive events that determines the lower limit of detection. For example, if the frequency of spuriously positive events is 1 in 5000 in the FMO negative control, it is impossible to use this assay to detect cells present at a frequency of 1 in 10 000, no matter how many events are acquired. It follows that there is a point of diminishing return beyond which acquiring a greater numbers of events will increase the precision of the rare event frequency estimate, but will not increase the sensitivity of the assay.

Two important factors bear on the signal to noise ratio: the difference in mean fluorescence intensity between negative and positive populations and their variances (usually expressed as the CV). Some membrane or cell-associated dyes give very bright signals and therefore place cells far from noise. When using combinations of fluorochrome-conjugated antibodies, we often reserve PE for the most critical measurement, because the absorption and emissions spectra are widely separated, and the extinction coefficient and quantum yield are high compared to other fluorochromes (Shapiro, 1995).

When autofluorescent myeloid cells, cellular debris or red blood cells interfere with rare event detection it is often possible to *move them out of the way* by targeting them with a specific antibody (e.g. CD14 for monocyte/macrophages). We have used this strategy to identify DC subsets that comprise a small proportion (1 in 10 000 to 1 in 100 000) of bronchoalveolar lavage cells (Donnenberg and Donnenberg, 2003). Cell doublets, either cells physically adherent to each other, or two or more cells erroneously detected as a single pulse, are also a source of concern for rare event detection. These can be gated from the analysis using doublet discrimination, a comparison of pulse height and pulse integral, or pulse height and pulse width (Wersto et al., 2001). An example of doublet discrimination will be given in Figure 20.4.

Another important aspect of the overall signal to noise is the number of parameters used to define the rare event of interest. Modern multi-laser, multi-PMT instruments permit detection strategies that make use of multiple parameters to define the rare event. In the case of DC1, the rare event of interest should be positively identified by more than one fluorescence parameter (CD4+, HLA-DR+ and CD11c+). Not quite so obvious is the importance of including one or more fluorescence parameters for which the rare event is negative (lineage negative, CD123 negative). In rare event detection, it is almost as important to specify where the rare event is *not*, as to specify where it is. This is especially helpful for defining a set of compound logical gates that assign the population of interest a unique location in multiparameter space. Such analyses are performed after the fact, on listmode datafiles. Compound gating strategies that maximize detection of events in the positive control while minimizing false positive events in the negative control can be determined empirically and applied to the experimental data. It is often helpful to use *color-eventing* to determine where the events of interest fall with respect to all of the measured parameters. From the clustering of colored events, it sometimes becomes apparent which are genuine and which are artifactual. Examples of *color-eventing* will be presented in Figures 20.1, 20.7 and 20.9.

Cellular autofluorescence, due primarily to the presence of native fluorescent intracellular molecules such as flavins are excited by the 488 nm laser line and can contribute to noise (Aubin, 1979). As long as the rare event of interest is not itself highly autofluorescent, autofluorescent cells can be eliminated from the analysis by acquiring an unstained or irrelevantly stained fluorescence parameter and including this in the dump gate. We are currently investigating the use of a green laser line to mitigate autofluorescence in cells stained with PE and PE-tandem dyes.

The use of a time parameter, the time that each event was acquired, will be illustrated in Figures 20.2, 20.3 and 20.4. Time, either saved as a listmode parameter or calculated offline, can be used to identify and eliminate episodic noise encountered during long sample acquisitions.

Reproducibility

The results of rare event experiments are often visually unimpressive. Against a denominator of a million or more acquired events are a small number of positive events that have been filtered through a series of logical gates defining the population of interest. Sometimes the events form a tight cluster in a two-parameter scatterplot (e.g. CD123 versus CD11c in Figure 20.1). Sometimes they are diffuse in two-parameter space but are unique in multiparameter space. The credibility of such results can be enhanced by performing replicate determinations. This will be illustrated in Figure 20.3, where six replicate determinations are used in the detection of T cells in a radically T-depleted hematopoietic stem cell graft. The frequency of rare events can then be reported as the mean value and the associated confidence interval and the CV can be calculated. For example, when we measured DC2 in the peripheral blood in triplicate, the intra-subject CV was only 6.9 per cent, indicating high reproducibility despite the relative rarity of the event being measured (Donnenberg and Donnenberg, 2003). The frequency of false positive events detected in the negative control sample (also collected in replicate with the same number of events as the experimental sample) should also be reported and a lower limit of detection may be calculated as the upper 99th percentile of negative control. In our DC studies the lower limits of detection for pDC was 0.0003 per cent (<1/300 000) (Donnenberg et al., 2001), whereas in our MHC tetramer studies it was only 0.0125 per cent (1/8000) (Hoffmann et al., 2000). This illustrates the critical importance of the FMO negative control for the interpretation of rare event data.

Example 1: Five-color simultaneous detection of DC1 and DC2

Immature dendritic cells are present in the peripheral blood at low frequency, but are easily visualized and resolved into myeloid and lymphoid subsets using multi-parameter cytometry, the gating strategy shown in Figure 20.1 (Donnenberg et al., 2001). A dump gate was used to actively define what the event of interest is not. In this example a *lineage cocktail* of antibodies directed against

CD3, CD14 and CD19 was used to eliminate T cells, monocytes and B cells during the first stage of analysis. Limiting the analysis to cells that coexpress CD4 and HLA-DR, a phenotype shared by myeloid and lymphoid DC, further narrowed the field. Finally, these subsets were distinguished by the expression of CD11c, unique on myeloid DCs, and CD123, unique on lymphoid DCs. *Backgating* the resulting DC1 and DC2 populations onto forward by side light scatter allowed these physical parameters to be compared between the two DC subsets.

Example 2: Cellular product monitoring

Flow cytometry plays a critical role in assessing the purity and, to some extent, the potency of products manufactured for cellular therapy. Release criteria for cellular products include limits for these two parameters, plus some assessment of product safety (often sterility and absence of endotoxin). In a recent NIH-sponsored trial conducted at the University of Pittsburgh, USA, patients with severe scleroderma, a systemic autoimmune disease, were treated with high dose anti-lymphocyte therapy followed by rescue with autologous hematopoietic progenitor cells. In order to avoid reintroduction of T and

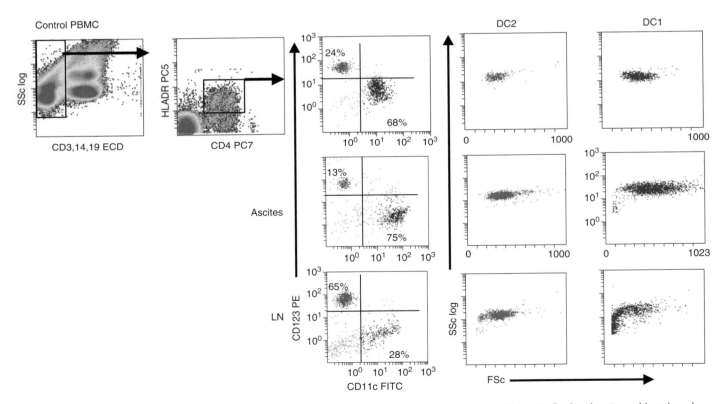

Figure 20.1 Detection of DC1 and DC2. DCs in the peripheral blood of a healthy subject are contrasted with ascitic fluid and peritoneal lymph node (LN) from a patient with newly diagnosed untreated ovarian cancer. Cell suspensions were stained with antibodies CD11c-FITC, CD123-PE, a cocktail of CD3, CD14 and CD19-PE, HLADR-PC5 and CD4-PC7. Cells were acquired on a Beckman-Coulter FC500 cytometer. In this analysis, lymphoid DCs have been color-evented red and myeloid DCs have been colored blue. The differences in scatter properties of these two populations are shown in the last column. In ovarian cancer, myeloid DCs are larger in ascites, compared to control peripheral blood. In LN, where lymphoid DCs predominate, the myeloid DC evidence a population with low forward and side scatter, consistent with apoptosis. **See colour plate 20.1.**

B lymphocytes that could reinitiate the disease process, peripheral blood progenitor cells were radically depleted in a two-step immunomagnetic separation process that included the positive selection of CD34+ progenitor cells followed by the negative selection of CD3+ T cells. In the starting product, T cells represent anywhere from 10 to 20 per cent of nucleated cells, whereas CD34 progenitor cells usually comprise 1 per cent or less. According to the release criteria of the study, a pure, potent and safe T-depleted product would have an adequate progenitor cell dose (5×10^6 CD34/kg), a 5-log or greater reduction in T cells and be negative for bacterial or fungal contamination. A single platform, bead-calibrated assay was used to assess CD34 purity, absolute CD34 content and CD34 viability (Figure 20.2), using the landmark gating strategy of Sutherland (Sutherland et al., 1996). Absolute white cell count (WBC) was also measured using CD45 to identify leukocytes. CD34 and WBC viability was determined by exclusion of the fluorescent agent 7-amino-actinomycin D (Donnenberg et al., 2002). This assay was modified for quantification of residual T cells in the product as rare events (Figure 20.3). The modifications included substitution of CD3 for CD34, an increase in the amount of product added per tube (from 100 μl to 200 μl)

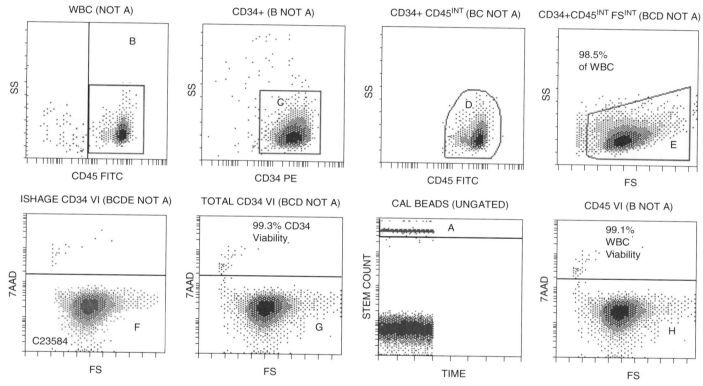

Figure 20.2 Single platform determination of CD34 content and viability of a CD34 selected, CD3 depleted peripheral hematopoietic progenitor cell graft. Graft aliquots (100 μl) were stained in duplicate with anti-CD45-FITC and anti-CD34-PE, in a bead-calibrated lyse/no wash assay (Beckman-Coulter StemKit). A sample stained with the same reagents plus great excess of unlabeled anti-CD34 was run as a negative *isoclonic* control. Cells were acquired on a Beckman-Coulter XL cytometer. StemCount beads are identified by their high fluorescence in FL4 versus time (Gate A). These are removed from subsequent analyses using a *not* gate. Collecting *time* as a parameter facilitates identification of fluidic and other instrument problems during sample acquisition. White blood cells are identified by CD45 expression (gate B). The WBC gate, compounded with the *not bead* gate is passed to a histogram of anti-CD34 versus side scatter. CD34+ events with low side scatter are identified (gate C). The compound gate of WBC, *not bead* and CD34+ is passed to a histogram of CD45 versus side scatter, where cells of intermediate CD45 expression are identified (gate D). The compound gate of WBC, *not bead*, CD34+ and intermediate CD45 expression is passed to a histogram of forward scatter versus side scatter (gate E), which is used to eliminate events with low forward scatter. The number of CD34+ cells obtained in gate E, taken as a percent of WBC identified in gate B, represents the percent CD34+ cells as defined by the International Society of Hematotherapy and Graft Engineering (ISHAGE, now the International Society of Cellular Therapy). For determination of the viability of CD34+ cells, as defined by ISHAGE, the compound gate of WBC, *not bead*, CD34+, intermediate CD45+ expression and intermediate to high forward scatter is passed to a histogram of forward scatter versus intracellular 7AAD concentration (FL3). Because 7AAD is excluded by viable cells, viable CD34+ cells are detected in region F. Even in samples with low overall viability, the proportion of dead cells within the F region is invariably low. This is because the majority of dead and dying cells have low forward scatter and are eliminated by gate E. It is for this reason that we measure and report CD34 viability using a compound gate of WBC, *not bead*, CD34+ and intermediate CD45 expression, where viable CD34+ cells are detected in region G and reported as a per cent of cells in gate D. Similarly, viable WBC are detected in region H and reported as a per cent of cells in gate B. Absolute WBC and CD34 counts are obtained by dividing the events in gates B and E, respectively, by the known StemCount bead concentration. In this sample, CD34+ cells represented more than 98 per cent of CD45+ events. The viability of total WBC (CD45+) and CD34+ cells exceeded 99 per cent. Prior to CD34 selection/CD3 depletion, CD34+ cells comprised 2.95% of CD45+ cells.

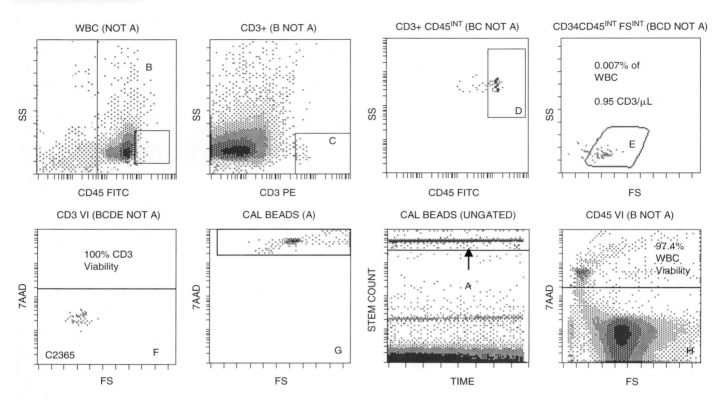

Figure 20.3 Detection of CD3+ T cells as rare events in a CD34 selected, CD3 depleted peripheral hematopoietic progenitor cell graft. The data are from the same product shown in Figure 20.2. In order to achieve maximum sensitivity, graft aliquots (200 μl) were stained with anti-CD45-FITC and anti-CD3-PE in 6-plicate and cells were acquired to exhaustion. Cells were acquired on a Beckman-Coulter XL cytometer. Analysis was similar to that used in Figure 20.2. CD3+ T cells were distinguished from noise by their bright expression of CD45 (Gate D). No events fitting these criteria were seen in the FMO control (not shown). CD3+ cells comprised only 0.007 ± 0.001 per cent (mean $\pm$ SEM) of nucleated cells in this sample and were present in the graft at a concentration of 0.950 ± 0.148 cells/μl, for a total of 1.3×10^5 T cells in the entire product. Prior to CD34 selection/CD3 depletion, CD3+ cells comprised 13 per cent of CD45+ cells for a total of 9.9×10^9 T cells in product. This represents a 5-log depletion.

and an increase in the number of replicate tubes from two to six. The samples were exhaustively acquired, such that every cell in 1.2 ml of product was counted, yielding a lower limit of detection of <500T cells/ml, several orders of magnitude lower than that of conventional assays. The replicate determinations also permit confidence intervals to be determined about the mean absolute count and per cent positive.

The *single-platform* nature of these assays also plays an important role in reducing the variability of this assay and bears some explanation. The first widely used absolute count application was the measurement of circulating CD4+ T cells. As recounted above, the accurate determination of CD4 count proved very useful for monitoring patients with HIV infection. The first efforts required dual platforms: the absolute lymphocyte count was determined by a hematology analyzer and the proportion of CD4+ cells, where the denominator was events falling within a lymphocyte light scatter gate, was determined by the flow cytometry. The absolute count (CD4 cells/μl of blood) was derived by multiplying these two values. This approach suffers from two faults: both assays contribute independent sources of variance and the two assays are not entirely consistent in identifying lymphocytes, especially in

abnormal samples. Single platform assays include those using a volumetric approach (O'Gorman and Gelman, 1997) and those that are calibrated with reference to beads of a known concentration. The latter approach was used in Figures 20.2 and 20.3. Undiluted product, added as precisely as possible using a positive displacement pipette, is incubated with antibodies. Red cells, if present, are lysed by addition of ammonium chloride. Before acquisition, a precise volume of uniform beads of known concentration (StemCount, Beckman-Coulter) is added. Since the sample is never washed, there is no possibility of cell loss. The number of events of interest counted (CD34+ cells or T cells) is compared to the number of beads counted. Since the concentration of the beads is known, the concentration of the events of interest can be inferred with accuracy and precision not attainable in dual platform assays.

Example 3: Measuring antigen specificity and T cell receptor repertoire in T cell subsets

MHC class I/peptide tetrameric complexes (tetramers) represent a powerful tool for detecting, quantifying and separating peptide-specific CD8+ T cells. Theoretically, cells binding a particular tetramer should be pauci-clonal (i.e. consisting of few clones), because they represent only those cells with T-cell receptors able to bind with sufficient avidity a particular nine-mer peptide in the context of a particular MHC class I allele. In this example, we used a strain-common influenza matrix protein peptide (GILGFVFTL) as a prototype recall peptide, because virtually all adult human subjects have experienced multiple exposures to influenza virus naturally or by vaccination. As part of our validation studies, we examined the V-beta usage in flu tetramer+ and flu tetramer negative CD8+ T cells. In unselected CD8+ T cells, individual V-beta families represent anywhere from 10 to 0.1 per cent. Even in highly immune individuals, flu tetramer positive cells represent 0.1–0.2 per cent of CD8+ T cells (Hoffmann et al., 2000). Evaluation of V-beta usage on tetramer+ T cells is therefore a quintessential rare event problem because the events of interest are the product of the tetramer and V-beta frequencies.

This analysis illustrates several principles of rare event analysis:

1 bulk staining
2 doublet discrimination
3 the use of a dump gate
4 live gating
5 the use of time as a gating parameter
6 high-speed sample acquisition.

To accomplish this, we stained approximately 200 million peripheral blood mononuclear cells obtained from an HLA A201+ volunteer donor under an IRB approved protocol. The cells (200×10^6) were first stained in bulk with APC conjugated Flu tetramer (Beckman-Coulter T20135), followed by anti-CD8 PE-Cy7 and anti-CD4 ECD (an internal negative control). When determining the amount of tetramer to use, it is important to remember that it is the final concentration of tetramer in the staining mixture and not the number of cells, that is the critical variable. The sample was then divided into 10 tubes (8 V-beta tubes representing 24 specificities, Beckman-Coulter BetaMark), plus alpha-beta/CD3 and isotype controls) and stained for V-beta. Each tube therefore contained about 20 million cells. The V-beta reagents occupied the FITC and PE channels, but covered 3 V-beta specificities per tube. This is possible because only one V-beta specificity is expressed on any given T cell. Thus for a mixture of antibodies to V-beta families X, Y and Z, X was FITC conjugated, Y was PE conjugated and Z was a mixture of FITC and PE conjugated antibodies. We resuspended the cells at approximately 30×10^6/ml and acquired the data on a Dako-Cytomation MoFlo cytometer. In order to keep the size of the data files under 2 megabytes each, 10–15 million events were collected and saved to a listmode file using a live gate that included only tetramer+ events (Figure 20.4). This reduced the number of events saved to the listmode file to about 50 000. For analysis tetramer+ events were

further gated on single cells, followed by lymphoid light scatter, CD8+, CD4− (Figure 20.4).

This reduced the number of true tetramer+ CD8+ T cells to approximately 2000 per tube, a number sufficient to perform V-beta analysis. At a rate of approximately 25 000 total events per second, acquisition required about 10 minutes per tube, or about 2 h for the entire data set. In order to compare V-beta usage in tetramer+ CD8+ T cells to that in total CD8+ T cells, we also acquired approximately 1 million events without the use of a live gate. The data clearly show that flu tetramer positive cells are heavily skewed toward the V-beta 16 family (Figure 20.4, panel H). Whereas only 1.2 per cent of total CD8+ T cells used this T-cell receptor sequence, fully 51.4 per cent of tetramer+ CD8+ T cells were V-beta 16 positive.

Example 4: Kinetic analysis of the multiple drug resistance transporter P-gp in T cell subsets

An aspect unique to multi-parameter flow cytometry is the ability to make functional measurements over time in defined subsets within a heterogeneous sample. The measurement of calcium flux in T cells immediately after T cell receptor binding (June et al., 1986) is an early and well-known application. In this present example we measured activity of the multiple drug resistance (MDR) transporter P-glycoprotein (P-gp) in freshly isolated peripheral blood CD8+ central memory/memory effector T cells. The probe, rhodamine 123 (R123) is a green fluorescent cationic lipophilic dye and a P-gp substrate. Cells can be pre-stained with monoclonal antibodies, so that P-gp activity can be determined individually in lymphocyte subsets. Conventionally, cells are loaded with R123 at 37°C in an incubator or water bath. The cells are washed and the R123 fluorescence is measured to determine the maximum brightness immediately after loading with the dye. The cells are then returned to the incubator for 30 min to 3 h and R123 fluorescence is determined again. R123 is not passively lost in this time frame and only cells actively transporting R123 from the plasma membrane will show a decrement in R123 fluorescence (Donnenberg et al., 2004). In the present example, we extended this assay by performing real-time measurement of R123 uptake and efflux in four circulating T cell populations subsetted by CD4, CD8 and CD45RA expression. Using a water-heated sample station, cells were maintained at 37°C while cells were acquired on the flow cytometer. Baseline data were acquired for 2 min, after which the cells were loaded with R123 and acquired continuously for 15 min. The sample was removed from the cytometer, washed at 4°C and returned to the cytometer for continuous measurement of R123 efflux for an additional 30 min. Kinetics of dye uptake and efflux were determined for each T cell subset and optimal loading and efflux times were determined. During uptake, R123 fluorescence increased rapidly and approached plateau by 10 min. The data for the

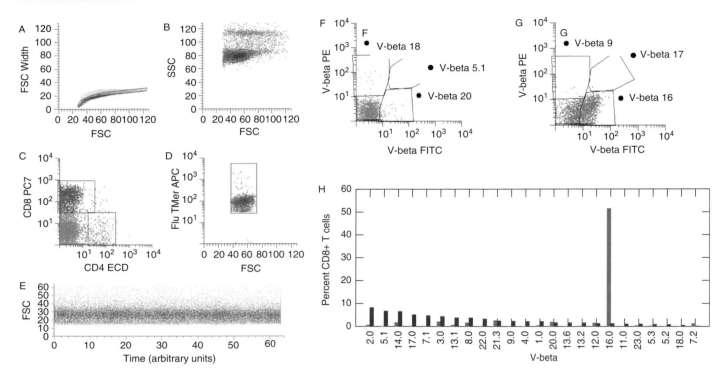

Figure 20.4 Rare event detection of TCR V-beta usage among Flu tetramer+ CD8+ T cells. In panel A, a gate is created on forward scatter pulse height and forward scatter pulse width, excluding doublets (high pulse width for a given pulse height). In panel B the analysis is limited to events displaying lymphoid forward and side light scatter properties. Panel C (*dump gate*) is used both to positively identify CD8+ T cells and to eliminate CD4+ T cells (and anything else appearing positive in the ECD channel). Panel D is the *live gate* on tetramer+ events. Only tetramer+ events falling within this gate were saved in the listmode file, greatly reducing the size of the datafile and increasing the speed of analysis. Forward scatter is shown versus Time (panel E), a calculated parameter that is used to identify and eliminate any spurious event bursts (none were detected here). Finally, panels F and G (from separately stained tubes) show the results of the application of this compound gating strategy. Panel F shows the usage of V-beta 18 (0.04 per cent), 5.1 (0.0 per cent) and 20 (1.9 per cent) among Flu tetramer+/CD8+/CD4− cells. Panel G shows that the majority of Flu tetramer+ T cells (51.4 per cent) are V-beta 16+. Panel H shows the final result, the V-beta repertoire of flu tetramer− and flu tetramer+ CD8+ T cells. Data from tetramer+ events were collected for 24 V-beta specificities. Data were acquired separately for determination of V-beta usage in tetramer negative T cells (without the use of the live gate D). The results are plotted in the order of frequency of V-beta usage in tetramer negative CD8+ T cells (blue bars). Common specificities such as V-beta 2, 5.1, 14 and 17 were very underrepresented in flu tetramer+ T cells (red bars), whereas V-beta 16, which comprised only 1.2 per cent of total CD8+ T cells, accounted for 51.4 per cent of flu tetramer+ T cells. These results are consistent with the clonality (or pauci-clonality) of the majority of influenza matrix peptide specific T cells in this sample. **See colour plate 20.4.**

CD8+ CD45RA− population, the population with the highest P-gp activity, is shown in Figure 20.5. All cell subsets tested achieved similar plateau levels. R123 efflux exhibited a biphasic profile. The initial slope over a 10-min interval (log-fluorescence channels/min) differed markedly among T cell subsets with CD8+ CD45RA+ evidencing the greatest slope. These results extend our previous static observations that the CD8 memory subset exhibits the greatest P-gp activity, which may have important pharmacological implications during cell-specific immune responses.

Example 5: Caspase 3 activity and plasma membrane phospholipid composition in early T cell apoptosis

Late apoptotic events can be visualized by flow cytometry in a variety of ways, including changes in light scatter (DC1 in Figure 20.1) and DNA laddering (Lyons et al., 1992). Many physical and biochemical changes take place

in the cell as it follows its program from initiation of apoptosis through cell death and, as Mario Roederer has commented, it is inadvisable to try to measure anything on a dead cell. If one wishes to perform analyses such as determination of apoptosis on specific subsets, it is therefore important to focus on the earliest phases of the apoptotic process, when cells are still technically alive by many criteria. In this example we combine two assays reported to reveal early aspects of apoptosis: activation of the protease caspase 3 (Hirata et al., 1998) and loss of plasma membrane phospholipid asymmetry (Aupeix et al., 1996). We were able to make inferences concerning the temporal sequence of these early events by the simultaneous analysis of changes in light scatter, a late apoptotic event. Caspase 3 activity was measured using the substrate Phi Phi Lux (OncoImmunin), which fluoresces green when cleaved. Plasma membrane phospholipid asymmetry was measured using PE-labeled Annexin V (BD-Pharmingen) binding to phosphatidyl serine. Phosphatidyl serine is

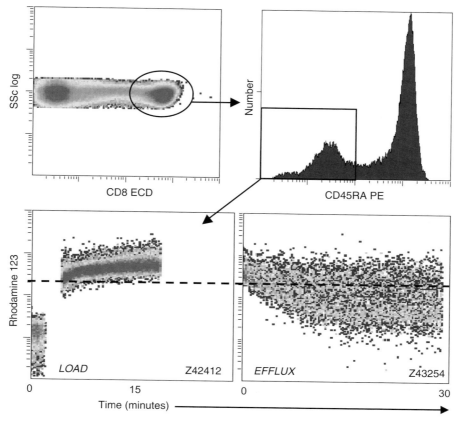

Figure 20.5 R123 load and efflux in CD45RA negative central memory/effector memory peripheral CD8+ T cells. Peripheral blood mononuclear cells were obtained from a normal healthy volunteer. Cells were stained with antibodies CD45RA-PE, CD8-ECD and CD4 plus CD3 PE-Cy5. Cells were acquired on a Beckman-Coulter XL cytometer. Cells were gated on CD3+ events (not shown). Low side scatter CD8+, CD45RA- T cells were identified using a compound gate (top panels). The lower panels show R123 fluorescence as a function of acquisition time. During the first 2 min of acquisition and prior to addition of R123, baseline autofluorescence was determined. R123 LOAD: Acquisition of R123 unstained sample was paused, R123 was added (0.13 μM final concentration) and acquisition was immediately resumed; cells were acquired continuously for an additional 15 min. R123 EFFLUX: Loaded cells were chilled and washed 2 times with 10 ml of ice cold PBS, resuspended in culture medium at 37°C and returned to the cytometer. Cells were maintained at 37°C and data acquired continuously for 30 min. R123 loading and efflux were also determined for CD3+ CD8+ CD45RA+ cells and for the analogous CD4+ T-cell subsets (not shown). **See colour plate 20.5**.

normally confined to the cytoplasmic side of the plasma membrane in T cells, but is exposed during the membrane perturbations associated with apoptosis. Exposure of phosphatidyl serine on the surface of T cells is a signal for phagocytosis by macrophages (Dini et al., 1996) and clearance from the circulation. Figure 20.6 illustrates the simultaneous measurement of caspase 3 activity, annexin V binding and forward light scatter in CD4+ CD45−CD27− effector memory cells in the ascitic fluid of an ovarian cancer patient. This subset is illustrated because it displayed the highest degree of early apoptosis among the subsets defined by CD45RA and CD27. A compound gate on CD4+, low side and intermediate side scatter, CD27−, CD45RA− (not shown) was applied to the data. We used color-eventing to identify temporal sequence of caspase activation and membrane perturbation, using loss of forward light scatter as an indication of late apoptosis. The data indicate that the earliest phase of apoptosis detectable with these parameters is marked

by a coordinate increase in caspase activity and annexin V binding.

Example 6: Measuring antigen-driven T cell activation and proliferation *in vitro*

One of the great puzzles in the dawning age of cellular immunology was the seemingly inert nature of circulating lymphocytes. With bland nuclear features and scant cytoplasm, they seemed ill suited for any real immunologic work. In 1960, Peter Nowell made a discovery that facilitated routine karyotyping when he determined that peripheral blood lymphocytes could be driven to mitogenesis *in vitro* when stimulated with the plant lectin phytohemagglutinin. In addition to solving an important practical problem, this observation was a milestone in the development of biomarkers of cellular immunity, paving the way for the development of the current battery of *in vitro* assays (Hirschhorn et al., 1963). Today, we recognize that

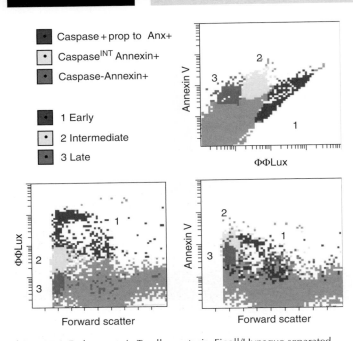

Caspase+prop to Anx+

Caspase^{INT} Annexin+

Caspase-Annexin+

1 Early

2 Intermediate

3 Late

Figure 20.6 Early events in T cell apoptosis. Ficoll/Hypaque separated mononuclear cells recovered from the ascitic fluid of an untreated ovarian cancer patient were stained with antibodies CD45RA-ECD, CD27-PC5 and CD4-PC5. Cells were washed and incubated with Phi Phi Lux-G1D2, washed again, resuspended in high calcium buffer and incubated with Annexin V-PE. Cells were acquired immediately on a Beckman-Coulter FC500 cytometer. CD4+ effector memory cells were identified by gating on CD4+, low and intermediate side scatter, CD27− and CD45RA− events (not shown). Color eventing was used to identify three populations of cells based on caspase 3 activity and annexin V binding. In the first population (blue), caspase activity and annexin V binding increase coordinately, forming a diagonal in the bivariate scatter plot. In the second population (yellow) annexin V binding remains high, but caspase activity, while still present, is reduced. In the third population (red), annexin binding is positive and somewhat decreased, but at this point caspase activity is lost. The temporal sequence of apoptotic events was confirmed by backgating on Phi Phi Lux versus forward light scatter, using color eventing to identify the three populations. Here, it can be seen that the first population (blue) forms an arc as it gains and then loses caspase activity as it collapses in forward scatter. The second population already has low light scatter and further loses caspase activity. The red population, the last in the sequence, consists of small annexin V low, caspase 3 negative cells. Note that a few red colored events have normal forward scatter characteristic. These represent annexin V- cells that were misclassified when the red color event gate was created in the top right panel. **See colour plate 20.6.**

T and B lymphocytes are far from inert. Ligation of their antigen receptors in conjunction with appropriate costimulatory signals results in striking physiologic alterations that can be measured by changes in the expression of a variety of physical, cell-surface and intracytoplasmic markers. One of the earliest assays to be applied to immune monitoring was the lymphocyte blast transformation assay (Curtis et al., 1970), later referred to as the lymphoproliferation assay. This was performed by stimulating isolated peripheral blood mononuclear cells (lymphocytes, monocytes and immature DC) with mitogens or soluble protein antigens. Proliferation was usually quantified by scintillation counting after a short pulse with tritiated thymidine. Our example is a modern day multiparameter variation in which Ficoll/Hypaque separated peripheral blood mononuclear cells are cultured for 5 days with a protein recall antigen (diphtheria toxoid) and proliferation is measured by expression of the transferrin receptor, CD71 (Shapiro, 2003). The multiparameter nature of flow cytometry allows us to measure an additional outcome, expression of the growth factor receptor IL-2 alpha (CD25), simultaneously on several subsets. In the present example, these outcomes have been measured on CD4+ cells subsetted into naive, memory and effector compartments based on CD45RA and CD27 expression (Figure 20.7). The gating strategy is first to determine which parameters are to be used to classify the cells into subsets, and then to measure outcome parameters in each subset.

In this example, we begin by plotting CD4 by log side scatter, rather than with the customary lymphocyte light scatter gate. This allows us to immediately resolve CD4+ cells. Had these been freshly isolated cells (see Figure 20.9), or unstimulated cultured cells, a monocyte population would have been clearly distinguishable and easily eliminated from the CD4+ T cell gate. In these activated cells, the CD4 bright cells with high log side scatter are activated T cells and if this were the only parameter that we wished to measure we could stop right here. Our sequential gating next proceeds to the scatter gate, which reveals much cleaner populations than we would have detected had we started with this gate. Late apoptotic cells, if present, can be identified as events with low forward scatter and relatively high log side scatter and eliminated at this step. Continuing with our classification parameters, we next divide non-apoptotic CD4+ T cells into four subsets based on CD45RA and CD27 expression. Here we used quadrant cuts based on unstimulated cells, but quadrants A and C seem to form a continuous population (this will be resolved in the next figure). Finally, we measured the outcome parameters, CD71 and CD25 expression in each subset. The majority of CD71/CD25 double positive cells are clearly in the CD45RA− population, but span CD27 negative and positive populations (quadrants A and C, respectively). A small proportion of responding cells can be seen in the naive (CD45RA+, CD27+) population, but many are positive for CD25 alone and have not entered the cell cycle as measured by CD71 expression. Once we have performed this analysis, we can now turn it inside out, starting with the outcome variable and proceeding to the classification parameters. Through the magic of color-eventing we will be able to visualize four parameters simultaneously in one histogram (Figure 20.8).

Using the quadrants determined in Figure 20.7 on the CD71 by CD25 histogram, we assign a unique color to the events in each quadrant. Thus, resting cells are green, CD25+/CD71− cells are red, CD25/CD71 double positive cells are gold and the rare CD25−/CD71+ cell is blue. These color-gated events are then projected to bivariate

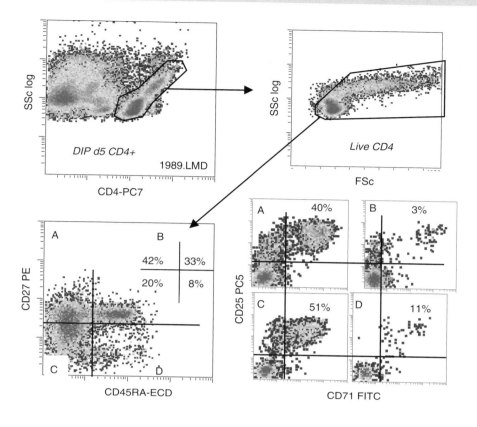

Figure 20.7 Antigen-driven upregulation of CD25 and CD71 in CD4+ T cell subsets. Peripheral blood mononuclear cells were obtained from a healthy subject and cultured for 5 days in the presence of diphtheria toxoid (2 μg/ml). Cultured cells were harvested and stained with antibodies CD71-FITC, CD27-PE, CD45RA-ECD, CD25-PC5 and CD4-PC7. Cells were acquired on a Beckman-Coulter FC500 cytometer. In the top left panel, responding cells can be visualized as CD4+ T cells with high log side scatter. CD4+ cells were filtered through a scatter gate (top right panel) used to eliminate late apoptotic cells, if present and subsetted on the basis of CD45RA and CD27 expression (A, B, C, D). The outcome parameters, CD71 and CD25 were determined in each subset. **See colour plate 20.7.**

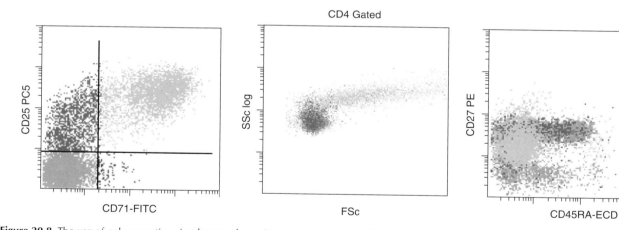

Figure 20.8 The use of color-eventing simultaneously to view outcome and classification parameters. The data are the same as those displayed in Figure 20.7. Here the outcome parameters CD71 and CD25 have been divided into quadrants and each quadrant used as a color-evented gate. For example, CD71/CD25 double positive cells were colored gold. These events are then displayed in bivariate scatter plots of forward by log side scatter and CD45RA by CD71 expression. Proliferating cells (gold) can clearly be visualized as CD45RA negative, CD27 intermediate cells with high forward scatter and high log side scatter. **See colour plate 20.8.**

scatter plots showing light scatter or CD4 subset. The particular colors that we have chosen create what we have termed the *flaming olive* pattern in forward by log side scatter. Resting cells (the olive) and CD25 single positive cells (the pimento) are small lymphocytes with low forward and side scatter. Proliferating CD25+/CD71+ cells (the flame) are heterogeneous with respect to forward scatter and high in side scatter. The subset distribution of

these populations can also be clearly delineated with color eventing. Resting cells (green) occupy all quadrants and look very similar to unstimulated cells (not shown). CD25+/CD71− cells (red) are confined to the CD27+ populations but span CD45RA expression, suggesting a transition in CD45 isoforms. Proliferating cells (gold) occupy a unique place in CD45RA/CD27 space, being CD45RA− but CD27 intermediate.

Example 7: Polychromatic flow cytometry

Recent improvements in cytometers and cytometry software have made multicolor (polychromatic) cytometry a reality for many laboratories (De Rosa et al., 2001, 2003). The advantages of polychromatic flow cytometry go beyond the convenience of multiplexing several determinations in a single tube. Most important is the resolution afforded by polychrome cytometry. Figure 20.9 illustrates the use of eight-color cytometry to resolve T cell subsets. Three solid-state lasers (violet 405, blue 488 and red 633) were used for this analysis of naive/memory markers on CD4+ and CD8+ cells. Five fluorochromes were detected off

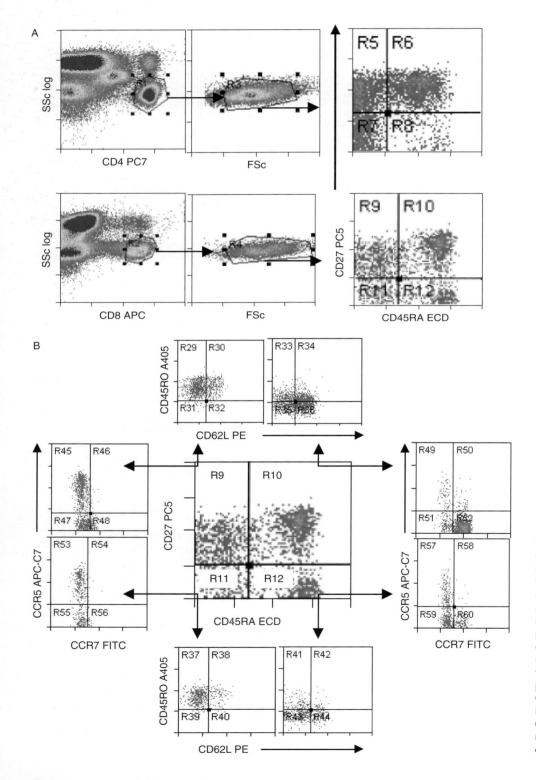

Figure 20.9 Polychromatic visualization of differentiation markers on CD4+ and CD8+ T cells. The gating strategy for this analysis begins in A in the same way as in Figure 20.7, this time with CD4+ and CD8+ populations identified and subsetted on CD45RA and CD27 in parallel. From here the 4 subpopulations each give rise to two bivariate plots (CD62L versus CD45RO and CCR7 versus CCR5). The data for the CD8+ population is shown in 9B. Note that CD8+ naive cells comprise a homogeneous population of CD45RA+, CD45RO−, CCR7+, CCD5− cells, the majority of which are CD62L+. **See colour plate 20.9.**

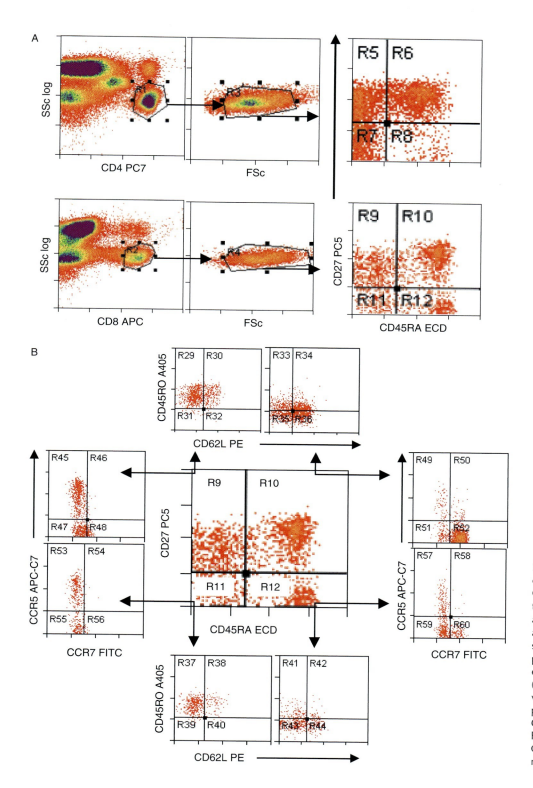

Figure 20.9 Polychromatic visualization of differentiation markers on CD4+ and CD8+ T cells. The gating strategy for this analysis begins in A in the same way as in Figure 20.7, this time with CD4+ and CD8+ populations identified and subsetted on CD45RA and CD27 in parallel. From here the 4 subpopulations each give rise to two bivariate plots (CD62L versus CD45RO and CCR7 versus CCR5). The data for the CD8+ population is shown in 9B. Note that CD8+ naive cells comprise a homogeneous population of CD45RA+, CD45RO−, CCr7+, CCD5− cells, the majority of which are CD62L+.

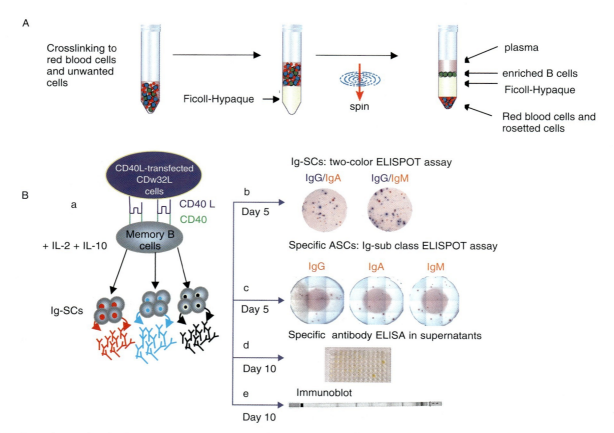

Figure 23.2 General procedure for detection and enumeration of circulating Ag-specific memory B cells. (A): Isolation of the derived peripheral B cells by eliminating unwanted cells and red blood cells using the tetrameric antibody complex reagent and gradient (Ficoll-Hypaque) centrifugation. (Ba): The purified B cells are cultured with CD40L-transfected CDW32L mouse fibroblasts and IL-2 plus IL-10. (Bb): Ig-SCs are enumerated by the two-color ELISPOT assay at day 5. (Bc): Inducible specific antibody-secreting cells are enumerated at day 5 by an ELISPOT. (Bd): Specific antibodies are detected in cell-free supernatants at day10 by ELISA. (Be): Antibody specificities are determined by immunoblotting. Ig-SCs, immunoglobulin secreting cells; ASCs, antibody secreting cells.

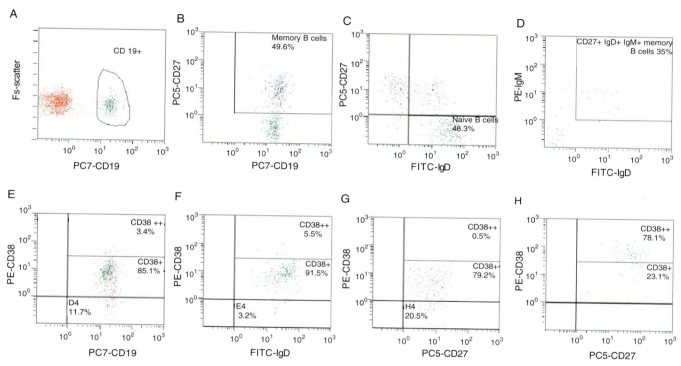

Figure 23.3 Circulating B cell subsets characterized according to membrane IgD, IgM, CD27, and CD38 receptor expression. After washing in RPMI, the blood is divided into two samples: one is incubated with a mixture of phycoerythrin-cyanin 7 (PC7) conjugated anti-CD19, phycoerythrin-cyanin 5 (PC5) conjugated anti-CD27, phycoerythrin (PE) conjugated anti-IgM and fluorescein isiothiocyanate (FITC) conjugated anti-IgD antibodies. The second is incubated with a mixture of PC7 conjugated anti-CD19, FITC conjugated anti-IgD, PC5 conjugated anti-CD27 and PE conjugated anti-CD38. (A) Memory B cells and naive B cells are enumerated on the basis of size and CD19 expression. (B) CD19$^+$ CD27$^+$ total memory B cells. (C) CD19$^+$ IgD$^+$CD27$^-$ naive B cells. (D) CD19$^+$ CD27$^+$ IgM$^+$ IgD$^+$ memory B cell subset. Using the second sample, subpopulations of circulating B cells are analyzed on the basis of their CD38 expression: (E) CD19$^+$ CD38$^+$; (F) naive B cells CD38$^+$ or CD38^{++}; (G) memory B cells CD38$^+$ or CD38^{++} and (H) activated memory B cells CD38$^+$ or CD38$^+$ $^+$. The horizontal line separates the CD38$^+$ negative and positive subpopulations defined using isotypic controls. The upper quadrant is divided into two subpopulations of CD19$^+$ cells expressing high CD38^{++} or low CD38$^+$ expression after CD40-CD40L B-cell activation *in vitro*. The number of B cells in each population is determined by using calibrated fluorospheres Kit (Flow Count™) according to the manufacturer's instructions (Beckman-Coulter).

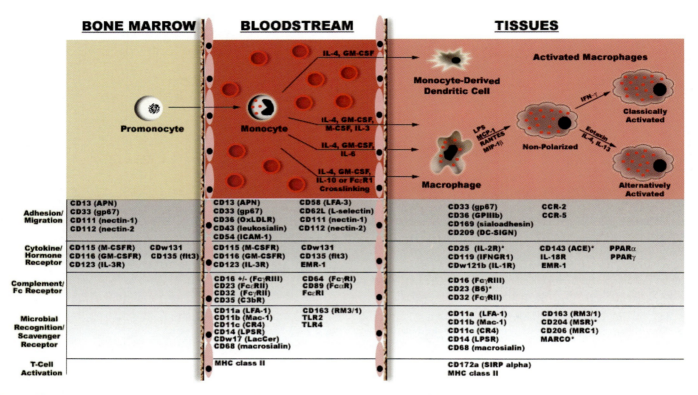

BONE MARROW **BLOODSTREAM** **TISSUES**

Promonocyte → Monocyte

IL-4, GM-CSF → Monocyte-Derived Dendritic Cell

IL-4, GM-CSF, M-CSF, IL-3

IL-4, GM-CSF, IL-6

IL-4, GM-CSF, IL-10 or FcεR1 Crosslinking → Macrophage

LPS, MCP-1, RANTES, MIP-1β → Non-Polarized

IFN-γ → Classically Activated

Eotaxin IL-4, IL-13 → Alternatively Activated

Activated Macrophages

	Bone Marrow		Bloodstream		Tissues		
Adhesion/ Migration	CD13 (APN) CD33 (gp67) CD111 (nectin-1) CD112 (nectin-2)		CD13 (APN) CD33 (gp67) CD36 (OxLDLR) CD43 (leukosialin) CD54 (ICAM-1)	CD58 (LFA-3) CD62L (L-selectin) CD111 (nectin-1) CD112 (nectin-2)	CD33 (gp67) CD36 (GPIIIb) CD169 (sialoadhesin) CD209 (DC-SIGN)	CCR-2 CCR-5	
Cytokine/ Hormone Receptor	CD115 (M-CSFR) CD116 (GM-CSFR) CD123 (IL-3R)	CDw131 CD135 (flt3)	CD115 (M-CSFR) CD116 (GM-CSFR) CD123 (IL-3R)	CDw131 CD135 (flt3) EMR-1	CD25 (IL-2R)* CD119 (IFNGR1) CDw121b (IL-1R)	CD143 (ACE)* IL-18R EMR-1	PPARα PPARγ
Complement/ Fc Receptor			CD16 +/- (FcγRIII) CD23 (FcεRII) CD32 (FcγRII) CD35 (C3bR)	CD64 (FcγRI) CD89 (FcαR) FcεRI	CD16 (FcγRIII) CD23 (B6)* CD32 (FcγRII)		
Microbial Recognition/ Scavenger Receptor			CD11a (LFA-1) CD11b (Mac-1) CD11c (CR4) CD14 (LPSR) CDw17 (LacCer) CD68 (macrosialin)	CD163 (RM3/1) TLR2 TLR4	CD11a (LFA-1) CD11b (Mac-1) CD11c (CR4) CD14 (LPSR) CD68 (macrosialin)	CD163 (RM3/1) CD204 (MSR)* CD206 (MRC1) MARCO*	
T-Cell Activation			MHC class II		CD172a (SIRP alpha) MHC class II		

Figure 25.1 Monocyte and macrophage antigen expression in bone marrow, blood or tissues. Promonocytes exit the bone marrow, mature into monocytes and express receptors important in phagocytosis and microbial recognition. Monocytes leave the circulation and take up residence in tissues where they differentiate into morphologically, phenotypically and functionally heterogeneous effector cells such as macrophages or dendritic cells. Macrophages become activated if exposed to antigens, pathogens and to substances such as lipopolysaccharide (LPS) via TLR and interferon-γ (IFN-γ) (classically activated) or IL-4, IL-13 (alternative activation). Antigens expressed on activated macrophages are denoted with asterisks (*).

A

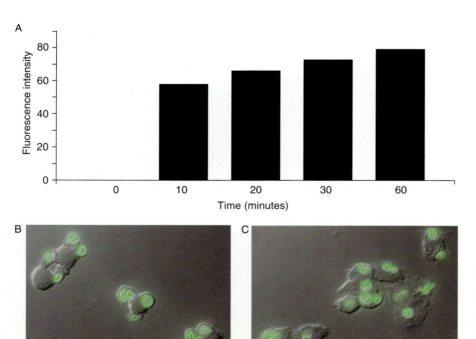

Figure 25.4 (A). Phagocytosis of FITC-labeled zymosan A particles by monocytes isolated by counterflow centrifugal elutriation and analyzed by FACS. A 20:1 zymosan A:monocyte ratio was used and samples harvested and analyzed by FACS at 10–60 min after the addition of particles. Photomicrographs of monocytes after a 10-min (B) and 60-min (C) incubation with FITC zymosan.

the blue laser (FITC, PE, ECD, PE-Cy5 and PE-C7), two by the red laser (APC and APC-Cy7) and one by the violet laser (Alexa 405). The matching of fluorochromes to antibodies was largely a matter of convenience and commercial availability, but care was taken to match a relatively dim marker in PE-Cy5 (CD27) with a bright marker in APC (CD8). This is advisable because PE-Cy5 is excited twice, once by the blue laser and again by the red laser. The latter signal emits at the same wavelength as APC and must be removed by cross-laser compensation. Once the data are acquired, the analysis begins by first identifying populations CD4+ or CD8+ T cells versus log side scatter. Note how beautifully the CD4 and CD8 populations stand out. This example shows freshly isolated PBMC, but in stimulated cells, the activated populations are very apparent with this gating strategy, owing to their higher side scatter and, in the case of CD4+ T cells, brighter CD4 expression (Figure 20.9). The gating proceeds as in Figure 20.7, except that this time, CD4+ and CD8+ are gated in parallel. Application of the *lymphocyte scatter gate* is far more informative when applied *after* the first classification gate (i.e. CD4 or CD8). Apoptotic cells having low forward scatter can be removed in this step and large activated cells, if present, can be gated separately for further analysis. Following this, the first subsetting cut is taken on the basis of CD45RA and CD27 expression. So far so good, but this is only four colors. If we want to look at all possible subsets in this panel, there are potentially 128 populations (counting the empty ones like CCR7+/CCR5+). This is clearly unfeasible and a strategy is required. In the example shown, we are using our primary subsetting antibodies (CD45RA and CD27) to divide our CD8+ T cells into central memory, naive effector/memory and effector populations and looking at CD62L, CD45RO, CCR7 and CCR5 expression on those four subsets. As an example, in naive CD8 T cells (CD45RA+/CD27+), we see that they are CD45RO−, largely (but not exclusively) CD62L+, CCR7+ and CCR5−. We could do the same sort of analysis for CD4+ T cells (not shown). As was shown in Figure 20.7, it is useful to think of markers as denoting either classification, or outcome. Outcome markers are determined on all meaningful permutations of classification markers.

FUTURE PROSPECTS

Surveying the newest cytometers and the voluminous catalogs of available reagents, it is clear that polychromatic cytometry will be available to a wide community of investigators by the time the currently deployed generation of four and five-color cytometers have finished their useful service lives. Other advances, such as the increasing speed of computers and the decreasing cost of mass data storage, will also remove barriers to multiparameter cytometry. As a result, we can expect to see more laboratories combine functional and phenotypic determinations

and increasingly apply these methods to rare events problems. As the number of parameters that can be measured increases, flow cytometry approaches cytomics, the integration of genomics, transciptomics and proteomics, all at the level of the single cell. Like proteomics (the study of the entire protein complement in a cell, tissue or organism), cytomics encompasses the activity, modification, localization and interaction of proteins. However, in cytomics the task of data reduction is even more daunting because the unit of analysis is the individual cell.

Among the areas for future applications identified by flow cytometry pioneer Leonard Herzenberg are, biochemical analysis of rare cells, multiparameter high-throughput screening and multidimensional assessment of cell signaling networks (Herzenberg et al., 2002). To this list, Howard Shapiro has added the use of flow cytometry to identify and characterize microorganisms (Shapiro, 2003). New analytical strategies and tools for exploratory data analysis will certainly be required to realize these goals. Although it is difficult to picture exactly what these tools will look like, they will help us cluster cell populations in multidimensional space better to identify and understand progenitor–progeny relationships, functional attributes and disease states.

REFERENCES

Ahmed, R. and Gray, D. (1996). Immunological memory and protective immunity: understanding their relation. Science *272*, 54–60.

Altman, J.D., Moss, P.A., Goulder, P.J. et al. (1996). Phenotypic analysis of antigen-specific T lymphocytes. Science *274*, 94–96.

Appay, V., Dunbar, P.R., Callan, M. et al. (2002). Memory CD8+ T cells vary in differentiation phenotype in different persistent virus infections. Nat Med *8*, 379–385.

Arulanandam, A.R., Kister, A., McGregor, M.J., Wyss, D.F., Wagner, G. and Reinherz, E.L. (1994). Interaction between human CD2 and CD58 involves the major beta sheet surface of each of their respective adhesion domains. J Exp Med *180*, 1861.

Aubin, J.E. (1979). Autofluorescence of viable cultured mammalian cells. J Histochem Cytochem *27*, 36–43.

Aupeix, K., Toti, F., Satta, N., Bischoff, P. and Freyssinet, J.M. (1996). Oyxsterols induce membrane procoagulant activity in monocytic THP-1 cells. Biochem J *314*, 1027–1033.

Baerlocher, G.M. and Lansdorp, P.M. (2003). Telomere length measurements in leukocyte subsets by automated multicolor flow-FISH. Cytometry *55A*, 1–6.

Barratt-Boyes, S.M., Zimmer, M.I., Harshyne, L.A. et al. (2000). Maturation and trafficking of monocyte-derived dendritic cells in monkeys: implications for dendritic cell-based vaccines. J Immunol *164*, 2487–2495.

Baumgarth, N. and Roederer, M. (2003). A practical approach to multicolor flow cytometry for immunophenotyping. J Immunol Methods *243*, 77–97.

Bergeron, M., Faucher, S., Minkus, T. et al. (1998). Impact of unified procedures as implemented in the Canadian Quality

Assurance Program for T lymphocyte subset enumeration. Participating Flow Cytometry Laboratories of the Canadian Clinical Trials Network for HIV/AIDS Therapies. Cytometry 33, 146–155.

Bradley, L.M., Bradley, J.S., Ching, D.L. and Shiigi, S.M. (1989). Predominance of T cells that express CD45R in the CD4+ helper/inducer lymphocyte subset of neonates. Clin Immunol Immunopathol 51, 426–435.

Brosterhus, H., Brings, S., Leyendeckers, H. et al. (1999). Enrichment and detection of live antigen-specific CD4(+) and CD8(+) T cells based on cytokine secretion. Eur J Immunol 29, 4053–4059.

Campbell, J.J., Murphy, K.E., Kunkel, E.J. et al. (2001).CCR7 expression and memory T cell diversity in humans. J Immunol 166, 877–884.

Cantor, H.. Simpson, E., Sato, V.L., Fathman, C.G. and Herzenberg, L.A. (1975). Characterization of subpopulations of T lymphocytes. I. Separation and functional studies of peripheral T-cells binding different amounts of fluorescent anti-Thy 1.2 (theta) antibody using a fluorescence-activated cell sorter (FACS). Cell Immunol 15, 180–196.

Centers for Disease Control. (1992). Guidelines for the performance of CD4+ T-cell determinations in persons with human immunodeficiency virus infection. MMWR. 41(No. RR-8).

Cossarizza, A., Baccarani-Contri, M., Kalashnikova, G. and Franceschi, C. (1993). A new method for the cytofluorimetric analysis of mitochondrial membrane potential using the J-aggregate forming lipophilic cation 5,5',6,6'-tetrachloro-1,1',3,3'-tetraethylbenzimidazolcarbocyanine iodide (JC-1). Biochem Biophys Res Commun 197, 40–45.

Curtis, J.E., Hersh, E.M., Harris, J.E., McBride, C. and Freireich, E.J. (1970). The human primary immune response to keyhole limpet haemocyanin: interrelationships of delayed hypersensitivity, antibody response and in vitro blast transformation. Clin Exp Immunol 6, 473–491.

Darzynkiewicz, Z., Traganos, F., Staiano-Coico, L., Kapuscinski, J. and Melamed, M.R. (1982). Interaction of rhodamine 123 with living cells studied by flow cytometry. Cancer Res 42, 799–806.

De Rosa, S.C., Herzenberg, L.A., Herzenberg, L.A. and Roederer, M. (2001). 11-color, 13-parameter flow cytometry: identification of human naive T cells by phenotype, function, and T-cell receptor diversity. Nat Med 7, 245–248.

De Rosa, S.C., Brenchley, J.M. and Roederer, M. (2003). Beyond six colors: a new era in flow cytometry. Nat Med 9, 112–117.

D'hautcourt, J.L. (1996). Quality control procedures for flow cytometric applications in the hematology laboratory. Hematol Cell Ther 38, 467–470.

Dini, L., Ruzittu, M.T. and Falasca, L. (1996). Recognition and phagocytosis of apoptotic cells. Scanning Microscop 10, 239–251.

Donnenberg, V.S. and Donnenberg, A.D. (2003). Identification, rare-event detection and analysis of dendritic cell subsets in broncho-alveolar lavage fluid and peripheral blood by flow cytometry. Frontiers Biosci 8, s1175–1180.

Donnenberg, A.D. and Meyer, E.M. (1999). Principles of rare event analysis by flow cytometry: detection of injected dendritic cells in draining lymphatic tissue. Clin Immunol Newslett 19, 124–128.

Donnenberg, A.D., Donnenberg, V.S. and Shen, H. (2003). Rare-event detection and analysis in flow cytometry. The Connection 5

Donnenberg, A.D., Koch, E.K., Griffin, D.L. et al. (2002). Viability of cryopreserved BM progenitor cells stored for more than a decade. Cytotherapy 4, 157–16.

Donnenberg, V.S., O'Connell, P.J., Logar, A.J., Zeevi, A., Thomson, A.W. and Donnenberg, A.D. (2001). Rare-event analysis of circulating human dendritic cell subsets and their presumptive mouse counterparts. Transplantation 72, 1946–1951.

Donnenberg, V.S., Wilson, J.W., Burckart, G.J., Zeevi, A., Iacono, A. and Donnenberg, A.D. (2004). Measurement of basal, substrate induced and total P-gp activity in broncho-alveolar lavage T-cell subsets. Cytometry. In press.

Drach, J., Gattringer, C., Glassl, H., Schwarting, R., Stein, H. and Huber, H. (1989). Simultaneous flow cytometric analysis of surface markers and nuclear Ki-67 antigen in leukemia and lymphoma. Cytometry 10, 743–749.

Gelman, R., Cheng, S.C., Kidd, P., Waxdal, M. and Kagan, J. (1993). Assessment of the effects of instrumentation, monoclonal antibody, and fluorochrome on flow cytometric immunophenotyping: a report based on 2 years of the NIAID DAIDS flow cytometry quality assessment program. Clin Immunol Immunopathol 66, 150–162.

Giorgi, J.V., Cheng, H.L., Margolick, J.B. et al. (1990). Quality control in the flow cytometric measurement of T-lymphocyte subsets: the multicenter AIDS cohort study experience. The Multicenter AIDS Cohort Study Group. Clin Immunol Immunopathol 55, 173–186.

Giorgi, J.V., Liu, Z., Hultin, L.E., Cumberland, W.G., Hennessey, K. and Detels, R. (1993). Elevated levels of CD38+ CD8+ T cells in HIV infection add to the prognostic value of low CD4+ T cell levels: results of 6 years of follow-up. The Los Angeles Center, Multicenter AIDS Cohort Study. J Acq Immune Defic Synd 6, 904–912.

Gratama, J.W., Bolhuis, R.L. and Van 't Veer, M.B. (1999). Quality control of flow cytometric immunophenotyping of haematological malignancies. Clin Lab Haematol 21, 155–160.

Guedez, L., Stetler-Stevenson, W.G., Wolff, L. et al. (1998). In vitro suppression of programmed cell death of B cells by tissue inhibitor of metalloproteinases-1. J Clin Invest 102, 2002–2010.

Hammerling, G.J., Lemke, H., Hammerling, U. et al. (1978). Monoclonal antibodies against murine cell surface antigens: anti-H-2, anti-Ia and anti-T cell antibodies. Curr Top Microbiol Immunol 81, 100–106.

Herzenberg, L.A., Parks, D., Sahaf, B., Perez, O., Roederer, M. and Herzenberg, L.A. (2002). The history and future of the fluorescence activated cell sorter and flow cytometry: a view from Stanford (Historical Article. Lectures). Clin Chem 48, 1819–1827.

Hirata, H., Takahashi, A., Kobayashi, S. et al. (1998). Caspases are activated in a branched protease cascade and control distinct downstream processes in Fas-induced apoptosis. J Exp Med 187, 587–600.

Hirschhorn, K., Bach, F., Kolodny, R.L., Firschein, I.L. and Hashem, N. (1963). Immune response and mitosis of human peripheral blood lymphocytes in vitro. Science 142, 1185.

Hoffmann, T.K., Donnenberg, V.S., Friebe-Hoffmann, U. et al. (2000). Competition of peptide-MHC class I tetrameric complexes with anti-CD3 provides evidence for specificity of peptide binding to the TCR complex. Cytometry 41, 321–328.

June, C.H., Ledbetter, J.A., Rabinovitch, P.S., Martin, P.J., Beatty, P.G. and Hansen, J.A. (1986). Distinct patterns of transmembrane calcium flux and intracellular calcium mobilization after differentiation antigen cluster 2 (E rosette receptor) or 3 (T3) stimulation of human lymphocytes. J Clin Invest 77, 1224–1232.

Kamentsky, (2003). In Practical Flow Cytometry, 3rd edn, Shapiro, H.M., ed. Hoboken, NJ: Wiley Liss, p. xivii.

Kedar, E. and Bonavida, B. (1975). Studies on the induction and expression of T cell-mediated immunity. IV. Non-overlapping populations of alloimmune cytotoxic lymphocytes with specificity for tumor-associated antigens and transplantation antigens. J Immunol 115, 1301–1308.

Kung, P., Goldstein, G., Reinherz, E.L. and Schlossman, S.F. (1979). Monoclonal antibodies defining distinctive human T cell surface antigens. Science 206, 347–349.

Landsteiner, K. and Chase, M.W. (1942). Experiments in transfer of cutaneous sensitivity to simple comounds. Proc Soc Exp Biol Med 49, 688–690.

Li, X. and Darzynkiewicz, Z. (1995). Labelling DNA strand breaks with BrdUTP. Detection of apoptosis and cell proliferation. Cell Prolif 28, 571–579.

Liu, L., Chahroudi, A., Silvestri, G. et al. (2002). Visualization and quantification of T cell-mediated cytotoxicity using cell-permeable fluorogenic caspase substrates. Nat Med 8, 185–189.

Loken, M.R. and Herzenberg, L.A. (1975). Analysis of cell populations with a fluorescence-activated cell sorter. Ann NY Acad Sci 254, 163–171.

Loken, M.R., Parks, D.R. and Herzenberg, L.A. (1977). Two-color immunofluorescence using a fluorescence-activated cell sorter. J Histochem Cytochem 25, 899–907.

Lyons, A.B., Samuel, K., Sanderson, A. and Maddy, A.H. (1992). Simultaneous analysis of immunophenotype and apoptosis of murine thymocytes by single laser flow cytometry. Cytometry 13, 809–821.

Mandy, F., Nicholson, J., Autran, B. and Janossy, G. (2002). T-cell subset counting and the fight against AIDS: reflections over a 20-year struggle. Cytometry 50, 39–45.

Mandy, F.F., Nicholson, J.K. and McDougal, J.S. (2003). Guidelines for Performing Single-Platform Absolute CD4+ T-Cell Determinations with CD45 Gating for Persons Infected with Human Immunodeficiency Virus. MMWR. 52(No. RR02): 1–13.

Margolick, J.B., Donnenberg, A.D., Munoz, A. et al. (1993). Changes in T and non-T lymphocyte subsets following seroconversion to HIV-1: stable CD3+ and declining CD3− populations suggest regulatory responses linked to loss of CD4 lymphocytes. The Multicenter AIDS Cohort Study. J Acq Immune Defic Synd 6, 153–161.

Margolick, J.B., Muñoz, A., Donnenberg, A.D. et al. for the multicenter AIDS cohort study. (1995). Failure of T-cell homeostasis preceding AIDS in HIV-1 infection. Nat Med 1, 674–681.

Margolick, J.B. and Donnenberg, A.D. (1997). T-cell homeostasis in HIV-1 infection. Sem Immunol 9, 381–388.

Mitchell, G.F., Chan, E.L., Noble, M.S., Weissman, I.L., Mishell, R.I. and Herzenberg, L.A. (1972). Immunological memory in mice. 3. Memory to heterologous erythrocytes in both T cell and B cell populations and requirement for T cells in expression of B cell memory. Evidence using immunoglobulin allotype and mouse alloantigen theta markers with congenic mice. J Exp Med 135, 165–184.

Morimoto, C., Letvin, N.L., Boyd, A.W. et al. (1985a). The isolation and characterization of the human helper inducer T cell subset. J Immunol 134, 3762–3769.

Morimoto, C., Letvin, N.L., Distaso, J.A., Aldrich, W.R. and Schlossman, S.F. (1985b). The isolation and characterization of

the human suppressor inducer T cell subset. J Immunol 134, 1508–1515.

Murphy, R.F. and Chused, T.M. (1984). A proposal for a flow cytometric data file standard. Cytometry 5, 553–555.

Noel, D.R., Witherspoon, R.P., Storb, R. et al. (1978). Does graft-versus-host disease influence the tempo of immunologic recovery after allogeneic human marrow transplantation? An observation on 56 long-term survivors. Blood 51, 1087–1105.

Nordon, R.E., Ginsberg, S.S. and Eaves, C.J. (1997). High-resolution cell division tracking demonstrates the FLt3-ligand-dependence of human marrow CD34+CD38− cell production in vitro. Br J Haematol 98, 528–553.

Nowell, P.C. (1960). PHA: An initiator of mitosis in cultures of normal human leukocytes. Cancer Res 20, 562.

O'Gorman, M.R. and Gelman, R. (1997). Inter- and intrainstitutional evaluation of automated volumetric capillary cytometry for the quantitation of CD4- and CD8-positive T lymphocytes in the peripheral blood of persons infected with human immunodeficiency virus. Site Investigators and the NIAID New CD4 Technologies Focus Group. Clin Diag Lab Immunol 4, 173–179.

Paxton, H., Kidd, P., Landay, A. et al. (1989). Results of the flow cytometry ACTG quality control program: analysis and findings. Clin Immunol Immunopathol 52, 68–84.

Pearson, T., Galfre, G., Ziegler, A. and Milstein, C. (1977). A myeloma hybrid producing antibody specific for an allotypic determinant on 'IgD-like' molecules of the mouse. Eur J Immunol 7, 684–690.

Perez, O.D. and Nolan, G.P. (2002). Simultaneous measurement of multiple active kinase states using polychromatic flow cytometry. Nat Biotechnol 20, 155–162.

Picker, L.J., Treer, J.R., Ferguson-Darnell, B., Collins, P.A., Buck, D. and Terstappen, L.W. (1993). Control of lymphocyte recirculation in man. I. Differential regulation of the peripheral lymph node homing receptor L-selectin on T cells during the virgin to memory cell transition. J Immunol 150, 1105–1121.

Reinherz, E.L., Geha, R., Wohl, M.E., Morimoto, C., Rosen, F.S. and Schlossman, S.F. (1981). Immunodeficiency associated with loss of T4+ inducer T-cell function. N Eng J Med 304, 811–816.

Roederer, M. (2001). Spectral compensation for flow cytometry: visualization artifacts, limitations, and caveats. Cytometry 45, 194–205.

Rosenblatt, J.I., Hokanson, J.A., McLaughlin, S.R. and Leary, J.F. (1997). Theoretical basis for sampling statistics useful for detecting and isolating rare cells using flow cytometry and cell sorting. Cytometry 27, 233–238.

Sallusto, F., Lenig, D., Forster, R., Lipp, M. and Lanzavecchia, A. (1999). Two subsets of memory T lymphocytes with distinct homing potentials and effector functions. Nature 401, 708–712.

Sanders, M.E., Makgoba, M.W., Sharrow, S.O. et al. (1988). Human memory T lymphocytes express increased levels of three cell adhesion molecules (LFA-3, CD2, and LFA-1) and three other molecules (UCHL1, CDw29, and Pgp-1) and have enhanced IFN-gamma production. J Immunol 140, 1401–1407.

Shapiro, H.M. (1995). Practical flow cytometry, 3rd edn. New York: Wiley-Liss, p. 276.

Shapiro, H.M. (ed.) (2003). Practical Flow Cytometry, 4th edn. Hoboken, NJ: John Wiley and Sons, pp. 565–566.

(2003). In Practical Flow Cytometry, 4th edn, Shapiro, H.M., ed. Hoboken, NJ: John Wiley and Sons, pp. 460.

Smith, S.H., Brown, M.H., Rowe, D., Callard, R.E. and Beverley, P.C. (1986). Functional subsets of human helper-inducer cells defined by a new monoclonal antibody, UCHL1. Immunology 58, 63–70.

Sutherland, D.R., Anderson, L., Keene, Y.M., Nayar, R. and Chin-Yee, I. (1996). The ISHAGE guidelines for CD34+ cell determination by flow cytometry. International Society of Hematotherapy and Graft Engineering. J Hematother 5, 213–226.

Tedder, T.F., Cooper, M.D. and Clement, L.T. (1985). Human lymphocyte differentiation antigens HB-10 and HB-11. II. Differential production of B cell growth and differentiation factors by distinct helper T cell subpopulations. J Immunol 134, 2989–2994.

Trowbridge, I.S. (1978). Interspecies spleen-myeloma hybrid producing monoclonal antibodies against mouse lymphocyte surface glycoprotein, T200. J Exp Med 148, 313–323.

Trowbridge, I.S. and Thomas, M.L. (1994). CD45: an emerging role as a protein tyrosine phosphatase required for lymphocyte activation and development. Annu Rev Immunol 12, 85–116.

van den Engh, G. (1993). New applications of flow cytometry. Curr Opin Biotechnol 4, 63–68.

Wersto, R.P., Chrest, F.J., Leary, J.F., Morris, C., Stetler-Stevenson, M.A. and Gabrielson, E. (2001). Doublet discrimination in DNA cell-cycle analysis. Cytometry 46, 296–306.

White, R.A., Mason, D.W., Williams, A.F., Galfre, G. and Milstein, C. (1978). T-lymphocyte heterogeneity in the rat: separation of functional subpopulations using a monoclonal antibody. J Exp Med 148, 664–673.

Winchester, R.J. and Ross, G. (1976). Methods for enumerating lymphocyte populations. In Manual of Clinical Immunology, Rose, N.R. and Friedman, H., eds. Washington DC: ASM Press, pp. 64–76.

Natural Killer Cells

Chapter 21

Bice Perussia and Matthew J. Loza

Jefferson Medical College, Department of Microbiology and Immunology, Kimmel Cancer Center, Philadelphia, PA, USA

The Master said: 'Yu, shall I tell you what it is to know? To say you know when you know, and to say you do not know when you do not, that is knowledge'

(Confucius, 551–479 BC) Lun Yü (Analects), II.17

INTRODUCTION

The existence of major histocompatibility complex (MHC)-non-restricted, spontaneously cytotoxic cells was originally proposed based on the observation that peripheral blood lymphocytes of any individual kill a variety of allogeneic and tumor target cells independently from previous sensitization. This was followed by the proposition that the putative effector cells might be involved in tumor immune surveillance (reviewed in Trinchieri, 1989). Appreciation of the existence of cells with immediate effector functions in viral infections (reviewed in Trinchieri, 1989) and in the rejection of parental hematopoietic transplants and 'hybrid resistance' (reviewed in Bennett, 1996), prompted studies that resulted in the physical separation and identification of natural killer (NK) cells as a leukocyte population, expressing receptors for the Fc portion of IgG (Fcγ R$^+$), mediating both spontaneous and antibody-dependent cytotoxicity and representing an average 15 per cent of peripheral lymphocytes, with high inter-donor variability (Perussia, 1998). Based on those studies, mature peripheral NK cells are now defined as a discrete lymphocyte subset expressing a characteristic combination of clusters of differentiation antigens (CD),

among which CD161 and CD16 and CD56 in humans, are most characteristic, in the absence of expression and gene rearrangement for T and B antigen (Ag)-specific receptors (i.e. the T cell receptor (TCR) and surface immunoglobulins (sIg)) (Lanier, 1986b). The following discussion focuses on the knowledge available in humans relevant to identifying NK cells in clinical settings.

NK CELL ROLE IN IMMUNE RESPONSES

NK cells mediate effector functions as a first line of defense in non-adaptive responses against virus-, intracellular bacteria-, and parasite-infected cells (reviewed in Trinchieri, 1989), especially those expressing low MHC class I molecule levels, primarily via cytotoxicity. However, they also regulate and modulate hematopoietic cell biology and the activity of other effector cells of the innate and adaptive systems of defense via cytokine production. In the mouse, interferon (IFN)-κ production by mature NK cells (Orange and Biron, 1996) directs the development of type 1 IFN-γ^+ cytotoxic T cells and thus effective adaptive cell-mediated responses to intracellular pathogens (reviewed in Trinchieri, 1989 and Coffman et al., 1991). Via production of granulocyte-macrophage-colony stimulating factor (GM-CSF), interleukin (IL)-3, IFN-γ and tumor necrosis factor (TNF)-α (reviewed in Perussia, 1996), NK cells also participate in the regulation of extra-medullary hematopoiesis (Hansson et al., 1988; Siefer et al., 1993) and activation of myeloid and monocytic cells (reviewed

Measuring Immunity, edited by Michael T. Lotze and Angus W. Thomson
ISBN 0-12-455900-X, London

in Trinchieri et al., 1993). Additionally, via production of IL-5 and possibly other factors likely also regulating humoral immune responses (Yuan et al., 1994), they play a significant role in *in vivo* models of asthma-associated eosinophilia (Walker et al., 1998; Korsgren et al., 1999). A minor subset(s) of IL-13- (Hoshino et al., 1999) and of IL-5-producing NK cells had been described in adult peripheral blood (Warren et al., 1995).

The possibility that production of type 1 and type 2 cytokines is a function of NK cells at different developmental stages was proposed based on the observation that immature IFN-γ^- CD161$^+$ NK cells in neonatal (umbilical cord) blood and in *in vitro* culture models for NK-cell differentiation are capable of producing IL-5 and IL-13 (Bennett et al., 1996a; Loza et al., 2002d). A possible equivalent DX5$^+$ population with phenotype distinct from that of mature NK, T or myeloid cells and reminiscent of that of human immature CD161$^+$CD56$^-$ NK cells, exists in the murine bone marrow, closely associated to immature B cells and protects them from B cell receptor engagement-induced apoptosis (Sandel et al., 2001).

Both T and NK cells are critical to support generation of inflammatory immune responses for successful pathogen eradication. Inflammatory mediators produced by accessory myeloid cells that first interact with the pathogen (monocytes and dendritic cells (DC)) induce rapid NK-cell activation. Among these, the major one affecting NK cells is IL-12, produced after the initial wave of IFN-α and TNF-α (reviewed in Trinchieri, 1998). IFN-α also plays several roles relevant to the initiation of inflammatory and type 1 responses, increasing expression of the signal transducing subunit of the IL-12R (IL-12Rβ2) (Wu et al., 2000), also regulated by IL-18 (Chang et al., 2000) and inducing production of IL-15 (Santini et al., 2000), a cytokine that allows proliferation or survival of both T and NK cells. The same monokines enhance NK cell cytotoxicity and IFN-γ production. The IFN-γ produced by NK cells in response to pathogen-induced IL-12 or IFN-α acts to increase IL-12 production and Ag-presentation by the monocytic cells and primes T cells to respond to IL-12, contributing to the generation of type 1 immune responses. TNF-α and GM-CSF, also produced by NK cells under these conditions, further contribute to the inflammatory milieu promoting generation, mobilization and activation of myeloid cells.

Aside from stimulation by cytokines, cytokine production is induced in mature NK cells by poorly characterized cellular interactions. An important regulatory effect of NK cells on the antigen-presenting/processing cells (APC) for adaptive responses, especially DC, has been identified, depending on a bi-directional activation of DC and NK cells during their interaction via specific 'NK cell-activating receptors' involved in DC recognition (Ferlazzo et al., 2002; Gerosa et al., 2002; Piccioli et al., 2002). These interactions are likely relevant to initiation and maintenance of immune responses, especially related to tumor immunity in tissues.

NK CELL DEVELOPMENT

NK cells originate and develop in the bone marrow from CD34$^+$ pluripotent stem cells that, under the influence of cytokines like IL-1 and IL-6, progress to the stage of self-renewing multipotent lymphoid progenitors. NK-cell differentiation is controlled by cytokines produced in an intact bone marrow microenvironment (reviewed in Sivakumar et al., 1998). In the mouse, these include Flt-3-ligand (L), c-*kit*-L (stem cell factor, SCF) and IL-15 acting, alone or together, on NK cells at different stages of differentiation (Williams et al., 1997). Flt-3-L and IL-15 also sustain differentiation of human CD34$^+$ cells to cells functionally and phenotypically similar to mature peripheral blood NK cells. Produced by stromal and monocytic/myeloid cells (Doherty et al., 1996), they likely act *in vivo* in physiologic conditions (reviewed in Carson and Caligiuri, 1996). Possible differential effects of these cytokines during NK cell differentiation have been analyzed at the level of the most immature precursor stages (Cavazzana-Calvo et al., 1996; Yu et al., 1998; Muench et al., 2000), when lineage-specific markers are not yet identifiable. In mouse (Delfino et al., 1991; Migliorati et al., 1992) and humans (Lotzova et al., 1992; Silva et al., 1994; Shibuya et al., 1995; Jaleco et al., 1997) IL-2 efficiently substitutes for IL-15 *in vitro* to support NK cell differentiation from CD34$^+$ or lineage negative (Lin$^-$) hematopoietic progenitor cells. The analysis of *in vitro* models of human NK cell differentiation from neonatal blood Lin$^-$ or CD34$^+$ hematopoietic progenitor cells (Bennett, 1996) served to establish that expression of CD161 (NKR-P1A) in the absence of other mature NK cell markers defines NK cells at a relatively immature phenotypic and functional stage of differentiation, at which the cells mediate TNF-related activation-induced ligand (TRAIL), but not FasL- or granule exocytosis-dependent cytotoxicity (Zamai et al., 1998) (see later) and express type 2 cytokines (Loza et al., 2002d), but not IFN-γ, even upon stimulation. Similar functional analysis in the mouse is yet to be performed.

TERMINAL NK CELL DEVELOPMENT IN THE PERIPHERY

Like for CD34$^+$, Ln$^-$ and myeloid cells, minor proportions of immature NK cells exist in the periphery (Loza et al., 2002c), with phenotypic characteristics similar to those of the immature CD161$^+$D56$^-$ cells generated in the *in vitro* cultures of hematopoietic progenitor cells. Like in those cells, their differentiation is induced, *in vitro*, in the presence of IL-12. Combined analysis of phenotype and cytokine production at the single cell level has provided direct evidence that immature peripheral NK cells proceed, transiting through an intermediate IL-13$^+$IFN-γ^+ stage, along a linear differentiation pathway from highly proliferative CD161$^+$ CD56$^-$ IL-13$^+$, to non- or minimally proliferative mature CD161$^+$CD56$^+$ IFN-γ^+ cells (Loza and Perussia, 2001).

This process is marked by sequential expression of functionally relevant differentiation antigens. Among these, the first ones expressed, independently from functional changes, are CD56 and, concomitantly, the CD94:NKG2A receptor capable of binding HLA-E and transducing signals inhibiting cytotoxicity upon engagement (Lopez-Botet et al., 1998). This is followed, concomitant to functional changes related to acquisition of ability to mediate granule exocytosis-dependent cytotoxicity and production of IFN-γ with loss of type 2 cytokine production, by expression of activating receptors, e.g. CD2 and NKp46 (Sivori et al., 1997) and finally CD16, CD8 on a proportion of the cells and the killer Ig-like receptors (KIR, both with inhibitory or activating functions) capable of binding relatively restricted MHC haplotypes (Colonna, 1997). The exact stage during development at which CD244 (2B4, an adhesion molecule of the CD2 family) (Mathew et al., 1993; Boles et al., 1999) and the (co)stimulatory/activating NKG2D molecule, expressed on most peripheral NK cells and recognizing the stress-induced MHC-like molecules MICA and B (Bauer et al., 1999), are expressed is yet to be defined. CD244 is expressed at early developmental stages both in mouse and humans (Rosmaraki et al., 2001; Sivori et al., 2002). It is likely that NKG2D is expressed, like most KIR, on cells at a relatively late stage, based on its expression concomitant with that of CD94 on NK cells derived in vitro from mouse embryonic stem cells (Lian et al., 2002) and association of the encoding genes to the NK locus, containing also CD94 (Sobanov et al., 1999). The sequence of acquisition of the distinct phenotypic markers is consistent with that, in the mouse, of functionally equivalent, though (with the exception of CD94 (Vance et al., 1997)) structurally distinct markers (Williams et al., 1997; Rosmaraki et al., 2001).

The developmental process of peripheral immature CD161$^+$CD56$^-$ human NK cells, which is accompanied by loss of GATA 3 (expressed in early lymphocytes (Hendriks et al., 1999)) and acquisition of T-bet expression (Loza and Perussia, 2001), is regulated by IL-12 and additional cytokines produced by accessory cells in the culture. It is momentarily retarded by IL-4 via induced proliferation of the immature cells and resumes as this cytokine is withdrawn from the microenvironment (Loza and Perussia, 2001). Like most differentiation processes, that of peripheral NK cells is irreversible. The terminally differentiated cells can then be further activated by IL-12 and other cytokines or ligands, some of which (e.g. immune complexes, IL-12, IL-2 (Azzoni et al., 1998; Perussia, 1998)) also modulate expression of specific markers (e.g. CD56, CD16, CD161, IL-12R, activating receptors) and finally produce IL-10 before undergoing activation-induced death by apoptosis (Loza and Perussia, 2001, discussed for its implications in Perussia and Loza, 2003). Thus, NK cell development involves at least two sequential phenotypically distinct (CD56$^-$ and CD56$^+$) stages functionally characterized by production of type 2 and type 1 cytokines (Loza and Perussia, 2001) and by the usage of distinct cytotoxic mechanisms (Zamai et al., 1998).

Interestingly, most T cells share NK cell differentiation antigen expression when, like NK cells at their latest differentiation stages, they lose ability to produce type 2 cytokines and to proliferate and gain that of producing IFN-γ (Loza et al., 2002a,b). IL-12 and monokines coordinately regulate a maturation pathway identical to that of NK cells also in T cells (including the CD1d-restricted invariant NKT cells recognizing α-galactosyl ceramide (α-GalCer) as surrogate antigen for mammalian glycolipids) and TCR stimulation modulates it via induced IL-12Rβ_2 expression (Loza et al., 2002a; Perussia and Loza, 2003). These data unravel the bases on which the CD1d-restricted invariant α-GalCer-activated NKT cells (and possibly, given the striking similarities between these cell types at their latest developmental stages, terminally differentiated (antigen)-activated T and NK cells) can alternatively regulate immune responses via production of type 1 or type 2 cytokines (Godfrey et al., 2000). Knowledge that CD56 expression by T cells correlates with an effector, IFN-γ^+ type 2 cytokine$^-$ phenotype may be of clinical, prognostic or diagnostic value in predicting the efficacy of responses to specific immune therapies.

NK CELLS IN PATHOLOGIC CONDITIONS

A primary in vivo role of NK cells has been established, based on a direct significant correlation between NK-cell status (number and cytotoxic functions) and disease progression in the eradication of murine cytomegalovirus infection (Orange et al., 1995; Andrews et al., 2003) and in the generation of type 1 immune responses to intracellular pathogens (reviewed in Trinchieri, 2003). This is confirmed in humans by the observations of recurrent viral and bacterial infections and death in patients with severe deficiencies in NK-cell numbers (Biron et al., 1989) or functions (Roder et al., 1980), also associated with increased tumor frequency (Targan and Oseas, 1983). Supporting this evidence, additional informative studies include:

1 association between decreased NK-cell numbers and cytotoxic function in patients with familial melanoma and their relatives (Hersey et al., 1979), suggesting a role for these cells in controlling tumor progression
2 association of disease state (tumor burden) with qualitative or quantitative alterations in signal transduction (Whiteside, 1999), the mechanistic bases for which are yet to be defined
3 possible role of NK cells in leukemia progression (Silla et al., 1995), given their cytotoxic potential against immature hematopoietic cells
4 presence of NK cells with 'activated' phenotype in inflammatory conditions associated with autoimmune diseases like rheumatoid arthritis (Dalbeth and Callan, 2002) and chronic hepatitis (Valiante et al., 2000), although it remains to be determined whether these are a consequence or cause of the disease.

PRINCIPLES

Based on the accumulated information on NK cell development, it is to be expected that, depending on the immunologic 'history' of an individual, peripheral CD161+CD56+ NK cells contain variable proportions of phenotypically distinct but developmentally related populations. Thus, determining whether NK cells participate in, or are altered in their numbers or functions in pathological conditions, involves determining the developmental stage of the cells with NK (CD3−CD161+) phenotype, after definitive exclusion that they are T cells based on combined phenotyping for TCR expression (CD3 as a surrogate). This may be difficult, because it is unlikely that their numbers and functions are established for comparison with those during disease, in the same individual before disease onset. Concomitant analysis of phenotype, cytotoxic potential and cytokine production at the single cell level is the sole means to ascribe specific functions to cells that are possibly at different developmental stages. NK cell phenotyping based solely on CD161, CD56 and CD16 detection is diagnostic only in rare total NK-cells deficiencies (Biron et al., 1989). However, in all other conditions, phenotypic analysis defining the developmental or 'activation' state of the detectable CD56+ CD16+/− NK cells can provide information on whether the cells may be involved (because of functional deficiencies) in the specific pathology and give indirect indication, based on expression levels of differentiation and activation antigens, of an inflammatory process and on whether innate effectors are available functionally relevant to modulating the responses.

APPLICATIONS

Surface phenotyping

The only marker, at present, detecting all peripheral cells defined as NK, including the immature CD56− ones, is CD161 (Table 21.1). Both in humans and mouse immature cells at a pre-CD161 stage may be recognizable based on CD244 (2B4) expression (Rosmaraki et al., 2001; Sivori et al., 2002), but lack of definitive characterization of the distribution of this marker on immature cells other than NK in the periphery precludes, at present, its use as a diagnostic marker. Further definition of the differentiation stage of NK cells relies on phenotypic analysis of the markers for which the sequence of appearance has been established in peripheral cells and clonal populations derived from them (Loza and Perussia, 2001) and in cells at sequential developmental stages in *in vitro* culture models for human (Bennett, 1996; Loza et al., 2002d) and mouse (Williams, 1997 et al.; Rosmaraki et al., 2001) NK-cell differentiation.

Both adult and neonatal NK cells are detectable in immunofluorescence (flow cytometry preferable) as cells with light scatter characteristics of lymphocytes, not expressing CD3 or other markers characteristic of B (sIg, CD19, CD20 or CD21), myeloid (CD15) and monocytic cells (CD14) (Figure 21.1). All NK cells in this population express CD161, but include both CD56+ (mature) and CD56− (immature) cells. Within the CD161+CD56+ cells, two populations are generally detected expressing CD56 at distinctly different levels. Most cells are CD56+lo; a variable, usually low, proportion of them is CD56+hi (Lanier et al., 1986a; Carson et al., 1997) and includes cells expressing either low or undetectable CD16 levels (Nagler et al., 1989). The CD56+hi cells have been proposed to represent a functionally 'unique' NK cell subset exerting low-to-null levels of granule exocytosis-mediated cytotoxicity (Nagler et al., 1989) (against the prototypic K562 target cells) and capable of producing both type1 and type 2 cytokines (Cooper et al., 2001). However, their definitive characterization as a more immature or distinct functionally 'specialized' subset, as proposed (Nagler et al., 1989; Cooper et al., 2001), awaits conclusive analysis at the single cell level. Indeed, the observations that these cells express differentiation antigens of mature NK cells, produce IL-10, detectable only in T and NK cells at the latest differentiation stages (Loza et al., 2001, 2002b) and can be present in significant proportions in the lymph node (Fehniger et al., 2003), where NK cells with mature resting phenotype are not detectable, are consistent with the hypothesis (and our preliminary unpublished data) that the CD56+hi NK cells are cells at the most terminally differentiated, mature and activated stage. Thus, their presence at higher proportions *in vivo* (e.g. systemically during IL-2 therapy (Caligiuri et al., 1990) and in inflamed tissues in autoimmune diseases like rheumatoid arthritis (Dalbeth and Callan, 2002)) likely witnesses occurred activation of effector functions in terminally differentiated cells.

Detection of CD161+ NK cells expressing only a partial combination of the markers of mature peripheral NK cells (e.g. lacking CD94, NKG2A (Wu et al., 1999), 'activating' receptors like NKp46 (Sivori et al., 1997) and NKp30 (Bottino et al., 1996) and CD244, all known to be expressed on most peripheral mature NK cells (Stepp et al., 1999)) may reflect alterations in NK-cell development, or *in vivo* conditions favoring their accumulation either directly, inducing their proliferation or inhibiting their differentiation, or indirectly, inducing terminal differentiation and death of the most mature cells, thus resulting in increased proportions of the immature ones. Distinguishing among these possibilities involves accurate evaluation of the absolute numbers of CD161+CD56+/− NK cells.

The lack, or reduced expression, of KIR and CD16 may instead be more difficult to interpret, given their late appearance during development (Loza and Perussia, 2001). In the absence of their expression, identification of the encoding specific mRNAs is needed before considering possible defects of accessory molecules necessary for their expression and signal transduction (e.g. CD3- and FcεRI-associated ζ and γ chains, or DAP family members).

Table 21.1 NK cell differentiation antigens and functions

Antigen/function		NK cell differentiation stage				
		CD161− CD56− CD16−	CD161+ CD56− CD16−	CD161+ CD56+ CD16−	CD161+ CD56+ CD16+	CD161+ CD56+hi CD16−/lo
Activating receptors	KIR, *activating*	−	−	?	?	?
	CD94:NKG2C	−	−	?	±	?
	NKG2D	?	?	?	+	?
	NKp30	?	?	?	+	?
	NKp44	−	−	−*	−*	+lo*
	NKp46	−	−	±	+	+hi
Inhibitory receptors	KIR, *inhibitory*	−	−	−	±	±
	CD94:NKG2A	−	−	±	+	+hi
Co-stimulatory/ adhesion molecules	CD2	−	−	±	+	+hi
	CD8	−	−	+	±	±
	CD11b	−	±	+	+	+
	CD62L	?	?	?	±	+
	CD162R (PEN5)	?	?	?	±	−
	CD244 (2B4)	?	+	+	+	+
	NKp80	?	?	?	+	?
Activation Ag	CD25	?	±	?	−*	+lo
	CD45RO	?	?	?	−	±
	HLA-DR	+/?	±	?	−	+lo/hi
Cytokines	GM-CSF	?	+	+	+	+
	IFN-γ	−	−	±	+lo/hi	+lo/hi
	IL-3**	?	?	?	?	?
	IL-5	?/+	±	−	−	−
	IL-10	?	−	−	−	−
	IL-13	?/+	+	±lo	−	−
	TNF-α	?	+	+	+	+
Cytotoxic mechanisms	TRAIL-L	?	+	?	−	−
	FasL	−	−	+	+	+
	Granule exocytosis	−	−	+	+	+

* Rapidly induced by IL-2 or IL-15.
** At present, mRNA demonstrated inducible only upon maximal non-specific stimulation.
? to be determined.
+lo, +hi, relatively low or high expression.
+lo/hi, distinct populations detectable expressing, respectively, relatively low and high levels.

Alternatively or in addition, the absence or low-to-undetectable expression of NK cell-specific markers on cells that are CD56+ may depend on their occurred downmodulation *in vivo* following ligand interaction or cytokine stimulation (e.g. CD16 is downmodulated upon immune-complex engagement, (Perussia, 1998); IL-12 enhances CD161 and CD56 expression while downmodulating that of CD16 (Azzoni et al., 1998)). Finally, constitutive expression of molecules like NKp44, MHC class II antigens (HLA-DR), CD68, CD25 (the high affinity IL-2R α chain) and CD62L on freshly *ex vivo*-derived NK cells likely reflects (*in vivo*) occurred activation. Thus, caution should be exerted in launching a definition of 'unique subsets' without a complete accurate phenotypic and functional characterization of the cells.

Cytokine production

Aside from GM-CSF and TNF-α, expressed during development at decreasing levels but by most NK cells (Loza et al., 2002d), most mature peripheral NK cells produce, upon stimulation, low levels of IFN-γ, whereas only a minor fraction produces high levels of IFN-γ or type 2 cytokines. Accurate determination of functional NK-cell competence requires identification of the cytokines produced at the single cell level and at least two of them can be detected by intracellular cytokine analysis combined with surface phenotyping by immunofluorescence to identify conclusively the cytokine-producing cells. A limitation of this analysis, possible only on fixed cells, is that it involves cell stimulation for a limited length of time and in the presence of inhibitors of secretion (e.g. brefeldin A). However, provided there are optimal controls (Loza et al., 2003), a significant positive correlation exists between cytokine expression levels (fluorescence intensity and per cent positive cells) and actual amount (pg/ml) of cytokines released and detectable in the supernatants of the same cells cultured for appropriately longer time-periods (Loza et al., 2002c). Thus, once alterations in secretion are excluded (unlike the case in patients with Chediak-Higashi

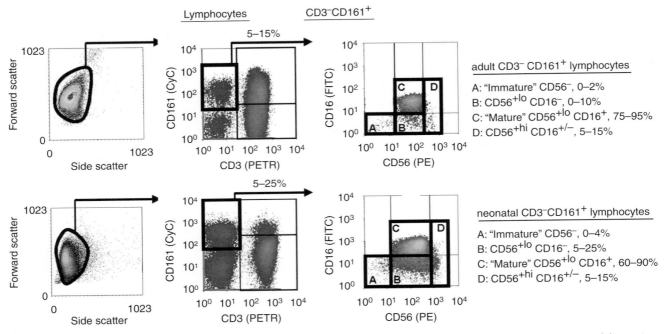

Figure 21.1 NK-cell detection in resting lymphocytes from healthy individuals. NK cells are identified, both in adult (top) and neonatal (bottom) lymphocytes, based on 4-color immunofluorescence detecting CD3, CD161 (x- and y-axis; middle panels, gated on cells with light scatter characteristics of lymphocytes, boxed regions in the density plots at the left), CD56 and CD16 (x- and y-axis; right panels, gated cells on CD3−CD161+ cells, boxed regions in the density plots in the middle). Middle:CD3−CD161− cells (bottom left) include B cells, few contaminant monocytes and possibly myeloid cells when neonatal samples are analyzed); CD3+CD161+ cells (top right) include T cells expressing NK cell markers and the invariant CD1d-restricted NKT cells; CD3+CD161− cells (bottom right) include most T cells; CD161+CD3− cells (top left) include all peripheral cells defined as NK. Right: the proportions and types of CD161+ NK cells (CD56±, CD16± and the relative expression of these markers) in each boxed quadrant are indicated at right. +lo, +hi, relatively low and high antigen density compared to the other populations within the NK cells identified by these markers.

syndrome or in Bg/Bg mice (reviewed in Spritz, 1998)), its results can be taken to reflect production of secreted cytokines. Other assays (ELISA or RIA), fail to give information on percentages of cells producing the cytokine of interest and ELISPOT, Northern blot or PCR analysis for mRNA expression, do not give information on actual levels of cytokine produced. Most importantly, none of these allows one to determine which cells, in the total population analyzed, produce which cytokines.

Constitutive production of specific cytokines is uncommon in resting non-stimulated PBL. However, constitutive, stimulation-independent production of type 2 cytokines (mostly IL-13) is observed in immature CD161+CD56− NK cells (Loza et al., 2002c), possibly depending on occurred activation *in vivo* by stimuli yet to be defined. The significant IL-13 levels produced by these cells are likely biologically relevant in clinical settings where, like in allergy, accumulation of immature CD56− NK (and T) cells can be demonstrated in the tissues affected by the pathological process (Table 21.2). The possibility of *in vivo* occurred stimulation, if suspected on this basis, is further supported if stimulation with NK cell-specific ligands (e.g. target cells, immune complexes, NK cell activating cytokines) induces cytokine levels and proportions of cytokine+ cells

similar to those detected upon maximal non-specific (PMA+Ca^{2+} ionophore+IL-2) stimulation.

Cytotoxicity

This is the result of an energy-dependent process involving a complex series of events including NK cell binding to the target cells via specific 'activating' receptors or combinations of adhesion molecules recognizing their ligands on the target cells; triggering of degranulation and release of preformed granules containing cytotoxic proteins (perforin and granzymes, serine-esterase family enzymes); and finally target cell death (reviewed in Trinchieri, 1989). Also, the cytotoxicity levels mediated by NK cells depend on the net result of positive (activation) and negative signals (KIR-mediated inhibition upon MHC binding) transduced in the NK cells (Renard et al., 1997). Alternatively, and in addition, NK cells induce apoptosis in susceptible target cells via binding, by constitutive or inducible ligands (FasL, TRAIL, membrane-bound TNF-α), of the respective receptors on the target (especially tumor) cells, all belonging to the TNF-R family of 'death receptors'. This occurs independently from active NK cell participation. Importantly, resting immature CD161+CD56− cells

Table 21.2 IL-13 production by NK cells in bronchoalveolar lavage from allergen-challenged atopic subjects

Stimulus Time, h	RWE Atopic A[a] None	RWE Atopic B		non-RWE Atopic C PMA+ion	non-RWE Atopic D	
		None	PMA+iono		None	PMA+iono
0	3.8[b]	0.5	0.5	ND[c]	0.0	0.2
24	ND	5.0	5.8	0.0	0.0	0.2

[a] Leukocytes from bronchoalveolar lavage (BAL) performed before (0), or 24 h after segmental allergen challenge with ragweed E (RWE) in two RWE-allergic (A, B) and two non-allergic (C, D) patients were cultured for 5 h with brefeldin A only (none), or in the presence of PMA and Ca^{2+} ionophore (PMA + iono). IL-13 and $CD3^-CD161^+$ NK cell detection was by 4-color intracellular immunofluorescence (flow cytometry) (Loza et al., 2003). Lymphocytes within BAL leukocytes were: A, time 0 = 40 per cent, 3 per cent of which NK cells; B, time 0 = 13 per cent, 24 h = 5 per cent, 3.3 per cent and 16.4 per cent of which, respectively, NK cells; C, 24 h = 6 per cent, 6.5 per cent of which NK cells; D, time 0 = 12 per cent, 24 h = 10 per cent, 9 per cent and 10 per cent of which, respectively, NK cells.
[b] Numbers are % $IL-13^+$ NK cells.
[c] Not done, insufficient cells for analysis.

are only capable of TRAIL-mediated cytotoxicity, whereas the mature cells, $CD56^+$, mediate both granule exocytosis and Fas-, but not TRAIL-dependent cytotoxicity (Zamai et al., 1998).

Cytotoxicity assays use the leukemic erythromyeloid K562 cell line, $Fas^-/TRAIL^-$ and expressing only low levels HLA-CW3 (Le Bouteiller et al., 2002), as prototype target cells for granule exocytosis-mediated cytotoxicity, which is completely abolished in the presence of Ca^{2+} chelators following inhibition of perforin assembly and thus pore formation, in the target cells; and the Jurkat T lymphoblastoid cell line, expressing Fas, TRAIL-R and TNF-R, as target for Fas-, TRAIL- and TNF-α-mediated cytotoxicity. The simplest assays rely on ^{51}Cr release from pre-labeled targets using serial effector cell dilutions to allow quantitation of cytotoxicity in a fixed time-period (3–4 h for the granule exocytosis, longer times for the Fas/TRAIL/TNF-α-mediated mechanisms). Easy to execute, these assays are informative of the functional capability of NK cells only if they allow:

1 quantitation of cytotoxicity levels
2 comparison with the pre-disease state.

The former is accomplished in assays with serial effector-to-target cell ratios upon determination of the absolute number of lytic units (LU) in the population under exam. These are defined as the numbers of effector cells needed to induce release of a predetermined percentage of ^{51}Cr equated, for practical reasons, to the proportion of target cells lysed (Pross et al., 1981) in the assay period. The second prerequisite is, in most cases, impossible to be met. However, comparison with cytotoxicity mediated by NK cells of 'healthy' control donors may provide some information. Given the high inter-donor variability of NK cell percentages and cytotoxic potential and the inter-experimental variability characteristic of ^{51}Cr release assays, quantitative comparison can only be made after normalizing LU of the patient to those of two constant control PBL samples of known cytotoxic potential used in each assay.

In general, cytotoxicity assays provide useful information only in cases of complete or significantly reduced cytotoxicity, like in NK cell-deficient patients, or patients with defects in granule exocytosis (Chediak-Higashi) (Spritz, 1998) or perforin (histiolymphocytic hemophagocytosis) (Stepp et al., 2000). Of some significance, however, may be the definition of cytotoxicity levels mediated after activation with cytokines known to enhance spontaneous cytotoxicity, based on which defects of response to cytokines may be defined.

Proliferative potential

Unlike immature $CD161^+CD56^-$ cells, most mature ($CD56^+$) NK cells are resting and have limited proliferative capability (Loza and Perussia, 2001). Analysis of the proliferative capability of the NK cells may serve to confirm detection of cells with an 'activated' phenotype (see above), possibly supported also by autonomous cytokine production, especially when cells actively cycling are detected in freshly ex vivo-derived cells in short-term culture in the absence of stimulating cytokines. This is best-accomplished using 5-bromo-2'-deoxyuridine (BrdU) incorporation by immunofluorescence with commercially available Ab (Mehta and Maino, 1997). For this, BrdU is added to freshly separated lymphocytes before short-term culture with or without exogenous cytokines (e.g. IL-2, IL-15, or IL-12), or in the presence of the G1-S transition inhibitor mimosine, to determine whether the cells were actively cycling (i.e. in S phase) in vivo, before culture. Combined surface phenotyping allows definition of the cycling cells, if any. Alternatively, carboxyfluorescein diacetate succinimidyl ester (CFSE) labeling combined with surface phenotyping and cytokine production (Loza and Perussia, 2001) can be used, although this assay is complicated by the larger numbers of cells needed. As discussed above for cytotoxicity, deficiencies of NK cells to respond to specific cytokines may be revealed with these assays.

MURINE BIOMARKERS FOR HUMAN APPLICATION

In vivo analysis of murine NK cells can be informative, but only provided its conclusions are accurately tested *in vitro* with human NK cells before any prediction is made on their translational potential. This is because of three considerations cautioning against the assumption that results in the murine system bear an identical significance in humans. First, murine biomarkers readily applicable to humans are not available. The murine CD161, NKR-P1C (Giorda and Trucco, 1991) has not been identified in humans and, unlike the apparently 'neutral' human NKR-P1A CD161 isoform, it transduces signals for activation; a murine homolog of human CD56 is missing; CD8, expressed on about 50 per cent of the mature human NK cells, is not expressed on murine NK cells; activating and inhibitory receptors are members of the Ly49 family (Raulet et al., 1997) and, although mediating functions similar to KIR and apparently expressed at similar developmental stages, are structurally distinct, belonging to the C-type lectin family, 'activating' receptors like NKp46 have not been identified yet. Second, reagents are missing, at present, for a complete NK-cell analysis. Most notably, the only anti-FcγRIII (CD16) mAb available (Unkeless, 1979) cross-reacts with the FcγRII (CD32) expressed on myeloid and B cells, making its detection on NK cells cumbersome; and anti-IL-13 mAb suitable for intracellular cytokine detection are yet to be produced. Finally, most analyses are performed, in the mouse, on splenic NK cells. Given the extremely low NK-cell numbers in this organ, frequently a direct analysis of freshly obtained cells is difficult and whether splenic NK cells are developmentally and functionally identical to those in peripheral blood is yet to be determined conclusively.

USEFULENESS OF TESTS ANALYZING NK CELLS IN PATHOLOGICAL CONDITIONS

It is now apparent that cytotoxicity, although used for a long time to detect NK cells and define their functional capabilities, may provide minimal and only descriptive information on NK cell functions in clinical settings, complete NK cell deficiencies excluded. As discussed in the previous sections, the most useful information on NK cells in pathological situations derives from their accurate surface phenotyping using in all cases both CD161 (as a pan-NK cell marker) and CD56 (as the only marker capable of distinguishing between immature and mature cells) and CD3 (to exclude T cells). This analysis, combined with cell counts, provides reliable information on the absolute NK-cell number and on the developmental and activation stage of the NK cells detected. This information should then guide more sophisticated analysis of cytokine production and proliferation to test well-defined hypotheses related to the specific pathology, e.g. like in the accurate

definition of large granular lymphocyte leukemias of NK and T cell origin (Lamy and Loughran, 1999).

FUTURE PROSPECTS

Consideration of the knowledge accumulated on NK cell biology and development will allow optimization of several lines of clinical application involving NK cells, because their complete characterization in clinical settings is now possible to provide conclusive information on their pathogenetic/protective roles in selected pathologies and on the status of innate immunity. The use of CD161 to identify NK cells at all developmental stages in tissues *in situ* is also expected possible and informative, pending production of mAb for use in immunohistochemistry. Definition of the homing potential, consequences of the interactions with the APC in the periphery and possibility of genetic manipulation of NK cells at distinct developmental stages may result in the possibility of using appropriate NK cell populations as a delivery system for factors involved in the initiation and maintenance of effective immune responses, especially in cancer treatment or prevention. Understanding the mechanisms involved in the survival advantage associated with KIR ligand incompatibility in hematopoietic stem cell transplantation (Ruggeri et al., 2002) will lead to a better management of graft-versus-host-disease.

On a translational standpoint, it is now possible to propose rational manipulation of NK cells at different stages of development to exploit their specific functions in therapeutic attempts. For example, immature NK cell infusion may be proposed for supportive therapy in immune reconstitution, or as effector cells against TRAIL-sensitive tumors, whereas primarily mature activated NK cells are preferred as cytotoxic effectors against TRAIL-insensitive ones. Provided efficient tumor localization, the latter cells, adoptively transferred, may induce fast and massive tumor lysis concomitant with self-limiting toxic side effects given their limited proliferative capabilities and beneficial effects related to cross-presentation of relevant epitopes to the tumor-specific T cells. Additionally, the IL-10 produced upon activation by the terminally differentiated cells may help in the same settings to halt uncontrolled inflammatory type 1 responses and allow generation of protective (B-cell mediated) immunity.

REFERENCES

Andrews, D.M., Scalzo, A.A., Yokoyama, W.M., Smyth, M.J. and Degli-Esposti, M.A. (2003). Functional interactions between dendritic cells and NK cells during viral infection. Nat Immunol 4, 175–181.

Azzoni, L., Zatsepina, O., Abebe, B., Bennett, I.M., Kanakaraj, P. and Perussia, B. (1998). Differential transcriptional regulation of CD161 and a novel gene, 197/15a, by IL-2, IL-15 and IL-12 in NK and T cells. J Immunol 161, 3493–3500.

Bauer, S.G.V., Wu, J., Steinle, A., Phillips, J.H., Lanier, L.L. and Spies T. (1999). Activation of NK cells and T cells by NKG2D, a receptor for stress-inducible MICA. Science Wash DC 285, 727–729.

Bennett, I.M., Zatsepina, O., Zamai, L., Azzoni, L., Mikheeva, T. and Perussia, B. (1996). Definition of a natural killer NKR-P1A+/CD56-/CD16- functionally immature human NK cell subset that differentiates in vitro in the presence of interleukin 12. J Exp Med 184, 1845–1856.

Bennett, M. (1996). Biology and genetics of hybrid resistance. Adv Immunol 41, 333–641.

Biron, C.A., Byron, K.S. and Sullivan, J.L. (1989). Severe herpesvirus infections in an adolescent without natural killer cells. N Engl J Med 89, 1731–1735.

Boles, K.S., Nakajima, H., Colonna, M. et al. (1999). Molecular characterization of a novel human natural killer cell receptor homologous to mouse 2B4. Tissue Antigens 54, 27–34.

Bottino, C., Sivori, S., Vitale, M. et al. (1996). A novel surface molecule homologous to the p58/p50 family of receptors is selectively expressed on a subset of human Natural Killer cells and induces both triggering of cell functions and proliferation. Eur J Immunol 26, 1816–1824.

Caligiuri, M.A., Zmuidzinas, A., Manley, T.J., Levine, H., Smith, K.A. and Ritz, J. (1990). Functional consequences of interleukin 2 receptor expression on resting human lymphocytes. Identification of a novel Natural Killer cell subset with high affinity receptors. J Exp Med 171, 1509–1526.

Carson, W. and Caligiuri, M. (1996). Natural killer cell subsets and development. Methods 9, 327–343.

Carson, W.E., Fehniger, T.A. and Caligiuri, M.A. (1997). CD56 bright natural killer cell subsets: characterization of distinct functional responses to interleukin-2 and the c-kit ligand. Eur J Immunol 27, 354–360.

Cavazzana-Calvo, M., Hacein-bey, S., de Saint Basile, G. et al. (1996). Role of interleukin-2 (IL-2), IL-7, and IL-15 in Natural Killer cell differentiation from cord blood hematopoietic progenitor cells and from gamma c transduced Severe Combined Immunodeficiency X1 bone marrow cells. Blood 88, 3901–3909.

Chang, J.T., Segal, B.M., Nakanishi, K., Okamura, H. and Shevach, E.M. (2000). The costimulatory effect of IL-18 on the induction of antigen-specific IFN-gamma production by resting T cells is IL-12 dependent and is mediated by up-regulation of IL-12 receptor beta 2 subunit. Eur J Immunol 30, 1113–1119.

Coffman, R.L., Varkila, K., Scott, P. and Chatelain, R. (1991). Role of cytokines in the differentiation of CD4+ T-cell subsets in vivo. Immunol Rev 123, 189–207.

Colonna, M. (1997). Specificity and function of immunoglobulin superfamily NK cell inhibitory and stimulatory receptors. Immunol Rev 155, 127–133.

Cooper, M.A., Fehniger, T.A., Turner, S.C. et al. (2001). Human natural killer cells: a unique innate immunoregulatory role for the CD56 bright subset. Blood 97, 3146–3151.

Dalbeth, N. and Callan, M.F.C. (2002). A subset of Natural Killer cells is greatly expanded within inflamed joints. Arthritis Rheum 46, 1763–1772.

Delfino, D., D'Adamio, F., Migliorati, G. and Riccardi, C. (1991). Growth of murine Natural Killer cells from bone marrow in vitro: role of TNF alpha and IFN gamma. Int J Immunopharmacol 13, 943–954.

Doherty, T.M.B., Seder, R.A. and Sher, A. (1996). Induction and regulation of IL-15 expression in murine macrophages. J Immunol 156, 735–741.

Fehniger, T.A., Cooper, M.A., Nuovo, G.J. et al. (2003). CD56 bright natural killer cells are present in human lymph nodes and are activated by T cell-derived IL-2: a potential link between adaptive and innate immunity. Blood 101, 3052–3057.

Ferlazzo, G., Tsang, M.L., Moretta, L., Melioli, G., Steinman, R. and Munz, C. (2002). Human dendritic cells activate resting natural killer (NK) cells and are recognized via the NKp30 receptor by activated NK cells. J Exp Med 195, 343–351.

Gerosa, F., Baldani-Guerra, B., Nisii, C., Marchesini, V., Carra, G. and Trinchieri, G. (2002). Reciprocal activating interaction between natural killer cells and dendritic cells. J Exp Med 195, 327–333.

Giorda, R. and Trucco, M. (1991). Mouse NKR-P1. A family of genes selectively coexpressed in adherent lymphokine-activated killer cells. J Immunol 91, 1701–1708.

Godfrey, D.I., Hammond, K.J., Poulton, L.D., Smyth, M.J. and Baxter, A.G. (2000). NKT cells: facts, functions and fallacies. Immunol Today 21, 573–583.

Hansson, M., Petersson, M., Koo, G.C., Wigzell, H. and Kiessling, R. (1988). In vivo function of natural killer cells as regulators of myeloid precursor cells in the spleen. Eur J Immunol 18, 485–488.

Hendriks, R.W., Nawijn, M.C., Engel, J.D., vanDoorninck, H., Grosveld, F. and Karis, A. (1999). Expression of the transcription factor GATA-3 is required for the development of the earliest T cell progenitors in the thymus and correlates with stages of cellular proliferation in the thymus. Eur J Immunol 29, 1912–1918.

Hersey, P., Edwards, A., Honeyman, M. and McCarthy, W.H. (1979). Low natural-killer-cell activity in familial melanoma patients and their relatives. Br J Cancer 40, 113–122.

Hoshino, T., Winkler-Pickett, R.T., Mason, A.T., Ortaldo, J.R. and Young, H.A. (1999). IL-13 production by NK cells: IL-13 producing NK and T cells are present in vivo in the absence of IFN-gamma. J Immunol 162, 51–59.

Jaleco, A.C., Blom, B., Res, P. et al. (1997). Fetal liver contains committed NK progenitors, but is not a site for development of CD34+ cells into T cells. J Immunol 159, 694–702.

Korsgren, M.C.G.P., Sundler, F., Bjerke, T.T.H. et al. (1999). Natural Killer cells determine development of allergen-induced eosinophilic airway inflammation in mice. J Exp Med 189, 553–562.

Lamy, T. and Loughran, T.P.J. (1999). Current concepts: large granular lymphocyte leukemia. Blood Rev 13, 230–240.

Lanier, L.L., Le, A.M., Civin, C.I., Loken, M.R. and Phillips, J.H. (1986a). The relationship of CD16 (Leu-11) and Leu-19 (NKH-1) antigen expression on human peripheral blood NK cells and cytotoxic T lymphocytes. J Immunol 86, 4480–4486.

Lanier, L.L., Phillips, J.H., Hackett, J., Jr, Tutt, M. and Kumar, V. (1986b). Natural killer cells: definition of a cell type rather than a function. J Immunol 86, 2735–2739.

Le Bouteiller, P., Barakonyi, A., Giustiniani, J. et al. (2002). Engagement of CD160 receptor by HLA-C is a triggering mechanism used by circulating natural killer (NK) cells to mediate cytotoxicity. Proc Natl Acad Sci USA 99, 16963–16968.

Lian, R.H., Maeda, M., Lohwasser, S. et al. (2002). Orderly and non stochastic acquisition of CD94/NKG2 receptors by developing NK cells derived from embryonic stem cells in vitro. J Immunol 168, 4980–4987.

Lopez-Botet, M., Carretero, M., Bellon, T., Perez-Villar, J.J., Llano, M. and Navarro, F. (1998). The CD94/NKG2 C-type lectin receptor complex. In Specificity, function, and development of NK cells, Karre, K. and Colonna, M. eds. Berlin: Springer Verlag, 41–52.

Lotzova, E., Savary, C.A. and Champlin, R.E. (1992). Genesis of human oncolytic Natural Killer cells from primitive CD34+CD33⁻ bone marrow progenitors. J Immunol 93, 5263–5269.

Loza, M., Faust, J.S. and Perussia, B. (2003). Multiple color immunofluorescence for cytokine detection at the single cell level. Mol Biotechnol 23, 245–258.

Loza, M.J., Metelitsa, L.M. and Perussia, B. (2002a). NKT and T cells: Coordinate regulation of NK-like phenotype and cytokine production. Eur J Immunol 32, 3543–3462.

Loza, M.J. and Perussia, B. (2001). Final steps of natural killer cells maturation: a general model for type 1-type 2 differentiation? Nat Immunol 2, 917–924.

Loza, M.J. and Perussia, B. (2002b). Peripheral immature CD2⁻/lo T cell development from type 2 to type 1 cytokine production. J Immunol 169, 3061–3068.

Loza, M.J., Peters, S.P., Zangrilli, J.G. and Perussia, B. (2002c). Distinction between IL-13⁺ and IFN-γ⁺ NK cells and regulation of their pool size by IL-4. Eur J Immunol 32, 413–423.

Loza, M.J., Zamai, L., Azzoni, L., Rosati, E. and Perussia, B. (2002d). Expression of type 1 (IFN-γ) and type 2 (IL-13, IL-5) cytokines at distinct stages of NK cell differentiation from progenitor cells. Blood 99, 1273–1281.

Mathew, P.A., Garni-Wagner, B.A., Land, K. et al. (1993). Cloning and characterization of the 2B4 gene encoding a molecule associated with non-MHC-restricted killing mediated by activated natural killer cells and T cells. J Immunol 93, 5328–5337.

Mehta, B.A. and Maino, V.C. (1997). Simultaneous detection of DNA synthesis and cytokine production in staphylococcal enterotoxin B activated CD4+ T lymphocytes by flow cytometry. J Immunol Methods 208, 49–59.

Migliorati, G., Moraca, R., Nicoletti, I. and Riccardi, C. (1992). IL-2-dependent generation of Natural Killer cells from bone marrow: role of MAC-1-, NK1-1- precursors. Cell Immunol 141, 323–331.

Muench, M.O., Humeau, L., Paek, B. et al. (2000). Differential effects of interleukin-3, interleukin-7, interleukin-15, and granulocyte-macrophage colony stimulating factor in the generation of natural killer and B cells from primitive human hematopoietic progenitors. Exp Hematol 28, 961–973.

Nagler, A., Lanier, L.L., Cwirla, S. and Phillips, J.H. (1989). Comparative studies of human FcRIII-positive and negative Natural Killer cells. J Immunol 143, 3183–3191.

Orange, J.S. and Biron, C.A. (1996). An absolute and restricted requirement for IL-12 in natural killer cell IFN-gamma production and antiviral defense. Studies of natural killer and T cell responses in contrasting viral infections. J Immunol 156, 1138–1142.

Orange, J.S., Wang, B., Terhorst, C. and Biron, C.A. (1995). Requirement for natural killer cell-produced interferon gamma in defense against murine cytomegalovirus infection and enhancement of this defense pathway by interleukin 12 administration. J Exp Med 95, 1045–1056.

Perussia, B. (1996). The cytokine profile of resting and activated NK cells. Methods 9, 370–378.

Perussia, B. (1998). Fc receptors on Natural Killer cells. Curr Top Microbiol Immunol 230, 63–88.

Perussia, B. and Loza, M.J. (2003). Linear '2-0-1' lymphocyte development: hypotheses on cellular bases for immunity. Trends Immunol 24, 235–242.

Piccioli, D., Sbrana, S., Melandri, E. and Valiante, N.M. (2002). Contact-dependent stimulation and inhibition of dendritic cells by natural killer cells. J Exp Med 195, 335–341.

Pross, H.F., Baines, M.G., Rubin, P., Shragge, P. and Patterson, M.S. (1981). Spontaneous human lymphocyte-mediated cytotoxicity against tumor target cells. IX. The quantitation of natural killer cell activity. J Clin Immunol 1, 51–63.

Raulet, D.H., Held, W., Correa, I., Dorfman, J.R., Wu, M.F. and Corral, L. (1997). Specificity, tolerance and developmental regulation of natural killer cells defined by expression of class I-specific Ly49 receptors. Immunol Rev 155, 41–52.

Renard, V., Cambiaggi, A., Vely, F. et al. (1997). Transduction of cytotoxic signals in natural killer cells: a general model of fine tuning between activatory and inhibitory pathways in lymphocytes. Immunol Rev 155, 205–221.

Roder, J.C., Haliotis, T., Klein, M. et al. (1980). A new immunodeficiency disorder in humans involving NK cells. Nature 284, 553–555.

Rosmaraki, E.E., Douagi, I., Roth, C., Colucci, F., Cumano, A. and Di Santo, J.P. (2001). Identification of committed NK cell progenitors in adult murine bone marrow. Eur J Immunol 31, 1900–1909.

Ruggeri, L., Capanni, M., Urbani, E. et al. (2002). Effectiveness of donor natural killer cell alloreactivity in mismatched hematopoietic transplants. Science 295, 2097–2100.

Sandel, P., Gendelman, M., Kelsoe, G. and Monroe, J.G. (2001). Definition of a novel cellular constituent of the bone marrow that regulates the response of immature B cells to B cell antigen receptor engagement. J Immunol 166, 5935–5944.

Santini, S., Lapenta, C., Logozzi, M. et al. (2000). Type 1 interferon as a powerful adjuvant for monocyte-derived dendritic cell development and activity in vitro and in Hu-PBL-SCID mice. J Exp Med 191, 1777–1788.

Shibuya, A., Nagayoshi, K., Nakamura, K. and Nakauchi, H. (1995). Lymphokine requirement for the generation of Natural Killer cells from CD34+ hematopoietic progenitor cells. Blood 85, 3538–3546.

Siefer, A.K., Longo, D.L., Harrison, C.L., Reynolds, C.W. and Murphy, W.J. (1993). Activated natural killer cells and interleukin-2 promote granulocytic and megakaryocytic reconstitution after syngeneic bone marrow transplantation in mice. Blood 82, 2577–2584.

Silla, L.M., Whiteside, T.L. and Ball, E.D. (1995). The role of natural killer cells in the treatment of chronic myeloid leukemia. J Hematother 4, 269–279.

Silva, M.R., Hoffman, R., Srour, E.F. and Ascensao, J.L. (1994). Generation of human Natural Killer cells from immature progenitors does not require marrow stromal cells. Blood 84, 841–846.

Sivakumar, P.V., Puzanov, I., Williams, N.S., Bennett, M. and Kumar, V. (1998). Ontogeny and differentiation of murine Natural Killer cells and their receptors. Curr Topics Microbiol Immunol 230, 161–190.

Sivori, S., Falco, M., Marcenaro, E. et al. (2002). Early expression of triggering receptors and regulatory 2B4 in human natural killer cell precursors undergoing in vitro differentiation. Proc Natl Acad Sci USA 99, 4526–4531.

Sivori, S., Vitale, M., Morelli, L. et al. (1997). p46, a novel natural killer cell-specific surface molecule that mediate cell activation. J Exp Med 186, 1129–1136.

Sobanov, Y., Glienke, J., Brostjaa, C., Lehrach, H., Francis, F. and Hofer, E. (1999). Linkage of the NKG2 and CD94 receptor genes to D12S77 in the human natural killer gene complex. Immunogenetics 49, 99–105.

Spritz, R.A. (1998). Genetic defects in Chediak-Higashi syndrome and the beige mouse. J Clin Immunol 98, 97–105.

Stepp, S.E., Mathew, P.A., Bennett, M., de Saint Basile, G. and Kumar, V. (2000). Perforin: more than just an effector molecule. Immunol Today 21, 254–256.

Stepp, S.E., Schatzle, J.D., Bennett, M., Kumar, V. and Mathew, P.A. (1999). Gene structure of the murine NK cell receptor 2B4: presence of two alternatively spliced isoforms with distinct cytoplasmic domains. Eur J Immunol 29, 2392–2399.

Targan, S.R. and Oseas, R. (1983). The 'lazy' NK cells of Chediak-Higashi syndrome. J Immunol 130, 2671–2674.

Trinchieri, G. (1989). Biology of Natural Killer cells. Adv Immunol 47, 187–376.

Trinchieri, G. (1998). Proinflammatory and immunoregulatory functions of interleukin-12. Int Rev Immunol 16, 365–396.

Trinchieri, G. (2003). Interleukin-12 and the regulation of innate resistance and adaptive immunity. Nat Rev Immunol 3, 133–146.

Trinchieri, G., Kubin, M., Bellone, G. and Cassatella, M.A. (1993). Cytokine cross-talk between phagocytic cells and lymphocytes: relevance for differentiation/activation of phagocytic cells and regulation of adaptive immunity. J Cell Biochem 53, 301–308.

Trinchieri, G. and Scott, P. (1994). The role of interleukin 12 in the immune response, disease and therapy. Immunol Today 15, 460–463.

Unkeless, J.C. (1979). Characterization of a monoclonal antibody directed against mouse macrophage and lymphocyte Fc receptors. J Exp Med 150, 580–596.

Valiante, N.M., D'Andrea, A., Crotta, S. et al. (2000). Life, activation and death of intrahepatic lymphocytes in chronic hepatitis C. Immunol Rev 174, 77–89.

Vance, R.E., Tanamachi, D.M., Hanke, T. and Raulet, D.H. (1997). Cloning of a mouse homolog of CD94 extends the family of C-type lectins on murine natural killer cells. Eur J Immunol 27, 3236–3241.

Walker, C., Checkel, J., Cammisuli, S., Leibson, P.J. and Gleich, G.J. (1998). IL-5 production by NK cells contributes to eosinophil infiltration in a mouse model of allergic inflammation. J Immunol 161, 1962–1969.

Warren, H.S., Kinnear, B.F., Phillips, J.H. and Lanier, L.L. (1995). Production of IL-5 by human NK cells and regulation of IL-5 secretion by IL-4, IL-10, and IL-12. J Immunol 154, 5144–5152.

Whiteside, T.L. (1999). Signaling defects in T lymphocytes of patients with malignancy. Cancer Immunol Immunother 48, 346–352.

Williams, N.S., Moore, T.A., Schatzle, J.D. et al. (1997). Generation of lytic natural killer 1.1+, Ly-49- cells from multipotential murine bone marrow progenitors in a stroma-free culture: definition of cytokine requirements and developmental intermediates. J Exp Med 186, 1609–1614.

Wu, C., Gadina, M., Wang, K., O'Shea, J. and Seder, R. (2000). Cytokine regulation of IL-12 receptor beta2 expression: differential effects on human NK and T cells. Eur J Immunol 30, 1364–1374.

Wu, J.S.Y., Bakker, A.B., Bauer, S., Spies, T., Lanier, L.L. and Phillips, J.H. (1999). An activating immunoreceptor complex formed by NKG2D and DAP10. Science, Wash DC 285, 730–732.

Yu, C.-R., Kirken, R.A., Malabarba, M.G., Young, H.A. and Ortaldo, J.R. (1998). Differential regulation of the Janus kinase-STAT pathway and biologic function of IL-13 in primary human NK and T cells: a comparative study with IL-4. J Immunol 161, 218–227.

Yuan, D., Koh, C.Y. and Wilder, J.A. (1994). Interactions between B lymphocytes and NK cells. FASEB J 8, 1012–1018.

Zamai, L., Ahmad, M., Bennett, I.M., Azzoni, L., Alnemri, E.S. and Perussia, B. (1998). Natural killer (NK) cell-mediated cytotoxicity: differential use of TRAIL and Fas ligand by immature and mature primary human NK cells. J Exp Med 188, 2375–2380.

Tetramer Analysis

Chapter 22

Peter P. Lee

Department of Medicine, Division of Hematology, Stanford University School of Medicine, Stanford, CA, USA

The idea that seeing life means going from place to place and doing a great variety of obvious things is an illusion natural to dull minds.

Charles Horton Cooley 1864–1929, American Sociologist

INTRODUCTION

Peptide/MHC (pMHC) tetramers were invented and first reported by Altman and Davis in 1996 (Altman et al., 1996). These novel reagents have revolutionized the study of T cell responses by allowing for accurate and rapid enumeration of antigen-specific T cells, the phenotypic characterization of such cells and their viable isolation for further analyses. Tetramers have been successfully used to gain new insights into the biology of T cell responses to viruses and cancer. Through their increasing availability from private, public and now commercial sources, tetramers are finding widespread use in many research and even clinical settings. However, due to significant differences in the biology of T cell receptor binding to pMHC versus antibody–antigen interactions, pMHC tetramers have significant special issues in their use. In this chapter, I will review some of these biological and practical issues and also discuss some of the more advanced uses of pMHC tetramers. While most work in the human setting has been done using MHC class I tetramers for analysis of CD8+ T cells, MHC class II tetramers are becoming available for the assessment of CD4+ T cell responses in humans (Kwok et al., 2000;

Meyer et al., 2000). The ability to monitor both CD4+ and CD8+ responses would be very powerful. However, MHC class II tetramers are generally more difficult to make and use, at least in the human setting (Nepom et al., 2002; Mallet-Designe et al., 2003), preventing their widespread use at this time. This chapter will focus on the use of MHC class I tetramers in humans.

BIOLOGY OF TCR-pMHC INTERACTIONS AND IMPLICATIONS IN TETRAMERS

Specificity of T cells is determined by each cell expressing a homogeneous population of T cell receptors (TCR). The ligand of the TCR is a complex made up of a peptide presented on the groove of a major histocompatibility complex (MHC) molecule. The affinity of the TCR-pMHC interaction in solution is much lower than that of an antibody–antigen interaction. Whereas the typical dissociation constant (Kd) of an antibody–antigen interaction is around 1 nM, a typical TCR-pMHC interaction may be in the range of 10 μM. This significant difference in affinity stems largely from the fact that antibodies are meant to bind their targets in solution, while TCRs bind their ligands in context of a cell surface. It is emerging that cell surface molecules interact with generally low affinities (Davis et al., 2003), with Kd in the range of 1–100 μM. This makes using soluble pMHC as a ligand to stain antigen-specific TCRs problematic. Due to the low affinity interaction, soluble pMHC complexes bound to a T cell would

Measuring Immunity, edited by Michael T. Lotze and Angus W. Thomson
ISBN 0-12-455900-X, London

fall off readily during washing. Hence, previous efforts to use soluble pMHC complexes as a staining reagent to identify antigen-specific T cells were unsuccessful. Altman and Davis came up with an ingenious solution of multimerizing pMHC complexes – making use of the biotin-steptavidin interaction to make 'tetramers'. Tetrameric complexes exist in a tetrahedral (pyramid) configuration, such that three pMHC molecules exist on one plane from any orientation (Figure 22.1). Potentially three pMHC complexes can interact with three TCRs simultaneously on a T cell surface, such that the avidity of this interaction becomes very strong, making staining possible. Others have shown that dimers of pMHC complexes (linked via an immunoglobulin framework) can also suffice in staining T cells (Schneck, 2000). These reagents are commercially available through Becton-Dickinson under the name DimerX (http://www.bdbiosciences.com/product_spotlights/dimerX_presentation_tools/).

COMPARISONS TO OTHER ASSAYS

Since the introduction of pMHC tetramers in 1996, a number of studies have extensively compared tetramer analysis to other methods of antigen-specific T cell analysis: limiting dilution assays (LDA), cytokine flow cytometry (CFC) and ELISPOT analyses (Dunbar et al., 1998; Gajewski, 2000; Clay et al., 2001; Whiteside et al., 2003). Typically, tetramer analyses have provided frequency estimates that exceed those detected using these alternate assay systems. The major reason is that these assays all entail a functional readout while tetramers is a reflection simply of TCR binding specificity. While this may be viewed as a limitation of tetramers, when combined with

a functional readout, this yields important additional information (see below). Tetramers could be used to mark T cells specific for an antigen while a functional readout could then be used to determine the fraction of the antigen-specific population which is functional. Such a combination was used successfully to demonstrate for the first time that a tumor-specific T cell population was anergic *in vivo* (Lee et al., 1999b).

PRODUCTION OF TETRAMERS

The production of tetramers is a time-consuming, labor-intensive process which requires skill and experience. Hence, this limited the widespread use of tetramers initially. However, tetramers are now widely available through public and commercial sources (Table 22.1) – the NIAID Tetramer Facility and Beckman Coulter Immunomics. The quality of tetramer reagents from both sources is excellent as they undergo rigorous quality control. Hence, there is now little reason for an individual laboratory to undertake the difficult task of making its own tetramers. Nonetheless, it is worth briefly discussing the basic process involved in tetramer production.

The basic components of a pMHC complex (class I) include the peptide, MHC class I molecule and beta-2-microglobulin (β2m). For subsequent tetramerization, the MHC class I molecule is engineered with a C-terminal substrate peptide for BirA-mediated biotinylation, biotin signal peptide (bsp). This MHC I-bsp recombinant protein (as well as β2m) is generally produced using *E. coli* in inclusion bodies. There are now numerous human and mouse MHC I alleles engineered with bsp in efficient *E. coli* expression vectors (generally BL21DE3 systems). For details of production, see the NIAID Tetramer Core Facility website (http://www.emory.edu/WHSC/TETRAMER/protocol.html) and protocols by Dr Dirk Busch from the Technical University Munich (http://www. mikrobio.med.tu-muenchen.de/ressourcen/repository/share/busch/tetprotocol.pdf).

Briefly, recombinant MHC I-bsp, β2m and the peptide of interest are mixed together in a folding reaction which generally goes over 48–72 h. During this time, refolding of the pMHC complex occurs. This is an inefficient process *in vitro*, resulting in a 1–5 per cent final yield. Properly folded pMHC complexes are extensively purified from unfolded materials via size exclusion columns (FPLC) and further cleaned up with anion exchange (MonoQ or ResourceQ). During this process, the biotinylation reaction is carried out via the addition of biotin-ligase (BirA enzyme), biotin and ATP. The efficiency

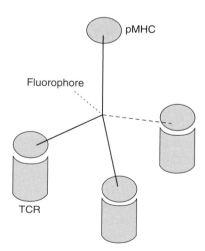

Figure 22.1 Cartoon of pMHC tetramer. Tetramers are a tetrahedral formation of four pMHC complexes linked via biotin to a central streptavidin. This configuration allows the simultaneous binding of three pMHC complexes to three TCRs on a T cell surface, thus enhancing avidity of binding. To facilitate flow cytometric analysis, streptavidin directly conjugated to fluorophores (such as PE or APC) are generally used.

Table 22.1 Sources for pMHC tetramers

NIAID Tetramer Core Facility	www.emory.edu/WHSC/TETRAMER/
Beckman Coulter Immunomics	www.immunomics.com/

of the biotinylation process is generally determined via a gel-shift assay using excess streptavidin to determine the fraction of pMHC complexes which bind streptavidin, hence biotinylated and the fraction that does not. Based on this information, a simple calculation is made to determine the amount of streptavidin to add to the purified, biotinylated pMHC complexes for a 1:4 molar ratio. Streptavidin directly conjugated to a fluorophore (generally phycoerythrin or APC) is used to facilitate their use in flow cytometry or sorting.

VALIDATION AND TITRATION

The first step when a new tetramer is made is to validate and titrate the reagent. Tetramers may fail for a number of reasons – peptides of very low MHC binding affinity do not fold into pMHC complexes well, incomplete purification or biotinylation of pMHC complexes, or bad batches of streptavidin-fluorophore. A T cell line or clone specific for the pMHC complex in the tetramer is needed for this process. These cells may be stained with serial twofold dilutions of tetramers (generally starting at 40 μg/ml), along with anti-CD8 antibodies. These data are then plotted with tetramer concentration versus median fluorescence intensity (MFI) of tetramer staining (Figure 22.2). When properly done, one should observe a sigmoidal curve where there is no staining below a certain threshold, followed by an exponential increase in MFI, then plateau staining above a certain tetramer concentration. The optimal staining concentration is a level just below the plateau, where there is a maximum spread between the specific staining (signal) and background staining (noise). It is important to use tetramers at optimal concentrations to maximize the signal-to-noise ratio determined via flow

cytometry, particularly when looking for rare T cell populations (<0.1 per cent). Under optimal conditions, the lower level of detection for tetramer-based assays is approximately 1/8000–1/10 000 (i.e. 0.01–0.0125 per cent) (He et al., 1999; Lee et al., 1999b; Molldrem et al., 1999). Since pMHC tetramers are non-covalent complexes, they 'degrade' at variable rates which depends in large part on the peptide-MHC affinity. Hence, a given batch of pMHC tetramers may be stable anywhere from 2 years (for many viral peptide antigens which bind MHC with high affinities) to as little as 3 months (for certain low-affinity 'self' peptides which bind MHC with low affinities). This necessitates periodic retesting of tetramers by retitration analyses on a regular (every 6–8 weeks) basis depending on the peptide used.

BASIC METHODOLOGY AND IMPORTANT FACTORS

Quality and numbers of cells

To ensure consistent results, roughly the same numbers of cells should be added per stain in all tetramer assays and these cells should be in an optimum state. T cells from peripheral blood (PBMC), lymph nodes or infiltrating tumors (TILs) may be used for tetramer analysis. Typically, one stains 1–2 million PBMCs per condition and collects as many events as possible (10^5–10^6) for each analysis. This is important especially when looking for rare T cell populations which may represent 0.01 per cent of CD8+ T cells. As an example, if one collects 5×10^5 events and CD8+ T cells represent 10 per cent of PBMC, then a 0.01 per cent antigen-specific population would represent five events. Of interest particularly for analysis of patient materials, frozen/thawed PBMC samples may be used without compromising the quality of tetramer staining data. This is important in allowing samples from a clinical trial to be collected, stored and analyzed in batches, or shipped to a reference laboratory. This also permits testing of patient materials collected longitudinally at different times to be analyzed together in single batches, thereby limiting variability associated with inter-assay assessment. The way in which cells are frozen and thawed may significantly impact on the quality of the resultant data. To maximize cell viability and quality, thawed cells may be 'rested' in complete media (containing human serum) for several hours to overnight and then enriched by discontinuous gradient centrifugation (Ficoll/Percoll) prior to staining. Of note, there is a theoretical concern that specific CD8+ T cells in cancer patients, particularly those with advanced stage disease, may undergo 'spontaneous' apoptosis ex vivo (Saito et al., 2000) during this 'resting' period and thereby not be detected in subsequent tetramer analysis. Hence, it may be advisable for each laboratory to undertake a direct comparison between fresh versus frozen/thawed samples before routinely using one or the other. Another consideration is that certain surface markers may not stain

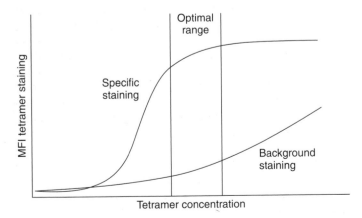

Figure 22.2 Titration of tetramers to determine optimal staining concentration. Varying concentrations of a tetramer (generally 1–40 μg/ml final) are stained against a specific T cell line or clone. The median fluorescence intensity (MFI) of tetramer staining of the antigen-specific and background populations is plotted. The optimal range is the region at which there is near plateau specific MFI staining but still minimal background MFI staining.

well in frozen/thawed samples. As an example, CD62L (an important marker for the distinction between naive versus memory T cells) contains glycosylations which may be cleaved during the freeze/thaw process (Mario Roederer, personal communication). Anti-CD62L antibodies require proper glycosylation of the protein for proper binding and may not bind CD62L+ cells from frozen/thawed samples.

Staining volume, temperature and time

To conserve reagents, it is advisable to stain in a small volume, generally 30–50 μl. This is adequate for 1–2 million PBMCs. If staining more cells, such as for sorting, it is necessary to scale up accordingly to 100–200 μl. All reagents (tetramers and antibodies) should be added to a desired final concentration based on the total staining volume. As an example, it may be convenient to make up a 3 × solution of tetramers and antibodies and add 10 μl of cells, 10 μl of tetramers and 10 μl of antibodies. The temperature at which the staining occurs may significantly impact the degree of specific tetramer staining (Whelan et al., 1999). Staining of T cells on ice (or at 4°C) allows for significant low avidity (frequently cross-reactive) tetramer binding, thus increasing the background. Staining at room temperature (23°C) or 37°C tends to favor higher avidity tetramer-TCR interactions and reduces background. The main reason to perform tetramer staining on ice rather than room temperature is to favor detection of low avidity tetramer–T cell interactions. However, the biological significance of low recognition efficiency T cells is unclear. The staining time is dependent on the temperature. At room temperature (23°C) or 37°C, tetramer staining generally saturates at 15–30 min, while on ice (or at 4°C) saturation does not occur until at least 2 h. Once staining is completed, cells should be washed and stored on ice until FACS analysis.

Tetramer concentration

As stated earlier, the concentration of tetramers used to stain cells is critical in obtaining the optimal signal-to-noise ratio. Staining with suboptimal tetramer concentrations may lead to an underestimate of antigen-specific T cell frequencies, while staining with excessive tetramer concentrations may lead to high backgrounds and overestimate of antigen-specific T cell frequencies. This is particularly important when making comparisons between samples or across multiple tetramers. For most tetramers, they are generally used at a 1–20 μg/ml final concentration. The optimal tetramer concentration can only be determined by careful titrations of each reagent against an antigen-specific T cell line or clone.

Anti-CD8 and other antibodies

Another important factor is the use of anti-CD8 antibodies. The MHC I molecule naturally has a low affinity for CD8 (Salter et al., 1990), such that MHC I tetramers may bind CD8+ T cells non-specifically at low temperature (4°C or on ice). The addition of anti-CD8 antibodies can block this interaction and several reports have suggested that tetramer staining may be affected by the concentration of anti-CD8 (or -CD3) antibodies used and even by the particular clone of antibody (Daniels and Jameson, 2000; Hoffmann et al., 2000). Indeed, depending on the CD8 determinant recognized by the antibody, anti-CD8 counterstaining may block, have little impact on, or even augment the intensity of pMHC tetramer staining of T cells (Whelan et al., 1999; Daniels and Jameson, 2000; Denkberg et al., 2001). In careful titration experiments, the percentage of tetramer+ events may vary depending on the concentration and type of anti-CD8 antibodies used. This could provide an additional variability when comparing data between experiments. The recent development of pMHC tetramers based on mutant class I heavy chains which do not bind CD8 should reduce such low-avidity or cross-reactive tetramer-T cell interactions based on CD8 binding and thereby further reduce background. Tetramers from Beckman Coulter Immunomics are made with such non-CD8 binding mutant MHC I molecules. In almost any bulk PBMC sample, there are cells which may non-specifically bind to staining reagents and thereby contribute to background. These are generally monocytes or dead/dying cells. The use of 'dump' antibodies to negatively gate out such non-specifically sticky cells may be quite useful in cleaning up data. For this purpose, one would use antibodies to markers not present on the cells of interest – for CD8+ T cells, useful 'dump' antibodies may include anti-CD4, 14, or 19.

Data interpretation

Lymphocytes are gated based on their forward and side-scatter, then dead and non-specifically 'sticky' cells are excluded based on propidium iodide staining and 'dump' (negative selecting) antibodies. The remaining cells are assessed for CD8 versus tetramer staining (Figure 22.3). Only cell populations that are well clustered and display a clear separation from the CD8+, tetramer-negative T cell population are considered to be 'real' events (Figure 22.4). If necessary, specific tetramer staining of T cells may be confirmed via competition with unlabeled pMHC monomers or anti-CD3 antibodies (Whelan et al., 1999; Hoffmann et al., 2000; Denkberg et al., 2001; Fong et al., 2001). As the percentage of CD8+ T cells in total PBMC can vary widely between samples, tetramer-positive events are generally 'normalized' as a percentage of total CD8+ T cells or data may be reported as the absolute number of tetramer+, CD8+ cells per amount (i.e. μl-ml) of blood.

ADVANCED USES OF TETRAMERS

In addition to the identification and enumeration of antigen-specific T cells within a heterogeneous cell sample,

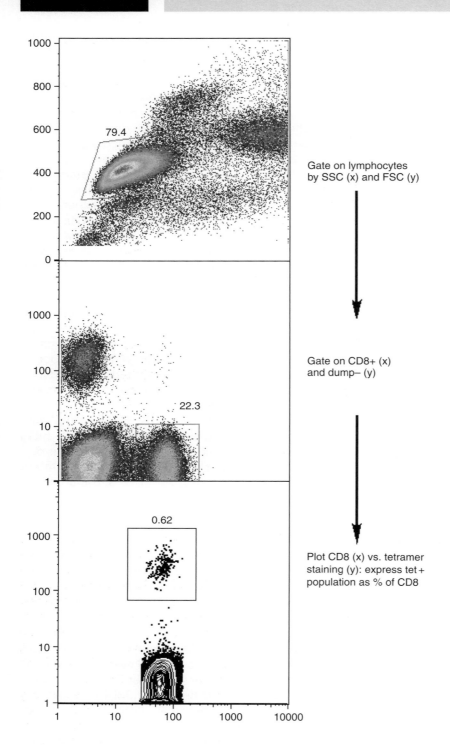

Gate on lymphocytes
by SSC (x) and FSC (y)

Gate on CD8+ (x)
and dump− (y)

Plot CD8 (x) vs. tetramer
staining (y): express tet+
population as % of CD8

Figure 22.3 Typical gating strategy for analysis of tetramer+ populations. Collected PBMC data are plotted first on SSC versus FSC with selection of the lymphocytes population. Gated cells are then plotted on CD8 versus dump (generally CD4, 14, 19) and further gated on CD8+ dump− cells. These are then plotted on CD8 versus tetramer staining. Tetramer+ populations are generally expressed as per cent of total CD8+ T cells.

tetramers may also be used to isolate such cells by sorting, thereby facilitating T cell cloning, TCR spectra-typing and microarray analyses (Dunbar et al., 1998; Lee et al., 1999b; Dietrich et al., 2001). Tetramers may also be used to discern the functional status of antigen-specific T cells using multi-parameter FACS to assess surface (acti-vation, memory, cytotoxic) markers and intracellular or secreted cytokines/chemokines (He et al., 1999; Lee et al., 1999b; Pittet et al., 2001).

Isolation by sorting and cloning

The viable isolation of antigen-specific T cells for cloning or further analyses is a powerful use of pMHC tetramers. This may be done routinely using a standard FACSort instru-ment (such as the BD FACS Vantage or the new Aria). For example, a tetramer+ T cell population may be isolated and directly tested *ex vivo* for cytolytic activity against tar-get cells in a standard chromium release assay. It is now

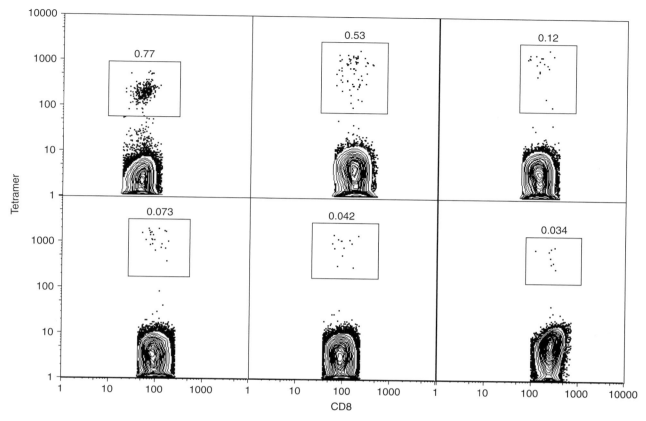

Figure 22.4 Examples of tetramer+ populations. With optimal staining conditions, a tetramer+ population should be well clustered and clearly separate from the bulk CD8+ population. The top three panels represent large populations (0.1–0.8 per cent). However, with careful titrations of reagents, even small populations (<0.1 per cent) may be clearly distinguishable (bottom panels).

well established that the tetramer staining and sorting process does not impair the cytolytic activity of T cells. Care should be taken to keep the cells cold and in serum-rich media to maximize their function before and after sorting. Furthermore, tetramer+ cells could be sorted singly into individual wells of a tissue culture plate and expanded in the presence of feeder cells and cytokines to create T cell clones. Such cells could then be analyzed for their TCR specificities and structural avidity (see below), or even expanded to high numbers for adoptive cellular immunotherapy (Yee et al., 2002). More recently, sorted T cells have also been analyzed for gene expression profiles using DNA microarray technology (Xu et al., 2003).

Phenotypic analysis by multi-color flow cytometry

The advent of multi-color flow cytometry allows the extensive phenotypic characterization of antigen-specific T cells on an individual cell basis. Even with three- or four-color FACS, the expression of several markers by an antigen-specific T cell population of interest may be determined by performing a few different stains. With the increasing availability of six- and even 10-color FACS (Table 22.2), large numbers of markers could be

determined from only a few stains (Lee et al., 1999b). This is important especially for rare populations and precious patient samples. In general, one channel is taken up by tetramers (usually PE) and another channel for anti-CD8. If cells are limiting, two channels could be devoted to two different tetramers (such as PE and APC) so that two separate antigen-specific T cell populations could be simultaneously assessed per stain. Not all antibodies work well in combination, so considerable effort must be made to optimize phenotypic panels which work well together (Table 22.2). For example, since anti-CD3 antibodies may compete with tetramers for binding to the TCR/CD3 complex (Hoffmann et al., 2000), it is advisable to not include this antibody in panels except for validation purposes. Panels could also be optimized for intracellular antigens (see below).

Intracellular staining

Tetramers can be combined successfully with intracellular staining to analyze expression of cytokines (e.g. IFN-γ, IL-2, IL-4, TNF-α) or cytolytic granules (perforin, granzyme A, granzyme B) by antigen-specific T cells. After routine surface staining with tetramers and other markers, cells are

Table 22.2 Sample antibodies panels for phenotypic analysis

FITC	PE	Cy5PE	APC	TR	Cy5.5 PE	Cy7PE	Cy5.5 APC	Cy7 APC	Cascade Blue
CD11a	Tetramer	CD38	CD8 beta	CD95 (Fas)	CD137 (4–1BB)	CD69	CD4	CD25	CD8
CD27	Tetramer	CD45RA	CCR7	CD80 (B7–1)	CD152 (CTLA4)	ICOS	CD4	CD28	CD8
CD44	Tetramer	HLA-DR	CD57	CD95L (FasL)	CD154 (CD40L)	CD134 (OX40)	CD4	CD56	CD8
CD3 zeta	Tetramer	IFN-γ	IL-4	TNF-α	IL-10	perforin	CD4	IL-2	CD8

These are 10-color FACS panels incorporating PE-labelled tetramers for the phenotypic analysis of antigen-specific T cell populations. The top three panels involve surface stains only; the bottom panel also includes intracellular stains.

fixed and permeabilized, then stained with antibodies against intracellular antigens (Lee et al., 1999b). As this process involves numerous washing steps, it is important to start with large numbers of cells to ensure sufficient cells remaining at the end to detect rare populations. It is also important to note that T cells generally downregulate the TCR complex upon activation. Since many intracellular cytokine staining protocols involve a non-specific cellular activation step with mitogens, the level of tetramer staining could go down substantially. To circumvent this problem, tetramer staining could be performed prior to cell activation such that tetramers are internalized (with the appropriate fluorophore) along with the TCR complex during the activation process.

Analysis of 'structural avidity'

'Functional avidity' or 'recognition efficiency' is emerging as a key factor in the effectiveness of an antigen-specific T cell response (Dutoit et al., 2002; Echchakir et al., 2002; Molldrem et al., 2003; Oh et al., 2003; Rubio et al., 2003). It is a measure of the sensitivity of a T cell to different peptide concentrations for stimulation (O'Connor et al., 2002). Recognition efficiency of a T cell reflects the cumulative effects of the intrinsic affinity of its TCRs for their cognate peptide displayed on the target cell, expression levels of TCR, CD4/8 and adhesion molecules, as well as redistribution of these molecules on the cell membrane and their recruitment efficacy of the signaling cascade (Margulies, 2001; Slifka and Whitton, 2001; Cawthon and Alexander-Miller, 2002). Identification of peptide-specific T cells using pMHC tetramers, ELISPOT or cytokine flow cytometry does not distinguish between cells of high or low recognition efficiency – at least not without careful reagent titration on each sample. While previous investigations have attempted to use the intensity of tetramer staining as a measure for binding strength (Crawford et al., 1998; Yee et al., 1999), recent evidence suggests that tetramer staining intensity alone does not directly correlate with recognition efficiency (Derby et al., 2001; Dutoit et al., 2002; Echchakir et al., 2002). Nonetheless,

the rate of dissociation of bound pMHC tetramers from antigen-specific T cells upon addition of a competing antibody (such as anti-TCR) may be used as a relative measure of the difference in TCR affinities between T cells (Savage et al., 1999); as such, this may be a useful assay to assess the 'structural avidity' of a T cell population.

Functional analysis

A number of assays which combine tetramer staining with a functional readout have been developed. As discussed above, these include staining for cytokine production, cytolytic granules and direct *ex vivo* testing for cytolytic activity after sorting. A novel flow cytometric method was recently developed (Betts et al., 2003; Rubio et al., 2003) which involves the quantification of the surface mobilization of CD107 – an integral membrane protein within cytolytic granules of cytotoxic T cells – as a marker for degranulation upon tumor stimulation. Mobilization of CD107 selectively identified T cells that were tumorcytolytic. CD107 mobilization could be combined with peptide/MHC tetramer staining to directly correlate antigen-specificity and cytolytic ability on a single-cell level.

In situ hybridization

There is significant interest in the use of tetramers for *in situ* hybridization to detect antigen-specific T cells within tissue sections. While several groups have achieved success (Skinner et al., 2000; Schrama et al., 2002), this is a technically challenging procedure which requires extensive optimization of staining conditions. As the TCR–pMHC interaction is of low affinity, any sample processing which may alter the conformation of TCRs on T cells – which may occur upon fixation of tissue specimens – could dramatically impact tetramer staining. Hence, most successful *in situ* tetramer staining has been achieved using fresh or frozen tissue sections, although some success has also been achieved with 'lightly fixed' tissue samples (Skinner et al., 2000).

USE IN CLINICAL TRIALS AND FUTURE PROSPECTS

Considerable experience has been accumulated over the past 5 years on the use of tetramers to analyze patient samples in clinical trials, both in viral infections (He et al., 1999, 2001) and cancer (Lee et al., 1999a, 2001; Molldrem et al., 1999). A good deal of knowledge has been derived on the size, kinetics and biology of these T cell responses. However, certain hurdles prevent the widespread use of tetramers in the clinical setting. In cancer vaccination, peptide-specific T cell responses as detected by tetramers have largely not correlated with clinical outcome (Lee et al., 1999a, 2001; Whiteside et al., 2003). However, this issue is not unique to tetramer analysis, but applies to all methods of detecting antigen-specific T cell responses, including ELISPOT and CFC. It is becoming clear that peptide-specificity does not necessarily guarantee tumor-reactivity of a T cell response – recognition efficiency of the T cells is a key factor (Rubio et al., 2003). Furthermore, T cells may be rendered non-functional or anergic in vivo, either as a consequence of direct contact with tumor cells or as part of a global immunosuppressive state (Lee et al., 1999b). Lastly, T cells may not home properly to tumor sites, and if so, may not function optimally due to the tumor microenvironment being hostile to lymphocytes. These issues illustrate clearly that one cannot simply rely on enumeration of antigen-specific T cells to predict clinical outcome in clinical trials. It is critical to be able to study the biology of such cells in terms of recognition efficiency, in vivo functional status and homing patterns. No currently available method can address all of these issues. It is likely that the immune assays in the future will involve identification, enumeration, phenotypic, functional, kinetic and gene expression analyses of T cell responses. Tetramers will likely play a prominent role in many of these assays.

REFERENCES

Altman, J.D., Moss, P.A., Goulder, P.J. et al. (1996). Phenotypic analysis of antigen-specific T lymphocytes. Science 274, 94–96.

Betts, M., Brenchley, J., Price, D. et al. (2003). Sensitive and viable identification of antigen-specific CD8+ T cells by a flow cytometric assay for degranulation. J Imm Methods in press.

Cawthon, A.G. and Alexander-Miller, M.A. (2002). Optimal colocalization of TCR and CD8 as a novel mechanism for the control of functional avidity. J Immunol 169, 3492–3498.

Clay, T.M., Hobeika, A.C., Mosca, P.J., Lyerly, H.K. and Morse, M.A. (2001). Assays for monitoring cellular immune responses to active immunotherapy of cancer. Clin Cancer Res 7, 1127–1135.

Crawford, F., Kozono, H., White, J., Marrack, P. and Kappler, J. (1998). Detection of antigen-specific T cells with multivalent soluble class II MHC covalent peptide complexes. Immunity 8, 675–682.

Daniels, M.A. and Jameson, S.C. (2000). Critical role for CD8 in T cell receptor binding and activation by peptide/major histocompatibility complex multimers. J Exp Med 191, 335–346.

Davis, S.J., Ikemizu, S., Evans, E.J., Fugger, L., Bakker, T.R. and van der Merwe, P.A. (2003). The nature of molecular recognition by T cells. Nat Immunol 4, 217–224.

Denkberg, G., Cohen, C.J. and Reiter, Y. (2001). Critical role for CD8 in binding of MHC tetramers to TCR: CD8 antibodies block specific binding of human tumor-specific MHC-peptide tetramers to TCR. J Immunol 167, 270–276.

Derby, M.A., Wang, J., Margulies, D.H. and Berzofsky, J.A. (2001). Two intermediate-avidity cytotoxic T lymphocyte clones with a disparity between functional avidity and MHC tetramer staining. Int Immunol 13, 817–824.

Dietrich, P.Y., Walker, P.R., Quiquerez, A.L. et al. (2001). Melanoma patients respond to a cytotoxic T lymphocyte-defined self-peptide with diverse and nonoverlapping T-cell receptor repertoires. Cancer Res 61, 2047–2054.

Dunbar, P.R., Ogg, G.S., Chen, J., Rust, N., van der Bruggen, P. and Cerundolo, V. (1998). Direct isolation, phenotyping and cloning of low-frequency antigen-specific cytotoxic T lymphocytes from peripheral blood. Curr Biol 8, 413–416.

Dutoit, V., Rubio-Godoy, V., Doucey, M.A. et al. (2002). Functional avidity of tumor antigen-specific CTL recognition directly correlates with the stability of MHC/peptide multimer binding to TCR. J Immunol 168, 1167–1171.

Echchakir, H., Dorothee, G., Vergnon, I., Menez, J., Chouaib, S. and Mami-Chouaib, F. (2002). Cytotoxic T lymphocytes directed against a tumor-specific mutated antigen display similar HLA tetramer binding but distinct functional avidity and tissue distribution. Proc Natl Acad Sci USA 99, 9358–9363.

Fong, L., Hou, Y., Rivas, A., Benike, C. et al. (2001). Altered peptide ligand vaccination with Flt3 ligand expanded dendritic cells for tumor immunotherapy. Proc Natl Acad Sci USA 98, 8809–8814.

Gajewski, T.F. (2000). Monitoring specific T-cell responses to melanoma vaccines: ELISPOT, tetramers, and beyond. Clin Diagn Lab Immunol 7, 141–144.

He, X.S., Rehermann, B., Boisvert, J. et al. (2001). Direct functional analysis of epitope-specific CD8+ T cells in peripheral blood. Viral Immunol 14, 59–69.

He, X.S., Rehermann, B., Lopez-Labrador, F.X. et al. (1999). Quantitative analysis of hepatitis C virus-specific CD8(+) T cells in peripheral blood and liver using peptide-MHC tetramers. Proc Natl Acad Sci USA 96, 5692–5697.

Hoffmann, T.K., Donnenberg, V.S., Friebe-Hoffmann, U. et al. (2000). Competition of peptide-MHC class I tetrameric complexes with anti-CD3 provides evidence for specificity of peptide binding to the TCR complex. Cytometry 41, 321–328.

Kwok, W.W., Liu, A.W., Novak, E.J. et al. (2000). HLA-DQ tetramers identify epitope-specific T cells in peripheral blood of herpes simplex virus type 2-infected individuals: direct detection of immunodominant antigen-responsive cells. J Immunol 164, 4244–4249.

Lee, K.H., Wang, E., Nielsen, M.B. et al. (1999a). Increased vaccine-specific T cell frequency after peptide-based vaccination correlates with increased susceptibility to in vitro stimulation but does not lead to tumor regression. J Immunol 163, 6292–6300.

Lee, P., Wang, F., Kuniyoshi, J. et al. (2001). Effects of interleukin-12 on the immune response to a multipeptide vaccine for resected metastatic melanoma. J Clin Oncol 19, 3836–3847.

Lee, P.P., Yee, C., Savage, P.A. et al. (1999b). Characterization of circulating T cells specific for tumor-associated antigens in melanoma patients. Nat Med 5, 677–685.

Mallet-Designe, V.I., Stratmann, T., Homann, D., Carbone, F., Oldstone, M.B. and Teyton, L. (2003). Detection of low-avidity CD4+ T cells using recombinant artificial APC: following the antiovalbumin immune response. J Immunol 170, 123–131.

Margulies, D.H. (2001). TCR avidity: it's not how strong you make it, it's how you make it strong. Nat Immunol 2, 669–670.

Meyer, A.L., Trollmo, C., Crawford, F. et al. (2000). Direct enumeration of Borrelia-reactive CD4 T cells ex vivo by using MHC class II tetramers. Proc Natl Acad Sci USA 97, 11433–11438.

Molldrem, J.J., Lee, P.P., Kant, S. et al. (2003). Chronic myelogenous leukemia shapes host immunity by selective deletion of high-avidity leukemia-specific T cells. J Clin Invest 111, 639–647.

Molldrem, J.J., Lee, P.P., Wang, C., Champlin, R.E. and Davis, M.M. (1999). A PR1-human leukocyte antigen-A2 tetramer can be used to isolate low-frequency cytotoxic T lymphocytes from healthy donors that selectively lyse chronic myelogenous leukemia. Cancer Res 59, 2675–2681.

Nepom, G.T., Buckner, J.H., Novak, E.J. et al. (2002). HLA class II tetramers: tools for direct analysis of antigen-specific CD4+ T cells. Arthritis Rheum 46, 5–12.

O'Connor, D.H., Allen, T.M., Vogel, T.U. et al. (2002). Acute phase cytotoxic T lymphocyte escape is a hallmark of simian immunodeficiency virus infection. Nat Med 8, 493–499.

Oh, S., Hodge, J.W., Ahlers, J.D., Burke, D.S., Schlom, J. and Berzofsky, J.A. (2003). Selective induction of high avidity CTL by altering the balance of signals from APC. J Immunol 170, 2523–2530.

Pittet, M.J., Zippelius, A., Speiser, D.E. et al. (2001). Ex vivo IFN-gamma secretion by circulating CD8 T lymphocytes: implications of a novel approach for T cell monitoring in infectious and malignant diseases. J Immunol 166, 7634–7640.

Rubio, V., Stuge, T.B., Singh, N. et al. (2003). Ex vivo identification, analysis, and isolation of tumor-cytolytic T cells. Nat Med in press.

Saito, T., Dworacki, G., Gooding, W., Lotze, M.T. and Whiteside, T.L. (2000). Spontaneous apoptosis of CD8+ T lymphocytes in peripheral blood of patients with advanced melanoma. Clin Cancer Res 6, 1351–1364.

Salter, R.D., Benjamin, R.J., Wesley, P.K. et al. (1990). A binding site for the T-cell co-receptor CD8 on the alpha 3 domain of HLA-A2. Nature 345, 41–46.

Savage, P.A., Boniface, J.J. and Davis, M.M. (1999). A kinetic basis for T cell receptor repertoire selection during an immune response. Immunity 10, 485–492.

Schneck, J.P. (2000). Monitoring antigen-specific T cells using MHC-Ig dimers. Immunol Invest 29, 163–169.

Schrama, D., Pedersen, L.O., Keikavoussi, P. et al. (2002). Aggregation of antigen-specific T cells at the inoculation site of mature dendritic cells. J Invest Dermatol 119, 1443–1448.

Skinner, P.J., Daniels, M.A., Schmidt, C.S., Jameson, S.C. and Haase, A.T. (2000). Cutting edge: In situ tetramer staining of antigen-specific T cells in tissues. J Immunol 165, 613–617.

Slifka, M.K. and Whitton, J.L. (2001). Functional avidity maturation of CD8(+) T cells without selection of higher affinity TCR. Nat Immunol 2, 711–717.

Whelan, J.A., Dunbar, P.R., Price, D.A. et al. (1999). Specificity of CTL interactions with peptide-MHC class I tetrameric complexes is temperature dependent. J Immunol 163, 4342–4348.

Whiteside, T.L., Zhao, Y., Tsukishiro, T., Elder, E.M., Gooding, W. and Baar, J. (2003). Enzyme-linked immunospot, cytokine flow cytometry, and tetramers in the detection of T-cell responses to a dendritic cell-based multipeptide vaccine in patients with melanoma. Clin Cancer Res 9, 641–649.

Xu, T., Shen, C., Dang, D., Ilsley, D., Holmes, S. and Lee, P.P. (2003). Subtle but consistent gene expression differences between T cells from melanoma patients and healthy subjects. Cancer Res in press.

Yee, C., Savage, P.A., Lee, P.P., Davis, M.M. and Greenberg, P.D. (1999). Isolation of high avidity melanoma-reactive CTL from heterogeneous populations using peptide-MHC tetramers. J Immunol 162, 2227–2234.

Yee, C., Thompson, J.A., Byrd, D. et al. (2002). Adoptive T cell therapy using antigen-specific CD8+ T cell clones for the treatment of patients with metastatic melanoma: in vivo persistence, migration, and antitumor effect of transferred T cells. Proc Natl Acad Sci USA 99, 16168–16173.

Peripheral Blood Naive and Memory B Cells

Chapter 23

Jean-Pierre Vendrell

Centre Hospitalier Régional et Universitaire de Montpellier, Institut National de la Santé et de la Recherche Médicale, Montpellier, France

The palest ink is better than the best memory.

Chinese Proverb

INTRODUCTION

Immunological memory is a defining feature of adaptive immunity and confers the ability to develop a more rapid and more vigorous humoral response after re-exposure to the antigen (Ag). It is characterized by the appearance of high-affinity antibodies in serum (Kocks and Rajewsky, 1989), 10- to 100-fold more Ag-specific B cells in the bone marrow and the spleen of immunized patients compared with the primary exposure (Ahmed and Gray, 1996; Mcheyzer-Williams et al., 2000; Pihlgren et al., 2001) and memory B cells. Ag-specific activation and differentiation of B cells occur in germinal centers (MacLennan et al., 1992; Liu and Arpin, 1997), where immature B cells expressing the preimmune B-cell repertoire undergo proliferation, somatic hypermutation of rearranged variable region genes, immunoglobulin isotype switching and subsequent selection by Ag (Banchereau and Rousset, 1992; MacLennan et al., 1997; Rajewsky, 1998) and mature into:

1 short-lived specific antibody-secreting cells (ASCs) producing low-affinity IgM antibodies (Ahmed and Gray, 1996; Smith et al., 1996)
2 ASCs producing IgG or IgA antibodies of high affinity (Thomson and Harris, 1977; Tarkoswki et al., 1985; Kantele et al., 1986; Czerkinsky et al., 1998)
3 long-lived plasma cells which secrete antibodies for extended periods of time (Slifka et al., 1995, 1998) and
4 memory B cells defined as long-living and non-dividing cells.

They recirculate in the body (Schittek and Rajewsky, 1990; Paramithiotis and Cooper, 1997; Klein et al., 1997, 1998) or join as resident cells more static lymphoid tissue microenvironments such as the marginal zone of the mucosal epithelium of tonsil (Liu et al., 1995), spleen (Dunn-Walters et al., 1998; Tangye et al., 1998), gut, peritoneal or pleural cavities. The transfer of B cells to other lymphoid compartments implies their migration through the blood and the lymphatic system. The analysis of peripheral blood B-cell subsets can provide information on the physiopathological phenomena under development in the lymphoid tissues.

Naive and memory B cells are defined by the expression of characteristic surface receptors (Agematsu et al., 1997; Klein et al., 1998). In human adults approximately 15–40 per cent of peripheral blood B cells are memory B cells (Odendahl et al., 2000; De Milito et al., 2001; Hansen et al., 2002). They possess an intrinsic advantage over naive B cells in both the time to initiate a response and the rate of generating rapidly dividing effector cells (Tangye et al., 2003a,b), differentiate into plasma cells and play a crucial role in the humoral immune response (Agematsu et al., 2000). Thus, the exposure and re-exposure to Ag or the development of acute benign infections generate transient ASCs in the blood detectable

Measuring Immunity, edited by Michael T. Lotze and Angus W. Thomson
ISBN 0-12-455900-X, London

only during several weeks or months (Stevens et al., 1979; Kerl and Fauci, 1983), whereas patients with chronic infections such as human immunodeficiency virus type 1 (HIV-1) have persistent specific ASCs (Amadori et al., 1988, 1989; Vendrell et al., 1991a; Morris et al., 1998).

In routine laboratory practice, several markers can be targeted to investigate the peripheral B cell subsets. The easiest approach consists of enumerating circulating naive and memory B cells on the basis of their membrane Ig and CD27, the key memory B cell marker (Agematsu et al. 2000). Circulating B cells can be identified by their capacity to secrete Ig and antibody spontaneously *in vitro*, a phenomenon called IVAP secretion. These rare cells, which result from the encounter *in vivo* of specific memory B cells with Ag, convert to cells that have not yet fully differentiated into plasma cells and then migrate to the bone marrow and other lymphoid tissues. The circulating memory B lymphocytes are usually non-functional *ex vivo*, however, they can be induced to synthesize Ig and specific antibodies when they are polyclonally activated *in vitro* by the CD40–CD40 ligand interaction in the presence IL-2 and IL-10 (Fondere et al., 2003, 2004). The Ig secreted by these cells can be characterized and enumerated by using a two-color ELISPOT assay to determine the IgG, IgM, IgA, κ and λ isotypes, whereas IgG-, IgA- or IgM-specific ASCs are enumerated by a specific antibody ELISPOT assay.

In vivo Ag re-exposure rapidly generates memory CD4$^+$ T and CD8$^+$ T lymphocytes and B cell effectors. Tests measuring circulating specific memory CD4$^+$ and CD8$^+$ T cells are based on T cell receptor interaction with an epitope resulting in IL-2 and IFN-γ production, respectively and they are enumerated by IL-2 and IFN-γ ELISPOT assays. In contrast, memory B cells cannot be activated through interaction between the B cell receptor and antigen, but they convert to cells that differentiate into early plasma cells when they are polyclonally activated *in vitro*. Under these conditions, nearly all memory B cells give immunoglobulin-secreting cells (Ig-SCs) and some of them are specific ASCs.

B-CELL SURFACE RECEPTORS

Background

Progress in B cell analysis has established that circulating B cells can be divided into IgD$^+$ CD27$^-$ CD19$^+$ or naive B cells (cB1) and IgD$^-$ CD27$^+$ CD19$^+$ or memory B cells (cB3) (Agematsu et al., 1997; Klein et al., 1998). A recent fine analysis of the human circulating memory B cell compartment clearly identified two subclasses of memory B cells showing similar ability to differentiate into plasma cells but with different phenotypes and functions (Shi et al., 2003). The majority of IgD$^-$ CD27$^+$ CD19$^+$ cells express membrane IgG or IgA and secrete IgG or IgA and

a minority express only surface IgM and secrete IgM (Klein et al., 1998). Another memory B cell subset phenotypically identified as IgM$^+$ IgD$^+$ CD27$^+$ CD19$^+$ (cB2) carries somatically mutated variable region genes (Klein et al., 1998) and secretes high levels of IgM (Agematsu et al., 1997); cB2 has been considered as unclass-switched and cB3 class-switched memory B cells (Klein et al., 1998). Other cell surface molecules, such as CD72 and HLA-DR markers, are expressed on many B cells. Expression of CD80 costimulatory molecules is higher on cB3 than on cB2 and is lacking on cB1, CD86 and CD95 are expressed predominantly on cB3, CD5 is weakly expressed on cB1 and cB2 but not on cB3 (Bar-Or et al., 2001; Shi et al., 2003), cB1 express CD38 but at low levels of intensity, CD23 are mainly expressed on cB1 and CD10 on only germinal center B cells (Bohnhorst et al., 2001). Predominant differentiation into plasma cells occurs at the same rate in all memory B cells that are IgD$^-$ CD27$^+$ (Agematsu et al., 1998) or IgD$^+$ CD27$^+$ (Shi et al., 2003). Thus, ASCs are circulating memory B cells which have not yet fully differentiated into plasma cells (Moir et al., 2001) and which express CD38 at high levels and CD19 at levels lower than memory B cells (Fournier et al., 2002a).

Clinical applications

B cell subsets in peripheral blood have been analyzed in individuals with various immunological disorders and diseases. In immunodeficiency diseases such as common variable immunodeficiency and X-linked hyper-IgM syndrome, IgD$^-$ CD27$^+$ CD19$^+$ cells are markedly reduced or absent but not IgD$^+$ CD27$^-$ CD19$^+$ cells (Agematsu et al., 2001; Warnatz et al., 2002). Patients with hyper-IgM syndrome type II present high amounts of cB2 but do not carry apparent immunoglobulin somatic hypermutation (Revy et al., 2000). A marked lymphocytopenia that affects CD27$^-$ CD19$^+$ naive B cells more than CD27$^+$ CD19$^+$ memory B cells has been identified in patients with systemic lupus erythematosus (Odendahl et al., 2000). Peripheral blood CD27$^+$ memory B cells are reduced in patients with Sjögren's syndrome and their accumulation/retention in the inflamed salivary glands has been suggested (Hansen et al., 2002). In patients with paroxysmal nocturnal hemoglobinuria, glycosylphosphatidylinositol-deficient B cells (CD48$^-$) are mainly naive cells with a CD27$^-$ IgM$^+$ IgD$^+$ CD19$^+$ phenotype and the majority of residual B cells (CD48$^+$) are not class switched CD27$^+$ IgM$^+$ IgD$^+$ CD19$^+$ memory B cells (Richards et al., 2000). In HIV-1, the peripheral blood memory B cells are significantly reduced (De Milito et al., 2000; Nagase et al., 2001) and the loss of humoral immunity correlates with B cell apoptosis and increased levels of FasL expression on B cells (Samuelson et al., 1997a,b). Memory B cells controlling *Streptococcus pnemoniae* infections require the spleen for their generation (Kruetzmann et al., 2003).

SPONTANEOUS B CELL IMMUNOGLOBULIN AND ANTIBODY SECRETION

Background

Circulating specific ASCs were initially measured by a limit dilution assay of peripheral blood mononuclear cells (PBMC) from HIV-1-infected patients and by the measure of HIV-1-specific antibodies in culture supernatants. Frequencies of HIV-1-specific ASCs have been evaluated at between 1/105 and 1/40 000 B cells and represent 22–100 per cent of Ig-SCs (Amadori et al., 1989). Morris et al. (1998) using ELISPOT assays detecting Ig-SCs and HIV-1 p24- and gp120-specific ASCs found Ig-SCs median frequencies of 2185/10^6 PBMC in HIV-1-infected patients and 177/10^6 in controls, whereas eight out of 11 patients had between 15 and 429 anti-gp120 ASCs/10^6 PBMCs, equivalent to 0.6–14.9 per cent of total Ig-SCs, the percentage of ASCs specific for p24 being lower than that for gp120. These secreting cells are highly differentiated B cells expressing a broad diversity of maturation markers such as $CD19^+$, $CD27^+$, $CD38^+$, $CD20^\pm$, $CD37^\pm$, $CD71^\pm$, HLA-$DQ^\pm$, $sIg^\pm$, but not sIgD, CD28, nor CD40. The phenotype and cytological aspects of purified B cells suggest strongly that Ig-SCs are early plasma cells originating from germinal centers in transit in the blood. Moreover, monocytes and natural killer cells enhance antibody secretion in vitro by cell-to-cell contacts, involving adhesion molecules such as CD11a, CD62L, CD27, CD50, CD54, CD80 costimulatory molecules and IL-6. CD40/CD40L, CD28/CD80 and CD27/CD70 in vivo interactions generate Ig-secreting peripheral B cells that, in the presence of IL-6, differentiate into early plasma cells in vitro (Fournier et al., 2002a).

An elegant application of the detection of circulating specific ASCs is the phenotypic characterization of circulating B cell subsets resulting from mucosal and non-mucosal immune responses by using a combination of cell sorting and an ELISPOT assay. Specific ASCs originating from mucosal and systemic sites are cells which are in fact in the process of differentiating into early plasma cells and express adhesion molecules such as CD44, CD62L and $\alpha4\beta7$-integrin, an intestinal homing receptor involved in the protective immunity for an intestinal pathogen (Quiding-Järbring et al., 1995, 1997; Williams et al., 1998). Characterization of circulating specific ASCs after systemic immunization with tetanus toxoid or cholera toxin B subunit for example, shows that they also express CD62L and $\alpha4\beta7$-integrin. Nearly all IgA- and IgG-specific ASCs detected after peroral and rectal immunization express $\alpha4\beta7$-integrin, with only a minor fraction of these cells expressing CD62L. In contrast to specific ASCs derived from enteric immunization, almost all circulating specific ASCs induced by nasal immunization coexpress CD62L and $\alpha4\beta7$-integrin. Thus, the immunization route rather than the nature of the immunogen determines the types of adhesion molecules expressed by the corresponding ASCs. In systemic and mucosal immunization, differential expression of adhesion molecules provides a cell surface receptor basis for the compartmentalization of the immune response. The CXCR4 receptor and CXCL12 play a critical role in precursor cell retention within the bone marrow (Hargreaves et al., 2001; Cyster et al., 2002) and splenic and bone marrow IgG-specific ASCs attract CXCL12 but fail to respond to CXCL13, CCL19 or CCL21 (Bowman et al., 2002; Hauser et al., 2002; Cyster, 2003).

Clinical applications

Immunization

The presence of ASCs has been described in subjects recently immunized with vaccinal antigens such as tetanus toxoid (Stevens et al., 1979; Fons et al., 1985), polio virus (Fons et al., 1985), pneumococcal polysaccharide (Kerhl and Fauci, 1983), Brucella abortus (Vendrell et al., 1992a) and hepatitis B virus (Ducos et al., 1996) and in subjects to whom cholera antigens (Czerkinsky et al., 1991, Quiding-Järbring et al., 1997) or attenuated Salmonella typhimurium (Forrest, 1992) has been administered orally. The specific ASC response is dominated by IgA-producing cells (Forrest, 1988, 1992; Kantele et al., 1991, 1994); these ASCs circulate 5 to 30 days after immunization, whereas the levels of specific antibodies in serum persist for several months or years as shown schematically in Figure 23.1.

Acute infections

ASCs have been detected during the course of mucosa-associated infections such as gastroenteritis (Kantele et al., 1988), lower urinary tract infections (Kantele et al., 1994), acute otitis media (Nieminen et al., 1995), cytomegalovirus (Vendrell et al., 1991b), rotavirus (Brown et al., 2000), bacterial (Vendrell et al., 1992a), Toxoplasma gondii acute infection (Vendrell et al., 1992b) and keratoconjunctivitis caused by Chlamydia trachomatis (Ghaem-Maghami et al., 1997). In acute infections, the circulation of specific ASCs is transient, detectable at the onset of clinical symptoms and disappears between 11 and 24 weeks after the seroconversion, as illustrated in Figure 23.1. Specific ASCs are not detectable in patients with chronic toxoplasmosis, suggesting that the very low levels of T. gondii Ag released by tissue cysts are not sufficient to stimulate the immune system; however, specific antibodies are detectable in serum for a long time.

Chronic infections

Human immunodeficiency virus-1

In HIV-1-infected patients, spontaneous in vitro secretion of anti-HIV-1 specific antibodies by PBMC has been

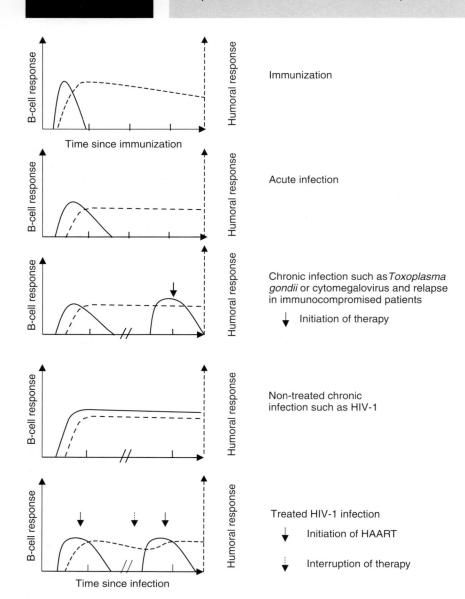

Figure 23.1 Characteristic patterns of the kinetics of circulating antibody-secreting cells *in vitro* and of the humoral immune response following immunization and in acute and chronic infections. The solid line represents the peripheral blood antibody-secreting cells and the dotted line represents the levels of specific antibodies.

observed in all untreated patients from the seroconversion to asymptomatic and symptomatic stages of HIV-1 infection, even if the rates of appearance of specific ASCs are very different from one patient to another (Amadori et al., 1988, 1989; Lee et al., 1989; Vendrell et al., 1991a). The levels of spontaneous *in vitro* Ig-SCs and HIV-1-specific ASCs decrease or become negative in patients receiving zidovudine (Pahwa et al., 1989, Conge et al., 1994, Pollack et al., 1994), or combined antiretroviral treatment (Morris et al., 1998; Fournier et al., 2002b). Changes in HIV-1-specific and non-specific B cell responses are striking and similar to those of the plasma viremia load, confirming that HIV-1 antigens generate B cell activation *in vivo*. In sustained responders to treatment, HIV-1-specific ASCs decrease significantly in parallel with the plasma viral load and levels of Ig-SCs become similar to those of controls, but in 66 per cent of responder patients residual HIV-1-specific ASCs persist. In incomplete responder patients, the number of HIV-1-specific ASCs also decreases

significantly; but these cells persist in all the patients, whereas the number of Ig-SCs returns to normal (Fournier et al., 2002b). In patients receiving an efficient antiretroviral therapy, discrepancies in modifications of circulating Ig-SCs and HIV-1-specific ASCs could be explained by *in vivo* polyclonal activation of B cells caused by interactions between HIV-1 superantigens (Berberian et al., 1993; Karray and Zouali, 1997) and B cells in lymphoid tissues, as observed *in vitro* when B cells from controls are cultured with high HIV-1 titers (Pahwa et al., 1986). Thus, a significant reduction in viral load dramatically decreases interactions between HIV-1 Ag and B cells and consequently abolishes polyclonal activation of B lymphocytes. However, a weak persistence of HIV-1-specific ASCs, as observed in sustained responder patients to therapy, might be due to the persistence of low amounts of HIV-1 antigens trapped in follicular dendritic cell networks in lymphoid tissues where the levels are sufficient to activate only HIV-1-specific memory B cells, leading to their differentiation into specific ASCs. Specific HIV-1 antibodies in serum persist in untreated HIV-1 patients, but their levels decline significantly in successfully treated patients (Notermans et al., 2001).

Relapse of Toxoplasma gondii infection in immunocompromised patients

In immunocompetent patients, circulating *T. gondii*-specific ASCs are observed only in acute toxoplasmosis and disappear when toxoplasmosis becomes chronic (Vendrell et al. 1992b); they are also detected in HIV-1-infected patients with toxoplasmic encephalitis at the onset of clinical symptoms and concomitantly with HIV-specific ASCs (Vendrell et al., 1993). A follow-up of 24 patients with encephalitis after initiation of anti-parasite treatment showed that *T. gondii*-specific ASCs disappeared in patients presenting clinical and radiological sustained responses to treatment ($n = 11$) but persisted in patients with an incomplete or transient therapeutic response, whereas no significant modifications of HIV-1-specific ASCs were observed. These findings strongly suggest that the circulation of *T. gondii*-specific ASCs is not generated by an *in vivo* polyclonal activation of B lymphocytes such as viral superantigens but caused by parasite antigens. The decrease or disappearance of these cells during therapy strengthens the hypothesis that the reduction of the parasite antigenic load *in vivo* results in a lower activation of *T. gondii*-specific B cells. In incomplete responders to parasite treatment in whom the *T. gondii*-specific ASCs decreased only moderately, persistent parasite antigens contributed to perpetuate circulating *T. gondii*-specific ASCs (Lacascade et al., 2000).

Cytomegalovirus infections

Cytomegalovirus (CMV) specific-ASCs have been demonstrated in patients with primary or recurrent CMV infections (Vendrell et al., 1991b). When the CMV is in a latent period, specific ASCs are not detectable, but they can reappear when the patients receive immunosuppressive therapies (Segondy et al., 1993) or in HIV-1-infected patients with reactivations of CMV symptomatic or asymptomatic (Segondy et al., 1990).

The transient, persistent, or recurrent character of circulating specific ASCs in representative infectious diseases is schematized in Figure 23.1 in comparison with the kinetics of antibody appearance in the serum. It should be noted that there is no correlation between ASCs and the levels of serum antibodies.

INDUCIBLE B-CELL IMMUNOGLOBULIN AND ANTIBODY SECRETION

Background

The ligation between B cell receptors of memory B cells and specific Ag causes B cell activation and differentiation into plasma cells that secrete antibodies, but methods investigating this basic function need to be developed for routine laboratory practice. Unmethylated single-stranded DNA natifs (CPG oligonucleotides) (Bernasconi et al., 2002), pocketweed mitogen and phosphothioated CPG ODN-2006 plus *Staphyolococcus aureus* Cowan (Crotty et al., 2003, 2004) and CD40-CD40L ligation, a key polyclonal B cell activation step, in the presence of IL-2 and IL-10 cytokines, induce memory B cells to differentiate into terminally differentiating B cells that have not yet fully differentiated into plasmocytes: they are plasmablasts secreting IgG, IgA or IgM (Arpin et al., 1995; Kindler and Zubler, 1997). Under these culture conditions, among the B cells converted to ASCs, a few specific memory B cells differentiate into early plasma cells secreting antibodies against antigens. The enumeration of these rare circulating B cells involves:

1 isolation of a sufficient number of B cells from the blood ($1-2 \times 10^6$ purified B cells)
2 controlled B cell cryopreservation and thawing procedures
3 culturing the B cells in the presence of the CD40L polyclonal activator, which is a delicate process
4 ELISPOT assays.

Clinical application

In vitro activated B lymphocytes from HIV-1-infected patients secrete anti-HIV-1-specific antibodies, whereas B cells from HIV-1-infected patients as well as those from controls chronically infected by *T. gondii* synthesize *T. gondii*-specific antibodies. In a study of 26 patients, HIV-1-specific IgG-, IgA-, or IgM-ASCs were found to represent 1×10^{-4} to 1×10^{-5} of total circulating B cells and 1×10^{-2} to 1×10^{-3} of Ig-SCs. HIV-1-specific memory B cells were found in all nine untreated patients and in only eight out of 17 patients receiving highly active antiretroviral therapy, although the number of Ig-SCs was similar for the two groups as well as the controls. Persistent low-level ongoing viral replication does not seem to be sufficient to maintain HIV-1-specific memory B cells (Fondere et al., 2003).

PHENOTYPING AND ENUMERATING B CELL SUBSETS

B cell enrichment and cultures

To detect a frequency of Ag-specific B cells of less than 1 per cent, several cell separation methods using antibodies directed against different membrane molecules have been described (Oshiba et al., 1994). The three main techniques used are:

1 capture on an antigen-coated solid matrix
2 staining with fluorescent antigen and isolation by fluorescence-activated cell sorting
3 rosetting with antigen-coated red blood cells or magnetic particles.

The preparation of an enriched fraction of a particular cell type and the purity of the cell suspension obtained are the key factors that determine the choice of the isolation technique. Important features of a good purification method are the maintenance of cell viability and function, reproducibility and general applicability. Each technique has its advantages and disadvantages, but Kodituwakku et al. (2003) concluded that, whereas there is no single method providing both high yield and very high purity, the most promising isolation methods use immunomagnetic sorting and multiparametric flow cytometric analysis. On the basis of our experience, a rosetting technique, the RosetteSep™ (StemCell, Meylan, France), has been found to be the most effective B cell isolation technique as compared with standard techniques using PBMC isolation on Ficoll-Hypaque and immunomagnetic B cell selection.

The B-cell purification procedure is schematized in Figure 23.2A. To prepare activated B cells, purified B cells are stimulated with CD40L-expressing mouse fibroblasts in the presence of IL-2 and IL-10 (Figure 23.2Ba).

At day five of culture, polyclonal B cell activation is measured by using a two-color ELISPOT assay (Figure 23.2Bb) and specific-ASCs are enumerated using ELISPOT assays (Figure 23.2Bc). In addition, antibodies secreted can be detected in cell-free supernatants by an ELISA and /or by immunoblotting (Figure 23.2Bd and Be, respectively). Despite the complex technical processing, between 55 and 98 per cent of circulating memory B cells can be satisfactorily recovered, cryopreserved and converted to Ig-SCs (Table 23.1).

Methods

Blood samples are incubated with a RosetteSep™ B cell enrichment cocktail (a cyclic tetramolecular complex of monoclonal antibodies against CD2, CD3, CD4, CD8, CD16, CD56, CD14 cell surface markers and red blood cell glycophorine A). Unwanted cells are cross-linked to red blood cells with the tetrameric complexes and mononuclear cells are discarded by sedimentation through Ficoll-Hypaque. Enriched B cell populations recovered at the density medium/plasma interphase are negatively selected, they contain more than 98 per cent of CD19+, as controlled by flow cytometry. Memory B cells can also be purified. Briefly enriched B cell

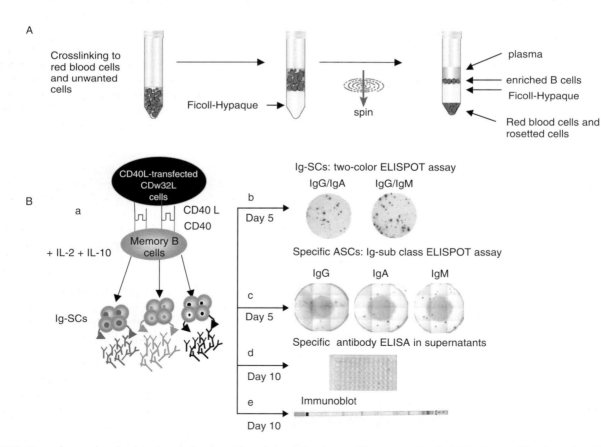

Figure 23.2 General procedure for detection and enumeration of circulating Ag-specific memory B cells. (A): Isolation of the derived peripheral B cells by eliminating unwanted cells and red blood cells using the tetrameric antibody complex reagent and gradient (Ficoll-Hypaque) centrifugation. (Ba): The purified B cells are cultured with CD40L-transfected CDW32L mouse fibroblasts and IL-2 plus IL-10. (Bb): Ig-SCs are enumerated by the two-color ELISPOT assay at day 5. (Bc): Inducible specific antibody-secreting cells are enumerated at day 5 by an ELISPOT. (Bd): Specific antibodies are detected in cell-free supernatants at day10 by ELISA. (Be): Antibody specificities are determined by immunoblotting. Ig-SCs, immunoglobulin secreting cells; ASCs, antibody secreting cells. **See colour plate 23.2.**

Table 23.1 Efficiency of the general procedure for enumeration of HIV-1-specific memory B cells

Subjects		Number[a] of circulating memory B cells/ 10^6 B cells	Number[b] of κ-+λ-L-chain SCs/ 10^6 B cells	Percentage of Ig-SCs[d]	Number[c] of anti-HIV-1-ASCs			Percentage of anti-HIV-1 IgG+IgA+IgM-SCs
					IgG	IgA	IgM	
Patients	1	86 000	60 000	69	10	100	190	0.500
	2	148 000	145 000	97	30	10	10	0.034
	3	99 000	81 000	81	30	10	60	0.123
	4	82 000	71 000	96	40	10	10	0.084
	5	241 000	142 000	60	70	10	30	0.077
	6	99 000	80 000	80	20	10	40	0.087
	7	240 000	142 600	59	20	10	10	0.028
	8	174 000	95 500	55	10	10	30	0.052
	9	89 700	83 700	93	10	10	40	0.071
	10	250 000	245 600	98	50	10	20	0.032
Controls	A	230 000	135 000	58	0	0	0	0
	B	300 000	284 000	94	0	0	0	0
	C	320 000	279 000	82	0	0	0	0

[a] Determined by flow cytometry.
[b] Determined by the two-color ELISPOT assay.
[c] Determined by the specific antibody ELISPOT assay.
[d] Ig-secreting memory B cells.
(Adapted from Fondere et al., 2004 with permission)

populations are incubated with anti-IgD human antibodies coupled via a short DNA fragment to magnetic beads. The purity and viability of both the naive and memory B cells subpopulations are greater than 95 per cent and their numbers are usually sufficient to detect Ag-specific memory B cells after *in vitro* polyclonal B cell activation (Fondere et al., 2004). Precisely, 1×10^5 purified B cells are cultured in 96-well tissue culture plates with 1×10^4 CD40L-expressing mouse fibroblasts treated with 0.1 μg mitomycine C in culture medium supplemented with fetal calf serum, 0.5 ng IL-2 and 1 ng IL-10. At day 5 of culture, cells are delicately recovered and seeded in the wells of ELISPOT microtiter plates.

Comments

B cell purification is not time-consuming and very easy to perform. B cells can be purified from as little as 5 ml of blood. The best option is to treat freshly recovered blood samples immediately, but blood samples conserved overnight at room temperature (20–23°C) also give satisfactory results. One major point concerning this elegant method is that purified B cells usually represent more than 98 per cent of the separated cells.

PHENOTYPING AND ENUMERATION OF B CELLS BY SURFACE MARKER EXPRESSION

In routine hospital laboratory practice, the number and percentage of B lymphocyte subsets in blood samples and in B cell enriched preparations are determined by flow cytometry (Beckman-Coulter, Villepinte, France). It is very important to note that free IgM and IgD are present in whole blood and they must be eliminated so as not to interfere with the anti-IgM and anti-IgD antibodies added to the blood samples for cytometry analysis. Free IgM and IgD molecules and IgM and IgD molecules passively adsorbed onto PBMC can be removed from the blood sample in a single step by incubation of the PBMC in RPMI for 10 min at room temperature (20–23°C) followed by centrifugation. An example of phenotyping all circulating B cell subsets is presented in Figure 23.3.

Methods

Only 1 ml of venous blood is needed to determine the number of circulating peripheral B cell subsets. Two hundred microlitres of blood collected in EDTA tubes are diluted in 4.8 ml of RPMI 1640, incubated for 10 min at room temperature (20–23°C), centrifuged (600 g) and washed twice with PBS. Each cell pellet is divided into two aliquots. The first is one incubated for 10 min with a mixture of phycoerythrin-cyanin 7 (PC7)-conjugated anti-CD19 antibodies, phycoerythrin-cyanin 5 (PC5)-conjugated anti-CD27 antibodies (Beckman-Coulter), phycoerythrin conjugated anti-IgM and fluorescein isothiocyanate (FITC)-conjugated anti-IgD antibodies (Tebu, Le Perray en Yvelines, France). The second sample is incubated with a mixture of PC5-conjugated anti-CD19 antibodies and FITC-conjugated anti-CD38 antibodies for 10 min. Then, the red cells are lysed and resting mononuclear cells are fixed by using an Immunoprep kit (Beckman-Coulter). Figure 23.3 shows the B cell subsets identified by flow cytometry.

Comments

Phenotyping of B cell subsets is not time-consuming and requires only 1 ml of venous blood. Blood samples are

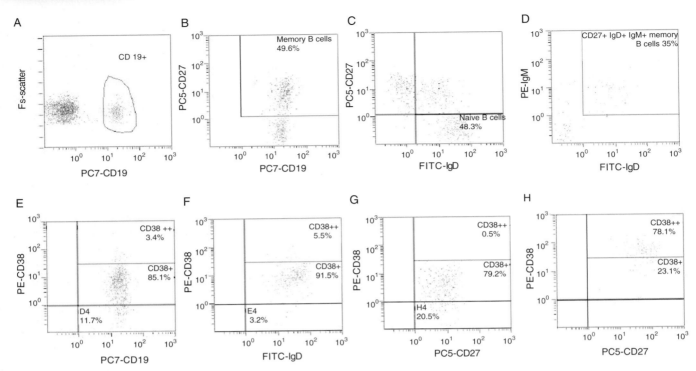

Figure 23.3 Circulating B cell subsets characterized according to membrane IgD, IgM, CD27, and CD38 receptor expression. After washing in RPMI, the blood is divided into two samples: one is incubated with a mixture of phycoerythrin-cyanin 7 (PC7) conjugated anti-CD19, phycoerythrin-cyanin 5 (PC5) conjugated anti-CD27, phycoerythrin (PE) conjugated anti-IgM and fluorescein isiothiocyanate (FITC) conjugated anti-IgD antibodies. The second is incubated with a mixture of PC7 conjugated anti-CD19, FITC conjugated anti-IgD, PC5 conjugated anti-CD27 and PE conjugated anti-CD38. (A) Memory B cells and naive B cells are enumerated on the basis of size and CD19 expression. (B) CD19$^+$ CD27$^+$ total memory B cells. (C) CD19$^+$ IgD$^+$CD27$^-$ naive B cells. (D) CD19$^+$ CD27$^+$ IgM$^+$ IgD$^+$ memory B cell subset. Using the second sample, subpopulations of circulating B cells are analyzed on the basis of their CD38 expression: (E) CD19$^+$ CD38$^+$; (F) naive B cells CD38$^+$ or CD38^{++}; (G) memory B cells CD38$^+$ or CD38^{++} and (H) activated memory B cells CD38$^+$ or CD38^{++}. The horizontal line separates the CD38$^+$ negative and positive subpopulations defined using isotypic controls. The upper quadrant is divided into two subpopulations of CD19$^+$ cells expressing high CD38^{++} or low CD38$^+$ expression after CD40-CD40L B-cell activation *in vitro*. The number of B cells in each population is determined by using calibrated fluorospheres Kit (Flow Count™) according to the manufacturer's instructions (Beckman-Coulter). **See colour plate 23.3.**

either analyzed immediately or conserved overnight at laboratory room temperature (20–23°C) before flow cytometry analysis within a week. One major aspect of this method is that B cell subsets in the blood sample are analyzed without preliminary PBMC isolation by Ficoll-Hypaque gradient sedimentation, which is not only time-consuming but also only allows for the determination of the percentage of the circulating B cell subsets. One minor drawback is that in a few cases the red cells are difficult to lyse and consequently a new blood sample has to be treated.

CHARACTERIZATION AND ENUMERATION OF FUNCTIONAL B CELLS

Spontaneous immunoglobulin and antibody secretion

Methods

The major characteristic of these cells is the spontaneous antibody production *in vitro* as measured in cell-free supernatants of PBMC cultured for 5–7 days. PBMC isolated by standard Ficoll-Hypaque density gradient centrifugation of heparinized blood samples are recovered and preincubated for 1 h at room temperature (20–23°C) with gentle shaking to remove cell-bound Ig (Vendrell et al.,1991a; Conge et al.,1994; Fournier et al., 2002b). Then, the cells are resuspended in culture medium supplemented with 10 per cent fetal calf serum at a final density of 2×10^6 cell/ml, washed three times and finally cultured without addition of mitogen or antigens for 5–7 days at 37°C in 5 per cent CO_2 humidified atmosphere. The amount of Ig is quantified in cell-free supernatants by ELISA and antibody levels are determined by using commercial ELISA kits and a standard reference serum pool containing arbitrary units/ml. *De novo* synthesis of Ig and antibodies is controlled by testing supernatants from PBMC initially incubated with cycloheximide (Fournier et al., 2002b). ELISPOT assays have also been used to enumerate Ag-specific ASCs. Nitrocellulose-bottom, 96-well microtiter plates (Millipore, Bedford, MA) are previously coated with Ag, as for example purified tetanus toxoid or cholera toxin (Quiding-Järbrink et al., 1997), chlamydial antigens (Ghaem-Maghami et al., 1997), or HIV-1 proteins such as recombinant gp120 or glutathione-S-transferase-p24 fusion protein (Morris et al., 1998). Serial dilutions of PBMC are then added and the plates are incubated overnight at 37°C. Solid phase-bound antibodies secreted by individual ASCs are detected as spots after stepwise addition of horseradish peroxidase (HRP)- or alkaline phosphatase (PA)-labeled anti-human IgG γ chain, IgA α chain or IgM μ chain antibodies and suitable chromogen substrates.

Comments

IVAP is a biomarker easy to evaluate, although freshly recovered venous blood is necessary and the procedure is time-consuming. Antibodies passively adsorbed onto the cell membrane are eluted in one step by preincubation of PBMC with mild shaking. This avoids adherence of monocytes onto the walls of the plastic flasks, monocytes being essential for optimal antibody production *in vitro*. IVAP measured in supernatants from cycloheximide-treated PBMC gives background levels of cell-bound antibodies passively released into the supernatant. HIV-1 ELISA detects a very large panel of HIV-1 antibodies because the wells of the microtiter plates are sensitized with HIV-1 peptides mimicking the immunodominant epitopes of the HIV-1 envelope glycoproteins and nucleocapsid recombinant proteins.

CHARACTERIZATION AND ENUMERATION OF B CELLS BY INDUCIBLE IG AND ANTIBODY SECRETION

Ig-SCs: two-color ELISPOT assay

Description

Ig-SCs can be enumerated by using a two-color ELISPOT assay (Czerkinsky et al., 1988) with slight modifications (Cordoba et al., 2000). Briefly, wells of Immunobilon-P flat bottomed 96-well microtiter plates (Millipore, Bedford, MA) are coated overnight at 4°C with goat polyclonal anti-human IgG, IgA, IgM, κ- and λ-L-chain antibodies (0.5 μg/100 ml in PBS, pH 7.4). The remaining binding sites are saturated with 5 per cent BSA in PBS for 2 h at 37°C. PBMC are added to each set of wells and incubated for 18 h at 37°C in a humidified atmosphere containing 5 per cent CO_2. After three washes, a mixture of AP- and HRP-conjugated goat antibodies to human IgG and IgA, IgG and IgM, and κ- and λ-L-chains Ig, respectively, is added. After washings, the AP chromogenic substrate solution, a mixture of 5-bromo-4-chloro-3 indolyl phosphate para-toluidine salt (B8503, Sigma Saint Louis, MO, USA) and para-nitroblue tetrazolium [2,2'-di-para-nitrophenyl-5,5'-diphenyl-3,3-(3,3'-dimethoxy-4,4'-diphenylen)-ditetrazolium chloride] (N 6876, Sigma, BCIP/NBT) is added. After 15 min, the 3-amino-9-ethyl carbazole HRP chromogenic substrate (AEC staining Kit, AEC-101, Sigma) is added. The reactions are stopped with distilled water after 20 min. Cells treated with

50 μg/ml of cycloheximide and wells without cells or coated antibody are used as controls. Spots of 0.05–0.2mm circular foci, densely granulated with a color decrease from the center to the periphery, are counted using an inverted microscope at a magnification of 40× or automatically using a KS ELISPOT reader (Carl Zeiss vision GmbH, Germany). Results are expressed as the number of immunospots/10^6 B lymphocytes.

Comments

The two-color ELISPOT as described above is easy to perform.

1. An important point concerns the preparation of the BCIP/NBT substrate; care must be taken to completely dissolve the NBT in the Tris buffer before adding the BCIP.
2. the number of cultured B cells added to each well must be adjusted to avoid an excess of secreted antibody by the specific ASCs which would mask the immunospots.

Antibody secretion: specific antibody ELISPOT assay

Description

An ELISPOT assay for enumerating Ag-specific ASC according to the isotype of the secreted antibody has also been developed (Fondere et al., 2004). Briefly, 96-well microtiter plates (Nunc, Roskilde, Denmark) using Immobilon-P membrane as solid phase (Millipore Corporation, Bedford, MA, USA) are coated overnight at 4°C with mouse monoclonal anti-human IgG (γ), IgA (α), or IgM (μ) (Tebu, Le Perray-en-Yvelines, France). Cultured B cells (5 × 10^4 per well) are incubated for 18 h and after extensive washings with PBS, purified horseradish peroxidase-labeled HIV-1 peptides mimicking the immunodominant epitopes of the HIV-1 envelope glycoproteins (Bio-Rad, Marnes-la-Coquette, France) are added for 5 h at 37°C or overnight at 4°C. After washing with PBS, 3-amino-9-ethyl-carbazol (Sigma) is added to each well, insoluble red-colored precipitates are obtained within 5–10 min and the immunoenzymatic reaction is stopped with distilled water.

Comments

Technical difficulties are minor for laboratories with expertise in routine ELISA assays. There are, however several drawbacks:

1. the test is time-consuming
2. the CD40L-transfected CDW32L cells must be used between the third and twelfth cell doubling.

FUTURE PROSPECTS

In humans, the circulating B cell subsets can be characterized by their surface markers and their capacity to secrete

Ig and specific antibodies. Phenotyping makes it possible to define and enumerate the different peripheral blood B cell subsets, including those circulating B cells activated *in vivo*. The proportion of peripheral blood B cell subpopulations is constantly being modified in many diseases such as common variable immunodeficiency, X-linked hyper-IgM syndrome, autoimmune disorders and HIV-1 infection which, in many patients, induces the decrease or the disappearance of certain B cell subsets, a disturbance in B cell trafficking, or increased circulation of activated B cells. Flow cytometry analysis renders it possible to identify and to enumerate all the peripheral blood B cell subsets including *ex vivo* or *in vitro* activated B cells. This test is performed on whole blood, necessitates only small amounts and is neither time-consuming nor expensive.

Peripheral B cells can also be investigated by analyzing their Ig and antibody production. Using the ELISPOT assay, even a very small number of specific spontaneous ASCs per million cells can be detected. Analysis of the specificities of the antibodies secreted in cell culture supernatants completes the results of the ELISPOT assay.

Human B cell investigations based on Ig and specific antibody secretion is adapted to enumerating circulating B cells which are terminally differentiating B cells that have not yet fully differentiated into plasma cells after encountering their Ag but secrete spontaneously antibodies *ex vivo*. The transient or persistent character of this cell trafficking reflects respectively temporary or continuous *in vivo* antigenic stimulation of the immune system and provides information as to the proliferation of pathogenic organisms in patients. Immunization effectiveness can be evaluated by analyzing the circulation of specific ASCs. The IVAP and ELISPOT assays could be surrogate markers to evaluate the efficiency of parenteral or oral vaccination. In addition, as the decrease or disappearance of ASCs in chronic infections is linked to temporary or continuous viral or bacterial reproduction *in vivo*, modifications in the number of circulating specific ASCs is highly indicative of the efficacy of drug regimens or of relapses.

Although circulating memory B cells can be identified by their phenotypic B cell surface characters, the real questions are: are antigen-specific memory B cells present in the peripheral blood and are the tests available able to detect these rare resting cells? Recent results suggest that peripheral B cells initially purified and polyclonally activated *in vitro* can be identified by their specific antibody production by ELISPOT assay and cell-free supernatant analyses (Bernasconi et al., 2002; Crotty et al., 2003, 2004; Fondere et al., 2003, 2004). Thus, the measurement of the establishment or the disappearance of an immune response is possible by the enumeration of rare circulating resting B cells able to secrete specific antibodies. Moreover, the isotype of the Ig secreted by these cells can be determined, thus giving important information on their potential role in the B cell response to antigens.

In some HIV-1 patients under highly active antiretroviral therapy, the persistent low-level ongoing viral antigen expression might not be sufficient to maintain HIV-1-specific memory B cells. This has implications for possible explanations of the mechanisms involved in the generation of HIV-1-specific memory B cells by HIV-1 antigens. The enumeration of circulating Ag-specific memory B cells could be a new surrogate marker:

1 in experimental protocols measuring immunization
2 in non-responder subjects to vaccination
3 for the follow-up of therapeutic vaccinations in chronic infections or cancer
4 in the investigation of anti-tumor immunity by the determination of the tumor Ag-specific B-cell response.

ACKNOWLEDGMENTS

We are indebted to Dr S. L. Salhi for critical review and editing of the manuscript.

REFERENCES

Agematsu, K., Nagumo, H., Yang, F.C. et al. (1997). B cell subpopulations separated by CD27 and crucial collaboration of CD27+ B cells and helper T cells in immunoglobulin production. Eur J Immunol 27, 2073–2079.

Agematsu, K., Nagumo, H., Oguchi, Y. et al. (1998). Generation of plasma cells from peripheral blood memory B cells: synergistic effect of interleukin-10 and CD27/CD70 interaction. Blood 91, 173–180.

Agematsu, K., Hokibara, S., Nagumo, H. and Komiyama, A. (2000). CD27: a memory B-cell marker. Immunol Today 21, 204–206.

Agematsu, K., Futatani, T., Hokibara, S. et al. (2002). Absence of memory B cells in patients with common variable immunodeficiency. Clin Immunol 103, 34–42.

Ahmed, R. and Gray, D. (1996). Immunological memory and protective immunity: understanding their relation. Science 272, 54–60.

Amadori, A., De Rossi, A., Faulkner-Valle, G.P. and Chieco-Bianchi, L. (1988). Spontaneous in vitro production of virus-specific antibody by lymphocytes from HIV-infected subjects. Clin Immunol Immunopathol 46, 342–351.

Amadori, A., Zamarki, R., Ciminale, V. et al. (1989). HIV-1 specific B cell activation. A major constituent of spontaneous B cell activation during HIV-1 infection. J Immunol 143, 2146–2152.

Arpin, C., Dechanet, J., Van Kooten, C. et al. (1995). Generation of memory B cells and plasma cells in vitro. Science 268, 720–722.

Banchereau, J. and Rousset, F. (1992). Human B lymphocytes: phenotype, proliferation, and differentiation. Adv Immunol 52, 125–262.

Bar-Or, A., Oliveira, E.M., Anderson, D.E. et al. (2001). Immunological memory: contribution of memory B cells expressing costimulatory molecules in the resting state. J Immunol 167, 5669–5677.

Berberian, L., Goodglick, L., Kipps, T.J. and Braun, J. (1993). Immunoglobulin VH3 gene products: natural ligands for HIV gp120. Science 261, 1588–1591.

Bernasconi, N., Traggiai, E. and Lanzavecchia, A. (2002). Maintenance of serological memory by polyclonal activation of human memory B cells. Science. 298, 2199–2202.

Bohnhorst, J.O., Bjorgan, M.B., Thoen, J.E., Natvig, J.B. and Thompson, K. M. (2001). Bm1-Bm5 classification of peripheral blood B cells reveals circulating germinal center founder cells in healthy individuals and disturbance in the B cell subpopulations in patients with primary Sjogren's syndrome. J Immunol 167, 3610–3618.

Bowman, E.P., Kuklin, N.A., Youngman, K.R. et al. (2002). The intestinal chemokine thymus-expressed chemokine (CCL25) attracts IgA antibody-secreting cells. J Exp Med 195, 269–275.

Brown, K.A., Kriss, J.A., Moser, C.A., Wenner, W.J. and Offit, P.A. (2000). Circulating rotavirus-specific antibody-secreting cells (ASCs) predict the presence of rotavirus-specific ASCs in the human small intestinal lamina propria. J Infect Dis 182, 1039–1043.

Conge, A.M., Reynes, J., Atoui, N. et al. (1994). Spontaneous in vitro anti-human immunodeficiency virus type 1 antibody secretion by peripheral blood mononuclear cells is related to disease progression in zidovudine-treated adults. J Infect Dis 170, 1376–1383.

Cordoba, F., Lavabre-Bertrand, T., Salhi, S.L. et al. (2000). Spontaneous monoclonal immunoglobulin-secreting peripheral blood mononuclear cells as a marker of disease severity in multiple myeloma. Br J Haematol 108, 549–558.

Crotty, S., Felgner, P., Davies, H. et al. (2003). Long-term B cell memory in humans after smallpox vaccination. J Immunol 171, 4969–4973.

Crotty, S., Albert, R., Glidewell, J. and Ahmed, R. (2004). Tracking human antigen-specific memory B cells: a sensitive and generalized ELISPOT system. J Immunol Methods 286, 111–122.

Cyster, J.G., Ansel, K.M., Ngo, V.N., Hargreaves, D.C. and Lu, T.T. (2002). Traffic patterns of B cells and plasma cells. Adv Exp Med Biol 512, 35–41.

Cyster, J.G. (2003). Homing of antibody secreting cells. Immunol Rev 194, 48–60.

Czerkinsky, C., Moldoveanu, Z., Mestecky, J., Nilsson, L.A. and Ouchterlony, O. (1988). A novel two colour ELISPOT assay. I. Simultaneous detection of distinct types of antibody-secreting cells. J Immunol Methods 115, 31–37.

Czerkinsky, C., Svennerholm, A.M., Quiding, M., Jonsson, R. and Holmgren, J. (1991). Antibody-producing cells in peripheral blood and salivary glands after oral cholera vaccination of humans. Infect Immun 59, 996–1001.

De Milito, A., Morch, C., Sonnerborg, A. and Chiodi, F. (2001). Loss of memory (CD27) B lymphocytes in HIV-1 infection. AIDS 15, 957–964.

Ducos, J., Bianchi-Mondain, A.M., Pageaux, G. et al. (1996). Hepatitis B virus (HBV)-specific in vitro antibody production by peripheral blood mononuclear cells (PBMC) after vaccination by recombinant hepatitis B surface antigen (rHBsAg). Clin Exp Immunol 103, 15–18.

Dunn-Walters, D.K., Dogan, A., Boursier, L., Macdonald, C.M. and Spencer, J. (1998). Base-specific sequences that bias somatic hypermutation deduced by analysis of out-of-frame human IgVH genes. J Immunol 160, 2360–2364.

Fondere, J.M., Huguet, M.F., Yssel, H. et al. (2003). Detection of peripheral HIV-1-specific memory B cells in patients untreated or receiving highly active antiretroviral therapy. AIDS 17, 2323–2330.

Fondere, J.M., Huguet, M.F., Macura-Biegun, A. et al. (2004). Detection and enumeration of circulating HIV-1-specific memory B cells in HIV-1-infected patients. J Acquir Immune Defic Syndr 35, 114–119.

Fons, C.M., Uytdehagg, M., Loggen, H.G. et al. (1985). Human peripheral blood lymphocytes from recently vaccinated individuals produce both type specific and intertypic cross reacting neutralizing antibody on in vitro stimulation with one type of poliovirus. J Immunol 135, 3094–3101.

Forrest, B.D. (1988). Identification of an intestinal immune response using peripheral blood lymphocytes. Lancet 1, 81–83.

Forrest, B.D. (1992). Indirect measurement of intestinal immune responses to an orally administered attenuated bacterial vaccine. Infect Immun 60, 2023–2029.

Fournier, A.M., Fondere, J.M., Alix-Panabieres, C. et al. (2002a). Spontaneous secretion of immunoglobulins and anti-HIV-1 antibodies by in vivo activated B lymphocytes from HIV-1-infected subjects: monocyte and Natural Killer cell requirement for in vitro terminal differentiation into plasma cells. Clin Immunol 103, 98–109.

Fournier, A.M., Baillat, V., Alix-Panabieres, C. et al. (2002b). Dynamics of spontaneous HIV-1 specific and non-specific B-cell responses in patients receiving antiretroviral therapy. AIDS 16, 1755–1760.

Ghaem-Maghami, S., Bailey, R.L., Mabey, D.C. et al. (1997). Characterization of B-cell responses to Chlamydia trachomatis antigens in humans with trachoma. Infect Immun 65, 4958–4964.

Hansen, A., Odendahl, M., Reiter, K. et al. (2002). Diminished peripheral blood memory B cells and accumulation of memory B cells in the salivary glands of patients with Sjogren's syndrome. Arthritis Rheum 46, 2160–2171.

Hargreaves, D.C., Hyman, P.L., Lu, T.T. et al. (2001). A coordinated change in chemokine responsiveness guides plasma cell movements. J Exp Med 194, 45–56.

Hauser, A.E., Debes, G.F., Arce, S. et al. (2002). Chemotactic responsiveness toward ligands for CXCR3 and CXCR4 is regulated on plasma blasts during the time course of a memory immune response. J Immunol 169, 1277–1282.

Kantele, A., Arvilommi, H. and Jokinen, I. (1986). Specific immunoglobulin-secreting human blood cells after peroral vaccination against Salmonella typhi. J Infect Dis 153, 1126–1131.

Kantele, A.M., Tanaken, R. and Arvilommi, R. (1988). Immune response to acute diarrhea seen as circulating antibody-secreting cells. J Infect Dis 158, 1011–1016.

Kantele, A., Kantele, J.M., Arvilommi, H. and Makela, P. H. (1991). Active immunity is seen as a reduction in the cell response to oral live vaccine. Vaccine 9, 428–431.

Kantele, A., Papunen, R., Virtanen, E. et al. (1994). Antibody-secreting cells in acute urinary tract infection as indicators of local immune response. J Infect Dis 169, 1023–1028.

Karray, S. and Zouali, M. (1997). Identification of the B cell super-antigen-binding site of HIV-1 gp120. Proc Natl Acad Sci USA 94, 1356–1360.

Kerhl, J. and Fauci, A.S. (1983). Activation of human B lymphocytes after immunization with pneumococcal polysaccharides. J Clin Invest 71, 1032–1040.

Kindler, V. and Zubler, R.H. (1997). Memory, but not naive, peripheral blood B lymphocytes differentiate into Ig-secreting cells after CD40 ligation and costimulation with IL-4 and the differentiation factors IL-2, IL-10, and IL-3. J Immunol 159, 2085–2090.

Klein, U., Kuppers, R. and Rajewsky, K. (1997). Evidence for a large compartment of IgM-expressing memory B cells in humans. Blood 89, 1288–1298.

Klein, U., Rajewsky, K. and Küppers, R. (1998). Human immunoglobulin (Ig)M+IgD+ peripheral blood B cells expressing the CD27 cell surface antigen carry somatically mutated variable region genes: CD27 as a general marker for somatically mutated (memory) B cells. J Exp Med 188, 1679–1689.

Kocks, C. and Rajewsky, K. (1989). Stable expression and somatic hypermutation of antibody V regions in B-cell developmental pathways. Annu Rev Immunol 7, 537–559.

Kodituwakku, A.P., Jessup, C., Zola, H. and Roberton, D.M. (2003). Isolation of antigen-specific B cells. Immunol Cell Biol 81, 163–170.

Kruetzmann, S., Rosado, M.M., Weber, H. et al. (2003). Human immunoglobulin M memory B cells controlling Streptococcus pneumoniae infections are generated in the spleen. J Exp Med 197, 939–945.

Lacascade, C., Conge, A.M., Baillat, V. et al. (2000). In vitro anti-Toxoplasma gondii antibody production by peripheral blood mononuclear cells in the diagnosis and the monitoring of toxoplasmic encephalitis in AIDS-related brain lesions. J Acquir Immune Defic Syndr 25, 256–260.

Lee, F.K., Nahmias, A.J., Lowery, S. et al. (1989). ELISPOT: a new approach to studying the dynamics of virus-immune system interaction for diagnosis and monitoring of HIV infection. AIDS Res Hum Retroviruses 5, 517–523.

Liu, Y.J., Barthelemy, C., De Bouteiller, O., Arpin, C., Durand, I. and Banchereau, J. (1995). Memory B cells from human tonsils colonize mucosal epithelium and directly present antigen to T cells by rapid up-regulation of B7-1 and B7-2. Immunity 2, 239–248.

Liu, Y.J. and Arpin, C. (1997). Germinal center development. Immunol Rev 156, 111–126.

Mcheyzer-Williams, L.J., Cool, M. and Mcheyzer-Williams, M.G. (2000). Antigen-specific B cell memory: expression and replenishment of a novel B 220(-) memory B cell compartment. J Exp Med 191, 1149–1166.

MacLennan, I.C., Liu, Y.J. and Johnson, G.D. (1992). Maturation and dispersal of B-cell clones during T cell-dependent antibody responses. Immunol Rev 126, 143–161.

MacLennan, I.C., Gulbranson-Judge, A., Toellner, K.M. et al. (1997). The changing preference of T and B cells for partners as T-dependent antibody responses develop. Immunol Rev 156, 53–66.

Moir, S., Malaspina, A., Ogwaro, K. et al. (2001). HIV-1.induces phenotypic and functional perturbations of B cells in chronically infected individuals. Proc Natl Acad Sci USA 98, 10362–10367.

Morris, L., Binley, J.M., Clas, B.A. et al. (1998). HIV-1 antigen-specific and -nonspecific B cell responses are sensitive to combination antiretroviral therapy. J Exp Med 188, 233–245.

Nagase, H., Agematsu, K., Kitano, K. et al. (2001). Mechanism of hypergammaglobulinemia by HIV infection: circulating memory B-cell reduction with plasmacytosis. Clin Immunol 100, 250–259.

Nieminen, T., Virolainen, A., Kayhty, H. et al. (1996). Antibody-secreting cells and their relation to humoral antibodies in serum and in nasopharyngeal aspirates in children with pneumococcal acute otitis media. J Infect Dis 173, 136–141.

Notermans, D.W., de Jong, J.J., Goudsmit, J. et al. (2001). Potent antiretroviral therapy initiates normalization of hyper-gammaglobulinemia and a decline in HIV type 1 specific antibody responses. AIDS Res Hum Retroviruses 17, 1003–1008.

Odendahl, M., Jacobi, A., Hansen, A. et al. (2000). Disturbed peripheral B lymphocyte homeostasis in systemic lupus erythematosus. J Immunol 165, 5970–5979.

Oshiba, A., Renz, H., Yata, J. and Gelfand, E.W. (1994). Isolation and characterization of human antigen-specific B lymphocytes. Clin Immunol Immunopathol 72, 342–349.

Pahwa, S., Pahwa, R., Good, R.A., Gallo, R.C. and Saxinger, C. (1986). Stimulatory and inhibitory influences of human immunodeficiency virus on normal B lymphocytes. Proc Natl Acad Sci USA 83, 9124–9128.

Pahwa, S., Chirmule, N., Leombruno, C. et al. (1989). In vitro synthesis of human immunodeficiency virus-specific antibodies in peripheral blood lymphocytes of infants. Proc Natl Acad Sci USA 86, 7532–7536.

Paramithiotis, E. and Cooper, M.D. (1997). Memory B lymphocytes migrate to bone marrow in humans. Proc Natl Acad Sci USA 94, 208–212.

Pihlgren, M., Schallert, N., Tougne, C. et al. (2001). Delayed and deficient establishment of the long-term bone marrow plasma cell pool during early life. Eur J Immunol 31, 939–946.

Pollack, H., Zhan, M.X., Moore, T. et al. (1994). Effects of antiviral therapy on the production of anti-human immunodeficiency virus-specific immunoglobulin in infants and children. J Infect Dis 170, 1003–1006.

Quiding-Jarbrink, M., Lakew, M., Nordstrom, I. et al. (1995). Human circulating specific antibody-forming cells after systemic and mucosal immunizations: differential homing commitments and cell surface differentiation markers. Eur J Immunol 25, 322–327.

Quiding-Jarbrink, M., Nordstrom, I., Granstrom, G. et al. (1997). Differential expression of tissue-specific adhesion molecules on human circulating antibody-forming cells after systemic, enteric, and nasal immunizations. A molecular basis for the compartmentalization of effector B cell responses. J Clin Invest 99, 1281–1286.

Rajewsky, K. (1998). Burnet's unhappy hybrid. Nature 394, 624–625.

Revy, P., Muto, T., Levy, Y. et al. (2000). Activation-induced cytidine deaminase (AID) deficiency causes the autosomal recessive form of the Hyper-IgM syndrome (HIGM2). Cell 102, 565–575.

Richards, S.J., Morgan, G.J. and Hillmen, P. (2000). Immunophenotypic analysis of B cells in PNH: insights into the generation of circulating naive and memory B cells. Blood 96, 3522–3528.

Samuelsson, A., Brostrom, C., Van Dijk, N., Sonnerborg, A. and Chiodi, F. (1997a). Apoptosis of CD4+ and CD19+ cells during human immunodeficiency virus type 1 infection – correlation with clinical progression, viral load, and loss of humoral immunity. Virology 238, 180–188.

Samuelsson, A., Sonnerborg, A., Heuts, N., Coster, J. and Chiodi, F. (1997b). Progressive B cell apoptosis and expression of Fas ligand during human immunodeficiency virus type 1 infection. AIDS Res Hum Retroviruses 13, 1031–1038.

Schittek, B. and Rajewsky, K. (1990). Maintenance of B-cell memory by long-lived cells generated from proliferating precursors. Nature 346, 749–751.

Segondy, M., Vendrell, J.P., Reynes, J. et al. (1990). Cytomegalovirus-specific B cell activation as a potential marker for the diagnosis of cytomegalovirus infection. Eur J Clin Microbiol Infect Dis 9, 745–750.

Segondy, M., Barat, L., Mourad, G., Huguet, M.F., Serre, A. and Vendrell, J.P. (1993). Cytomegalovirus-specific in vitro antibody production by peripheral blood lymphocytes from renal transplant recipients with CMV infection. J Med Virol 40, 200–203.

Shi, Y., Agematsu, K., Ochs, H.D. and Sugane, K. (2003). Functional analysis of human memory B-cell subpopulations: IgD+CD27+ B cells are crucial in secondary immune response by producing high affinity IgM. Clin Immunol 108, 128–137.

Slifka, M.K., Matloubian, M. and Ahmed, R. (1995). Bone marrow is a major site of long-term antibody production after acute viral infection. J Virol 69, 1895–1902.

Slifka, M.K., Antia, R., Whitmire, J.K. and Ahmed, R. (1998). Humoral immunity due to long-lived plasma cells. Immunity 8, 363–372.

Smith, D.S., Creadon, G., Jena, P.K., Portanova, J.P., Kotzin, B.L. and Wysocki, L.J. (1996). Di- and trinucleotide target preferences of somatic mutagenesis in normal and autoreactive B cells. J Immunol 156, 2642–2652.

Stevens, R.H., Macy, E., Morrow, C. and Saxon, A. (1979). Characterization of a circulating subpopulation of spontaneous antitetanus toxoid antibody producing B cells following in vivo booster immunization. J Immunol 122, 2498–2504.

Tangye, S.G., Liu, Y.J., Aversa, G., Phillips, J.H. and De Vries, J.E. (1998). Identification of functional human splenic memory B cells by expression of CD148 and CD27. J Exp Med 188, 1691–1703.

Tangye, S.G., Avery, D.T. and Hodgkin, P.D. (2003a). A division-linked mechanism for the rapid generation of Ig-secreting cells from human memory B cells. J Immunol 170, 261–269.

Tangye, S.G., Avery, D.T., Deenick, E.K. and Hodgkin, P.D. (2003b). Intrinsic differences in the proliferation of naive and memory human B cells as a mechanism for enhanced secondary immune responses. J Immunol 170, 686–694.

Tarkowski, A., Czerkinsky, C. and Nilsson, L.A. (1985). Simultaneous induction of rheumatoid factor- and antigen-specific antibody-secreting cells during the secondary immune response in man. Clin Exp Immunol 61, 379–387.

Thomson, P.D. and Harris, N.S. (1977). Detection of plaque-forming cells in the peripheral blood of actively immunized humans. J Immunol 118, 1480–1482.

Vendrell, J.P., Segondy, M., Ducos, J. et al. (1991a). Analysis of the spontaneous in vitro anti-HIV-1 antibody secretion by peripheral blood mononuclear cells in HIV-1 infection. Clin Exp Immunol 83, 197–202.

Vendrell, J.P., Segondy, M., Fournier, A.M. et al. (1991b). Spontaneous in vitro secretion of antibody to cytomegalovirus (CMV) by human peripheral blood mononuclear cells: a new approach to studying the CMV-immune system interaction. J Infect Dis 164, 1–7.

Vendrell, J.P., Conge, A.M., Segondy, M. et al. (1992a). In vitro antibody secretion by peripheral blood mononuclear cells as an expression of the immune response to Brucella spp. in humans. J Clin Microbiol 30, 2200–2203.

Vendrell, J.P., Pratlong, F., Decoster, A. et al. (1992b). Secretion of Toxoplasma gondii-specific antibody in vitro by peripheral blood mononuclear cells as a new marker of acute toxoplasmosis. Clin Exp Immunol 89, 126–130.

Vendrell, J.P., Reynes, J., Huguet, M.F. et al. (1993). In-vitro synthesis of antibodies to Toxoplasma gondii by lymphocytes from HIV-1-infected patients. Lancet 342, 22–23.

Warnatz, K., Denz, A., Drager, R. et al. (2002). Severe deficiency of switched memory B cells (CD27(+)IgM(−)IgD(−)) in subgroups of patients with common variable immunodeficiency: a new approach to classify a heterogeneous disease. Blood 99, 1544–1551.

Williams, M.B., Rose, J.R., Rott, L.S., Franco, M.A., Greenberg, H.B. and Butcher, E.C. (1998). The memory B cell subset responsible for the secretory IgA response and protective humoral immunity to rotavirus expresses the intestinal homing receptor, alpha4beta7. J Immunol 161, 4227–4235.

Dendritic Cells

Chapter 24

Kenneth Field, Slavica Vuckovic and Derek N.J. Hart

Mater Medical Research Institute, South Brisbane, QLD, Australia

Honest differences are often a healthy sign of progress.

Mahatma Gandhi

INTRODUCTION

Surrogate markers to measure adaptive T cell immunity include cytotoxic T lymphocyte responses, cytokine production by T lymphocytes and more recently, antigen-specific T lymphocytes determined by tetramer/monomer technology. However, T lymphocyte responses are dependent on antigen-presenting cells, notably dendritic cells (DC), which in their various forms have been shown to initiate and direct T lymphocyte responses. DC also contribute to B lymphocyte and natural killer (NK) cell responses. Thus, fundamental to the complete measurement of immunity is the ability to accurately assess DC numbers and function along with other effector cells. Therefore, the requirement for reliable and rapid methods to assess DC numbers and function as clinical research tools has become an imperative. One can assume that the on-going technical evolution in these methods will be a stimulus for an exponential increase in data covering DC counts and function in a broad range of disease states. Wherever possible, available functional DC data have been correlated with absolute DC count data. DC counting and DC function are predicted to become clinically relevant biomarkers that correlate with clinical responses.

DC COUNTING: CAVEATS AND DIFFICULTIES

Flow cytometric methods for DC enumeration have progressed slowly. This has been primarily due to a lack of monoclonal antibodies (mAb) specific for DC cell surface markers and the relative low frequency of this leukocyte population in blood and other tissues (Hart, 1997; Banchereau and Steinman, 1998). Human research is limited by access, requiring a focus on peripheral blood DC rather than bone marrow, spleen, thymus or lymph node DC, which are readily available for murine studies.

Many studies have measured blood DC counts in both healthy donors and patients, but a lack of consistency in the DC isolation procedures and the phenotypic criteria used to define DC has led to considerable variability in reported DC counts (Macey et al., 1998; Fagnoni et al., 2001; Vuckovic, et al., 2001; Hock et al., 2002; Szabolcs et al., 2003). A further issue is DC viability after isolation from blood (Ho et al., 2002). The lack of DC specific reference standards is another technical obstacle that makes validation of any DC counting assay difficult. Direct comparison of DC counts between studies is currently very difficult. The two key contributions to improve peripheral blood DC counting have been the evolution of mAb to help identify DC and their subsets, plus the better standardization of the flow cytometric methodology.

Measuring Immunity, edited by Michael T. Lotze and Angus W. Thomson
ISBN 0-12-455900-X, London

TOOLS FOR DC COUNTING

Defining DC as CMRF-44$^+$ or CMRF-56$^+$ cells

Pioneering studies identifying and quantifying peripheral blood DC utilized the mAb CMRF-44 (Fearnley et al., 1999). Similarly, the CMRF-56 mAb can be used as an additional marker to identify blood DC (Hock et al., 1999; Lopez et al., 2003). Directly isolated blood DC lack both the CMRF-44 and the CMRF-56 antigens, but they are upregulated on DC during in vitro culture (Hock et al., 1994, 1999). Therefore, this approach quantified blood DC that undergo spontaneous maturation during in vitro culture, which may not represent the entire blood DC population. Nonetheless, it indicated the utility of blood DC counting and that blood DC counts changed in different clinical circumstances (Fearnley et al., 1999). To exclude monocyte or B lymphocyte subpopulations, which express detectable, but lesser amounts of these antigens, the method also includes labeling with mAb specific for CD14 and CD19 antigens, so that DC were determined as CMRF-44$^+$CD14$^-$CD19$^-$ or CMRF-56$^+$CD14$^-$CD19$^-$ cells. Forward scatter (FSC) and side scatter (SSC) light characteristics were used to gate the 'live' cells and exclude debris and dead cells. The use of propidium iodide (PI) or 7-aminoactinomycin D (7-AAD) as a viability marker was recommended, due to the cell death observed during the culture of isolated peripheral blood mononuclear cells (PBMC). Absolute DC counts were calculated by multiplying the number of PBMC (as determined by an automated cell counter) by the flow cytometers determined percentage of DC in the CMRF-44$^+$CD14$^-$CD19$^-$ or CMRF-56$^+$CD14$^-$CD19$^-$ gate (dual-platform approach).

Defining DC as Lin$^-$HLA-DR$^+$ cells

Initially, directly isolated blood DC were defined as leukocytes, which lack differentiation antigens associated with T, B, monocyte and NK lineages, but express the HLA-DR antigen (referred to as Lin$^-$HLA-DR$^+$ cells) (Egner et al., 1993). In this method, ficoll-density gradient isolated PBMC or whole blood is labeled with a cocktail of mAb specific for T lymphocytes, B lymphocytes, monocytes, NK cells and HLA-DR antigen. The choice of mAb that comprise the lineage cocktail is critical. Routinely, mAb specific for CD3, CD14, CD19, CD20, CD34 and CD56 are present in the mix and frequently mAb specific for CD16 is added to the mix to facilitate NK cell recognition. Due to the low cell surface antigen expression of CD19 antigen, the use of mAb specific for both CD19 and CD20 is recommended for the exclusion of B lymphocytes. DC are determined as Lin$^-$HLA-DR$^+$ cells. FSC and SSC characteristics are used to gate the 'live' cells and exclude debris and dead cells. Decisions regarding the margins of the Lin$^-$HLA-DR$^+$ gate remain an important issue

(Ho et al., 2001). It is relevant that the key discriminator regarding monocytes is completely dependent on the expression of the CD14 antigen, which is not ideal. Absolute DC counts are determined using a dual-platform approach, where the number of PBMC (as determined by an automated cell counter) is multiplied by the percentage of DC in the Lin$^-$HLA-DR$^+$ gate.

Defining DC as CD11c$^+$DC (M-DC) and CD123^{hi} DC (P-DC)

Distinct DC subsets have now been defined within Lin$^-$HLA-DR$^+$ cells with the CD11c$^+$DC (known as myeloid DC or M-DC) and the CD123^{hi}DC (known as plasmacytoid monocytes or P-DC) (Olweus et al., 1997; Cella et al., 1999; Siegal et al., 1999) now well accepted as having differing precursors and functional characteristics (Robinson et al., 1999; Kadowaki et al., 2001). The terms DC1 (M-DC, originally monocyte-derived DC) and DC2 (P-DC) were introduced, attempting to indicate the capacity of DC1 or DC2 cells to induce Th1 or Th2 responses, respectively (Rissoan et al., 1999). The plasticity of M-DC and P-DC has meant these terms are now less favored (Cella et al., 2000; Reis e Sousa, 2004). Commercial reagent systems for enumerating the blood M-DC and P-DC subsets are available. Four color 'dendritic value bundles' include a fluorescein isothiocyanate (FITC) conjugated lineage cocktail (anti-CD3, anti-CD14, anti-CD16, anti-CD19, anti-CD20 and anti-CD56), peridinin chlorophyll protein (PerCP) conjugated anti-HLA-DR, allophycocyanin (APC) conjugated anti-CD11c and R-phycoerythrin (PE) conjugated anti-CD123 mAb. The manufacturer's recommended gating strategy is to draw a region around all leukocytes in a FSC versus SSC dot plot, while excluding debris and dead cells. From this initial region all Lin$^-$ events are gated and then displayed in a dot plots of anti-CD11c versus anti-HLA-DR or anti-CD123 versus anti-HLA-DR, where M-DC are identified as CD11c$^+$HLA-DR$^+$ and P-DC as CD123^{hi}HLA-DR$^+$ cells, respectively. These two subsets account for the majority of Lin$^-$HLA-DR$^+$ cells in blood samples from healthy donors. It is important to realize that we are still dealing with uncertainties regarding human blood DC subpopulations. Thus, it is possible that the CD14$^+$CD16$^+$ subset contributes directly to the DC pool (Ho et al., 2002) and an additional new CD11c$^-$CD123$^-$Lin$^-$HLA-DR$^+$ subpopulation has been noted previously (Hagendorens et al., 2003). This is known colloquially in our laboratory as the 'gap population' (Ho et al. in preparation). This 'gap population' may rise in pathological circumstances but is not formally included in most current DC analyses. Absolute DC counts are determined using a dual-platform approach, where the number of PBMC (as determined by an automated cell counter) is multiplied by the percentage of DC in either the CD11c$^+$ HLA-DR$^+$ or CD123^{hi}HLA-DR$^+$ gate.

Defining DC as CD1c$^+$, BDCA-3$^+$ and BDCA-2$^+$ cells

More recently, the blood M-DC subset was further subdivided into three subsets, demarcated by CD16, CD1c and BDCA-3 expression (MacDonald et al., 2002). The antibody BDCA-1 was shown in Human Leukocyte Differentiation Antigen Workshop (HLDAW) studies to identify CD1c, while BDCA-3 recognizes a distinct subset of high density CD11c$^+$M-DC (MacDonald et al., 2002). Production of the mAb BDCA-2 and BDCA-4 (Dzionek et al., 2000) further reinforced the identity of the P-DC and helped avoid the pitfall of classifying M-DC, which express lower levels of CD123, as P-DC. A commercial blood DC enumeration kit that identifies CD1c$^+$DC, BDCA-3$^+$DC and BDCA-2$^+$DC either in PBMC or in whole blood has recently become available. To exclude monocytes and B lymphocytes, which react with the mAb CD1c, the kit includes labeling with mAb specific for CD14 and CD19 antigens. Using this kit, cells are labeled with a cocktail of FITC-conjugated BDCA-2, PE-conjugated anti-CD1c, APC-conjugated BDCA-3, R-phycoerythrin-cyanine 5 (PE-Cy5) conjugated anti-CD14 and PE-Cy5-conjugated anti-CD19 mAb, as well as a dead cell discriminator dye. An advantage with this approach compared to previous approaches, is that fewer mAb are required providing a significant cost benefit. However, potential problems include the loss of cells due to the inclusion of a washing step and complex compensation issues due to the use of the tandem conjugate PE-Cy5 in combination with APC.

DC counting using single-platform TruCOUNT™ technology

Most DC counting methods utilized labor-intensive cell isolation protocols to prepare PBMC, including ficoll-density separation and washing/centrifugation steps. The enumeration of human blood DC subsets, utilizing TruCOUNT™ bead technology, was introduced recently by Vuckovic et al. (2004) as a clinically applicable test for diagnostic work. This technology employs a whole blood lyse/no-wash protocol to eliminate centrifugation and washing steps, which are potential sources of variability and cell loss. DC counts are determined on a single-platform, which eliminates the requirement for automated cell counts. The small sample volume required facilitates the routine clinical use of this technology for both pediatric and patient samples, where the collection of large volumes of blood is problematic. This is an important step forward that could lead to the global standardization of DC counting for physiological, diagnostic and prognostic applications in clinical practice. Briefly, each TruCOUNT™ tube contains a known number of fluorescent beads to which a known quantity of whole blood sample is added. The absolute number of DC in the sample is determined by comparing total bead events to cellular events in the particular DC gating region. Vuckovic

et al. (2004) use a CD45 versus SSC primary gate, which is currently the predicate method or 'gold standard' for absolute counting of both CD4$^+$ T lymphocytes (Gratama et al., 2002; Schnizlein-Bick et al., 2002) and CD34$^+$ hematopoietic stem cells (HSC) (Gratama et al., 2003). This gating clearly distinguishes between cellular debris and all leukocyte populations. The DC population is subsequently determined using a cocktail of mAb specific for HLA-DR and lineage antigens. The Lin$^-$HLA-DR$^+$DC population is further differentiated into M-DC and P-DC subsets, as has been described previously. Szabolcs et al. (2003) used TruCOUNT™ technology to count DC in peripheral blood, cord blood and bone marrow. Their gating strategy required a subjective determination of HLA-DR^{dim} cells and this decision may account for the significantly lower absolute blood DC counts described by them.

It is also relevant that, when Vuckovic et al. (2004) determined the absolute DC counts in 10 normal adult donors, using the single platform technique and compared the DC counts obtained using ficoll-density gradient isolated PBMC, the latter counts were three- to fourfold lower. This discrepancy between counting methods can in part be attributed to the formation of DC-CD3$^+$ T lymphocyte conjugates during density gradient isolation as well as multiple washing steps. Whether these conjugate formations are a result of specific DC-CD3$^+$ T lymphocyte interactions or occur non-specifically due to enhanced cell adhesion is unclear. However, now that it has been demonstrated that ficoll-density gradient cell isolation adversely affects absolute DC counts in peripheral blood, this method can no longer be recommended for DC counting.

TOOLS FOR DC FUNCTION

Stimulation of allogeneic MLR by DC

It is known that DC are potent inducers of proliferation of allogeneic naive lymphocytes in a mixed leukocyte reaction (MLR) and this functional property distinguishes them from other leukocytes (Hart, 1997; Banchereau and Steinman, 1998). This potent allostimulatory capacity is related to their high constitutive expression of MHC class II and costimulatory molecules CD40, CD80 and CD86 (Lu and Thomson, 2001). Multiple factors influence the number and type of effector cells generated in the allogeneic MLR including the DC type, DC produced cytokines and DC:T lymphocyte ratio (Tanaka et al., 2000). McDonald et al. (2002) demonstrated clear differences between DC subsets, with the CD1c$^+$ subset exhibiting the greatest allostimulatory MLR capacity. Our data indicate that monocyte-derived DC (Mo-DC) may stimulate greater allogeneic proliferative responses than blood M-DC, though it is difficult to draw definite conclusions due to the inconsistency in MLR responses and inherent technical variability in the MLR assay (Osugi et al., 2002). Monitoring relative allostimulatory capacity compared to a control preparation using the same responders is essential, but logistically very difficult.

Cytokine production by DC

DC can discriminate between various types of micro-organisms by toll-like receptors and are capable of producing different inflammatory cytokines in response to various microbial stimuli (Kadowaki et al., 2001). A functional definition of cytokines distinguishes between type-1 cytokines, which induce cell-mediated immunity and type-2 cytokines, which promote humoral immunity against tumors and/or tolerance (Belardelli and Ferrantini, 2002). M-DC after stimulation with lipopolysaccharide (LPS), poly I:C or CD40 ligand produce IL-12, a critical Th1 polarizing cytokine (Langenkamp et al., 2000). P-DC after stimulation with virus produce large amounts of IFN-α, a critical cytokine for humoral immunity (Chehimi et al., 1989). However, cytokine production by P-DC may vary considerably depending on external stimuli (Hart, 2001). Nonetheless, it is now relatively easy to sort DC subsets from patients and analyse their cytokine production to a defined stimulus. This may be used more as a quality control assay rather than an investigational/diagnostic assay.

Phagocytic capacity of DC

Immature DC possess the capacity for phagocytosis, macropinocytosis and endocytosis of soluble or particulate antigen (Banchereau and Steinman, 1998). M-DC possess a similar phagocytic capacity as monocytes, whereas P-DC have less phagocytic capacity (Robinson et al., 1999; Stent et al., 2002). M-DC have been reported to phagocytose large particles such as whole cells, bacteria and synthetic beads (Hart, 1997). Apoptotic cells phagocytosed by DC are broken down and apoptotic cell-derived antigens are presented in the context of MHC class I (cross-presentation) or MHC class II on the cell surface (Zinkernagel, 2002). Flow cytometry based methods allow some of these, e.g. fluid phase (lucifer yellow), phagocytosis FITC-dextran or particle (FITC beads), to be readily investigated.

Spontaneous apoptosis of DC

Apoptosis regulates many aspects in immunological homeostasis and DC express surface receptors that are known to mediate cell death (Matsue and Takashima, 1999). In vitro experiments have shown DC to undergo rapid apoptosis during antigen-specific interaction with CD4$^+$ lymphocytes, requiring a class II-dependent DC-T lymphocyte interaction and this serves as a mechanism to downregulate cellular immune responses (Matsue et al., 1999).

Indoleamine 2,3-dioxygenase production by DC

Activated DC produce the enzyme indoleamine 2,3-dioxygenase (IDO), which causes tryptophan depletion and inhibition of T lymphocyte proliferation (Hwu et al., 2000). A recent study established that IDO$^+$ DC constituted a discrete subset of DC, identified by the expression of CD123 and CCR6 (Munn et al., 2002). It would appear that this minor subset of plasmacytoid DC plays a significant role in immune regulation. An increase in IDO production and an accumulation of IDO$^+$ cells has been described in infection, autoimmunity, allergy and cancer patients (Grohmann et al., 2003; von Bubnoff et al., 2003). Murine studies have shown that IDO producing mononuclear cells invade tumors and tumor-draining lymph nodes and this may be one of the mechanisms by which tumors evade rejection by the immune system (Friberg et al., 2002).

CLINICAL UTILIZATION OF DC COUNTS AND FUNCTION

Whereas initial DC studies focused primarily on functional and phenotypic characterization of DC and their subpopulations, there was a paucity of data detailing changes in absolute counts. Subsequently, there has been some correlation between studies showing alterations in DC counts in certain disease states (Fearnley et al., 1999; Vuckovic, et al., 2004), though methodology differences prohibit direct comparison of absolute DC counts. While early observations would indicate significant clinical relevance, comprehensive longitudinal studies need to be established to define DC count changes in the context of clinical pathophysiology. The true value of DC counting and function will be how well it helps clinicians to understand and manipulate immune responses in disease.

DC counts in age

While it is well known that total white blood cell counts decline with age (Hulstaert et al., 1994), it has only recently been observed that DC counts also follow this pattern of decline with age (Shodell and Siegal, 2002; Teig et al., 2002; Vakkila et al., 2004; Vuckovic et al., 2004). Our studies have shown significantly higher M-DC and P-DC counts in children compared to adults (Vuckovic et al., 2004). These observations raise the important issue that DC counts change in normal individuals with age, either because of host physiological factors or as a result of immune experience (Figure 24.1). These data emphasize the need to use normal age-matched controls when investigating alterations in absolute DC counts in disease patients, especially in infants. One can imagine that more comprehensive reports of the kinetics of these age-related changes in DC counts will be forthcoming.

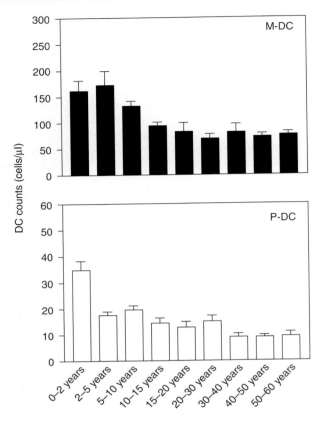

Figure 24.1 Age related changes of absolute DC counts. Absolute DC counts obtained by the single-platform TruCOUNT assay in newborn (age range 0–2 years, $n = 7$), children (age range 2–5 years, $n = 5$; age range 5–10 years, $n = 13$; age range 10–15 years, $n = 13$) and adult blood samples (age range 15–20 years, $n = 4$; age range 20–30 years, $n = 15$; age range 30–40 years, $n = 6$; age range 40–50 years, $n = 22$ and age range 50–60 years, $n = 12$). The absolute M-DC (solid bars) and the P-DC (open bars) counts are shown (mean +/−SEM, cells/μl).

DC counts and function in physical stress

Exercise and surgical stress have been demonstrated to cause a rapid rise in DC numbers (Upham et al., 2000; Ho et al., 2001) and that this *in vivo* rise during surgical stress, but not exercise, is independent of monocyte counts. This would indicate that blood DC and monocytes, considered by some to be an *in vivo* precursor of DC, are regulated differently depending on the physiological conditions. Ho et al. (2001) also noted that 2–3 day postoperative DC counts showed a temporary decrease of 25 per cent compared to pre-operative counts and if pronounced, these changes may potentially be an important factor in infection risk following major surgery. Routine monitoring of peripheral blood DC numbers may have prognostic value after surgery and the potential to assist in patient management.

Functionally, no corresponding increase in the ability of DC collected during surgical stress to stimulate an allogeneic MLR, or measurable upregulation of the activation

and costimulatory molecules CMRF-44, CD40 and CD86 was evident (Ho et al., 2001).

DC counts and function in autoimmune disease and infection

It has been shown that P-DC are preferentially increased in the peripheral blood of atopic patients compared to age-matched controls (Matsuda et al., 2002; Reider et al., 2002). The increase in P-DC counts in these atopic patients also positively correlated with serum IgE levels and eosinophil counts (Uchida et al., 2001). Alterations in DC counts have also been noted in systemic lupus erythematosus (SLE) patients (Blanco et al., 2001; Scheinecker et al., 2001). Chronic liver disease patients (hepatitis B, hepatitis C, hepatocellular carcinoma, primary biliary cirrhosis and autoimmune hepatitis) showed a significant reduction in the number of circulating M-DC with disease progression (Kunitani et al., 2002). A significant decrease in M-DC counts, inversely correlated with virus replication, has also been observed in HIV patients, while P-DC counts are also significantly reduced in HIV patients irrespective of viral load (Grassi et al., 1999; Chehimi et al., 2002).

Functional studies have shown that Mo-DC from hepatitis B and hepatitis C patients have significantly lower allostimulatory capacity in MLR compared to healthy donors and this functional impairment may indicate a contributory mechanism for viral persistence in chronic viral infection (Kanto et al., 1999; Auffermann-Gretzinger et al., 2001; Bain et al., 2001; Beckebaum et al., 2002). Interestingly, DC from HIV patients are not impaired in their ability to stimulate allogeneic T lymphocytes (Cameron et al., 1992; Chehimi et al., 2002). In patients with inflammatory bowel disease, blood M-DC show an activation phenotype, with high levels of surface expression of CD40 and CD86 compared to normal age matched controls (Vuckovic et al., 2001). Monitoring the activation state of blood DC in inflammatory disease may yield prognostic information. Mo-DC from atopic patients produce significantly less IL-12 than those from healthy donors in response to maturation agents (Reider et al., 2002). Histamine, a mediator released by allergen-stimulated mast cells, inhibits IL-12 production and consequently the Th1 response (Caron et al., 2001). This release of histamine and potentially other mediators, in conjunction with the increased P-DC counts in atopic patients may contribute to the enhanced Th2-type immune responses seen in these disease states. SLE patients, though having markedly reduced numbers of circulating blood P-DC, produce similar levels of IFN-α as normal controls. These defects may contribute to the pathological mechanisms involved in the autoimmune response seen in this disease (Cederblad et al., 1998; Blanco et al., 2001; Palucka et al., 2002). IFN-α has been proposed as a potential target for therapeutic intervention in SLE (Dzionek et al., 2001; Blomberg et al., 2003).

DC counts and function in cancer

Controversial findings have been reported on the number of blood DC in cancer patients. Decreased numbers of blood DC in multiple myeloma (MM) patients have been described (Ratta et al., 2002). Our data suggested that, although the numbers of P-DC are significantly reduced in MM patients, M-DC numbers are only slightly reduced in early disease (Vuckovic et al., 2004) (Figure 24.2). CMRF-44[+] DC counts are relatively unaffected in early stage MM patients (Brown et al., 2001). CMRF-44[+] DC numbers in breast cancer appear to decline in early stage disease (Ho et al. in preparation). Likewise, a study by Almand et al. (2000) demonstrated reduced DC counts in head and neck squamous cell carcinoma patients, which positively correlated with disease stage. Surgical excision of the tumours resulted in increased counts of circulating blood DC. This might be attributed to the effects of vascular endothelial growth factor on DC hematopoiesis (Gabrilovich et al., 1996; Almand et al., 2000) but data needs to be reproduced using the latest counting systems. Conversely, significantly higher DC counts have been observed in acute myeloid leukemia patients (Mohty et al., 2001). A study conducted on a limited cohort of patients with solid tumors (gastrointestinal, lung, breast, renal cell and uterine carcinoma) indicated that blood DC numbers are substantially decreased in patients with metastatic disease, but not in locally limited disease (Lissoni et al., 1999). For DC based cancer immunotherapy, DC count monitoring may well become a critical marker for mobilization schedules, in much the same way as CD34[+] HSC counting in bone marrow transplantation (Arpinati et al., 2000; Vuckovic et al., 2003). It has been shown that the administration of cytokines can expand blood DC numbers. For example, Flt-3-ligand significantly increased both M-DC and P-DC counts in peripheral blood of healthy donors (Pulendran et al., 2000) and cancer patients (Marroquin et al., 2002), while granulocyte-colony stimulating factor (G-CSF) preferentially increased the P-DC counts in healthy donors, MM patients and to a lesser extent in non-Hodgkin lymphoma. This increase in P-DC counts may be due to their inability to home to secondary lymphoid tissues (Vuckovic et al., 2003). Other DC mobilizing factors, e.g. MIP-1 alpha (Zhang et al., 2004), are likely to be investigated and careful monitoring of blood DC counts will be needed to optimize the dose of mobilization agents and timing of apheresis for DC collection.

DC function is also affected by cancers, for example, MM patients show impaired induction of allogeneic T lymphocyte proliferation due to the failure of CD80 upregulation after human CD40 ligand stimulation (Brown et al., 2001). Tumor-associated DC in transitional cell carcinoma of the bladder and kidney have also been shown to be minimally activated (Troy et al., 1998, 1999). Aberrant antigen presenting functions in blood DC from advanced stage breast cancer patients have been observed (Gabrilovich et al., 1996, 1997) and a lack of activated DC has been noted within breast tumors (Bell et al., 1999; Coventry et al., 2002). Another report demonstrated reduced phagocytic ability of DC from breast cancer patients (Pockaj et al., 2004).

DC counts and function in transplantation

DC counting may also have implications for the monitoring of patients following allogeneic hematopoietic stem cell transplantation. Clarke et al. (2003) have demonstrated that patients with chronic graft-versus host disease (cGVHD) had significantly higher numbers of P-DC than patients without this complication. No differences were observed in the DC phenotype between these two patient groups, however, chimerism studies established that the DC in patients with cGVHD were exclusively of donor origin. It has also been observed that an increase in CMRF-44[+] DC counts coincides with GVHD episodes (Vuckovic and Hart, 2002).

Given the fundamental role DC play in allograft rejection, there would appear to be a justification for the monitoring of DC counts and their activation status in solid organ (renal, liver and heart) transplantation.

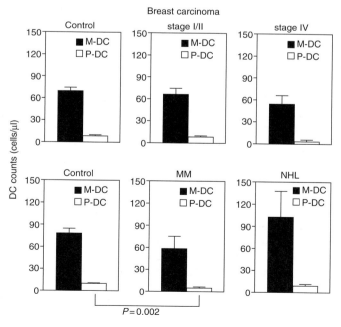

Figure 24.2 Absolute DC counts in patients with neoplastic diseases. Absolute DC counts obtained by the single-platform TruCOUNT assay in breast carcinoma patients (stage I/II, $n = 11$; stage IV, $n = 6$), multiple myeloma (MM) patients ($n = 7$), non-Hodgkin lymphoma (NHL) patients ($n = 5$) and in age matched control adult blood samples. The absolute M-DC (solid bars) and the P-DC (open bars) counts are shown (mean +/−SEM, cells/μl).

CONCLUDING REMARKS

Rapid technological advances in the field of flow cytometry, e.g. instrumentation, software and fluorochrome chemistry, will have profound effects on the future of measuring DC numbers and function. We are currently seeing a range of techniques being adapted to whole blood, which include the ability to test some DC functions. One can envisage that, in the near future, multiplexing assays that simultaneously measure a range of clinically meaningful blood DC biomarkers in a small volume of whole blood will be commonplace in measuring immunity.

ACKNOWLEDGEMENTS

The authors gratefully acknowledge Dr David Munster and Adam McKinlay for their assistance in the editing of this manuscript.

REFERENCES

Almand, B., Resser, J.R., Lindman, B. et al. (2000). Clinical significance of defective dendritic cell differentiation in cancer. Clin Cancer Res 6, 1755–1766.

Arpinati, M., Green, C.L., Heimfeld, S., Heuser, J.E. and Anasetti, C. (2000). Granulocyte-colony stimulating factor mobilizes T helper 2-inducing dendritic cells. Blood 95, 2484–2490.

Auffermann-Gretzinger, S., Keeffe, E.B. and Levy, S. (2001). Impaired dendritic cell maturation in patients with chronic, but not resolved, hepatitis C virus infection. Blood 97, 3171–3176.

Bain, C., Fatmi, A., Zoulim, F., Zarski, J.-P., Trepo, C. and Inchauspe, G. (2001). Impaired allostimulatory function of dendritic cells in chronic hepatitis C infection. Gastroenterology 120, 512–524.

Bancereau, J. and Steinman, R.M. (1998). Dendritic cells and the control of immunity. Nature 392, 245–252.

Beckebaum, S., Cicinnati, V.R., Dworacki, G. et al. (2002). Reduction in the circulating pDC1/pDC2 ratio and impaired function of ex vivo-generated DC1 in chronic hepatitis B infection. Clin Immunol 104, 138–150.

Belardelli, F. and Ferrantini, M. (2002). Cytokines as a link between innate and adaptive antitumor immunity. Trends Immunol 23, 201–208.

Bell, D., Chomarat, P., Broyles, D. et al. (1999). In breast carcinoma tissue, immature dendritic cells reside within the tumor, whereas mature dendritic cells are located in peritumoral areas. J Exp Med 190, 1417–1426.

Blanco, P., Palucka, A.K., Gill, M., Pascual, V. and Bancereau, J. (2001). Induction of dendritic cell differentiation by IFN-alpha in systemic lupus erythematosus. Science 294, 1540–1543.

Blomberg, S., Eloranta, M.L., Magnusson, M., Alm, G.V. and Ronnblom, L. (2003). Expression of the markers BDCA-2 and BDCA-4 and production of interferon-alpha by plasmacytoid dendritic cells in systemic lupus erythematosus. Arthritis Rheum 48, 2524–2532.

Brown, R.D., Pope, B., Murray, A. et al. (2001). Dendritic cells from patients with myeloma are numerically normal but functionally defective as they fail to up-regulate CD80 (B7–1) expression after huCD40LT stimulation because of inhibition by transforming growth factor-beta1 and interleukin-10. Blood 98, 2992–2998.

Cameron, P.U., Forsum, U., Teppler, H., Granelli-Piperno, A. and Steinman, R.M. (1992). During HIV-1 infection most blood dendritic cells are not productively infected and can induce allogeneic CD4+ T cells clonal expansion. Clin Exp Immunol 88, 226–236.

Caron, G., Delneste, Y., Roelandts, E. et al. (2001). Histamine polarizes human dendritic cells into Th2 cell-promoting effector dendritic cells. J Immunol 167, 3682–3686.

Cederblad, B., Blomberg, S., Vallin, H., Perers, A., Alm, G.V. and Ronnblom, L. (1998). Patients with systemic lupus erythematosus have reduced numbers of circulating natural interferon-alpha- producing cells. J Autoimmun 11, 465–470.

Cella, M., Facchetti, F., Lanzavecchia, A. and Colonna, M. (2000). Plasmacytoid dendritic cells activated by influenza virus and CD40L drive a potent TH1 polarization. Nat Immunol 1, 305–310.

Cella, M., Jarrossay, D., Facchetti, F. et al. (1999). Plasmacytoid monocytes migrate to inflamed lymph nodes and produce large amounts of type I interferon. Nat Med 5, 919–923.

Chehimi, J., Starr, S.E., Kawashima, H. et al. (1989). Dendritic cells and IFN-alpha-producing cells are two functionally distinct non-B, non-monocytic HLA-DR+ cell subsets in human peripheral blood. Immunology 68, 488–490.

Chehimi, J., Campbell, D.E., Azzoni, L. et al. (2002). Persistent decreases in blood plasmacytoid dendritic cell number and function despite effective highly active antiretroviral therapy and increased blood myeloid dendritic cells in HIV-infected individuals. J Immunol 168, 4796–4801.

Coventry, B.J., Lee, P.L., Gibbs, D. and Hart, D.N. (2002). Dendritic cell density and activation status in human breast cancer – CD1a, CMRF-44, CMRF-56 and CD-83 expression. Br J Cancer 86, 546–551.

Dzionek, A., Fuchs, A., Schmidt, P. et al. (2000). BDCA-2, BDCA-3, and BDCA-4: three markers for distinct subsets of dendritic cells in human peripheral blood. J Immunol 165, 6037–46.

Dzionek, A., Sohma, Y., Nagafune, J. et al. (2001). BDCA-2, a novel plasmacytoid dendritic cell-specific type II C-type lectin, mediates antigen capture and is a potent inhibitor of interferon {alpha}/{beta} induction. J Exp Med 194, 1823–1834.

Egner, W. and Hart, D.N. (1995). The phenotype of freshly isolated and cultured human bone marrow allostimulatory cells: possible heterogeneity in bone marrow dendritic cell populations. Immunology 85, 611–620.

Egner, W., Andreesen, R. and Hart, D.N. (1993). Allostimulatory cells in fresh human blood: heterogeneity in antigen-presenting cell populations. Transplantation 56, 945–950.

Fagnoni, F.F., Oliviero, B., Zibera, C. et al. (2001). Circulating CD33+ large mononuclear cells contain three distinct populations with phenotype of putative antigen-presenting cells including myeloid dendritic cells and CD14+ monocytes with their CD16+ subset. Cytometry 45, 124–132.

Fearnley, D.B., Whyte, L.F., Carnoutsos, S.A., Cook, A.H. and Hart, D.N. (1999). Monitoring human blood dendritic cell numbers in normal individuals and in stem cell transplantation. Blood 93, 728–736.

Friberg, M., Jennings, R., Alsarraj, M. et al. (2002). Indoleamine 2,3-dioxygenase contributes to tumor cell evasion of T cell-mediated rejection. Int J Cancer 101, 151–155.

Gabrilovich, D.I., Corak, J., Ciernik, I.F., Kavanaugh, D. and Carbone, D.P. (1997). Decreased antigen presentation by dendritic cells in patients with breast cancer. Clin Cancer Res 3, 483–490.

Gabrilovich, D.I., Chen, H.L., Girgis, K.R. et al. (1996). Production of vascular endothelial growth factor by human tumors inhibits the functional maturation of dendritic cells. Nat Med 2, 1096–1103.

Grassi, F., Hosmalin, A., McIlroy, D., Calvez, V., Debre, P. and Autran, B. (1999). Depletion in blood CD11c-positive dendritic cells from HIV-infected patients. Aids 13, 759–766.

Gratama, J.W., Kraan, J., Keeney, M., Granger, V. and Barnett, D. (2002). Reduction of variation in T-cell subset enumeration among 55 laboratories using single-platform, three or four-color flow cytometry based on CD45 and SSC-based gating of lymphocytes. Cytometry 50, 92–101.

Gratama, J.W., Kraan, J., Keeney, M., Sutherland, D.R., Granger, V. and Barnett, D. (2003). Validation of the single-platform ISHAGE method for CD34(+) hematopoietic stem and progenitor cell enumeration in an international multicenter study. Cytotherapy 5, 55–65.

Grohmann, U., Fallarino, F. and Puccetti, P. (2003). Tolerance, DCs and tryptophan: much ado about IDO. Trends Immunol 24, 242–248.

Hagendorens, M.M., Ebo, D.G., Schuerwegh, A.J. et al. (2003). Differences in circulating dendritic cell subtypes in cord blood and peripheral blood of healthy and allergic children. Clin Exp Allergy 33, 633–639.

Hart, D.N. (1997). Dendritic cells: unique leukocyte populations which control the primary immune response Blood 90, 3245–3287.

Hart, D.N. (2001). Dendritic cells and their emerging clinical applications. Pathology 33, 479–492.

Ho, C.S., Munster, D., Pyke, C.M., Hart, D.N. and Lopez, J.A. (2002). Spontaneous generation and survival of blood dendritic cells in mononuclear cell culture without exogenous cytokines. Blood 99, 2897–2904.

Ho, C.S., Lopez, J.A., Vuckovic, S., Pyke, C.M., Hockey, R.L. and Hart, D.N. (2001). Surgical and physical stress increases circulating blood dendritic cell counts independently of monocyte counts. Blood 98, 140–145.

Hock, B.D., Starling, G.C., Daniel, P.B. and Hart, D.N. (1994). Characterization of CMRF-44, a novel monoclonal antibody to an activation antigen expressed by the allostimulatory cells within peripheral blood, including dendritic cells. Immunology 83, 573–581.

Hock, B.D., Haring, L.F., Ebbett, A.M., Patton, W.N. and McKenzie, J.L. (2002). Differential effects of G-CSF mobilisation on dendritic cell subsets in normal allogeneic donors and patients undergoing autologous transplantation. Bone Marrow Transplant 30, 733–740.

Hock, B.D., Fearnley, D.B., Boyce, A. et al. (1999). Human dendritic cells express a 95 kDa activation/differentiation antigen defined by CMRF-56. Tissue Antigens 53, 320–334.

Hulstaert, F., Hannet, I., Deneys, V. et al. (1994). Age-related changes in human blood lymphocyte subpopulations. II. Varying kinetics of percentage and absolute count measurements. Clin Immunol Immunopathol 70, 152–158.

Hwu, P., Du, M.X., Lapointe, R., Do, M., Taylor, M.W. and Young, H.A. (2000). Indoleamine 2,3-dioxygenase production by human dendritic cells results in the inhibition of T cell proliferation. J Immunol 164, 3596–3599.

Kadowaki, N., Ho, S., Antonenko, S. et al. (2001). Subsets of human dendritic cell precursors express different toll-like receptors and respond to different microbial antigens. J Exp Med 194, 863–869.

Kanto, T., Hayashi, N., Takehara, T. et al. (1999). Impaired allostimulatory capacity of peripheral blood dendritic cells recovered from hepatitis C virus-infected individuals. J Immunol 162, 5584–5591.

Kunitani, H., Shimizu, Y., Murata, H., Higuchi, K. and Watanabe, A. (2002). Phenotypic analysis of circulating and intrahepatic dendritic cell subsets in patients with chronic liver diseases. J Hepatol 36, 734–741.

Langenkamp, A., Messi, M., Lanzavecchia, A. and Sallusto, F. (2000). Kinetics of dendritic cell activation: impact on priming of TH1, TH2 and nonpolarized T cells. Nat Immunol 1, 311–316.

Lissoni, P., Vigore, L., Ferranti, R. et al. (1999). Circulating dendritic cells in early and advanced cancer patients: diminished percent in the metastatic disease. J Biol Regul Homeost Agents 13, 216–219.

Lopez, J.A., Bioley, G., Turtle, C.J. et al. (2003). Single step enrichment of blood dendritic cells by positive immunoselection. J Immunol Methods 274, 47–61.

Lu, L. and Thomson, A.W. (2001). Dendritic cell tolerogenicity and prospects for dendritic cell-based therapy of allograft rejection and autimmune disease. In Dendritic cells, 2nd edn, Lotze, M. and Thomson, A., eds. London: Academic Press, pp. 587–607.

MacDonald, K.P., Munster, D.J., Clark, G.J., Dzionek, A., Schmitz, J. and Hart, D.N. (2002). Characterization of human blood dendritic cell subsets. Blood 100, 4512–4520.

Macey, M.G., McCarthy, D.A., Vogiatzi, D., Brown, K.A. and Newland, A.C. (1998). Rapid flow cytometric identification of putative CD14- and CD64- dendritic cells in whole blood. Cytometry 31, 199–207.

Marroquin, C.E., Westwood, J.A., Lapointe, R. et al. (2002). Mobilization of dendritic cell precursors in patients with cancer by flt3 ligand allows the generation of higher yields of cultured dendritic cells. J Immunother 25, 278–288.

Matsuda, H., Suda, T., Hashizume, H. et al. (2002). Alteration of balance between myeloid dendritic cells and plasmacytoid dendritic cells in peripheral blood of patients with asthma. Am J Respir Crit Care Med 166, 1050–1054.

Matsue, H. and Takashima, A. (1999). Apoptosis in dendritic cell biology. J Dermatol Sci 20, 159–171.

Matsue, H., Edelbaum, D., Hartmann, A.C. et al. (1999). Dendritic cells undergo rapid apoptosis in vitro during antigen-specific interaction with CD4+ T cells. J Immunol 162, 5287–5298.

Mohty, M., Jarrossay, D., Lafage-Pochitaloff, M. et al. (2001). Circulating blood dendritic cells from myeloid leukemia patients display quantitative and cytogenetic abnormalities as well as functional impairment. Blood 98, 3750–3756.

Munn, D.H., Sharma, M.D., Lee, J.R. et al. (2002). Potential regulatory function of human dendritic cells expressing indoleamine 2,3-dioxygenase. Science 297, 1867–1870.

Olweus, J., BitMansour, A., Warnke, R. et al. (1997). Dendritic cell ontogeny: a human dendritic cell lineage of myeloid origin. Proc Natl Acad Sci USA 94, 12551–12556.

Osugi, Y., Vuckovic, S. and Hart, D.N.J. (2002). Myeloid blood CD11c+ dendritic cells and monocyte-derived dendritic cells differ in their ability to stimulate T lymphocytes. Blood 100, 2858–2866.

Palucka, A.K., Banchereau, J., Blanco, P. and Pascual, V. (2002). The interplay of dendritic cell subsets in systemic lupus erythematosus. Immunol Cell Biol 80, 484–488.

Pockaj, B.A., Basu, G.D., Pathangey, L.B. et al. (2004). Reduced T-cell and dendritic cell function is related to cyclooxygenase-2 overexpression and prostaglandin E2 secretion in patients with breast cancer. Ann Surg Oncol 11, 328–339.

Pulendran, B., Banchereau, J., Burkeholder, S. et al. (2000). Flt3-ligand and granulocyte colony-stimulating factor mobilize distinct human dendritic cell subsets in vivo. J Immunol 165, 566–572.

Ratta, M., Fagnoni, F., Curti, A. et al. (2002). Dendritic cells are functionally defective in multiple myeloma: the role of inter-leukin-6. Blood 100, 230–237.

Reider, N., Reider, D., Ebner, S. et al. (2002). Dendritic cells contribute to the development of atopy by an insufficiency in IL-12 production. J Allergy Clin Immunol 109, 89–95.

Reis e Sousa, C. (2004). Toll-like receptors and dendritic cells: for whom the bug tolls. Semin Immunol 16, 27–34.

Rissoan, M.-C., Soumelis, V., Kadowaki, N. et al. (1999). Reciprocal control of T helper cell and dendritic cell differentiation. Science 283, 1183–1186.

Robinson, S.P., Patterson, S., English, N., Davies, D., Knight, S.C. and Reid, C.D. (1999). Human peripheral blood contains two distinct lineages of dendritic cells. Eur J Immunol 29, 2769–2778.

Scheinecker, C., Zwolfer, B., Koller, M., Manner, G. and Smolen, J.S. (2001). Alterations of dendritic cells in systemic lupus erythematosus: phenotypic and functional deficiencies. Arthritis Rheum 44, 856–865.

Schnizlein-Bick, C.T., Mandy, F.F., O'Gorman, M.R. et al. (2002). Use of CD45 gating in three and four-color flow cytometric immunophenotyping: guideline from the National Institute of Allergy and Infectious Diseases, Division of AIDS. Cytometry 50, 46–52.

Shodell, M. and Siegal, F.P. (2002). Circulating, interferon-producing plasmacytoid dendritic cells decline during human ageing. Scand J Immunol 56, 518–521.

Siegal, F.P., Kadowaki, N., Shodell, M. et al. (1999). The nature of the principal type 1 interferon-producing cells in human blood. Science 284, 1835–1837.

Stent, G., Reece, J.C., Baylis, D.C. et al. (2002). Heterogeneity of freshly isolated human tonsil dendritic cells demonstrated by intracellular markers, phagocytosis, and membrane dye transfer. Cytometry 48, 167–176.

Szabolcs, P., Park, K.D., Reese, M., Marti, L., Broadwater, G. and Kurtzberg, J. (2003). Absolute values of dendritic cell subsets in bone marrow, cord blood, and peripheral blood enumerated by a novel method. Stem Cells 21, 296–303.

Tanaka, H., Demeure, C.E., Rubio, M., Delespesse, G. and Sarfati, M. (2000). Human monocyte-derived dendritic cells induce naive T cell differentiation into T helper cell type 2 (Th2) or Th1/Th2 effectors. Role of stimulator/responder ratio. J Exp Med 192, 405–412.

Teig, N., Moses, D., Gieseler, S. and Schauer, U. (2002). Age-related changes in human blood dendritic cell subpopulations. Scand J Immunol 55, 453–457.

Troy, A.J., Davidson, P.J., Atkinson, C.H. and Hart, D.N. (1999). CD1a dendritic cells predominate in transitional cell carcinoma of bladder and kidney but are minimally activated. J Urol 161, 1962–1967.

Troy, A.J., Summers, K.L., Davidson, P.J., Atkinson, C.H. and Hart, D.N. (1998). Minimal recruitment and activation of dendritic cells within renal cell carcinoma. Clin Cancer Res 4, 585–593.

Uchida, Y., Kurasawa, K., Nakajima, H. (2001). Increase of dendritic cells of type 2 (DC2) by altered response to IL-4 in atopic patients. J Allergy Clin Immunol 108, 1005–1011.

Upham, J.W., Lundahl, J., Liang, H., Denburg, J.A., O'Byrne, P.M. and Snider, D.P. (2000). Simplified quantitation of myeloid dendritic cells in peripheral blood using flow cytometry. Cytometry 40, 50–59.

Vakkila, J., Thomson, A.W., Vettenranta, K., Sariola, H. and Saarinen-Pihkala, U.M. (2004). Dendritic cell subsets in childhood and in children with cancer: relation to age and disease prognosis. Clin Exp Immunol 135, 455–461.

von Bubnoff, D., Koch, S. and Bieber, T. (2003). New jobs for an old enzyme: the revival of IDO. Trends Immunol 24, 296–297; author reply 8.

Vuckovic, S., Florin, T.H., Khalil, D. et al. (2001). CD40 and CD86 upregulation with divergent CMRF44 expression on blood dendritic cells in inflammatory bowel diseases. Am J Gastroenterol 96, 2946–2956.

Vuckovic, S., Gardiner, D., Field, K. et al. (2004). Monitoring dendritic cells in clinical practice using a new whole blood single-platform TruCOUNT assay. J Immunol Methods 284, 73–87.

Vuckovic, S., Kim, M., Khalil, D. et al. (2003). Granulocyte-colony stimulating factor increases CD123hi blood dendritic cells with altered CD62L and CCR7 expression. Blood 101, 2314–2317.

Vuckovic, S. and Hart, D.N.J. (2002). Dendritic cells versus macrophages as antigen presenting cells: common and unique features. In The Macrophage as Therapeutic Target. Oxford: Springer, pp. 337–352.

Zhang, Y., Yoneyama, H., Wang, Y. et al. (2004). Mobilization of dendritic cell precursors into the circulation by administration of MIP-1alpha in mice. J Natl Cancer Inst 96, 201–209.

Zinkernagel, R.M. (2002). On cross-priming of MHC class I-specific CTL: rule or exception? Eur J Immunol 32, 2385–2392.

Monocytes and Macrophages

Chapter 25

Salvador Nares and Sharon M. Wahl

Oral Infection and Immunity Branch, National Institute of Dental and Craniofacial Research, National Institutes of Health, Bethesda, MD, USA

> What lies behind us and what lies before us are tiny matters compared to what lies within us.
>
> Ralph Waldo Emerson

INTRODUCTION

In 1908 Élie Metchnikoff was awarded the Nobel Prize for Physiology or Medicine based on his discovery of amoeboid-like cells in animals capable of engulfing foreign bodies. While investigating the digestive system in starfish larvae, he noted cells converging on and then appearing to eat inert dye particles and splinters. Metchnikoff then infected transparent water fleas with viable yeast spores and observed mobile cells migrating towards and internalizing these invading pathogens. He called these cells 'phagocytes' (i.e. devouring cells) and noted their critical nature in host defense when the phagocytes did not respond fast enough to the invading microbes, allowing the spores to multiply and kill the water flea. His discoveries spawned the fundamental tenet of phagocytosis and ushered in the principles underlying innate immunity. Undoubtedly, Metchnikoff was witness to phagocytosis by the amoeba-like white corpuscles, the macrophage and its precursor, the monocyte.

Monocytes represent circulating members of the myeloid cell lineage, give rise to tissue dendritic cells and macrophages and are functionally active in innate and adaptive immunity. These multifaceted cells are capable of performing various functions of vital importance to the host, serving as important and usually effective sentinels strategically poised against foreign invaders. In addition to phagocytic clearance of microbes, mononuclear phagocytes orchestrate immune responses within tissues at sites of antigen deposition and/or pathogen invasion by processing and presenting antigen in the context of MHC class II molecules to effector cells, as well as amplifying the immune response via the production of mediators, cytokines and chemokines. Phagocytes contribute to debridement during tissue injury and foster wound healing by orchestrating the homeostatic processes involved in tissue turnover and repair via the production and secretion of numerous bioactive molecules. However, beyond its essentiality in tissue remodeling and host defense, the macrophage has also been implicated in the evolution of pathological processes including atherosclerosis, cancer and autoimmunity.

MONOCYTE/MACROPHAGE BIOLOGY

Monocytes are derived from monoblast precursors in the bone marrow that originate as pleuripotent stem cells (Figure 25.1) which are highly influenced by their microenvironment (van Furth, 1976). In this regard, in high concentrations of granulocyte macrophage-colony stimulating factor (GM-CSF), these progenitor cells differentiate into granulocytes, while low concentrations of GM-CSF favor differentiation into monocytes. Further induction of

Measuring Immunity, edited by Michael T. Lotze and Angus W. Thomson
ISBN 0-12-455900-X, London

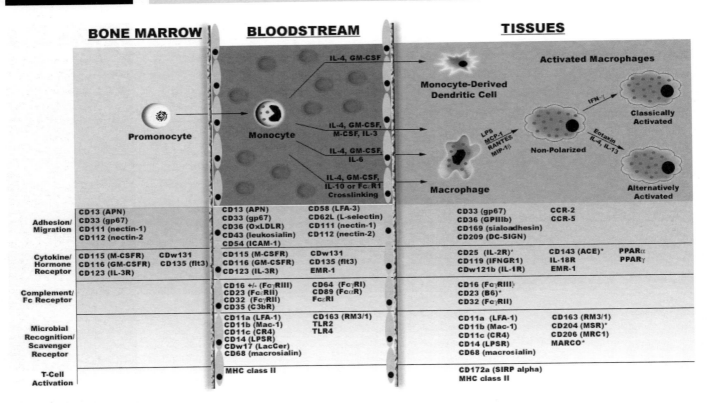

Figure 25.1 Monocyte and macrophage antigen expression in bone marrow, blood or tissues. Promonocytes exit the bone marrow, mature into monocytes and express receptors important in phagocytosis and microbial recognition. Monocytes leave the circulation and take up residence in tissues where they differentiate into morphologically, phenotypically and functionally heterogeneous effector cells such as macrophages or dendritic cells. Macrophages become activated if exposed to antigens, pathogens and to substances such as lipopolysaccharide (LPS) via TLR and interferon-γ (IFN-γ) (classically activated) or IL-4, IL-13 (alternative activation). Antigens expressed on activated macrophages are denoted with asterisks (*). **See colour plate 25.1**.

differentiation along the monocytic lineage occurs in the presence of macrophage-colony stimulating factor (M-CSF).

Once released from the bone marrow, monocytes circulate in the blood, but after monocyte-derived dendritic cells and macrophages enter and move around in the tissues, they do not typically re-enter the circulation (Hume et al., 2002). Thus, in measuring surrogate biomarkers of immunity and disease, the focus is, of necessity, on circulating monocyte populations. Morphologically, monocytes measure 10–18 μm in diameter with a high nucleus/cytoplasm ratio and an eccentrically placed U-shaped or round nucleus. Mononuclear phagocytes have limited proliferation potential and circulate in the blood as monocytes with a half-life of 12–100 h. Peripheral blood monocyte counts in adults are normally between 1 and 6 per cent of the total white blood cell count (an absolute monocyte count of between 300 and 700 cells per microliter of blood) and rarely exceed 10 per cent. Monocytosis may occur in non-infectious and infectious conditions (Table 25.1), often in association with neutrophilia, particularly in the recovery phase of many acute infections, while monocytopenia is not a frequent typical clinical problem. Monocytes eventually emigrate to take up residence in virtually every tissue in the body where

Table 25.1 Conditions associated with monocytosis (non-leukemic)

Infectious diseases	Non-infectious conditions	Drugs	Poisons
Subacute bacterial endocarditis	Ulcerative colitis	Griseofulvin	Carbon disulfide
Pulmonary tuberculosis	Regional enteritis	Haloperidol	Phosphorus
Brucellosis	Sarcoidosis	Methsuximide	Tetrachloroethane
Typhoid fever	Collagen diseases	Corticosteroids	
Rickettsial infections	Hodgkin's disease		
Kala-azar	Non-Hodgkin's lymphomas		
Trypanosomiasis	Gaucher's disease		
Leishmaniasis	SLA, RA		
	Asplenia		
	Pregnancy		
	Depression		
	Trauma		

they differentiate into morphologically and functionally heterogeneous effector cells such as macrophages, microglia, Kupffer cells, dendritic cells and osteoclasts (Hume et al., 2002).

Macrophages, which differ morphologically and functionally between tissues, also exhibit unique characteristics between normal and pathologic states. Macrophages are typically large cells (10–30 μm in diameter) and are one of the few cell types that can traverse among and between body compartments, which is dependent upon their capacity to degrade basement membranes and other extracellular matrices by the production of collagenolytic, elastinolytic and gelatinolytic hydrolases (Takemura and Werb, 1984). Virtually any local disturbance of tissue homeostasis including infection, wounding, immune response or malignancy, will result in a rapid recruitment and differentiation of monocytes and tissue macrophages (Hume et al., 2002). Ultrastructurally, macrophages possess a round or indented eccentrically poised nucleus, a well-developed Golgi apparatus, abundant endocytotic vacuoles, lysosomes, phagolysosomes and a complex ruffled microvillous plasma membrane equipping the cell for phagocytosis and pinocytosis.

In innate immunity to infectious pathogens, mononuclear phagocytes are among the earliest responders, recognizing pathogens through a family of toll-like receptors (TLR) (Beutler et al., 2003) which engage signals driving host defense (reviewed in Chapter 6). Monocytes triggered via TLR exhibit a repertoire distinct from resting monocytes which can be monitored by changes in recognizable biomarkers (see Figure 25.1). The activation profile can be measured at the molecular level and/or by protein analysis (Greenwell-Wild et al., 2002). Most commonly monitored are changes in cell surface expression of a variety of receptors and antigenic markers (Figure 25.2) as well as the inflammatory cytokines, TNFα and IL-1β (see Figure 25.3), which can be detected intracellularly (RNA or protein), in cell culture supernatants and also in serum. Similarly, in an adaptive immune response, products from antigen-activated Th1 lymphocytes, most notably IFNγ interacting with its receptor on monocytes, drive changes in monocytes associated with an activation phenotype, referred to as M1 (classically activated) macrophages whereas Th2 cytokines, including IL-4 and/or IL-10, alternatively activate macrophages (M2) and may dampen function. Other inflammatory and/or tumor products, i.e. transforming growth factor beta (TGF-β) can also profoundly alter monocyte behavior and may polarize macrophages into the M2 phenotype (Mantovani et al., 2002).

Compared to monocytes, macrophages represent a more functionally and phenotypically diverse population of cells stemming from the needs, architecture and biochemical signals of the local microenvironment (Gordon et al., 1992). Thus, macrophages in different tissues may respond uniquely in terms of cell surface antigens, inflammatory mediators, proteases and cytokines to identical stimuli. Even within a single tissue, the macrophage population can vary functionally and phenotypically depending upon maturity and activation status. Fully mature and activated macrophages may respond vigorously to a gram-negative bacterial infection (Zisman et al., 1997), whereas they may be unresponsive when faced with

tumor cells (Dinapoli et al., 1996). Among the inducible antimicrobial armamentarium, macrophages produce nitric oxide (NO), reactive oxygen species (O_2^-, HO^-) and cytokines. Tumor-associated macrophages (TAMs) begin as cells mobilized in defense against neoplastic cells. On their best behavior, they destroy tumor cells and present their antigens for the initiation of a targeted immune response. Unfortunately, repetitive and chronic recruitment and stimulation of TAMs can promote metastasis and proliferation of neoplastic cells via the production of macrophage-derived cytokines, growth factors and proteases. How these cells become 'realigned' in support of the tumor is not yet fully understood. Moreover, macrophage differentiation may be suppressed by the tumor since cytotoxicity has been shown to be higher in mature macrophages compared to monocytes (Andreesen et al., 1983) and in inflammatory macrophages compared to resident macrophages (Hauptmann et al., 1993).

Although dendritic cells are maximally effective in antigen presentation (see Chapter 24), macrophages also acquire antigen and present antigen in the context of MHC class II molecules to T and B lymphocytes. Thus quick mobilization, active phagocytosis and antigen presentation are among the many virtues of these cells. However, in certain complex diseases such as cancer and atherosclerosis, the mononuclear phagocytes play a contributory role in the onset and progression of these pathological processes. Discriminating self versus nonself is one of the most important and fundamental tasks of the immune system and macrophages are involved in induction of T cell tolerance. Failure to tolerate self antigens, as well as an unchecked response to foreign antigens can result in equally disastrous outcomes. The cellular infiltrate accompanying the end-organ damage in arthritis (VanderBorght et al., 2001), multiple sclerosis (Izikson et al., 2002) and a multitude of other immune disorders are often laden with macrophages spewing out tissue-damaging proteases, reactive oxygen and nitrogen intermediates and excess cytokines. In atherosclerosis one of the earliest detectable events leading to plaque formation is the adhesion of circulating monocytes to endothelium (see Chapter 54). Thereafter monocytes and monocyte-derived macrophages phagocytize large quantities of lipids and produce cytokines, proteases, inflammatory mediators and growth factors typical of chronic inflammatory lesions.

Macrophages are not always proinflammatory and in fact, these cells can be potent instruments of immune suppression. In receptor-mediated phagocytosis of apoptotic cells, the release of anti-inflammatory mediators such as IL-10, PGE2 and particularly, TGFβ by the phagocytosing macrophages may create an immunosuppressive local milieu (Wahl and Chen, 2003; Fadok and Henson, 2003). Moreover, in the presence of IgG immune complexes, macrophage Fc receptors (FcγRIII-CD16) are engaged, triggering production of high levels of IL-10 and virtually no IL-12 upon exposure to endotoxin, thereby favoring a Th2-like immune response (Anderson et al., 2002). Thus monocytes and macrophages are not only instrumental in surveillance, initiation and the development of inflammation and immune responses, they are also pivotal in the restoration of homeostasis. Given the host of monocyte/macrophage functions and their roles in both normal and pathological processes, the study of these cells is important in elucidating the underlying cellular and molecular mechanisms of disease and in the development of novel therapeutic targets.

CHARACTERIZATION OF CLINICAL SAMPLES

Overview

Many clinical protocols require the collection and analysis of data in real time to monitor an individual's hematologic inflammatory and/or immune status, as well as a patient's response to therapies and for further evaluation during and/or after completion of a study (AACTG, 2001). Although monocytes and tissue macrophages are essential in host defense, identification of biomarkers for monocyte/macrophage activation and their association with disease remains problematic due to their small numbers in the circulation, their short time in the blood and their natural propensity to exit the circulation during times of immune stress. Moreover, changes in phenotype and function in circulating monocytes may not reflect events associated with tissue macrophages. Nonetheless, phenotypic (Table 25.2) and functional changes in circulating monocytes have been associated with a variety of disease entities, documenting the utility of characterizing these cells as surrogate markers in health, disease and during therapeutic interventions. As increasingly sophisticated techniques are developed, additional genomic and proteomic analyses will likely become standard as clinical correlates of disease.

In order to measure changes in phenotypic and functional parameters, we describe mechanisms by which monocytes can be isolated from peripheral blood and then characterized as to their constitutive expression of surface markers and their cellular, biochemical and molecular profile, which may reflect *in vivo* influences associated with immunopathogenesis as well as responsiveness to stimuli *in vitro*. Typically, monocytes are isolated from peripheral blood mononuclear cells (PBMC) obtained by density gradient sedimentation (Ficoll-Hypaque) from whole blood samples. Once PBMC are collected, monocytes can be further purified by a number of methods, which generally rely on their unique sedimentation properties, adherence and/or the use of cell surface markers. Collectively, these assessments can provide an evaluation of this population consonant with evidence of activation or suppression with the potential to recognize targets that can be monitored as surrogate biomarkers during clinical intervention.

Table 25.2 Changes in mononuclear phagocyte phenotype in disease

Condition	Marker antigen	References
Asthma	CD23↑	Mouri, 1993; Viksman et al., 2002
	HLA-DR↑	Mazzarella et al., 2000; Viksman et al., 2002
	CD14↓↑	Mazzarella et al., 2000; Viksman et al., 2002
Autoimmunity Rheumatoid arthritis	CD23↑	Huissoon et al., 2000
	HLA-DR↑	Koller et al., 1999
	CD16↑	Wahl et al., 1992; Masuda et al., 2003a,b; Wijngaarden et al., 2003
	CD32↑	Wijngaarden et al., 2003
	CD163↑↓	Matsushita et al., 2002; Fonseca et al., 2002
Inflammatory bowel disease	CD68↑	Nielsen et al., 2003; Fujino et al., 2003
	HLA-DR↓	Dijkstra et al., 2002
Multiple sclerosis	CD16↑	Bergh et al., 2004
	CD11c↑	Alpsoy et al., 2003
Behçet's	CD64↑	Alpsoy et al., 2003
Cancer	CD23↑	Schoppmann et al., 2002
	HLA-DR↓	Ugurel et al., 2004
	CD163↑	Møller et al., 2002, 2004
	CD16↑	Mytar et al., 2002
	CD68↑	Bingle et al., 2002; Schoppmann et al., 2002
Cardiovascular	CD163↑	Goldstein et al., 2003
	CD14↓	Sbrana et al., 2004
	HLA-DR↓	Sbrana et al., 2004
	CD14↑	Fingerle-Rowson et al., 1998b
	CD16↑	Fingerle-Rowson et al., 1998b
Glucocorticoids	HLA-DR↑↓	Oehling et al., 1997; Caulfield et al., 1999
	CD14↓	Fingerle-Rowson et al., 1998c; Scherberich JE, 2003
	CD16↓	Fingerle-Rowson et al., 1998c
	CD163↑	Buechler et al., 2000
Infection Bacterial	HLA-DR↓	Shumilla et al., 2004
	CD14↑	Kolb-Maurer et al., 2004
	CD14↓	Lin and Rinkihisa, 2004
	TLR2↓	Lin and Rinkihisa, 2004
	TLR4↓	Lin and Rinkihisa, 2004
HIV	CD23↓	Miller et al., 2001; Swingler et al., 2003
	HLA-DR↓↑	Rakoff-Nahoum et al., 2001; Gascon et al., 2002
	CD16↑	Allen et al., 1991; Pulliam et al., 1997
	CD14↑	Pulliam et al., 1997; Gascon et al., 2002
	CD25↑	Allen et al., 1990
Protozoan	CD23↑	Vouldoukis et al., 1994; Cabrera et al., 2003
	HLA-DR↓	De Almeida et al., 2003
Trauma	HLA-DR↓	Kampalath et al., 2003; Lendemans et al., 2004
	CD14↑	Kampalath et al., 2003;
	CD4↓	Kampalath et al., 2003
	CD16↓	Kampalath et al., 2003
Surgery	CD14↓	Fingerle-Rowson et al., 1998a
	CD163↑	Goldstein et al., 2003; Philippidis et al., 2004

For evaluation of macrophage function, monocyte-derived macrophages can be differentiated from adherent monocytes after 7–10 days culture. If tissue samples/biopsies are available, macrophages can be isolated following proteolytic and/or mechanical disruption followed by isolation using standard methods. Macrophages have also been obtained from sputum samples as well as bronchiolar lavage (Mazzarella et al., 2000). Assays that measure macrophage phenotypic markers, phagocytosis, secretion and/or production of cytokines and other products, and gene expression can be performed using techniques similar to those for monocytes.

MONOCYTE ISOLATION

Purification of monocytes can be readily accomplished by adherence of PBMC to glass and/or plastic (Wahl and Smith, 1997), magnetic separation, size sedimentation or counterflow centrifugal elutriation (Wahl et al, 1984; Wahl and Smith, 1997). Yields and activation state vary between isolation techniques and caution must be taken to avoid endotoxin contamination which independently activates these cells. The quantity and purity of monocytes will vary between individual donors.

Preparation of PBMC

This easy and rapid technique for isolating PBMC relies on the differences in densities between blood components. Fresh EDTA, heparin or citrate-anticoagulated whole blood is diluted in an equal volume of phosphate buffered saline (PBS, pH 7.4) and carefully overlayed onto a cushion of Ficoll (Lymphocyte Separation Media, ICN Biomedicals, Aurora, OH) in 15 ml conical centrifuge tubes (i.e. layer 8 ml diluted blood over 4 ml Ficoll). Centrifuge at 2000 rpm (900 × g) for 20 min at 18–25°C with no brake. Using a sterile transfer pipette, transfer the mononuclear cell layer evident at the interface between the Ficoll and plasma/PBS to a fresh centrifuge tube, wash with three volumes of PBS, centrifuge 10 min at 1200 rpm and repeat wash to decrease contaminating platelets. The mononuclear cells (PBMC) can be resuspended in PBS for further purification of monocytes (adherence, magnetic separation, counterflow centrifugal elutriation) or for staining prior to flow cytometry.

Isolation by adherence

Isolation of monocytes from PBMC using adherence is a relatively quick and easy option but may result in potential cell activation and contamination of ≤10 per cent non-monocytic cells (Wahl and Smith, 1997). PBMC are resuspended in serum-free DMEM or RPMI (supplemented with 2 mM L-glutamine, 10–50 μg/ml gentamicin) and seeded in tissue culture flasks, plates or on cover slips at 2×10^6 cell/ml for 1–2 h in a 37°C, 5 per cent CO_2 humidified incubator. Non-adherent cells are removed by gently aspirating or decanting the media followed by washing remaining adherent monocytes twice with pre-warmed media. Monocytes can be analyzed while in this adherent condition or if removal of adherent cells is desired, gently scrape with a plastic scraper or rubber policeman or incubate in ice-cold 0.02 per cent EDTA/PBS solution for 10 min then firmly tap the flask (Wahl and Smith, 1997). Alternatively, disassociation buffers are available commercially (InVitrogen, Carlsbad, CA). Cell counts and viability are determined by trypan blue exclusion. For long-term cultures to enable differentiation and maturation of monocytes into macrophages, heat-inactivated fetal calf serum (FCS) is added to the culture medium at 1–10 per cent after adherence.

Magnetic separation

Magnetic separation using coated iron beads coupled with antibodies to CD14 or other antigens is another method to isolate monocytes from both large and small volumes of whole blood. CD14, which recognizes the complex of lipopolysaccharide (LPS) and the LPS-binding protein (Wright et al., 1990), is highly expressed on monocytes, but not on immature monocytic cells. Magnetic bead separation technologies isolate monocytes by either positive (i.e. CD14+ microbeads) or negative (depletion) selection. Positive selection involves the magnetic labeling of target cells using antibody-coated magnetic beads against a specific cellular antigen followed by isolation from other populations using special columns and magnets. Because positive selection of monocytes can potentially activate these cells, this method is not appropriate for some types of studies. Negative selection involves the elimination of unwanted cells (T and B cells, NK cells, granulocytes) by magnetically labeling and depleting them from the cell mixture to enrich the population of naive monocytes. Antibody-labeled magnetic beads are available from several commercial suppliers (Dynal Biotech, Oslo, Norway; Miltenyi Biotec Inc., Auburn, CA).

Isolation by counterflow centrifugal elutriation

Counterflow centrifugal elutriation relies on the principles of cell size and density to separate monocytes from PBMC. Although specialized equipment is required (Beckman Avanti® Series centrifuge or equivalent and J-6M rotor, Beckman Coulter, Inc., Fullerton, CA), highly purified and non-activated monocytes can be recovered in large quantities (Wahl et al., 1984; Wahl and Smith, 1997). In this method, PBMC flow within the separation chamber of a centrifuge rotor counter to the centrifugal force of the spinning rotor resulting in the stratification of cells where the sedimentation rate of the cell is balanced by the flow rate. Therefore, the flow rate counters the force of gravity and the smaller (less dense) cells are the first to exit the separation chamber and rotor as the flow rate is increased. Because the mononuclear cell subsets differ in size, B cells exit the chamber first followed by T cells and monocytes (Wahl et al., 1984). We routinely obtain large quantities of non-activated monocytes (1×10^8–2×10^9) from 300 ml of blood obtained by leukapheresis. However, in the absence of leukapheresis, approximately 2×10^8–4×10^8 monocytes can still be recovered from 1 unit of whole blood. Small volumes of blood (<100 ml) will require careful monitoring of exiting cell populations during elutriation in order to obtain appreciable quantities of monocytes.

DIFFERENTIATION OF MONOCYTES INTO MACROPHAGES

If analysis of macrophage biomarkers is of interest, macrophages can be derived from in-vitro culture of monocytes isolated by the above methods. In our laboratory, we routinely culture elutriated monocytes in DMEM or RPMI supplemented with 2 mM L-glutamine and 50 μg/ml gentamicin in plates or flasks. Monocytes and macrophages grown in culture have a very limited proliferative potential and are thus seeded at high density (400 000 cells/cm^2 of culture area). Adherence of monocytes to the plating surface can be improved by first incubating these cells in serum-free media. After 1–2 h, 2–10 per cent FCS or human AB$^-$ serum is added to the culture media. Monocytes adhere well to both plastic and glass and differentiate into macrophages in about 7–10 days depending on donor and culture conditions. In situations where only limited quantities of blood are available, monocyte yields from PBMC (obtained by Histopaque-Ficoll gradient centrifugation) can be improved by collection of both the interface and more than half of the overlaying supernatant followed by culturing cells in the presence of M-CSF at low FCS concentration (1 per cent). In studies where higher serum concentrations may interfere with antigen uptake, processing and presentation on HLA molecules, the generation of macrophages by this method may prove useful (Plesner, 2003). For nucleic acid or protein analysis, lysis of macrophage monolayers is best performed on the plating surface (Greenwell-Wild et al., 2002). FACS analysis of macrophage monolayers requires detachment using mechanical or chemical treatment. A sterile rubber policeman, disassociation in ice-cold 0.02 per cent EDTA/PBS or commercially available disassociation buffer treatment is recommended to detach cells. Trypsinization of macrophage monolayers is ineffective.

Monocyte/macrophage phenotype characterization

Once isolated, monocytes can be characterized phenotypically by flow cytometry using monocyte-specific antibodies tagged with fluorochromes. If an insufficient quantity of blood is available to isolate monocytes, then whole blood or PBMC can be used. In these mixed cell populations, monocytes can be gated (isolated from other cell populations using software, e.g. CellQuest, Becton Dickinson, San Jose, CA) for specific analysis. One of the most common antigenic markers for identifying monocytes is CD14, which can be detected with a fluorescently labeled antibody to CD14 and is highly expressed in monocytes but not on immature monocytic cells (see Figure 25.1). In addition to quantitation of CD14+ cells, the relative median fluorescent intensity, an indicator of the number of detected CD14 molecules on an individual cell, which may change with maturation/activation can also be measured. CD14 is often used in dual fluorescence analyses and combined with intracellular cytokine staining (discussed below).

A number of surface antigens change on monocytes depending on activation status associated with maturation and with immunopathogenesis in the host, some of which are exemplified in Table 25.2. In addition, in vitro stimulation of cells from patient populations may result in differential expression of select phenotypic markers. Among the cell surface antigens which may be discriminatory, HLA-DR is a commonly detected activation marker antigen (see Table 25.2). Additional antigens altered by activation/differentiation of monocytes include CD163, a member of the group B scavenger receptor cysteine-rich family expressed exclusively on monocytes and macrophages (Møller, et al., 2002). CD163 is an acute phase-regulated and signal-inducing transmembrane receptor for the hemoglobin–haptoglobin (Hb:Hp) complexes (Kristiansen et al., 2001), important in countering Hb-induced oxidative tissue damage after hemolysis via induction of IL-10 and heme oxygenase-1 synthesis. CD163 surface expression is increased by glucocorticoids, IL-6 and IL-10 and downregulated by LPS, TNF-α and IFN-γ (Högger et al., 1998; Buechler et al., 2000; Sulahian et al., 2000). Moreover, elevated levels of CD163 were noted on circulating monocytes in post-surgical cardiac patients during the resolution phase of the systemic inflammatory response to cardiopulmonary bypass graft surgery (Goldstein et al., 2003; Philippidis et al., 2004). Conversely, in rheumatoid arthritis (RA) patients, reduced surface expression of CD163 was found on macrophages in the CD4+ T lymphocyte-rich microenvironment within the RA synovium (Fonseca et al., 2002), whereas elevated soluble CD163 was detected within patient synovial fluid and sera (Matsushita et al., 2002). Furthermore, the soluble form of CD163 was also recently identified in the plasma of patients with Gaucher's disease, Crohn's disease and acute myelomonocytic leukemia (Møller et al., 2002, 2004) as well as in plasma of patients undergoing coronary bypass graft surgery (Goldstein et al., 2003). Thus CD163 represents an informative marker or clue of macrophage aberrancies associated with pathogenesis. Resting monocytes do not typically express IL-2R, but following activation and/or in infections, IL-2Rα chain (CD25) is expressed on monocytes (Allen et al., 1990, 1991). Changes in FcγRIII (i.e. CD16) (Allen et al., 1991; Wahl et al., 1992), HLA-DR and other cell surface antigens have also been reported in disease (representative markers shown in Table 25.2) and can be detected by flow cytometry.

Of interest, CD68 (see Figure 25.1, Table 25.2) is a lysosomal marker, which can be used to identify mononuclear phagocytes in blood and in tissues. In cancer, CD68 detects TAM number/density and serves as a prognostic indicator of different human malignancies including breast, prostate, ovary, cervical, stomach, lung and bladder (Bingle et al., 2002). In these circumstances, increased CD68 expression is associated with poor prognosis. Moreover, in the tumor types with high TAM density and poor prognosis, strong evidence has been presented demonstrating a correlation with the overexpression of macrophage growth factors or chemokines (Pollard, 2004).

Analysis of monocyte surface antigens using fluorescence activated cell sorting (FACS)

FACS analysis can be used to characterize the monocyte population in whole blood, PBMC, or elutriated monocytes using cell surface marker antigens, such as CD14, in numerous disease states (see Table 25.2). Antibodies to numerous monocyte antigens directly conjugated to various fluorochromes are available commercially. If a secondary detection antibody is needed, it is recommended to use F(ab')$_2$ fragments to prevent binding of the Fc region of an antibody to monocyte FcγR. Non-specific antibody binding of detection antibody can also be minimized by pre-incubating the cells with normal serum or IgG from the same species as the secondary antibody for 30 min in the dark on ice.

The assay

1 Pipette 50–100 µl of blood, 1×10^6 PBMC, or isolated (elutriated) monocytes to 12×75-mm polystyrene tubes and add appropriate fluorescently-labeled marker antibody (i.e. anti-CD14) or isotypic control antibody (typically 10 µg/ml) and incubate for 30 min in the dark on ice. If using whole blood, add 2 ml of lysing solution (ACK lysing solution, Cambrex, East Rutherford, NJ) after the incubation period for an additional 10 min at 4°C in the dark to lyse red blood cells. Centrifuge for 5 min at $500 \times$ g and remove supernatant.

2 Wash with 2 ml of PBS containing 2 per cent BSA and 0.01 per cent NaN$_3$ then centrifuge for 5 min at $500 \times$ g. Add 500 µl of 1 per cent paraformaldehyde/PBS prior to analysis by FACS. If a secondary detection antibody is required, add fluorescently-labeled F(ab')$_2$ antibody and incubate for an additional 30 min in the dark on ice then wash the cells and add 500 µl of 1 per cent paraformaldehyde prior to FACS analysis.

3 Analysis of data can be accomplished using FACS-specific software (e.g. CellQuest, Becton Dickinson,

San Jose, CA). Samples incubated with isotypic control antibodies are used to establish non-specific staining for subtraction of background noise. Unlabeled cells are used to determine autofluorescence. Monocytes can be gated from other cell populations in PBMC for analysis (Figure 25.2A, C) or assessed directly in elutriated monocyte populations (Figure 25.2B, D). Once these parameters are established, staining can be assessed to determine the percentage of positive cells (Figure 25.2C, D) and relative median fluorescence intensity for comparison of patient and control populations (Table 25.2).

Intracellular cytokine production in monocytes

Intracellular detection of cytokines by flow cytometry in conjunction with positive identification of monocytes enables analysis of potential changing cytokine expression profiles in whole blood, PBMC or isolated monocyte preparations. Using whole blood and FACS analysis is ideal for small clinical samples and may more closely reflect the in vivo response compared to isolated cells, as the effects of the other blood components on the experimental variable are conserved (West and Heagy, 2002). Intracellular cytokine levels may reflect in vivo stimulation and/or response to stimulation in vitro, but the presence of intracellular cytokines does not guarantee their secretion (Crucian and Widen, 1998) which can be quantified in the culture supernatants.

In this method, surface staining of monocytes in mixed populations using a fluorescently-labeled anti-CD14 or other relevant antibody is followed by fixation/permeabilization to introduce a second fluorescently-labeled antibody which recognizes a cytokine of interest. Whole blood, PBMC or purified monocytes can be used in this assay. PBMC can be isolated after stimulation of whole blood cultures or isolated then incubated directly with stimulant (i.e. LPS, drug, etc.) directly. Additional details for detection of intracellular cytokines can be found in Chapter 28.

The assay

1 To evaluate intracellular cytokine production in resting and/or activated monocytes, add PBS (control) or activating agent (i.e. LPS, bacteria, drug) to 1 ml of heparinized whole blood, 6×10^6 isolated PBMC (in culture media) or purified monocytes and incubate at 37°C for 4–24 h. Treatment of cells with brefeldin A, a protein transport inhibitor, at 10 µg/ml or monensin, a carboxylic ionophore, at 3 µM for the final 4–5 h is required to increase the detection capabilities of FACS analysis. These agents result in an accumulation of intracellular protein without altering de novo synthesis (Crucian and Widen, 1998).

2 Using intracellular TNFα as an example, label 5 tubes as follows: 1. cells only; 2. CD14-FITC (fluorescein

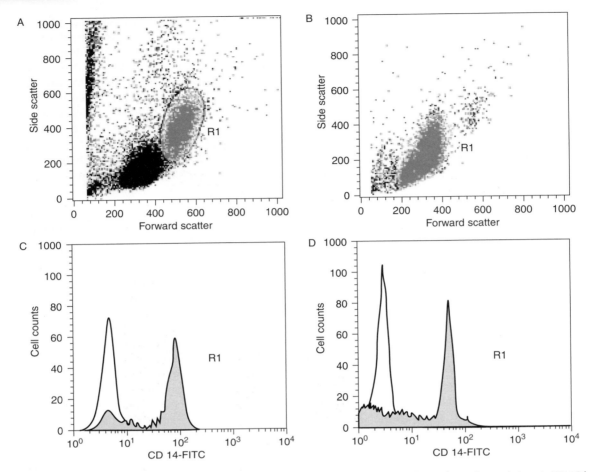

Figure 25.2 FACS analysis of CD14 positive monocytes. (A) Monocytes can be identified (gated-R1) from other cell populations in PBMC based on forward (size) and side (granularity) scatter and FACS software (e.g. CellQuest, Becton Dickinson, San Jose, CA) for specific analysis. (B) Typical forward and side scatter distribution of elutriated monocytes. (C) Histograms from analysis of gated (R1) PBMC and (D) elutriated monocytes demonstrating that the majority of cells stain positively for CD14 FITC. Open histogram: isotypic control (IgG1), filled histogram: CD-14-FITC (IgG1).

isothiocyanate-green); 3. TNFα-PE (phycoerythrin-red); 4. CD14-FITC/TNFα-PE; 5. CD14-FITC isotype/ TNFα-PE isotype. Pipette 100 μl of blood, or 100 μl of PBMC or monocytes (1×10^6 cells) to 12 × 75-mm polystyrene tubes and add appropriate fluorescently-labeled surface antigen-specific antibody (i.e. CD14) or isotypic control antibody (10 μg/ml) and incubate on ice for 30 min in the dark. If using whole blood, add 2 ml of lysing solution (ACK lysing solution, Cambrex, East Rutherford, NJ) after the incubation period for an additional 10 min on ice in the dark to lyse red blood cells. Centrifuge for 5 min at 500 × g and remove supernatant.

3 Resuspend cells in 250 μl Cytofix/Cytoperm (BD Pharmingen, San Diego, CA) solution for 20 min on ice in the dark. Wash cells twice in 1 ml of 1X Perm/Wash (PW) permeabilization buffer (stock:10X, BD Pharmingen) then resuspend fixed/permeabilized cells in 50 μl of PW buffer along with 2–5 μl (0.5–2.0 μg/ml) of intracellular cytokine detection antibodies (i.e. anti-TNFα) and incubate in the dark for 30 min on ice. Wash in 2 ml PW buffer then resuspend cells in 0.5 ml of 1 per cent paraformaldehyde prior to FACS analysis.

Following a 4-h exposure of elutriated monocytes to 1μg/ml of *E. coli* LPS, FITC-labeled anti-CD14 and PE-labeled anti-TNFα antibodies revealed differential expression of intracellular TNFα between stimulated and unstimulated populations with a 25-fold increase in CD14+ cells expressing TNFα (Figure 25.3A, B). Moreover, differential intracellular TNFα expression can be detected in unstimulated and stimulated patient monocyte populations (data not shown).

Measurement of cytokine secretion (inflammatory mediators)

In order to monitor cytokine secretion, the supernatants/plasma of stimulated and unstimulated whole blood cultures, isolated PBMC or monocytes can be monitored for cytokine proteins by ELISA and/or Luminex (see Chapter 18). As evident in Figure 25.3C, differential cytokine expression can be detected in stimulated whole blood cultures from control and patient populations (autoimmune patient with rheumatoid arthritis shown). Supernatants, as well as sera and biological fluids can

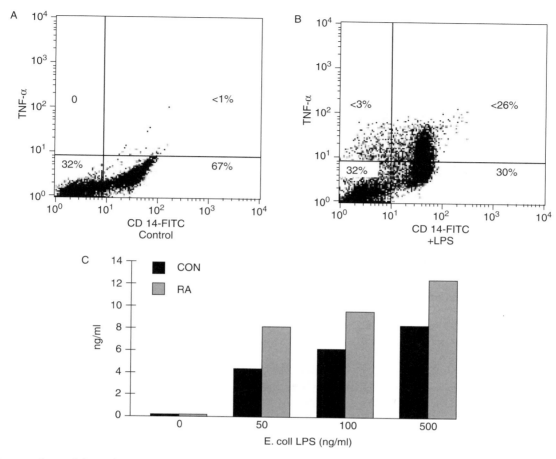

Figure 25.3 Monocyte intracellular and secreted TNF-α. One microgram of *E. coli* LPS was added to elutriated monocytes for 4 h and intracellular TNF-α measured in CD14 positive monocytes by FACS. (A) Control cells without LPS demonstrating positive CD14 staining only and (B) LPS treated cells staining positive for both CD14 and TNFα. A 25-fold increase in TNFα positive staining was noted on monocytes exposed to LPS compared to controls. C. Comparison of cytokine production in whole blood cultures. Luminex measurement of plasma TNFα levels from healthy (CON) and rheumatoid arthritis (RA) patient in whole blood culture plasma aliquots demonstrating increased levels of TNFα in response to increasing amounts of *E. coli* LPS after 24 h *in vitro*.

also be tested for additional monocyte-derived inflammatory mediators including reactive oxygen and nitrogen intermediates, proteases, prostaglandins and other secreted products which may be discriminatory between healthy subjects and patient populations. At the RNA level, changes in expression profiles of these biological mediators as well as other genes of interest can be performed using real-time PCR, RNase protection assays and microarrays (Greenwell-Wild et al., 2002; see Chapter 60).

Phagocytosis

Recurrent and chronic bacterial and fungal infections are often associated with aberrant phagocytic function and clearance of pathogenic organisms (Gallin, 1992; Perticarari et al., 1994; Lehmann, et al., 2000). From the time of Metchnikoff, we have known that phagocytosis is the primary means through which invading pathogenic organisms are eliminated by the host. Microorganisms such as heat killed *S. aureus* and yeast can be labeled with FITC (Perticarari et al., 1991) or alternatively, fluorescently-labeled

microorganisms are commercially available (Molecular Probes, Eugene, OR). Fluorochrome-labeled microorganisms must be sonicated and accurately quantitated microscopically, by cell counter, or by FACS (Stewart and Steinkamp, 1982) prior to and after dilution to obtain a particle to cell ratio of 1:1–1:100 for accurate quantification of phagocytosis (Bassøe et al., 2000).

For limited volumes of blood, Nacimento et al. (2003) described a method using a 96-well microassay to determine sequentially the oxidative burst (H_2O_2), nitric oxide production and MHC II (IA^k) expression in bacillus Calmette-Guérin-activated macrophages (2×10^5/well). Adaptation of this method may be useful for high throughput evaluation, but if limited blood volume is not an issue, FACS determination of phagocytosis is optimal.

The assay

1 To evaluate phagocytosis in whole blood preparations, PBMC, or isolated monocytes in suspension, add 20 μl of diluted fluorescently-labeled *E. coli*, *S. aureus*, or

zymosan A particles to 100 μl of heparinized whole blood or 1×10^6 cells and place in a shaking 37°C water bath for 15–60 min in the dark. For adherent macrophage cultures, add particles directly into culture media (i.e. 6 well plates or culture slides) and shake in a 37°C incubator.

2   For analysis of phagocytic uptake in whole blood, add 2 ml of RBC lysing solution (ACK solution) and incubate for 10 min at 4°C in the dark. Centrifuge for 5 min at $500 \times g$ and remove supernatant before fixation in 500 μl of 1 per cent paraformaldehyde for FACS. For adherent macrophage cultures, free particles can be removed by washing cells three times in ice-cold PBS and analyzed by microscopy (Figure 25.4) or FACS. FACS analysis of macrophages requires the detachment of cells as previously described using ice-cold 0.02 per cent EDTA/PBS or commercially available disassociation buffer.

As demonstrated in Figure 25.4, when isolated monocytes were incubated with FITC-labeled zymosan A particles for up to 10–60 min and analyzed by FACS (Figure 25.4A) and/or microscopy (Figure 25.4B, C), an increase in zymosan uptake was noted. After 10 min, zymosan particles were largely adhered to monocytes membranes and by 60 min, the particles had been internalized. Using this assay, in combination with measurements of oxidative burst (Lehmann et al., 2000), it is possible to compare monocyte populations for adherence, phagocytosis and reactive oxygen intermediates, key determinants of host defense and/or if aberrant, important contributors to pathogenesis.

FUTURE PROSPECTS AND CONCLUSIONS

Monocytes and macrophages are central to innate immunity and in the transition to adaptive immune responses, as well as in the resolution of immune responses and restoration of homeostasis. While access to monocyte populations in the peripheral blood provides opportunities to monitor molecular, phenotypic and functional parameters associated with disease, often their dominant contributions to host defense and/or pathogenesis occur in tissues sites of inflammation, infection and or neoplasia. The study of these cells in tissue specimens can be a slow and tedious process hindered by the limited access to normal and diseased tissues, the heterogeneous nature of tissues and the small numbers of localized tissue macrophages. The advent of laser-capture microdissection (LCM) has provided a powerful means to study the genomic and proteomic landscape of newly recruited monocytes, resident and recruited macrophages and dendritic cells in both normal and pathological specimens (Simone et al., 2000). Typical macrophage markers used to identify macrophages for LCM are CD68 and CD163 enabling detection of macrophage specific HIV-1 DNA in brain tissue with HIV-1 encephalitis (Trillo-Pazos et al., 2003) and in other tissues (Frungieri et al., 2002). LCM has been successfully used to extract macrophages from tissue biopsy specimens which have been fresh frozen in OCT (optimal cutting temperature) media (Tuomisto et al., 2003) with subsequent extraction of high quality RNA for microarray or real-time PCR analysis. Recently, new protocols and products have been introduced for interrogation of gene expression from

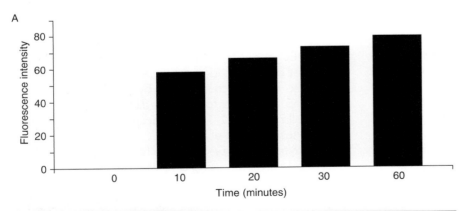

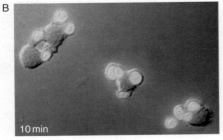

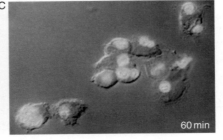

Figure 25.4 (A). Phagocytosis of FITC-labeled zymosan A particles by monocytes isolated by counterflow centrifugal elutriation and analyzed by FACS. A 20:1 zymosan A:monocyte ratio was used and samples harvested and analyzed by FACS at 10–60 min after the addition of particles. Photomicrographs of monocytes after a 10-min (B) and 60-min (C) incubation with FITC zymosan. **See colour plate 25.4.**

paraffin-embedded samples using LCM (Arcturus, Mountain View, CA) and gene arrays (Affymetrix, Santa Clara, CA), which will now allow for reproducible comparison of gene expression between paraffin-embedded samples from autopsy or biopsy of patient tissues and those of normal tissue.

Monocytes and macrophages are involved in a remarkably diverse array of homeostatic processes ranging from host defense to tissue turnover. However, beyond their essentiality in host defense, monocytes and macrophages have also been implicated in the evolution of pathological processes including atherosclerosis, cancer and autoimmunity. This 'split personality' presents unique challenges in the study of monocytes and macrophages and the dissection of their essential roles in host defense from their ignoble functions in immunopathology. Understanding their roles in both normal and pathological processes will be vital in elucidating the underlying cellular and molecular mechanisms of disease and in developing therapeutic strategies.

REFERENCES

AACTG – The Adult AIDS Clinical Trials Group (2001). ACTG Specimen Processing Guide Index, 15 June (Online). US Department of Health and Human Services, Division of AIDS, National Institute of Allergy and Infectious Diseases, National Institutes of Health, USA. Available: http://aactg.s-3.com/pub/download/SpecimenProcessingGuide.pdf (2004, 15 Feb).

Allen, J.B., Wong, H.L., Guyre, P.M., Simon, G.L. and Wahl, S.M. (1991). Association of circulating receptor Fc gamma RIII-positive monocytes in AIDS patients with elevated levels of transforming growth factor-beta. J Clin Invest 87, 1773–1779.

Allen, J.B., McCartney-Francis, N., Smith, P.D. et al. (1990). Expression of interleukin 2 receptors by monocytes from patients with acquired immunodeficiency syndrome and induction of monocyte interleukin 2 receptors by human immunodeficiency virus in vitro. J Clin Invest 85, 192–199.

Alpsoy, E., Kodelja, V., Goerdt, S., Orfanos, C.E. and Zouboulis, Ch.C. (2003). Serum of patients with Behcet's disease induces classical (pro-inflammatory) activation of human macrophages in vitro. Dermatology 206, 225–232.

Anderson, C.F., Gerber, J.S. and Mosser, D.M. (2002). Modulating macrophage function with IgG immune complexes. J Endotox Res 8, 477–481.

Andreesen, R., Osterholz, J., Bross, K.J., Schulz, A., Luckenbach, G.A. and Lohr, G.W. (1983). Cytotoxic effector cell function at different stages of human monocyte-macrophage maturation. Cancer Res 43, 5931–5936.

Bassøe, C.F., Smith, I., Sørnes, S., Halstensen, A. and Lehmann, A.K. (2000). Concurrent measurement of antigen- and antibody-dependent oxidative burst and phagocytosis in monocytes and neutrophils. Methods 2, 203–220.

Bergh, F.T., Dayyani, F. and Ziegler-Heitbrock, L. (2004). Impact of type-I-interferon on monocyte subsets and their differentiation to dendritic cells. An in vivo and ex vivo study in multiple sclerosis patients treated with interferon-beta. J Neuroimmunol 146, 176–188.

Beutler, B., Hoebe, K., Du, X. and Ulevitch, R.J. (2003). How we detect microbes and respond to them: the Toll-like receptors and their transducers. J Leukoc Biol 74, 479–485.

Bingle, L., Brown, N.J. and Lewis, C.E. (2002). The role of tumour-associated macrophages in tumour progression: implications for new anticancer therapies. J Pathol 196, 254–265.

Buechler, C., Ritter, M., Orso, E., Langmann, T., Klucken, J. and Scmitz, G. (2000). Regulation of scavenger receptor CD163 expression in human monocytes and macrophages by pro- and anti-inflammatory stimuli. J Leukoc Biol 67, 97–103.

Cabrera, M., Rodriguez, O., Monsalve, I., Tovar, R. and Hagel, I. (2003). Variations in the serum levels of soluble CD23, nitric oxide and IgE across the spectrum of American cutaneous leishmaniasis. Acta Trop 88, 145–151.

Caulfield, J.J., Fernandez, M.H., Sousa, A.R., Lane, S.J., Lee, T.H. and Hawrylowicz, C.M. (1999). Regulation of major histocompatibility complex class II antigens on human alveolar macrophages by granulocyte-macrophage colony-stimulating factor in the presence of glucocorticoids. Immunology 98, 104–110.

Crucian, B.E. and Widen, R.H. (1998). The use of flow cytometry to detect intracellular cytokine production in individual cells. In Flow Cytometry Protocols, Jaroszeski, M.J. and Heller, H., eds. Totowa, New Jersey: Humana Press, pp. 37–55.

De Almeida, M.C., Cardoso, S.A. and Barral-Netto, M. (2003). Leishmania (Leishmania) chagasi infection alters the expression of cell adhesion and costimulatory molecules on human monocyte and macrophage. Int J Parasitol 33, 153–162.

Dijkstra, G., Zandvoort, A.J., Kobold, A.C. et al. (2002). Increased expression of inducible nitric oxide synthase in circulating monocytes from patients with active inflammatory bowel disease. Scand J Gastroenterol 37, 546–554.

Dinapoli, M.R., Calderon, C.L. and Lopez, D.M. (1996). The altered tumoricidal capacity of macrophages isolated from tumor-bearing mice is related to reduce expression of the inducible nitric oxide synthase gene. J Exp Med 183, 1323–1329.

Fadok, V.A. and Henson, P.M. (2003). Apoptosis: giving phosphatidylserine recognition an assist – with a twist. Curr Biol 13, R655–R657.

Fadok, V.A., Bratton, D.L., Konowal, A., Freed, P.W., Westcott, J.Y. and Henson, P.M. (1998). Macrophages that have ingested apoptotic cells in vitro inhibit proinflammatory cytokine production through autocrine/paracrine mechanisms involving TGF-beta, PGE2, and PAF. J Clin Invest 101, 890–898.

Fingerle-Rowson, G., Auers, J., Kreuzer, E. et al. (1998a). Down-regulation of surface monocyte lipopolysaccharide-receptor CD14 in patients on cardiopulmonary bypass undergoing aorta-coronary bypass operation. J Thorac Cardiovasc Surg 115, 1172–1178.

Fingerle-Rowson, G., Auers, J., Kreuzer, E., Fraunberger, P., Blumenstein, M. and Ziegler-Heitbrock, L.H. (1998b). Expansion of CD14+CD16+ monocytes in critically ill cardiac surgery patients. Inflammation 22, 367–379.

Fingerle-Rowson, G., Angstwurm, M., Andreesen, R. and Ziegler-Heitbrock, H.W. (1998c). Selective depletion of CD14+ CD16+ monocytes by glucocorticoid therapy. Clin Exp Immunol 112, 501–506.

Fonseca, J.E., Edwards, J.C.W., Blades, S. and Goulding, N.J., (2002). Macrophage subpopulations in rheumatoid synovium. Reduced CD163 expression in CD4+ T lymphocyte-rich microenvironments. Arthritis Rheum 46, 1210–1216.

Frungieri, M.B., Calandra, R.S., Lustig, L. et al. (2002). Number, distribution pattern, and identification of macrophages in the testes of infertile men. Fertil Steril 78, 298–306.

Fujino, S., Andoh, A., Bamba, S. et al. (2003). Increased expression of interleukin 17 in inflammatory bowel disease. Gut 52, 65–70.

Gallin, J.I. (1992). Phagocytic cells: disorders of function. In Inflammation: Basic Principles and Clinical Correlates, Gallin, J.I., Goldstein, I.M. and Snyderman R., eds. New York: Raven Press, p. 859.

Gascon, R.L., Narvaez, A.B., Zhang, R. et al. (2002). Increased HLA-DR expression on peripheral blood monocytes in subsets of subjects with primary HIV infection is associated with elevated CD4 T-cell apoptosis and CD4 T-cell depletion. J Acquir Immune Defic Syndr 30, 146–153.

Goldstein, J.I., Goldstein, K.A., Wardell, K. et al. (2003). Increase in plasma and surface CD163 levels in patients undergoing coronary artery bypass graft surgery. Atherosclerosis 170, 325–332.

Gordon, S., Lawson, G.S., Rabinowitz, S., Crocker, P.R., Morris, L. and Perry, V.H. (1992). Antigen markers of macrophage differentiation in murine tissues. Curr Top Microbiol Immunol 181, 1–37.

Greenwell-Wild, T., Vazquez, N., Sim, D. et al. (2002). Mycobacterium avium infection and modulation of human macrophage gene expression. J Immunol 169, 6286–6297.

Hauptmann, S., Zwaldo-Klarwasser, G., Jansen, M., Klosterhalfen, B. and Kirkpatrick, C.J. (1993). Macrophages and multicellular tumor spheroids in co-culture: a three dimensional model to study tumor-host interactions. Evidence for macrophage-mediated tumor cell proliferation and migration. Amer J Pathol 143, 1406–1415.

Högger, P., Dreier, J., Droste, A., Buck, F. and Sorg, C. (1998). RM3/1 on human monocytes as a glucocorticoid-inducible member of the scavenger receptor cysteine-rich family (CD163). J Immunol 161, 1883–1905.

Huissoon, A.P., Emery, P., Bacon, P.A., Gordon, J. and Salmon, M. (2000). Increased expression of CD23 in rheumatoid synovitis. Scand J Rheumatol 29, 154–159.

Hume, D.A., Ross, I.L., Himes, S. R., Sasmono, R.T., Wells, C.A. and Ravus, T. (2002). The mononuclear phagocyte system revisited. J Leuk Biol 72, 621–627.

Izikson, L., Klein, R.S., Luster, A.D. and Weiner, H.L. (2002). Targeting monocyte recruitment in CNS autoimmune disease. Clin Immunol 103, 125–131.

Kampalath, B., Cleveland, R.P., Chang, C.C. and Kass, L. (2003). Monocytes with altered phenotypes in posttrauma patients. Arch Pathol Lab Med 127, 1580–1585.

Kolb-Maurer, A., Weissinger, F., Kurzai, O., Maurer, M., Wilhelm, M. and Goebel, W. (2004). Bacterial infection of human hematopoietic stem cells induces monocytic differentiation. FEMS Immunol Med Microbiol 40, 147–153.

Koller, M., Aringer, M., Kiener, H. et al. (1999). Expression of adhesion molecules on synovial fluid and peripheral blood monocytes in patients with inflammatory joint disease and osteoarthritis. Ann Rheum Dis 58, 709–712.

Kristianson, M., Graverson, J., Jacobsen, J. et al. (2001). Identification of the haemoglobin scavenger receptor. Nature 409, 198–201.

Lehmann, A.K., Sørnes, S. and Halstensen, A. (2000). Phagocytosis: measurement by flow cytometry. J Immunol Methods 243, 229–242.

Lendemans, S., Kreuzfelder, E., Waydhas, C., Nast-Kolb, D. and Flohe, S. (2004). Clinical course and prognostic significance of immunological and functional parameters after severe trauma. Unfallchirurg 107, 203–210.

Lin, M. and Rikihisa, Y. (2004). Ehrlichia chaffeensis downregulates surface Toll-like receptors 2/4, CD14 and transcription factors PU.1 and inhibits lipopolysaccharide activation of NF-kappa B, ERK 1/2 and p38 MAPK in host monocytes. Cell Microbiol 6, 175–186.

Mantovani, A., Sozzani, S., Locati, M., Allavena, P. and Sica, A. (2002). Macrophage polarization: tumor-associated macrophages as a paradigm for polarized M2 mononuclear phagocytes. Trends Immunol 23, 549–555.

Masuda, M., Morimoto, T., De Haas, M. et al. (2003a). Increase of soluble FcgRIIIa derived from natural killer cells and macrophages in plasma from patients with rheumatoid arthritis. J Rheumatol 30, 1911–1917.

Masuda, M., Morimoto, T., Kobatake, S. et al. (2003b). Measurement of soluble Fcgamma receptor type IIIa derived from macrophages in plasma: increase in patients with rheumatoid arthritis. Clin Exp Immunol 132, 477–484.

Matsushita, N., Kashiwagi, M., Wait, R. et al. (2002). Elevated levels of soluble CD163 in sera and fluids from rheumatoid arthritis patients and inhibition of the shedding of CD163 by TIMP-3. Clin Exp Immunol 130, 156–161.

Mazzarella, G., Grella, E., D'Auria, D. et al. (2000). Phenotypic features of alveolar monocytes/macrophages and IL-8 gene activation by IL-1 and TNF-alpha in asthmatic patients. Allergy 55 Suppl 61, 36–41.

Miller, L.S., Atabai, K., Nowakowski, M et al. (2001). Increased expression of CD23 (Fc(epsilon) receptor II) by peripheral blood monocytes of aids patients. AIDS Res Hum Retroviruses 17, 443–452.

Møller, H.J., de Fost, M., Aerts, H., Hollak, C. and Moestrup, S.K. (2004). Plasma level of the macrophage-derived soluble CD163 is increased and positively correlates with severity in Gaucher's disease. Eur J Haematol 72, 135–139.

Møller, H.J., Aerts, H., Grønbæk, H. et al. (2002). Soluble CD163: a marker for monocyte/macrophage activity in disease. Scan J Clin Lab Invest 62 Suppl, 29–34.

Mouri, T. (1993). Induction of IgE-Fc receptor (FcRII/CD23) expression on stimulated monocytes by mite allergen in patients with asthma. Jpn J Allergol 42, 1683–1691.

Mytar, B., Baran, J., Gawlicka, M., Ruggiero, I. and Zembala, M. (2002). Immunophenotypic changes and induction of apoptosis of monocytes and tumour cells during their interactions in vitro. Anticancer Res 22, 2789–2796.

Nascimento, F.R.F., Rodríquez, D., Gomes, E., Fernvik, E.C. and Russo, M. (2003). A method for multiple sequential analysis of macrophage functions using a small single cell sample. Braz J Med Bio Res 36, 1221–1226.

Nielsen, O.H., Kirman, I., Rudiger, N., Hendel, J. and Vainer, B. (2003). Upregulation of interleukin-12 and -17 in active inflammatory bowel disease. Scand J Gastroenterol 38, 180–185.

Oehling, A.G., Akdis, C.A., Schapowal, A., Blaser, K., Schmitz, M. and Simon, H.U. (1997). Suppression of the immune system by oral glucocorticoid therapy in bronchial asthma. Allergy 52, 144–154.

Perticarari, S., Presani, G. and Banfi, E. (1994). A new flow cytometric assay for the evaluation of phagocytosis and the oxidative burst in whole blood. J Immunol Methods 170, 117–124.

Perticarari, S., Presani, G., Mangiarotti, M.A. and Banfi, E. (1991). Simultaneous flow cytometric method to measure phago-cytosis and oxidative products by neutrophils. Cytometry 12, 687–693.

Philippidis, P., Mason, J.C., Evans, B.J. et al. (2004). Hemaglobin scavenger receptor CD163 mediates interleukin release and heme oxygenase-1 synthesis. Antiinflammatory monocyte-macrophage responses in vitro, in resolving skin blisters in vivo, and after cardiopulmonary bypass surgery. Circ Res 94, 119–126.

Plesner, A. (2003). Increasing the yield of human mononuclear cells and low serum concentrations for in vitro generation of macrophages with M-CSF. J Immunol Methods 279, 287–295.

Pollard, J.W. (2004). Tumour-educated macrophages promote tumour progression and metastasis. Nat Rev Cancer 4, 71–78.

Pulliam, L., Gascon, R., Stubblebine, M., McGuire, D. and McGrath, M.S. (1997). Unique monocyte subset in patients with AIDS dementia. Lancet 349, 692–695.

Rakoff-Nahoum, S., Chen, H., Kraus, T. et al. (2001). Regulation of class II expression in monocytic cells after HIV-1 infection. J Immunol 167, 2331–2342.

Sbrana, S., Parri, M.S., De Filippis, R., Gianetti, J. and Clerico, A. (2004). Monitoring of monocyte functional state after extra-corporeal circulation: A flow cytometry study. Cytometry 58, 17–24.

Scherberich, J.E. (2003). Proinflammatory blood monocytes: main effector and target cells in systemic and renal disease; background and therapeutic implications. Int J Clin Pharmacol Ther 41, 459–464.

Schoppmann, S.F., Birner, P., Stockl, J. et al. (2002). Tumor-asso-ciated macrophages express lymphatic endothelial growth factors and are related to peritumoral lymphangiogenesis. Am J Pathol 161, 947–956.

Shumilla, J.A., Lacaille, V., Hornell, T.M et al. (2004). Bordetella pertussis infection of primary human monocytes alters HLA-DR expression. Infect Immun 72, 1450–1462.

Simone, N.L., Paweletz, C.P., Charboneau, L., Petricoin, E.F., 3rd and Liotta, L.A. (2000). Laser capture microdissection: beyond functional genomics to proteomics. Mol Diagn 5, 301–307.

Stewart, C.C. and Steinkamp, J.A. (1982). Quantitation of cell concentration using the flow cytometer. Cytometry 2, 238–243.

Sulahian, T.H., Högger, P., Wahner, A.E. et al. (2000). Human monocytes express CD163, which is upregulated by IL-10 and identical to p155. Cytokine 12, 1312–1321.

Swingler, S., Brichacek, B., Jacque, J.M., Ulich, C., Zhou, J. and Stevenson, M. (2003). HIV-1 Nef intersects the macrophage CD40L signalling pathway to promote resting-cell infection. Nature 424, 213–219.

Takemura, R. and Werb, Z. (1984). Secretory products of macrophages and their physiological functions. Amer J Physiol 246, C1–C9.

Trillo-Pazos, G., Diamanturos, A., Rislove, L. et al. (2003). Detection of HIV-1 DNA in microglia/macrophages, astro-cytes and neurons isolated from brain tissue with HIV-1 encephalitis by laser capture microdissection. Brain Pathol 13, 144–154.

Tuomisto, T.T., Korleela, A., Rutanen, J. et al. (2003). Gene expression in macrophage-rich inflammatory infiltrates in human atherosclerotic lesions as studied by laser microdis-section and DNA array. Arterioscler Thromb Vasc Biol 23, 2235–2240.

Ugurel, S., Uhlig, D., Pfohler, C., Tilgen, W., Schadendorf, D. and Reinhold, U. (2004). Down-regulation of HLA class II and cos-timulatory CD86/B7-2 on circulating monocytes from melanoma patients. Cancer Immunol Immunother Jan 16 (Epub ahead of print).

van Furth, R. (1976). Macrophage activity and clinical immun-ology. Origin and kinetics of mononuclear phagocytes. Ann NY Acad Sci 278, 161–175.

VanderBorght, A., Geusens, P., Raus, J. and Stinissen, P. (2001). The autoimmune pathogenesis of rheumatoid arthritis: role of autoreactive T cells and new immunotherapies. Semin Arthritis Rheum 31, 160–175.

Viksman, M.Y., Bochner, B.S., Peebles, R.S., Schleimer, R.P. and Liu, M.C. (2002). Expression of activation markers on alveolar macrophages in allergic asthmatics after endobronchial or whole-lung allergen challenge. Clin Immunol 104, 77–85.

Vouldoukis, I., Issaly, F., Fourcade, C. et al. (1994). CD23 and IgE expression during human immune response to cutaneous leishmaniasis: possible role in monocyte activation. Res Immunol 145, 17–27.

Wahl, L.M. and Smith, P.D. (1997). Isolation of monocyte/macrophage populations. In Current Protocols in Immunology. Indianapolis: John Wiley & Sons, Inc., 2: 7.6.1–7.6.8.

Wahl, L.M., Katona, R.L., Winter, C.C., Haraoui, B., Scher, I. and Wahl, S.M. (1984). Isolation of human mononuclear cells subsets by counterflow centrifugal elutriation (CCE). I. Characterization of B-lymphocyte-, T-lymphocyte-, and monocyte-enriched frac-tions. Cell Immunol 85, 373–383.

Wahl, S.M. and Chen, W. (2003). TGF-beta: how tolerant can it be? Immunol Res 28, 167–179.

Wahl, S.M., Allen, J.B., Welch, G.R. and Wong, H.L. (1992). Transforming growth factor-beta in synovial fluids modulates Fc gamma RII (CD16) expression on mononuclear phagocytes. J Immunol 148, 485–490.

West, M.A. and Heagy, W. (2002). Endotoxin tolerance: A review. Crit Care Med 30, 64–73.

Wijngaarden, S., van Roon, J.A., Bijlsma, J.W., van de Winkel, J.G. and Lafeber, F.P. (2003). Fcgamma receptor expression levels on monocytes are elevated in rheumatoid arthritis patients with high erythrocyte sedimentation rate who do not use anti-rheumatic drugs. Rheumatology (Oxford) 42, 681–688.

Wright, S.D., Ramos, R.A., Tobias, P.S., Ulevitch, R.J. and Mathison, J.C. (1990). CD14, a receptor for complexes of lipopolysaccharide (LPS) and LPS binding protein. Science 249, 1431–1433.

Zisman, D.A., Kunkel, S.L., Streiter, R.M. et al. (1997). Anti-interleukin-12 therapy protects mice in lethal endotoxemia but impairs bacterial clearance in murine Escherichia coli peritoneal sepsis. Shock 8, 349–356.

Tumor Cells

**Hans Loibner, Gottfried Himmler, Andreas Obwaller
and Patricia Paukovits**
IGENEON Krebs-Immuntherapie Forschungs- und Entwicklungs-AG Vienna, Austria

Truth is ever to be found in the simplicity, and not in the
multiplicity and confusion of things.

Sir Isaac Newton (1642–1727)

INTRODUCTION

Despite advances in conventional cancer management,
the probability of relapse and death from cancer remains
increased in certain tumors (Agarwala and Kirkwood,
1998; Midgley and Kerr, 2000). The high mortality relates
mainly to the early spread of malignant cells from a
primary tumor to distant organs and to the fact that viable
single tumor cells may remain after a course of treatment (Klein, 2000). The metastatic process consists of
several consecutive steps (Woodhouse et al., 1997).
Disseminated tumor cells (DTCs) enter the circulation via
bloodstream or lymphatic vessels and migrate to new
sites where they extravasate into the surrounding tissue.
There, they may either exist as single cells or develop into
micrometastases. In both cases, the cells must initiate and
maintain growth until angiogenesis forms vascularized
metastases. For a review of the metastatic process see
Chambers et al. (2002). Some cancer types show an
organ-specific pattern of metastatic spread, such as
epithelial tumors, that preferentially mestastasize to
bone. This organ specificity is most probably depending
on the compatibility of molecular interactions of those
cells with the new tissue that enables organ-specific
growth (Chambers et al., 2002). The characteristics of

DTCs can be very different from that of the primary tissue
they originate from. Some primary tumors and metastatic
cell clones have been reported to independently diverge
in such a way that the primary neoplasm disappears and
only the metatases remain detectable (Bell et al., 1989).
Generally, the progression from a primary tumor to a
metastasis is not linear and much is unclear about which
cells survive in the new site and what mechanism triggers
the development of a metastasis. The process of dissemination is generally occult and may already have occurred
by the time of primary diagnosis (Poste and Fidler, 1980;
Fidler, 1999). In the new site, DTCs or micrometastases
may enter a dormant state in which they barely divide
(Pantel et al., 1993a). During this time, they are invisible to
currently used diagnostic methods such as nuclear and
radiological imaging techniques and often refractory to
cancer therapies that target actively dividing cells (Braun
et al., 2000a). Increasing knowledge of the molecular biology of cancer evolution has provided evidence that DTCs
can be appropriate targets for treatment forms that aim
both at dormant and proliferating cells, such as cancer
immunotherapies (Pantel and Otte, 2001). In contrast to
solid metastases, circulating tumor cells are more accessible for immunomodulatory substances and antibodies
(Klein, 2000).

Initial research concentrated on the detection of DTCs
in bone marrow (BM) aspirates from carcinoma patients
(Schlimok et al., 1987), but occult tumor cells were also
detected in BM of patients with primary tumors that generally do not metastasize to the bone (Pantel et al., 1999).

Further advantages of BM as an indicator organ were considered good accessibility, vascularization and lack of epithelial cells (Pantel et al., 1995a). Blood as well is an important compartment for DTC research because the hematogenous route is fundamental for the process of dissemination to distant organs. Peripheral blood is easy to sample and advantageous when several samples are needed to decrease sampling error (Wharton et al., 1999). The clinical relevance of DTCs in blood remains ambiguous, although there is some evidence that these cells may reflect the stage of growth and spread of cancer (Z'graggen et al., 2001). Methods for detection of DTCs are mainly designed to recognize certain tumor associated antigens or specific markers. Regarding cancer screening and immunotherapy, the identification of tumor antigens that elicit an immune response is thought to be useful. Yet of the large array of tumor antigens that has been identified so far, only a small number has shown to be capable of inducing an immune response in patients (Lloyd, 1993). A clinically effective immune response to a tumor antigen is generally expected to be a T cell response, but also the humoral immunity could be involved, for example when the antigen is carbohydrate-based (Keilholz et al., 2002). Thus, the assessment of tumor-specific immune responses should include analysis of cellular and humoral immune responses, both involving techniques that are covered elsewhere in this book. Therapeutic success of a therapy aimed at DTCs could be assessed by monitoring such cells and their properties. To develop efficient therapeutics to target DTCs we need to learn about mechanisms that trigger dissemination, migration, dormancy and metastatic outgrowth – properties reflected by the genotypic and phenotypic characteristics of the cells. The characterization of DTCs has therefore become a major goal in DTC research. In this chapter, we report on existing methods for detection and characterization of DTCs in blood and bone marrow of patients with epithelial tumors, clinical implications and suitability of DTCs as surrogate markers for therapeutic success.

CHARACTERIZATION OF DISSEMINATED TUMOR CELLS

Phenotyping and genotyping of DTCs is useful to confirm the malignant nature and to learn about the immunogenic potential of those cells and their proliferative capacity. Genomic analyses have been developed in recent years by combining either immunostaining methods or immunofluorescence with in situ hybridization (Muller et al., 1996; Litle et al., 1997). The studies confirmed the malignant character of DTCs and demonstrated heterogeneity between disseminated cells found at different sites and their primary tumor (Klein et al., 1999; Tortola et al., 2001). Phenotypic features such as growth factor receptors and adhesion molecules can

be identified by immunocytological double labeling of cells. Studies using these techniques revealed tumor-associated characteristics, such as downregulation of MHC-I antigen in colorectal and gastric carcinomas (Pantel et al., 1991), expression of growth factor receptors in metastatic breast cancer (Schlimok et al., 1990) and expression of the epithelial cell adhesion molecule E-cadherin in breast and gastric cancer (Funke et al., 1996). Tumor cell lines established from BM of patients with carcinomas revealed an invasive phenotype reflected by consistent expression of metastasis-associated adhesion molecules (Putz et al., 1999). Expression of proliferative markers was found to be low (Pantel et al., 1993a; Mueller et al., 1998) substantiating DTC dormancy. The ineffectiveness of conventional chemotherapeutic approaches in eliminating cytokeratine-positive cells in BM (Braun et al., 2000a) is likely to be caused by this state of dormancy. Long-term follow-up of breast cancer patients has revealed tumor dormancy periods of up to 20–25 years (Karrison et al., 1999). In vitro experiments with viable tumor cells from BM of patients with epithelial cancers revealed differences in proliferative capacity of tumor cells (Solakoglu et al., 2002). Further evidence that the local microenvironment of the organ site, to which the DTCs have migrated, influences whether metastases develop or not has been provided by Tarin et al. (1984).

Recent reports indicate that cancer cells acquire their metastatic potential early during tumor development (van't Veer et al., 2002; Kang et al., 2003) and not, as assumed, in late tumorigenesis. Subpopulations of cells may even display tissue-specific expression profiles determining the site of metastasis (Kakiuchi et al., 2003; van't Veer and Weigelt, 2003). Fluorescent-labeled human breast cancer cell lines with differential metastatic potential were inoculated into the mammary glands of nude mice and cell dissemination from resulting tumors was visually tracked (Goodison et al., 2003). DTCs were found in lungs, where they did not generate metastases but remained dormant for months, even when they were derived from a clone with high metastatic potential. In vitro and reinoculation experiments revealed that these cells had not lost their proliferative capacity or tumorigenicity but that their quiescence had been induced by the surrounding host organ. Analysis of metastatic and non-metastatic cells of the primary tumor revealed that these cells differed in their intravasation behavior. Non-metastatic cells demonstrated fragmentation when they got in contact with vessels, while metastatic cells exhibited orientation towards blood vessels indicating intravasive behavior (Wyckoff et al., 2000).

METHODS OF DETECTION

Over the past 20 years, different immunocytological and molecular methods have been developed to detect individual disseminated tumor cells in bone marrow, peripheral blood and lymph nodes (Pantel and Ahr, 1998; Noack et al., 2000; Lacroix and Doeberitz, 2001; Zehentner, 2002; Ambros et al., 2003). Whereas PCR, flow cytometry and fluorescence *in situ* hybridization (FISH) have become standard techniques for the detection of DTCs in hematopoietic malignancies, the standardization of methods for detection of DTCs in solid tumors is still in process (Kostler et al., 2000). Using immunocytochemical analyses, cells are usually centrifuged onto microscope slides (cytospins); several protocols and devices for processing and analysis of cell suspensions have been developed. Using molecular methods, DNA is extracted either from plasma or from tumor cells that occur in fractions that also contain mononuclear cells. Extraction of mRNA and amplification via reverse transcriptase polymerase chain reaction (RT-PCR) analysis is the preferred method of practice. Immunocytochemical methods have a long tradition in the detection of DTCs and are considered as the gold standard for the detection of DTCs in bone marrow aspirates, although non-specific staining or masking of non-malignant cells by epithelial antigens may produce false positive results and morphological criteria need to be included in the evaluation (Ambros et al., 2003).

The microscopic screening of large sample volumes can be time-consuming. To reduce the effort of manual sample evaluation, several semi-automated, computer-aided detection devices have been developed, which allow for digital storage for later visual evaluation (Gross et al., 1995; Kraeft et al., 2000). Although molecular methods are less arduous, morphological evaluation of the sample is not possible. Cells found in these assays are generally designated as tumor cells, but these should more accurately be described as simply epithelial cells in a non-epithelial environment, since most methods do not differentiate between tumor cells and normal cells. Several consecutive work steps are required for the detection of DTCs including sample collection, preparation of tumor cell containing fractions, staining/PCR and the analysis of results. An overview of steps and methods is shown in Figure 26.1.

Sample collection

Blood samples are taken by venous blood puncture, whereas bone marrow is aspirated by puncture of the iliac crest (spina iliaca posterior superior). To avoid contamination of blood with epithelial cells during venepuncture, the first 3 ml of blood are discarded. To reach sufficient sensitivity, at least 5 ml of peripheral blood should be used for analysis. If bone marrow is used, at least 2×10^6 cells should be prepared for analysis. Regardless of the type of the sample or mode of detection, tumor cell-containing fractions of nucleated cells must initially be separated from red blood cells. This can be achieved either by density centrifugation using a ficoll gradient, or

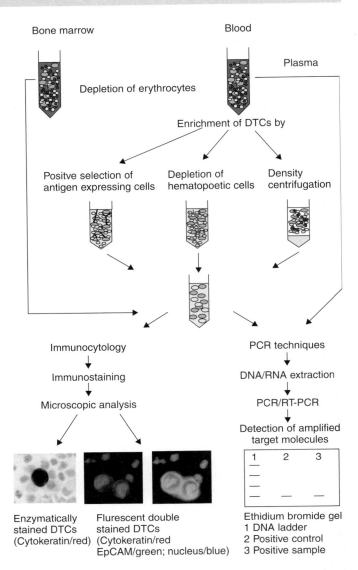

Figure 26.1 Illustration of methods for the detection of disseminated tumor cells in blood and bone marrow. **See colour plate 26.1.**

by hypotonic lysis of red blood cells using ammonium chloride buffer.

Enrichment of disseminated tumor cells from peripheral blood

As the detection of DTCs in blood is limited by the low frequency of the cells, tumor cells must be enriched first. Enrichment of DTCs can be achieved after depletion of red blood cells by negative or positive selection of tumor cells or by density centrifugation. In positive enrichment of epithelial cells, the cellular fraction is first incubated with magnetic particles (beads or ferrofluid systems) coated with antibodies directed against epithelial antigens and then separated magnetically (Racila et al., 1998; Meye et al., 2002). Most authors use antibodies against the epithelial cell adhesion antigen EpCAM, ErbB-2, or against members of the cytokeratin molecule family which are components of the cytoskeleton. In negative selection techniques, normal blood cells are first depleted using beads coated with antibodies against hematopoietic cell antigens (CD45) (Naume et al., 1998). This negative selection has a major advantage of providing antigen independent enrichment of DTCs, which is very useful since some epithelial antigens may be poorly expressed or, in some cases, even missing (Kasimir-Bauer et al., 2003; Thurm et al., 2003).

A further antigen independent enrichment method is density centrifugation that uses a gradient which facilitates the separation of mononuclear cells, including tumor cells, from normal non-malignant cells. Such a density gradient is employed by the OncoQuick® (Rosenberg et al., 2002) system which is composed of a centrifugation tube with a liquid density separation medium. This method does not require a primary step in which red blood cells are eliminated. DTC-enriched fractions will be centrifugated onto microscope slides for immunocytochemical analysis (ICC), stained in suspension (alternative cytometric approaches) or lysed for DNA or RNA-preparation (PCR, RT-PCR).

Techniques for detection

Immunocytochemistry

Immunocytochemical methods are based on the staining of tumor cells using specific antibodies against tissue (tumor) specific antigens. Target antigens include EpCAM, members of the cytokeratin family or other antigens, which are overexpressed on tumor cells (HER2-neu or MUC-1) but not on hematopoietic cells (Braun et al., 2001). These antibodies are either directly labeled with horseradish peroxidase, alkaline phosphatase or fluorescent proteins, or the antigen– antibody complex is visualized by a labeled second antibody as in the commonly used alkaline phosphatase anti-alkaline phosphatase (APAAP) method (Cordell et al., 1984). The sensitivity of the assay is examined by spiking experiments, in which cells from different cancer cell lines are spiked into blood from healthy donors.

To discriminate between DTCs and non-specifically stained non-malignant cells, an additional evaluation step that includes morphological criteria and/or an additional counterstaining, is necessary (Ambros et al., 2003). This step employs a second tumor cell-specific antigen as inclusion criterion or an antibody against a marker of hematopoietic cells (CD45) (Pantel et al., 1994). During the last years several computer-aided search-systems have been developed (MetaSystems, RCDetect®; Chroma Vision, ACIS®), which are used for scanning of microscope slides and image analysis. Enriched fractions are commonly centrifuged onto microscope slides (cytospins) for immunohistochemical detection and evaluation of DTCs. Due to the absence of morphologic evaluation of labeled cells, FACS analysis has not become a standard tool in the

detection of DTCs. However, cytometric methods have been recently developed, which combine an 'in suspension staining protocol' with a microscopic evaluation of the cells (Tibbe et al., 1999, 2002a,b; Pachmann et al., 2001).

The specificity of immunocytological assays can be increased by FISH. After identification and storage of pictures of immunopositive tumor cells, the slide can be removed from the microscope and the same sample can be used for examination of genetic aberrations. The cell proteins are enzymatically digested and aberrant genetic markers are hybridized with fluorescent DNA probes. Immunopositive cells can now be relocated and the immunocytologic result can be verified by the presence of fluorescent genetic aberrations. For this approach, additional devices such as automated image analysis systems are useful, with the help of which an exact relocation of the immunopositive cell is feasible.

Alterations in nucleic acids

Specific mutations of defined sequences within the DNA of tumor cells, which are not present on non-transformed cells, permit the identification of micrometastases (Hayashi et al., 1995). Since the earliest reports of tumors derived from oncogene mutations (K-ras), a number of DNA and RNA markers have been identified by means of oncogene amplification, microsatellite alteration and gene rearrangements (Silva et al., 2002a,b; Anker et al., 2003). Epigenetic alterations, such as promoter methylations of oncogene suppressor genes, have been reported as well (Goessl et al., 2002; Widschwendter and Jones, 2002; Widschwendter et al., 2004b). Thus, investigations of nucleic acids as tumor markers in plasma or in DTCs recently acquired interest.

Detection of DNA/mRNA alterations in plasma

Circulating DNA can be detected in plasma from normal individuals and, to a greater extent, in plasma from tumor patients. Some investigations have reported an increase in the number of genetic alterations in circulating DNA from tumor patients, including mutations of proto-oncogenes, tumor suppressor genes or methylated tumor suppressor genes (Goessl et al., 2002; Johnson and Lo, 2002; Widschwendter and Jones, 2002; Anker et al., 2003; Goessl, 2003; Widschwendter et al., 2004a,b).

DNA is extracted from plasma using standard methods and subjected to PCR using primers specific for mutated tumor DNA, genetic rearrangements or sequences of oncogenic viruses. Another approach is the detection of methylated (inactivated) tumor suppressor genes. A list of methylated genes was published by Issa (2004). In this approach, DNA is modified by sodium bisulfite treatment, which converts unmethylated, but not methylated cytosines to uracil. This DNA is then used as a template in two PCR reactions. One is specific for DNA, where the gene of interest is methylated (using primers containing the cytosins) and one is specific for unmethylated original

DNA using primers that contain uracil instead of cytosine. PCR products are separated on 6–8 per cent non-denaturing polyacrylamide gels and the bands are visualized by staining with ethidium bromide. The presence of a band of the appropriate molecular weight indicates the presence of unmethylated and/or methylated targets in the original sample.

Tumor-cell specific mRNA in cell lysates

For RT-PCR, RNA is extracted from DTC-containing mononuclear cell fractions using standard methods. Then, mRNA is randomly transcribed into cDNA. The cDNA is then used as a template for PCR-reactions that use primers specific for tissue specific markers, similar to protein markers used in immunostaining approaches. The most frequently targeted sequences are cytokeratins, mucins, HER2 and others (Raynor et al., 2002; Huang et al., 2003; Vlems et al., 2003a; Weber et al., 2003; Rosenberg et al., 2004; Schuster et al., 2004; Ady et al., 2004). Further target sequences are listed in Table 26.1.

To increase sensitivity, a second PCR approach (nested PCR) with different primers located within the first primer pair can be appended, using the PCR-product of the first PCR-reaction as template. The quality of the PCR-components is controlled by co-amplification of housekeeping genes such as ribosomal RNA or β-actin. PCR products are then separated on agarose gels and stained with ethidium bromide. The sensitivity of the assay is examined by spiking of cancer cell lines into the blood of healthy donors. Using standard PCR protocols, only a qualitative determination of the presence of target cDNA-templates is possible. A PCR-approach which combines a semi-quantitative determination of target cDNA with increased sensitivity, is real time PCR technique. By testing a number of samples from healthy donors, a background level can be determined and a cut-off level can be established. Molecular techniques make quantification of DTCs very difficult or even impossible since the transcription rate of target mRNA molecules (expression of target antigens) varies within and between samples and individuals. One cannot differentiate between one tumor cell that highly expresses the target molecule and several tumor cells that express the target molecule to a lower extent. Therefore, the conclusion that a high number of copies in the PCR product correlates with a high number of tumor cells is illegitimate.

Clonogenic assays

This method has gained importance in testing of hematopoietic autografts for tumor cell contamination and in optimization of autologous tumor cell vaccines (Pantel et al., 1995b). Several attempts have been made to establish tissue-culture assays to detect and expand disseminated tumor cells (Kruger et al., 2003). In many cases, the tumor cells could be propagated and used for further immunological and molecular examination. Tumor colonies are identified by immunocytochemical methods and may be also tested for growth capacity (Ross et al., 1993). However, there is a possibility of biased cultivation and false positive results due to the clonogenic growth of non-malignant cells such as Epstein-Barr virus transformed lymphoblastoid cells.

Limitations of the assays

Sensitivity

Spiking experiments of both immunocytochemical and nucleic acid based methods, could recover one tumor cell in up to 10^6 mononucleated cells when DTCs were not enriched first (bone marrow samples) and one tumor cell in up to 10^8 mononucleated cells after enrichment of DTC-containing fractions. Although it is generally accepted that marker genes are expressed on most DTCs, several authors report great heterogeneity in the expression of these marker genes (Zippelius et al., 1997; Braun et al., 1999; Kasimir-Bauer et al., 2003). It was even indicated that a high fraction of DTCs is apoptotic (Mehes et al., 2001) and therefore susceptible to damage and loss during the procedure of enrichment. Considering these facts, a multiparameter detection of marker genes or proteins could help to increase the sensitivity of the assays. This can be achieved by either using a panel of antibodies with different specificities or a multi-marker PCR (multiplex-PCR).

Specificity

Although the expression of epithelial antigens is mostly limited to epithelial cells, antibodies used for detection of these proteins may cross-react with non-specific antigens as well. Several attempts have been made to standardize the detection protocols. Since immunocytochemical and PCR methods aim at the detection of tissue specific markers, which are not necessarily tumor cell specific, the interpretation of results has to be considered carefully. Epithelial cells shed during inflammatory responses or chemotherapy may yield false positive

Table 26.1 Frequently used epithelial cell markers

Marker	Technique
Pan Cytokeratin	ICC
Cytokeratins 7 and 8	ICC
Cytokeratins 8, 18 and 19	ICC
Cytokeratin 19	ICC, RT-PCR
Cytokeratin 20	RT-PCR
Cytokeratin c-erbB2	ICC, RT-PCR
EpCAM	ICC
MUC-1	ICC, RT-PCR
EGFR	RT-PCR
Mammaglobin	RT-PCR
MAGE-A3	RT-PCR
β-human chorionic gonadotropin (β-HCG)	RT-PCR

ICC, immunocytochemistry.

results. Furthermore, transcription of cytokeratin 19 and carcinoembryonic antigen could be observed in mononuclear, normal cells during inflammatory responses and neutropenia (Jung et al., 1998; Ring et al., 2004), leading to false positive results. The illegitimate transcription of pseudogenes can generate false positive results as well. Therefore, the International Society for Hematotherapy and Graft Engineering (ISHAGE) has issued a guideline for the detection and evaluation of DTCs in blood and bone marrow (Borgen et al., 1998). It has to be taken into account that DNA fragments amplified by PCR could have been released from decaying tumor cells anywhere in the organism and do not point to the presence of viable cells. The latter can only be reliably demonstrated by immunocytological detection.

CLINICAL RELEVANCE

Over the years several reports could show that the detection of DTCs in BM is not only associated with increased risk of relapse and decreased overall survival, but it could also be proved by large clinical trials that monitoring of DTCs constitutes an independent prognostic factor (Cote et al., 1991; Mansi et al., 1991; Schlimok et al., 1991; Lindemann et al., 1992; Pantel et al., 1993b; Diel et al., 1996; Jauch et al., 1996). It was therefore proposed that detection and quantification of DTCs could help to assess disease progression and therapeutic success and may thus constitute a surrogate marker for estimation of prognosis and therapeutic efficacy (Kostler et al., 2000).

Though numerous studies have tried to link the presence of DTCs to prognostic significance, the findings are contradictory and hard to compare (Vlems et al., 2003b). Some of the results are listed in Table 26.2. First of all, the percentage of DTC positive patients varies between the studies. For instance, studies that employed nucleic-acid-based techniques found DTCs in the blood of 0–88 per cent of patients with operable breast cancer and

in 0–100 per cent of patients with metastatic disease (Ring et al., 2004). Different detection rates have been published in studies that used cytometric assays to identify circulating tumor cells in the blood, ranging for instance in mammary carcinoma from 4 to 45 per cent (Osborne and Rosen, 1994). In colorectal cancer, the percentages of patients positive for DTCs ranged from about 39 to 100 per cent in blood and from 9 to 52 per cent in bone marrow (Vlems et al., 2003b). The reports differ also considerably with regard to the number of analysed cells. For a comparison of reports see Pantel and von Knebel Doeberitz (2000).

The discordance in results is mainly due to substantial methodological differences. These differences, ranging from variations in sample handling, location of sampling, and time of sampling to discrepancies in the numerous antibodies directed against different epitopes applied in different staining protocols, have led to confusing results rather than to an improvement of the assays. In many studies that employed antibodies directed against epithelial antigens, an inclusion of control patients that could reduce false positive results caused by non-specific staining, was omitted. On the other hand, bone marrow samples from healthy donors did stain positive for cytokeratins, most probably due to unspecific binding of dyes and antibodies (Pantel et al., 1996). Furthermore does the choice of the sample size, which varies greatly between studies, influence the statistical power of the results (Funke and Schraut, 1998), particularly when only a small number of patients is tested for DTCs. Also the composition of the patient population could influence the results. In some studies for example, different disease stages were pooled in one analysis (de Cremoux et al., 2000; Silva et al., 2001). Preoperative chemoradiation of patients was also shown to influence the number of DTCs detected in BM and blood (Kienle et al., 2003). It is still unclear whether DTCs detected in blood and bone marrow can be compared regarding clinical relevance (Z'graggen et al., 2001). Studies that compared the frequency of DTCs in BM and blood samples from the same

Table 26.2 Prognostic relevance of DTCs in blood and bone marrow of patients with epithelial cancers

Detection site	Detection technique; target	Tumor type	Number of patients/controls	Detection rate (%)	Prognostic significance	Median follow-up (months)	Reference
BM	ICC; EMA	breast	285/0	27	RFS, OS	29	(Berger et al., 1988)
BM	ICC; CK	breast	49/0	37	DFS a	30	(Cote et al., 1991)
BM	ICC; EMA	breast	350/0	25	RFS, OS	76	(Mansi et al., 1991)
BM	ICC; EMA, CK	breast	100/0	38	RFS, OS a	34	(Harbeck et al., 1994)
BM	ICC; TAG12	breast	727/0	43	DFS, OS a	36	(Diel et al., 1996)
BM	ICC; CK	breast	552/191	36	DFS, OS a	38	(Braun et al., 2000b)
BM	ICC; CK18	colorectal	88/102	32	DFS a	35	(Lindemann et al., 1992)
Blood, BM	ICC; CK, 17-1A	pancreatic	105/66	26	none a	27	(Z'graggen et al., 2001)
Blood	RT-PCR; CEA	colorectal	95/0	41	none	41	(Bessa et al., 2001)
Lymph nodes	ICC; 17-1A	esophageal	68/24	62	RFS, OS	21	(Izbicki et al., 1997)
Lymph nodes	RT-PCR; CEA	colorectal	26/0	54	RFS, OS	73 (mean)	(Liefers et al., 1998)

BM, bone marrow; CK, cytokeratins; EMA, epithelial membrane antigen; GP, glycoproteins; ICC; immunocytochemistry; DFS, disease-free survival; OS, overall survival; RFS, relapse-free survival; a, Prognostic value tested by multivariate analysis.

patient showed that the detection rate was higher in BM than in the corresponding blood investigation (Melchior et al., 1997; Soeth et al., 1997). A standardization of preanalytical and analytical procedures is therefore essential to ensure reproducibility of results and to enable prediction of prognoses.

Future prospects

Identification of patients with poor prognosis based on the presence of DTCs will only be feasible when reproducible detection methods are established. A current study that employed a semiautomated sample preparation system, was able to link the presence of circulating tumor cells in blood to progression-free and overall survival in patients with metastatic breast cancer (Cristofanilli et al. 2004). Long-term observations including repeated bone marrow and peripheral blood examination of a large number of patients is required to monitor whether a therapy is able to reduce DTCs and to ascertain whether this reduction correlates with improved prognosis.

Cancer therapy still lacks suitable surrogate markers acceptable to the regulatory authorities that provide both indication of metastatic risk following treatment of the primary tumor together with a basis for reliable comparisons of effects of particular therapies. In cancer studies using survival time as the primary endpoint, tumor response or time to progression are frequently used as surrogate endpoints since these events occur earlier. Surrogate markers used today are markers that have the property of mirroring the disease state (e.g. tumor markers). Information regarding the success of an adjuvant therapy can be only obtained after an observation period of several years. Should tumor cells (into disseminated bone marrow or circulating in blood) prove suitable as biological surrogate markers that could predict therapeutic benefit and be sufficiently correlated with the primary endpoint, conventional staging systems may be refined and evaluation of new therapies could be accelerated.

REFERENCES

Ady, N., Morat, L., Fizazi, K. et al. (2004). Detection of HER-2/neu-positive circulating epithelial cells in prostate cancer patients. Br J Cancer 90, 443–448.

Agarwala, S.S. and Kirkwood, J.M. (1998). Adjuvant therapy of melanoma. Semin Surg Oncol 14, 302–310.

Ambros, P.F., Mehes, G., Ambros, I.M. and Ladenstein, R. (2003). Disseminated tumor cells in the bone marrow – chances and consequences of microscopical detection methods. Cancer Lett 197, 29–34.

Anker, P., Mulcahy, H. and Stroun, M. (2003). Circulating nucleic acids in plasma and serum as a noninvasive investigation for cancer: time for large-scale clinical studies? Int J Cancer 103, 149–152.

Bell, C.W., Pathak, S. and Frost, P. (1989). Unknown primary tumors: establishment of cell lines, identification of chromosomal abnormalities, and implications for a second type of tumor progression. Cancer Res 9, 4311–4315.

Berger, U., Bettelheim, R., Mansi, J.L., Easton, D., Coombes, R.C. and Neville, A.M. (1988). The relationship between micrometastases in the bone marrow, histopathologic features of the primary tumor in breast cancer and prognosis. Am J Clin Pathol 90, 1–6.

Bessa, X., Elizalde, J.I., Boix, L. et al. (2001). Lack of prognostic influence of circulating tumor cells in peripheral blood of patients with colorectal cancer. Gastroenterology 120, 1084–1092.

Borgen, E., Beiske, K., Trachsel, S. et al. (1998). Immunocytochemical detection of isolated epithelial cells in bone marrow: non-specific staining and contribution by plasma cells directly reactive to alkaline phosphatase. J Pathol 185, 427–434.

Braun, S., Hepp, F., Sommer, H.L. and Pantel, K. (1999). Tumor-antigen heterogeneity of disseminated breast cancer cells: implications for immunotherapy of minimal residual disease. Int J Cancer 84, 1–5.

Braun, S., Kentenich, C., Janni, W. et al. (2000a). Lack of effect of adjuvant chemotherapy on the elimination of single dormant tumor cells in bone marrow of high-risk breast cancer patients. J Clin Oncol 18, 80–86.

Braun, S., Pantel, K., Muller, P. et al. (2000b). Cytokeratin-positive cells in the bone marrow and survival of patients with stage I, II, or III breast cancer. N Engl J Med 342, 525–533.

Braun, S., Schlimok, G., Heumos, I. et al. (2001). ErbB2 overexpression on occult metastatic cells in bone marrow predicts poor clinical outcome of stage I-III breast cancer patients. Cancer Res 61, 1890–1895.

Chambers, A.F., Groom, A.C. and MacDonald, I.C. (2002). Dissemination and growth of cancer cells in metastatic sites. Nat Rev Cancer 2, 563–572.

Cordell, J.L., Falini, B., Erber, W.N. et al. (1984). Immunoenzymatic labeling of monoclonal antibodies using immune complexes of alkaline phosphatase and monoclonal anti-alkaline phosphatase (APAAP complexes). J Histochem Cytochem 32, 219–229.

Cote, R.J., Rosen, P.P., Lesser, M.L., Old, L.J. and Osborne, M.P. (1991). Prediction of early relapse in patients with operable breast cancer by detection of occult bone marrow micrometastases. J Clin Oncol 9, 1749–1756.

Cristofanilli, M., Budd, G.T., Ellis, M.J. et al. (2004). Circulating tumor cells, disease progression, and survival in metastatic breast cancer. N. Engl. J Med 351, 781–791.

de Cremoux, P., Extra, J.M., Denis, M. G. et al. (2000). Detection of MUC1-expressing mammary carcinoma cells in the peripheral blood of breast cancer patients by real-time polymerase chain reaction. Clin Cancer Res 6, 3117–3122.

Diel, I.J., Kaufmann, M., Costa, S.D., Holle, R. et al. (1996). Micrometastatic breast cancer cells in bone marrow at primary surgery: prognostic value in comparison with nodal status. J Natl Cancer Inst 88, 1652–1658.

Fidler, I.J. (1999). Critical determinants of cancer metastasis: rationale for therapy. Cancer Chemother Pharmacol 43 Suppl, S3–10.

Funke, I., Fries, S., Rolle, M. et al. (1996). Comparative analyses of bone marrow micrometastases in breast and gastric cancer. Int J Cancer 65, 755–761.

Funke, I. and Schraut, W. (1998). Meta-analyses of studies on bone marrow micrometastases: an independent prognostic impact remains to be substantiated. J Clin Oncol 16, 557–566.

Goessl, C., Muller, M., Straub, B. and Miller, K. (2002). DNA alterations in body fluids as molecular tumor markers for urological malignancies. Eur Urol 41, 668–676.

Goessl, C. (2003). Diagnostic potential of circulating nucleic acids for oncology. Expert Rev Mol Diagn 3, 431–442.

Goodison, S., Kawai, K., Hihara, J. et al. (2003). Prolonged dormancy and site-specific growth potential of cancer cells spontaneously disseminated from nonmetastatic breast tumors as revealed by labeling with green fluorescent protein. Clin Cancer Res 9, 3808–3814.

Gross, H.J., Verwer, B., Houck, D., Hoffman, R.A. and Recktenwald, D. (1995). Model study detecting breast cancer cells in peripheral blood mononuclear cells at frequencies as low as 10(−7). Proc Natl Acad Sci USA 92, 537–541.

Harbeck, N., Untch, M., Pache, L. and Eiermann, W. (1994). Tumour cell detection in the bone marrow of breast cancer patients at primary therapy: results of a 3-year median follow-up. Br J Cancer 69, 566–571.

Hayashi, N., Ito, I., Yanagisawa, A. et al. (1995). Genetic diagnosis of lymph-node metastasis in colorectal cancer. Lancet 345, 1257–1259.

Huang, P., Wang, J., Guo, Y. and Xie, W. (2003). Molecular detection of disseminated tumor cells in the peripheral blood in patients with gastrointestinal cancer. J Cancer Res Clin Oncol 129, 192–198.

Issa. J.P. (2004). Genes affected by promoter CpG island methylation in aging and/or cancer (online). M.D. Anderson Cancer Center, The University of Texas. Available from: http://www.mdanderson.org/departments/methylation/dIndex.cfm?pn = D02B3250–57D7–4F61–88358636A8073A08 (accessed March 2004).

Izbicki, J.R., Hosch, S.B., Pichlmeier, U. et al. (1997). Prognostic value of immunohistochemically identifiable tumor cells in lymph nodes of patients with completely resected esophageal cancer. N Engl J Med 337, 1188–1194.

Jauch, K.W., Heiss, M.M., Gruetzner, U. et al. (1996). Prognostic significance of bone marrow micrometastases in patients with gastric cancer. J Clin Oncol 14, 1810–1817.

Johnson, P.J. and Lo, Y.M. (2002). Plasma nucleic acids in the diagnosis and management of malignant disease. Clin Chem 48, 1186–1193.

Jung, R., Kruger, W., Hosch, S. et al. (1998). Specificity of reverse transcriptase polymerase chain reaction assays designed for the detection of circulating cancer cells is influenced by cytokines in vivo and in vitro. Br J Cancer 78, 1194–1198.

Kakiuchi, S., Daigo, Y., Tsunoda, T., Yano, S., Sone, S. and Nakamura, Y. (2003). Genome-wide analysis of organ-preferential metastasis of human small cell lung cancer in mice. Mol Cancer Res 1, 485–499.

Kang, Y., Siegel, P.M., Shu, W. et al. (2003). A multigenic program mediating breast cancer metastasis to bone. Cancer Cell 3, 537–549.

Karrison, T.G., Ferguson, D.J. and Meier, P. (1999). Dormancy of mammary carcinoma after mastectomy. J Natl Cancer Inst 91, 80–85.

Kasimir-Bauer, S., Otterbach, F., Oberhoff, C., Schmid, K.W., Kimmig, R. and Seeber, S. (2003). Rare expression of target antigens for immunotherapy on disseminated tumor cells in breast cancer patients without overt metastases. Int J Mol Med 12, 969–975.

Keilholz, U., Weber, J., Finke, J.H. et al. (2002). Immunologic monitoring of cancer vaccine therapy: results of a workshop sponsored by the Society for Biological Therapy. J Immunother 25, 97–138.

Kienle, P., Koch, M., Autschbach, F. et al. (2003). Decreased detection rate of disseminated tumor cells of rectal cancer patients after preoperative chemoradiation: a first step towards a molecular surrogate marker for neoadjuvant treatment in colorectal cancer. Ann Surg 238, 324–330; discussion 330–321.

Klein, C.A., Schmidt-Kittler, O., Schardt, J.A., Pantel, K., Speicher, M.R. and Riethmuller, G. (1999). Comparative genomic hybridization, loss of heterozygosity, and DNA sequence analysis of single cells. Proc Natl Acad Sci USA 96, 4494–4499.

Klein, C.A. (2000). The biology and analysis of single disseminated tumour cells. Trends Cell Biol 10, 489–493.

Kostler, W.J., Brodowicz, T., Hejna, M., Wiltschke, C. and Zielinski, C.C. (2000). Detection of minimal residual disease in patients with cancer: a review of techniques, clinical implications, and emerging therapeutic consequences. Cancer Detect Prev 24, 376–403.

Kraeft, S.K., Sutherland, R., Gravelin, L. et al. (2000). Detection and analysis of cancer cells in blood and bone marrow using a rare event imaging system. Clin Cancer Res 6, 434–442.

Kruger, W.H., Lange, A., Badbaran, A., Gutensohn, K., Kroger, N. and Zander, A.R. (2003). Detection of disseminated epithelial cancer cells by liquid culture – factors interfering with the standardization of assays. Cytotherapy 5, 252–258.

Lacroix, J. and Doeberitz, M.K. (2001). Technical aspects of minimal residual disease detection in carcinoma patients. Semin Surg Oncol 20, 252–264.

Liefers, G.J., Cleton-Jansen, A.M., van de Velde, C.J. et al. (1998). Micrometastases and survival in stage II colorectal cancer. N Engl J Med 339, 223–228.

Lindemann, F., Schlimok, G., Dirschedl, P., Witte, J. and Riethmuller, G. (1992). Prognostic significance of micrometastatic tumour cells in bone marrow of colorectal cancer patients. Lancet 340, 685–689.

Litle, V.R., Warren, R.S., Moore, D., 2nd and Pallavicini, M.G. (1997). Molecular cytogenetic analysis of cytokeratin 20-labeled cells in primary tumors and bone marrow aspirates from colorectal carcinoma patients. Cancer 79, 1664–1670.

Lloyd, K.O. (1993). Tumor antigens known to be immunogenic in man. Ann NY Acad Sci 690, 50–58.

Mansi, J.L., Easton, D. and Berger, U. (1991). Bone marrow micrometastases in primary breast cancer: prognostic significance after 6 years' follow-up. Eur J Cancer 27, 1552–1555.

Mehes, G., Witt, A., Kubista, E. and Ambros, P.F. (2001). Circulating breast cancer cells are frequently apoptotic. Am J Pathol 159, 17–20.

Melchior, S.W., Corey, E., Ellis, W.J. et al. (1997). Early tumor cell dissemination in patients with clinically localized carcinoma of the prostate. Clin Cancer Res 3, 249–256.

Meye, A., Bilkenroth, U., Schmidt, U. et al. (2002). Isolation and enrichment of urologic tumor cells in blood samples by a semi-automated CD45 depletion autoMACS protocol. Int J Oncol 21, 521–530.

Midgley, R. and Kerr, D. (2000). Immunotherapy for colorectal cancer: a challenge to clinical trial design. Lancet Oncol 1, 159–168.

Mueller, P., Carroll, P., Bowers, E. et al. (1998). Low frequency epithelial cells in bone marrow aspirates from prostate carcinoma patients are cytogenetically aberrant. Cancer 83, 538–546.

Muller, P., Weckermann, D., Riethmuller, G. and Schlimok, G. (1996). Detection of genetic alterations in micrometastatic cells in bone marrow of cancer patients by fluorescence in situ hybridization. Cancer Genet Cytogenet *88*, 8–16.

Naume, B., Borgen, E., Nesland, J.M. et al. (1998). Increased sensitivity for detection of micrometastases in bone-marrow/peripheral-blood stem-cell products from breast-cancer patients by negative immunomagnetic separation. Int J Cancer *78*, 556–560.

Noack, F., Schmitt, M., Bauer, J. et al. (2000). A new approach to phenotyping disseminated tumor cells: methodological advances and clinical implications. Int J Biol Markers *15*, 100–104.

Osborne, M.P. and Rosen, P.P. (1994). Detection and management of bone marrow micrometastases in breast cancer. Oncology (Huntingt) *8*, 25–31; discussion 26–35, 39–42.

Pachmann, K., Heiss, P., Demel, U. and Tilz, G. (2001). Detection and quantification of small numbers of circulating tumour cells in peripheral blood using laser scanning cytometer (LSC). Clin Chem Lab Med *39*, 811–817.

Pantel, K. and Ahr, A. (1998). Immunocytochemical and molecular strategies for the detection of micrometastases in patients with solid epithelial tumours: a review. Nucl Med Commun *19*, 521–527.

Pantel, K., Schlimok, G., Kutter, D. et al. (1991). Frequent down-regulation of major histocompatibility class I antigen expression on individual micrometastatic carcinoma cells. Cancer Res *51*, 4712–4715.

Pantel, K., Schlimok, G., Braun, S. et al. (1993a). Differential expression of proliferation-associated molecules in individual micrometastatic carcinoma cells. J Natl Cancer Inst *85*, 1419–1424.

Pantel, K., Braun, S., Schlimok, G. and Riethmuller, G. (1993b). Micrometastatic tumour cells in bone marrow in colorectal cancer. Lancet *341*, 501.

Pantel, K., Schlimok, G., Angstwurm, M. et al. (1994). Methodological analysis of immunocytochemical screening for disseminated epithelial tumor cells in bone marrow. J Hematother *3*, 165–173.

Pantel, K., Aignherr, C., Kollermann, J., Caprano, J., Riethmuller, G. and Kollermann, M.W. (1995a). Immunocytochemical detection of isolated tumour cells in bone marrow of patients with untreated stage C prostatic cancer. Eur J Cancer *31A*, 1627–1632.

Pantel, K., Dickmanns, A., Zippelius, A. et al. (1995b). Establishment of micrometastatic carcinoma cell lines: a novel source of tumor cell vaccines. J Natl Cancer Inst *87*, 1162–1168.

Pantel, K., Izbicki, J., Passlick, B. et al. (1996). Frequency and prognostic significance of isolated tumour cells in bone marrow of patients with non-small-cell lung cancer without overt metastases. Lancet *347*, 649–653.

Pantel, K., Cote, R.J. and Fodstad, O. (1999). Detection and clinical importance of micrometastatic disease. J Natl Cancer Inst *91*, 1113–1124.

Pantel, K. and Otte, M. (2001). Disseminated tumor cells: diagnosis, prognostic relevance, and phenotyping. Recent Results Cancer Res *158*, 14–24.

Pantel, K. and von Knebel Doeberitz, M. (2000). Detection and clinical relevance of micrometastatic cancer cells. Curr Opin Oncol *12*, 95–101.

Poste, G. and Fidler, I.J. (1980). The pathogenesis of cancer metastasis. Nature *283*, 139–146.

Putz, E., Witter, K., Offner, S. et al. (1999). Phenotypic characteristics of cell lines derived from disseminated cancer cells in bone marrow of patients with solid epithelial tumors: establishment of working models for human micrometastases. Cancer Res *59*, 241–248.

Racila, E., Euhus, D., Weiss, A.J. et al. (1998). Detection and characterization of carcinoma cells in the blood. Proc Natl Acad Sci USA *95*, 4589–4594.

Raynor, M., Stephenson, S.A., Walsh, D.C., Pittman, K.B. and Dobrovic, A. (2002). Optimisation of the RT-PCR detection of immunomagnetically enriched carcinoma cells. BMC Cancer *2*, 14.

Ring, A., Smith, I.E. and Dowsett, M. (2004). Circulating tumour cells in breast cancer. Lancet Oncol *5*, 79–88.

Rosenberg, R., Gertler, R., Friederichs, J. et al. (2002). Comparison of two density gradient centrifugation systems for the enrichment of disseminated tumor cells in blood. Cytometry *49*, 150–158.

Rosenberg, R., Friederichs, J., Gertler, R. et al. (2004). Prognostic evaluation and review of immunohistochemically detected disseminated tumor cells in peritumoral lymph nodes of patients with pN0 colorectal cancer. Int J Colorectal Dis.

Ross, A.A., Cooper, B.W., Lazarus, H.M. et al. (1993). Detection and viability of tumor cells in peripheral blood stem cell collections from breast cancer patients using immunocytochemical and clonogenic assay techniques. Blood *82*, 2605–2610.

Schlimok, G., Funke, I., Holzmann, B. et al. (1987). Micrometastatic cancer cells in bone marrow: *in vitro* detection with anti-cytokeratin and *in vivo* labeling with anti-17-1A monoclonal antibodies. Proc Natl Acad Sci USA *84*, 8672–8676.

Schlimok, G., Funke, I., Bock, B., Schweiberer, B., Witte, J. and Riethmuller, G. (1990). Epithelial tumor cells in bone marrow of patients with colorectal cancer: immunocytochemical detection, phenotypic characterization, and prognostic significance. J Clin Oncol *8*, 831–837.

Schlimok, G., Funke, I., Pantel, K. et al. (1991). Micrometastatic tumour cells in bone marrow of patients with gastric cancer: methodological aspects of detection and prognostic significance. Eur J Cancer *27*, 1461–1465.

Schuster, R., Max, N., Mann, B. et al. (2004). Quantitative real-time RT-PCR for detection of disseminated tumor cells in peripheral blood of patients with colorectal cancer using different mRNA markers. Int J Cancer *108*, 219–227.

Silva, J.M., Dominguez, G., Silva, J. et al. (2001). Detection of epithelial messenger RNA in the plasma of breast cancer patients is associated with poor prognosis tumor characteristics. Clin Cancer Res *7*, 2821–2825.

Silva, J.M., Rodriguez, R., Garcia, J.M. et al. (2002a). Detection of epithelial tumour RNA in the plasma of colon cancer patients is associated with advanced stages and circulating tumour cells. Gut *50*, 530–534.

Silva, J.M., Silva, J., Sanchez, A. et al. (2002b). Tumor DNA in plasma at diagnosis of breast cancer patients is a valuable predictor of disease-free survival. Clin Cancer Res *8*, 3761–3766.

Soeth, E., Vogel, I., Roder, C. et al. (1997). Comparative analysis of bone marrow and venous blood isolates from gastrointestinal cancer patients for the detection of disseminated tumor cells using reverse transcription PCR. Cancer Res *57*, 3106–3110.

Solakoglu, O., Maierhofer, C., Lahr, G. et al. (2002). Heterogeneous proliferative potential of occult metastatic cells in bone marrow of patients with solid epithelial tumors. Proc Natl Acad Sci USA 99, 2246–2251.

Tarin, D., Price, J.E., Kettlewell, M.G., Souter, R.G., Vass, A.C. and Crossley, B. (1984). Mechanisms of human tumor metastasis studied in patients with peritoneovenous shunts. Cancer Res 44, 3584–3592.

Thurm, H., Ebel, S., Kentenich, C. et al. (2003). Rare expression of epithelial cell adhesion molecule on residual micrometastatic breast cancer cells after adjuvant chemotherapy. Clin Cancer Res 9, 2598–2604.

Tibbe, A.G., de Grooth, B.G., Greve, J., Liberti, P.A., Dolan, G.J. and Terstappen, L.W. (1999). Optical tracking and detection of immunomagnetically selected and aligned cells. Nat Biotechnol 17, 1210–1213.

Tibbe, A.G., de Grooth, B.G., Greve, J., Dolan, G.J., Rao, C. and Terstappen, L.W. (2002a). Magnetic field design for selecting and aligning immunomagnetic labeled cells. Cytometry 47, 163–172.

Tibbe, A.G., de Grooth, B.G., Greve, J., Dolan, G.J. and Terstappen, L. W. (2002b). Imaging technique implemented in CellTracks system. Cytometry 47, 248–255.

Tortola, S., Steinert, R., Hantschick, M., Peinado, M.A. et al. (2001). Discordance between K-ras mutations in bone marrow micrometastases and the primary tumor in colorectal cancer. J Clin Oncol 19, 2837–2843.

van't Veer, L.J., Dai, H., van de Vijver, M.J. et al. (2002). Gene expression profiling predicts clinical outcome of breast cancer. Nature 415, 530–536.

van't Veer, L.J. and Weigelt, B. (2003). Road map to metastasis. Nat Med 9, 999–1000.

Vlems, F.A., Diepstra, J.H., Cornelissen, I.M. et al. (2003a). Investigations for a multi-marker RT-PCR to improve sensitivity of disseminated tumor cell detection. Anticancer Res 23, 179–186.

Vlems, F.A., Ruers, T.J., Punt, C.J., Wobbes, T. and van Muijen, G. N. (2003b). Relevance of disseminated tumour cells in

blood and bone marrow of patients with solid epithelial tumours in perspective. Eur J Surg Oncol 29, 289–302.

Weber, T., Lacroix, J., Worner, S. et al. (2003). Detection of hematogenic and lymphogenic tumor cell dissemination in patients with medullary thyroid carcinoma by cytokeratin 20 and preprogastrin-releasing peptide RT-PCR. Int J Cancer 103, 126–131.

Wharton, R.Q., Jonas, S.K., Glover, C. et al. (1999). Increased detection of circulating tumor cells in the blood of colorectal carcinoma patients using two reverse transcription-PCR assays and multiple blood samples. Clin Cancer Res 5, 4158–4163.

Widschwendter, M. and Jones, P.A. (2002). DNA methylation and breast carcinogenesis. Oncogene 21, 5462–5482.

Widschwendter, A., Ivarsson, L., Blassnig, A. et al. (2004a). CDH1 and CDH13 methylation in serum is an independent prognostic marker in cervical cancer patients. Int J Cancer 109, 163–166.

Widschwendter, A., Muller, H.M., Fiegl, H. et al. (2004b). DNA methylation in serum and tumors of cervical cancer patients. Clin Cancer Res 10, 565–571.

Woodhouse, E.C., Chuaqui, R.F. and Liotta, L.A. (1997). General mechanisms of metastasis. Cancer 80, 1529–1537.

Wyckoff, J.B., Jones, J.G., Condeelis, J.S. and Segall, J.E. (2000). A critical step in metastasis: in vivo analysis of intravasation at the primary tumor. Cancer Res 60, 2504–2511.

Zehentner, B.K. (2002). Detection of disseminated tumor cells: strategies and diagnostic implications. Expert Rev Mol Diagn 2, 41–48.

Z'graggen, K., Centeno, B.A., Fernandez_del_Castillo, C., Jimenez, R. E., Werner, J. and Warshaw, A. L. (2001). Biological implications of tumor cells in blood and bone marrow of pancreatic cancer patients. Surgery 129, 537–546.

Zippelius, A., Kufer, P., Honold, G. et al. (1997). Limitations of reverse-transcriptase polymerase chain reaction analyses for detection of micrometastatic epithelial cancer cells in bone marrow. J Clin Oncol 15, 2701–2708.

Regulatory T. Cells

Chapter 27

Zoltán Fehérvari and Shimon Sakaguchi

Department of Experimental Pathology, Institute for Frontier Medical Sciences, Kyoto University, Sakyo-ku, Kyoto, Japan

All truth passes through three stages. First, it is ridiculed. Second, it is violently opposed. Third, it is accepted as being self-evident.

Arthur Schopenhauer (1788–1860)

INDUCTION AND MAINTENANCE OF IMMUNOLOGICAL SELF-TOLERANCE

Self-tolerance is defined as a failure to respond to specific autoantigens and its efficient maintenance is essential for the prevention of destructive autoimmunity. Self-tolerance is attained through a number of processes. Initially, autoreactive cells are purged in the thymus during the process of negative selection (Palmer, 2003). This critical component of self-tolerance, referred to as *central tolerance*, is dependent upon the expression of self-antigens within the thymus. Although of unsurpassed importance, central tolerance is not infallible since either not all self-antigens are represented in the thymus, or if they are, then they may be at too low a level to trigger deletion. Either scenario could allow the escape of autoreactive clones from the thymus and there is abundant experimental evidence to suggest that potentially destructive T cells do in fact exist in the periphery of animals and humans. Their presence can be readily demonstrated by the triggering of aggressive autoimmunity following the administration of an autoantigen plus adjuvant e.g. EAE (experimental autoimmune encephalitis) or CIA (collagen-induced arthritis) (Weigle, 1980; Holmdahl, 1998). Despite

the presence of these potentially harmful cells in the periphery, self-tolerance is generally still maintained and individuals remain healthy through the action of *peripheral tolerance* mechanisms (Arnold, 2002).

Peripheral tolerance appears to be maintained by a number of mechanisms, including:

1 immune ignorance
2 peripheral deletion/anergy and
3 active suppression by regulatory T cells.

While all these mechanisms play roles of varying importance, this chapter will focus on regulatory cells in the maintenance of immunological self-tolerance and the control of immune responses in general.

REGULATORY CELLS IN THE MAINTENANCE OF SELF-TOLERANCE

Introduction

The existence of a specific cell type that could control immune responses was first proposed by Gershon and Kondo in 1970 (Gershon and Kondo, 1970). The concept arose from some early observations suggesting that normal self-tolerance could be broken by the elimination of immunocytes and, more specifically, T cells. Nishizuka and Sakakura were able to demonstrate that neonatal thymectomy (especially 2–4 days post-parturition) of normal mice resulted in autoimmune destruction of their

Measuring Immunity, edited by Michael T. Lotze and Angus W. Thomson
ISBN 0-12-455900-X, London

ovaries (Nishizuka and Sakakura, 1969). Subsequent cell depletion studies could elicit autoimmunity (in this case thyroiditis) in adult animals as well, as long as the thymectomy was followed by scheduled doses of sublethal irradiation (Penhale et al., 1973). Collectively, such data appeared to suggest that a cell population playing a crucial role in maintaining self-tolerance was resident within the normal T lymphocyte pool. However, the support for a T-cell-mediated mechanism for maintaining self-tolerance gradually waned for a number of reasons. First, many of the proposed models of regulation became overly complex and the Th1-Th2 paradigm, which emerged in 1989, appeared to more simply subsume most of the observed suppression phenomena (Benacerraf et al., 1982; Dorf and Benacerraf, 1984; Mosmann and Coffman, 1989; Green and Webb, 1993). Second, difficulties in cloning any actual suppressive cells or identifying functionally important molecules associated with them called into question their existence as a discrete cell type (e.g. Green and Webb, 1993). Recent years have, however, witnessed a dramatic revival of interest in regulatory cells following the publication of some key experiments (Powrie and Mason, 1990; Powrie et al., 1993; Sakaguchi et al., 1995; Saoudi et al., 1996; Groux et al., 1997). Subsequent detailed phenotypic evidence now leaves no doubt as to the existence of regulatory T cells as crucial mediators of self-tolerance in both animal models and humans. Broadly speaking, T cells with regulatory properties can be divided into two types: 'naturally occurring' thymically-generated regulatory cells defined here as 'T$_R$ cells', and those generated by antigenic stimulation under special conditions in the periphery; referred to variously as 'Th3', 'Tr1 cells' or 'adaptive regulatory cells' (e.g. Bluestone and Abbas, 2003).

Thymically produced T$_R$ cells

A discrete molecular description of T$_R$ cells has been an important issue in this field and was a major stumbling block to their original exposition. Early demonstrations of the existence of T$_R$ cells relied on the induction of some form of lymphopenia, e.g. by the thymectomy described above or by the use of an immunosuppressive treatment regimen (Sakaguchi et al., 1985, 1994a,b; Sakaguchi and Sakaguchi, 1989). Depending on the strain background, experimental manipulations of this kind result in a variety of autoimmune diseases such as thyroiditis, gastritis, oophoritis and orchitis. It was subsequently shown that induction of such autoimmunity could be prevented by the transfer of normal CD4$^+$ splenocytes or CD4$^+$CD8$^-$ thymocytes (Kojima et al., 1976; Sakaguchi et al., 1982, 1994a; Seddon and Mason, 1999). Collectively, the evidence therefore suggested that T$_R$ cells resided within the T helper subset.

Attempts were then made to more specifically phenotype putative T$_R$ cells by isolating the T lymphocyte subset that harbored regulatory activity. Sakaguchi and

co-workers managed first to identify the CD5 molecule as a marker for T$_R$ cells by demonstrating that otherwise normal lymphocytes depleted of CD5^{high}CD4$^+$ cells induced broad-spectrum autoimmunity when transferred into athymic nude mice (Sakaguchi et al., 1985). Unfractionated CD4$^+$ cells (which contain CD5^{high} expressers) prevented the induction of autoimmunity when co-transferred along with the CD5^{low} cells, implying that the T$_R$ cells were confined specifically to the CD5^{high} compartment. Subsequent experiments aimed at homing-in yet further on T$_R$ cell-specific markers have identified a number of other potential candidate molecules. For instance, CD45RB appears to divide T cells into two distinct functional subsets (Powrie et al., 1993). Lymphopenic mice transferred with CD45RB^{high} cells develop a lethal wasting disease characterized by severe IBD (inflammatory bowel disease), whereas unfractionated T cells or CD45RB^{low} cells alone cause no disease. Importantly, co-transfer of the CD45RB^{low} and CD45RB^{high} populations results in protection of the mice from colitis. Currently, the most useful surface marker for T$_R$ cells has proven to be the IL-2 receptor α-chain, CD25 (Sakaguchi et al., 1995). Approximately 5–10 per cent of CD4$^+$ T cells and less than 1 per cent of CD8$^+$ peripheral T cells constitutively express CD25 in normal naive mice and such cells are found in the CD5^{high} and CD45RB^{low} T cell fractions. Many lines of evidence have now demonstrated the potent regulatory abilities of the constitutive CD25$^+$ T cell subset both in vivo and in vitro (Takahashi and Sakaguchi, 2003).

A comprehensive characterization of the T$_R$ cell surface profile has revealed them to be quite distinct from conventional naive effector T cells. Aside from the constitutive expression of CD25, T$_R$ cells show elevated levels of adhesion molecules such as CD11a (LFA-1), CD44, CD54 (ICAM-1), CD103 ($\alpha_E\beta_7$ integrin) in the absence of any apparent exogenous antigenic stimulation (Itoh et al., 1999; McHugh et al., 2002). Naturally occurring CD25$^+$CD4$^+$ cells additionally express CD152 (CTLA4), a molecule classically only expressed following T cell activation (Read et al., 2000; Salomon et al., 2000; Takahashi et al., 2000). Most recently, several groups have demonstrated that GITR (glucocorticoid-induced tumor necrosis factor family related protein) is predominantly expressed both at the RNA and protein level by CD25$^+$CD4$^+$ cells (Gavin et al., 2002; McHugh et al., 2002; Shimizu et al., 2002). In vivo administration of the anti-GITR mAb, DTA-1, elicits autoimmune disease without actually depleting the T$_R$ cells suggesting that this molecule plays an important functional role in maintaining T$_R$ cell suppression (Shimizu et al., 2002).

The surface marker profile of T$_R$ cells is thus quite different from that of naive T cells. However, it should be noted that most, if not all, of their apparently characteristic molecules are upregulated during conventional T cell activation. This similarity to otherwise normal but primed T cells is potentially problematic when trying to identify/isolate true T$_R$ cells and precludes the use of CD25 alone (or any

Table 27.1 Comparison of the basic constitutive phenotype and biological properties of conventional naive CD4$^+$ T cells and CD25$^+$CD4$^+$ T$_R$ cells

Conventional naive helper T cell	Natural regulatory (T$_R$) cell
CD5^{low}, CD11a^{low}, CD25^{low}, CD38^{low}, CD44^{low}, CD45RB^{high}, CD54^{low}, CD103ε^{low}, GITR^{low}	CD5^{high}, CD11a^{high}, CD25^{high}, CD38^{high}, CD44^{high}, CD45RB^{low}, CD54^{high}, CD103^{high}, GITR^{high}
~90–95% of splenic CD4$^+$ T cells	~5–10% of splenic CD4$^+$ T cells
Responsive to conventional T cell stimuli	Anergic to conventional *in vitro* TCR cell stimuli
Non-suppressive	Suppressive *in vitro* and *in vivo*

other surface molecule found to date) as an infallible marker. With this caveat aside, a number of important distinctions still remain between the surface phenotype of T$_R$ and primed T cells, but they are more relative than absolute. For example, although both primed conventional T cells and T$_R$ cells express CD25, the latter does so to a higher level and more stably. Indeed when stimulation of normal T cells ceases, CD25 expression is lost, whereas T$_R$ cells revert back to their original constitutive expression level (Kuniyasu et al., 2000). In addition, CD25$^+$ cells generated from originally CD25$^-$CD4$^+$ cells show no suppressive ability either *in vitro* or *in vivo* (Kuniyasu et al., 2000). As a component of the high-affinity IL-2R, CD25 itself is essential for the survival of T$_R$ cells and they are exquisitely sensitive to an absence of signaling through this receptor (Almeida et al., 2002). Clear evidence for this can be seen by the almost total absence of CD25$^+$CD4$^+$ cells in IL-2 deficient mice. In conclusion, the similarities between T$_R$ cells and primed T cells are therefore likely only a reflection of a shared activation state.

Foxp3 as a lineage-specific marker for T$_R$ cells

The Scurfy mutant mouse exhibits a fatal X-linked lymphoproliferation characterized by a multi-organ immunopathology very similar to the human disease IPEX (immune dysregulation, polyendocrinopathy, enteropathy, X-linked syndrome) (Lyon et al., 1990; Godfrey et al., 1991; Blair et al., 1994). The gene, *Foxp3* (*FOXP3* in humans), which underlies both syndromes, encodes the forkhead/winged-helix family transcriptional repressor Scurfin (Bennett et al., 2001; Brunkow et al., 2001; Schubert et al., 2001; Wildin et al., 2002). The overt similarities seen between mutations in *Foxp3/FOXP3* and depletion of CD25$^+$CD4$^+$ cells prompted several groups to investigate the relationship of this gene to T$_R$ cell development and function. Experiments demonstrated *Foxp3* mRNA and Scurfin protein to be expressed specifically in CD25$^+$CD4$^+$ T cells and, in contrast to the cell surface markers used to date, was never observed in conventional T cells following activation or differentiation into Th1/Th2 (Fontenot et al., 2003; Hori et al., 2003;

Khattri et al., 2003). Furthermore, Scurfy mutant mice, or those with a targeted deletion of *Foxp3* were unable to support the development of T$_R$ cells, although they contained large numbers of chronically activated CD25$^+$ T cells (Fontenot et al., 2003; Khattri et al., 2003). In contrast, CD25$^+$CD4$^+$ cells increased significantly in number in transgenic mice over-expressing *Foxp3* (Khattri et al., 2003). Critically, retroviral transduction of *Foxp3* into *Foxp3$^-$* conventional CD4$^+$ cells apparently converted them into fully-fledged T$_R$, i.e. they became anergic, expressed the appropriate surface markers and could mediate suppression both *in vitro* and *in vivo* (Fontenot et al., 2003; Hori et al., 2003). These, and subsequent experiments, have also revealed the existence of a small population (1–2 per cent of CD4$^+$ cells) of CD25$^-$CD4$^+$ cells with intermediate levels of *Foxp3* mRNA expression which also exhibited T$_R$-like functions (Hori et al., 2003; M. Ono, manuscript in preparation). The relevance of these CD25$^-$ *Foxp3$^+$* cells to immunohomeostasis and their placement in T$_R$ cell ontogeny remains to be determined, but highlights the existence of regulatory cells outside the more usual CD25$^+$ compartment. Collectively the *Foxp3* data demonstrate it to be not only a seemingly unambiguous marker for naturally occurring T$_R$ cells, whose genetically programmed expression is sufficient to drive their development and function, but also shows T$_R$ cells to be a genuinely distinct lineage rather than simply a specialized activation state of conventional T cells.

More recently, selective *FOXP3* expression has been reported in human T$_R$ cells (Walker et al., 2003; H. Yagi et al., submitted). However, even at these very early stages of analysis some fundamental differences seem to be emerging between the patterns of human and mouse *FOXP3/Foxp3* expression (Walker et al., 2003). For instance *FOXP3* appears to be induced after the activation of normal CD25$^-$ human T cells, which is a behavior never observed in murine cells. If the human T cell data are supported, then it would suggest that normal human CD4$^+$ T cell activation results in a number of lineage decisions with peripheral differentiation potentially into effector cells and/or true regulatory cells. It should however be noted that these are still very early reports and it may be premature to draw any firm conclusions regarding the relative roles of human and murine *FOXP3/Foxp3* and its relationship to T$_R$ cells.

Extra-thymically generated regulatory cells: e.g. Tr1, Th3 and related cells

The previous section concentrated on thymically-produced regulatory cells or T$_R$ cells, but there is also an abundance of evidence for the extra-thymic induction of regulatory CD4$^+$ cells (Chen et al., 1994; Groux et al., 1997; Sato et al., 2003b; Wakkach et al., 2003; Groux, 2003). These cells, commonly termed Tr1 or Th3, can be generated using a variety of approaches, but most of them have in common a requirement for some form of 'suboptimal' signaling to the nascent regulatory cell, e.g. activation in the presence of immunomodulating cytokines or repetitive stimulation with non-professional antigen presenting cells. Tr1 cells were initially generated by chronic stimulation of normal non-regulatory T cells in the presence of immunomodulatory IL-10 (Groux et al., 1997). These cells secrete a pattern of cytokines distinct from that of the more usual Th1/2 profile and are characterized by high levels of IL-10 and generally low levels of TGF-β and IL-5 (Groux et al., 1997). Moreover, Tr1 cells are functionally suppressive *in vivo* and able to prevent the development of Th1 autoimmune diseases such as gastritis (Groux et al., 1997; Groux, 2003).

Another form of peripherally generated regulatory cells are Th3 cells, which can be cloned-out from the mesenteric lymph nodes of mice orally tolerized with MBP (myelin basic protein) (Chen et al., 1994). The majority of such cells produce TGF-β and varying levels of Th2 cytokines and are able to suppress the induction of EAE. *In vitro* treatment with the immunosuppressants vitamin D$_3$ plus dexamethasone has also resulted in the generation of regulatory cells but with properties somewhat distinct from those reported for Tr1 or Th3 cells in that they secreted only detectable amounts of IL-10 and retained a robust proliferative capacity, the latter property being useful for any putative clinical regimen (Barrat et al., 2002). There is also a report suggesting that signaling through the complement receptor, CD46 concomitant to more conventional TCR activation, can trigger the peripheral induction of human CD4$^+$ regulatory cells (Kemper et al., 2003).

Attention has also focused on the influence that DC may have on the extra-thymic development of regulatory cells. Stimulation with both immature (i.e. low levels of costimulatory molecules) and cytokine modified DC (occasionally referred to as 'regulatory DC' or 'tolerogenic DC') have been shown to result in the induction of anergic cells with suppressive capabilities *in vitro* and *in vivo* (Jonuleit et al., 2000; Sato et al., 2003a,b). Under normal conditions, i.e. in the absence of microbial 'danger' signals, DC would assume an immature state and be engaged in the physiological presentation of autologous-peptides to self-reactive T cells. Antigen presentation in such a context could thus be a way of maintaining peripheral tolerance through the systematic generation of regulatory cells (Lutz and Schuler, 2002; Steinman et al., 2003). The qualities of a tolerogenic DC that enable it to generate regulatory cells are only partially understood, but is at least partly related to low costimulatory molecule expression coupled to high MHC class II (Chen et al., 1994, Sato et al., 2003a,b). Novel molecular interactions may also be important, such as Notch-ligand or some, as yet, uncharacterized molecule(s) (Hoyne et al., 2001; Vigouroux et al., 2003). The various characteristics of extra-thymic and thymically produced regulatory cells are summarized in Table 27.2.

Although certainly suppressive in nature, the various forms of extra-thymically generated regulatory T cells are probably fundamentally distinct from thymically produced CD25$^+$CD4$^+$ T$_R$ cells in that the former generally employ cytokines (typically IL-10 or TGF-β) and not contact-dependent mechanisms of suppression. As described above, extra-thymically generated regulatory cells also differ somewhat in their properties according to the means of their production. Evidence of a genuine lineage continuity between Tr1 (or related cells) and thymically

Table 27.2 Comparison of thymically and peripherally produced regulatory cells. Regulatory cells can be divided into two broad types depending principally on the means of their generation: those produced in the thymus (commonly referred to as CD25$^+$CD4$^+$ T$_R$ cells) and those produced extra-thymically or *ex vivo* under specialized conditions (e.g. Tr1, Th3)

	Thymic TR	Extra-thymic regulatory cell (e.g. Tr1, Th3)
Phenotype	CD25, CTLA4, GITR Anergic *Foxp3*$^+$	CD25, CTLA4 Usually anergic *Foxp3*$^+$?
Developmental signal(s)	B7-CD28 interactions (?) CD40-CD40L interactions (?) IL-2 (?) Endogenous TCR-α chain ligation Novel molecules/ mediators (?)	Cytokines (TGF-β, IL-4, IL-10) Vitamin D$_3$- Dexamethasone Immature DC *In vivo* anti-CD4 Vitamin D$_3$/ Dexamethasone Complement receptor ligation (CD46) Oral tolerance induction protocols
Suppression mechanism		
In vitro	Contact dependent	IL-10 and/or TGF-β
In vivo	Contact dependent? IL-4, IL-10, TGF-β	IL-10 and/or TGF-β

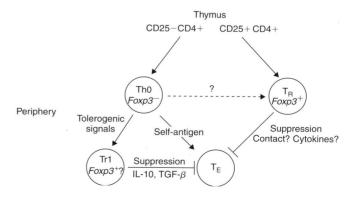

Figure 27.1 T cells emerge from the thymus as either regulatory cells (T$_R$) or conventional naive T cells. The pathological responses of autoreactive effector cells (T$_E$) can be suppressed by the action of both thymically (T$_R$) and peripherally (e.g. Tr1) generated regulatory cells. Most evidence seems to suggest different mechanisms of suppression between the two groups of regulatory cells, furthermore their precise developmental relationships to each other are still not entirely clear.

produced T_R cells is lacking but *Foxp3* expression could be used to address this. It should be emphasized though, that there is yet no clear consensus as to the ontogenic relationship of Tr1 (or related cells) to thymically-produced $CD25^+CD4^+$ T_R cells nor, indeed, whether the former have a natural role in immunohomeostasis. However, these unknowns do not undermine the therapeutic possibilities of extra-thymically generated regulatory cells, as their proven suppressive abilities and the potential to produce large numbers *ex vivo* may represent great hope for the control of immune responses.

MODELLING REGULATORY CELLS

A number of approaches can be used to model the normal suppressive behavior of regulatory cells both *in vitro* and *in vivo*.

In vitro modeling of T_R cells

The suppressive function of T_R cells can be examined by the use of an *in vitro* technique commonly referred to as a 'Treg assay' or 'suppression assay'. The technique is essentially a simple modification of a standard *in vitro* proliferation assay and has been described by a number of different groups (Takahashi et al., 1998; Thornton and Shevach, 1998; Kuniyasu et al., 2000). Purified responder T cells (e.g. normal $CD25^-CD4^+$ cells) are plated out in a round-bottom 96-well format with antigen presenting cells (APC) in the form of bulk splenocytes or purified

B cells, plus a TCR stimulus such as anti-CD3. The $CD25^-$ responder cells are then mixed with titrated doses of highly purified $CD25^+CD4^+$ T_R cells, typically in a $CD25^-$:$CD25^+$ ratio ranging from 1:1 to 1:0.125. The effects of the $CD25^+CD4^+$ T_R cells on the proliferation and/or IL-2 production of the responder $CD25^-$ T cells can then be ascertained. A basic summary of the technique is shown in Figure 27.2A.

The functional response (e.g. proliferation or cytokine production) by the $CD25^-$ cells is effectively inhibited by the presence of T_R cells in a dose-dependent manner, but the suppressive effects are often negligible when 25^-:25^+ ratios of >10:1 are used (Kuniyasu et al., 2000). The technique can be further altered by changing the T cell stimulus from anti-CD3 to an allogeneic response using MHC disparate APCs or, in the case of TCR-transgenic T cells, by the addition of specific peptide (Takahashi et al., 1998; Thornton and Shevach, 1998). Under normal activation conditions, e.g. splenic APC plus anti-CD3, the T_R cells themselves are anergic, showing little or no proliferation and undetectable IL-2 production, which conveniently allows analysis of the $CD25^-$ response in effective isolation (Takahashi et al., 1998; Thornton and Shevach, 1998). This T_R cell *in vitro* anergy and, indeed, their ability to suppress, can be broken by a sufficiently strong stimulus such as the addition of either anti-CD28, high doses of exogenous IL-2, or by using professional APCs in the form of DC (Thornton and Shevach, 1998; Takahashi et al., 1998; Yamazaki et al., 2003; Fehervari and Sakaguchi, submitted). On withdrawal of such stimuli, T_R cells revert once more to their anergic and suppressive status (Kuniyasu

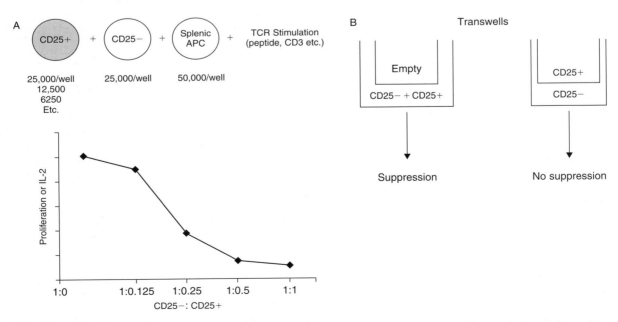

Figure 27.2 *In vitro* modeling of regulatory cells. (A) The suppressive function of T_R cells can be demonstrated by mixing titrated doses of T_R cells, responder $CD25^-$ cells, APC and a TCR stimulus. The functional response (IL-2 production or proliferation) is inhibited in a T_R cell dose-dependent manner. (B) The role of soluble suppressive factors can be assessed by the use of Transwells which separate the $CD25^-$ and $CD25^+$ fractions by a semi-permeable membrane. Such analysis demonstrates the importance of contact for T_R cell-mediated suppression.

et al., 2000). Anergy (at least *in vitro*) therefore appears to be a fundamental property of T_R cells, which is closely entwined with their suppressive functions.

The regulatory mechanisms of T_R cells *in vitro* can also be examined by using a Transwell system (Figure 27.2B). Under these conditions it is possible to separate the $CD25^-$ and $CD25^+$ cells by a semi-permeable membrane, which prevents cell–cell contact but allows the transmission of potentially suppressive cytokines making an assessment of the role of humoral factors possible (Figure 27.2B). Along with the use of neutralizing antibodies (anti-IL-10 and anti-TGF-β), such analyses have been instrumental in demonstrating T_R cell suppression to be mediated exclusively by cell–cell contact (Takahashi et al., 1998; Thornton and Shevach, 1998, 2000).

In summary then, a number of important parameters of T_R cell behavior have been revealed by *in vitro* studies:

1 T_R cells are anergic *in vitro* and this property is related to their suppressive functions. Anergy and suppression can be broken by sufficiently strong TCR stimuli such as the addition of costimulation, IL-2, or by using professional APC such as DC.
2 T_R cell suppression is dependent on close cell–cell contact, therefore suppression is more pronounced when using round-bottom plates.
3 Activation of T_R cell suppressive functions requires TCR stimulation but without a breakage of their anergy and once activated suppression is antigen-independent.
4 T_R cell suppression acts in an APC-independent manner.

In vivo modeling of T_R cells

Evidence for the existence of T_R cells first came to light through various *in vivo* methodologies and some were briefly described in the previous sections. All such *in vivo* approaches share some means of selectively eliminating T_R cells or abrogating their suppressive function (Table 27.3) (Fowell and Mason, 1993; Sakaguchi et al., 1994a,b; Barrett et al., 1995; Asano et al., 1996; Tung et al., 1998; Toh et al., 2000).

Many of the experimental methods of inducing autoimmunity described in Table 27.3 can be readily interpreted by invoking the involvement of T_R cells. For instance, the various approaches involving neonatal thymectomy could be inducing autoimmunity by removing the thymus prior to its export of self-tolerogenic T_R cells, which emerge from the thymus at a stage slightly later than autoreactive T cells. The use of immunosuppressive treatments such as cyclophosphamide, cyclosporin or irradiation may also act by specifically targeting T_R cells in the periphery (Sakaguchi and Sakaguchi, 1989; Sakaguchi et al., 1994a, 1995, Barrett et al., 1995). This specific targeting seems likely since, in contrast to their *in vitro* behavior, T_R cells show active proliferation in the periphery which would render them sensitive to an immunosuppressive treatment such as cyclophosphamide (Almeida et al., 2002; Walker et al., 2003; Yamazaki et al., 2003). When coupled to thymectomy, immunosuppression is thus a very effective method of triggering autoimmunity since it not only targets any peripheral T_R cells but also prevents their

Table 27.3 The importance of T_R cells for the maintenance of immunological self-tolerance and the control of autoimmunity can be demonstrated by a variety of manipulations *in vivo*. Such approaches operate by either eliminating/reducing T_R cell numbers or perturbing their function

Procedure	Mouse or rat strain	Autoimmune disease(s) induced (% incidence)	Reference(s)
Neonatal Tx	BALB/c A SWR NFS/sld	Gast. (40%), Ooph. (80%), Thy. (20%), Orch. (50%), Ooph. (40%), Gast. (30%) Sial. (70%)	(Nishizuka and Sakakura, 1969; Asano et al., 1996; Tung et al., 1998; Toh et al., 2000)
Anti-CD25, -IL-2, CTLA-4, -GITR treatment	BALB/c	Gast.(100%)	(Read et al., 2000; Takahashi et al., 2000; Shimizu et al., 2002)
Neonatal CsA treatment	BALB/c	Gast.(30%)	(Sakaguchi and Sakaguchi, 1989)
Adult Tx and cyclophosphamide treatment	BALB/c	Gast.(50%)	(Barrett et al., 1995)
Total lymphoid irradiation	BALB/c	Gast.(90%)	(Sakaguchi et al., 1994a)
Neonatal MTLV infection	BALB/c	Gast.(30%)	(Sakaguchi et al., 1994a)
Transgenic TCR-α chain transgenic mice	BALB/c A SWR	Gast. (60%) Ooph. (80%), Gast. (30%), Thy. (20%) Orch. (50%), Ooph. (40%), Gast. (40%)	(Sakaguchi et al., 1994b)
Tx followed by fractionated irradiation	PVG/c PVG-R1^U	Thy. (80%), T1D(10–50%) Thy. (70%) T1D(100%)	(Fowell and Mason, 1993)

CsA, cyclosporin A; Gast., gastritis; Ooph., oophoritis; Thy., thyroiditis; Sial., sialodentitis; Orch., orchitis; T1D, type-1 diabetes; MTLV, mouse T lymphotropic virus; Tx, thymectomy.

renewal from the thymus. Using such a combination approach, autoimmunity can be induced even in adult (6–8 weeks) mice (Barrett et al., 1995).

The *in vivo* administration of antibodies to the T_R cell-associated molecules CD25, CTLA4, or GITR induces autoimmune gastritis in otherwise normal mice or accelerates diabetes in autoimmune-prone NOD mice (Read et al., 2000; Salomon et al., 2000; Takahashi et al., 2000; McHugh et al., 2002; Shimizu et al., 2002). Interestingly, in the case of GITR, the antibodies do not seem to act by simple depletion of T_R cells, rather they appear to transmit an agonistic signal responsible for inactivating suppressive functions (Shimizu et al., 2002).

An effective method for inducing a variety of autoimmune diseases and demonstrating the importance of CD25$^+$CD4$^+$ cells is described in Figure 27.3 (Sakaguchi et al., 1995). This approach involves depleting CD25$^+$ cells from the splenocytes of normal mice and adoptively transferring them into nude mice (T cell deficient) recipients. Depending on the cell dose, multiple autoimmune pathologies were seen to develop from 3 months post-transfer. Importantly, co-transfer with relatively small numbers of unfractionated splenocytes (which contain T_R cells) or purified CD25$^+$CD4$^+$ T_R cells very efficiently prevented disease manifestation (Sakaguchi et al., 1995).

REGULATORY CELL FUNCTIONAL MECHANISMS

The suppression mechanism of activation-induced regulatory cells such as Tr1 cells, is primarily based on the secretion of anti-inflammatory cytokines such as IL-10 and TGF-β (Groux, 2003). However, the story with naturally occurring T_R cells is not nearly so clear-cut and despite

intense interest the answer remains largely equivocal. The *in vitro* characteristics of T_R cell-suppression were briefly described above but this section will go into more detail with what is currently known about this area.

Potential T_R cell suppression mechanisms can be basically divided into those mediated by secreted factors or those requiring intimate cell–cell contact. Most of the *in vivo* experiments examining T_R cell suppression have been based on the murine IBD model described above and have, as with Tr1 cells, highlighted the importance of IL-10 and TGF-β. By blocking IL-10 signaling *in vivo* with anti-IL-10 receptor monoclonal antibodies (mAb), Asseman and co-workers were able to abrogate the normal IBD-preventative action of CD45RB^{low} T cells (Asseman et al., 1999). The same group were also able to show that CD45RB^{low} T cells from IL-10-deficient mice were unable to prevent colitis and, moreover, were even colitogenic themselves (Asseman et al., 1999). The importance of IL-10 in the control of IBD is also implied by the observation that IL-10-/- mice spontaneously develop IBD even though these mice are not lymphopenic (Berg et al., 1996).

Similarly, several groups have shown that a mAb-mediated blockade of TGF-β abrogated T_R cell suppressive functions both *in vivo* and *in vitro* (Powrie et al., 1996; Nakamura et al., 2001). Interestingly, TGF-β may not necessarily have to act as a soluble factor but can be expressed exclusively on the surface of CD25$^+$CD4$^+$ cells following TCR stimulation and therefore may mediate its effects in a membrane proximal manner (Nakamura et al., 2001). It should be cautioned, however, that the importance of cell-surface TGF-β was not corroborated by another group and thus still remains somewhat controversial (Piccirillo et al., 2002). The level at which these anti-inflammatory cytokines operate to maintain tolerance

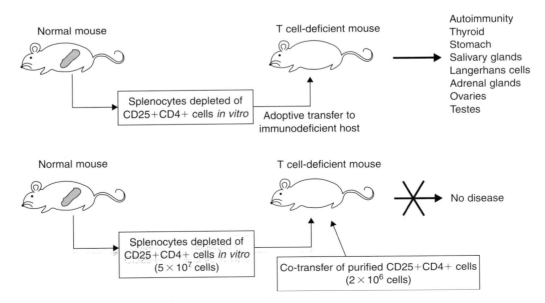

Figure 27.3 Induction of autoimmune diseases in T cell-deficient mice by transferring CD4$^+$ splenocyte suspensions depleted of CD25$^+$ cells to T cell deficient mice. Co-transfer of purified CD25$^+$CD4$^+$ T cells prevents the induction of autoimmunity.

is also uncertain, but it may be via inhibition of APC/pathogenic T cells, maintenance of the T_R cell population and/or enhancement of their function (Takahashi and Sakaguchi, 2003).

Elucidation of the mechanism of T_R cell suppression is complicated by the fact that the bulk of *in vitro* evidence shifts the emphasis of suppression to solely cell contact-based mechanisms. First, anti-IL-10 or anti-TGF-β mAb fail to perturb the suppressive activity of CD25$^+$CD4$^+$ cells *in vitro* (Takahashi and Sakaguchi, 2003), although use of soluble IL-10R appears to have a partial effect (Zhang et al., 2001). A study showing successful neutralization of suppression using anti-TGF-β mAb at the same time also demonstrated the TGF-β to be cell-surface bound (Nakamura et al., 2001). Secondly, culture supernatants from activated CD25$^+$CD4$^+$ cells show no inherent suppressive ability nor is any suppression observed across a semi-permeable membrane (Takahashi et al., 1998; Thornton and Shevach, 1998). Collectively the *in vitro* data thus appear to obviate the role of not just IL-10/TGF-β but also soluble factors in general, suggesting that T_R cell suppression is dependent on close cell–cell contact, although it is still not possible to discount completely suppression mediated in an extreme paracrine fashion. The membrane events that occur during cell contact-dependent suppression are entirely unclear, but presumably an, as yet uncharacterized, inhibitory molecule is expressed on the surface of activated T_R cells. Another mechanism of cell contact-mediated suppression could proceed via simple competition for APC and specific MHC-peptide antigenic complexes. The high level of adhesion molecules and chemokine receptors present on the surface of T_R cells would make them particularly well suited at homing to and stably interacting with APCs and therein physically exclude normal CD25$^-$CD4$^+$ effector cells. Furthermore, the constitutive expression of the high-affinity IL-2 receptor would make T_R cells into an effective sink for IL-2, depriving potential autoreactive cells of this essential growth factor. A final, conceptually attractive model of suppression would

be T_R cell-mediated inhibition/alteration of APC function. Supporting this model is the observation that CD25$^+$CD4$^+$ cells could alter the antigen-presenting function of DC by downregulating their expression levels of CD80/86 (Cederbom et al., 2000) or, as has been recently demonstrated, by triggering the immunosuppressive catabolism of tryptophan by DC (Fallarino et al., 2003). While APC perturbation may well occur *in vivo*, it is not essential since T_R cells are able to suppress effectively even in the absence of any APCs, such as occurs during stimulation with MHC-peptide tetramers (Piccirillo and Shevach, 2001). Potential suppressive mechanisms of T_R cells are depicted in Figure 27.4.

ROLE OF T_R CELLS IN IMMUNOLOGICAL PROCESSES OTHER THAN THE MAINTENANCE OF SELF-TOLERANCE

As described above, there is an abundance of experimental evidence demonstrating the role of T_R cells in the control of self-tolerance. The potent immunomodulatory properties of these cells could, however, impact on a number of other clinically important areas such as tumor immunity, transplantation biology and infectious diseases.

T_R cells and tumor immunity

It is now clear that many tumor-associated antigens recognized by autologous T cells are normal self-constituents and thus presumably within the remit of control by T_R cells. In such a way the desirable elimination of tumors by cytotoxic effector T cells may be impeded by the action of T_R cells and evidence is accumulating that this does in fact appear to be the case (Sakaguchi, 2000; Takahashi and Sakaguchi, 2003). Experiments suggest that the simple elimination of T_R cells from splenocyte preparations by treatment with anti-CD25 mAbs results in productive responses to syngeneic tumors when

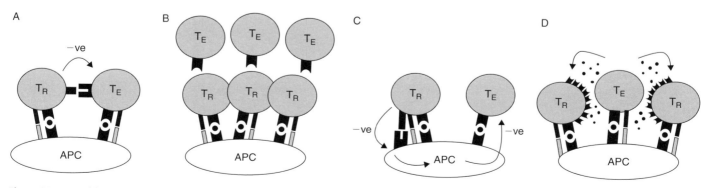

Figure 27.4 Possible mechanisms of T_R cell suppression. These mechanisms are not necessarily mutually exclusive and potentially two or more may act in concert. (A) APC activated T_R cells transduce an unidentified *active* negative signal to nearby effector T (T_E) cells located on the same or adjacent APC. (B) T_R cells out-compete T_E cells for stimulatory ligands on the APC surface by virtue of their high expression of adhesion molecules. (C) T_R cells modulate the behavior of the APC so that they become ineffective or suppressive stimulators of T_E cells. (D) CD25 expression by the T_R cells acts as an IL-2 sink and hinders autocrine/paracrine stimulation of T_E cells.

transferred to lymphopenic recipients (Onizuka et al., 1999; Shimizu et al., 1999; Sutmuller et al., 2001). Similarly beneficial effects are seen with the *in vivo* administration of antibodies and it appears this result is attributable to a reduction of CD25⁺CD4⁺ T_R cell numbers and a subsequent enhancement of cytolytic T cell responses (Onizuka et al., 1999; Shimizu et al., 1999). One potential side effect of such treatment is the possible induction of autoimmunity. The costs and benefits of such an outcome need to be weighed carefully if such a treatment is to ever be implemented clinically.

T_R cells and organ transplantation

The ultimate goal for organ transplantation would be to establish tolerance to the foreign graft as effectively as that to self-tissues, but without the need for generalized immunosuppression (Cobbold and Waldmann, 1998; Zhai and Kupiec-Weglinski, 1999; Wood and Sakaguchi, 2003). One way in which this could be realized is through the exploitation of T_R cells. BALB/c nude mice transplanted with B6 skin and subsequently reconstituted with normal BALB/c T cells show robust graft rejection, which is accelerated by the removal of CD25⁺ cells from the reconstituting T cell population (Sakaguchi et al., 1995). This finding suggests that the small population (5–10 per cent) of T_R cells resident in the BALB/c T cell transfer is able to retard somewhat the normal allogeneic response and therefore increasing the numbers (or function) of transferred T_R cells may engender a permanent state of allograft survival. This does indeed appear to be the case, since the transfer of highly purified CD25⁺CD4⁺ cells to nude recipients, either prior or simultaneous to reconstitution with naïve T cells, significantly prolongs graft survival (Figure 27.6A) (Sakaguchi et al., 2001). Furthermore, permanent allograft survival may be established by the transfer of large doses of T_R cells. The scarcity of T_R cells means that obtaining large numbers (as would be required for clinical applications) is highly problematic.

However, it is possible to expand *in vitro*, purified CD25⁺ T_R cells on donor-specific splenocytes (plus IL-2 to break T_R cell *in vitro* anergy) prior to *in vivo* transfer (Figure 27.6B) (Sakaguchi et al., 2001; Trenado et al., 2003; Nishimura et al., submitted). As well as generating large numbers of T_R cells facilitating *in vivo* use, such expansion can have the additional advantage of selectively expanding the donor-responsive cells and hence improving the suppressive outcome (Sakaguchi et al., 2001; Trenado et al., 2003).

A large number of studies have also been able to induce prolonged graft survival by the administration of mAbs to various T cell- and APC-associated molecules such as CD4, CD8, CD40, CD40L, CD80 and CD86 (Waldmann and Cobbold, 1998; Hara et al., 2001; Taylor et al., 2001; Graca et al., 2002; Takahashi and Sakaguchi, 2003). Many such studies employing mAbs implicate the role of regulatory cells in maintaining graft tolerance, although it is generally unclear whether the mAbs act by inducing T_R cells *de novo* or by enhancement of their function. One way such mAb-induced tolerance to allografts could operate is by restraining the destructive action of effector T cells which would allow time for the expansion of alloreactive and protective T_R cells on the graft *in situ*. Such a scenario is therefore an *in vivo* analogy to that summarized in Figure 27.6B. Bone marrow transplantation for the treatment of hematological malignancies presents particular clinical problems. Such treatments must carefully balance the immunosuppression of potentially lethal graft versus host disease (GVHD), yet permit a robust and beneficial graft versus tumor (GVT) response. T_R cells have also been shown to be potentially effective in such a setting. Initially, studies demonstrated that the transfer of donor-type CD25⁺CD4⁺ T_R cells with bone marrow precursor cells could markedly protect from lethal GVHD and this effect was dependent in part on IL-10 production (Hoffmann et al., 2002). In subsequent related studies, it was shown that T_R cells were able not only to protect from GVHD following bone marrow transplantation, but also

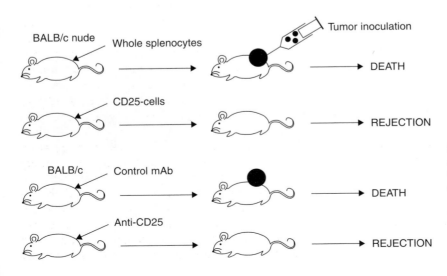

Figure 27.5 Induction of tumor immunity by manipulation of T_R cells. BALB/c nude mice reconstituted with BALB/c T cells depleted of CD25⁺ cells reject otherwise fatal inoculated tumor cells. In contrast, mice reconstituted with whole spleen cells (which contain CD25⁺ cells) show no tumor rejection due to immunosuppression mediated by the T_R cells. Effective tumor immunity can also be elicited *in vivo* by elimination of resident CD25⁺ cells with anti-CD25 mAb.

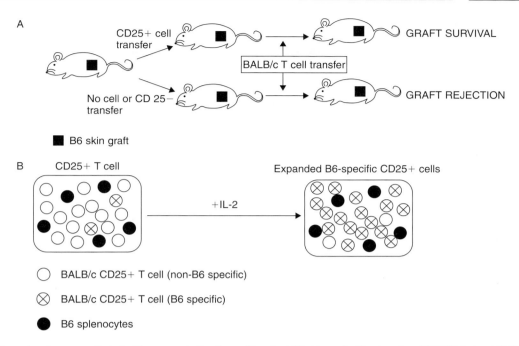

Figure 27.6 (A) BALB/c nude mice reconstituted with syngeneic T cells readily reject B6 skin grafts. The transfer of CD25$^+$ but not CD25$^-$ T cells can suppress the activation of graft specific cells and prevent rejection. (B) The number of graft (B6) specific 25$^+$ T$_R$ cells can be expanded *in vitro* prior to transfer. Only a subset of a normal BALB/c T$_R$ cell population contains B6-specific cells, however, their numbers can be expanded *in vitro* by mixing purified CD25$^+$CD4$^+$ cells with donor-specific splenocytes plus IL-2 to support T$_R$ cell expansion.

retain strong enough immunity for an effective GVT response (Edinger et al., 2003; Trenado et al., 2003). Similarly encouraging results for the facilitation/suppression of GVT/GVHD, have been achieved with the transfer of the tolerogenic DC described above (Sato et al., 2003b). These DC appear to act by the *in vivo* generation of regulatory cells, whose precise identity is as yet unclear. T$_R$ cells thus appear to offer the flexibility of function and potency required for bone marrow transplantation, by balancing the conflicting requirements of immunosuppression and immunopermissiveness.

T$_R$ cells and microbial immunity

T$_R$ cells also seem to play an important role in the suppression of excessive immune responses to pathogens or inappropriate responses to commensal/mutualistic microbes. It is well known for example, that SCID mice transferred with CD25$^-$CD45RB^{hi}CD4$^+$ cells develop IBD, whereas similarly treated mice lacking intestinal microbes under germ-free conditions show no such immunopathology (Singh et al., 2001). The sensitivity of the gut in general to perturbation of T$_R$ cell number or function hints at the fundamental involvement of these cells in the control of immune responses to otherwise harmless symbiotes. The finding that T$_R$ cells express toll-like receptors and their functions are affected by a 'dangerous environment', is further evidence for their direct involvement with microbes, whether harmful or beneficial (Yamazaki et al., 2003; Pasare and Medzhitov, 2003; Caramalho et al., 2003; Fehervari and Sakaguchi, submitted).

T$_R$ cells also have a role to play in infectious diseases by blunting overactive and damaging immune responses to pathogens. Evidence for this comes from the rapid and fatal pulmonary inflammation seen following CD25$^+$CD4$^+$ T$_R$ cell depletion during chronic infection with *Pneumocystis carinii* (Hori et al., 2002). In this model, the immunopathology was mediated by CD25$^-$CD4$^+$ effector T cells and their damage could be prevented by the presence of CD25$^+$CD4$^+$ T$_R$ cells. Another study has examined the role of T$_R$ cells during chronic infection with *Leishmania major* (Belkaid et al., 2002). This model suggested that the long-term persistence of *L. major* is maintained through the action of T$_R$ cells and the removal of CD25$^+$CD4$^+$ cells resulted in complete elimination of the parasite. Interestingly, eradication of the microbe in this way prevented immunity to subsequent re-infection and so demonstrated the importance of T$_R$ cells for the support of long-term immunological memory. The perseverance of immunological memory has been long suspected to be mediated by the presence of a small 'antigen depot' and the action of T$_R$ cells thus provides a hitherto unappreciated mechanism by which this could occur. As with many such host–parasite interactions, it is often difficult to disentangle which party benefits from a particular immune response; i.e. is dampening down immunity beneficial to the host through the prevention of immunopathology or is the parasite 'co-opting' the T$_R$ cells to ensure its survival/transmission? More data implicating the roles of T$_R$ cells in microbial immune responses will surely come to light over the coming years and will serve to deepen our understanding of the evolutionary arms race which has shaped our immune systems over the millennia.

FUTURE PERSPECTIVES AND THE POTENTIAL CLINICAL APPLICATIONS OF REGULATORY CELLS

Abundant evidence now strongly supports the once controversial existence of T_R cells as key controllers of self-tolerance. It also now seems that their roles can be expanded to many areas of immunology, in fact potentially to any scenario where the suppression and/or tuning of an immune response is required. A strategic manipulation of T_R cells to either dampen or enhance their functions, e.g. in tumor or transplantation immunity respectively, may prove to have great clinical benefit. As evidenced by bone marrow transplantation, T_R cells also seem to offer a flexible and adaptive form of immunological control apparently not achievable with standard small molecule immunosuppression.

Recent advances in our understanding of T_R cell development and important functional markers such as the association with *Foxp3/FOXP3* has permitted the accurate isolation and manipulation of these cells in ways previously not possible. Furthermore, understanding the events both upstream and downstream of *Foxp3/FOXP3* may enable us to 'tailor-make' large numbers of T_R cells for the specific suppression of immune responses in autoimmunity and allergy. The potential clinical focus though need not just be on thymically produced T_R cells since peripherally generated regulatory cells (e.g. Tr1), with their potent immunomodulatory capacity, may also hold great therapeutic promise. An identification of the molecular triggers of T_R and Tr1 cell development and/or stimulation will be key to any potential exploitation of these potentially powerful immunological allies.

ACKNOWLEDGEMENTS

The authors would like to thank all their colleagues at Kyoto University for years of engaging discussion and the permission to cite pre-publication work.

REFERENCES

Almeida, A.R., Legrand, N., Papiernik, M. and Freitas, A.A. (2002). Homeostasis of peripheral CD4+ T cells: IL-2R alpha and IL-2 shape a population of regulatory cells that controls CD4+ T cell numbers. J Immunol 169, 4850–4860.

Arnold, B. (2002). Levels of peripheral T cell tolerance. Transpl Immunol 10, 109–114.

Asano, M., Toda, M., Sakaguchi, N. and Sakaguchi, S. (1996). Autoimmune disease as a consequence of developmental abnormality of a T cell subpopulation. J Exp Med 184, 387–396.

Asseman, C., Mauze, S., Leach, M.W., Coffman, R.L. and Powrie, F. (1999). An essential role for interleukin 10 in the function of regulatory T cells that inhibit intestinal inflammation. J Exp Med 190, 995–1004.

Barrat, F.J., Cua, D.J., Boonstra, A. et al. (2002). *In vitro* generation of interleukin 10-producing regulatory CD4(+) T cells is induced by immunosuppressive drugs and inhibited by T helper type 1 (Th1)- and Th2-inducing cytokines. J Exp Med 195, 603–616.

Barrett, S.P., Toh, B.H., Alderuccio, F., van Driel, I.R. and Gleeson, P.A. (1995). Organ-specific autoimmunity induced by adult thymectomy and cyclophosphamide-induced lymphopenia. Eur J Immunol 25, 238–244.

Belkaid, Y., Piccirillo, C.A., Mendez, S., Shevach, E.M. and Sacks, D.L. (2002). CD4+ CD25+ regulatory T cells control Leishmania major persistence and immunity. Nature 420, 502–507.

Benacerraf, B., Greene, M.I., Sy, M.S. and Dorf, M.E. (1982). Suppressor T cell circuits. Ann NY Acad Sci 392, 300–308.

Bennett, C.L., Christie, J., Ramsdell, F. et al. (2001). The immune dysregulation, polyendocrinopathy, enteropathy, X-linked syndrome (IPEX) is caused by mutations of FOXP3. Nat Genet 27, 20–21.

Berg, D.J., Davidson, N., Kuhn, R. et al. (1996). Enterocolitis and colon cancer in interleukin-10-deficient mice are associated with aberrant cytokine production and CD4(+) TH1-like responses. J Clin Invest 98, 1010–1020.

Blair, P.J., Bultman, S.J., Haas, J.C., Rouse, B.T., Wilkinson, J.E. and Godfrey, V.L. (1994). CD4+ CD8− T cells are the effector cells in disease pathogenesis in the scurfy (sf) mouse. J Immunol 153, 3764–3774.

Bluestone, J.A. and Abbas, A.K. (2003). Natural versus adaptive regulatory T cells. Nat Rev Immunol 3, 253–257.

Brunkow, M.E., Jeffery, E.W., Hjerrild, K.A. et al. (2001). Disruption of a new forkhead/winged-helix protein, scurfin, results in the fatal lymphoproliferative disorder of the scurfy mouse. Nat Genet 27, 68–73.

Caramalho, I., Lopes-Carvalho, T., Ostler, D., Zelenay, S., Haury, M. and Demengeot, J. (2003). Regulatory T cells selectively express toll-like receptors and are activated by lipopolysaccharide. J Exp Med 197, 403–411.

Cederbom, L., Hall, H. and Ivars, F. (2000). CD4+ CD25+ regulatory T cells down-regulate co-stimulatory molecules on antigen-presenting cells. Eur J Immunol 30, 1538–1543.

Chen, Y., Kuchroo, V.K., Inobe, J., Hafler, D.A. and Weiner, H.L. (1994). Regulatory T cell clones induced by oral tolerance: suppression of autoimmune encephalomyelitis. Science 265, 1237–1240.

Cobbold, S. and Waldmann, H. (1998). Infectious tolerance. Curr Opin Immunol 10, 518–524.

Dorf, M.E. and Benacerraf, B. (1984) Suppressor cells and immunoregulation. Annu Rev Immunol, 2, 127–157.

Edinger, M., Hoffmann, P., Ermann, J. et al. (2003). CD4+ CD25+ regulatory T cells preserve graft-versus-tumor activity while inhibiting graft-versus-host disease after bone marrow transplantation. Nat Med 9, 1144–1150.

Fallarino, F., Grohmann, U., Hwang, K.W. et al. (2003). Modulation of tryptophan catabolism by regulatory T cells. Nat Immunol 4, 1206–1212.

Fontenot, J.D., Gavin, M.A. and Rudensky, A.Y. (2003). Foxp3 programs the development and function of CD4+ CD25+ regulatory T cells. Nat Immunol 4, 330–336.

Fowell, D. and Mason, D. (1993). Evidence that the T cell repertoire of normal rats contains cells with the potential to cause diabetes. Characterization of the CD4+ T cell subset that inhibits this autoimmune potential. J Exp Med 177, 627–636.

Gavin, M.A., Clarke, S.R., Negrou, E., Gallegos, A. and Rudensky, A. (2002). Homeostasis and anergy of CD4(+)CD25(+) suppressor T cells in vivo. Nat Immunol 3, 33–41.

Gershon, R. K. and Kondo, K. (1970). Cell interactions in the induction of tolerance: the role of thymic lymphocytes. Immunology 18, 723–737.

Godfrey, V.L., Wilkinson, J.E., Rinchik, E.M. and Russell, L.B. (1991). Fatal lymphoreticular disease in the scurfy (sf) mouse requires T cells that mature in a sf thymic environment: potential model for thymic education. Proc Natl Acad Sci USA 88, 5528–5532.

Graca, L., Cobbold, S.P. and Waldmann, H. (2002). Identification of regulatory T cells in tolerated allografts. J Exp Med 195, 1641–1646.

Green, D.R. and Webb, D.R. (1993). Saying the 'S' word in public. Immunol Today 14, 523–525.

Groux, H. (2003). IL-10 is required for regulatory T cells to mediate tolerance to alloantigens in vivo. Transplantation 75, 8S–12S.

Groux, H., O'Garra, A., Bigler, M. et al. (1997). A CD4+ T-cell subset inhibits antigen-specific T-cell responses and prevents colitis. Nature 389, 737–742.

Hara, M., Kingsley, C.I., Niimi, M. et al. (2001). IL-10 is required for regulatory T cells to mediate tolerance to alloantigens in vivo. J Immunol 166, 3789–3796.

Hoffmann, P., Ermann, J., Edinger, M., Fathman, C.G. and Strober, S. (2002). Donor-type CD4(+)CD25(+) regulatory T cells suppress lethal acute graft-versus-host disease after allogeneic bone marrow transplantation. J Exp Med 196, 389–399.

Holmdahl, R. (1998). Genetics of susceptibility to chronic experimental encephalomyelitis and arthritis. Curr Opin Immunol 10, 710–717.

Hori, S., Carvalho, T.L. and Demengeot, J. (2002). CD25+ CD4+ regulatory T cells suppress CD4+ T cell-mediated pulmonary hyperinflammation driven by Pneumocystis carinii in immunodeficient mice. Eur J Immunol 32, 1282–1291.

Hori, S., Nomura, T. and Sakaguchi, S. (2003). Control of regulatory T cell development by the transcription factor Foxp3. Science 299, 1057–1061.

Hoyne, G.F., Dallman, M.J., Champion, B.R. and Lamb, J.R. (2001). Notch signalling in the regulation of peripheral immunity. Immunol Rev 182, 215–227.

Itoh, M., Takahashi, T., Sakaguchi, N. et al. (1999). Thymus and autoimmunity: production of CD25+ CD4+ naturally anergic and suppressive T cells as a key function of the thymus in maintaining immunologic self-tolerance. J Immunol 162, 5317–5326.

Jonuleit, H., Schmitt, E., Schuler, G., Knop, J. and Enk, A.H. (2000). Induction of interleukin 10-producing, nonproliferating CD4(+) T cells with regulatory properties by repetitive stimulation with allogeneic immature human dendritic cells. J Exp Med 192, 1213–1222.

Kemper, C., Chan, A.C., Green, J.M., Brett, K.A., Murphy, K.M. and Atkinson, J.P. (2003). Activation of human CD4+ cells with CD3 and CD46 induces a T-regulatory cell 1 phenotype. Nature 421, 388–392.

Khattri, R., Cox, T., Yasayko, S.A. and Ramsdell, F. (2003). An essential role for Scurfin in CD4+ CD25+ T regulatory cells. Nat Immunol 4, 337–342.

Kojima, A., Tanaka-Kojima, Y., Sakakura, T. and Nishizuka, Y. (1976). Prevention of postthymectomy autoimmune thyroiditis in mice. Lab Invest 34, 601–605.

Kuniyasu, Y., Takahashi, T., Itoh, M., Shimizu, J., Toda, G. and Sakaguchi, S. (2000). Naturally anergic and suppressive CD25(+)CD4(+) T cells as a functionally and phenotypically distinct immunoregulatory T cell subpopulation. Int Immunol 12, 1145–1155.

Lutz, M.B. and Schuler, G. (2002). Immature, semi-mature and fully mature dendritic cells: which signals induce tolerance or immunity? Trends Immunol 23, 445–449.

Lyon, M.F., Peters, J., Glenister, P.H., Ball, S. and Wright, E. (1990). The scurfy mouse mutant has previously unrecognized hematological abnormalities and resembles Wiskott-Aldrich syndrome. Proc Natl Acad Sci USA 87, 2433–2437.

McHugh, R.S., Whitters, M.J., Piccirillo, C.A. et al. (2002). CD4(+)CD25(+) immunoregulatory T cells: gene expression analysis reveals a functional role for the glucocorticoid-induced TNF receptor. Immunity 16, 311–323.

Mosmann, T.R. and Coffman, R.L. (1989). TH1 and TH2 cells: different patterns of lymphokine secretion lead to different functional properties. Annu Rev Immunol 7, 145–173.

Nakamura, K., Kitani, A. and Strober, W. (2001). Cell contact-dependent immunosuppression by CD4(+)CD25(+) regulatory T cells is mediated by cell surface-bound transforming growth factor beta. J Exp Med 194, 629–644.

Nishizuka, Y. and Sakakura, T. (1969). Thymus and reproduction: sex-linked dysgenesia of the gonad after neonatal thymectomy in mice. Science 166, 753–755.

Onizuka, S., Tawara, I., Shimizu, J., Sakaguchi, S., Fujita, T. and Nakayama, E. (1999). Tumor rejection by in vivo administration of anti-CD25 (interleukin-2 receptor alpha) monoclonal antibody. Cancer Res 59, 3128–3133.

Palmer, E. (2003). Negative selection – clearing out the bad apples from the T-cell repertoire. Nat Rev Immunol 3, 383–391.

Pasare, C. and Medzhitov, R. (2003). Toll pathway-dependent blockade of CD4+ CD25+ T cell-mediated suppression by dendritic cells. Science, 299, 1033–1036.

Penhale, W.J., Farmer, A., McKenna, R.P. and Irvine, W.J. (1973). Spontaneous thyroiditis in thymectomized and irradiated Wistar rats. Clin Exp Immunol 15, 225–236.

Piccirillo, C.A., Letterio, J.J., Thornton, A.M. et al. (2002). CD4(+)CD25(+) regulatory T cells can mediate suppressor function in the absence of transforming growth factor beta1 production and responsiveness. J Exp Med 196, 237–246.

Piccirillo, C.A. and Shevach, E.M. (2001). Cutting edge: control of CD8 + T cell activation by CD4+ CD25+ immunoregulatory cells. J Immunol 167, 1137–1140.

Powrie, F., Carlino, J., Leach, M.W., Mauze, S. and Coffman, R.L. (1996). A critical role for transforming growth factor-beta but not interleukin 4 in the suppression of T helper type 1-mediated colitis by CD45RB(low) CD4+ T cells. J Exp Med 183, 2669–2674.

Powrie, F., Leach, M.W., Mauze, S., Caddle, L.B. and Coffman, R.L. (1993). Phenotypically distinct subsets of CD4+ T cells induce or protect from chronic intestinal inflammation in C. B-17 scid mice. Int Immunol 5, 1461–1471.

Powrie, F. and Mason, D. (1990). OX-22high CD4+ T cells induce wasting disease with multiple organ pathology: prevention by the OX-22low subset. J Exp Med 172, 1701–1708.

Read, S., Malmstrom, V. and Powrie, F. (2000). Cytotoxic T lymphocyte-associated antigen 4 plays an essential role in the function of CD25(+)CD4(+) regulatory cells that control intestinal inflammation. J Exp Med 192, 295–302.

Sakaguchi, N., Miyai, K. and Sakaguchi, S. (1994a). Ionizing radiation and autoimmunity. Induction of autoimmune disease in mice by high dose fractionated total lymphoid irradiation and its prevention by inoculating normal T cells. J Immunol 152, 2586–2595.

Sakaguchi, S. (2000). Regulatory T cells: key controllers of immunologic self-tolerance. Cell 101, 455–458.

Sakaguchi, S., Ermak, T. H., Toda, M. et al. (1994b). Induction of autoimmune disease in mice by germline alteration of the T cell receptor gene expression. J Immunol 152, 1471–1484.

Sakaguchi, S., Fukuma, K., Kuribayashi, K. and Masuda, T. (1985). Organ-specific autoimmune diseases induced in mice by elimination of T cell subset. I. Evidence for the active participation of T cells in natural self-tolerance; deficit of a T cell subset as a possible cause of autoimmune disease. J Exp Med 161, 72–87.

Sakaguchi, S. and Sakaguchi, N. (1989). Organ-specific autoimmune disease induced in mice by elimination of T cell subsets. V. Neonatal administration of cyclosporin A causes autoimmune disease. J Immunol 142, 471–480.

Sakaguchi, S., Sakaguchi, N., Asano, M., Itoh, M. and Toda, M. (1995). Immunologic self-tolerance maintained by activated T cells expressing IL-2 receptor alpha-chains (CD25). Breakdown of a single mechanism of self-tolerance causes various autoimmune diseases. J Immunol 155, 1151–1164.

Sakaguchi, S., Sakaguchi, N., Shimizu, J. et al. (2001). Immunologic tolerance maintained by CD25+ CD4+ regulatory T cells: their common role in controlling autoimmunity, tumor immunity, and transplantation tolerance. Immunol Rev 182, 18–32.

Sakaguchi, S., Takahashi, T. and Nishizuka, Y. (1982). Study on cellular events in post-thymectomy autoimmune oophoritis in mice. II. Requirement of Lyt-1 cells in normal female mice for the prevention of oophoritis. J Exp Med 156, 1577–1586.

Salomon, B., Lenschow, D. J., Rhee, L. et al. (2000). B7/CD28 costimulation is essential for the homeostasis of the CD4+ CD25+ immunoregulatory T cells that control autoimmune diabetes. Immunity 12, 431–440.

Saoudi, A., Seddon, B., Fowell, D. and Mason, D. (1996). The thymus contains a high frequency of cells that prevent autoimmune diabetes on transfer into prediabetic recipients. J Exp Med 184, 2393–2398.

Sato, K., Yamashita, N., Baba, M. and Matsuyama, T. (2003a). Modified myeloid dendritic cells act as regulatory dendritic cells to induce anergic and regulatory T cells. Blood 101, 3581–3589.

Sato, K., Yamashita, N., Baba, M. and Matsuyama, T. (2003b). Regulatory dendritic cells protect mice from murine acute graft-versus-host disease and leukemia relapse. Immunity 18, 367–379.

Schubert, L.A., Jeffery, E., Zhang, Y., Ramsdell, F. and Ziegler, S.F. (2001). Scurfin (FOXP3) acts as a repressor of transcription and regulates T cell activation. J Biol Chem 276, 37672–37679.

Seddon, B. and Mason, D. (1999). Regulatory T cells in the control of autoimmunity: the essential role of transforming growth factor beta and interleukin 4 in the prevention of autoimmune thyroiditis in rats by peripheral CD4(+)CD45RC-cells and CD4(+)CD8(-) thymocytes. J Exp Med 189, 279–288.

Shimizu, J., Yamazaki, S. and Sakaguchi, S. (1999). Induction of tumor immunity by removing CD25+ CD4+ T cells: a common basis between tumor immunity and autoimmunity. J Immunol 163, 5211–5218.

Shimizu, J., Yamazaki, S., Takahashi, T., Ishida, Y. and Sakaguchi, S. (2002). Stimulation of CD25(+)CD4(+) regulatory T cells through GITR breaks immunological self-tolerance. Nat Immunol 3, 135–142.

Singh, B., Read, S., Asseman, C. et al. (2001). Control of intestinal inflammation by regulatory T cells. Immunol Rev 182, 190–200.

Steinman, R.M., Hawiger, D. and Nussenzweig, M.C. (2003). Tolerogenic dendritic cells. Annu Rev Immunol 21, 685–711.

Sutmuller, R.P., van Duivenvoorde, L.M., van Elsas, A. et al. (2001). Synergism of cytotoxic T lymphocyte-associated antigen 4 blockade and depletion of CD25(+) regulatory T cells in antitumor therapy reveals alternative pathways for suppression of autoreactive cytotoxic T lymphocyte responses. J Exp Med 194, 823–832.

Takahashi, T., Kuniyasu, Y., Toda, M et al. (1998). Immunologic self-tolerance maintained by CD25+ CD4+ naturally anergic and suppressive T cells: induction of autoimmune disease by breaking their anergic/suppressive state. Int Immunol 10, 1969–1980.

Takahashi, T. and Sakaguchi, S. (2003). The role of regulatory T cells in controlling immunologic self-tolerance. Int Rev Cytol 225, 1–32.

Takahashi, T., Tagami, T., Yamazaki, S. et al. (2000). Immunologic self-tolerance maintained by CD25(+)CD4(+) regulatory T cells constitutively expressing cytotoxic T lymphocyte-associated antigen 4. J Exp Med 192, 303–310.

Taylor, P.A., Noelle, R.J. and Blazar, B.R. (2001). CD4(+)CD25(+) immune regulatory cells are required for induction of tolerance to alloantigen via costimulatory blockade. J Exp Med 193, 1311–1318.

Thornton, A.M. and Shevach, E.M. (1998). CD4+ CD25+ immunoregulatory T cells suppress polyclonal T cell activation in vitro by inhibiting interleukin 2 production. J Exp Med 188, 287–296.

Thornton, A.M. and Shevach, E.M. (2000). Suppressor effector function of CD4+ CD25+ immunoregulatory T cells is antigen nonspecific. J Immunol 164, 183–190.

Toh, B.H., Sentry, J.W. and Alderuccio, F. (2000). The causative H+/K+ ATPase antigen in the pathogenesis of autoimmune gastritis. Immunol Today 21, 348–354.

Trenado, A., Charlotte, F., Fisson, S. et al. (2003). Recipient-type specific CD4+ CD25+ regulatory T cells favor immune reconstitution and control graft-versus-host disease while maintaining graft-versus-leukemia. J Clin Invest 112, 1688–1696.

Tung, K., Lou, Y., Garza, K. and Teuscher, C. (1998). Autoimmune ovarian disease: mechanism of disease induction and prevention. Curr Opin Immunol 10, 839–845.

Vigouroux, S., Yvon, E., Wagner, H. J. et al. (2003). Induction of antigen-specific regulatory T cells following overexpression of a Notch ligand by human B lymphocytes. J Virol 77, 10872–10880.

Wakkach, A., Fournier, N., Brun, V., Breittmayer, J. P., Cottrez, F. and Groux, H. (2003). Characterization of dendritic cells that induce tolerance and T regulatory 1 cell differentiation in vivo. Immunity 18, 605–617.

Waldmann, H. and Cobbold, S. (1998). How do monoclonal antibodies induce tolerance? A role for infectious tolerance? Annu Rev Immunol 16, 619–644.

Walker, L.S., Chodos, A., Eggena, M., Dooms, H. and Abbas, A.K. (2003). Antigen-dependent proliferation of CD4+ CD25+ regulatory T cells *in vivo*. J Exp Med *198*, 249–258.

Wather, M.R., Kasprowicz, D.J., Gersuk, V.H. et al. (2003). Induction of FoxP3 and acquisition of T regulatory activity by stimulated human CD4+ CD25- T cells. J Clin Invest *112*, 1437–1443.

Weigle, W.O. (1980). Analysis of autoimmunity through experimental models of thyroiditis and allergic encephalomyelitis. Adv Immunol *30*, 159–273.

Wildin, R.S., Smyk-Pearson, S. and Filipovich, A.H. (2002). Clinical and molecular features of the immunodysregulation, polyendocrinopathy, enteropathy, X linked (IPEX) syndrome. J Med Genet *39*, 537–545.

Wood, K.J. and Sakaguchi, S. (2003). Regulatory T cells in transplantation tolerance. Nat Rev Immunol *3*, 199–210.

Yamazaki, S., Iyoda, T., Tarbell, K. et al. (2003). Direct expansion of functional CD25+ CD4+ regulatory T cells by antigen-processing dendritic cells. J Exp Med *198*, 235–247.

Zhai, Y. and Kupiec-Weglinski, J.W. (1999). What is the role of regulatory T cells in transplantation tolerance? Curr Opin Immunol *11*, 497–503.

Zhang, X., Izikson, L., Liu, L. and Weiner, H.L. (2001). Activation of CD25(+)CD4(+) regulatory T cells by oral antigen administration. J Immunol *167*, 4245–4253.

Intracellular Cytokine Assays

Chapter
28

Amy C. Hobeika, Michael A. Morse, Timothy M. Clay, Takuya Osada, Paul J. Mosca and H. Kim Lyerly

Program in Molecular Therapeutics, Departments of Surgery, Pathology, Immunology, and Medicine, Duke University Medical Center, Durham, NC, USA

> Whenever you are asked if you can do a job, tell 'em, 'Certainly I can!' Then get busy and find out how to do it.
>
> Theodore Roosevelt (1858–1919)

INTRODUCTION

Progress in the field of immunotherapy for human disease has increasingly relied upon the ability to detect immunity based on the assumption that effective immunotherapy leads to a measurable immune response. As a result, a variety of cell-based assays are now available for measuring cellular responses to different types of immunogens. The choice of immune assay used depends on the expected mediator of the response. The most potent immune therapies will simultaneously activate multiple pathways and effectors that play complementary roles. T cells are believed to be important effector cells in protecting the body against a wide range of threats and *in vitro* T cell assays are particularly useful in detecting antigen specific responses. Functional assays that measure T cell activity in response to a specific stimulus typically include cellular proliferation, cytokine secretion and cytolytic function. These assays show promise for quantifying and characterizing antigen specific immune responses and can be performed on specimens stimulated *in vitro* with antigen and cytokines as well as directly on PBMC or whole blood.

Antigen specific immune responses are regulated by cytokine production. The profile of cytokines secreted by T cells is a primary means by which these cells mediate the host defense. For this reason, cytokine production by T cells responding to a specific antigen is often used as a measure of a functional immune response. Although it can illustrate the relationship between T cell phenotype and function in response to antigen, analysis of cytokine secretion by T cells using traditional bulk measurement techniques such as ELISA is not strictly quantitative (Picker et al., 1995; Prussin and Metcalfe, 1995; Altman et al., 1996; Morita et al., 1998). In addition, methods that estimate total secreted cytokine levels do not allow for a direct correlation between a cytokine producing T cell and surface marker expression.

Flow cytometric methods are increasingly being employed to assess both the phenotypical and functional state of lymphocytes. Intracellular cytokine assays are a relatively new method of identifying cytokine production by individual T cells and have the ability to correlate cytokine expression with cell surface phenotype without cell separation (Waldrop et al., 1997; Suni et al., 1998). In addition, this highly sensitive flow cytometric method allows for the rapid detection of low frequency T cells expressing cytokine in response to specific antigen stimulation. The unique capabilities of this method make it a model assay for clinical and research applications.

BASIC PRINCIPLES OF INTRACELLULAR CYTOKINE ASSAYS

The overall premise of intracellular cytokine assays is direct detection of intracellular cytokine expression in response to antigen stimulation. Several reports initially

Measuring Immunity, edited by Michael T. Lotze and Angus W. Thomson
ISBN 0-12-455900-X, London

described methods for intracellular detection of cytokines using flow cytometry (Jung et al., 1993; Picker et al., 1995; Prussin and Metcalfe, 1995; Jason and Larned, 1997) and it has become a common technique for enumerating cytokine-producing T cells. The basic protocol described by these studies consists of an initial stimulation step, followed by permeabilization, staining with intracellular antibodies of interest and flow cytometric analysis. The details and versatility of this assay are described below.

Intracellular cytokine assays can be performed using various sources of cells and antigen depending upon the target(s) of interest. T cell stimulation can be performed directly on whole blood, PBMC, in vitro manipulated lymphocytes, isolated cells and lymph nodes, although it has been suggested that using whole blood for these assays provides a more physiological environment and may have an effect on the T cell response to stimulation (Picker et al., 1995; Suni et al., 1998, Nomura et al., 2000). The antigens used for stimulation include mitogens, peptide antigens, whole protein preparations, bacterial and viral proteins and cellular lysates. Because these assays are most often used to detect very low frequency events, appropriate control antigens are particularly important to ensure clear antigen specific responses.

Most intracellular cytokine assays involve a short period of in vitro T cell activation. This short-term incubation with antigen, usually 4–6 h, avoids the disadvantages associated with long-term culture of T cells (e.g. proliferation, media changes) and minimizes artifacts (Maecker et al., 2000). In addition, an incubation time of 6 h is optimal for achieving measurable levels of cytokine-secreting cells for specific cytokines, therefore achieving maximal cytokine staining intensity (Nomura et al., 2000). However, longer incubation times may be required under certain circumstances with unusual cell types or stimuli. At least 3–4 h of the incubation time with antigen is done in the presence of a protein secretion inhibitor to aid in the detection of weakly expressed proteins like cytokines. Brefeldin A (BFA) is an appropriate reagent for this purpose because it blocks protein secretion by disassembling the Golgi complex and redistributing it in the endoplasmic reticulum (Openshaw et al., 1995; Chardin and McCormick, 1999). BFA has also been shown to be a potent and effective protein secretion inhibitor with minimal toxicity during the short incubation time used in intracellular cytokine assays (Nylander and Kalies, 1999).

Cells are fixed using paraformaldehyde or similar agents following the stimulation period. At this stage of the assay, the stimulated cells may be cryopreserved for permeabilization and antibody staining at a later time (Nomura et al., 2000). Once fixed, the cell membrane can be permeabilized using a non-ionic detergent such as saponin (Jung et al., 1993; Prussin and Metcalfe, 1995). Proper permeabilization combined with quality antibodies that can withstand fixation conditions is required for successful staining of low frequency antigen specific

events. Antibodies used for intracellular staining techniques must be highly specific and possess considerable affinity for the markers of interest (Keilholz et al., 2002). Highly purified antibody-fluorochrome conjugates are also essential for minimizing background staining. Another option is to stain surface markers prior to the fixation and permeabilization steps.

Clearly a variety of surface markers and cytokine specific antibodies can be used for staining stimulated T cells. For most standard T cell intracellular cytokine protocols, fluorochrome-conjugated anti-CD4 and anti-CD8 antibodies are used to allow gating on T cells, along with anti-CD69 to monitor activation of T cells and an antibody to the cytokine of interest. Three or four color flow cytometry is performed and the percentage of CD4(+) or CD8(+) CD69(+) cytokine(+) T cells is enumerated (Suni et al., 1998; Nomura et al., 2000). Typical T cell percentages in response to antigen stimulation range from 0.1 (measles or mumps antigen) to 5 per cent (CMV antigen) or more (Maino and Picker, 1998). Reproducibility of the antigen-specific responses detected by intracellular cytokine methods has also been studied. Intra-assay variability has been reported to be within 5 per cent coefficient of variation in a CMV specific intracellular cytokine assay and within 20 per cent in a multi-site study (Nomura et al., 2000; Keilholz et al., 2002).

T CELL SUBSETS

The critical evaluation of an effective T cell assay requires an understanding of the complexity of T cell subsets and their different impacts upon immune responses. Recently, studies of T cell clones, first in the mouse and subsequently recapitulated in the human, have led to the characterization of specialized subsets of T helper cells (CD4+) and cytotoxic T cells (CD8+). Specific cytokine secretion profiles now permit the subdivision of T helper cells into T helper type 1 (Th1) and T helper type 2 (Th2) subsets. Th1 are interleukin-2 (IL-2) and interferon-gamma (IFNγ) producing cells while Th2 are IL-4 and IL-5 producers (Del Prete et al., 1991; Street and Mosmann, 1991; Swain et al., 1991; Wierenga et al., 1991; Paul and Seder, 1994). Th1 cells are associated with induction of CTL responses, while Th2 cells are involved in promoting antibody responses. The cytokines produced by each cell type regulate the other cell type. Indeed, the effect of IL-4 on Th1 cells and IFNγ on Th2 cells is antagonistic, such that each subset essentially suppresses the proliferation of the other subset. Consequently, Th2 cells could negatively impact CTL generation and the maintenance of CTL responses that are the objective of some immunotherapeutics. For example, because some cancer patients have a predominant Th2 bias, evidence is mounting that Th2 cells could also play a role in cancer growth (Lauerova et al., 2002; Tatsumi et al., 2002). Immunologic monitoring of cancer vaccine clinical trials until very recently has concentrated on CTL responses. Now emphasis is also being placed on examining Th2 type responses and cytokines. T helper cell subsets have led to similar definitions being drawn for cytotoxic T cells, specifically Tc1 and Tc2, based on cytokine profiles similar to Th1 and Th2 cells (Vukmanovic-Stejic et al., 2000). Again, type 1 cells are involved with promoting CTL responses and type 2 cells are involved in the generation of antibody responses.

In addition to the above CD8+ and CD4+ T cell subclassifications, protective T cell immunity has also been found to be dependent upon the functional activity of immune memory/effector cell subsets. The ability to secrete many of the key suppressor and effector cytokines including IL-2, IL-4, IL-5, IL-10 and IFNγ is restricted to these populations that are described using several surface markers. Effector CD8+ cells (CD45RA+ CCR7−) are cytolytic and produce IFNγ (Cho et al., 1999; Valmori et al., 2002). CD4+ regulatory cells (CD4+ CD25+) produce IL-10 and TGFβ and suppress different aspects of the immune system (Ng et al., 2001; Liyanage et al., 2002). Immune effector cells are identified by virtue of their cytokine production upon short-term *in vitro* incubation with antigen, though intracellular cytokine assays can also be dominated by memory cell responses (Suni et al., 1998). Immune cell subset definitions such as effector/memory and Th1/Th2 phenotypes are continually evolving, emphasizing the need to identify cytokine production along with surface marker expression.

CLINICAL RELEVANCE

One of the most valuable features of an *in vitro* immune assay is correlation with clinical outcome. Several clinical studies have now used intracellular cytokine assays to evaluate the immune response to cancer therapy. In a phase I/II study of immunization with SRL 172 in patients with stage IV malignant melanoma, lymphocyte activation was assayed prior to each vaccine administration using an intracellular cytokine assay (Maraveyas et al., 1999). Induction of intracellular IL-2 production was associated with improved survival. Surprisingly, induction of IFNγ or both IL-2 plus IFNγ was not associated with improved survival, demonstrating the complexities in choosing surrogate markers. Reinartz et al. (1999) followed intracellular cytokine production in T cells obtained at various time points during immunization of ovarian cancer patients with the anti-idiotype vaccine ACA125. Early in the immunizations, predominantly IL-2 and interferon alpha were observed but later a Th2 pattern was observed. This correlated with generation of anti-anti-idiotype antibodies and prolonged survival.

COMPARISON TO OTHER IMMUNE ASSAYS

Prior to choosing an assay to monitor an immune response, it is important to consider the performance characteristics of the assay in detecting a response and what magnitude of the immune response should be considered a positive response. Important features for detecting a T cell response consist of:

1 adequate sensitivity, specificity, reliability and reproducibility
2 measurement of the true state of *in vivo* T cell activity without introducing significant distortions
3 simple and rapid to perform
4 requirement for only small quantities of specimen
5 close correlation with clinical data.

As compared to older methods of immune response analysis such as delayed type hypersensitivity (DTH) response, chromium release assays (^{51}Cr), limiting dilution assays (LDA) and tritiated thymidine incorporation, new immunologic monitoring techniques more closely fit these guidelines and, in general, are more robust and reproducible. In addition to intracellular cytokine assays, these highly sensitive *in vitro* methods include peptide-MHC tetramers and ELISPOT.

An increase in the number of defined tumor and viral antigens along with a more detailed understanding of T cell antigen recognition and the character of peptides presented in the major histocompatibitiy complex (MHC) has resulted in the development of peptide-MHC tetramers that specifically bind antigen specific CD8+ cells via the T cell receptor (TCR) (Altman et al., 1996). While tetramer analysis is quick to perform (less than 2–3 h) and highly sensitive, tetramers are restricted to a purely phenotypic measurement of the T cell response and rely on known MHC restricted peptide epitopes. Further, in our experience, the reliability of peptide-MHC tetramers varies with some preparations and, because not all peptides form functional tetramers, those with an untried peptide must be tested empirically. Similar to intracellular cytokine assays, ELISPOT assays also have the capability to measure multiple cytokines from an individual cell with the major difference being ELISPOTs measure secreted cytokines in response to antigen stimulation (Czerkinsky et al., 1983; Hutchings et al., 1989). The ELISPOT has been shown reliably to measure antigen specific T cell frequency and is a highly quantitative method (Schmittel et al., 1997). However, the ELISPOT assay requires a longer incubation time than intracellular cytokine assays (24–48 h) and requires computerized plate readers for optimal readings (Vaquerano et al., 1998).

There are a number of studies that have directly compared the various assays for their performance in evaluating immune responses. Most of the data come from studies against viral antigens (Kuzushima et al., 1999; Tan et al., 1999). Kuzushima et al. observed intracellular cytokine analysis detected a higher percentage of antigen specific cells than LDA and ELISPOT. Other reports have suggested the sensitivity of intracellular cytokine assays are superior to ELISPOT in studies looking at CMV and mycobacteria. ELISPOT and LDA assays detected in the order of 1/1000 to 1/10 000 CMV and mycobacteria specific T cells compared to the 1/1000 to 2/100 CD4+ cells indicated by intracellular assays (Brett, 1987; Clouse et al., 1989; Lolli et al., 1993; Surcel et al., 1994).

Intracellular cytokine assays in part have an advantage over other assays due to the use of flow cytometry. Flow cytometry offers a number of advantages such as the speed with which the assays may be performed, the ability to analyze cytokine secretion on an individual cell basis while simultaneously determining other characteristics of the cell phenotype (such as CD4/CD8 expression or memory versus naive phenotypic markers), the lack of interference with measurements by variability in the concentration of cellular or free cytokine receptors that can occur with ELISAs by reducing the cytokine content of the culture supernatant and the capacity to measure a variety of cytokines for quantitating Th1 and Th2 cytokines

In contrast to these characteristics, although the ELISPOT assay can analyze multiple cytokines, it does not have the ability to measure T cell phenotypes in conjunction with cytokine expression without cell separation techniques being employed. Intracellular cytokine methods are also superior to peptide-MHC tetramer staining because only a portion of T cells stained by tetramers have been found to function in response to antigen stimulation. The principal issue with the use of intracellular cytokine assays is that they can be technically demanding, though with adequate experience it can be reliably reproducible. Rapidity of flow cytometric intracellular cytokine assays as well as the widespread availability of the reagents used such as surface staining antibodies makes this a useful assay with broad clinical and research applications.

CONCLUSION

Optimization of immunotherapeutic strategies for human disease is dependent on reliable and sensitive assays that permit comparison of the immune responses induced. Standards are needed for performing the assays and interpreting the results to allow different clinical trials to be more directly compared. Because the various assays yield estimates of antigen-specific T cells that sometimes differ in magnitude, it is critical to compare the immune response detected by a particular assay in a particular patient with the specific immune response for a well-established, immunogenic antigen, such as EBV or CMV peptide. It is also important to determine what constitutes an effective level of immunologic response. For example, it is not currently known what level of immunity would be sufficient to eradicate established tumor or prevent recurrence of microscopic disease in humans. Estimates from transgenic mouse experiments (Hanson et al., 2000) suggest that protection from tumor challenge

requires relatively small numbers of tumor specific CTL, in the 12–30 000 cell range, which would be in the 35–100 million range for humans based upon simple extrapolation of blood volumes, suggesting 10–30 per cent of CD8+ T cells would need to be tumor specific. Clearly, rapidly growing mouse tumors are not comparable to a naturally arising human tumor, so these simple calculations are speculative, but they do suggest that levels seen in viral diseases are not unreasonable targets.

Currently, several highly specific immune assays are available to monitor immune responses, but it has not yet been established which will correlate best with clinical outcome. Intracellular cytokine assays are rapid, quantitative and provide valuable information on functional role of T cells in various diseases. One disadvantage of this assay compared to simple phenotypical analysis is due to the permeabilization step required to stain intracellularly. The permeabilized cells are no longer viable and cannot be sorted for culturing and further analysis or cloning. However, intracellular staining is essential to detect the cytokine production pattern of individual antigen-stimulated cells. This assay presently offers the best method for directly correlating cell phenotype with cytokine production.

REFERENCES

Altman, J.D., Moss, P.A., Goulder, P.J. et al. (1996). Phenotypic analysis of antigen-specific T lymphocytes. Science 274, 94–96.

Brett, S.J. (1987). Regulatory interactions between macrophages and T cells in Mycobacterium lepraemurium-specific T-cell activation. Cell Immunol 110, 379–390.

Chardin, P. and McCormick, F. (1999). Brefeldin A: the advantage of being uncompetitive. Cell 97, 153–155.

Cho, B.K., Wang, C., Sugawa, S., Eisen, H.N. and Chen, J. (1999). Functional differences between memory and naive CD8 T cells. Proc Natl Acad Sci USA 96, 2976–2981.

Clouse, K.A., Adams, P.W. and Orosz, C.G. (1989). Enumeration of viral antigen-reactive helper T lymphocytes in human peripheral blood by limiting dilution for analysis of viral antigen-reactive T-cell pools in virus-seropositive and virus-seronegative individuals. J Clin Microbiol 27, 2316–2323.

Czerkinsky, C.C., Nilsson, L.A., Nygren, H., Ouchterlony, O. and Tarkowski, A. (1983). A solid-phase enzyme-linked immunospot (ELISPOT) assay for enumeration of specific antibody-secreting cells. J Immunol Methods 65, 109–121.

Del Prete, G.F., De Carli, M., Ricci, M. and Romagnani, S. (1991). Helper activity for immunoglobulin synthesis of T helper type 1 (Th1) and Th2 human T cell clones: the help of Th1 clones is limited by their cytolytic capacity. J Exp Med 174, 809–813.

Hanson, H.L., Donermeyer, D.L., Ikeda, H. et al. (2000). Eradication of established tumors by CD8+ T cell adoptive immunotherapy. Immunity 13, 265–276.

Hutchings, P.R., Cambridge, G., Tite, J.P., Meager, T. and Cooke, A. (1989). The detection and enumeration of cytokine-secreting cells in mice and man and the clinical application of these assays. J Immunol Methods 120, 1–8.

Jason, J. and Larned, J. (1997). Single-cell cytokine profiles in normal humans: comparison of flow cytometric reagents and stimulation protocols. J Immunol Methods 207, 13–22.

Jung, T., Schauer, U., Heusser, C., Neumann, C. and Rieger, C. (1993). Detection of intracellular cytokines by flow cytometry. J Immunol Methods 159, 197–207.

Keilholz, U., Weber, J., Finke, J.H. et al. (2002). Immunologic monitoring of cancer vaccine therapy: results of a workshop sponsored by the Society for Biological Therapy. J Immunother 25, 97–138.

Kuzushima, K., Hoshino, Y., Fujii, K. et al. (1999). Rapid determination of Epstein-Barr virus-specific CD8(+) T-cell frequencies by flow cytometry. Blood 94, 3094–3100.

Lauerova, L., Dusek, L., Simickova, M. et al. (2002). Malignant melanoma associates with Th1/Th2 imbalance that coincides with disease progression and immunotherapy response. Neoplasma 49, 159–166.

Liyanage, U.K., Moore, T.T., Joo, H.G. et al. (2002). Prevalence of regulatory T cells is increased in peripheral blood and tumor microenvironment of patients with pancreas or breast adenocarcinoma. J Immunol 169, 2756–2761.

Lolli, F., Sundqvist, V.A., Castagna, A. et al. (1993). T and B cell responses to cytomegalovirus antigens in healthy blood donors and bone marrow transplant recipients. FEMS Immunol Med Microbiol 7, 55–62.

Maecker, H.T., Maino, V.C. and Picker, L.J. (2000). Immunofluorescence analysis of T-cell responses in health and disease. J Clin Immunol 20, 391–399.

Maino, V.C. and Picker, L.J. (1998). Identification of functional subsets by flow cytometry: intracellular detection of cytokine expression. Cytometry 34, 207–215.

Maraveyas, A., Baban, B., Kennard, D. et al. (1999). Possible improved survival of patients with stage IV AJCC melanoma receiving SRL 172 immunotherapy: correlation with induction of increased of intracellular interleukin-2 in peripheral blood lymphocytes. Ann Oncol 10, 817–824.

Morita, Y., Yamamura, M., Kawashima, M. et al. (1998). Flow cytometric single-cell analysis of cytokine production by CD4+ T cells in synovial tissue and peripheral blood from patients with rheumatoid arthritis. Arthritis Rheum 41, 1669–1676.

Ng, W.F., Duggan, P.J., Ponchel, F. et al. (2001). Human CD4(+)CD25(+) cells: a naturally occurring population of regulatory T cells. Blood 98, 2736–2744.

Nomura, L.E., Walker, J.M. and Maecker, H.T. (2000). Optimization of whole blood antigen-specific cytokine assays for CD4(+) T cells. Cytometry 40, 60–68.

Nylander, S. and Kalies, I. (1999). Brefeldin A, but not monensin, completely blocks CD69 expression on mouse lymphocytes: efficacy of inhibitors of protein secretion in protocols for intracellular cytokine staining by flow cytometry. J Immunol Methods 224, 69–76.

Openshaw, P., Murphy, E.E., Hosken, N.A. et al. (1995). Heterogeneity of intracellular cytokine synthesis at the single-cell level in polarized T helper 1 and T helper 2 populations. J Exp Med 182, 1357–1367.

Paul, W.E. and Seder, R.A. (1994). Lymphocyte responses and cytokines. Cell 76, 241–251.

Picker, L.J., Singh, M.K., Zdraveski, Z. et al. (1995). Direct demonstration of cytokine synthesis heterogeneity among human memory/effector T cells by flow cytometry. Blood 86, 1408–1419.

Prussin, C. and Metcalfe, D.D. (1995). Detection of intracytoplasmic cytokine using flow cytometry and directly conjugated anticytokine antibodies. J Immunol Methods 188, 117–128.

Reinartz, S., Boerner, H., Koehler, S., Von Ruecker, A., Schlebusch, H. and Wagner, U. (1999). Evaluation of immunological responses in patients with ovarian cancer treated with the anti-idiotype vaccine ACA125 by determination of intracellular cytokines – a preliminary report. Hybridoma 18, 41–45.

Schmittel, A., Keilholz, U. and Scheibenbogen, C. (1997). Evaluation of the interferon-gamma ELISPOT-assay for quantification of peptide specific T lymphocytes from peripheral blood. J Immunol Methods 210, 167–174.

Street, N.E. and Mosmann, T.R. (1991). Functional diversity of T lymphocytes due to secretion of different cytokine patterns. FASEB J 5, 171–177.

Suni, M.A., Picker, L.J. and Maino, V.C. (1998). Detection of antigen-specific T cell cytokine expression in whole blood by flow cytometry. J Immunol Methods 212, 89–98.

Surcel, H.M., Troye-Blomberg, M., Paulie, S. et al. (1994). Th1/Th2 profiles in tuberculosis, based on the proliferation and cytokine response of blood lymphocytes to mycobacterial antigens. Immunology 81, 171–176.

Swain, S.L., Bradley, L.M., Croft, M. et al. (1991). Helper T-cell subsets: phenotype, function and the role of lymphokines in regulating their development. Immunol Rev 123, 115–144.

Tan, L.C., Gudgeon, N., Annels, N.E. et al. (1999). A re-evaluation of the frequency of CD8+ T cells specific for EBV in healthy virus carriers. J Immunol 162, 1827–1835.

Tatsumi, T., Kierstead, L.S., Ranieri, E. et al. (2002). Disease-associated bias in T helper type 1 (Th1)/ Th2 CD4(+) T cell responses against MAGE-6 in HLA-DRB10401(+) patients with renal cell carcinoma or melanoma. J Exp Med 196, 619–628.

Valmori, D., Scheibenbogen, C., Dutoit, V. et al. (2002). Circulating tumor-reactive CD8(+) T cells in melanoma patients contain a CD45RA(+)CCR7(−) effector subset exerting ex vivo tumor-specific cytolytic activity. Cancer Res 62, 1743–1750.

Vaquerano, J.E., Peng, M., Chang, J.W., Zhou, Y.M. and Leong, S. P. (1998). Digital quantification of the enzyme-linked immunospot (ELISPOT). Biotechniques 25, 830–834, 836.

Vukmanovic-Stejic, M., Vyas, B., Gorak-Stolinska, P., Noble, A. and Kemeny, D.M. (2000). Human Tc1 and Tc2/Tc0 CD8 T-cell clones display distinct cell surface and functional phenotypes. Blood 95, 231–240.

Waldrop, S.L., Pitcher, C.J., Peterson, D.M., Maino, V.C. and Picker, L.J. (1997). Determination of antigen-specific memory/effector CD4+ T cell frequencies by flow cytometry: evidence for a novel, antigen-specific homeostatic mechanism in HIV-associated immunodeficiency. J Clin Invest 99, 1739–1750.

Wierenga, E.A., Snoek, M., Jansen, H.M., Bos, J.D., van Lier, R.A. and Kapsenberg, M.L. (1991). Human atopen-specific types 1 and 2 T helper cell clones. J Immunol 147, 2942–2949.

Section IV

Cellular function and physiology

Cytolytic Assays

Stephen E. Winikoff, Herbert J. Zeh, Richard DeMarco and Michael T. Lotze

University of Pittsburgh School of Medicine, Pittsburgh, PA, USA

Chapter 29

DEATH be not proud, though some have called thee
Mighty and dreadfull, for, thou art not so,
For, those, whom thou think'st, thou dost overthrow,
Die not, poore death, nor yet canst thou kill me.

John Donne (1572–1631)

INTRODUCTION

Early observations made during the period of initial understanding of the critical role in immune responses of lymphocytes (Hellstrom et al., 1965, 1968; Brown et al., 1976) suggested that they had the ability to induce killing of cells. Many of these early studies of tumor cytolysis, thought to be mediated by specific T cells, were subsequently shown to be mediated by NK cells (Herberman et al., 1977; Alvarez et al., 1978; Djeu et al., 1979; Riccardi et al., 1979; Santoni et al., 1979) or cytokine (lymphokine) activated killer cells (Lotze et al., 1980a,b, 1981, 1985, 1988; Lotze and Rosenberg, 1981; Strausser et al., 1981; Rayner et al., 1985a,b) mediated by a mixture of NK and T cells. Although the initial notion of cell death was one of osmotic death driven by delivery of pore-forming structures, it was subsequently clear that most of the death pathways involved a form of apoptosis (Kerr et al., 1972; Danilevicius, 1973). Currently our understanding of cell biology is that intrinsic pathways of cell death are induced by genomic damage from mutagens, ultraviolet or gamma irradiation and mediated through mitochondrial sensors; extrinsic pathways are mediated by death domain-containing cell

surface receptors for either cellular or soluble ligands (TNF, lymphotoxin, TRAIL, FasL, etc.) which trigger caspase-dependent pathways (Ashkenazi, 2002); and cytolytic pathways, although capable of mediating the extrinsic pathway, primarily through perforin-mediated delivery of granzymes (Grossman et al., 2003; Lieberman, 2003; Smyth et al., 2003; Veugelers et al., 2004). T cells with high avidity for the target of interest can be distinguished using these strategies (Lotze et al., 1992a,b; Zeh et al., 1993, 1994, 1999).

AVAILABLE ASSAY METHODOLOGY

The earliest means to assess cytotoxicity were those related to trypan blue exclusion of non-viable cells and projection of a microscopic field onto a screen for direct visual counting. This has been supplanted by a variety of radioactive and fluorescent strategies to facilitate higher throughput and accuracy. These are briefly introduced below.

CHROMIUM RELEASE ASSAY

Since 1968, the chromium release microcytotoxicity assay (CRA) has been the standard and most frequently used assay for assessment of cell-mediated cytotoxicity in vitro. In this assay, target cells are loaded with $Na^{51}Cr$, which passively enters the cells and binds to intracellular proteins. Upon target cell lysis, ^{51}Cr is released into the

Measuring Immunity, edited by Michael T. Lotze and Angus W. Thomson
ISBN 0-12-455900-X, London

Table 29.1 Advantages and disadvantages of available assay methods

Assay method	Advantages	Disadvantages
Chromium release	Reproducibility Ease of operation Extensively validated in literature	Poor labeling of cells with low cytoplasm:nucleus ratio High spontaneous release in longer assays Delay between cell damage and measurable release Limitations of using radioactivity Need to pre-stimulate cells Lack of correlation with clinical response
Europium release	High rate of early release Non-radioactive Fewer target and effector cells needed High sensitivity and specificity Performs well with non-adherent tumor cell targets	Requires fluorimeter Daudi, certain targets give high spontaneous release
Modified microcytotoxicity assay	Reflects specific mechanism of killing (TNF family ligands) Useful for measuring NK activity	Not extensively validated in literature
MTT assay	Easily and rapidly performed Reproducible Good correlation to *in vivo* testing. Useful for cytotoxic drug testing	Change in culture medium accompanied by decrease in MTT-formazan MTT reduction takes place in apoptotic cells at early stages Drugs may alter mitochondrial activity
FATAL assay	Variations in incubation period allowed due to long retention of dyes Immediate, unambiguous readout Low spontaneous readout Good correlation with chromium release	Not standardized, requires specific experience and reagents
CFSE/7-AAD	Tracks effector and target cells alike Allows measurement of intracellular molecules involved in apoptosis Sensitive, especially at low E:T ratios	Results may be affected by debris
Calcein release	Sensitive Safe Ease of performance May combine with other fluorescent markers	Requires fluorescence scanner
Monoclonal Ab assays	May use multiple labels to identify cells of interest	Not readily adaptable from one system to next
FCC assays	Reflects molecular activity of apoptotic pathway Real time assay Allows visualization of individual cells May study effector cells and target cells More sensitive than CRA	
CD 107a flow assay	Identifies effector cells *ex vivo* Useful for clinical assays	
Cell transfection assays.	Continuous expression No loss of expression during cell division Exquisitely sensitive. High correlation with CRA May incubate for short time interval	Specific reagents needed.

supernatant and the amount of ^{51}Cr is quantified using a gamma counter. Since the spontaneous release of chromium is relatively low, depending in part on the cell type, rapid release of chromium into the cytoplasm reflects breakdown of the cell membrane accompanying cell death.

The application of this method is exemplified by the measurement of CD8+ CTL activity. It is thought that the ability of CTLs to lyse tumor is a relevant marker for *in vivo* antitumor activity. Surrogate targets are often used for autologous tumor, such as HLA-matched allogeneic cell lines or dendritic cell targets loaded with the antigen of interest. Targets sensitive to natural killer cell lysis such as K562 or Daudi are also included to determine the level of non-specific lytic activity. Using different effector:target cell ratios, it is possible to derive a value for the potency of cytotoxicity measured in lytic units, the number of T cells needed to achieve a stated amount of lysis.

In theory, various CTL preparations can be compared in this way.

The assay is reproducible and relatively easy to perform, but has several drawbacks. These include difficulty in labeling cells possessing a low cytoplasm-nucleus ratio; increasing spontaneous release of ^{51}Cr from target cells over time, especially relevant in long-term assays; and a delay between actual cell damage and release of ^{51}Cr -bound intracellular proteins into the supernatant. There is also a need for specific care and handling associated with radioactive usage, with attendant health risks, high cost and practical limitations due to the short half-life of the radioisotope (Zarcone et al., 1986; Ozdemir et al., 2003).

While such cytotoxicity assays have been used for immune monitoring in studies of immunotherapy, the assay is relatively insensitive, lacking precise quantitation of cellular activity at the single cell level. In addition, often there is a need to stimulate cells several times before testing their lytic activity. These stimulations may distort the composition and activity of the T cell population from its original state. Furthermore, it only measures a subset of memory/effector cells capable of proliferating following lengthy *in vitro* stimulation. Surrogate targets for autologous tumor may not reflect the ability of cells to lyse autologous tumor cells *in vivo*, especially in the complex tumor microenvironment. Mechanisms of immune escape may not be accounted for and antigen levels present on the targets may not reflect those of the *in situ* tumor. Questions concerning the lack of correlation with clinical response have been raised (Lyerly, 2003).

An alternative method, using limiting dilution analysis, involves serial dilution of T cells in a large number of wells, followed by *in vitro* stimulation and assessment of target cell lysis. Using Poisson distribution analysis, the number of antigen-specific precursor T cells can be determined and a frequency calculated, based on the number of positive wells at successively higher dilutions of the original T cell population. This technique has been described as being technically demanding and operator dependent. It rests on the assumption that a single antigen-specific T cell can be expanded during the stimulation phase to generate a detectable signal and, in actuality, measures only a subset of memory/effector cells capable of proliferating during the lengthy *in vitro* stimulation. Such limiting dilution analysis results have not been well correlated with clinical benefit (Clay et al., 2001; Hobeika et al., 2001; Lyerly et al., 2001; Lyerly, 2003).

EUROPIUM RELEASE ASSAY

The Europium release method was introduced as an alternative to the standard CRA. This method, described by Blomberg et al. and colleagues (Blomberg et al., 1986; Lovgren and Blomberg, 1994), is based on the release into the supernatant of a non-radioactive substance, europium, which is measurable by time-resolved fluorescence. Due to

the high rate of release compared to that of ^{51}Cr, europium released from the target is detectable long before lysis is complete. Consequently, fewer target and effector cells are needed to perform the assay. This assay is sensitive and specific and performs well with non-adherent tumor cell targets. Additional advantages are the reduced health risk and radioactive waste and lower cost per assay. The assay does require the availability of a fluorimeter and certain targets such as Daudi give unacceptable high spontaneous release values. The europium release assay was compared with the standard ^{51}Cr release assay using the peripheral blood mononuclear cells from patients with cervical carcinoma, using fresh and IL-2 activated effector cells, with K562 as targets. Assays using ^{51}Cr and europium gave comparable results (von Zons et al., 1997).

MODIFIED MICROCYTOXICITY ASSAY

Another alternative to the standard ^{51}Cr release assay is the modified microcytotoxicity assay (MCA). The assay is performed in microwells, with adherent tumor cell targets. Following exposure to cytotoxic immune cells, dead cells become non-adherent and are removed by washing of the wells. Remaining adherent cells are fixed, stained and optically counted. This method has been used successfully for quantitation of NK cell activity (Vujanovic et al., 1996; Wahlberg et al., 2001). These investigators found that solid tumor cell targets such as the BT-20 breast cancer, which were selectively susceptible to killing by cell membrane bound TNF family ligands and resistant to killing by secreted perforin/granzymes of freshly isolated non-activated NK cells, were readily killed in MCA by peripheral blood mononuclear cells as well as purified NK cells. They were not, however, lysed by the same effectors in a 4 h ^{51}Cr release assay (CRA). They concluded that MCA showed better reliability, reproducibility and sensitivity than CRA, while measuring an activity of NK cells different from that measured by CRA.

MTT (3-(4,5-DIMETHYLTHIAZOL-2-YL)-2,5-DIPHENYLTETRAZOLIUM BROMIDE) ASSAY

The MTT assay relies on the cellular reduction of tetrazolium salts to their formazan crystals. The range of cell concentrations in which there is a direct relationship between optical density and the number of cells counted should be determined. The cell number at the beginning and end of the incubation period should fall within the linear range of the calibration curve. Towards the end of the incubation period for a given assay, the MTT solution is added and the plate is incubated for an additional time period. The formazan crystals are then dissolved in an acid/alcohol solution and the plate is read on a multiwell scanning spectrophotometer (ELISA reader). Optical density values of the treated cells are compared with the optical density values of the control cells and results are presented as a percentage of cell survival. Cell number is then calculated based on the calibration curve.

The advantages of the MTT assay include ease and rapidity of performance, reproducibility of the results and observed clinical correlation between *in vitro* and *in vivo* testing (Pieters et al., 1988; Isselt et al., 1989; Colangelo et al., 1992; Jiao et al., 1992). There are several limitations, however, to the MTT assay. A decrease in the concentration of D-glucose, NADH or NADPH in the culture medium may be accompanied by a decrease in MTT-formazan production. In cells undergoing apoptosis, there may be some MTT reduction at early stages, since mitochondria remain intact. Drug effects may also result in changes in mitochondrial activity that could influence the results. Modifications to the original assay have been made to increase homogeneity of the solubilized formazan and other tetrazolium-based compounds have been substituted.

The MTT assay has been most widely applied in the assessment of cytotoxic drug therapy. Because implementation of the MTT protocol is technically easier in cell cultures grown in suspension, the assay has been tested for its ability to serve as a predictive tool for selection of chemotherapy for leukemia (Jiao et al., 1992). The assays can predict drug resistance with high accuracy and, in some cases, drug sensitivity. A detailed review of modifications of this assay as well as the application in leukemic patients and fresh tumor specimens has been recently performed (Hayon et al., 2003; Sargent 2003).

FLOW CYTOMETRIC ASSAYS

Because of the disadvantages of CRAs, a number of flow cytometry based killing assays have been developed. In most of these assays, target cells are stained with individual markers and after incubation with effector cells, target cell lysis is measured. In early efforts, dead or apoptotic cells were identified by the use of fluorescent dyes such as propidium iodide (PI) or annexin V (Sheehy et al., 2001). This method has been criticized as being unreliable.

The FATAL assay (fluorometric assessment of T-lymphocyte antigen-specific lysis), described by Sheehy and colleagues (Sheehy et al., 2001), utilizes two fluorescent dyes to track the target cell population. The first PKH-26 associates with cell membranes, the second, carboxy-fluorescein diacetate succinidyl ester (CFSE) is internalized by target cells. The dyes are retained longer than ^{51}Cr, allowing for variations in the incubation period and CFSE fluorescence occurs in a single step, providing an unambiguous measure of cytolytic activity. The CFSE binds intracellular proteins and produces a signal that halves with each mitotic division and does not interfere with cell function. The percentage of specific lysis is calculated based upon the disappearance of the CFSE-positive target cell population after incubation with effector cells. The FATAL assay has a 40-fold lower spontaneous leakage rate than CRA,

permitting a more accurate assessment of the effector:target (E:T) ratio while sensitively detecting low levels of CTL-mediated lysis. A strong correlation is noted between CRA and FATAL when performed in parallel.

A second method, the CFSE/7-AAD assay is able simultaneously to track effector cells and target cells. This assay uses CFSE to label effector cells and the DNA intercalating dye 7-AAD to stain target cells (Lecoeur et al., 2001). Because the 7-AAD staining is resistant to fixation and permeabilization procedures required for intracellular staining of target cells, it allows the concomitant detection of intracellular molecules involved in the apoptotic processes, such as caspase-3.

The assay is also more sensitive than ^{51}Cr, particularly at low E:T ratios, probably because of detection by 7-AAD staining of early apoptotic cells that exhibit weak membrane alteration and do not release ^{51}Cr. One limitation is that it does not take into account the debris discarded during the cytometric analysis.

A number of dyes have been used to label target cells and several groups have developed flow cytometry-based methods using these dyes. In the calcein release assay (Lichtenfels et al., 1994; Papadopoulos et al., 1994; Giacomello et al., 1999; Roden et al., 1999), the probe used is a lipid soluble diester that passively diffuses into the cell and is cleaved by intracellular esterases to induce fluorescence and render the compound lipid insoluble, trapping the probe inside the cell. The release of the marker into the supernatant is measured by an automated fluorescence scanner and correlates with the number of lysed cells. In another variation, extracellular fluorescence is excluded with a quenching reagent. Fluoro-quench is used to extinguish fluorescence outside viable cells, since it is unable to penetrate viable plasma membranes but is able to enter dead or dying cells with compromised membranes.

One approach to overcoming the problem of dyes leaking and labeling other cells in the environment involves the use of monoclonal antibodies. Zamai developed an assay using preculture with a CD56 antibody and light scatter changes for detection of cytotoxicity against K562 (Zamai et al., 2002, 2004). Unfortunately, this is not easily adaptable to other systems. Another method developed, by Ozdemir (Ozdemir et al., 2003), utilizes mAB staining of either effector or target cells to evaluate cytotoxicity and employs the use of fluorospheres for calibration. The strategy involves labeling effector or target cells with specific fluorochrome conjugated mAbs, in addition to staining with annexin V and PI to identify apoptotic/dead cells. The integration of fluorospheres allows determination of the absolute number of events and the assay correlates well with the CRA.

THE FLOW CYTOMETRY CASPASE (FCC) ASSAY

The flow cytometry caspase (FCC) assay (Chahroudi et al., 2003; Jayaraman, 2003; Jerome et al., 2003; Telford et al.,

2004) detects activation of caspase enzymes within target cells. This assay reveals the processes responsible for target-cell killing. Caspase activation occurs early in the process of CTL killing and is critical in apoptosis mediated via both perforin and granzymes as well as the Fas/Fas ligand pathway. The method utilizes fluorogenic caspase substrates that detect caspase activation within individual target cells. The substrates are composed of two covalently linked fluorophores that are cleaved by caspases. The uncleaved substrates form dimers, quenching the fluorescence, whereas the cleaved substrates produce detectable fluorescence. Cells can also be visualized at the single-cell level using confocal microscopy. The FCC assay, therefore, allows monitoring of cells undergoing apoptosis in real time at the individual cell level. Effector cells as well as target cells can also be studied using this methodology.

In a direct comparison with the ^{51}Cr release assay, the FCC assay is more sensitive than the CRA in detecting eptiope specific CTL response. This method additionally allowed direct visualization of the CTL killing process. The FCC assay enables monitoring of cellular immune responses in real time. It can be used to study CTL-mediated lysis of primary host target cells and not only immortalized cell lines.

Quantitative studies based on functional activity have been likewise applied to the identification of effector cells. Peter Lee described a flow cytometric technique to identify tumor cytolytic T cells *ex vivo*, based on identification of CD107a (Betts et al., 2003; Rubio et al., 2003). CD107a is an integral membrane protein in cytolytic granules and serves as a marker of degranulation upon interaction with tumor cells. This method identifies functional tumor reactive T cells with high recognition efficiency directly from PBMCs of cancer patients after vaccination, based on their clonal expansion and ability to kill tumor cells.

Another simple fluorescence based assay utilizes transfection of targets with a plasmid expressing enhanced green fluorescent protein (eGFP) (Kienzle et al., 2002). Unlike other fluorochrome-based methods, the expression of the transfected eGFP protein was continuous, hence leakage or loss of the fluorochrome was prevented during subsequent cell divisions. This exquisitely sensitive method measures the cytolytic activity of less than or equal to two T cells, enabling the detection of CTL in very small clones and in small numbers of T cells activated *in vivo*. Similarly, eGFP transfection can be used to test NK cell cytotoxicity against eGFP-transfected K562 target cells with high correlation to the standard ^{51}Cr assay. A 2 h incubation time gives comparable results to the optimal 4 h assay (Kantakamalakul et al., 2003).

PROSPECTS FOR THE FUTURE

While this brief review of techniques for measuring cytotoxicity is by no means exhaustive, it is evident that newer

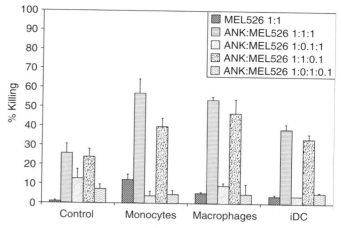

Figure 29.1 Measurement of melanoma cytotoxicity by NK:monocyte/macrophage/iDC co cultures using Yoyo-1. Activated NK:monocyte/macrophage/iDC co-cultures and MEL526 cytotoxicty. Activated NK cells (ANK) were cultured for 2 days in the presence of 1000 IU/ml IL-2 at 1×10^6 cells/ml. Monocytes were purified by CD14+ selection with CD14 MACS microbeads. Macrophages were cultured from MACS isolated CD14+ cells (1×10^6 cells/ml) for 6 days in the presence of 1000 IU/ml M-CSF. Immature dendritic cells (iDC) were cultured from MACS isolated CD14+ cells (1×10^6 cells/ml) for 6 days in the presence of 500 IU/ml GM-CSF and 250 IU/ml IL-4. Cells were added at ratios of 5×10^4 cells or 5×10^3 and incubated for 12 h. 1×10^6 MEL526 were labeled with 1 µg/ml Hoechst 33342 for 20 min at 37°C, washed and then added at 10 000 cells per well in a flat-bottom 96-well Falcon plate with various co-culture ratios. At 12 h, a final concentration of 100 nM Yoyo-1 was added to each well and incubated for 15 min at 37°C. The plate was read on the ArrayScan HCS Reader using the Target Activation assay. The algorithm parameters were set to identify Hoechst 33342 in the primary channel and Yoyo-1 in the secondary channel using a FITC-specific filter. The average fluorescence intensity/cell/well was measured for Yoyo-1. Controls were either MEL526 alone or MEL526 incubated with 0.1 per cent NP-40 for 15 min at 37°C. Per cent killing is reported as the mean of 3 replicates of ((sample−min)/(max−min)) × 100, where min = the average fluorescence intensity/cell/well for MEL526 alone and max = average fluorescence intensity/cell/well for MEL526 + 0.1 per cent NP-40.

methods offer the opportunity to study functional activity of effectors and target cells in real time, with increasing sensitivity, sometimes at the single cell level. The opportunity to study multiple parameters simultaneously is also offered by newer methodologies. Results from a novel method currently under investigation at the University of Pittsburgh are illustrated in Figure 29.1.

We are currently developing strategies to utilize eGFP-HMGB1 (Scaffidi et al., 2002) adenoviral transfected targets as a means to distinguish apoptotic and necrotic death, given the increasingly apparent importance of this distinction (Lotze and DeMarco, 2003; Vakkila et al., 2004. Standardization of measurement of cytotoxicity in the context of clinical investigations awaits the correlation of laboratory assays to a measurable clinical response.

REFERENCES

Alvarez, J.M., de Landazuri, M.O., Bonnard, G.D. and Herberman, R.B. (1978). Cytotoxic activities of normal cultured human T cells. J Immunol 121, 1270–1275.

Ashkenazi, A. (2002). Targeting death and decoy receptors of the tumour-necrosis factor superfamily. Nat Rev Cancer 2, 420–430.

Betts, M.R., Brenchley, J.M., Price, D.A. et al. (2003). Sensitive and viable identification of antigen-specific CD8+ T cells by a flow cytometric assay for degranulation. J Immunol Methods 281, 65–78.

Blomberg, K., Granberg, C., Hemmila, I. and Lovgren, T. (1986). Europium-labelled target cells in an assay of natural killer cell activity. I. A novel non-radioactive method based on time-resolved fluorescence. J Immunol Methods 86, 225–229.

Brown, J.P., van Belle, G. and Hellstrom, I. (1976). Design of experiments using the microcytotoxicity assay. Int J Cancer 18, 230–235.

Chahroudi, A., Silvestri, G. and Feinberg, M.B. (2003). Measuring T cell-mediated cytotoxicity using fluorogenic caspase substrates. Methods 31, 120–126.

Clay, T.M., Hobeika, A.C., Mosca, P.J., Lyerly, H.K. and Morse, M.A. (2001). Assays for monitoring cellular immune responses to active immunotherapy of cancer. Clin Cancer Res 7, 1127–1135.

Colangelo, D., Guo, H.Y., Connors, K.M., Silvestro, L. and Hoffman, R.M. (1992). Noncolorimetric measurement of cell activity in three-dimensional histoculture using the tetrazolium dye 3-(4,5-dimethylthiazol-2-yl)-2,5-diphenyltetrazolium bromide: the pixel image analysis of formazan crystals. Anal Biochem 205, 8–13.

Danilevicius, Z. (1973). Apoptosis: a factor in neoplastic growth? J Am Med Assoc 223, 434–435.

Djeu, J.Y., Heinbaugh, J.A., Vieira, W.D., Holden, H.T. and Herberman, R. B. (1979). The effect of immunopharmacological agents on mouse natural cell-mediated cytotoxicity and on its augmentation by poly I:C. Immunopharmacology 1, 231–244.

Giacomello, E., Neumayer, J., Colombatti, A. and Perris, R. (1999). Centrifugal assay for fluorescence-based cell adhesion adapted to the analysis of ex vivo cells and capable of determining relative binding strengths. Biotechniques 26, 758–762, 764–766.

Grossman, W.J., Revell, P.A., Lu, Z.H. et al. (2003). The orphan granzymes of humans and mice. Curr Opin Immunol 15, 544–552.

Hayon, T., Dvilansky, A., Shpilberg, O. and Nathan, I. (2003). Appraisal of the MTT-based assay as a useful tool for predicting drug chemosensitivity in leukemia. Leuk Lymphoma 44, 1957–1962.

Hellstrom, K.E., Hellstrom, I. and Bergheden, C. (1965). Allogeneic inhibition of tumour cells by in vitro contact with cells containing foreign H-2 antigens. Nature 208, 458–460.

Hellstrom, I., Hellstrom, K.E., Pierce, G.E. and Yang, J.P. (1968). Cellular and humoral immunity to different types of human neoplasms. Nature 220, 1352–1354.

Herberman, R.B., Bartram, S., Haskill, J.S. et al. (1977). Fc receptors on mouse effector cells mediating natural cytotoxicity against tumor cells. J Immunol 119, 322–326.

Hobeika, A.C., Clay, T. M., Mosca, P.J., Lyerly, H.K. and Morse, M.A. (2001). Quantitating therapeutically relevant T-cell responses to cancer vaccines. Crit Rev Immunol 21, 287–297.

Iselt, M., Holtei, W. and Hilgard, P. (1989). The tetrazolium dye assay for rapid in vitro assessment of cytotoxicity. Arzneimittelforschung 39, 747–749.

Jayaraman, S. (2003). Intracellular determination of activated caspases (IDAC) by flow cytometry using a pancaspase inhibitor labeled with FITC. Cytometry 56A, 104–112.

Jerome, K.R., Sloan, D.D. and Aubert, M. (2003). Measurement of CTL-induced cytotoxicity: the caspase 3 assay. Apoptosis 8, 563–571.

Jiao, H., Soejima, Y., Ohe, Y. et al. (1992). Differential macrophage-mediated cytotoxicity to P388 leukemia cells and its drug-resistant cells examined by a new MTT assay. Leuk Res 16, 1175–1180.

Kantakamalakul, W., Jaroenpool, J. and Pattanapanyasat, K. (2003). A novel enhanced green fluorescent protein (EGFP)-K562 flow cytometric method for measuring natural killer (NK) cell cytotoxic activity. J Immunol Methods 272, 189–197.

Kerr, J.F., Wyllie, A.H. and Currie, A.R. (1972). Apoptosis: a basic biological phenomenon with wide-ranging implications in tissue kinetics. Br J Cancer 26, 239–257.

Kienzle, N., Olver, S., Buttigieg, K. and Kelso, A. (2002). The fluorolysis assay, a highly sensitive method for measuring the cytolytic activity of T cells at very low numbers. J Immunol Methods 267, 99–108.

Lecoeur, H., Fevrier, M., Garcia, S., Riviere, Y. and Gougeon, M.L. (2001). A novel flow cytometric assay for quantitation and multiparametric characterization of cell-mediated cytotoxicity. J Immunol Methods 253, 177–187.

Lichtenfels, R., Biddison, W.E., Schulz, H., Vogt, A.B. and Martin, R. (1994). CARE-LASS (calcein-release-assay), an improved fluorescence-based test system to measure cytotoxic T lymphocyte activity. J Immunol Methods 172, 227–239.

Lieberman, J. (2003). The ABCs of granule-mediated cytotoxicity: new weapons in the arsenal. Nat Rev Immunol 3, 361–370.

Lotze, M.T. and Rosenberg, S.A. (1981). In vitro growth of cytotoxic human lymphocytes. III. The preparation of lectin-free T cell growth factor (TCGF) and an analysis of its activity. J Immunol 126, 2215–2220.

Lotze, M.T., Line, B.R., Mathisen, D.J. and Rosenberg, S.A. (1980a). The in vivo distribution of autologous human and murine lymphoid cells grown in T cell growth factor (TCGF): implications for the adoptive immunotherapy of tumors. J Immunol 125, 1487–1493.

Lotze, M.T., Strausser, J.L. and Rosenberg, S.A. (1980b). In vitro growth of cytotoxic human lymphocytes. II. Use of T cell growth factor (TCGF) to clone human T cells. J Immunol 124, 2972–2978.

Lotze, M.T., Grimm, E.A., Mazumder, A., Strausser, J.L. and Rosenberg, S.A. (1981). Lysis of fresh and cultured autologous tumor by human lymphocytes cultured in T-cell growth factor. Cancer Res 41, 4420–4425.

Lotze, M.T., Rayner, A.A. and Grimm, E.A. (1985). Problems with the isolation of lymphoid clones with reactivity to human tumors. Behring Inst Mitt 105–114.

Lotze, M.T., Ross, W.G., Tomita, S. and Custer, M.C. (1988). Cells invading tumors: strategies for the identification and expansion of tumor reactive lymphocytes. Transplant Proc 20, 326–331.

Lotze, M.T., Rubin, J.T. and Zeh, H.J. (1992a). New biologic agents come to bat for cancer therapy. Curr Opin Oncol 4, 1116–1123.

Lotze, M.T., Zeh, H.J., Elder, E.M. et al. (1992b). Use of T-cell growth factors (interleukins 2, 4, 7, 10, and 12) in the evaluation of T-cell reactivity to melanoma. J Immunother 12, 212–217.

Lotze, M.T. and DeMarco, R.A. (2003). Dealing with Death: HMGB1 As a Novel Target for Cancer Therapy. Curr Opin Investig Drugs.

Lovgren, J. and Blomberg, K. (1994). Simultaneous measurement of NK cell cytotoxicity against two target cell lines labelled with fluorescent lanthanide chelates. J Immunol Methods *173*, 119–125.

Lyerly, H.K. (2003). Quantitating cellular immune responses to cancer vaccines. Semin Oncol *30*, 9–16.

Lyerly, H.K., Morse, M.A. and Clay, T.M. (2001). Surrogate markers of effective anti-tumor immunity. Ann Surg Oncol *8*, 190–191.

Ozdemir, O., Ravindranath, Y. and Savasan, S. (2003). Cell-mediated cytotoxicity evaluation using monoclonal antibody staining for target or effector cells with annexinV/propidium iodide colabeling by fluorosphere-adjusted counts on three-color flow cytometry. Cytometry *56A*, 53–60.

Papadopoulos, N.G., Dedoussis, G.V., Spanakos, G. et al. (1994). An improved fluorescence assay for the determination of lymphocyte-mediated cytotoxicity using flow cytometry. J Immunol Methods *177*, 101–111.

Pieters, R., Huismans, D.R., Leyva, A. and Veerman, A.J. (1988). Adaptation of the rapid automated tetrazolium dye based (MTT) assay for chemosensitivity testing in childhood leukemia. Cancer Lett *41*, 323–332.

Rayner, A.A., Grimm, E.A., Lotze, M.T., Wilson, D.J. and Rosenberg, S.A. (1985a). Lymphokine-activated killer (LAK) cell phenomenon. IV. Lysis by LAK cell clones of fresh human tumor cells from autologous and multiple allogeneic tumors. J Natl Cancer Inst *75*, 67–75.

Rayner, A.A., Grimm, E.A., Lotze, M.T., Chu, E.W. and Rosenberg, S.A. (1985b). Lymphokine-activated killer (LAK) cells. Analysis of factors relevant to the immunotherapy of human cancer. Cancer *55*, 1327–1333.

Riccardi, C., Puccetti, P., Santoni, A. and Herberman, R.B. (1979). Rapid in vivo assay of mouse natural killer cell activity. J Natl Cancer Inst *63*, 1041–1045.

Roden, M.M., Lee, K.H., Panelli, M.C. and Marincola, F.M. (1999). A novel cytolysis assay using fluorescent labeling and quantitative fluorescent scanning technology. J Immunol Methods *226*, 29–41.

Rubio, V., Stuge, T.B., Singh, N. et al. (2003). Ex vivo identification, isolation and analysis of tumor-cytolytic T cells. Nat Med *9*, 1377–1382.

Santoni, A., Herberman, R.B. and Holden, H.T. (1979). Correlation between natural and antibody-dependent cell-mediated cytotoxicity against tumor targets in the mouse. II. Characterization of the effector cells. J Natl Cancer Inst *63*, 995–1003.

Sargent, J.M. (2003). The use of the MTT assay to study drug resistance in fresh tumour samples. Recent Results Cancer Res *161*, 13–25.

Scaffidi, P., Misteli, T. and Bianchi, M.E. (2002). Release of chromatin protein HMGB1 by necrotic cells triggers inflammation. Nature *418*, 191–195.

Sheehy, M.E., McDermott, A.B., Furlan, S.N., Klenerman, P. and Nixon, D.F. (2001). A novel technique for the fluorometric assessment of T lymphocyte antigen specific lysis. J Immunol Methods *249*, 99–110.

Smyth, M.J., Street, S.E. and Trapani, J.A. (2003). Cutting edge: granzymes A and B are not essential for perforin-mediated tumor rejection. J Immunol *171*, 515–518.

Strausser, J.L., Mazumder, A., Grimm, E.A., Lotze, M.T. and Rosenberg, S.A. (1981). Lysis of human solid tumors by autologous cells sensitized in vitro to alloantigens. J Immunol *127*, 266–271.

Telford, W.G., Komoriya, A. and Packard, B.Z. (2004). Multiparametric analysis of apoptosis by flow and image cytometry. Methods Mol Biol *263*, 141–160.

Vakkila, J., DeMarco, R.M. and Lotze, M.T. (2004). Rapid assessment of blood-derived dendritic cell activation by imaging cytometry.

Veugelers, K., Motyka, B., Frantz, C. et al. (2004). The granzyme B-serglycin complex from cytotoxic granules requires dynamin for endocytosis. Blood.

von Zons, P., Crowley-Nowick, P., Friberg, D. et al. (1997). Comparison of europium and chromium release assays: cytotoxicity in healthy individuals and patients with cervical carcinoma. Clin Diagn Lab Immunol *4*, 202–207.

Vujanovic, N.L., Nagashima, S., Herberman, R.B. and Whiteside, T.L. (1996). Nonsecretory apoptotic killing by human NK cells. J Immunol *157*, 1117–1126.

Wahlberg, B.J., Burholt, D.R., Kornblith, P. et al. (2001). Measurement of NK activity by the microcytotoxicity assay (MCA): a new application for an old assay. J Immunol Methods *253*, 69–81.

Zamai, L., Canonico, B., Gritzapis, A. et al. (2002). Intracellular detection of Bcl-2 and p53 proteins by flow cytometry: comparison of monoclonal antibodies and sample preparation protocols. J Biol Regul Homeost Agents *16*, 289–302.

Zamai, L., Burattini, S., Luchetti, F. et al. (2004). In vitro apoptotic cell death during erythroid differentiation. Apoptosis *9*, 235–246.

Zarcone, D., Tilden, A.B., Cloud, G. et al. (1986). Flow cytometry evaluation of cell-mediated cytotoxicity. J Immunol Methods *94*, 247–255.

Zeh, H.J. 3rd, Hurd, S., Storkus, W.J. and Lotze, M.T. (1993). Interleukin-12 promotes the proliferation and cytolytic maturation of immune effectors: implications for the immunotherapy of cancer. J Immunother *14*, 155–161.

Zeh, H.J., Leder, G.H., Lotze, M.T. et al. (1994). Flow-cytometric determination of peptide-class I complex formation. Identification of p53 peptides that bind to HLA-A2. Hum Immunol *39*, 79–86.

Zeh, H.J. 3rd, Perry-Lalley, D., Dudley, M.E., Rosenberg, S.A. and Yang, J.C. (1999). High avidity CTLs for two self-antigens demonstrate superior in vitro and in vivo antitumor efficacy. J Immunol *162*, 989–994.

Mixed Leukocyte Reactions

Chapter
30

Stella C. Knight, Penelope A. Bedford and Andrew J. Stagg

Antigen Presentation Research Group, Northwick Park Institute for Medical Research, Imperial College Faculty of Medicine, Harrow, UK

There is very little difference between one man and another; but what little there is, *is very important.*

An unlearned carpenter's comment reported by William James (1842–1910)

INTRODUCTION

In 1949 Li and Osgood reported the use of a saline extract of the red kidney bean, *Phaseolus vulgaris*, (called phyto-haemagglutinin, PHA) in a rapid method for separating leukocytes from blood or bone marrow; PHA caused red cell agglutination and rapid sedimentation and left leuko-cyte rich plasma that could be decanted. However, large blast cells appeared in the mononuclear cells separated in this way. Later Nowell showed formally that the bean extract PHA stimulated the formation of large 'primitive-looking' blast cells (Nowell, 1960). Shortly afterwards these cells were shown to be lymphoblasts derived from small lymphocytes (Carstairs, 1962). At the time when these first formal reports of lymphocyte transformation were appearing in the literature, Schrek and Donnelly noted that when leucocytes from two individuals were mixed – accidentally – large blast-like cells appeared in the cultures as assessed by phase contrast microscopy (Schrek and Donnelly, 1961). This mixed reaction was investigated using cells from human peripheral blood and significant increases in numbers of blast cells were shown routinely on mixing leukocytes from unrelated individuals (Bain and Lowenstein, 1964; Bain et al., 1964).

The degree of transformation was diminished if the cell donors were related or were from monozygotic twins as estimated not only by morphological observation but also from tritiated thymidine labeling followed by auto-radiography or scintillation counting (Hirschhorn et al., 1964; Oppenheim et al., 1965). Increased lymphocyte proliferation was reported in mixtures of cells taken from donors and recipients at the time of skin graft rejection; this activity was the result particularly of the proliferation of lymphocytes from the graft recipient (Oppenheim et al., 1965). This phenomenon of stimulation in mixtures of allogeneic cells was originally described as a 'mixed lymphocyte reaction' and became established rapidly as the *in vitro* counterpart to homograft recognition *in vivo*. It is still accepted that the activation in mixed cell cultures is a reflection of likely allograft recognition *in vivo*, although there have been many refinements in the practi-cal and theoretical knowledge of this allogeneic lympho-cyte stimulation.

In comparatively early work it was observed that 'macrophages' both of stimulator and of responder type contributed to the stimulation of allogeneic lymphocytes (Alter and Bach, 1970; Twomey et al., 1970; Mann and Abelson, 1980; Weinberger et al., 1982). The late 1970s and early 1980s saw the discovery that the major stimula-tors of the allogeneic proliferation using either mouse or human cells were dendritic antigen presenting cells (DC) (Steinman and Witmer, 1978; Crow and Kunkel, 1982). What had been known as the mixed lymphocyte reaction then became termed the mixed leukocyte reaction (MLR)

Measuring Immunity, edited by Michael T. Lotze and Angus W. Thomson
ISBN 0-12-455900-X, London

since this name more accurately reflected the cellular interactions that underlie the response. More recently, there is evidence that a proportion of the stimulatory capacity in the mixed leukocyte reaction may be indirect presentation of alloantigens via DC syngeneic with responder cells (Bedford et al., 1999). Both stimulator and responder DC may, therefore, be involved in the generation of the responses to allogeneic antigens in the mixed leukocyte reaction. The situation in the MLR *in vitro* reflects closely the practical observation of *in vivo* homograft rejection. In the *in vivo* homograft rejection it was originally believed that direct stimulation of immune response by alloantigens on DC was the major route of activation of alloreactivity (Knight et al., 1983; Lechler and Batchelor, 1982). However, despite evidence that direct stimulation by allogeneic DC may occur (Song et al., 1999) it has become apparent that a major route *in vivo* is via secondary presentation of alloantigens by dendritic cells of the recipient type (Benichou et al., 1997).

APPLICATIONS

MLR as a measure of homograft reactivity

From the introductory comments it is apparent that the MLR has multiple applications. One area is still in assessing histocompatibility between the donor and recipient of a graft in order to gauge the likely immunological stimulation on grafting. The main histocompatibility differences can be assessed from tissue typing but the responses observed in MLR will include additional effects. The relevance of disparities in major histocompatibility antigens and others induced by minor antigens, not generally assessed by tissue typing, can be more directly assessed by using an MLR (Jeras, 2002). Increased stimulation, due to presensitization of recipients to donor antigens caused by earlier grafting, may also contribute to the MLR.

MLR as a surrogate primary T cell stimulation

There were two major anomalies initially recognized between the MLR and normal primary responses to exogenous antigens. First, a high proportion of lymphocytes was stimulated in response to alloantigens compared with the proportion responding to specific antigens (Chalmers et al., 1966). Thus, primary proliferative responses were not identified when antigens were added to populations of naive T cells containing antigen-presenting cells *in vitro*. However, when antigen-pulsed DC are added to responder populations, there are specific primary proliferative and cytotoxic T cell responses *in vitro* (Macatonia et al., 1989). Exogenous antigens can, thus, be acquired by DC, processed via the MHC class I pathway and presented to cause a primary proliferative response *in vitro*. This stimulation indicates that that more cells than originally believed are able to respond to individual antigens if the culture conditions are appropriate. The identification of specific responder cells using tetramer technology confirms that

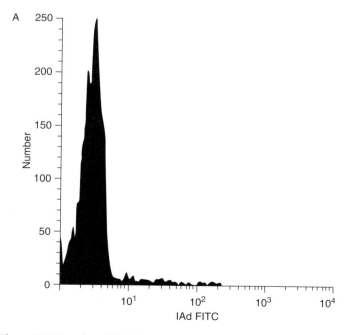

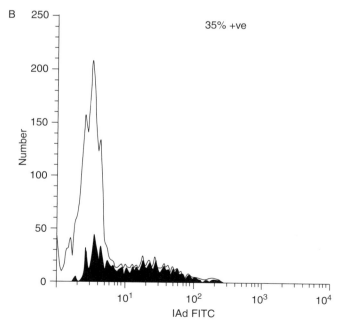

Figure 30.1 Transfer of MHC class II antigens between allogeneic dendritic cells. Dendritic cells were separated from the spleens of CBA and BALB/c mice. Cells were mixed in culture and incubated for 2 h at 37°C or mixed on ice and immediately labeled with antibodies to I-A^k and I-A^d. Using 2-color flow cytometry, the I-A^k positive cells were gated and then the 1-A^d labeling of these cells measured. Double labeling for both class II molecules was assessed by subtracting the I-A^d labelling of the 0 h mix (A) from the I-A^d labelling of the 2 h mix (B). Using the super-enhanced Dmax method in Winlist (Verity Software House, Topsham ME) 35 per cent of the DC were shown to have become positive for both class II molecules.

substantially more T cells than originally believed can recognize individual T cell epitopes (Klenerman et al., 2002). Although the proportions of cells responding in an MLR are still high – up to 5 per cent of cells may respond – the numbers responding to individual T cell epitopes can reach in the order of a tenth of that number.

Second, in normal syngeneic stimulation of primary immune responses to antigens there is restriction of the responses associated with responder type MHC (Zinkernagel and Doherty, 1997); the stimulation of an MLR occurring across an allogeneic boundary (Song et al., 1999) was therefore again considered unusual. Restriction of cytotoxic T cell responses to the MHC of the stimulator type reinforces the idea that there is direct stimulation of allogeneic T cells by DC. However, there is increasing evidence of transfer of alloantigens between DC in the MLR. The antigen transfer between allogeneic DC is significant and has been identified using specific anti-class II antibodies in the mouse (Bedford et al., 1999). In Figure 30.1 the transfer of alloantigens between lymph node DC from BALB/c and CBA mice after a 2-h incubation is shown.

The MHC is transferred in such a way that conformation is maintained since the transferred MHC antigens are still recognized by antibodies to the strain specific MHC molecules. Any subsequent presentation of alloantigens via DC syngeneic with responder cells means that the stimulation is more compatible with the syngeneic presentation seen in normal primary immune responses to exogenous antigens. However, since there is no evidence of restriction to responder type MHC, the relative importance of syngeneic (indirect) versus allogeneic (direct) presentation of MHC molecules in the MLR remains difficult to establish. Nevertheless, transfer of antigens between DC and indirect presentation of antigens to T cells may be more prevalent than has been appreciated. Exogenously acquired antigens are transferred between syngeneic DC in stimulation of primary T cell responses *in vitro* (Knight et al., 1998). Thus antigen-pulsed DC transfer processed antigens to DC not directly exposed to antigen. Indirect stimulation may form an integral part of primary T cell stimulation either in the MLR or in primary presentation of exogenous antigens (Knight et al., 2002). The MLR also reprises the *in vivo* events of primary T cell responses to antigens since a major route of presentation *in vivo* can also be indirect presentation. When syngeneic DC exposed to exogenous antigen *in vitro* are given *in vivo*, DC of the recipient participate in the generation of a primary immune response (Lambrecht et al., 2000; Kleindienst and Brocker, 2003). The reason for the potency of DC in stimulating a primary MLR may be questioned in the light of observations showing that the stimulation can occur not only by direct stimulation but also by indirect presentation. It may be expected that any cells bearing MHC molecules could 'donate' these antigens to DC of responder type to stimulate primary responses. However, the high levels of MHC molecules expressed by DC and the extraordinary effectiveness of DC in both

donating and acquiring MHC antigens demonstrated in Figure 30.1 is probably one of the factors that underlie their potency at stimulation of an MLR. All in all the MLR may be an entirely appropriate surrogate test for the capacity of DC to stimulate normal primary immune responses since, in each case, there is evidence both for direct and indirect stimulation by DC. Further understanding of the different roles of both direct antigen bearing (stimulator DC) and those DC acquiring the antigens secondarily and presenting them (responder type DC) in the MLR should allow the assessment of different mechanisms for alteration or deficiency in immune function.

MLR as a functional test for DC

The MLR has also become the standard functional test to identify DC; DC are the only cells known to be potent stimulators of primary T cell responses (Knight and Stagg, 1993). The experimental assessment of primary stimulation using the MLR will indicate the functional capacity of DC that is in turn affected by many genetic and environmental aspects of the DC. Factors affecting stimulatory capacity of DC include their state of maturity; immature DC may be poor stimulators of allogeneic T cells and may even have tolerogenic effects. The subtype of DC, the types of antigens to which they have been exposed and the consequent cytokine profile of the stimulatory DC will all influence the outcome of primary stimulation by DC (Banchereau et al., 2000). Thus, the MLR can be used to assess the basic capacity of DC, including those produced for various forms of immunotherapy, to stimulate primary immune responses. The types of T cells stimulated and the type of response elicited (e.g. the cytokine production) may also be assessed to give a picture of the stimulatory effects of different DC populations on the lymphocytes activated in primary stimulation.

THE ASSAY

In the 1960s the proliferative responses in lymphocytes in an MLR were already measured using tritiated thymidine uptake. Over the next decade thymidine uptake was shown to occur in the form of bell-shaped response curves with time, dose of stimulator cells and dose of responder cells all interacting. Therefore simply describing 'higher' or 'lower' responses or percentage change in counts per minute from scintillation counting of the radioactivity, which is still often done, is likely to give a false picture of stimulation. There is a need to define the position on the response curves in order to interpret responses. Some of the practical issues of interpretation of the mixed leukocyte reaction will be discussed in detail in this chapter since this technique is arguably one of the most abused and inappropriately applied techniques. We shall draw mainly on work from our own laboratory accrued over four decades to demonstrate these practical issues.

The elements of the MLR

The main elements that interact during the development of a primary MLR are shown in the cartoon at the top of Figure 30.2.

Dendritic cells of the stimulator type express antigens that are allogeneic to those of the responder. Since there is evidence that at least part of the response is an indirect simulation, the stimulator type DC must interact with the responder DC and transfer of MHC molecules occurs. This interaction appears most efficient with cell-cell contact, although supernatant material from allogeneic DC may substitute for the live DC-DC contact. In our hands, this latter system is comparatively ineffective and the secreted material that can stimulate an MLR is labile and short lived (Bedford et al., 1999). It could be that direct nibbling of

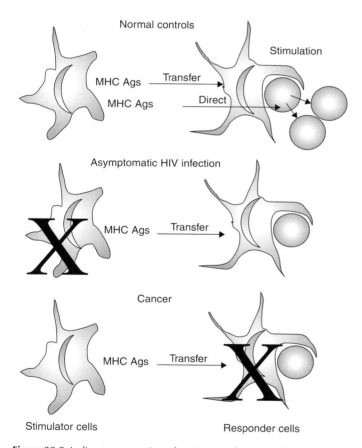

Figure 30.2 Indirect presentation of antigens in the MLR. This cartoon shows the contributions of stimulator (left) and donor (right) dendritic cells in the mixed leukocyte reaction. In the normal MLR (top) direct and indirect mechanisms of stimulation of allogeneic T-cells are depicted. If a major contribution of the indirect pathway is present (see text), then the suggestions made for the defects that occur in asymptomatic HIV and for cancer become relevant. Thus, in asymptomatic HIV infection (in patients with no lymphadenopathy and without treatment) the DC from patients are defective and fail to stimulate but their cells give normal MLR responses; the latter finding means that both the lymphocytes and DC within responder cell populations must be functioning normally. Conversely, responder DC in patients with cancer can block ongoing responsiveness in MLR reactions.

MHC molecules from live cells by allogeneic DC through scavenger receptor molecules (Harshyne et al., 2003) is the major route of antigen transfer. By contrast other work suggests that MHC class II molecules are shed into the supernatants of DC in the form of exosomes and that this material can be acquired and presented by other DC to stimulate immune responses (Thery et al., 2002; Vincent-Schneider et al., 2002). The use of such materials as novel vaccine candidates has been postulated (Zitvogel et al., 1998) Thus, there is a number of ways in which antigens may be acquired indirectly so that DC of responder type can present the alloantigens to syngeneic T cells. Direct allogeneic presentation of antigen is indicated since there is residual T cell stimulation after responder type DC have been removed. However, it is difficult to rule out the presence of small numbers of residual responder type DC, which may contribute to residual T cell stimulation observed.

The numbers and proportion of stimulator and responder DC, the numbers and proportion of responder lymphocytes and the total cell density dictated by the surface area of the culture vessel together with the time allowed for the cells to interact will all be factors influencing the cellular interactions required for the development of the proliferative activity. These factors all contribute to bell-shaped response curves, so the simple designations of higher or lower responses often presented may only reflect the true situation over a narrow range of conditions.

The use of tritiated thymidine

Thymidine is an alternative pathway nucleotide precursor and in mixed leukocyte cultures the cells are likely to contribute insignificant amounts of thymidine so what is added is virtually all that is present. Thymidine is also broken down by the cells to thymine and after a few hours in culture may become unavailable (Cleaver, 1967). Thus a major feature in many MLR protocols is that the thymidine is initially limiting, or becomes limiting or unavailable during the pulse period. Uptake then reflects not only the DNA synthesis itself but also the availability of the thymidine. Unavailability will be more apparent in highly stimulated cultures where more of the precursor is removed by uptake into dividing cells. For this reason, the concentration of thymidine present for a high stimulation may need to be as much as 0.5–1 μg/ml if it is to be freely available, whereas low level responses may plateau with as little as 0.1–0.2 μg/ml (Thorpe and Knight, 1974). The breakdown of the thymidine to thymine becomes significant after 6 h (and possibly after 2 h) (Farrant et al., 1980) so that a pulse time longer than 6 h with the thymidine may be inappropriate. Since more thymidine can sometimes be added at the beginning of a long pulse time without affecting the uptake in stimulated cultures it may seem logical to believe that the thymidine remains in flooding conditions (Thorpe and Knight, 1974); however, for longer pulse times addition of more thymidine 6 h or more after the initial pulse increases the uptake demonstrating the increasing unavailability of thymidine with time (Farrant et al., 1980). If the amount of thymidine is in excess throughout the pulse time then small inaccuracies in the addition of the thymidine make no difference to the uptake measured. Too great an addition of thymidine – in the order of >10 μg/ml – blocks the cells in the G1 phase of cell cycle and has been used in protocols aimed at synchronizing cells (Cooper, 2003).

The next consideration is the use of the tritiated precursor. The radiation emission path of tritium is so small that only the cells that incorporate the tritiated thymidine are subject to significant irradiation and are damaged preferentially. This damaging effect contrasts with that seen when using other radioactive isotopes in culture which, because of their longer emission path lengths, will effectively irradiate all the cells in the culture equally. The specific activity of the thymidine that is taken into the DNA, i.e. the proportion that is radioactive, rather than the total amount of radioactivity added to the culture will influence the amount of radioactive exposure and consequent damage received by the cells. Increases in the specific activity of the tritiated thymidine cause more cell damage but these effects are proportional and do not interact with other culture variables such as time, dose of stimulant or cell concentration. Thus accurate reflection of DNA synthesis can theoretically be obtained with thymidine over a range of different specific activities. However, use of excess tritiated thymidine that has a specific activity of greater than 6 Ci/mM may mean that radiation damage to the cells causes greater loss of counts through cell damage than any increased counts due to greater radioactivity added (Thorpe and Knight, 1974). Thymidine of specific activities around 10 Ci/mM can be used specifically to kill dividing cells. In those papers where thymidine of 21 Ci/mM has been used to measure thymidine incorporation into dividing cells only a low amount of thymidine has been added so that insufficient radioactive material is taken up into the cells to cause damage. Under these conditions high counts of radioactivity are obtained but the limited availability of the precursor in addition to the DNA synthesis influences the counts. Strangely, these facts mean that those stimulation assays that are measured in hundreds of thousands of counts are often those where the conditions of thymidine incorporation particularly reflect the lack of availability of the precursor as well as uptake into DNA. This situation of using small amounts of hot thymidine may be useful as a sensitive test for assessing whether or not there is a response since small amounts of incorporated thymidine give high counts. Under these conditions, counts in cultures with different levels of DNA synthesis will give values in a pecking order related to the relative amounts of DNA synthesis but the discrimination between different levels of DNA synthesis will be reduced due to the limiting thymidine (Thorpe and Knight, 1974). In our laboratory, for measuring relative amounts of DNA synthesis, we use thymidine at 1 μg/ml to ensure its free availability, a pulse time of 2 h to be certain that thymidine

remains in excess during the pulse time and a specific activity of 2 Ci/mM to ensure that radioactive damage is minimal (Knight, 1987). Despite concern that uptake of tritiated thymidine that we report can be lower than the background counts in some other studies, this type of protocol produces results that reflect closely the relative amounts of DNA synthesis in the cultures.

Influence of culture variables on thymidine uptake

The proportion of a lymphocyte population that responds to alloantigens in the mixed leukocyte reaction varies and is not usually known. The proportion of specific responder cells within the whole lymphocyte population is also critical in determining the total number of cells required to see primary T cell stimulation (Thorpe and Knight, 1974). Figure 30.3 shows the thymidine uptake seen in different numbers of peripheral blood mononuclear cells when stimulated with different numbers of allogeneic cells; there are two stimulator cell populations homozygous for different D locus antigens. For demonstrating the interactive variables affecting the MLR, cells from two B cell lines are used as the stimulator cells in these experiments since activated B cells may also stimulate primary immune responses (Metlay et al., 1989). The cell line used on the right shares a D locus antigen with the responder cells (DR2). The counts per minute from triplicate cultures of five concentrations of responder lymphocytes were each stimulated with six concentrations of allogeneic cells. The stimulator cells were treated with mitomycin C (Sigma) at 40 μg/ml for 25 min to allow the maintenance of stimulatory capacity while blocking the capacity of the cells to proliferate thus ensuring a unidirectional stimulation. (An alternative way of preventing cells from within the stimulator cell population from contributing to the thymidine uptake is to irradiate 1000–2000 rads.) The results are expressed in two-dimensional graphs (Figure 30.3A and B) showing the uptake of tritiated thymidine in different numbers of peripheral blood lymphocytes with single response curves for each dose of stimulator cells.

Alternatively, the responses in different numbers of responder cells on stimulation with different numbers of stimulator cells were used as a matrix to provide a stable response surface with contours joining points at 500 counts per minute intervals (Figure 30.3C and D). The peak response in each case is similar (9000–9500 counts per minute) but the conditions of cell concentration required to produce this maximum response are dramatically different between the stimuli tested. On the left the individual responses required fewer total responder and stimulator cells in culture to produce responses reflecting the presence of a larger proportion of cells responding to the stimulation. There is often a preoccupation in producing the correct ratio of responder and stimulator cells and the graphs show that this ratio is important. However, surprisingly, if there are higher numbers of responder cells then better responses are obtained with lower numbers

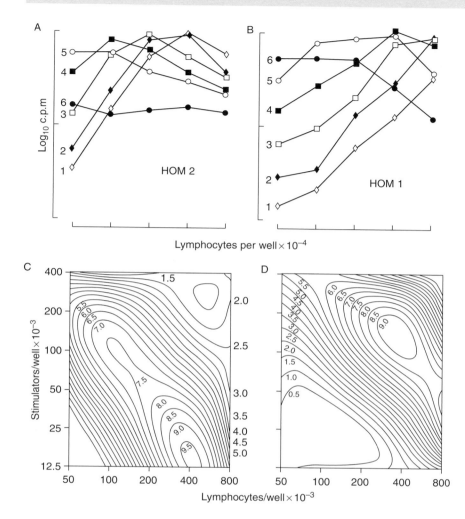

Figure 30.3 The effects of concentration of stimulator and responder cells in the MLR. In this experiment stimulator cells were different concentrations of cells from B cell lines homozygous for DR1 (Hom 2, A, C) and for DR2 (Hom 1, B, D). An MLR was stimulated in different numbers of normal peripheral blood lymphocytes from an individual that expressed DR2 but not DR1. Thus the graphs on the right represent responses where there was partial histocompatibility for the MHC antigens between the stimulator and responder cells. The uptake of tritiated thymidine is shown in the upper graphs as different response curves for each concentration of stimulator cells where the stimulator concentrations $\times 10^{-3}$ were 1,12.5; 2, 25; 3, 50; 4, 100; 5, 200; and 6, 400. The lower graphs show the counts per minute in a three-dimensional graph form where the responses were used to generate a response matrix and contours were drawn for responses at 500 count intervals. The peak response where there was partial histocompatibility required higher numbers of both stimulator and responder cells.

of stimulator cells and vice versa. This relationship probably reflects the requirement to have appropriate numbers of cells that can contact one another in the time available to interact within the confines of the culture vessel. For each ratio of responder to stimulator cells there is an optimal total cell number to produce the maximal response. If the same cells are put onto a smaller surface area then peak responses occur at lower total cell numbers (Thorpe and Knight, 1974). The interpretation of this stimulation data is that lymphocytes, despite the fact that they are non-adherent, make cell contacts and generally exhibit contact inhibition of growth at higher concentrations of specific responder cells (Knight, 1982).

In most MLR studies it is likely that responses are measured either on the up-slope or on the plateau of the response with lower total cell numbers (Figure 30.3A and C). Thus, under these fixed conditions, responses requiring more cells will be seen as low or negative and 'typing' reactions can be undertaken to determine the degree of histo-incompatibility. Figure 30.4 shows single point responses of cells from normal controls and from individuals with multiple sclerosis to stimulation with cells from the cell lines homozygous for HLA-DR antigens.

A single set of 'optimized' culture conditions was chosen. Cells from a high proportion of the multiple sclerosis patients show 'low' responses to cells bearing this antigen under the single set of conditions chosen reflecting the high proportion of patients expressing DR2. It is often on this type of single point data that lymphocyte responsiveness is assessed.

The data in Figures 30.2, 30.3 and 30.4 show results obtained only at a single time point in culture. Figure 30.5 shows information for stimulating mixed leukocyte reactions for different lengths of culture.

Cells initially enter the response at early times in culture as seen for mouse cells (Figure 30.5A). With longer times in culture, lower concentrations of cells have time to interact and enter the response so that the peak response is seen at progressively lower cell concentrations as time proceeds (Figure 30.5A, mouse and Figure 30.5B, human cells) before, finally, the response declines (Knight and Burman, 1981). There is, however, a close correlation between the time in culture when peak responses are obtained and the number of responder lymphocytes present with higher numbers of responder cells resulting in earlier peak responses. The fallacy of comparisons at single cell concentrations or time points, as indicated from Figures 30.2–30.5, comes when lower counts per minute are designated as lower responses on the basis of single point data without the knowledge of the position on the curves. Lower responses can reflect the presence of too many or too few responder or stimulator cells at

that time in culture. Optimized conditions may also be inappropriate where individuals may have different total proportions of responder T cells and DC for example as a result of disease processes or from lower lymphocyte counts in blood resulting from habitual exercise or higher numbers following a brief unusual bout of exercise. The sideways shift on the cell concentration axis of a response curve in relation to a control curve will give variable comparative results depending on the total cell concentration in culture chosen for that comparison.

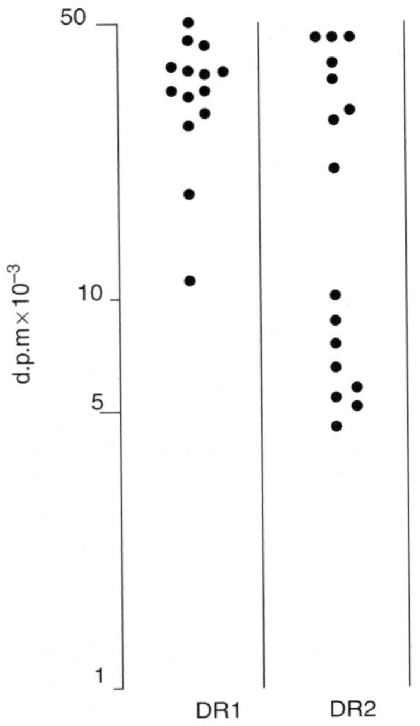

Assessment of 'suppressor' or 'regulatory' effects of cell populations can also be misinterpreted. Increased suppression can merely reflect the addition of a population of cells with a high proportion of responder cells contributing to the cell concentration curves with the consequent rapid decline in responses at higher cell concentrations. These multi-parameter data demonstrate the pitfalls of interpreting in vitro lymphocyte stimulation assays and invoking the concept of suppressor or regulatory cells when simple cell concentration studies and kinetics have not been worked out. The argument is given that 'regulatory' cells in vivo also produce inhibitory effects. However, cell contact inhibition is presumably as effective as a growth control mechanism within the limited confines of immune organs in vivo. However, for in vitro stimulation of an MLR using cells from normal individuals, comparison of responses using a single set of conditions in the early phase of a response curve can show variability that is, over a narrow range, linearly related to the number of cells entering the response. Such results can give information reflecting the level of responsiveness and degree of compatibility. However, particularly in disease situations or under experimental conditions using separated cells, differences under optimized conditions will require time,

Figure 30.4 Tissue typing reactions using MLR. Peripheral blood lymphocytes (2×10^5) from patients with multiple sclerosis were stimulated in an MLR with cells from the cell lines homozygous for DR1 and DR2 (2.5×10^4). Under these conditions cells from a group of patients gave low responses to the DR2 positive cell line reflecting the presence of DR2 in a high proportion of the patients.

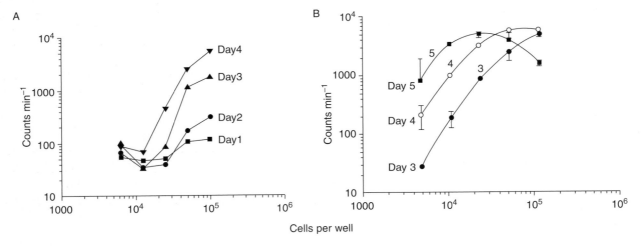

Figure 30.5 The effect of time in culture on thymidine uptake in the MLR. Different numbers of responder lymphocytes from mouse lymph node (A) or from human peripheral blood (B) were stimulated with fixed stimulator cell concentration (125 allogeneic DC or 2.5×10^3 B cell line cells respectively). These cells were cultured for different culture periods before pulsing for 2 h with tritiated thymidine and processing for liquid scintillation counting. The cells slowly entered the response and increased during the early time period (A). With longer times in culture, responses were seen progressively in the cultures initially containing smaller numbers of responder cells which were given time to respond (B).

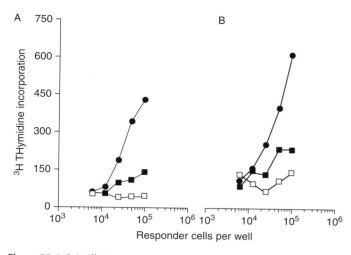

Figure 30.6 Scintillation counting versus imaging for measuring uptake of tritiated thymidine. An MLR was set up in 20 μl hanging drop cultures in Terasaki plates. Responder cells were different numbers of CBA lymph node cells (○) stimulated with 500 (■) or 1000 (●) allogeneic BALB/c splenic DC. After 3 days of culture the cells were pulsed for 2 h with tritiated thymidine (1 μg/ml, 2 Ci/mM). The cells were then blotted onto filters and washed with saline, trichloracetic acid to precipitate the DNA and methanol to decolorize and dry the filters. The filter was either cut into individual filter discs and counted individually in a scintillation counter (A), or the whole filter was exposed to a tritium screen for 4 h and imaged on a phosphor imager and the counts for the areas corresponding to the individual cultures were quantified (B). Means from triplicate cultures are shown. There was a good correlation between the counts obtained by the two methods (r = 0.967).

dose and cell concentration studies in order fully to interpret the differences in responses.

In our own laboratory we have addressed the problems of comparing lymphocyte stimulation in different samples by miniaturizing the system so that cultures are performed in 20 μl hanging drops in Terasaki plates with a range of stimulator and responder cell concentrations. Uptake of tritiated thymidine is assessed by liquid scintillation counting of samples blotted onto filter discs (Knight, 1987). More recently, instead of measuring counts in individually cut filter discs, we have been blotting the 60 20 μl cultures onto a single filter that is then imaged on a phosphor imager with a tritium screen. There is a close correlation between the counts per minute obtained from scintillation counting of the filter discs and the counts obtained on a phosphor imager after a 4 h exposure of the tritium screen (Figure 30.6).

In these small cultures it is easier to vary responder and stimulator lymphocyte and dendritic cell numbers within individual experiments. Analysis of variance then allows us to assess the effects of different variables in culture and the significance of differences between different samples and culture conditions (Knight, 1987).

Use of CFSE to assess proliferation

Flow cytometry based methods are being developed as alternatives to ³H-thymidine incorporation for measuring

MLR. These approaches offer the advantages that they avoid the use of radioisotopes and provide scope for obtaining additional information about the proliferating cells. In one such approach the responder cell population is labeled with the dye 5- (and 6-) carboxyfluorescein diacetate succinimidyl ester (CFSE; Molecular Probes, Eugene OR) prior to setting up the MLR assay. Staining with this cytoplasmic dye is rapid and the labeling is stable for prolonged periods *in vitro* and *in vivo* with little or no adverse effects on the cells. Upon cell division the dye partitions equally between daughter cells and these can be visualized on the flow cytometer (Givan et al., 1999). When fluorescence is plotted on a logarithmic scale undivided cells appear at the far right and to the left of these are a series of peaks corresponding to cells that have gone though one, two, three and so on, cell divisions (Figure 30.7).

Figure 30.7A illustrates the technique using responses to stimulation with anti-CD3. The left-hand panel shows a dose response curve using ³H-thymidine incorporation to measure cell proliferation. The next two panels show parallel flow cytometry data using CFSE labeled cells. The middle shows cells cultured for 3 days without stimulation and shows the level of labeling in undivided cells; the right hand panel shows cells cultured for 3 days with anti-CD3 (4 mg/ml). The same approach can be used to measure responses to allogeneic stimulation in an MLR; Figure 30.7B illustrates the proliferation of CFSE labeled BALB/c T cells stimulated for 6 days with dendritic cells from CBA mice. In this instance, the longer culture period has meant that most of the cells have gone through a similar number of divisions.

To quantify the proliferative response in CFSE assays the proportion of cells that have undergone one or more cell divisions can readily be determined. However, this analysis makes the assumption that non-dividing cells survive, at least in a form detectable with the 'gate' used for cytometric analysis and that this survival and detection is not influenced by the presence or absence of proliferating cells. This assumption may not be valid since cytokines in stimulated cultures may influence survival of non-dividing cells or removal of dying cells by macrophages. Therefore, in a modification of the original method we have added fluorescent beads to the flow cytometry tubes so that absolute numbers of dividing cells, rather than the proportion of dividing cells, can be assessed (Stagg et al., 2002).

Extending this absolute number calculation further it is possible to obtain an estimate of the frequency of cells responsive to a particular stimulus present at the start of the culture. This precursor frequency (pf) can be estimated by the formula:

$$pf = \left[\sum_{k=1}^{k=\max} N/2^k \right] / I$$

where N is the absolute number of cells per well in generation 'k' at the time of the assay and I is the total number

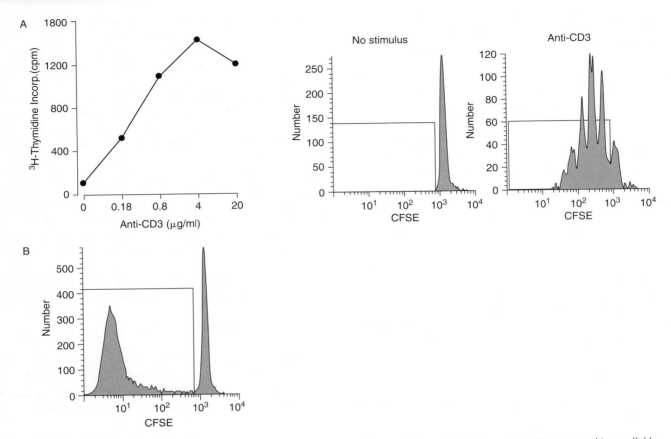

Figure 30.7 (A) Proliferative responses of lymph node cells (LNC) from BALB/c mice to soluble anti-CD3 (clone 145-2C11) assessed in parallel by ^{3}H-thymidine incorporation (left hand panel) and by flow cytometry using CFSE labeled cells (right hand panel). CFSE labeled LNC cultured with medium alone are shown in the center panel. For the ^{3}H-thymidine assay, 5×10^4 LNC were cultured in 20 μl hanging drop cultures for 3 days with 0–20 μg/ml anti-CD3 and proliferation assessed by liquid scintillation counting. For the flow cytometry assay, LNC were labeled with 5 μM CFSE and cultured, with 4 μg/ml anti-CD3 or medium alone, for 3 days at a concentration of 4×10^5 LNC per well in flat-bottomed microtiter plates. At this timepoint, the contents of each well were harvested and examined by flow cytometry. Histogram peaks in the marked regions indicate cells that had undergone one or more cell divisions; cells to the right of the region had not divided. (B) Measurement of an MLR by flow cytometry. LNC from BALB/c mice were labeled with 5 μM CFSE and cultured at a concentration of 4×10^5 per well in a flat-bottomed microtiter plate with 8×10^3 lymph node dendritic cells from CBA mice. The contents of the wells were harvested after 6 days of culture and examined by flow cytometry. By this time, all responsive cells have undergone multiple rounds of division.

of input cells added per well at initiation of the culture. For the parental generation, k = 0 and for the maximum number of generations detectable in the experiment k = max.

Estimates of precursor frequency can also be obtained using ^{3}H-thymidine in limiting dilution assays (LDA). LDA uses the zero term of the Poisson distribution to estimate frequency from multiple replicate wells at different input cell concentrations, each of which are scored positive or negative for a response (Waldmann and Lefkovits, 1984). These are large assays, separate from the standard MLR and can be difficult to perform.

One advantage of the CFSE approach is that, in multicolor flow cytometers, staining with antibodies in the remaining channels can be used to determine the phenotype of responding cells and to measure other functional characteristics such as cytokine production.

The response measured in the CFSE assay is a cumulative one with the measurement made over the entire culture period. Therefore one source of variability in the ^{3}H-thymidine assay is eliminated, namely the timing of the pulse of thymidine relative to the proliferation in culture. However, it should be cautioned that variability associated with different cell concentrations, proportions and densities will still contribute to the calculated number of cells responding. These issues have not been explored experimentally in the CFSE system.

FUTURE PROSPECTS

Separate effects of stimulator- and responder-type DC

The recognition that both stimulator- and responder-type DC are involved in the generation of an MLR means that the separate effects of the two DC populations contributing to the development of a primary immune response can be studied. This separation of the two types of DC is already providing additional information about the nature of defects in immunity in different conditions. One example is in infection with human immunodeficiency virus type 1 (HIV). The DC from untreated patients with asymptomatic HIV infection, without evidence of lymphadenopathy, stimulate only low levels of MLR. By contrast, lymphocytes taken from the same patients respond normally to stimulation with normal allogeneic DC (Macatonia et al., 1990). This observation indicates that the defect in DC in this condition may be in the capacity of the DC to donate appropriately processed antigen to other DC (see Figure 30.1B).

The reverse picture is seen using cells from patients with cancers of the head and neck. DC from these individuals can block the response of their own T cells in the MLR (Almand et al., 2001). In this example the defect appears to be in the endogenous DC in the responding cells from the patients. Such endogenous DC are required in the generation of an effective response to tumour antigen delivered by DC. Under these conditions the use of antigen pulsed DC bearing tumor antigens for therapy may be ineffective (Kleindienst and Brocker, 2003).

Flow-based techniques

The use of flow-based techniques as described above opens the way to more analytical approaches to the assessment of activities of cells participating in the MLR. With the aid of multicolor flow cytometry, the phenotyping of different lymphocyte and DC populations plus the intracellular measurement of proteins that they produce (e.g. cytokines, chemokines or molecules of different signaling pathways), the functional attributes of the different participating cells may be measured. Much more information may thus be obtained about the potential effects of DC produced for immunotherapy.

CONCLUSIONS

The MLR can be used to assess the histocompatibility differences between two individuals by the recognition of histocompatibility antigens differentially expressed on DC of stimulator and responder type. The test also assesses *in vitro* the ability of DC to initiate primary immune responses either directly or indirectly. The MLR will also measure the capacity of different lymphocyte populations to respond to primary stimulation. The practicalities of the major test system of measuring responses using tritiated thymidine uptake appear to be mainly lost in the pre-computerized literature. Some of these practicalities are revisited here. These problems include the method for utilization of tritiated thymidine as a reflection of DNA synthesis without the complications of decreasing availability of the precursor in culture and ways of minimizing the effects of radiation-induced damage specifically to dividing cells. In addition, the effects of numbers and densities of stimulator and

responder DC/lymphocytes at different times in culture described provide information allowing the MLR to be used more accurately to reflect the differences between different samples. The dangers of assuming that specific suppressor or regulator cells are the reason that lower responses are obtained on addition of different cell populations are demonstrated from the curves showing cell contact inhibition at high densities of responder cells. Kinetic/cell concentration experiments may be required to interpret differences obtained in the MLR under a set of optimized conditions. Flow based techniques, such as the use of CFSE for measurement of an MLR, are being developed and allow assessment of the numbers and types of cells dividing in the MLR. There is a need to be able to measure with an *in vitro* test the function of both DC and lymphocytes in the stimulation of primary immune responses. However, there is still much to be gained from a more critical approach to the measurement of lymphocyte stimulation in the MLR as a test system reflecting primary immune responses.

ACKNOWLEDGEMENTS

We would like to thank Alison Scoggins for her administrative assistance in the production of this chapter.

REFERENCES

Almand, B., Clark, J.I., Nikitina, E. et al. (2001). Increased production of immature myeloid cells in cancer patients: a mechanism of immunosuppression in cancer. J Immunol 166, 678–689.
Alter, B.J. and Bach, F.H. (1970). Lymphocyte reactivity in vitro. Cellular reconstitutuion of the purified lymphocyte response. Cell Immunol 1, 207–218.
Bain, B. and Lowenstein, L. (1964). Genetic studies on the mixed reaction. Science 145, 1315.
Bain, B., Vas, M.R. and Lowenstein, L. (1964). The development of large immature mononuclear cells in mixed leucocyte cultures. Blood 23, 108.
Bancereau, J., Briere, F., Caux, C. et al. (2000). Immunobiology of dendritic cells. Annu Rev Immunl 18, 767–811.
Bedford, P., Garner, K. and Knight, S.C. (1999). MHC class II molecules transferred between allogeneic dendritic cells stimulate primary mixed leukocyte reactions. Int Immunol 11, 1739–1744.
Benichou, G., Tam, R.C., Soares, L.R. and Fedoseyeva, E.V. (1997). Indirect T-cell allorecognition: perspectives for peptide-based therapy in transplantation 4. Immunol Today 18, 67–71.
Carstairs, K. (1962). The human small lymphocyte – its possible pluripotential quality. Lancet 1, 829.
Chalmers, D.G., Coulson, A.S., Evans, C. and Yealland, S. (1966). Immunologically stimulated human peripheral blood lymphocytes 'in vitro' II. Mixed lymphocyte cultures with related and unrelated donors. Int Arch Allergy 30, 177.
Cleaver, J.E. (1967). Thymidine metabolism and cell kinetics. Amsterdam: North Holland.

Cooper, S. (2003). Rethinking synchronization of mammalian cells for cell cycle analysis. Cell Mol Life Sci 60, 1099–1106.

Crow, M.K. and Kunkel, H.G. (1982). Human dendritic cells: major stimulators of the autologous and allogeneic mixed leucocyte reactions 4. Clin Exp Immunol 49, 338–346.

Farrant, J., Clark, J.C., Lee, H., Knight, S.C. and O'Brien, J. (1980). Conditions for measuring DNA synthesis in PHA stimulated human lymphocytes in 20 ml hanging-drops with various cell concentrations and periods of culture. J Immunol Methods 33, 301–312.

Givan, A.L., Fisher, J.L., Waugh, M., Ernstoff, M.S. and Wallace, P.K. (1999). A flow cytometric method to estimate the precursor frequencies of cells proliferating in response to specific antigens. J Immunol Methods 230, 99–112.

Harshyne, L.A., Zimmer, M.I., Watkins, S.C. and Barratt-Boyes, S.M. (2003). A role for class A scavenger receptor in dendritic cell nibbling from live cells. J Immunol 170, 2302–2309.

Hirschhorn, K., Bach, F., Rapaport, F.T., Converse, J.M. and Lawrence, H.S. (1964). The relationship of 'in vitro' lymphocyte compatibility to homograft sensitivity in man. Ann NY Acad Sci 120, 303.

Jeras, M. (2002). The role of in vitro alloreactive T-cell functional tests in the selection of HLA matched and mismatched haematopoietic stem cell donors. Transpl Immunol 10, 205–214.

Kleindienst, P. and Brocker, T. (2003). Endogenous dendritic cells are required for amplification of T cell responses induced by dendritic cell vaccines in vivo. J Immunol 170, 2817–2823.

Klenerman, P., Cerundolo, V. and Dunbar, P.R. (2002). Tracking T cells with tetramers: new tales from new tools. Nat Rev Immunol 2, 263–272.

Knight, S.C. (1982). Control of lymphocyte stimulation in vitro: 'Help' and 'suppression' in the light of lymphoid population dynamics. J Immunol Methods 50, R51–R63.

Knight, S.C. (1987). Lymphocyte proliferation assays. In Lymphocytes: A Practical Approach, Klaus, G.G.B. ed. Oxford: IRL Press. pp. 189–207.

Knight, S.C., Burke, F. and Bedford, P.A. (2002). Dendritic cells, antigen distribution and the initiation of primary immune responses to self and non-self antigens. Semin Cancer Biol 12, 301–308.

Knight, S.C. and Burman, S. (1981). Control of mixed lymphocyte reactions by cellular concentration: Studies in 20 ml hanging droplet cultures. Trans Proc 8, 1637–1641.

Knight, S.C., Iqball, S., Roberts, M.S., Macatonia, S. and Bedford, P.A. (1998). Transfer of antigen between dendritic cells in the stimulation of primary T cell proliferation. Eur J Immunol 28, 1636–1644.

Knight, S.C., Mertin, J., Stackpoole, A. and Clarke, J.B. (1983). Induction of immune responses in vivo with small numbers of veiled (dendritic) cells. Proc Nat Acad Sci USA 80, 6032–6035.

Knight, S.C. and Stagg, A.J. (1993). Antigen-presenting cell types. Curr Opin Immunol 5, 374–382.

Lambrecht, B.N., Pauwels, R.A. and Fazekas De St Groth, B. (2000). Induction of rapid T cell activation, division, and recirculation by intratracheal injection of dendritic cells in a TCR transgenic model (In Process Citation). J Immunol 164, 2937–2946.

Lechler, R.I. and Batchelor, J.R. (1982). Restoration of immunogenicity to passenger cell-depleted kidney allografts by the addition of donor strain dendritic cells 3. J Exp Med 155, 31–41.

Li, J.G. and Osgood, E.E. (1949). A method for the rapid separation of leukocytes and nucleated erythrocytes from blood or marrow with a phytohemagglutinin from red beans (Phaseolus vulgaris). Blood 4, 670.

Macatonia, S.E., Lau, R., Patterson, S., Pinching, A.J. and Knight, S.C. (1990). Dendritic cell infection, depletion and dysfunction in HIV-infected individuals. Immunology 71, 38–45.

Macatonia, S.E., Taylor, P.M., Knight, S.C. and Askonas, B.A. (1989). Primary stimulation by dendritic cells induces antiviral proliferative and cytotoxic T cell responses in vitro. J Exp Med 169, 1255–1264.

Mann, D.L. and Abelson, L. (1980). Monocyte function in mixed lymphocyte reactions 2. Cell Immunol 56, 357–364.

Metlay, J.P., Pure, E. and Steinman, R.M. (1989). Control of the immune response at the level of antigen-presenting cells: A comparison of the function of dendritic cells and B lymphocytes. Advan Immunol 47, 45–116.

Nowell, P.C. (1960). Phytohaemagglutinin an inhibitor of mitosis in cultures of normal human leucocytes. Cancer Res 20, 462.

Oppenheim, J.J., Whang, J. and Frei, E. (1965). The effect of skin homograft rejection on recipient and donor mixed leukocyte cultures. J Exp Med 122, 651.

Schrek, R. and Donnelly, W.J. (1961). Differences between lymphocytes of leukemic and non-leukemic patients with respect to morphologic features, motility and sensitivity to guinea pig serum. Blood 18, 561–571.

Song, H.K., Noorchashm, H., Lieu, Y.K. et al. (1999). Cutting edge: alloimmune responses against major and minor histocompatibility antigens: distinct division kinetics and requirement for CD28 costimulation. J Immunol 162, 2467–2471.

Stagg, A.J., Kamm, M.A. and Knight, S.C. (2002). Intestinal dendritic cells increase T cell expression of $\alpha4\beta7$ integrin. Eur J Immunol 32, 1445–1454.

Steinman, R.M. and Witmer, M.D. (1978). Lymphoid dendritic cells are potent stimulators of the primary mixed leukocyte reaction in mice. Proc Natl Acad Sci USA 75, 5132–5136.

Thery, C., Zitvogel, L. and Amigorena, S. (2002). Exosomes: composition, biogenesis and function. Nat Rev Immunol 2, 569–579.

Thorpe, P.E. and Knight, S.C. (1974). Microplate culture of mouse lymph node cells. Quantitation of responses to allogeneic lymphocytes, endotoxin and phytomitogens. J Immunol Methods 5, 387.

Twomey, J.J., Sharkey, O., Brown, J.A., Laughter, A.H. and Jordan, P.H. (1970). Cellular requirements for the mitotic response in allogeneic mixed leucocyte cultures. J Immunol 104, 845–853.

Vincent-Schneider, H., Stumptner-Cuvelette, P., Lankar, D. et al. (2002). Exosomes bearing HLA-DR1 molecules need dendritic cells to efficiently stimulate specific T cells. Int Immunol 14, 713–722.

Waldmann, H. and Lefkovits, I. (1984). Limiting dilution analysis of cells of the immune system: what can be learnt. Immunol Today 5, 259–298.

Weinberger, O., Germain, R.N., Springer, T. and Burakoff, S.J. (1982). Role of syngeneic Ia+ accessory cells in the generation of allospecific CTL responses 1. J Immunol 129, 694–697.

Zinkernagel, R.M. and Doherty, P.C. (1997). The discovery of MHC restriction. Immunol Today 18, 14–17.

Zitvogel, L., Regnault, A., Lozier, A. et al. (1998). Eradication of established murine tumors using a novel cell-free vaccine: dendritic cell-derived exosomes. Nat Med 4, 594–600.

Antigen/Mitogen-Stimulated Lymphocyte Proliferation

Chapter 31

Theresa L. Whiteside

Departments of Pathology, Immunology and Otolaryngology, University of Pittsburgh School of Medicine and University of Pittsburgh Cancer Institute, Pittsburgh, PA, USA

> All we know is still infinitely less than all that still remains unknown.
>
> William Harvey (1578–1657) *De Motu Cordis et Sanguinis* (1628)

INTRODUCTION

Lymphocytes, like other cells, respond to appropriate environmental stimuli by activation and proliferation. The proliferative potential of a T cell, for example, is an important parameter for evaluating its immune status. Upon leaving the thymus, naive T cells have the capacity to expand and give rise to effector/memory cells (Lanzavecchia and Sallusto, 2000; Champagne et al., 2001; Kaech et al., 2002). T cells that constitute the memory pool acquire a high proliferative potential and are able to mount a rapid secondary immune response. These T cells progressively lose the capacity for clonal expansion after terminal differentiation into effector cells and then die. The host maintains immune competence through the homeostatic balance of lymphocyte expansion, death and survival. In this context, assessments of the proliferative potential of T cell populations can provide useful information about their differentiation, maturation and overall immune function. However, populations of immune cells contain multiple clonally-expanded cells, each clone programmed to respond to a unique antigen upon stimulation. Thus, it is often more important and informative to evaluate antigen-specific T cell proliferation rather than responses to non-specific stimuli, with a caveat that the identity of the relevant antigen is known. While a decade or so ago, lymphocyte proliferation was measured largely by quantitating mitogen-driven responses, newer technologies have recently emerged which permit evaluation of antigen-specific immune cell proliferation, including the determination of the precursor frequencies of such antigen-specific cells in the population.

In its simplest form, a proliferation assay measures the numbers of cells surviving in culture following stimulation. Such a measurement could be made by counting of the cells in a light microscope using a vital dye. However, counting of cells by eye is very labor intensive and has been replaced by methods utilizing flow cytometry to determine the number of blasts or, more frequently, by estimating new DNA production. The proliferative response can be measured using cultures of whole blood or separated mononuclear cells as well as subsets of lymphocytes. In this latter case, it is important to remember that, in many cases, more than one cell type is necessary for a response to occur. Specifically, a response to an antigen will involve not only the responding T or B cells but also an accessory cell (monocyte, macrophage, dendritic cell) expressing a required HLA molecule on its surface.

This chapter will first briefly describe the methods used for measuring non-specific expansion of immune cells. The antigen-specific proliferation will then be considered in a greater depth, with the priority given to flow cytometry-based techniques. The flow cytometry-based proliferation assays have recently revolutionized our approaches to measuring immunity in health as well as disease and

Measuring Immunity, edited by Michael T. Lotze and Angus W. Thomson
ISBN 0-12-455900-X, London

have provided a novel and simpler way of quantifying antigen-specific responses, including proliferation at both the population and single-cell levels. The objective of the chapter is to introduce these various methodologies and, focusing largely on T cell responses, to comment on their overall usefulness as tools for monitoring of patients with immune-mediated diseases as well as those treated with biologic therapies.

PROLIFERATION IN RESPONSE TO MITOGENS

Lymphocytes respond to a variety of plant mitogens, such as phytohemagglutinin (PHA), concanavalin A (ConA) and pokeweed mitogen (PWM), as well as to mitogens of bacterial origin such as *Staphylococcus* enterotoxin or *S. aureus* Cowan 1, a B cell stimulant. Lymphocytes also respond to various chemicals, e.g. phorbol myristate acetate (PMA) and ionomycin (Miyamoto et al., 2000; Barten et al., 2001). Specific interactions between a surface receptor on lymphocytes and the ligand can trigger intracellular signals that culminate in cell division and expansion. Because lymphocytes obtained from patients who are immunologically compromised (e.g. patients with HIV-1, congenital immune abnormalities or cancer) often have poor responses to mitogens, this assay can be informative about the functional capacity of lymphocytes and may be of value in the assessment of the immune status of patients with a variety of disorders. Responses to mitogens are, of course, non-antigen specific, but for many years they have served as a measure of general functionality of immune cells obtained from tissue sites or those present in the peripheral circulation. While PHA and ConA are considered to be T cell mitogens, PWM has been commonly used for B cell stimulation. Mitogen stimulation is seldom used today, having been largely replaced by antigen-specific assays or by the assessment of T cell receptor-mediated responses. Nevertheless, the value of mitogen stimulation assays as classical monitors of T cell or B cell abilities to respond to an external signal by activation and proliferation remains unchanged.

Method

The assay involves plating of a defined number of mononuclear cells (e.g. 5×10^4) in triplicate wells of a 96-well U-bottom microtiter plate in the presence of various concentrations of a mitogen. Control wells contain cells in the medium but no mitogen. The culture medium can be RPMI-1640 supplemented with heat-inactivated fetal bovine serum (FBS; 10 per cent v/v) and containing penicillin (10 000 µg/ml) and streptomycin (10 000 µg/ml). The mitogen concentrations are adjusted to cover a desired range, e.g. from 4 to 64 µg PHA/ml or 12.5 to 200 µg Con A/ml. The rationale for using a range of mitogen concentrations is that lymphocytes obtained from different subjects have a distinct response profile, which becomes

important when normal versus abnormal responses are to be distinguished. The plates containing mitogen-stimulated cells are incubated in a humidified CO_2 incubator at 37°C for 3 days. On day 3, cells in individual wells are pulsed with ^{3}H-thymidine solution (20 µl/well) in the assay medium (specific activity 6 Ci/mmol, 1 mCi/ml), using an Eppendorf repeating pipettor and a sterile 0.5 ml combitip. The plates are then incubated for 18 h in a humidified 37°C incubator in the atmosphere of 5 per cemt CO_2 in air. The incorporation of radioactive nucleoside (^{3}H-thymidine) into cellular DNA being synthesized in proliferating lymphocytes is the basis for this assay. Following incubation with labeled nucleoside, cells are harvested onto filter mats using a harvester, non-incorporated nucleoside is washed away, the filters are placed in individual scintillation vials and radioactivity is counted in a beta counter.

Result calculations

The results of mitogen proliferation assays reflect the amount of ^{3}H-thymidine in cpm incorporated into cellular DNA during the 18 h incubation. The results are expressed in one of the following ways:

$$\text{SI (stimulation index)} = \frac{\text{experimental (stimulated) mean cpm}}{\text{control (unstimulated) mean cpm}}$$

$$\text{RPI (relative proliferation index)} = \frac{\text{mean cpm of individual tested}}{\text{mean cpm of 3 normal subjects tested simultaneously}}$$

$$\text{TPR (total proliferative response)} = \frac{\text{net cpm MC1} + \text{net cpm MC2} + \text{net cpm MC3}}{3}$$

MC = mitogen concentration

The SI is the commonest way of expressing results of proliferation assays. However, it is also the least accurate, especially when comparisons are made between cells of different individuals, which often have disparate background levels of ^{3}H-thymidine incorporation. Thus, patients' cells may have higher background counts than control cells, contributing to the variability of SI. The RPI normalizes proliferation of the experimental sample against three controls and if the same cryopreserved control cells are used repeatedly, it offers a reliable way of comparing changes over time in serially acquired specimens. Finally, the TPR is probably the optimal way of evaluating the proliferation data, because it summarizes the responses at three (or more) mitogen concentrations and gives the overall magnitude of response, which can then be compared to the TPR of controls set up at the same mitogen concentrations in the same assay. In essence, this approach compares area under the curve established in the same assay for a patient and a control.

Controls

The utility of all proliferation assays is dependent on the comparison of patient response values to those obtained from immunologically competent matched controls. Each laboratory is responsible for establishing its own range of normal values that reflect age, ethnicity and gender of the investigated populations. Controls are an essential component of any proliferation assay. In the author's laboratory three frozen normal controls are run with each mitogen assay. These frozen cells are selected to represent high, medium and low responders. The selected donors donate 100 ml of blood and the cells are cryopreserved, using a late-controlled device (cryomed), in cryovials containing 10×10^6 cells/vial and stored in liquid N_2 vapors. The vials are thawed as needed to provide control cells for daily assays. The mean SI $\pm$ 2 SD is determined for each control cell and these values are used to set control limits for the assay. In addition, the laboratory has established normal ranges $\pm$ SD for mitogen responses of cells obtained from over 30 normal individuals. This range is used as a guide to define whether a patient's cells give high, medium or low response to a mitogen. If the assay is performed with fresh rather than cryopreserved cells, freshly harvested normal control cells have to be used to establish the assay range and a coefficent of variation (CV).

Result interpretation/clinical utility

Proliferation following stimulation by mitogens has been used as a general measure of lymphocyte capability to recognize a stimulatory signal and mount a functional response. As such, it is best used for distinguishing large differences and discriminating patients who are severely immunodepressed from those with normal immune competence. For example, proliferation assays are helpful in establishing a diagnosis of congenital immune abnormalities (Fletcher et al., 1987). They are not particularly helpful in distinguishing conditions associated with partial immune dysfunctions, including infections or cancer, because lymphocytes of most patients with these diseases respond to mitogens at some level and quantitation of such responses cannot be related to clinical symptoms. Similarly, mitogen stimulation assays are of little use in monitoring responses to therapy in clinical trials, because the discrimination between levels of *in vitro* proliferative responses cannot be correlated to clinical responses or to distinguish responders from non-responders to therapy. Currently, mitogen stimulation assays are most widely used in a research setting, especially in murine models of disease, where proliferation, viewed as a general functional attribute of a lymphocyte population, often provides the initial indication for further studies.

PROLIFERATION IN RESPONSE TO ANTIGENS

Proliferative responses to antigens occur following an interaction of the cognate epitope presented by a restricting HLA molecule on the surface of antigen-presenting cells (APC) with the T cell receptor (TCR) on responder T cells. Measuring of antigen-specific responses is considered to be more useful than mitogen stimulation, because it focuses attention on responses that may be, and often are, relevant to the disease process or to the therapeutic intervention at hand. There are a variety of systems for measuring antigen-specific responses and the most widely used rely upon the incorporation of ^{3}H-thymidine into cellular DNA, as described above. The systems that are flow-cytometry based offer a welcome departure from radioactive labeling of cells and a possibility to identify the proliferating T lymphocyte subsets by their phenotypes (Lyons and Parish, 1994; Allsopp et al., 1998).

Radioactivity-based methods

These methods generally use ^{3}H-thymidine incorporation and follow the procedure described above for mitogen stimulation. The T cells used as responders in these assays may or may not be separated into subsets prior to the assays and APC have to be present when the separated T cells are responders. Responses to recall antigens (e.g. tetanus toxoid or *Candida albicans*) are frequently assessed in these assays, as are responses to allogeneic lymphocytes, cytokines and monoclonal antibodies to cell surface receptors, such as CD3 or CD2. The mixed lymphocyte reaction (MLR) is perhaps the most widely used assay in this category today.

Proliferation in response to alloantigens (MLR)

The MLR measures the ability of lymphocytes to respond to foreign alloantigens present on the surface of stimulator cells. The stimulatory determinants are predominantly disparate HLA class II molecules expressed on B cells, monocytes or dendritic cells. The first descriptions of this assay as a measure of cellular immunity, together with the development of a one-way method of stimulation by irradiating the stimulator cells, allowed for the assessment of proliferative responses between siblings for transplantation (Bach and Hirschhorn, 1964). In MLR, responders which proliferate are multiple clones of alloactivated T lymphocytes. This proliferation is measured by incorporation of ^{3}H thymidine into replicating DNA during the logarithmic phase of cell growth, usually on the fifth day of culture. The degree of response in MLR correlates with the degree of antigenic disparity between responding and stimulating cells.

Method

The MLR is similar to the mitogen stimulation assay. However, instead of stimulating responders with mitogens, an MLR pool of cells is used. In the author's laboratory, the MLR pool is composed of lymphocytes obtained from six normal donors selected to represent most of the known HLA specificities. To make up the pool, normal individuals are screened for HLA and recruited to serve as donors of lymphocytes for the MLR pool. The pool is cyropreserved and vials are thawed as needed, cells are washed and irradiated at 7500 rads or treated with mitomycin C to prevent their proliferation. Next, the responder and stimulator cells are micropipetted into triplicate U-bottom wells of 96-well microtiter plates (e.g. 5×10^4 responders and 5×10^4 stimulators). Control wells include responder cells alone, stimulator cells alone and a mix of autologous responder and irradiated stimulators from the same cell donor. The cultures are incubated in a 37°C humidified incubator in an atmosphere of 5 per cent CO_2inair for 5 days. Cells are pulsed with ^{3}H-thmidine on day 5 and are incubated for the additional 18 h. The samples are harvested and counted as described above.

Results interpretations/clinical utility of MLR

MLR results obtained as mean cpm are computed and presented as the SI or RPI. MLR has been used clinically for donor selection, predominantly for bone marrow transplantation. Today, MLR is used most often for monitoring of the immune status of transplant organ recipients after transplantation. In this context, anti-donor MLR responses of the graft recipient are measured and pre-transplant versus post-transplant responses are compared to define changes. This is clinically important because such changes (increases or decreases) predict the onset of immunologic complications, such as acute or chronic rejection episodes in solid organ recipients (Reinsmoen et al., 1990; Reinsmoen and Matas, 1993). Also, it may be possible to differentiate immune rejections from other forms of dysfunction such as infection or primary graft dysfunction. Further, MLR might assist in evaluations of patients' responses to anti-rejection therapies and thus help in preventing excessive immune suppression (Reinsmoen and Matas, 1993).

In addition to monitoring the immune status of transplant recipients, MLR assays have been used to gauge the functional potential of human dendritic cells (DC) generated in 6-day cultures for vaccine-based therapy of patients with cancer. In this type of MLR assays, *ex vivo*-generated DC serve as stimulators and populations of human PBMC (again, available as a pool of cryopreserved cells with different HLA specificities) as responders. The rationale for this MLR assay is that functionally competent DC should be able effectively to present allogeneic determinants to T cells. However, aside from logistical problems with the preparation of suitable responders pools, it appears that MLR is not the optimal assay for functional evaluation of immature DC, largely because of the absence of well-defined criteria for qualifying a response and also because other characteristics, e.g. cytokine production in response to selected activating stimuli seem to provide a more relevant assessment of DC functions.

A mixed lymphocyte-tumor culture (MLTC) is a variety of MLR assay, in which irradiated autologous tumor cells serve as stimulators and lymphocyte populations isolated from the cancer patient's blood or tissue are responders.

This assay follows the procedure described above, except that responses to antigens that are expressed by the tumor and recognized by the autologous T cells are measured. The MLTC assay has been used to demonstrate the lack of reactivity to autologous tumor cells in many patients with advanced malignant diseases (Vose et al., 1977; Whiteside, 1993). In humans, autologous tumor cells are seldom available in numbers sufficient for monitoring of anti-tumor responses and, for this reason, other assays requiring fewer cells have replaced MLTC.

Proliferation in response to primary versus recall antigens

Responses to primary and recall antigens are usually determined by performing a delayed type hypersensitivity (DTH) *in vivo* test (Black, 1999). Proliferation assays represent an *in vitro* correlate of skin testing for DTH and they have an advantage of providing a quantitative estimate of the response. The antigens selected for measuring primary responses are those not usually encountered by the immune system of most individuals (e.g. certain chemicals or bacteriophages). These antigens have to be presented by APC in order to induce activation and proliferation of naive T lymphocytes. The assay usually requires a relatively long (7–14 day) incubation period in the presence of APC and low doses of IL-2 and is, therefore, more complex to perform than a recall antigen assay. Testing for primary immune responses is used for diagnosis in patients with immunodeficiencies to establish the potential of naive T cells to expand as well as the ability of APC to present the antigen not previously seen by the subject's immune system.

Recall antigens are those that most individuals are exposed to, such as tetanus toxoid or *Candida albicans*. This type of antigen-specific proliferation is dependent on the presence and functionality of memory T cells. The assay measures competence in mounting a secondary immune response to previously encountered antigens and it only requires a short-term incubation (5 days). These assays are useful in defining general immune competence and in evaluating responses to vaccines. In this latter setting, pre- and post-vaccination blood specimens are tested in the same assay for responses to the vaccinating antigen.

In vitro sensitization (IVS) assays have been used in monitoring of responses to vaccines in order to expend clonal populations of T lymphocytes able to recognize immunizing antigens. Such antigen-specific T lymphocytes are rare and may be present in the blood at frequencies that are too low to be detected by 'single cell' assays such as ELISPOT or intracytoplasmic cytokine (ICC) expression. *In vitro* stimulation with the relevant antigen or antigenic epitope leads to expansion of T cell clones able to recognize and respond to the stimulant. Following expansion in the presence of IL-2, the culture is harvested and tested in 'single cell' assays to determine the number of T cells able to express or produce a cytokine (e.g. IFN-γ) upon a brief (24–48 h) exposure to the relevant antigen. Cells in pre- and post-vaccination samples expanded in the same assay upon IVS with an immunizing component of the vaccine can thus be compared for the content of the immunogen-specific T cells. This version of a proliferation assay is used to amplify the response that is then quantified in another assay. IVS has been useful in detecting low responses to vaccines with complex protein antigens, such as PSA or CA125, in patients with cancer (Meidenbauer et al., 2000; Schultes and Whiteside, 2003). As these antigens require processing and presentation, autologous DC are used in IVS assays, adding to their complexity. Furthermore, while allowing for quantification of antigen-responsive T cells in a subsequent ELISPOT or ICC and for estimating the difference between pre- versus post-vaccination samples, IVS cannot be equated with the frequency estimate of antigen-responsive T cells in the peripheral circulation. It only allows for the frequency estimate of T cell proliferating in culture in response to the antigen. Because not every antigen-specific pre-tumor cell will proliferate in culture and some will proliferate and die, IVS only helps in measuring the difference between antigen-specific proliferating T cells and *not* the difference in the actual frequency of precursor T cells between pre- and post-therapy peripheral blood samples. Thus, the interpretation of IVS assays as well as selection of conditions for optimal amplification of antigen-specific responses are difficult and require considerable experimental acumen.

Limiting dilution analysis (LDA)

This method determines the frequency of T cell precursors in a population. Antigen-responding cells are plated at limiting dilutions in wells of 96-well microtiter plates. Multiple wells per dilution are necessary to ensure an accurate measurement of the frequency. The proliferating microcultures are scored microscopically or assayed for ^{3}H-thymidine incorporation to determine the proportion of responders (Letkovits and Waldmann, 1972; Sharrock et al., 1990). In contrast to MLR, which measures the bulk response, LDA is a quantitative method, which implies that every precursor T cell able to recognize a cognate antigen will respond by proliferation and form a clone (Moretta et al., 1983). Clearly, this assay must be done under conditions favorable to clonal expansion, usually in the presence of feeder cells, which supply essential cytokines, including IL-2 and serve as APC. The responders are plated in limiting numbers and cultured with constant numbers of irradiated stimulator cells or APC presenting antigens. Exogenous IL-2 is added to the assay on days 3 and 6 and cultures are incubated for 10–25 days. Wells (microcultures) containing proliferating cells are microscopically scored against those that do not proliferate and the frequency of proliferating T cell precursors in the population of plated cells is determined by the minimum x^2 method from the Poisson distribution

relationship between the responding cell number and the logarithm of the percentage of non-responding (negative) microcultures. Various modifications of this 'single cell' assay have been developed in order to test functional activities of proliferating responder microcultures (cytokine production, cytotoxicity, extent of proliferation; Lefkovits and Waldmann, 1992). For example, helper T lymphocytes (HTL) are detected by their ability to produce IL-2, using the murine IL-2 dependent cell line, CTLL2. Constant numbers of CTLL2 cells are added to plated and irradiated microcultures of responders, with control wells containing responders alone and CTLL2 cells alone. The plates are incubated for 72 h at 37°C in a 5 per cent CO_2 environment. An aliquot (1 mci/well) of ^{3}H-thymidine is then added and after 12 h the microcultures are harvested for counts of incorporated radioactivity. CTLL2 cells proliferate only if irradiated responders produce IL-2. The positive wells are those that show [^{3}H] thymidine incorporation greater than the mean + 3 SD of 24 control wells. The frequency of responding cells is determined based on a maximum likelihood estimation using a computer program (Kaminski et al., 1989a). Cytotoxic T lymphocytes (CTL) can be detected by adding ^{51}Cr-labeled targets to microcultures of proliferating responder cells and assessing the release of ^{51}Cr in supernatants. A computer program (Kaminski et al., 1989b) is used to calculate the frequency of CTL in the plated population.

LDA has been widely used for cloning of antigen-specific T lymphocytes from blood, lymph nodes or diseased tissue sites and for estimations of the frequency of antigen-specific T cells in patients with various diseases. Although laborious in execution, LDA has remained as a 'benchmark' for single-cell analysis of T lymphocytes and their functions. While newly introduced single-cell assays have largely replaced LDA today, the performance characteristics of these new assays and especially their specificity and sensitivity are nearly always compared to those of LDA.

Non-radioactive proliferation assays

The use of labeled nucleosides to measure their incorporation into cellular DNA limits the application of proliferation assays to laboratories certified to handle radioactivity and equipped with scintillation counters. More recently, several non-radioactive systems have become available and practically replaced ^{3}H-thymidine incorporation. Examples include MTT and MTS; Almar Blue dye- or antibody-based assays as well as flow cytometry-based technologies.

A non-radioactive colormetric system, which measures cellular proliferation by estimating the level of oxidative respiration, is based on the use of tetrazolium substrates. These substrates become converted to a blue formazan dye in the presence of products secreted during cellular respiration. The assay measures activity of mitochondrial enzymes and reflects the number of metabolically active cells present in culture. The MTT, a yellow aqueous solution, is taken up by viable cells and reduced in the mitochondria to a blue formazan dye. Distinct spectrophotometric properties of formazan allow for quantification of the cellular response based on the principle that more cells produce more respiratory intermediates and give more intense blue color. Two different substrates MTT (3–4, 5-dimethylthiazol-2-yl)-2,5 diphenyl tetrazolium bromide salt and MTS (3–4,5 dimethylthiazol-2-yl)-5(carboxymethoxyphenyl)-2-(4-sulfophenyl) tetrazolium, which differ in their solubilization requirements, are available (Mosmann, 1983; Riss and Morabec, 1992). These assays are simply set up by adding different numbers of cells into wells of microtiter plates in the presence of the substrate and they can be easily automated. For this reason, they are frequently used for screening of large libraries of compounds for the ability to inhibit or stimulate cellular proliferation.

An Almar Blue dye-based proliferation assay is available in the enzyme-linked immunosorbent format and has been used to monitor lymphocyte proliferation (Ahmed et al., 1994). The degree of change in the dye color reflects the extent of cellular proliferation.

Flow cytometry-based proliferation assays

Flow cytometry has been used to measure cellular proliferation for many years. For example, bromodeoxyuridine (BRDU)-based methods were commonly employed in lymphocyte studies (Kovacs et al., 2001; Savitskiy et al., 2003; Dionigi et al., 2004). BRDU is a thymidine analog which is incorporated into cellular DNA during chromosomal replication. The system utilizes an anti-BRDU-specific monoclonal antibody to detect this base after it becomes incorporated into cellular DNA. Following incubation with BRDU, lymphocytes are permeabilized and stained with fluorescently-labeled anti-BRDU antibody. The amount of the analog incorporated into DNA can then be quantified by flow cytometry (Savitskiy et al., 2003).

More recently, a variety of fluorescent dyes has become available which stain the cytoplasm or the cell membrane and can be used to quantitate the expansion of a cell population by flow cytometry (Lyons and Parish, 1994). The principle of the method is that the amount of the dye taken up by a cell is equally partitioned between daughter cells during mitosis and, therefore, decreased by half at each cell division. Dyes such as carboxyfluorescein diacetate succinimidyl ester (CFSE) diffuse into a cell and are cleaved by intracellular esterases into compounds that are fluorescent and react with amino groups of intracytoplasmic proteins (Fulcher and Wong, 1999; Lyons, 1999). Other dyes, such as long-chain aliphatic PKH26 dye, become stably integrated into the lipid bilayer of the outer cellular membrane (Horan and Slezak, 1989). The ability to determine the proliferative history of a specific cell population, which can be identified by combining surface staining with CFSE or PKH26 dyes, is a particularly important advantage of these assays. In addition to assessing total proliferation of cells with a particular phenotype in the population, this method allows for calculating the precursor frequency of lymphocyte populations responding to specific antigen (Givan et al., 1999).

Of the two tracking dyes used for the flow cytometric method, CSFE is perhaps more popular, largely because CFSE-stained cells show better intensity resolution between daughter generations than do PKH26-stained cells (Givan et al., 1999). CFSE diffuses into cells and is non-fluorescent until cellular esterases cleave carboxyl groups from the molecule, rendering it non-permanent and fluorescent. The succinimidyl moiety of CFSE covalently attaches to the cytoplasmic amine groups. The covalently bound CFSE is divided equally between the daughter cells, allowing for resolution of up to eight cell division cycles. The CFSE staining in combination with immunophenotyping makes it possible to compare the kinetics of proliferation in various cell populations. By analysis of the flow cytometric histogram plots, using software deconvolution algorithms (Bagwell, 1993), a quantitative assessment of cells that have undergone any particular number of divisions is obtained. The number of precursors that divided can be extrapolated and summed to derive the number of cells in the population that responded to the antigen. By comparing the number of cells that divided with those that did not divide, a precursor frequency values can be derived. A flow dye dilution assay that can be used to calculate the precursor frequency and expansion potential of antigen-specific T cells has been described and shown to give 100-fold higher values than the traditional LDA method (Givan et al., 1999). Newer modifications of this method allow for simultaneous assessments of other T cell functions, i.e. proliferation, cytokine synthesis or tetramer-binding, by multiparameter flow cytometry (Bercovici et al., 2003).

Method

The method requires that four-color flow cytometer and CellQuest software be available. Culture media, cell separation and washing buffers are the same as for the MLR procedure described above. CFSE is dissolved in dimethyl sulfoxide and aliquots stored at −20°C in the dark. For staining of cells, the optimal dilution of CFSE needs to be determined. For lymphocytes, this may vary from 0.25 μM to 1.0 μM. Higher concentrations of CFSE should be avoided because of the potential dye-induced inhibitory effects. Responder cells ($<1 \times 10^7$/ml) suspended in PBS-0.1 per cent bovine serum albumin (BSA) are incubated with CFSE for 5–15 min at room temperature, washed in medium containing 5–10 per cent (v/v) of human AB serum and cultured with a stimulatory agent or stimulator cells under conditions described for the MLR, including positive and negative controls, for an optimal time to be determined by the investigator. The harvested and washed cells are then stained with the appropriate antibodies for immunophenotyping. Flow cytometry analysis is the most important step in this procedure and green fluorescence (i.e. CFSE) is collected with a 525 nm band-pass filter. Forward/side scatter gating, which defines resting lymphocytes and lymphoblasts, is used in all analyses. Proliferation of responder cells results in sequential CFSE dilution, which is accompanied by increasing forward scatter of the cells, consistent with blast formation of activated lymphocytes. CFSE fluorescence is plotted against forward scatter. Resting cells retain bright CFSE staining consistent with no proliferation response to the stimulator. Among responding cells, a substantial population of cells should be detected that had lost CFSE fluorescence indicative of stimulator-induced proliferation. This type of CFSE dye dilution and analysis of flow cytometric histogram plots, using CellQuest software, provides quantitative assessments of the cells within each CFSE fluorescent peak. A series of calculations need to be performed to calculate the total number of proliferating cells or the number of precursors that divided (Givan et al., 1999).

Results interpretation/clinical utility of CFSE

The critical aspect of the method is labeling with CFSE. The staining should be bright, but excess staining can cause problems with cell viability and compensation during data acquisition and analysis. The optimal conditions for CFSE labeling should be pre-determined for each cell type. With lymphocytes, it may be helpful to set the conditions by stimulating with anti-CD3 antibodies or a recall antigen such as tetanus toxoid. An advantage of the method is that it can determine the proportion of proliferating cells in the population and characterize further the responding cells by concomitant subset analysis based on their phenotype. For example, it might be of interest to determine which T cell subsets proliferate in response to specific helper epitopes that are candidates for vaccines. Also, in monitoring responses of patients to vaccines, it may be important to determine which lymphocyte subsets are responding and also to estimate the precursor frequency of responding cells prior to and after vaccination. The ability to ask questions about the potential responses to specific antigen of lymphocytes in naive versus memory compartments is likely to contribute to the general body of knowledge about these immune cells. In general, antigen-specific proliferating cells represent a small subset of the original plated population. The high level of sensitivity of the flow-based assays is an advantage in this respect, as is its simplicity, particularly *vis a vis* radioactivity-based proliferation assays. The assay can be performed in a single well or tube. The number of generations that have occurred among the proliferating cells can be determined and the doubling time can be calculated with multiple readings over time. The new generation of multiparameter CFSE-based assays (Bercovici et al., 2003) offers an even greater advantage of defining the phenotype as well as

other functional capabilities of the proliferating cell subset (Bercovici et al., 2000). This approach might prove to be particularly useful in dissecting the diversity of the T cell populations in patients with various diseases and particularly those undergoing transplantation, vaccination or other therapy targeting the host immune system. It is expected that this flow-based methodology will assume a prominent place in routine testing and monitoring of cellular proliferation in the fields of autoimmunity, cancer immunotherapy, transplantation and allergy in the near future.

CONCLUSIONS

Assays for cellular proliferation are useful clinical and monitoring tools. Today, a broad selection of such assays is available and the investigator faced with a choice must determine the utility of the particular assay in answering the question(s) being posed. It is important to remember that flow cytometry-based proliferation assays, for example, may be unnecessary for evaluations of general capability of T cells to respond to mitogens or for screening of multiple agents for the ability to induce lymphocyte proliferation. On the other hand, analyses of individual lymphocyte subsets for responses to specific epitopes have been greatly facilitated by the flow cytometry-based assays. The clinical significance of profiling the responsive T cell repertoire is not clear at present. However, preliminary results emerging from a number of laboratories indicate that it may be useful to define such profiles in health and in disease. An additional opportunity exists for defining the proliferating profiles of individual immune cell subsets before and after therapy, including vaccinations or organ replacement procedures. As our understanding of the complexities associated with T cell responses *in vivo* expands and the available assays become more sensitive and specific as well as simpler in execution, the functional assessments of lymphocyte subsets, including proliferation, are likely to gain importance for routine evaluations of the immune system in the clinical laboratory.

REFERENCES

Ahmed, S.A., Gogal, R.M. and Walsh, J.E. (1994). A new rapid and simple non-radioactive assay to monitor and determine the proliferation of lymphocytes: an alternative to [3H]thymidine incorporation assay. J Immunol Methods 170, 211–224.

Allsopp, C.E.M., Nicholls, S.J. and Langjorne, J. (1998). A flow cytometric method to assess antigen-specific proliferative responses of different subpopulations of fresh and cryopreserved human peripheral blood mononuclear cells. J Immunol Methods 214, 175–186.

Bach, R.H. and Hirschhorn, K. (1964). Lymphocyte interaction: a potential histocompatibility rest *in vitro*. Science 143, 813–814.

Bagwell, C.B. (1993). Theoretical aspects of data analysis. In Clinical Flow Cytometry, Bauer, K.D., Duque, R.E., Shankey, T.V., eds. Baltimore: Williams and Wilkins, p. 41.

Barten, M.J., Gummert, J.F., van Gelder, T., Shorthouse, R. and Morris, R.E. (2001). Flow cytometric quantitation of calcium-dependent and –independent mitogen-stimulation of T cell functions in whole blood; inhibition by immunosuppressive drugs in vitro. J Immunol Methods 253, 95–112.

Bercovici, N., Duffour, M.T., Agarwal, S., Salacedo, M. and Abastado, J.P. (2000). New methods for assessing T-cell responses. Clin Diagn Lab Immunol 7, 859–237.

Bercovici, N., Givan, A.L., Waugh, M.G. et al. (2003). Multiparameter precursor analysis of T-cell responses to antigen. J Immunol Methods 276, 5–17.

Black, C.A. (1999). Delayed type hypersensitivity: current theories with an historic perspective. J Dermatol Online Review 5, 7.

Champagne, P., Ogg, G.S., King, A.S. et al., (2001). Skewed maturation of memory HIV-specific CD8+ T lymphocytes. Nature 410, 106–111.

Dionigi, P., Ferrari, A., Jemos, V. et al. (2004). Tumor cell proliferation in early gastric cancer: biological and clinical behavior. Hepatogastroenterology 51, 264–268.

Fletcher, M.A., Baron, G.A., Ashman, M.A. and Klimas, N.G. (1987). Use of whole blood methods in assessment of immune parameters in immunodeficiency syndromes. Clin Diag Immunol 5, 69–81.

Fulcher, D. and Wong, S. (1999). Carboxyfluorescein succinimidyl ester-based proliferative assays for assessment of T cell function in the diagnostic laboratory. Immunol Cell Biol 77, 559–564.

Givan, A.L., Fisher, J.L., Waugh, M., Ernstoff, M.S. and Wallace, P.K. (1999). A flow cytometric method to estimate the precursor frequencies of cells proliferating in response to specific antigens. J Immunol Methods 230, 99–112.

Horan, P.K. and Slezak, S.E. (1989). Stable cell membrane labeling. Nature 340, 167–168.

Kaech, S.M., Wherry, E.J. and Ahmed, R. (2002). Effector and memory T-cell differentiation: implications for vaccine development. Nat Rev Immunol 2, 251–262.

Kaminski, E., Hows, J., Brookes, P. et al. (1989a). Alloreactive cytotoxic T-cell frequency analysis and HLA matching for bone marrow transplants from HLA matched unrelated donors. Transplant Proc 21, 2976–2977.

Kaminski, E., Hows, J., Man, S. et al. (1989b). Prediction of graft versus host disease by frequency analysis of cytotoxic T cells after unrelated donor bone marrow transplantation. Transplantation 48, 608–613.

Kovacs, J.A., Lempicki, R.A., Sidorov, I.A. et al. (2001). Identification of dynamically distinct subpopulations of T lymphocytes that are differentially affected by HIV. J Exp Med 194, 1731–1741.

Lanzavecchia, A. and Sallusto, F. (2000). Dynamics of T lymphocyte responses: intermediates, effectors, and memory cells. Science 290, 92–97.

Lefkovits, I. and Waldmann, H. (1999). Limiting dilution analysis of cells in the immune system. Cambridge: Cambridge University Press.

Lyons, A.B. and Parish, C.R. (1994). Determination of lymphocyte division by flow cytometry. J Immunol Meth 171, 131–137.

Lyons, A.B. (1999). Divided we stand: tracking cell proliferation with carboxyfluorescein diacetate succinimidyl ester. Immunol Cell Biol 77, 509–515.

Meidenbauer, N., Harris, D.T., Spitler, L.E. and Whiteside, T.L. (2000). Generation of PSA-reactive effector cells after vaccination with a PSA-based vaccine in patients with prostate cancer. Prostate 43, 88–100.

Miyamoto, S., Kimball, S.R. and Safer, B. (2000). Signal transduction pathways that contribute to increased protein synthesis during T-cell activation. Biochim Biophys Acta 1494, 28–42.

Moretta, A., Pantaleo, G., Moretta, M., Cerottini, J-C. and Mingari, C.M. (1983). Direct demonstration of the clonogenic potential of every human peripheral blood T cell. Clonal analysis of HLA-DR expression and cytolytic activity. J Exp Med 157, 743–754.

Mosmann, T. (1983). Rapid colorimetric assay for cellular growth and survival: application to proliferation and cytotoxicity assays. J Immunol Methods 65, 55–63.

Reinsmoen, N.L., Kaufman, D., Sutherland, D., Matas, A.J., Najarian, J.S. and Bach, F.H. (1990). A new in vitro approach to determine acquired tolerance in long-term kidney allograft recipients. Transplantation 50, 783–789.

Reinsmoen, N.L. and Matas, A.J. (1993). Evidence that improved late renal transplant outcome correlates with the development of in vitro donor antigen-specific hypo-reactivity. Transplantation 55, 1017–1023.

Riss, T.L. and Moravec, R.A. (1992). Comparison of MTT, XTT and a novel tetrazolium compound MTS for in vitro proliferation and chemosensitivity assays. Mol Biol Cell 3, 184a.

Savitskiy, V.P., Shman, T.V. and Potapnev, M.P. (2003). Comparative measurement of spontaneous apoptosis in pediatric acute leukemia by different techniques. Cytometry 56, 16–22.

Schultes, B. and Whiteside, T.L. (2003). Monitoring of immune responses to CA125 with an IFN-γ ELISPOT assay. J Immunol Methods 279, 1–15.

Sharrock, C.E.M., Kaminski, E. and Man, S. (1990). Limiting dilution analysis of human T cells: a useful clinical tool. Immunol Today 11, 281–283.

Vose, B.M., Vanky, F. and Klein, E. (1977). Human tumour-lymphocyte interactions in vitro. V. Comparison of the reactivity of tumour-infiltrating, blood and lymph-node lymphocytes with autologous tumor cells. Int J Cancer 20, 895–899.

Whiteside, T.L. (1993). Tumor-infiltrating lymphocytes in human malignancies. Austin, TX: Medical Intelligence Unit, R.G. Lands Co.

Monitoring Cell Death

Chapter 32

Deborah Braun and Matthew L. Albert

Laboratory of Dendritic Cell Immunobiology, Pasteur Institute, Paris, France

The Way of the Samurai is found in death. When it comes to either/or, there is only the quick choice of death. It is not particularly difficult. Be determined and advance. To say that dying without reaching one's aim is to die a dog's death.

Hagakure by Yamamoto Tsunetomo (1979)

INTRODUCTION

Apoptosis is widely recognized as the primary mechanism whereby physiologic and pathologic cell death occurs. It has become increasingly clear that dying cells have an influence on the immune system through the modulation of cytokine production and the delivery of antigen for MHC presentation. In order to dissect the ways in which dying cells influence the regulation of immune activation versus tolerance, we must clearly define the path taken as a cell moves from among the living to its final resting place within the phagosome. This chapter will examine principles of and methods for monitoring cell death.

Multicellular organisms have evolved genetic and epigenetic mechanisms of programmed cell death for the elimination of cells that are no longer needed or have become damaged. In this chapter, we provide an overview of the ways in which cells die and discuss the methods employed for asking the following set of *in vitro* and *in vivo* questions: are my cells dying? and what death effector pathways are responsible for their demise? While we cannot provide an exhaustive review nor do we offer detailed technical protocols, it is our hope that this overview will assist in the choice of methodology for

monitoring apoptotic cell death. We have subdivided the chapter into *in vitro* and *in vivo* methodologies – in each, we consider morphologic, biochemical and functional assays for monitoring cell death. Attention will be given to those methods that provide insight into what may be occurring during homeostatic and inflammatory cell death.

DEFINITIONS OF CELL DEATH

In the late nineteenth century Ruldolf Virchow characterized the morphologic features of cell death (Virchow, 1978). Necrosis (from the Greek word *nekroun*, meaning 'to make dead') was defined by localized death of living tissue as noted by the change in color, the refraction of light and by evidence of inflammation. On a cellular level, Virchow noted cell swelling and the loss of membrane integrity. In current day scientific literature, necrosis (or primary necrosis) is defined as passive death, triggered by noxious stimuli including extreme temperatures, toxins and hypotonic conditions (Raff, 1998; Savill et al., 2002). Such triggers typically affect large numbers of cells in a tissue microenvironment and result in the diffusion of cellular contents, which in turn provokes the release of inflammatory signals from surrounding, living cells (Zimmerman and Green, 2001). This loss of membrane integrity results in the release of lysosomal and nuclear contents, which triggers death in adjacent cells and initiates an inflammatory process in those that survive. Importantly, necrotic cell death is *not* under genetic control and death by necrosis does not result in the utilization of energy (e.g. ATP). In fact, these two criteria constitute the operational definition of necrosis that will be used herein as it provides a clear distinction from apoptosis.

To avoid confusion we distinguish necrosis from 'secondary necrosis': in the former, loss of membrane integrity is the mechanism of death; in contrast, 'secondary necrosis' connotes a cell that died an apoptotic death, but due to a defect in clearance the dying cell undergoes autolysis, thus compromising membrane integrity.

The term apoptosis (again from the Greek, *apo* meaning 'off' and *ptosis* meaning 'a falling of' as in autumn leaves) was first used to describe controlled cell deletion by Kerr et al. in 1972 (Kerr et al., 1972; Wylie et al., 1980). As in Virchow's time, it was characterized morphologically: 'nuclear and cytoplasmic condensation and breaking up of the cell into a number of membrane-bound, ultrastructurally well-preserved fragments' in the first stage; and later by the shedding of 'apoptotic bodies... from epithelial lined-surfaces' or internalization by 'other cells, where they undergo a series of changes resembling *in vitro* autolysis within phagosomes' (Kerr et al., 1972). Based on these microscopic observations in the adrenal gland following hormone withdrawal, it was concluded that apoptosis is an active, programmed phenomenon that is involved in cell turnover. The last 30 years of research suggest that their intellectual leap was correct and that programmed cell death (PCD) does indeed offer a counterpoint to mitosis in the regulation of tissue homeostasis. Note, while some

distinguish the terms 'apoptosis' and 'programmed cell death,' with the former referring to the morphologic characterization and the latter the biochemical features of active cell death, we will use these terms interchangeably with the operational definition being the requirement for energy (in the form of broken phosphate bonds).

While apoptotic cell death is a complex biochemical process involving multiple signaling pathways, the program has been conserved throughout evolution. In fact, it was work on the metazoan *Caenorhabditis elegans* (*C. elegans*) which resulted in the first reports on cell death abnormal (*ced*) genes (Ellis and Horvitz, 1986; Yuan et al., 1993). Based on these early studies and now more recent biochemical analysis, apoptosis has been divided into four stages: initiation, execution (early phase apoptosis), degradation (late phase apoptosis) and disposal (typically mediated by phagocytes) (Kim et al., 2003). Most of the death stimuli that have been studied (e.g. TNF-SF mediated, UV induced, serum starvation) will result in apoptosis with all four stages being evident (as based on morphology and biochemical analysis). It is important to point out, however, that some death stimuli (e.g. Granzyme B) and some cell types (e.g. neurons) will not display some of the characteristic features of apoptosis (Barry et al., 2000; Mektar et al., 2003). This points out the need for multiple assays for monitoring death and the need for kinetic studies/time courses in order to characterize the type of cell death and the molecular pathways responsible for cellular demise (Figure 32.1).

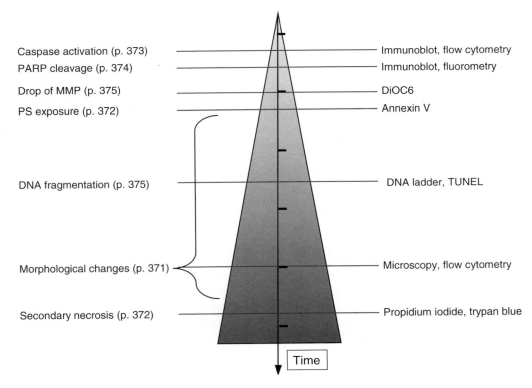

Figure 32.1 Monitoring the kinetics of apoptotic cell death. This figure illustrates the kinetic course of key apoptotic events and a subset of techniques that are available for their monitoring. Of note, the time course varies depending on the cell type and the mode of apoptosis induction. Detection of multiple events may help distinguish apoptosis from necrosis, as well as differentiate some of the known apoptotic pathways.

OVERVIEW OF CELL DEATH PATHWAYS

Currently, two distinct yet molecularly intertwined pathways are believed to play a role in programmed cell death – caspase activation and mitochondrial membrane permeabilization (MMP). Briefly, caspases constitute a family of aspartic acid-specific proteases that coordinate as well as execute the apoptotic process (Thornberry and Lazebnik, 1998). Caspases are synthesized as inactive precursors (zymogens) and are typically activated via proteolysis at an internal aspartic acid residue to become fully active. There are fourteen known mammalian caspases (Borner and Monney, 1999). The group of caspases involved in apoptosis can be divided in several ways. Initiator caspases, responsible for phase 1 of the death process include caspases -2, -8, -9, -10 (Salvesen and Dixit, 1999). These caspases activate effector caspases that are responsible for triggering the molecular pathways that control the biochemical and morphologic features characteristic of apoptosis. For example, activation of caspase-3 results in the cleavage of ICAD (inhibitor of CAD), in turn permitting the endogenous endonuclease CAD (caspase-3 activated DNAse) entry into the nucleus where it mediates nuclear fragmentation (Sakahira et al., 1998). The formation of apoptotic bodies and blebs occurs secondary to caspase-3 cleavage and the activation of gelsolin, p21-activated kinase-2 and fodrin, which together, facilitate dissociation of the cytoskeleton (Martin et al., 1995; Kothakota et al., 1997).

Over the past 10 years, a caspase-centric view of programmed cell death has emerged, in part due to the essential role for CED-3 in *C. elegans* and the aforementioned definition of caspase-mediated molecular pathways that control the biochemical and morphologic features of apoptosis. Recent studies using caspase knockout mice or pan-caspase inhibitors such as z-VAD-fmk offer a strikingly different perspective – evidence suggests that caspases are not essential for achieving cell death in mammalian cells (Perfettini and Kroemer, 2003). In fact, in some models, caspase inhibition resulted in higher levels of tumor necrosis factor (TNF-α) mediated apoptosis (Luschen et al., 2000). One such caspase-independent mechanism involves the generation of intracellular reactive oxygen species (ROS) secondary to death receptor engagement, which results in mitochondrial membrane permeability (MMP) (Cauwels et al., 2003). Such intracellular signals may induce pro-apoptotic Bcl-2 family members to translocate from the cytosol to the mitochondria, where they trigger release of cytochrome-c (cyt-c) (Green and Reed, 1998; Kroemer and Reed 2000). It is known that cyt-c in the cytosol may oligomerize apoptotic protease activating factor-1 (APAF-1) thus activating caspase-9 and in turn caspase-3 (Li et al., 1997; Zou et al., 1997). However, in the presence z-VAD-fmk, the cascade is interrupted – yet the cell does die, albeit a different kind of programmed cell death. While some have called these caspase-independent pathways 'sub-apoptosis' or even necrosis due to the absence of the classical morphologic features of apoptosis, these death effector pathways are energy dependent and *in vivo* phagocytes likely capture these cells without release of their intracellular contents.

While the biochemical details of these cell death pathways are beyond the scope of this chapter (and can be found detailed elsewhere), the critical point that has emerged from this complexity is that there exist distinct pathways for death and corpse removal. These may be distinguished by the apoptotic trigger, the cell-type undergoing programmed cell death and the phagocyte responsible for clearance. For a detailed discussion of this subject, please refer to the many excellent reviews that map the known execution pathways within a cell.

IN VITRO METHODS FOR MONITORING PROGRAMMED CELL DEATH

Morphologic characterization of apoptosis

Microscopic evaluation

Cell death by apoptosis is characterized by a series of morphological changes distinguishing them from healthy cells. Morphological examination of cells undergoing apoptosis by microscopy is still a standard method to study this phenomenon (Leist and Jaattela, 2001). The first evidence for apoptosis is chromatin condensation as visualized by electron microscopy (Figure 32.2, left). Compact globular or crescent-shaped figures accumulate at the edge of the nucleus, which to the careful observer can also be seen by light microscopy as change in refraction or by the visualization of dense structures using nucleic acid-binding dyes such as hematoxylin, acridine orange or propidium iodide (Figure 32.2, right) (Foglieni et al., 2001). Next, cell shrinkage may be observed, and in adherent cultures detachment from neighboring cells may be evident. Depending on the cell type, late-stage apoptosis features the formation of cytoplasmic blebs and apoptotic bodies, the former are 0.2–1.0 μm vesicles containing membrane from the endoplasmic reticulum (ER), RNA and RNA binding proteins, while the latter are 0.8–6.0 μm in size and contain nuclear fragments (Figure 2, bottom) (Casciola-Rosen et al., 1994; Rosen et al., 1995). Time-lapse studies show that these changes take place in the course of a few hours.

While light microscopic evaluation permits rapid assessment of cultured cells, this method is qualitative and does not permit classification based on the triggering of distinct death pathways. As will be discussed below, the use of vital dyes (e.g. trypan blue) allows for assessment of membrane integrity. Electron microscopy is much more sensitive, however, it is not as readily available and again, quantification is difficult to achieve.

Flow cytometry

Morphologic assessment may also be performed using flow cytometric analysis (Vermes et al., 2000). We may

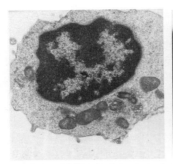
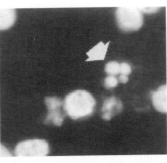
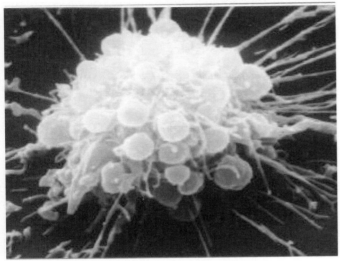

Figure 32.2 Morphologic characteristics of apoptotic cell death. Apoptotic cells may be visualized by transmission electron microscopy (top left), light microscopy (top right) or scanning EM (bottom). The progressive stages of apoptotis: chromatin condensation; nuclear fragmentation (visualized using Hoescht staining); body and bleb formation can be seen here (clockwise). (From www.cyto.purdue.edu/cdroms/flow/vol14/15_apop/data/malorni/malorni.htm)

distinguish healthy cells from late apoptotic cells by taking advantage of the fact that incident light can be used to determine a cell's size (forward scatter, FSC) and granularity (side scatter, SSC). Shrinkage of the cytoplasm and condensation of the nucleus results in decreased FSC and increased SSC. One consideration in using this method is that classical nuclear condensation is a feature of late stage (phase 3) cell death. An obvious advantage to using cytometry is the rapid and quantitative assessment of large numbers of cells. As discussed below, evaluation of these morphologic changes may be combined with FACS-based assays for biochemical events occurring during cell death. Our experience suggests that SSC changes correspond to nuclear fragmentation as monitored by TUNEL staining (see below).

Apoptosis versus necrosis

Chromatin condensation and maintenance of cell membrane integrity help differentiate apoptosis from necrosis (Leist and Jaattela, 2001). This may be evaluated by light

and electron microscopy – necrosis is characterized by mitochondrial swelling, nuclear flocculation and disruption of the plasma membrane. As a consequence of this latter point, necrotic cells lose their capacity to exclude vital dyes such as trypan blue. One caveat is that necrosis and 'secondary necrosis' (autolysis as a terminal event in programmed cell death) cannot be distinguished by this method, again highlighting the importance of kinetic studies.

The morphologic diversity of apoptotic cell death

While it is agreed that apoptotic cell death is characterized by chromatin condensation, cell shrinkage and the maintenance of plasma membrane integrity, there exist many variants (depending on the cell type, the death effector pathways and possibly, the observer). Thus, as recently catalogued (Zitvogel et al.), cells may die from apoptosis (Kerr et al., 1972), apoptosis-like programmed cell death (Leist and Jaattela, 2001), necroapoptosis (Jaeschke and Lemasters, 2003), oncosis (Majno and Joris, 1995), paraptosis (Sperandio et al., 2000), limoktonia (Xue et al., 2001), autoschizis (Jamison et al., 2002), autophagic cell death (Bursch, 2001), mitotic catastrophe (Roninson, 2002) or terminal senescence (Roninson and Dokmanovic, 2003). While we cannot underestimate the importance of looking at cultured cells, the diversity of phenotypes reported in the literature and the subjective nature of morphologic analysis demands that we also pursue biochemical analysis of our dying cells.

Molecular/biochemical features of apoptosis

Cell surface changes

While much is known regarding the triggers and signal transduction cascades responsible for apoptosis, less is known about changes in the plasma membrane of the dying cell. Investigations employing a variety of cell types imply that changes may include carbohydrate motifs (e.g. N-acetyl glucosamine), distinct patterns of surface phospholipid exposure, as well as subtle structural changes (Savill et al., 2002).

One of the best characterized changes in the plasma membrane occurs during early apoptotic death. Caspase-3 has been shown to inactivate a flipase (also called the aminophospholipid translocase) that is responsible for maintaining anionic phospholipids exclusively within the inner leaflet of the plasma membrane (Schlegel and Williamson, 2001; Williamson and Schlegel, 2002). Additionally, there is the activation of a lipid scramblase, which effectively scrambles the lipid bilayers of the dying cell. Together, these two events result in loss of membrane asymmetry throughout the cell, including the plasma membrane. One of the newly exposed phospholipids is phosphatidylserine (PS), and it has been proposed that this may serve as a ligand for engagement with the phagocyte (Fadok and Henson, 1998; Savill and Fadok, 2000).

Competition experiments employing either liposomes containing PS, or soluble phosphoserine salts suggest that this indeed constitutes a means of phagocyte recognition of the dying cell. Supporting these data is the observation that externalized PS may bind soluble proteins to form a molecular complex that is recognized by relevant phagocytic receptors.

Exposure of PS can be detected by the use of an endogenous Ca^{2+}-dependent phospholipid binding protein, annexin V (Koopman et al., 1994; van Engeland et al., 1996). Several commercial vendors sell recombinant annexin V conjugated to fluorescent or biotin moieties, thus allowing for rapid detection of PS. For example, the high affinity of annexin V for PS renders it a sensitive probe for apoptotic cell analysis by flow cytometry (Vermes et al., 2000). Staining is commonly used in conjunction with DNA intercalating dye such as PI (or 7-AAD). Indeed sole use of annexin V cannot distinguish between early, late apoptotic and secondary necrotic cells. Typically, live cells are annexin V and PI negative. After apoptosis induction, they become annexin V positive but stay impermeable to PI. At later stages, due to the loss of membrane integrity, they finally become annexin V positive and PI positive, which render them indistinguishable from necrotic cells. As cell death in a cell population may not be synchronous, kinetic studies are necessary to ensure that cell death occurs by apoptosis. Of note, other PS-binding opsonins such as C3bi may be used, however, they are less specific than annexin V (Verbovetski et al., 2002).

Another detectable change of physiologic relevance is a conformational shift in ICAM-3 (CD50) (Moffatt et al., 1999). During cell death, the shape of this leukocyte-restricted protein changes so that the distal extracellular domain of the protein (domain 1) may now interact with CD14, a receptor on macrophages that mediates recognition of apoptotic cells. Antibodies specific for domain 1 seem capable of detecting this conformation shift and may prove useful for the monitoring of cell death.

Recent studies have shown that phagocytosis of apoptotic cells is not only driven by the expression of 'eat-me' signals displayed by the dying cell, but also respond to the loss of 'don't eat me' signals. CD31 (PECAM-1) constitutes such a receptor and signaling through CD31 has been shown to prevent phagocyte engulfment of viable cells (Brown et al., 2002). Disruption of CD31 signaling promotes tight binding and ingestion by the phagocytes. CD31 is a widely expressed adhesion receptor involved in cell–cell contact through homotypic interactions. While the mechanism by which CD31 signaling is altered in dying cells is unknown, Brown et al. have shown that both CD31 tyrosine phosphorylation and SHP-1/2 recruitment are altered in apoptotic leukocytes. These changes in the CD31 signaling pathway may thus be used as markers of apoptosis.

Other surface changes include the display of increased amounts of fucose residues. This has been reported for apoptosis secondary to dexamethasone, gliotoxin and thepsigargin treatment (Staudacher et al., 1999). Finally, it

bears mention that as a result of caspase-3 activation, an acid pH-dependent sphingomyelinase (ASMase) is triggered, which in turn catabolizes sphingomyelin (SM) present in the outer leaflet of the plasma membrane and results in the generation of ceramide and sphingosine 1-phosphate (S1p) (Pena et al., 1997). Decreased SM also results in the loss of cholesterol from the plasma membrane, thought to be a mechanism by which increased membrane curvature is achieved (a requisite for being eaten and degraded by phagocytes). Rapid, user-friendly assays do not exist for these sets of surface changes, however, a complete characterization of different death pathways may require the establishment of such experimental techniques.

Cytoplasmic changes – caspase effector pathways

While apoptosis is mostly triggered by external stimuli (cross-linking of death receptors), the initial changes may be followed by assaying biochemical events in the cytosol. Classical apoptosis is characterized by the activation of a set of cysteine proteases called caspases (Thornberry and Lazebnik, 1998). As is true for many proteases, caspases are synthesized as enzymatically inert zymogens. Caspase activation is, in most cases, achieved by proteolytic cleavage of the pro-enzyme by upstream caspases. Exceptions include caspase-8, caspase-9 (and likely caspase-10). For caspase-8 and caspase-10, aggregation results in allosteric regulation of basal activity, leading to self-proteolysis. For caspase-9, cleavage has very little effect; activation requires its association with two other proteins, Apaf-1 and cytochrome c, which together form the apoptosome (Adams and Cory, 2002).

As we have suggested, the term 'apoptosis' encompasses diverse death-initiating programs that share similar morphologic features. With recently developed assays, it is possible to monitor differential usage of caspases and map them to a given apoptotic trigger. For example, death receptor engagement (e.g. TNF-RI and FAS) induces a program that employs caspase-8 and, depending on the cell type, activates caspase-3 directly or via a mitochondrial pathway (Nagata, 1997); CTLs kill via secretion of granzyme B, which bypasses initiator caspases and results in the activation of caspase-2, caspase-3 or direct cleavage of Bid, a bcl-2 family member capable of triggering mitochondrial-mediated cell death (again depending on the cell type) (Barry et al., 2000; Lord et al., 2003; Metkar et al., 2003); ER stress responses, such as those provoked by oxidative stress, glycosylation inhibitors or calcium ionophores, involve caspase-12 (Nakagawa and Yuan, 2000; Nakagawa et al., 2000); external stress such as induced by UV, gamma irradiation or serum withdrawal mediate death via altered mitochondrial membrane potential and the activation of caspase-9 (Green and Read, 1998). Thus, monitoring the activation of specific caspase molecules (and the order in which they are triggered) may reveal characteristic patterns indicating the type of stimulus and may turn out to correlate with downstream immunologic outcomes of death (Albert, 2004).

Caspase activation may be monitored in several ways. Using immunoblot analysis, it is possible to detect cleaved/active forms of the caspases themselves, or cleavage products of defined substrates. This is a widely used method by which the processing of a particular procaspase is studied by detecting (with a specific antibody) the appearance of a small or large subunit of the mature caspase, or caspase target. To date, more than 280 targets have been identified (Fischer et al., 2003). These have been detailed with the precise cleavage site identified and careful choice of substrate analysis may help define the precise apoptotic pathway triggered during programmed cell death. Standard Western blot or two-dimensional gel immunoblot protocols may be used for monitoring these cleavage events and many antibodies are now commercially available. While sensitive, these assays are not specific for cell death as processed caspases or cleaved caspase substrates may be found in living cells (Alam et al., 1999). Furthermore, these assays are qualitative and do not provide per cell analysis of caspase activity.

An alternative strategy to detect caspase activity is through the use of defined synthetic substrates (e.g. PARP, α-fodrin) (Green, 1998). Cell lysates may be prepared, re-suspended in appropriate buffer and exposed to known substrates containing the tetrapeptide consensus sequences (Table 32.1). The synthetic substrate can be evaluated by immunoblot as above. Alternatively, substrates conjugated to chromophores or fluorochromes may be employed. In this way, cleavage can be monitored using a spectrophotometer or a fluorescence microtiter plate reader, respectively (Garcia-Calvo et al., 1998; Kohler et al., 2002). To determine the activity of a specific caspase, substrates containing restricted consensus motifs may be used. For example, LETD containing substrates will selectively test for activated caspase-8 and Granzyme B. The advantage of this technique is that it is quantitative and highly sensitive and, as mentioned above, the use of different peptide substrates offers the possibility of discriminating/comparing the activity of different caspases. Still, this method does not achieve per cell analysis of cell death.

A recent advance has been the use of cell-permeable caspase inhibitors for detection of apoptotic cell death. As an important technical point, it should be noted that these inhibitors can themselves be toxic to cells so one must always run live cell controls with the experimental samples. Caspase inhibitors were first identified in pox virus (CrmA) and baculovirus (p35); elucidation of their mechanism of action demonstrated that the pseudosubstrate site (LVAD and DQMD, respectively) effectively bound and inhibited activated caspase molecules (Clem et al., 1991; Miura et al., 1993). Derivative three- and four-amino acid substrates have been characterized and via chemical linkage to reactive organic moieties, they bind and inhibit

Table 32.1 Polypetidic probes for detection of active caspases. Polypetidic sequences used for monitoring active caspases are listed. These peptides may be used as fluorogenic substrates when coupled to AMC (aminomethylcoumarin), AFC (aminotrifluoromethylcoumarin) or other fluorophores. When conjugates to an aldehyde group (reversible binding) or a ketone derivative (irreversible binding), they function as potent inhibitors of caspase activity. The consensus peptide sequence are primarily recognized by caspases indicated in bold; weaker binding by caspases is indicated by italics.

Peptide sequence	Target for Caspases
VAD	1, 2, 3, 4, 5, 6, 7, 8, 9,
YVAD	*1*, 4
VDVAD	2
DEVD	**3**, *6, 7, 8, 10*
VEID	**6**, *3, 7, 8*
IETD	*8*, granzyme B
LETD	*8*, granzyme B
LEHD	**9**, *4, 5, 6*
LEED	13
AAD	granzyme B
Aspartic acid	generic

caspase activity. Functional groups that have been employed include aldehyde (CHO), fluoro-methylketone (FMK), chloromethylketone (CMK) and fluoroacyloxymethylketone (FAOM) – screening your specific cell type in question may identify the appropriate reagent as based on minimal cell toxicity. One additional consideration is that probes conjugated with CHO are reversible inhibitors, while those with CMK, FMK or FAOM are irreversible (Salgado et al., 2002). Many of the known caspase inhibitors (see Table 32.1) are commercially available, both unconjugated (for functional studies) and conjugated to fluorochromes (for detection). Alternatively, cell permeable tetrameric peptides coupled to quenched fluorochromes permit detection of real-time caspase activation – cleavage of these substrates releases the fluorochome, detectable via cytometry. FACS based and immunofluorescent studies are advantageous as both allow for evaluation of cell death on a per cell basis. Such analysis also facilitates identification (and even isolation) of small populations of apoptotic cells. Finally, dissection of the caspase activation pathways may be possible using combinations of these reagents (Hirata et al., 1998).

Cytoplasmic changes – mitochondrial effector pathways

While the use of caspase-selective inhibitors may help identify the cell death pathway employed, it is also worth considering analysis of mitochondrial changes that are known to occur during cell death. The mitochondria play a major role in the apoptotic processes and the effort to characterize relevant changes may be critical for illuminating the specific cell death pathways utilized. In caspase-dependent pathways, the mitochondria are the source of cytochrome c, known to activate the apoptosome in turn facilitating pro-caspase-3 cleavage (Li et al., 1997). The mitochondria are also the source for apoptosis inducing factor (AIF), which may play a role in caspase-independent cell death (Susin et al., 1999, 2000). Moreover, a number of pro- and counter-apoptotic molecules, belonging to the Bcl-2 family, are localized to the mitochondrial membrane and regulate cell death (Chao and Korsmeyer, 1998).

Although there still exists some controversy, a drop in mitochondrial transmembrane potential ($\Delta \Psi m$) is likely one of the first measurable events (Green and Read, 1998). It is also possible to detect alterations in oxidation-reduction potential. Changes in the transmembrane potential are presumed to occur due to the opening of pores and channels, resulting in the equilibration of ions, interruption of the electron transport chain and release of cytochrome c into the cytosol. Assays have been developed to monitor each of these steps.

The drop in $\Delta \Psi m$ can be revealed through the use of potential-sensitive probes which include (but are not limited to) 3,3-dihexyloxacarbocyanine iodide (DiOC6), 5,5',6,6'-tetrachloro-1,1',3,3'-tetraethylbenzimidazolcarbocyanine iodide (JC-1) and tetramethulrosamine derivatives (CMXRos) (Gilmore and Wilson, 1999; Ozgen et al., 2000; Rasola and Geuna, 2001; Kalbacova et al., 2003; Zuliani et al., 2003). Each works slightly differently but, in all cases, a drop in membrane potential translates in a shift in fluorescence that may be analyzed by flow cytometry or fluorescence microscopy. As with other assays, it is useful to exclude necrotic cells from the analysis (Zuliani et al., 2003). This may be possible by combining the potential-sensitive probes with Hoescht (UV detector is required), TOTO-3 or TOPRO-3.

Cytochrome c release can also be monitored as a marker of cell death. This is possible through the use of available anti-cytochrome c antibodies. Diffusion of the protein in the cytosol is evaluated by immunofluorescence. Alternatively, transduction of target cells with a construct expressing cytochome c-GFP fusion protein allows for real time imaging of cytochrome c release (Goldstein et al., 2000).

Other cytosolic changes that can be monitored include: bax translocation to the nucleus, p53 upregulation, increased acidification and actin cytoskeleton rearrangement.

Nuclear changes

One of easiest features of apoptotic cells to monitor is the break-up of the genomic DNA by cellular nucleases. This late and characteristic event in apoptosis is a result of the activation of CAD and other endonucleases, creating extensive double-stranded and single-stranded breaks in DNA (Sakahira et al., 1998). This process yields mono- and oligonucleosomes, effectively reducing the higher order chromatin structure. These cleavage events may be assessed by electrophoresis using extracted DNA, run on

an agarose gel. The DNA of non-apoptotic cells remains intact and does not enter the gel, while the DNA from apoptotic cells displays the classic appearance of 'DNA laddering'. Although straightforward, this assay cannot distinguish subpopulations of cells.

A more quantitative method involves the use of flow cytometry to monitor a sub-diploid peak in a cell population undergoing cell death (Vermes et al., 2000). Propidium iodide (PI), a DNA intercalating agent that may be excited at the 488 nm line of an argon-ion laser, fluoresces at 617 nm, making it useful for such a FACS-based assay for DNA content. Briefly, cells are fixed and permeabilized with a mild saponin solution (Nicoletti et al., 1991). After washing, the cells are resuspended in a solution of 50–100 μg/ml PI and cells are analyzed by FACS. The amount of PI fluorescence is proportional to the amount of double-stranded DNA present in the cell. It thus enables the detection of cells undergoing DNA fragmentation (as well as cells in the S and G2 phases of the cell cycle). The cells undergoing late-stage apoptosis will show up in a sub-diploid (G0–G1) peak. While quite easy to perform, the emission spectrum of PI overlaps with both phycoerythrin (FL2) and Cy5 (FL3), thus partially limiting the possibilities for simultaneous surface staining. An alternative DNA-binding agent is 7-aminoactinomycin D (7-AAD), a fluorescent nucleoside analog, which intercalates between cytosine and guanosine bases. It fluoresces in the far red and may be used in conjunction with FITC and PE, allowing for surface staining and identification of subpopulations undergoing cell death.

Another method often used to detect fragmented DNA utilizes a reaction catalyzed by terminal deoxynucleotidyl transferase (TdT), often referred to as TUNEL (TdT dUTP nick-end labeling). In TUNEL assays, TdT catalyzes a template-independent addition of labeled deoxyuridine triphosphates (X-dUTP) to the 3'-hydroxyl (OH) termini of double- and single-stranded DNA. dUTP is typically conjugated to a fluorochrome, biotin moiety (detected with streptavidin-conjugated fluorochromes) or a bromine molecule (detected with anti-BrdU antibodies). After incorporation, cells may be monitored by cytometry. Alternatively, labeled DNA may be assessed using a peroxidase-based reporter assay. This enzyme is typically used to catalyze a substrate for the generation of a colored signal, read out on a spectrophotometer.

A similar assay uses the Klenow fragment of the DNA polymerase instead of TdT. This assay is called in situ end-labeling (ISEL) and is comparable, although slightly less sensitive than TUNEL (Mundle et al., 1995). Decreased sensitivity is due to the fact that ISEL labels only 3' recessed ends, whereas TdT can label 3' recessed, 5' recessed or blunt ends of DNA.

Functional assays

The final outcome of cell death is clearance of the apoptotic corpse/bodies/blebs by phagocytes. As discussed above, the dying cell exposes novel and altered surface markers on its plasma membrane, thus facilitating recognition and rapid internalization. Strikingly, some studies indicate that phagocytosis precedes the earliest markers of apoptosis; instead, it is suggested that the loss of 'life-signals', which had held the phagocyte at bay, offers the trigger for clearance (Brown et al., 2002). This is an attractive idea given the extreme difficulty in observing TUNEL positive apoptotic cells in situ under physiologic and even pathologic conditions. An alternative possibility would simply be that the 'eat-me' signals detected by the phagocyte are more sensitive than our earliest markers for cell death. In either case, it suggests that functional assays monitoring phagocytosis may be employed as an early means of detecting cell death.

Several microscopic- and FACS-based assays have been established for phagocytosis (Albert et al., 1998; Jersmann et al., 2003). Given the need for quantification, we favor cytometric based assays. Briefly, it is possible to dye label apoptotic cells and phagocytes with cytosolic esters (e.g. CFSE, CMFDA) or lipid intercalating dyes (e.g. PKH-26, -67) and upon co-culture monitor the percentage of phagocytes that have become double positive. It is important to control for cell aggregates being scored as double positive cells. Incubation in 5–10 mM EDTA followed by rigorous vortexing should dissociate clusters (with the notable exception of antibody opsonized apoptotic cells binding Fc receptors). Phagocytosis may be validated through use of inhibitors such as cytochalasins or incubation at low temperature. Another important consideration is that phagocytic or non-phagocytic populations can be further characterized (e.g. cytokine production) using additional probes and multicolor cytometric analysis.

IN VIVO DETECTION OF CELL DEATH

Ex vivo approaches

Most of the described methodology can be applied to ex vivo purified cells to assess for death occurring in vivo. Such methods have for example been applied to HIV and cancer patients. Notably, Whiteside and colleagues have been able to correlate T cell apoptosis with prognosis of head and neck as well as ovarian carcinoma (Bauernhofer et al., 2003; Tsukishiro et al., 2003).

Histologic analysis

The rapidity with which apoptotic cells are phagocytosed in vivo renders their detection in histologic section difficult. Furthermore, early apoptotic cells often cannot be distinguished from living cells. A few techniques, however, are useful to detect apoptotic cells in tissue sections. Careful imaging should be performed to determine if the dying cells are extracellular or within the phagolysosome of a neighboring cell or professional phagocytes. Several of the methods discussed above are useful for

such analysis. These include use of probes for monitoring active caspase molecules, detection of nick-end labeled DNA using TUNEL staining and the subcellular localization of translocated molecules (e.g. p53, bax).

One assay unique to tissue section is the detection of tissue transglutaminase (tTG) (Grabarek et al., 2002; Volokhina et al., 2003). This enzyme is activated during the clearance phase of apoptosis and is considered critical for the formation of apoptotic bodies. It catalyzes the cross-linking of intracellular proteins and facilitates assembly of a protein scaffold that prevents leakage of intracellular contents. Notably, the cross-linkage itself is not degraded by the phagocyte but instead released and thus detectable in the extracellular space. In this way, it offers a sign of a prior apoptotic event. In situ hybridization may allow detection of tTG mRNA, upregulated during cell death. Alternatively, it is possible to monitor tTG by immunocytochemistry or immunoelectron microscopy using anti-tTG antibodies, by identification of glutamyl-lysine cross-links in apoptotic cells or by use of detergents to reveal insoluble cross-linked proteins.

Imaging dying cells

One recent advance in the field has been the use of non-invasive imaging techniques for monitoring cell death in vivo. This technology has thus far been applied to the detection of cardiac allograft rejection as well as other transplanted organs, monitoring of atherosclerotic lesions and imaging of cell death in solid tumors (Narula et al., 2001; Blankenberg et al., 2003; Petrovsky et al., 2003). Briefly, technetium-99m-labeled annexin-V has been infused intravenously into human subjects and used as a non-invasive means of assessing apoptosis (Narula et al., 2001). Serial gamma imaging may be performed and through radiographic image analysis uptake of the annexin-V by a specific tissue may be evaluated. One convincing use of this technology was in a population of cardiac allotransplant patients. Myocardial uptake of annexin-V correlated with TUNEL staining and active caspase molecules in endomyocardial biopsy specimens. The high affinity of annexin-V for PS ($Ka = 7$ nm) makes this analysis feasible, however, the rapid internalization of dying cells and the recent evidence that PS may be present on the outer leaflet of activated macrophages as well as other cell types introduces the possibility of false positives. For this reason, careful consideration must be given to the clinical setting used for this technique. Of note, intravital study in animals has also been performed using annexin-V conjugated to Oregon Green (Dumont et al., 2001).

WHY SO MANY ASSAYS FOR MONITORING CELL DEATH?

We now know that antigen derived from internalized apoptotic cells may be processed and presented by dendritic cells for the engagement of CD4$^+$ and CD8$^+$ T cells (Albert, 2001; Albert et al., 2001). Defects in clearance may result in autoimmunity whereas phagocytosis by macrophages that have been recruited as part of the tumor stroma may be a mechanism of tumor antigen sequestration and/or TGF-α secretion. As such, the dying cell is influencing immunity. With respect to the different types of cell death, we expect that, as we uncover the intricacy of programmed cell death pathways, we will also discover subtle ways in which the specific trigger of apoptosis is influencing the immunologic microenvironment. As it is increasingly important to be precise about the specific death effector pathways triggered and the class of proteins upregulated, multiple parameters for monitoring are required. Furthermore, we predict that in vivo imaging of apoptosis will improve and help clinicians identify early events in tumorigenesis, graft rejection and sites of chronic inflammation. This added level of complexity will synergize with the growing insights from the field of clearance and the importance of how receptor utilization influences immunity. In this way, we may decipher the complex and active signals that are transmitted by the newly dead and the phagocytes interested in eating them.

REFERENCES

Adams, J.M. and Cory, S. (2002). Apoptosomes: engines for caspase activation. Curr Opin Cell Biol 14, 715–720.

Alam, A., Cohen, L.Y., Aouad, S. and Sekaly, R.P. (1999). Early activation of caspases during T lymphocyte stimulation results in selective substrate cleavage in nonapoptotic cells. J Exp Med 190, 1879–1890.

Albert, M.L. (2001). Resurrecting the dead: phagocytosis of apoptotic cells by dendritic cells results in the cross-presentation of exogenous antigen. In Dendritic Cells: Biology and Clinical Applications, Lotze, M., ed. Academic Press.

Albert, M.L. (2004). Death-defying immunity: do apoptotic cells influence antigen processing and presentation? Nat Rev Immunol 4, 223–231.

Albert, M.L., Pearce, S.F., Francisco, L.M. et al. (1998). Immature dendritic cells phagocytose apoptotic cells via alphavbeta5 and CD36, and cross-present antigens to cytotoxic T lymphocytes. J Exp Med 188, 1359–1368.

Albert, M.L., Jegathesan, M. and Darnell, R.B. (2001). Dendritic cell maturation is required for the cross-tolerization of CD8+ T cells. Nat Immunol 2, 1010–1017.

Barry, M., Heibein, J.A., Pinkoski, M.J. et al. (2000). Granzyme B short-circuits the need for caspase 8 activity during granule-mediated cytotoxic T-lymphocyte killing by directly cleaving Bid. Mol Cell Biol 20, 3781–3794.

Bauernhofer, T., Kuss, I., Henderson, B., Baum, A.S. and Whiteside, T.L. (2003). Preferential apoptosis of CD56dim natural killer cell subset in patients with cancer. Eur J Immunol 33, 119–124.

Blankenberg, F., Mari, C. and Strauss, H.W. (2003). Imaging cell death in vivo. Q J Nucl Med 47, 337–348.

Borner, C. and Monney, L. (1999). Apoptosis without caspases: an inefficient molecular guillotine? Cell Death Differ 6, 497–507.

Brown, S., Heinisch, I., Ross, E. et al. (2002). Apoptosis disables CD31-mediated cell detachment from phagocytes promoting binding and engulfment. Nature 418, 200–203.

Bursch, W. (2001). The autophagosomal-lysosomal compartment in programmed cell death. Cell Death Differ 8, 569–581.

Casciola-Rosen, L.A., Anhalt, G. and Rosen, A. (1994). Autoantigens targeted in systemic lupus erythematosus are clustered in two populations of surface structures on apoptotic keratinocytes (see comments). J Exp Med 179, 1317–1330.

Cauwels, A., Janssen, B., Waeytens, A., Cuvelier, C. and Brouckaert, P. (2003). Caspase inhibition causes hyperacute tumor necrosis factor-induced shock via oxidative stress and phospholipase A2. Nat Immunol 4, 387–393.

Chao, D.T. and Korsmeyer, S.J. (1998). BCL-2 family: regulators of cell death. Annu Rev Immunol 16, 395–419.

Clem, R.J., Fechheimer, M. and Miller, L.K. (1991). Prevention of apoptosis by a baculovirus gene during infection of insect cells. Science 254, 1388–1390.

Dumont, E.A., Reutelingsperger, C.P., Smits, J.F. et al. (2001). Real-time imaging of apoptotic cell-membrane changes at the single-cell level in the beating murine heart. Nat Med 7, 1352–1355.

Ellis, H.M. and Horvitz, H.R. (1986). Genetic control of programmed cell death in the nematode C. elegans. Cell 44, 817–829.

Fadok, V.A. and Henson, P.M. (1998). Apoptosis: getting rid of the bodies. Curr Biol 8, R693–695.

Fischer, U., Janicke, R.U. and Schulze-Osthoff, K. (2003). Many cuts to ruin: a comprehensive update of caspase substrates. Cell Death Differ 10, 76–100.

Foglieni, C., Meoni, C. and Davalli, A.M. (2001). Fluorescent dyes for cell viability: an application on prefixed conditions. Histochem Cell Biol 115, 223–229.

Garcia-Calvo, M., Peterson, E.P., Leiting, B. et al. (1998). Inhibition of human caspases by peptide-based and macromolecular inhibitors. J Biol Chem 273, 32608–32613.

Gilmore, K. and Wilson, M. (1999). The use of chloromethyl-X-rosamine (Mitotracker red) to measure loss of mitochondrial membrane potential in apoptotic cells is incompatible with cell fixation. Cytometry 36, 355–358.

Goldstein, J.C., Waterhouse, N.J., Juin, P., Evan, G.I. and Green, D.R. (2000). The coordinate release of cytochrome c during apoptosis is rapid, complete and kinetically invariant. Nat Cell Biol 2, 156–162.

Grabarek, J., Ardelt, B., Kunicki, J. and Darzynkiewicz, Z. (2002). Detection of in situ activation of transglutaminase during apoptosis: correlation with the cell cycle phase by multiparameter flow and laser scanning cytometry. Cytometry 49, 83–89.

Green, D.R. (1998). Apoptotic pathways: the roads to ruin. Cell 94, 695–698.

Green, D.R. and Reed, J.C. (1998). Mitochondria and apoptosis. Science 281, 1309–1312.

Hirata, H., Takahashi, A., Kobayashi, S. et al. (1998). Caspases are activated in a branched protease cascade and control distinct downstream processes in Fas-induced apoptosis. J Exp Med 187, 587–600.

Jaeschke, H. and Lemasters, J.J. (2003). Apoptosis versus oncotic necrosis in hepatic ischemia/reperfusion injury. Gastroenterology 125, 1246–1257.

Jamison, J.M., Gilloteaux, J., Taper, H.S., Calderon, P.B. and Summers, J.L. (2002). Autoschizis: a novel cell death. Biochem Pharmacol 63, 1773–1783.

Jersmann, H.P., Ross, K.A., Vivers, S. et al. (2003). Phagocytosis of apoptotic cells by human macrophages: analysis by multi-parameter flow cytometry. Cytometry 51A, 7–15.

Kalbacova, M., Vrbacky, M., Drahota, Z. and Melkova, Z. (2003). Comparison of the effect of mitochondrial inhibitors on mitochondrial membrane potential in two different cell lines using flow cytometry and spectrofluorometry. Cytometry 52A, 110–116.

Kerr, J.F., Wyllie, A.H. and Currie, A.R. (1972). Apoptosis: a basic biological phenomenon with wide-ranging implications in tissue kinetics. Br J Cancer 26, 239–257.

Kim, S.J., Gershov, D., Ma, X., Brot, N. and Elkon, K.B. (2002). Opsonization of apoptotic cells and its effect on macrophage and T cell immune responses. Ann NY Acad Sci 987, 68–78.

Kohler, C., Orrenius, S. and Zhivotovsky, B. (2002). Evaluation of caspase activity in apoptotic cells. J Immunol Methods 265, 97–110.

Koopman, G., Reutelingsperger, C.P., Kuijten, G.A. et al. (1994). Annexin V for flow cytometric detection of phosphatidylserine expression on B cells undergoing apoptosis. Blood 84, 1415–1420.

Kothakota, S., Azuma, T., Reinhard, C. et al. (1997). Caspase-3-generated fragment of gelsolin: effector of morphological change in apoptosis. Science 278, 294–298.

Kroemer, G. and Reed, J.C. (2000). Mitochondrial control of cell death. Nat Med 6, 513–519.

Leist, M. and Jaattela, M. (2001). Four deaths and a funeral: from caspases to alternative mechanisms. Nat Rev Mol Cell Biol 2, 589–598.

Li, P., Nijhawan, D., Budihardjo, I. et al. (1997). Cytochrome c and dATP-dependent formation of Apaf-1/caspase-9 complex initiates an apoptotic protease cascade. Cell 91, 479–489.

Lord, S.J., Rajotte, R.V., Korbutt, G.S. and Bleackley, R.C. (2003). Granzyme B: a natural born killer. Immunol Rev 193, 31–38.

Luschen, S., Ussat, S., Scherer, G., Kabelitz, D. and Adam-Klages, S. (2000). Sensitization to death receptor cytotoxicity by inhibition of fas-associated death domain protein (FADD)/caspase signaling. Requirement of cell cycle progression. J Biol Chem 275, 24670–24678.

Majno, G. and Joris, I. (1995). Apoptosis, oncosis, and necrosis. An overview of cell death. Am J Pathol 146, 3–15.

Martin, S.J., O'Brien, G.A., Nishioka, W.K. et al. (1995). Proteolysis of fodrin (non-erythroid spectrin) during apoptosis. J Biol Chem 270, 6425–6428.

Metkar, S.S., Wang, B., Ebbs, M.L. et al. (2003). Granzyme B activates procaspase-3 which signals a mitochondrial amplification loop for maximal apoptosis. J Cell Biol 160, 875–885.

Miura, M., Zhu, H., Rotello, R., Hartwieg, E.A. and Yuan, J. (1993). Induction of apoptosis in fibroblasts by IL-1 beta-converting enzyme, a mammalian homolog of the C. elegans cell death gene ced-3. Cell 75, 653–660.

Moffatt, O.D., Devitt, A., Bell, E.D., Simmons, D.L. and Gregory, C.D. (1999). Macrophage recognition of ICAM-3 on apoptotic leukocytes. J Immunol 162, 6800–6810.

Mundle, S.D., Gao, X.Z., Khan, S. et al. (1995). Two in situ labeling techniques reveal different patterns of DNA fragmentation during spontaneous apoptosis in vivo and induced apoptosis in vitro. Anticancer Res 15, 1895–1904.

Nagata, S. (1997). Apoptosis by death factor. Cell 88, 355–365.

Nakagawa, T. and Yuan, J. (2000). Cross-talk between two cysteine protease families. Activation of caspase-12 by calpain in apoptosis. J Cell Biol 150, 887–894.

Nakagawa, T., Zhu, H., Morishima, N. et al. (2000). Caspase-12 mediates endoplasmic-reticulum-specific apoptosis and cytotoxicity by amyloid-beta. Nature 403, 98–103.

Narula, J., Acio, E.R., Narula, N. et al. (2001). Annexin-V imaging for noninvasive detection of cardiac allograft rejection. Nat Med 7, 1347–1352.

Nicoletti, I., Migliorati, G., Pagliacci, M.C., Grignani, F. and Riccardi, C. (1991). A rapid and simple method for measuring thymocyte apoptosis by propidium iodide staining and flow cytometry. J Immunol Methods 139, 271–279.

Ozgen, U., Savasan, S., Buck, S. and Ravindranath, Y. (2000). Comparison of DiOC(6)(3) uptake and annexin V labeling for quantification of apoptosis in leukemia cells and non-malignant T lymphocytes from children. Cytometry 42, 74–78.

Pena, L.A., Fuks, Z. and Kolesnick, R. (1997). Stress-induced apoptosis and the sphingomyelin pathway. Biochem Pharmacol 53, 615–621.

Perfettini, J.L. and Kroemer, G. (2003). Caspase activation is not death. Nat Immunol 4, 308–310.

Petrovsky, A., Schellenberger, E., Josephson, L., Weissleder, R. and Bogdanov, A. Jr (2003). Near-infrared fluorescent imaging of tumor apoptosis. Cancer Res 63, 1936–1942.

Raff, M. (1998). Cell suicide for beginners. Nature 396, 119–122.

Rasola, A. and Geuna, M. (2001). A flow cytometry assay simultaneously detects independent apoptotic parameters. Cytometry 45, 151–157.

Roninson, I.B. (2002). Oncogenic functions of tumour suppressor p21(Waf1/Cip1/Sdi1): association with cell senescence and tumour-promoting activities of stromal fibroblasts. Cancer Lett 179, 1–14.

Roninson, I.B. and Dokmanovic, M. (2003). Induction of senescence-associated growth inhibitors in the tumor-suppressive function of retinoids. J Cell Biochem 88, 83–94.

Rosen, A., Casciola-Rosen, L. and Ahearn, J. (1995). Novel packages of viral and self-antigens are generated during apoptosis. J Exp Med 181, 1557–1561.

Sakahira, H., Enari, M. and Nagata, S. (1998). Cleavage of CAD inhibitor in CAD activation and DNA degradation during apoptosis. Nature 391, 96–99.

Salgado, J., Garcia-Saez, A.J., Malet, G., Mingarro, I. and Perez-Paya, E. (2002). Peptides in apoptosis research. J Pept Sci 8, 543–560.

Salvesen, G.S. and Dixit, V.M. (1999). Caspase activation: the induced-proximity model. Proc Natl Acad Sci USA 96, 10964–10967.

Savill, J. and Fadok, V. (2000). Corpse clearance defines the meaning of cell death. Nature 407, 784–788.

Savill, J., Dransfield, I., Gregory, C. and Haslett, C. (2002). A blast from the past: clearance of apoptotic cells regulates immune responses. Nat Rev Immunol 2, 965–975.

Schlegel, R.A. and Williamson, P. (2001). Phosphatidylserine, a death knell. Cell Death Differ 8, 551–563.

Sperandio, S., de Belle, I. and Bredesen, D.E. (2000). An alternative, nonapoptotic form of programmed cell death. Proc Natl Acad Sci USA 97, 14376–14381.

Staudacher, E., Altmann, F., Wilson, I.B. and Marz, L. (1999). Fucose in N-glycans: from plant to man. Biochim Biophys Acta 1473, 216–236.

Susin, S.A., Daugas, E., Ravagnan, L. et al. (2000). Two distinct pathways leading to nuclear apoptosis. J Exp Med 192, 571–580.

Susin, S.A., Lorenzo, H.K., Zamzami, N. et al. (1999). Molecular characterization of mitochondrial apoptosis-inducing factor. Nature 397, 441–446.

Thornberry, N.A. and Lazebnik, Y. (1998). Caspases: enemies within. Science 281, 1312–1316.

Tsukishiro, T., Donnenberg, A.D. and Whiteside, T.L. (2003). Rapid turnover of the CD8(+)CD28(−) T-cell subset of effector cells in the circulation of patients with head and neck cancer. Cancer Immunol Immunother 52, 599–607.

van Engeland, M., Ramaekers, F.C., Schutte, B. and Reutelingsperger, C.P. (1996). A novel assay to measure loss of plasma membrane asymmetry during apoptosis of adherent cells in culture. Cytometry 24, 131–139.

Verbovetski, I., Bychkov, H., Trahtemberg, U. et al. (2002). Opsonization of apoptotic cells by autologous iC3b facilitates clearance by immature dendritic cells, down-regulates DR and CD86, and up-regulates CC chemokine receptor 7. J Exp Med 196, 1553–1561.

Vermes, I., Haanen, C. and Reutelingsperger, C. (2000). Flow cytometry of apoptotic cell death. J Immunol Methods 243, 167–190.

Virchow, R. (1978). Cellular Pathology. Birmingham: The Classics of Medicine Library.

Volokhina, E.B., Hulshof, R., Haanen, C. and Vermes, I. (2003). Tissue transglutaminase mRNA expression in apoptotic cell death. Apoptosis 8, 673–679.

Williamson, P. and Schlegel, R.A. (2002). Transbilayer phospholipid movement and the clearance of apoptotic cells. Biochim Biophys Acta 1585, 53–63.

Wyllie, A.H., Kerr, J.F. and Currie, A.R. (1980). Cell death: the significance of apoptosis. Int Rev Cytol 68, 251–306.

Xue, L., Fletcher, G.C. and Tolkovsky, A.M. (2001). Mitochondria are selectively eliminated from eukaryotic cells after blockade of caspases during apoptosis. Curr Biol 11, 361–365.

Yuan, J., Shaham, S., Ledoux, S., Ellis, H.M. and Horvitz, H.R. (1993). The C. elegans cell death gene ced-3 encodes a protein similar to mammalian interleukin-1 beta-converting enzyme. Cell 75, 641–652.

Zimmermann, K.C. and Green, D.R. (2001). How cells die: apoptosis pathways. J Allergy Clin Immunol 108, S99–103.

Zitvogel, L., Casores, N., Pequignot, M.O. et al. (2004). Immune response against dying tumor cells. Adv Immunol 84, 131–179.

Zou, H., Henzel, W.J., Liu, X., Lutschg, A. and Wang, X. (1997). Apaf-1, a human protein homologous to C. elegans CED-4, participates in cytochrome c-dependent activation of caspase-3. Cell 90, 405–413.

Zuliani, T., Duval, R., Jayat, C. et al. (2003). Sensitive and reliable JC-1 and TOTO-3 double staining to assess mitochondrial transmembrane potential and plasma membrane integrity: interest for cell death investigations. Cytometry 54A, 100–108.

Cytokine Enzyme Linked Immunosorbent Spot (ELISPOT) Assay

Chapter 33

Donald D. Anthony, Donald E. Hricik and Peter S. Heeger

Departments of Medicine and Pathology, Case Western Reserve University, Cleveland, OH and Department of Immunology and The Glickman Urologic Institute, The Cleveland Clinic Foundation, Cleveland, OH, USA

. . . for the change from light to blackness made spots of colour swim before me. . .

H.G. Wells, *The Time Machine*, 1898

The focus of this chapter will be one such promising approach, the cytokine enzyme linked immunosorbent spot (ELISPOT) assay.

INTRODUCTION

As illustrated by the clinical expression of inherited and acquired immune deficiency syndromes in humans, T lymphocytes play a central role in host defense directed against infectious agents and certain malignancies (Bielorai et al., 2002; Church, 2002; O'Driscoll and Jeggo, 2002; Quartier and Prieur, 2002; Subauste, 2002; Ward et al., 2002; Brewer et al., 2003; Jain et al., 2003; Wolff and O'Donnell, 2003). At the other end of the disease spectrum, as exemplified by transplant rejection (Suthanthiran and Strom, 1994; Benichou et al., 1999; Heeger, 2003) and organ-specific autoimmune disease (Kong et al., 2003; Medina et al., 2003; von Herrath and Harrison, 2003; Weetman, 2003; Yu et al., 2003), uncontrolled T cell immune responses can be pathogenic. Despite significant progress, the cellular and molecular mechanisms that mediate these disease states are only partially understood. Thus, the development of methods to describe and quantify T cell immunity in humans may provide novel insights into our basic understanding of human disease. Such methodology will aid in developing strategies directed at improving clinical outcomes in a wide range of disorders. As discussed throughout this textbook, a number of laboratory techniques are being evaluated for just these reasons.

T CELL IMMUNITY

To interpret cytokine ELISPOT analyses, it is first necessary to review some of the fundamental characteristics of T cell immune responses. T cell immunity begins with low frequency naive T cell precursors that utilize heterodimeric T cell receptors (TCRs) to recognize peptides bound to major histocompatibility (MHC) molecules (Garcia et al., 1999). To become fully activated, a naive T cell must interact with this ligand when the ligand is expressed on a professional antigen-presenting cell (APC) in a secondary lymphoid organ (Picker et al., 1993; Lakkis et al., 2000) and in the context of appropriate co-stimulatory signals (Croft et al., 1994; Carreno and Collins, 2002). Under these highly regulated circumstances, the naive T cell initially produces only IL-2 and then differentiates into an effector T cell, a process that occurs over the course of several days (Matesic et al., 1998a; Gudmundsdottir et al., 1999; Wells et al., 2000; Salomon and Bluestone, 2001) (Figure 33.1). During effector cell differentiation T lymphocytes clonally expand and alter gene expression patterns so as to be able to circulate to peripheral organs (Xie et al., 1999; Zimmermann et al., 1999; Masopust et al., 2001), produce cytokines (i.e. IFNγ, IL-4, IL-5) and ultimately mediate effector functions such as cytotoxicity, delayed type

Measuring Immunity, edited by Michael T. Lotze and Angus W. Thomson
ISBN 0-12-455900-X, London

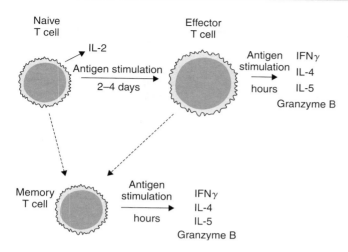

Figure 33.1 Schematic of T cell differentiation emphasizing the difference in kinetics for cytokine secretion of naive versus effector or memory T cells. Naive T cells initially produce only IL-2 and require several days of differentiation in order to produce effector cytokines such as IFNγ. In contrast, effector and memory T cells rapidly secrete effector cytokines upon re-encountering their antigen on a target cell. Memory T cells may derive from a population of effector cells or may derive directly from a subgroup of naive T cells (dashed arrows).

hypersensitivity and provision of help for antibody isotype switching (Mosmann and Coffman, 1989; Oxenius et al., 1996; Russell and Ley, 2002). Upon resolution/control of the inciting stimulus, the majority of antigen-specific T cells undergo apoptosis leaving a residual number of memory T lymphocytes capable of rapidly and effectively responding to a second stimulus of the same specificity (Swain, 1994; Dutton et al., 1998).

This paradigm highlights important features common to any T cell immune response that determine whether and how the response is effective, ineffective or inappropriately pathogenic. Clearly, clonal size (the number of antigen-specific cells induced) is a core characteristic, as low frequency responses may be inadequate to control certain infections and therapy might be aimed at boosting the frequency (Valdez et al., 2000; Buseyne et al., 2002; Lauer et al., 2002a). In contrast, high frequency pathogenic T cell immune responses may mediate more severe pathology and therapy should be directed at inhibiting the function of these cells (Matesic et al., 1998a; Benichou et al., 1999; Heeger et al., 2000a; Pelfrey et al., 2000). The specificity and functional avidity of the responding T cells are also relevant characteristics (Lehmann et al., 1989, 1998; Targoni and Lehmann, 1998; Hesse et al., 2001). Delineating the fine specificity for antigen-reactive T cells could provide specific targets for immunotherapy aimed at appropriately manipulating the quality and quantity of the response, so as ultimately to improve clinical outcome. Independent of clonal size and specificity, the cytokine secretion pattern, as well as the ability to mediate alternate effector functions such as cytotoxicity, can have a large impact on the outcome of T cell immunity (Mosmann et al., 1986;

Mosmann and Coffman, 1989; Locksley and Scott, 1991; Nicholson and Kuchroo, 1996; Rodrigues et al., 2000). While a type 1 cytokine-secreting phenotype (IFNγ-dominated) may protect against certain intracellular infections, a T cell immune response of similar specificity and frequency, but producing IL-4 or IL-5, may not be able to control the same pathogen. Finally, discerning whether the antigen-reactive T cells are activated *in vivo* and function as effector or memory cells versus being naive T cell precursors is an essential characteristic that could influence how therapeutic interventions are ultimately designed (Croft et al., 1994; Zimmermann et al., 1999; Masopust et al., 2001). Developing assays capable of precisely, reproducibly, rapidly and repeatedly measuring all of these features is one goal of the immunologic community. If such tests were available then the results could potentially permit physicians to guide treatments based upon functional measures of T cell immunity.

THE ELISPOT ASSAY

Assay procedure

Versions of the ELISPOT assay have been used for ~20 years to detect antibody-secreting B cells (Czerkinsky et al., 1983, 1988; Tarkowski et al., 1984) and more recently, cytokine-secreting lymphocytes (Forsthuber et al., 1996; Matesic et al., 1998a; Tary-Lehmann et al., 1998; Benichou et al., 1999; Heeger et al., 1999; Hricik et al., 2003). Several technical advances, including development of synthetic membranes and computer-assisted image analysis hardware and software, have improved the reliability and reproducibility of the assay and have facilitated the data analysis (Forsthuber et al., 1996; Matesic et al., 1998a; Tary-Lehmann et al., 1998; Benichou et al., 1999; Heeger et al., 1999; Hricik et al., 2003).

To detect cytokine-secreting lymphocytes, commercially available 96-well ELISPOT plates that have a white synthetic membrane as a floor are coated with a primary antibody specific for the cytokine to be detected (Figure 33.2). Responding lymphocytes, in most clinical situations peripheral blood lymphocytes (PBLs) or purified peripheral blood T cells (or T cell subsets), are added to the wells at varying dilutions. Syngeneic antigen-presenting cells, for example T cell depleted PBLs, can be added if needed. Stimulating antigens with appropriate controls are then added to selected wells. The antigens to be used may be proteins, synthetic peptides or allogeneic cells (see below for details) depending on the specific question being asked. If soluble peptides or proteins are being tested, PBLs (containing T cells, B cells and monocytes) rather than purified T cells must be tested as responders so as to provide a population of antigen-presenting cells capable of presenting the antigens to the T cells in the culture. Under such conditions, the exogenously added antigens are processed *in vitro* (in the ELISPOT wells) by the APCs

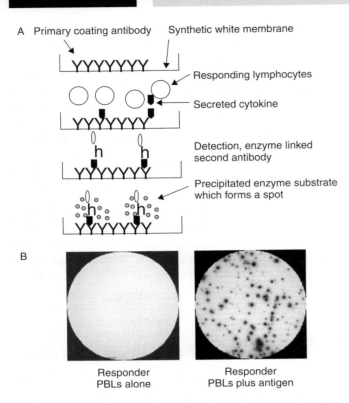

A Primary coating antibody   Synthetic white membrane

Responding lymphocytes

Secreted cytokine

Detection, enzyme linked second antibody

Precipitated enzyme substrate which forms a spot

B

Responder PBLs alone

Responder PBLs plus antigen

Figure 33.2 The ELISPOT procedure. A. Schematic representation of the steps involved in performing an ELISPOT assay. See text for details. B. Representative individual wells of an IFNγ ELISPOT assay in which human PBLs from a tuberculin skin test positive subject were cultured with PPD antigen (right) and without PPD antigen (left). Reproduced with permission from Valujskikh and Heeger, 2000.

within the PBL mixture and are subsequently presented to the T cells. The ELISPOT plates are incubated for 18–24 h (for some cytokines such as IL-4 or IL-5 longer times may be required) to permit the responder cells in the culture to recognize their specific antigen(s) and subsequently to release cytokine. As the antigen-specific lymphocytes recognize their specific ligands they produce cytokines, which are captured directly at their source, before they are diluted, degraded or absorbed to receptors on bystander cells. At the end of the culture period the cells are washed off the plates leaving behind only the cytokines bound to the capture antibody. A second, enzyme linked detecting antibody is then added to the wells. Typically the enzymes used are either horseradish peroxidase or alkaline phosphatase. This second antibody will only bind to the captured cytokine and recognizes a different epitope on the cytokine than the primary capture antibody. The plates are then developed using a chromogen substrate for the antibody-linked enzyme, resulting in spots at the site of cytokine secretion (Forsthuber et al., 1996; Matesic et al., 1998a; Tary-Lehmann et al., 1998; Benichou et al., 1999; Heeger et al., 1999; Hricik et al., 2003).

Once developed, the results can be rapidly quantified by computer-assisted image analysis, thus providing reproducible information on frequency, spot size, antigen

specificity and cytokine-producing quality of the induced polyclonal immune response. The plates can be maintained for years without loss of signal if kept away from direct light, providing a 'permanent' record that can be reassessed at later times if the need arises (Forsthuber et al., 1996; Matesic et al., 1998a; Tary-Lehmann et al., 1998; Benichou et al., 1999; Heeger et al., 1999; Hricik et al., 2003).

Sensitivity of the ELISPOT assay

To determine the sensitivity of the ELISPOT assay a number of experiments using both murine and human T cell lines and clones were performed (Heeger et al., 1999; Karulin et al., 2000; Rininsland et al., 2000). This approach permitted independent verification of the number of antigen-specific T cells added to a given culture. Such studies demonstrated that both the mouse and human ELISPOT assays have the capability to assess cytokine production by individual T cells among several hundred thousand bystander cells. The assay is sufficiently sensitive to detect as few as 1 in 5×10^5–1×10^6 cytokine-secreting lymphocytes (Forsthuber et al., 1996; Heeger et al., 1999; Yip et al., 1999; Hesse et al., 2001; Karulin et al., 2000; Rininsland et al., 2000). Direct comparisons between ELISPOT assays and either flow cytometry or cytokine detection in culture supernatants by standard enzyme linked immunosorbent assays (ELISA) showed that the ELISPOT assay is 100–1000 times more sensitive than either of these other approaches (Matesic et al., 1998a; Heeger et al., 1999; Gebauer et al., 2002). The ELISPOT is sufficiently sensitive to permit analysis of cytokine-secreting organ-infiltrating lymphocytes (Targoni et al., 2001) as well as lymphocytes obtained from blood or secondary lymphoid organs. Accuracy and reproducibility of the assay has also been carefully documented. In experienced hands, the well-to-well variability of a given assay is 10–30 per cent (Gebauer et al., 2002). Therefore, any detected differences in frequency between one time point and another of <20 per cent is likely to fall within the error of the assay.

Differentiating naive from effector/memory T cells by ELISPOT

Effector or memory T cells can rapidly produce IFNγ, IL-4 or IL-5, but naive T cells cannot (Dutton et al., 1998; Matesic et al., 1998a; Zimmermann et al., 1999). Naive T cells require several days of differentiation *in vivo* or *in vitro* to become type 1 or type 2 cytokine-secreting effector cells. The ELISPOT assay should therefore be able to differentiate naive from primed T cells based on the ability to detect effector cytokines over a <24 h time period. Consistent with this contention, PBLs from normal human volunteers who were purified protein derivative (PPD) skin test positive produced PPD-specific IFNγ (but not IL-4 or IL-5) ELISPOTs, while PBLs from volunteers who were not PPD skin test negative did not (Figure 33.3)

(Heeger et al., 1999). The specific secretion of IFNγ under these conditions is consistent with the proinflammatory type 1 immunity required to protect an individual from active tuberculosis (an intracellular pathogen). Analogously, PBLs isolated from patients allergic to cats produce IL-4 and IL-5 (but not IFNγ) ELISPOTs in response to cat pelt antigen, while non-allergic individuals do not (Figure 33.3) (Heeger et al., 1999). The type 2 cytokine profile of this latter response is consistent with what would be anticipated for an allergic phenotype. In additional studies memory and naive T cells from single patients were separated based on the differential expression of characteristic cell surface markers (CD45RA versus CD45RO) and individually tested for reactivity to recall antigens (Gebauer et al., 2002). These data formally demonstrated that only effector/ memory CD45RO+ T cells from antigen-experienced volunteers (i.e. PPD skin test positive) produced the anticipated cytokine in response to the specific antigen. Overall, these fundamental results showed that the ELISPOT assay can provide the investigator with a reliable *ex vivo* 'fingerprint' of the *in vivo* antigen-specific frequency and cytokine quality of a given immune response at high resolution and at the time point evaluated.

Advantages of the ELISPOT approach

From a technical standpoint, the ELISPOT assay is relatively easy to set up and in contrast to limiting dilution assays, for example, requires a minimum amount of labor. Because

ELISPOT assays are high-resolution and are performed in 96-well plates, it is possible to adapt the assay for high throughput to test for immunity to large numbers of antigens. One example of this application is comprehensive determinant mapping, in which PBLs from a given patient are tested against large numbers of peptides (several hundred can be tested at once) derived from candidate antigenic proteins, in an effort to determine the relevant immunogenic peptides for that subject (Anthony et al., 2002). This comprehensive determinant mapping approach has been used in both mice and humans (Figure 33.4) to define novel epitopes relevant to vaccines for infections, autoimmune diseases and transplant rejection (Heeger et al., 2000b; Anthony et al., 2002). A further refinement of the assay permits the detection of two different cytokines at once (Karulin et al., 2000). As explained in more detail below, it is anticipated that such information will be useful for improving our understanding of disease pathogenesis as well as for clinical decision-making and directing novel therapies for a variety of T cell-mediated processes in humans.

The above explanations show that the ELISPOT can provide information on the frequency, cytokine profile and antigen specificity of a primed immune response. In addition, within a polyclonal population of T cells specific for a given antigen the responding T cells have varying affinities. Although determining the true affinity of a given TCR for its peptide/MHC ligand can be difficult, one can reliably use an ELISPOT approach to estimate the relative

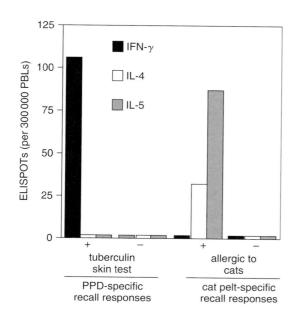

Figure 33.3 Effector/memory T cells produce cytokines in short-term assays but naive cells do not. PBLs isolated from a tuberculin skin test positive subject and from a skin test negative subject were tested for PPD-specific recall responses in IFNγ, IL-4 and IL-5 ELISPOT assays (left). PBLs isolated from a subject known to be allergic to cats and from a non-allergic subject were tested for cat pelt antigen-specific recall responses in IFNγ, IL-4 and IL-5 ELISPOT assays (right). Reproduced with permission from Valujskikh and Heeger, 2000.

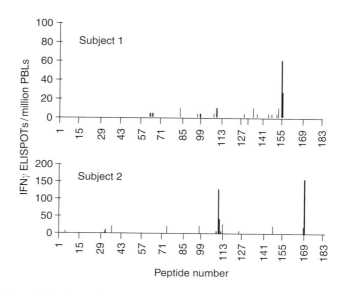

Figure 33.4 Comprehensive determinant mapping by ELISPOT. PBLs from two different subjects previously infected with hepatitis C virus (anti-HCV antibody titers in serum were positive, but HCV RNA was not detectable) were tested in IFNγ ELISPOT assays against > 180 overlapping nonamer peptides derived from the hepatitis C core protein. Quantitative results as assessed by computer assisted image analysis are shown for each subject. No responses were detected in uninfected subjects (not shown). Reproduced with permission from Anthony et al., 2002.

functional avidity of a polyclonal T cell response (Targoni and Lehmann, 1998; Hesse et al., 2001; Anthony et al., 2002). Polyclonal immunity with high functional avidity is characterized by higher numbers of antigen-specific ELISPOTs elicited at lower concentrations of antigens when compared with low avidity responses (Figure 33.5). Understanding the functional avidity of a given immune response provides information about its relative strength that could be compared from one time point to another in a given patient and could be useful for quantifying effects of therapeutic interventions.

Finally, the size of the individual spots in each ELISPOT well can provide some insight into the quantity of cytokine produced by each cell. On average, larger spot sizes imply more cytokine produced per cell. However, it is important to remember that the size of a given spot can also be influenced by other factors, including the length of time that T cell produced cytokine within the study period, potentially confounding such interpretations regarding the amount of cytokine produced per cell (Hesse et al., 2001).

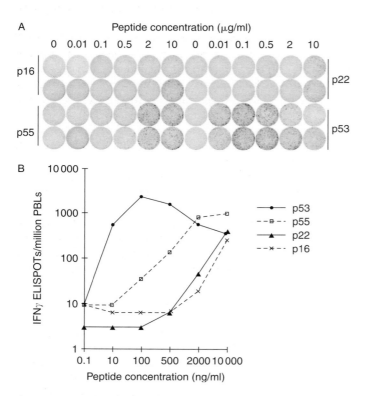

Figure 33.5 Measuring functional avidity by ELISPOT. PBLs from a subject previously infected with hepatitis C virus (anti-HCV antibody titers in serum were positive, but HCV RNA was not detectable) were tested in IFNγ ELISPOT assays for their ability to respond to varying concentrations of four different HCV derived peptides. A. Photograph of IFNγ ELISPOT plate illustrating duplicate wells for responses to each of the four different peptides tested over the concentration range shown. B. Quantitative comparison of responses to each peptide. Note that the detected response to peptide 53 (p53, closed circles) peaked at significantly lower concentrations of peptide compared to the other three peptides, consistent with a higher functional avidity.

Limitations of ELISPOT analysis

While the ELISPOT assay has many advantages compared to other tests, it is important also to understand its limitations. First, the ELISPOT only detects the specific cytokines being tested and does not provide direct information on the ability of antigen-specific lymphocytes to mediate other effector functions. There may be a population of antigen-reactive cells in an individual that do not produce cytokines but instead mediate cytotoxicity, for example. Secondly, in contrast to flow cytometry, there is presently no ability to co-stain the responding immune cells to determine whether a given subtype of lymphocyte within the culture is producing the cytokine. In the ELISPOT approach, the only way to ascertain this information would be to test individual purified T cell subpopulations (i.e. isolated CD4 T cells), to deplete T cell subtypes and/or to add blocking antibodies to the individual test wells (Matesic et al., 1998a,b; Tary-Lehmann et al., 1998; Benichou et al., 1999; Yip et al., 1999; Anthony et al., 2002). Similarly, the assay provides the investigator with a 'shadow' of a given T cell's function after that cell has been removed from the culture, so that that it is not possible to 'pick out' the individual responding cell for additional study. Finally, the high sensitivity of the assay and the fact that non-T cells in a culture can release cytokine can occasionally lead to results that may be difficult to interpret. IFNγ produced by a T cell can lead to bystander production of IL-4 by nearby APCs (Karulin et al., 2002). Thus, the produced IL-4 in an ELISPOT may appear to be antigen-specific, but may be an artifact of the *in vitro* system and not relevant to the *in vivo* immunity. In general, IL-5 is not produced by APCs, so that using IL-5 ELISPOTs as a prototypic cytokine for type 2 immunity may lead to less confusion than using IL-4 for this purpose (Forsthuber et al., 1996; Karulin et al., 2000, 2002). Overall, our view is that the ELISPOT assay should be considered one of several approaches used within a comprehensive armamentarium for evaluating T cell immunity.

MEASURING IMMUNITY IN DISEASE STATES BY ELISPOT

The ELISPOT assay is being used as one of several candidate immune monitoring tools, largely in research settings and within a number of different clinical contexts. Many studies suggest that the ELISPOT approach may eventually become clinically useful for evaluation of immune responses to infectious agents, transplant antigens, tumor antigens and autoantigens. The following sections will summarize highlights of the published studies addressing the use of ELISPOTs for these purposes.

Measuring immunity in the context of infectious disease

Developing effective T cell immunity is essential for eliminating certain invading pathogens from a host and thereby preventing or curing the infection. In the clinical arena, state-of-the-art testing for evaluating protective immunity against a pathogen has largely occurred through the determination of specific antibody titers, an approach that provides no direct assessment of T cell immunity. Additional measurements specifically assessing the magnitude and quality of a pathogen-specific T cell immune response by ELISPOT in susceptible or infected persons therefore has the potential to provide insight into the pathogenesis of certain disease states as well as to facilitate diagnosis and to assess prognosis for these patients.

Evaluating immunity in chronic viral infections

Of particular interest are the studies performed in patients chronically infected with disease-producing viruses such as human immunodeficiency virus (HIV) and hepatitis C virus (HCV), where ineffective antiviral T cell immunity is thought to contribute to the inability to resolve the infection. In initial studies aimed at attempting to understand why such chronic viral infections are not resolved, a number of investigators described the naturally developing antiviral T cell immune response in infected patients. Because the specific antigenic peptide determinants of a virus cannot be reliably predicted for any given patient using HLA binding motifs (Anthony et al., 2002; Lauer et al., 2002b), ELISPOT-based determinant mapping, using as many as 500 different peptides per assay, was used to assess comprehensively the magnitude and fine specificity of the virus-specific T cells in individual patients (Altfeld et al., 2001; Goulder et al., 2001a,b; Currier et al., 2002; Addo et al., 2003; Cao et al., 2003b). Studies in HIV-infected individuals have not surprisingly shown that the frequency of HIV peptide-specific T cells varies widely from subject to subject (280–25 860 /million PBLs) (Addo et al., 2003), that the mean frequency of IFN-γ producing CD8 T cells often correlates with the number of epitopes recognized and that the antigen specificity of the immune repertoire broadens over time (Cao et al., 2003a). Similar complex relationships between the magnitude and fine specificity of viral-specific immunity and the chronicity of disease have been documented in HCV-infected patients (Lechner et al., 2000; Valdez et al., 2000; Gruener et al., 2001; Thimme et al., 2001; Anthony et al., 2002; Lauer et al., 2002a,b).

In addition to providing some basic insight into how the immune system responds to these viral infections, such studies describing the magnitude and specificity of antiviral immunity provide important baseline information that could be clinically useful. For example, there is some evidence that the frequency of detected antiviral T cells as determined by ELISPOT correlates with disease outcome and thus might be useful to provide prognostic information in infected patients. Cross-sectional and longitudinal studies of cohorts of HCV-infected patients have suggested that successful resolution of viremia is associated with the natural development of a high frequency of HCV-specific,

IFNγ-producing CD8 T cells (Lechner et al., 2000; Thimme et al., 2001). A number of studies have also revealed a relative paucity of HCV-specific effector T cells in freshly prepared PBLs isolated from subjects with chronic HCV infection (Valdez et al., 2000, 2002; Gruener et al., 2001; Lauer et al., 2002a; Wedemeyer et al., 2002) suggesting that the *inability* to respond to viral antigens correlates with disease state.

Analogous studies performed in HIV-infected individuals revealed differences between those individuals with acute versus chronic infection (Goulder et al., 2001b). The HIV Nef, Tat and Vpr antigens appeared to be preferentially targeted by the host's immune system over other HIV-derived proteins during early infection (Cao et al., 2003a). In addition, some studies showed that the frequency of peripheral viral antigen-specific T cells correlated inversely with the HIV viral load, although this remains controversial (Altfeld et al., 2001; Goulder et al., 2001b; Buseyne et al., 2002; Edwards et al., 2002; Addo et al., 2003; Cao et al., 2003a). While certainly intriguing, it remains to be determined through the use of controlled trials whether any of these observations will eventually lead to routine ELISPOT-based determinant mapping as a clinical guide to prognosis.

Serial evaluation of virus-specific immunity by ELISPOT has provided some insight into the efficacy of antiviral therapy (Altfeld et al., 2001). For HIV infections, however, anti-retroviral therapy is directed at the virus itself, rather than being directed at enhancing the antiviral T cell immune repertoire. Thus alterations in peripheral immunity might not be anticipated during the course of therapy. This has largely been found to be the case, although selected studies suggested that the frequency of anti-HIV-specific T cells directly correlated with successful pharmacologic treatment in both early and late HIV infection (Altfeld et al., 2001). In HCV-infected patients, however, IFN-α treatment is thought in part to be directed at enhancing the antiviral T cell immune response. Increases in detectable frequencies of HCV-specific T cell immunity were correlated with successful clinical responses to treatment in this disease, although again the results are controversial (Barnes et al., 2002; Kamal et al., 2002). Overall, these types of studies suggest that serial analysis of antiviral immunity during the course of therapy might act as a surrogate marker for clinical responses. One could envision ultimately making therapeutic decisions based on results of such kinetic analyses in individual patients, but the present data are too premature to reach definitively this conclusion.

As a byproduct of studies investigating virus-specific immunity in the HCV and HIV infections, we have also learned about the functional relationships between of IFNγ-secreting T cells as assessed by ELISPOT and the detection of antiviral immunity by other methods (intracellular cytokine staining, cytotoxicity assays and tetramer analysis). These comparisons have indicated that the frequency of IFNγ-producing cells by ELISPOT does not always correlate well with the total number of tetramer-specific T cells and/or detected cytotoxic capability (Goepfert et al., 2000; Mwau et al., 2002; Sun et al., 2003), thereby underscoring the need to perform ELISPOT analyses as one of many monitoring approaches to assess human immunity to infectious agents.

Tuberculin testing

For some pathogens, including tuberculosis, induction of pathogen-specific cellular immunity can be assessed by *in vivo* skin delayed type hypersensitivity reactions (the tuberculin skin test), but the sensitivity and specificity of this approach, particularly in chronically ill patients, is less than ideal (Bilen et al., 2003; Bugiani et al., 2003). Recent literature supports the clinical use of ELISPOT-based testing of tuberculosis (TB) antigen-reactive T cell immunity as being superior to the tuberculin skin test for detecting previous exposure to TB (Ewer et al., 2003). A prospective analysis of peripheral immunity in 50 healthy contacts with varied degrees of exposure to tuberculosis revealed a strong direct correlation between the frequency of tuberculin antigen-specific, IFNγ-producing PBLs as determined by ELISPOT and the intensity of exposure to TB (odds ratio 9.0 per unit increase in level of exposure, $P = 0.001$) (Ewer et al., 2003). In contrast, the tuberculin skin test had only a weak relationship to the intensity of exposure (odds ratio 1, $P = 0.05$) (Lalvani et al., 2001; Ewer et al., 2003). Notably, this ELISPOT assay tested for reactivity to ESAT-6, an antigen found in *Mycobacterium tuberculosis* and not the Bacillus Calmette-Guerin (BCG) strain. The ELISPOT diagnostic approach was able to differentiate individuals truly exposed to TB from those immunized with the BCG vaccine, a feature that is not true of standard tuberculin skin tests (Bugiani et al., 2003; Ewer et al., 2003). Perhaps more impressive are the emerging data that suggest that the ELISPOT assay can be more sensitive and specific than tuberculin skin testing for detection of both active and latent TB in chronically ill, HIV infected individuals (Chapman et al., 2002).

Assessing vaccine efficacy

Vaccines have been or are being developed to prevent disease from infection with a large number of infectious pathogens, including HIV. While the ultimate test of efficacy for any vaccine will be the prevention of infection in large scale controlled trials, surrogate markers of vaccine efficacy should include tests to determine the effects of the vaccine on antigen-specific cellular immunity. In studies of simian immunodeficiency virus (SIV), a primate model of HIV infection, ELISPOT analyses confirmed that therapeutic vaccination of infected macaques induced the expansion of SIV-specific IFNγ producing T cells (Tryniszewska et al., 2002). Importantly, the frequency of the induced virus-specific T cells correlated inversely with detected viral load during a critical period in the course of

infection, providing proof of principle that therapeutic vaccines may be useful in treating SIV and that ELISPOT analysis of virus specific immunity can potentially function as a surrogate marker for vaccine efficacy (Tryniszewska et al., 2002).

There are some limited data evaluating vaccine-induced immunity by ELISPOT in humans as well. ELISPOT analysis of immune response to tetanus vaccine administered to 22 healthy control subjects revealed that tetanus-reactive IFNγ-producing CD4 cells were detectable in all subjects and that these responses were stable over several months of repeated testing (Mayer et al., 2002). Similarly, measles vaccination induced detectable cellular immunity by ELISPOT (Ovsyannikova et al., 2003). Measles-vaccine-induced virus-specific IFNγ-producing CD8 T cells were detectable in all subjects and the responses were more vigorous in subjects who had previously been exposed to the vaccine. ELISPOTs have similarly been used to detect anticipated increases in herpes zoster specific immunity after booster immunizations (Smith et al., 2003).

In the context of HIV vaccines, peripheral cellular immunity in two small cohorts of HIV-seronegative (non-infected) subjects was evaluated by ELISPOT. Immunization with either a DNA-based or a canarypox-based HIV vaccine elicited virus-specific T cell immunity as detected by ELISPOT (MacGregor et al., 2002; Cao et al., 2003a). The ELISPOT approach was more sensitive than standard cytotoxicity assays when they were compared in head-to-head analyses (MacGregor et al., 2002; Cao et al., 2003a). Neither of these studies was designed to evaluate vaccine efficacy using protection from disease as an endpoint, so the physiologic relevance of the detected responses remains unknown. Overall, the data still provide support for the continued use of ELISPOT-based monitoring of peripheral blood cells as one approach for evaluating vaccine efficacy in research settings.

MEASURING IMMUNITY TO TRANSPLANT ANTIGENS

T cell recognition of transplant antigens

Before discussing the measurement of immunity in transplantation by ELISPOT it is necessary to clarify several concepts that are specific to the immunology of transplantation. Alloreactive T lymphocytes recognize and respond to donor antigens via two distinct allorecognition pathways. Recipient CD4 and CD8 T cells can recognize donor MHC peptide complexes expressed directly on donor cells through the direct pathway of allorecognition (Heeger, 2003). The relatively high frequency of T cells capable of responding through the direct pathway must be related to cross-reactivity, because recipient T cells have not been trained to recognize allogeneic MHC molecules. Studies in animal models and in humans show that donor-reactive T cells responding through the direct pathway are associated with acute T cell-mediated rejection. These pathogenic lymphocytes derive from both naive and memory T cell pools. The finding that memory alloreactive T cells exist in individuals that have not received a transplant, suggests that a proportion of alloreactive T cells are primed to environmental antigens (for example viruses) that happen to cross-react with alloantigens (Heeger et al., 1999; Pantenburg et al., 2002; Heeger, 2003). This, and the fact that memory/effector cells are more resistant to immunosuppression and tolerance induction than naive cells (Pantenburg et al., 2002; Valujskikh et al., 2002), raises the hypothesis that the frequency of alloreactive memory T cells detected in an individual could represent a surrogate marker for transplant outcome (see below).

In addition to responding through the direct pathway, recipient T cells can recognize and respond to donor-derived peptide determinants that have been processed and presented by recipient MHC molecules through the indirect pathway (Benichou et al., 1999; Heeger, 2003). Many of such peptides derive from the polymorphic regions of allogeneic MHC molecules found on donor cells. T cells responding through the indirect pathway may preferentially participate in the development of chronic graft injury. Several studies in animal models and observations in human transplant recipients carrying a diagnosis of 'chronic rejection' are consistent with this hypothesis (see below), but conclusive data are lacking.

Measuring transplant reactive T cells by ELISPOT in mouse models

The frequencies and cytokine profiles of alloreactive T cells responding to donor antigens after skin and cardiac transplantation in mice were evaluated using the ELISPOT assay (Benichou et al., 1999; Valujskikh et al., 1999, 2002). Donor spleen cells or synthetic donor derived peptides were used to detect recipient T cells responding through the direct versus indirect pathways respectively. Overall, these data confirmed results of studies using other methodologies, including limiting dilution analysis, flow cytometry and standard proliferation assays and additionally provided more detailed information at higher resolution. The studies showed an anticipated high frequency of alloreactive T cells responding through the direct pathway (1000–5000 per million cells or up 1 in 200 T cells) with a 10–20-fold less frequent response to indirectly presented peptides and/or minor antigenic determinants. In wild type animals, T cell alloreactivity was dominated by IFNγ production consistent with naturally developing type 1 cytokine profile (Matesic et al., 1998a; Benichou et al., 1999; Valujskikh et al., 2002; Heeger, 2003). Cell separation experiments confirmed that IFNγ detected by ELISPOT derived from alloreactive T cells with a memory or effector cell surface phenotype and not from naive T cells (Matesic et al., 1998a).

A related relevant finding was that the frequency of donor-reactive T cells directly correlated with the speed of skin graft rejection. That is, high frequency responses to fully MHC-disparate skin resulted in rejection by day 11–13 while lower frequency responses induced to minor antigen disparate skin grafts led to rejection that occurred by day 15–25 depending on the strain combination tested (Valujskikh et al., 1999). Moreover, higher frequencies of donor-reactive T cells developed during rejection of a second allograft consistent with the presence of memory T cells prior to the transplantation (Valujskikh et al., 1999, 2002). No type 1 or type 2 cytokine-producing T cells were detectable in animals made tolerant to skin or heart grafts via co-stimulatory blockade (Valujskikh et al., 1999, 2002). Overall, these strong associations based on well-controlled animal models suggested that monitoring frequencies and cytokine profiles of alloreactive T cells could act as a surrogate marker for transplant outcome in humans. That is, the frequency of donor-reactive effector or memory IFNγ-producing T cells in a given human allograft recipient was hypothesized to correlate with the risk for poor short- or long-term function of the transplanted organ.

Measuring transplant reactive immunity in humans

Based on this foundation and on a series of studies performed in other animal models it was hypothesized that testing anti-donor immunity by ELISPOT in humans would be a clinically useful surrogate marker for transplant outcome. In order to evaluate this hypothesis, it was necessary to design reliable, reproducible and clinically applicable methods of measuring donor-reactive T cell immunity by ELISPOT. To test for anti-donor immunity, recipient PBLs or purified T cells were tested against donor cells in 24-h ELISPOT assays, analogous to a standard mixed lymphocyte reaction (Heeger et al., 1999; Gebauer et al., 2002; Hricik et al., 2003). Donor stimulator cells were obtained from the peripheral blood of living donors or spleen cells from cadaver donors. When standard proliferative mixed lymphocyte reactions are performed, donor cells are irradiated or treated with mitomycin C to prevent the donor cells from proliferating against the responder cells. In an ELISPOT assay, the readout is cytokine production, not proliferation and irradiation/mitomycin C treatment is insufficient to prevent cytokine release, even in a short-term assay (Gebauer et al., 2002). However, T cell depletion of the donor cells essentially eliminates cytokine secretion by the stimulator cells permitting the responder cells to secrete cytokine in a 'one-way' response (Gebauer et al., 2002). The T cell depletion procedure does not affect antigen presentation capability; in fact it seems to enhance the efficiency of antigen presentation. T cell depleted lymphocytes can function as well as activated dendritic cells to induce recall responses using alloreactive T cell lines, if sufficient numbers of T cell depleted donor cells are used (Gebauer et al., 2002). Controlled analyses showed that 300 000–400 000 T cell depleted stimulator cells were sufficient to provide a maximal response

(Gebauer et al., 2002). From a practical standpoint, aliquots of the T cell depleted stimulators can be frozen and thawed for use at later times without loss of function or without additional treatments, thereby facilitating recurrent post-transplant monitoring (Gebauer et al., 2002).

Indirect alloreactivity can theoretically be measured by stimulating recipient PBLs with synthetic peptides derived from polymorphic regions of donor HLA molecules. Because of the polygenic, co-dominant inheritance and expression pattern of HLA alleles in recipients, it is not possible reliably to predict which donor-derived peptides will be immunogenic in a given patient. Still, because the ELISPOT assay is highly sensitive and requires relatively few responder cells, repeatedly testing large numbers of candidate peptides for responses is feasible. Such an approach has been used successfully to detect indirect alloreactivity in a small number of transplant recipients (Najafian et al., 2002; Salama et al., 2003) and may prove to be a useful clinical tool for diagnostic and prognostic purposes (see below).

Peripheral blood lymphocytes isolated from immuno-suppressed human transplant recipients responded to donor antigens through the direct and indirect pathways by predominantly producing IFNγ and IL-2 with little IL-4 or IL-5 (Heeger et al., 1999; Gebauer et al., 2002; Hricik et al., 2003). Consistent with work published by others, ELISPOT-based results also showed that PBLs from many normal (non-transplanted) individuals who had not been previously exposed to known alloantigens still contained IFNγ-producing memory T cells reactive to allogeneic stimulator cells (Heeger et al., 1999; Gebauer et al., 2002; Hricik et al., 2003). Because such alloreactive T cells were presumably primed to environmental antigens (i.e. viral infection, vaccines, etc.) that happened to cross-react with alloantigens, the frequency of IFNγ-producing allo-reactive T cells did not correlate with the number of HLA mismatches between responder and stimulator (Heeger et al., 1999). The frequency of donor-reactive IFNγ-producers, as assessed by ELISPOT, might therefore inde-pendently correlate with or predict outcome in humans.

Clinical utility of ELISPOT in transplantation

ELISPOT measurements of transplant-reactive cellular immunity could theoretically be useful in several settings so as to guide clinical decision-making. There are however, no prospective clinical trials yet published specifically evaluat-ing ELISPOT-based immune monitoring for such purposes. All of the reported studies were performed in limited research settings and much additional work needs to be done before physicians can reliably use the ELISPOT assay for clinical decision-making. Nonetheless, preliminary work suggests that ELISPOT-based monitoring of donor-reactive immunity is a promising one. The following discussion will describe how such an immune monitoring approach might be used theoretically and will point out specific instances where supporting data in humans have been published.

Pretransplantation assessment of post-transplant outcome

Donor-reactive alloantibodies detected prior to trans-plantation represent a significant risk to graft outcome (Patel and Terasaki, 1969; Jeannet et al., 1970). Because of the high risk for hyperacute and acute rejection associ-ated with the detection of such donor-reactive anti-bodies, serum from all potential transplant recipients is tested against donor cells in a pretransplant 'cross-match'. Patients with a positive pretransplant cross-match are gen-erally not transplanted with a graft from that donor. Additionally, as noted above, PBLs from non-transplanted humans can contain alloreactive memory T cells. These memory T cells were presumably activated in response to cross-reactive environmental antigens and their fre-quency cannot be predicted based on the number of HLA matches or mismatches between recipient and potential donor. Since effector/memory T cells, when compared to naive T cells, are relatively resistant to tolerance induction and immunosuppression, it was hypothesized that the pretransplant frequency of donor-reactive IFNγ-producing (effector/ memory) PBLs might provide a surrogate marker for post-transplant outcome, independent of other known risk factors. This in fact appears to be the case.

Analogous to a positive antibody cross-match, early results suggest that the pretransplant presence of donor-reactive memory T cells also portend a worse prognosis for the transplanted allograft (Heeger et al., 1999). In renal allograft recipients treated with a calcineurin inhibitor, mycophenolic and corticosteroids as immunosuppres-sants, the pretransplant frequency of donor-reactive immu-nity as defined by IFNγ ELISPOT was significantly higher in those individuals who developed a post-transplant episode of acute rejection compared to those who did not (Figure 33.6). Moreover, those individuals with the highest pretransplant frequencies had the worst overall outcome as defined by graft loss or early chronic rejection (Patel and Terasaki, 1969; Jeannet et al., 1970). The number of patients evaluated in this study was too small to perform multivariate analysis and to determine whether the pre-transplant frequencies would predict outcome independ-ent of other risk factors such as race, pretransplant panel of reactive antibody positivity, delayed graft function, etc. However, similar findings were published in preliminary forms by others (Reinsmoen, 2002) and this type of work is the subject of ongoing investigation by a number of labora-tories. Therefore it appears that pretransplant assessment of anti-donor immunity by ELISPOT can act as a surrogate marker for post-transplant graft function/survival, a finding that merits further investigation.

Post-transplant prediction and evaluation of acute rejection in renal allograft recipients

There are no easily performed reliable methods capable of predicting acute rejection before it is clinically evident. Early work in this field is beginning to show that the

ELISPOT-detected frequencies of donor-reactive PBLs are higher in patients who have experienced acute rejection than in those that have not (Gebauer et al., 2002; Najafian et al., 2002). However, these preliminary cross-sectional associations have not been properly performed in a prospective manner. Clearly, more rigorous prospective analyses are needed to determine if the ELISPOT assay may play an important role in determining this important clinical outcome.

All acute rejection episodes are not equivalent. From a clinical standpoint, defined histologic criteria (Gaber et al., 1998) and the presence or absence of C4d staining (Collins et al., 1999; Watschinger and Pascual, 2002), among other factors, are used to stratify acute allograft rejections episodes into various grades. It is hoped that such gradation, along with emerging data from molecular studies (Sarwal et al., 2003) and potentially ELISPOT analysis, will not only predict outcome but will ultimately guide tailored therapy specific for the individual mechanisms involved in that particular rejection episode. Preliminary studies of peripheral blood immunity suggest that the ELISPOT may be helpful in this regard. IFNγ and IL-5 production by recipient PBLs in renal allograft recipients was studied at the time of diagnosis of acute rejection but prior to therapy (Tary-Lehmann et al., 1998). Those individuals with high IFNγ to IL-5 ratios (a dominance of 'type 1' immunity) had poor outcomes (graft failure) 3 months following rejection compared to those individuals with low IFNγ to IL-5 ratios (Tary-Lehmann et al., 1998). Again, additional, larger prospective studies will be required in order to ascertain whether this approach will be reliably useful as a prognostic test.

Predicting chronic graft dysfunction

Perhaps more important than diagnosing and prognosticating the outcome of acute rejection is the looming problem of chronic graft injury and failure. So-called 'chronic rejection', characterized by slowly deteriorating transplant function with scarring/fibrosis and transplant vasculopathy (or its equivalent in non-renal allografts), is a complex pathophysiologic process with multiple contributing etiologic factors (Gourishankar and Halloran, 2002; Halloran, 2002). There is clear evidence that immune factors, including both donor-reactive antibodies and donor-reactive T cells, contribute to the development of chronic graft injury (Gourishankar and Halloran, 2002; Halloran, 2002). It is important to understand, however, that there are no published studies providing any evidence that detection of such immune reactivity can be used to diagnose or predict chronic graft injury.

One study provided support for using serial post-transplant monitoring of donor-reactive immunity by ELISPOT to provide prognostic information about long-term renal function in kidney transplant recipients (Hricik et al., 2003). This study evaluated the average post-transplant frequency of donor-reactive IFNγ-producing PBLs over the first 6 months after transplantation and correlated it with renal function at 12 months, in a cohort of living and cadaver renal allograft recipients (Figure 33.7, Table 33.1). The results revealed a direct and independent correlation between the two variables, providing the first suggestive evidence that post-transplant monitoring could be used to stratify patients into low versus high risk subgroups at an early time point post-transplant (Hricik et al., 2003). Future studies will need to verify these preliminary findings and will need to determine whether a therapeutic intervention in the identified higher-risk subgroup will

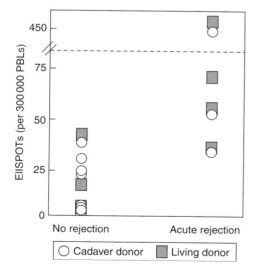

Figure 33.6 Pretransplant frequency of donor-reactive IFNγ-producing PBLs correlates with post-transplant outcome. PBLs from each patient were obtained prior to renal allograft transplantation and tested in IFNγ ELISPOT assays against donor stimulator cells. The detected frequencies were plotted against the presence or absence of biopsy proven acute renal allograft rejection. Circles: cadaver donors, Squares: living donors. Reproduced with permission from Valujskikh and Heeger, 2000.

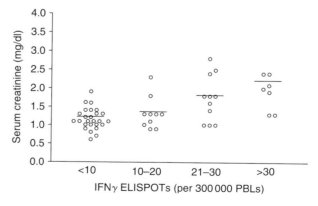

Figure 33.7 Post-transplant frequency of donor-reactive immunity by ELISPOT correlates with renal function. PBLs from 55 renal allograft recipients were studied in serial donor-reactive IFNγ ELISPOT assays over the first 6 months following transplantation and average values for each patient were determined. The graph depicts a scatterplot of 6-month serum creatinine concentrations versus category of post-transplant alloreactivity as defined by the average of the serial post-transplant donor-reactive IFNγ-ELISPOTs per 300 000 PBLs. Reproduced with permission from Hricik et al., 2003.

Table 33.1 The average number of IFNγ ELISPOTs post-transplant independently correlates with renal function at 6 and 12 months in renal allograft recipients

Serum creatinine at 6 months			Serum creatinine at 12 months		
Variable	Beta Coefficient	P	Variable	Beta Coefficient	P
Delayed graft function	0.570	<0.001	Acute rejection in 1st 6 months	0.437	0.001
Average IFN-ELISPOTS	0.465	0.001	African American ethnicity	0.338	0.014
PRAs (class 2)	0.516	0.007	Average IFN-ELISPOTS	0.287	0.03
PRAs (class 1)	0.388	0.041	Male gender	0.287	0.03
Acute rejection in 1st 6 months	0.268	0.048			
Age, gender, HLA match, HLA mismatch, ethnicity, body weight		NS	Age, HLA match, HLA mismatch, body weight, delayed graft function		NS

Reproduced with permission from Hricik et al., 2003.
55 renal allograft recipients were monitored by IFNγ ELISPOT to assess the frequency of donor-reactive and third party-reactive PBLs post-transplant. The average value for each patient for months 0–6 was determined (average IFN-ELISPOTS). Linear regression analysis was used to determine independent correlations between this value and serum creatinine at 6 and 12 months post-transplant.
Using serum creatinine at 6 months: $R^2 = 0.648$; $F = 10.7$; $P < 0.001$;
Using serum creatinine at 12 months: $R^2 = 0.483$; $F = 9.6$; $P < 0.001$;
NS = not significant; PRA = pretransplant panel reactive antibodies.

decrease the number of detectable anti-donor T cells and alter the purported risk by preventing/diminishing the long-term functional damage.

Potential for guiding withdrawal of immunosuppressant medications

Therapy with potent immunosuppression has made transplantation feasible and the development of novel immunosuppressant medications clearly has improved short- and long-term graft survival over the last decade. Nonetheless, immunosuppressants have multiple side effects, not the least of which is that many such agents contribute to graft fibrogenesis and ultimately failure of transplanted organs (Halloran, 2002). Thus, using the minimum amount of immunosuppression required to prevent immune-mediated injury is desirable. Presently, such medications are dosed empirically, based on predefined pharmacodynamic parameters. Withdrawal of immunosuppression in stable graft recipients is becoming a routine procedure, despite the fact that such drug withdrawal can lead to late acute rejection episodes and in some cases graft loss (Hricik and Heeger, 2001). Again, having a means to measure functional donor-reactive immunity under such conditions would be desirable, so as to guide withdrawal of immunosuppression in the appropriate groups of patients. There are no published data using any defined immune monitoring analysis for this purpose. Nonetheless, it is possible that high resolution, non-invasive approaches such as ELISPOT-based monitoring could be useful in this regard. Ongoing studies are directly addressing whether these hypothetical parameters will provide clinically useful information.

Potential for defining and monitoring immune tolerance

Induction of immune tolerance is the ultimate goal of transplantation (Heeger et al., 2000a; Hricik and Heeger, 2001; Thomson et al., 2001). Clinical allograft tolerance can be defined as an absence of pathogenic immunity directed towards the allograft while immunity directed at all other foreign antigens remains intact. Studies in animal models have shown that tolerance can be mediated through deletion, anergy, alteration in cytokine profiles and/or active regulation of donor-reactive T cells. Due to the multifactorial nature of the tolerant state and the difficulty in defining tolerant patients in the clinic, it is very unlikely that any single test will be able to be used to define tolerance. The detection of donor-specific hyporesponsiveness or responsiveness using IFNγ, IL-10 or TGFβ ELISPOT assays may ultimately provide useful information in this regard (Thomson et al., 2001; Heeger and Hricik, 2002).

Recent studies have further suggested that CD25$^+$ CD4$^+$ regulatory T cells may be pertinent mediators of tolerance under certain conditions (Francois Bach, 2003; Wood and Sakaguchi, 2003). One study provided evidence in a small number of stable patients that ELISPOT monitoring may be able to detect regulation by these T cells (Salama et al., 2003). Assays were performed using untreated PBLs or PBLs that were depleted of CD25$^+$ cells using magnetic beads. The samples derived from a proportion of the stable patients exhibited a significant increase in IFNγ-producing, peptide-reactive PBLs after elimination of the purported CD25$^+$ regulatory cells, providing one approach to assessing whether active regulatory tolerance may be occurring in vivo. These types of assays and approaches represent a good start but much work is yet to be done. A number of controlled trials evaluating the ability to induce tolerance in the clinic as well as underlying mechanisms and tests to detect the tolerant state are being performed in conjunction with the National Institutes of Health-sponsored Immune Tolerance Network. It is anticipated that these studies will provide new insight into the utility of ELISPOT and other approaches as the results unfold over the next 5 years.

TUMOR IMMUNITY

T cell immunity is thought to play a key role in host defense against tumor growth and metastasis, although the interactions between the immune system and tumor are complex (Ochsenbein et al., 2001; Pardoll, 2001). The ELISPOT technique has been widely accepted among tumor immunologists as a powerful method for analysis of tumor or tumor vaccine immunity (Clay et al., 2001). The frequency and cytokine profiles of tumor antigen specific T cells have been quantified in malignancies such as acute myelogenous leukemia, colorectal cancer, breast cancer and melanoma (Wierda et al., 2000; Zier et al., 2000; Scheibenbogen et al., 2002a,c; Nagorsen et al., 2003; Slager et al., 2003). Additionally, a large number of tumor vaccines have been developed over the past 5 years and the use of these vaccines in small clinical trials for prostate cancer, multiple myeloma and melanoma have heavily utilized the ELISPOT method for monitoring the effects of the vaccines on tumor specific immunity (Meidenbauer et al., 2000; Belli et al., 2002; Scheibenbogen et al., 2002b; Yi et al., 2002; Peterson et al., 2003). These data provide evidence that those patients with clinical responses to the vaccines also developed detectable increases in the frequency of tumor specific immunity (Meidenbauer et al., 2000; Belli et al., 2002; Scheibenbogen et al., 2002b; Yi et al., 2002; Peterson et al., 2003), suggesting that the ELISPOT-based results could function as surrogate markers for outcome. Larger studies need to be conducted and analyzed before conclusive statements can be made regarding routine clinical utility of this assay in these settings.

AUTOIMMUNE DISEASE

Similarly, ELISPOT assays have been widely utilized in the investigation of a number of autoimmune diseases. Most of these studies have been directed towards understanding the pathogenesis of disease and have involved analysis of

clonal size and cytokine-secretion profiles of autoantigen-specific T cells in the peripheral blood of patients with active autoimmune disease. This work has provided descriptive and, in some cases, comprehensive epitope mapping analysis of immune reactivity to putative autoantigens in patients with multiple sclerosis (Hellings et al., 2001; Pelfrey et al., 2000, 2002; Vandenbark et al., 2001), ankylosing spondylitis (Fiorillo et al., 2000), autoimmune sensory neural hearing loss (Lorenz et al., 2002), idiopathic thrombocytopenic purpura (Kuwana et al., 2002) systemic lupus erythematosus (Hagiwara et al., 1996), diabetes (Meierhoff et al., 2002) and rheumatoid arthritis (Lampa et al., 2002). It is important to reiterate, however, that there have not yet been any controlled trials to show that ELISPOT-based immune monitoring is useful for making clinical decisions regarding prognosis, diagnosis or for guiding alterations in therapy.

CONCLUDING REMARKS

Cytokine ELISPOT analysis of T cell immunity has multiple advantages over many other approaches for accurately measuring the multiple relevant features of T cell immunity in animal models and in humans. This high-resolution assay has already proven to be invaluable in the research setting as one approach to delineating immune responses to infectious agents, tumor antigens, autoantigens and transplant antigens. As clinical medicine moves into the twenty-first century, it is possible to envision an era in which serial immunologic monitoring analyses will rationally guide the day-to-day clinical care of patients with a variety of disorders. Drug doses could be individually optimized, preemptive therapies could be instituted for patients with high-risk profiles, vaccine efficacy could be readily monitored and early treatment could be instituted, all based on the results of simple yet reliable studies of antigen-reactive immunity performed with peripheral blood samples. The implications of such an approach, including the cost savings, the avoidance of side effects related to the optimization of drug use and the clinical benefit of anticipated improved outcome are enormous. It is hoped that over the next several years cooperative, prospective, multicenter trials will be designed to address these important questions and that the findings from such studies will ultimately result in improved patient care. Until then, it is our view that the ELISPOT analyses of human immunity should continue to be utilized within the context of research protocols as part of a compendium of immune monitoring tools aimed at comprehensively and repeatedly assessing immune function to clinically relevant antigens.

REFERENCES

Addo, M.M., Yu, X.G., Rathod, A. et al. (2003). Comprehensive epitope analysis of human immunodeficiency virus type 1

(HIV-1)-specific T-cell responses directed against the entire expressed HIV-1 genome demonstrate broadly directed responses, but no correlation to viral load. J Virol 77, 2081–2092.

Altfeld, M., Rosenberg, E.S., Shankarappa, R. et al. (2001). Cellular immune responses and viral diversity in individuals treated during acute and early HIV-1 infection. J Exp Med 193, 169–180.

Anthony, D.D., Valdez, H., Post, A.B., Carlson, N.L., Heeger, P.S. and Lehmann, P.V. (2002). Comprehensive determinant mapping of the hepatitis-C-specific CD8 cell repertoire reveals unpredicted immune hierarchy. Clin Immunol 103, 264–276.

Barnes, E., Harcourt, G., Brown, D. et al. (2002). The dynamics of T-lymphocyte responses during combination therapy for chronic hepatitis C virus infection. Hepatology 36, 743–754.

Belli, F., Testori, A., Rivoltini, L. et al. (2002). Vaccination of metastatic melanoma patients with autologous tumor-derived heat shock protein gp96-peptide complexes: clinical and immunologic findings. J Clin Oncol 20, 4169–4180.

Benichou, G., Valujskikh, A. and Heeger, P.S. (1999). Contributions of direct and indirect T cell alloreactivity during allograft rejection in mice. J Immunol 162, 352–358.

Bielorai, B., Golan, H., Rechavi, G. and Toren, A. (2002). Stem-cell transplantation for primary immunodeficiencies. Isr Med Assoc J 4, 648–652.

Bilen, C.Y., Inci, K., Erkan, I. and Ozen, H. (2003). The predictive value of purified protein derivative results on complications and prognosis in patients with bladder cancer treated with bacillus Calmette-Guerin. J Urol 169, 1702–1705.

Brewer, D.D., Brody, S., Drucker, E. et al. (2003). Mounting anomalies in the epidemiology of HIV in Africa: cry the beloved paradigm. Int J STD AIDS 14, 144–147.

Bugiani, M., Borraccino, A., Migliore, E. et al. (2003). Tuberculin reactivity in adult BCG-vaccinated subjects: a cross-sectional study. Int J Tuberc Lung Dis 7, 320–326.

Buseyne, F., Scott-Algara, D., Porrot, F. et al. (2002). Frequencies of ex vivo-activated human immunodeficiency virus type 1-specific gamma-interferon-producing CD8+ T cells in infected children correlate positively with plasma viral load. J Virol 76, 12414–12422.

Cao, H., Kaleebu, P., Hom, D. et al. (2003a). Immunogenicity of a recombinant human immunodeficiency virus (HIV)-canarypox vaccine in HIV-seronegative Ugandan volunteers: results of the HIV Network for Prevention Trials 007 Vaccine Study. J Infect Dis 187, 887–895.

Cao, J., McNevin, J., Holte, S., Fink, L., Corey, L. and McElrath, M.J. (2003b). Comprehensive analysis of human immunodeficiency virus type 1 (HIV-1)-specific gamma interferon-secreting CD8+ T cells in primary HIV-1 infection. J Virol 77, 6867–6878.

Carreno, B.M., and Collins, M. (2002). The B7 family of ligands and its receptors: new pathways for costimulation and inhibition of immune responses. Annu Rev Immunol 20, 29–53.

Chapman, A.L., Munkanta, M., Wilkinson, K.A. et al. (2002). Rapid detection of active and latent tuberculosis infection in HIV-positive individuals by enumeration of Mycobacterium tuberculosis-specific T cells. Aids 16, 2285–2293.

Church, A.C. (2002). X-linked severe combined immunodeficiency. Hosp Med 63, 676–680.

Clay, T.M., Hobeika, A.C., Mosca, P.J., Lyerly, H.K. and Morse, M.A. (2001). Assays for monitoring cellular immune responses to active immunotherapy of cancer. Clin Cancer Res 7, 1127–1135.

Collins, A.B., Schneeberger, E.E., Pascual, M.A. et al. (1999). Complement activation in acute humoral renal allograft rejection: diagnostic significance of C4d deposits in peritubular capillaries. J Am Soc Nephrol 10, 2208–2214.

Croft, M., Bradley, L.M. and Swain, S.L. (1994). Naive versus memory CD4 T cell response to antigen. Memory cells are less dependent on accessory cell costimulation and can respond to many antigen-presenting cell types including resting B cells. J Immunol 152, 2675–2685.

Currier, J.R., deSouza, M., Chanbancherd, P., Bernstein, W., Birx, D.L. and Cox, J.H. (2002). Comprehensive screening for human immunodeficiency virus type 1 subtype-specific CD8 cytotoxic T lymphocytes and definition of degenerate epitopes restricted by HLA-A0207 and -C(W)0304 alleles. J Virol 76, 4971–4986.

Czerkinsky, C., Andersson, G., Ekre, H.P., Nilsson, L.A., Klareskog, L., and Ouchterlony, O. (1988). Reverse ELISPOT assay for clonal analysis of cytokine production. I. Enumeration of gamma-interferon-secreting cells. J Immunol Methods 110, 29–36.

Czerkinsky, C.C., Nilsson, L.A., Nygren, H., Ouchterlony, O. and Tarkowski, A. (1983). A solid-phase enzyme linked immunospot (ELISPOT) assay for enumeration of specific antibody-secreting cells. J Immunol Methods 65, 109–121.

Dutton, R.W., Bradley, L.M. and Swain, S.L. (1998). T cell memory. Annu Rev Immunol 16, 201–223.

Edwards, B.H., Bansal, A., Sabbaj, S., Bakari, J., Mulligan, M.J. and Goepfert, P.A. (2002). Magnitude of functional CD8+ T-cell responses to the gag protein of human immunodeficiency virus type 1 correlates inversely with viral load in plasma. J Virol 76, 2298–2305.

Ewer, K., Deeks, J., Alvarez, L. et al. (2003). Comparison of T-cell-based assay with tuberculin skin test for diagnosis of Mycobacterium tuberculosis infection in a school tuberculosis outbreak. Lancet 361, 1168–1173.

Fiorillo, M.T., Maragno, M., Butler, R., Dupuis, M.L. and Sorrentino, R. (2000). CD8(+) T-cell autoreactivity to an HLA-B27-restricted self-epitope correlates with ankylosing spondylitis. J Clin Invest 106, 47–53.

Forsthuber, T., Yip, H.C. and Lehmann, P.V. (1996). Induction of TH1 and TH2 immunity in neonatal mice. Science 271, 1728–1730.

Francois Bach, J. (2003). Regulatory T cells under scrutiny. Nat Rev Immunol 3, 189–198.

Gaber, L.W., Moore, L.W., Gaber, A.O. et al. (1998). Utility of standardized histological classification in the management of acute rejection. 1995 Efficacy Endpoints Conference. Transplantation 65, 376–380.

Garcia, K.C., Teyton, L., and Wilson, I.A. (1999). Structural basis of T cell recognition. Annu Rev Immunol 17, 369–397.

Gebauer, B.S., Hricik, D.E., Atallah, A. et al. (2002). Evolution of the enzyme linked immunosorbent spot assay for post-transplant alloreactivity as a potentially useful immune monitoring tool. Am J Transplant 2, 857–866.

Goepfert, P.A., Bansal, A., Edwards, B.H. et al. (2000). A significant number of human immunodeficiency virus epitope-specific cytotoxic T lymphocytes detected by tetramer binding do not produce gamma interferon. J Virol 74, 10249–10255.

Goulder, P.J., Addo, M.M., Altfeld, M.A. et al. (2001a). Rapid definition of five novel HLA-A*3002-restricted human immunodeficiency virus-specific cytotoxic T-lymphocyte Epitopes by Elispot and intracellular cytokine staining assays. J Virol 5, 1339–1347.

Goulder, P.J., Altfeld, M.A., Rosenberg, E.S. et al. (2001b). Substantial differences in specificity of HIV-specific cytotoxic T cells in acute and chronic HIV Infection. J Exp Med 193, 181–194.

Gourishankar, S. and Halloran, P.F. (2002). Late deterioration of organ transplants: a problem in injury and homeostasis. Curr Opin Immunol 14, 576–583.

Gruener, N.H., Lechner, F., Jung, M.C. et al. (2001). Sustained dysfunction of antiviral CD8+ T lymphocytes after infection with hepatitis C virus. J Virol 75, 5550–5558.

Gudmundsdottir, H., Wells, A.D. and Turka, L.A. (1999). Dynamics and requirements of T cell clonal expansion in vivo at the single-cell level: effector function is linked to proliferative capacity. J Immunol 162, 5212–5223.

Hagiwara, E., Gourley, M.F., Lee, S. and Klinman, D.K. (1996). Disease severity in patients with systemic lupus erythematosus correlates with an increased ratio of interleukin-10: interferon-gamma-secreting cells in the peripheral blood. Arthritis Rheum 39, 379–385.

Halloran, P.F. (2002). Call for revolution: a new approach to describing allograft deterioration. Am J Transplant 2, 195–200.

Heeger, P.S. (2003). T-cell allorecognition and transplant rejection: a summary and update. Am J Transplant 3, 525–533.

Heeger, P.S., Forsthuber, T., Shive, C. et al. (2000a). Revisiting tolerance induced by autoantigen in incomplete Freund's adjuvant. J Immunol 164, 5771–5781.

Heeger, P.S., Greenspan, N.S., Kuhlenschmidt, S. et al. (1999). Pretransplant frequency of donor-specific, IFN-gamma-producing lymphocytes is a manifestation of immunologic memory and correlates with the risk of posttransplant rejection episodes. J Immunol 163, 2267–2275.

Heeger, P.S., and Hricik, D. (2002). Immune monitoring in kidney transplant recipients revisited. J Am Soc Nephrol 13, 288–290.

Heeger, P.S., Valujskikh, A. and Lehmann, P.V. (2000b). Comprehensive assessment of determinant specificity, frequency, and cytokine signature of the primed CD8 cell repertoire induced by a minor transplantation antigen. J Immunol 165, 1278–1284.

Hellings, N., Baree, M., Verhoeven, C. et al. (2001). T-cell reactivity to multiple myelin antigens in multiple sclerosis patients and healthy controls. J Neurosci Res 63, 290–302.

Hesse, M.D., Karulin, A.Y., Boehm, B.O., Lehmann, P.V. and Tary-Lehmann, M. (2001). A T cell clone's avidity is a function of its activation state. J Immunol 167, 1353–1361.

Hricik, D.E. and Heeger, P.S. (2001). Minimization of immunosuppression in kidney transplantation. The need for immune monitoring. Transplantation 72, S32–35.

Hricik, D.E., Rodriguez, V., Riley, J. et al. (2003). Enzyme linked immunosorbent spot (ELISPOT) assay for interferon-gamma independently predicts renal function in kidney transplant recipients. Am J Transplant 3, 878–884.

Jain, M.K., Skiest, D.J., Cloud, J.W., Jain, C.L., Burns, D. and Berggren, R.E. (2003). Changes in mortality related to human immunodeficiency virus infection: comparative analysis of inpatient deaths in 1995 and in 1999–2000. Clin Infect Dis 36, 1030–1038.

Jeannet, M., Pinn, V.W., Flax, M.H., Winn, H.J. and Russell, P.S. (1970). Humoral antibodies in renal allotransplantation in man. N Engl J Med 282, 111–117.

Kamal, S.M., Fehr, J., Roesler, B., Peters, T. and Rasenack, J.W. (2002). Peginterferon alone or with ribavirin enhances HCV-specific CD4 T- helper 1 responses in patients with chronic hepatitis C. Gastroenterology 123, 1070–1083.

Karulin, A.Y., Hesse, M.D., Tary-Lehmann, M. and Lehmann, P.V. (2000). Single-cytokine-producing CD4 memory cells predominate in type 1 and type 2 immunity. J Immunol 164, 1862–1872.

Karulin, A.Y., Hesse, M.D., Yip, H.C. and Lehmann, P.V. (2002). Indirect IL-4 pathway in type 1 immunity. J Immunol 168, 545–553.

Kong, P.L., Odegard, J.M., Bouzahzah, F. et al. (2003). Intrinsic T cell defects in systemic autoimmunity. Ann NY Acad Sci 987, 60–67.

Kuwana, M., Okazaki, Y., Kaburaki, J., Kawakami, Y. and Ikeda, Y. (2002). Spleen is a primary site for activation of platelet-reactive T and B cells in patients with immune thrombocytopenic purpura. J Immunol 168, 3675–3682.

Lakkis, F.G., Arakelov, A., Konieczny, B.T. and Inoue, Y. (2000). Immunologic 'ignorance' of vascularized organ transplants in the absence of secondary lymphoid tissue. Nat Med 6, 686–688.

Lalvani, A., Pathan, A.A., Durkan, H. et al. (2001). Enhanced contact tracing and spatial tracking of Mycobacterium tuberculosis infection by enumeration of antigen-specific T cells. Lancet 357, 2017–2021.

Lampa, J., Klareskog, L. and Ronnelid, J. (2002). Effects of gold on cytokine production in vitro; increase of monocyte dependent interleukin 10 production and decrease of interferon-gamma levels. J Rheumatol 29, 21–28.

Lauer, G.M., Nguyen, T.N., Day, C.L. et al. (2002a). Human immunodeficiency virus type 1-hepatitis C virus coinfection: intraindividual comparison of cellular immune responses against two persistent viruses. J Virol 76, 2817–2826.

Lauer, G.M., Ouchi, K., Chung, R.T. et al. (2002b). Comprehensive analysis of CD8(+)-T-cell responses against hepatitis C virus reveals multiple unpredicted specificities. J Virol 76, 6104–6113.

Lechner, F., Wong, D.K.H., Dunbar, P.R. et al. (2000). Analysis of successful immune responses in persons infected with hepatitis C virus. J Exp Med 191, 1499–1512.

Lehmann, P.V., Cardinaux, F., Appella, E. et al. A. (1989). Inhibition of T cell response with peptides is influenced by both peptide-binding specificity of major histocompatibility complex molecules and susceptibility of T cells to blocking. Eur J Immunol 19, 1071–1077.

Lehmann, P.V., Targoni, O.S. and Forsthuber, T.G. (1998). Shifting T-cell activation thresholds in autoimmunity and determinant spreading. Immunol Rev 164, 53–61.

Locksley, R.M. and Scott, P. (1991). Helper T-cell subsets in mouse leishmaniasis: induction, expansion and effector function. Immunol Today 12, A58–61.

Lorenz, R.R., Solares, C.A., Williams, P. et al. (2002). Interferon-gamma production to inner ear antigens by T cells from patients with autoimmune sensorineural hearing loss. J Neuroimmunol 130, 173–178.

MacGregor, R.R., Ginsberg, R., Ugen, K.E. et al. (2002). T-cell responses induced in normal volunteers immunized with a DNA-based vaccine containing HIV-1 env and rev. Aids 16, 2137–2143.

Masopust, D., Vezys, V., Marzo, A.L. and Lefrancois, L. (2001). Preferential localization of effector memory cells in non-lymphoid tissue. Science 291, 2413–2417.

Matesic, D., Lehmann, P.V. and Heeger, P.S. (1998a). High-resolution characterization of cytokine-producing alloreactivity in naive and allograft-primed mice. Transplantation 65, 906–914.

Matesic, D., Valujskikh, A., Pearlman, E., Higgins, A.W., Gilliam, A.C. and Heeger, P.S. (1998b). Type 2 immune deviation has differential effects on alloreactive CD4+ and CD8+ T cells. J Immunol 161, 5236–5244.

Mayer, S., Laumer, M., Mackensen, A., Andreesen, R. and Krause, S.W. (2002). Analysis of the immune response against tetanus toxoid: enumeration of specific T helper cells by the Elispot assay. Immunobiology 205, 282–289.

Medina, J., Garcia-Buey, L. and Moreno-Otero, R. (2003). Review article: immunopathogenetic and therapeutic aspects of autoimmune hepatitis. Aliment Pharmacol Ther 17, 1–16.

Meidenbauer, N., Harris, D.T., Spitler, L.E. and Whiteside, T.L. (2000). Generation of PSA-reactive effector cells after vaccination with a PSA-based vaccine in patients with prostate cancer. Prostate 43, 88–100.

Meierhoff, G., Ott, P.A., Lehmann, P.V. and Schloot, N.C. (2002). Cytokine detection by ELISPOT: relevance for immunological studies in type 1 diabetes. Diabetes Metab Res Rev 18, 367–380.

Mosmann, T.R., Cherwinski, H., Bond, M.W., Giedlin, M.A. and Coffman, R.L. (1986). Two types of murine helper T cell clone. I. Definition according to profiles of lymphokine activities and secreted proteins. J Immunol 136, 2348–2357.

Mosmann, T.R. and Coffman, R.L. (1989). TH1 and TH2 cells: different patterns of lymphokine secretion lead to different functional properties. Annu Rev Immunol 7, 145–173.

Mwau, M., McMichael, A.J., and Hanke, T. (2002). Design and validation of an enzyme linked immunospot assay for use in clinical trials of candidate HIV vaccines. AIDS Res Hum Retroviruses 18, 611–618.

Nagorsen, D., Scheibenbogen, C., Schaller, G. et al. (2003). Differences in T-cell immunity toward tumor-associated antigens in colorectal cancer and breast cancer patients. Int J Cancer 105, 221–225.

Najafian, N., Salama, A.D., Fedoseyeva, E.V., Benichou, G. and Sayegh, M.H. (2002). Enzyme linked immunosorbent spot assay analysis of peripheral blood lymphocyte reactivity to donor HLA-DR peptides: potential novel assay for prediction of outcomes for renal transplant recipients. J Am Soc Nephrol 13, 252–259.

Nicholson, L.B. and Kuchroo, V.K. (1996). Manipulation of the Th1/Th2 balance in autoimmune disease. Curr Opin Immunol 8, 837–842.

Ochsenbein, A.F., Sierro, S., Odermatt, B. et al. (2001). Roles of tumour localization, second signals and cross priming in cytotoxic T-cell induction. Nature 411, 1058–1064.

O'Driscoll, M. and Jeggo, P. (2002). Immunological disorders and DNA repair. Mutat Res 509, 109–126.

Ovsyannikova, I.G., Dhiman, N., Jacobson, R.M., Vierkant, R.A. and Poland, G.A. (2003). Frequency of measles virus-specific CD4(+) and CD8(+) T cells in subjects seronegative or highly seropositive for measles vaccine. Clin Diagn Lab Immunol 10, 411–416.

Oxenius, A., Campbell, K.A., Maliszewski, C.R. et al. (1996). CD40-CD40 ligand interactions are critical in T-B cooperation but not for other anti-viral CD4+ T cell functions. J Exp Med 183, 2209–2218.

Pantenburg, B., Heinzel, F., Das, L., Heeger, P.S. and Valujskikh, A. (2002). T cells primed by Leishmania major infection cross-react with alloantigens and alter the course of allograft rejection. J Immunol 169, 3686–3693.

Pardoll, D. (2001). T cells and tumours. Nature 411, 1010–1012.

Patel, R. and Terasaki, P.I. (1969). Significance of the positive crossmatch test in kidney transplantation. N Engl J Med 280, 735–739.

Pelfrey, C.M., Cotleur, A.C., Lee, J.C. and Rudick, R.A. (2002). Sex differences in cytokine responses to myelin peptides in multiple sclerosis. J Neuroimmunol 130, 211–223.

Pelfrey, C.M., Rudick, R.A., Cotleur, A.C., Lee, J.C., Tary-Lehmann, M. and Lehmann, P.V. (2000). Quantification of self-recognition in multiple sclerosis by single-cell analysis of cytokine production. J Immunol 165, 1641–1651.

Peterson, A.C., Harlin, H. and Gajewski, T.F. (2003). Immunization with Melan-A peptide-pulsed peripheral blood mononuclear cells plus recombinant human interleukin-12 induces clinical activity and T-cell responses in advanced melanoma. J Clin Oncol 21, 2342–2348.

Picker, L.J., Treer, J.R., Ferguson-Darnell, B., Collins, P.A., Buck, D. and Terstappen, L.W. (1993). Control of lymphocyte recirculation in man. I. Differential regulation of the peripheral lymph node homing receptor L-selection on T cells during the virgin to memory cell transition. J Immunol 150, 1105–1121.

Quartier, P. and Prieur, A.M. (2002). Immunodeficiency and genetic conditions that cause arthritis in childhood. Curr Rheumatol Rep 4, 483–493.

Reinsmoen, N.L. (2002). Cellular methods used to evaluate the immune response in transplantation. Tissue Antigens 59, 241–250.

Rininsland, F.H., Helms, T., Asaad, R.J., Boehm, B.O. and Tary-Lehmann, M. (2000). Granzyme B ELISPOT assay for ex vivo measurements of T cell immunity. J Immunol Methods 240, 143–155.

Rodrigues, M.M., Ribeirao, M. and Boscardin, S.B. (2000). CD4 Th1 but not Th2 clones efficiently activate macrophages to eliminate Trypanosoma cruzi through a nitric oxide dependent mechanism. Immunol Lett 73, 43–50.

Russell, J.H. and Ley, T.J. (2002). Lymphocyte-mediated cytotoxicity. Annu Rev Immunol 20, 323–370.

Salama, A.D., Najafian, N., Clarkson, M.R., Harmon, W.E. and Sayegh, M.H. (2003). Regulatory CD25(+) T Cells in human kidney transplant recipients. J Am Soc Nephrol 14, 1643–1651.

Salomon, B. and Bluestone, J.A. (2001). Complexities of CD28/B7: CTLA-4 costimulatory pathways in autoimmunity and transplantation. Annu Rev Immunol 19, 225–252.

Sarwal, M., Chua, M.S., Kambham, N. et al. (2003). Molecular heterogeneity in acute renal allograft rejection identified by DNA microarray profiling. N Engl J Med 349, 125–138.

Scheibenbogen, C., Letsch, A., Thiel, E. et al. (2002a). CD8 T-cell responses to Wilms tumor gene product WT1 and proteinase 3 in patients with acute myeloid leukemia. Blood 100, 2132–2137.

Scheibenbogen, C., Nagorsen, D., Seliger, B. et al. (2002b). Long-term freedom from recurrence in 2 stage IV melanoma patients following vaccination with tyrosinase peptides. Int J Cancer 99, 403–408.

Scheibenbogen, C., Sun, Y., Keilholz, U. et al. (2002c). Identification of known and novel immunogenic T-cell epitopes from tumor antigens recognized by peripheral blood T cells from patients responding to IL-2-based treatment. Int J Cancer 98, 409–414.

Slager, E.H., Borghi, M., van der Minne, C.E. et al. (2003). CD4+ Th2 cell recognition of HLA-DR-restricted epitopes derived from CAMEL: a tumor antigen translated in an alternative open reading frame. J Immunol 170, 1490–1497.

Smith, J.G., Levin, M., Vessey, R. et al. (2003). Measurement of cell-mediated immunity with a Varicella-Zoster Virus-specific interferon-gamma ELISPOT assay: responses in an elderly population receiving a booster immunization. J Med Virol 70 Suppl 1, S38–41.

Subauste, C.S. (2002). CD154 and type-1 cytokine response: from hyper IgM syndrome to human immunodeficiency virus infection. J Infect Dis 185 Suppl 1, S83–89.

Sun, Y., Iglesias, E., Samri, A. et al. (2003). A systematic comparison of methods to measure HIV-1 specific CD8 cells. J Immunol Methods 272, 23–34.

Suthanthiran, M. and Strom, T.B. (1994). Renal transplantation. N Engl J Med 331, 365–376.

Swain, S.L. (1994). Generation and in vivo persistence of polarized Th1 and Th2 memory cells. Immunity 1, 543–552.

Targoni, O.S., Baus, J., Hofstetter, H.H. et al. (2001). Frequencies of neuroantigen-specific T cells in the central nervous system versus the immune periphery during the course of experimental allergic encephalomyelitis. J Immunol 166, 4757–4764.

Targoni, O.S. and Lehmann, P.V. (1998). Endogenous myelin basic protein inactivates the high avidity T cell repertoire. J Exp Med 187, 2055–2063.

Tarkowski, A., Czerkinsky, C., Nilsson, L.A., Nygren, H. and Ouchterlony, O. (1984). Solid-phase enzyme linked immunospot (ELISPOT) assay for enumeration of IgG rheumatoid factor-secreting cells. J Immunol Methods 72, 451–459.

Tary-Lehmann, M., Hricik, D.E., Justice, A.C., Potter, N.S. and Heeger, P.S. (1998). Enzyme linked immunosorbent assay spot detection of interferon-gamma and interleukin 5-producing cells as a predictive marker for renal allograft failure. Transplantation 66, 219–224.

Thimme, R., Oldach, D., Chang, K.M., Steiger, C., Ray, S.C. and Chisari, F.V. (2001). Determinants of viral clearance and persistence during acute hepatitis C virus infection. J Exp Med 194, 1395–1406.

Thomson, A.W., Mazariegos, G.V. and Reyes, J. (2001). Monitoring the patient off immunosuppression. Conceptual framework for a proposed tolerance assay study in liver transplant recipients. Transplantation 72, S13–22.

Tryniszewska, E., Nacsa, J., Lewis, M.G. et al. (2002). Vaccination of macaques with long-standing SIVmac251 infection lowers the viral set point after cessation of antiretroviral therapy. J Immunol 169, 5347–5357.

Valdez, H., Anthony, D., Farukhi, F. et al. (2000). Immune responses to hepatitis C and non-hepatitis C antigens in hepatitis C virus infected and HIV-1 coinfected patients. Aids 14, 2239–2246.

Valdez, H., Carlson, N.L., Post, A.B. et al. (2002). HIV long-term non-progressors maintain brisk CD8 T cell responses to other viral antigens. Aids 16, 1113–1111.

Valujskikh, A. and Heeger, P. (2000). A closer look at cytokine-secreting T lymphocytes. Graft 3, 250–258.

Valujskikh, A., Matesic, D. and Heeger, P.S. (1999). Characterization and manipulation of T cell immunity to skin grafts expressing a transgenic minor antigen. Transplantation 68, 1029–1036.

Valujskikh, A., Pantenburg, B. and Heeger, P.S. (2002). Primed allospecific T cells prevent the effects of costimulatory blockade on prolonged cardiac allograft survival in mice. Am J Transplant 2, 501–509.

Vandenbark, A.A., Finn, T., Barnes, D. et al. (2001). Diminished frequency of interleukin-10-secreting, T-cell receptor peptide-reactive T cells in multiple sclerosis patients might allow expansion of activated memory T cells bearing the cognate BV gene. J Neurosci Res 66, 171–176.

von Herrath, M.G. and Harrison, L.C. (2003). Antigen-induced regulatory T cells in autoimmunity. Nat Rev Immunol 3, 223–232.

Ward, D.M., Shiflett, S.L. and Kaplan, J. (2002). Chediak-Higashi syndrome: a clinical and molecular view of a rare lysosomal storage disorder. Curr Mol Med 2, 469–477.

Watschinger, B. and Pascual, M. (2002). Capillary C4d deposition as a marker of humoral immunity in renal allograft rejection. J Am Soc Nephrol 13, 2420–2423.

Wedemeyer, H., He, X.S., Nascimbeni, M. et al. (2002). Impaired effector function of hepatitis C virus-specific CD8+ T cells in chronic hepatitis C virus infection. J Immunol 169, 3447–3458.

Weetman, A.P. (2003). Autoimmune thyroid disease: propagation and progression. Eur J Endocrinol 148, 1–9.

Wells, A.D., Walsh, M.C., Sankaran, D. and Turka, L.A. (2000). T cell effector function and anergy avoidance are quantitatively linked to cell division. J Immunol 165, 2432–2443.

Wierda, W.G., Cantwell, M.J., Woods, S.J., Rassenti, L.Z., Prussak, C.E. and Kipps, T.J. (2000). CD40-ligand (CD154) gene therapy for chronic lymphocytic leukemia. Blood 96, 2917–2924.

Wolff, A.J. and O'Donnell, A.E. (2003). HIV-related pulmonary infections: a review of the recent literature. Curr Opin Pulm Med 9, 210–214.

Wood, K.J. and Sakaguchi, S. (2003). Regulatory T cells in transplantation tolerance. Nat Rev Immunol 3, 199–210.

Xie, H., Lim, Y.C., Luscinskas, F.W. and Lichtman, A.H. (1999). Acquisition of selectin binding and peripheral homing properties by CD4(+) and CD8(+) T cells. J Exp Med 189, 1765–1776.

Yi, Q., Desikan, R., Barlogie, B. and Munshi, N. (2002). Optimizing dendritic cell-based immunotherapy in multiple myeloma. Br J Haematol 117, 297–305.

Yip, H.C., Karulin, A.Y., Tary-Lehmann, M. et al. (1999). Adjuvant-guided type-1 and type-2 immunity: infectious/noninfectious dichotomy defines the class of response. J Immunol 162, 3942–3949.

Yu, C.C., Mamchak, A.A. and DeFranco, A.L. (2003). Signaling mutations and autoimmunity. Curr Dir Autoimmun 6, 61–88.

Zier, K., Johnson, K., Maddux, J.M. et al. (2000). IFNgamma secretion following stimulation with total tumor peptides from autologous human tumors. J Immunol Methods 241, 61–68.

Zimmermann, C., Prevost-Blondel, A., Blaser, C. and Pircher, H. (1999). Kinetics of the response of naive and memory CD8 T cells to antigen: similarities and differences. Eur J Immunol 29, 284–290.

Testing Natural Killer Cells

Chapter 34

Nikola L. Vujanovic

University of Pittsburgh Department of Pathology and Cancer Institute, Pittsburgh, PA, USA

> A fact in itself is nothing. It is valuable only for the idea attached to it, or for the proof which it furnishes.
>
> Claude Bernard

INTRODUCTION

Natural killer (NK) cells are essential effectors of the innate anticancer immunity which spontaneously kill transformed cells, eliminate bloodborne metastases and characteristically respond to cancer. Consequently, NK cells reflect both host ability to fight cancer and cancer development and thus sense cancer outcome. The present chapter reviews and discusses studies that have correlated numbers and functions of peripheral blood, cancer tissue or regional lymph node NK cells with prognosis of cancer patients. The reviewed data show that NK cell status may be a reliable marker of cancer prognosis.

Accurate cancer staging and prognostic are essential for adequate treatment of cancer. A number of cancer prognosis markers have been identified and evaluated in clinical practice. Several of them, including cancer histological type, mitotic index and invasion of surrounding normal tissues, size of primary tumor, lymph node metastases and distant metastases, have been proven to be useful. However, the available markers can fail in more than 30 per cent of early stage cancer patients (Naruke et al., 1998). Therefore, more sensitive and reliable cancer prognosis markers are needed.

Multiple cell types of the immune system, including NK cells, dendritic cells (DC) and tumor-specific T cells and B cells, can recognize, interact with and characteristically respond to cancer. Thus, cancer-dependent changes in the immune system may represent sensitive and reliable markers for cancer prognosis. NK cells are among the most sensitive spontaneous immune cell responders to cancer and their numbers and functions have been frequently evaluated as markers for cancer prognosis. The present chapter reviews the supporting evidence for and discusses the relevance of NK cells to cancer resistance and cancer prognosis.

NK CELLS: CONSTITUTIVE SENSORS AND KILLERS OF CANCER CELLS

NK cells are essential effector cells of the innate immunity that spontaneously and rapidly recognize and lyse transformed and infected cells and therefore represent the first line of the host immune defense against cancer and invading pathogens (Trinchieri, 1989; Vujanovic et al., 1996a; Biron et al., 1999). NK cells utilize two major constitutive mechanisms to recognize and kill cancer cells: the secretory/necrotic mechanism, which is mediated by secretion and cytolytic activity of perforin/granzymes and the non-secretory/apoptotic mechanism, which is mediated by transmembrane proapoptotic TNF family ligands (Vujanovic, 2001).

The secretory/necrotic mechanism is selectively operative against target cells that both express ligands for killer cell activating receptors (KARs) and lack MHC class I molecules. The killing mechanism is triggered in

NK cells by balanced signaling via engaging KARs (i.e. NKp30, NKp44, NKp46 and NKG2D) with KAR ligands (e.g. the MHC class I homologues MICA and MICB) and disengaging killer cell inhibitory receptors (KIRs) in the absence of MHC class I molecules (Lanier, 1998; Moretta et al., 2000; Yokoyama and Plougastel, 2003). Both the acquisition of KAR ligands and loss of KIR ligands are induced in cells by acute stress/danger signals such as malignant transformation, heat-shock or invading pathogens and function as signals of cellular stress (Vivier and Biron, 2002; Gleimer and Parham, 2003).

The non-secretory/apoptotic killing mechanism is triggered by a simultaneous engagement of multiple transmembrane TNF family ligands (i.e. TNF, FasL and LT-$\alpha 1\beta 2$), constitutively expressed by NK cells, with the corresponding transmembrane TNF family receptors (i.e. TNFR1, TNFR2, Fas and LT-βR) preferentially expressed by cancer cells and probably infected and stressed cells (Vujanovic et al., 1996b; Kashii et al., 1999; Vujanovic, 2001).

Both NK cell cytotoxic mechanisms are selective for tumor cells and ineffective against most normal cells, because normal cells, in contrast to cancer cells, express relatively high levels of MHC class I molecules and low levels or none of KAR ligands (Vivier and Biron, 2002; Gleimer and Parham, 2003) and do not express the major proapoptotic TNF family receptors TNFR1, TRAILR1 and TRAILR2 (Lu et al., 2002). Using these constitutive and cancer-specific cytotoxic mechanisms, NK cells spontaneously and rapidly mediate in vivo elimination of newly formed cancer cells and bloodborne metastases and thus prevent development of both primary tumors and metastases (Trinchieri, 1989; Vujanovic et al., 1996a).

In addition to KIRs and KARs, NK cells express a variety of other biologically important receptors, including the receptors for Fc portions of immunoglobulin G (FcγRIII and FcγRII) (Sulika et al., 2001) and inflammatory cytokines. Therefore, NK cells respond to not only acute stress/danger signals but also to immune complexes and inflammation by the increases of their constitutive tumoricidal activities and de novo development of proliferation and production of immunoregulatory cytokines (e.g. IFN-γ, IFN-α, TNF and GM-CSF) and chemochines (e.g. IL-8, MIP-1α, MIP-1β and RANTES) (Trinchieri, 1989; Robertson and Ritz, 1990; Lanier and Philips, 1992; Vitolo et al., 1993; Vujanovic et al., 1996a; Peritt et al., 1998; Oliva et al., 1998; Cooper et al., 2001). The newly acquired functions may lead to the augmentation of NK cell anticancer activities and direct elimination of cancer cells (Vujanovic et al., 1996a) and induction of cancer-specific Th1 adaptive immune responses (Kos and Engleman, 1995, 1996), which in concert can control growth of primary tumors and metastases.

NK cells also cooperate with dendritic cells (DC) and polarize, promote and regulate effective innate and adaptive antitumor immune functions by reciprocal induction of the central Th1-type cytokines IFN-γ and IL-12 (Fernandez et al., 1999; Gerosa et al., 2002; Piccioli et al., 2002; Ferlazzo et al., 2002). The interactions of NK cells and DC are promoted by acute stress/danger signals (e.g. bacterial endotoxins) and their activation/maturation cytokines (e.g. IL-2 and TNF). NK cells activated by DC become not only potent killers of tumor cells but they also acquire the ability to kill immature DC expressing low levels of MHC class I molecules via engagement of KARs and provide a 'control switch' for the immune system (Fernandez et al., 1999; Gerosa et al., 2002; Piccioli et al., 2002; Ferlazzo et al., 2002; Moretta 2002). This killing of DC by NK cells might be an important immune mechanism that regulates quality and magnitude of an evolving immune response by eliminating DC that are unsuitable for antigen presentation (Moretta, 2002; Ruggeri et al., 2002). In vivo studies in experimental murine tumor models have suggested that the NK cell–DC interactions and their functional consequences might be critical for the host anticancer immune defense against both non-immunogenic (MHC class I−, NK-susceptible) (Fernandez et al., 1999) and immunogenic (MHC class I+, NK-resistant) tumors (Peron et al., 1998).

In contrast to the above-described stimulatory signals that induce activation of NK cells, chronic emotional or physical stress through increased and prolonged secretion of corticosteroids and endorphins, as well as some cancer cell products, such as TGF-β, FasL, oncoproteins (Whiteside and Rabinowich, 1998) and soluble MIC ligands (Gleimer and Parham, 2003), provide inhibitory signals for NK cells and counteract NK cell anticancer functions.

NK cells represent a relatively small population of immune cells and, in order optimally to mediate their functions, are strategically distributed in the blood, lymphoid tissues, parenchymal organs and tissues bordering the external environment (Vujanovic et al., 1996a; Li et al., 2003). NK cells represent 5–20 per cent of peripheral blood mononuclear leukocytes, 2–7 per cent of lymph node lymphocytes, 3–10 per cent of splenic lymphocytes, 20–40 per cent of liver-resident lymphoid cells, 15–30 per cent of lung-resident lymphoid cells and an appreciable proportion of lymphoid cells in the skin, intestine and placental subepithelia. Importantly, NK cells also infiltrate stromal tissues of various solid tumors, where they may make up 8–30 per cent of tumor infiltrating lymphocytes (TILs).

The constitutive distribution and functions of NK cells are dramatically and characteristically changed by developing cancer, invading pathogens and systemic treatments with cytokines (i.e. IL-2, IL-12, IL-15, IL-18, interferons and Flt3-ligand) or cytotoxic drugs (Vujanovic et al., 1996a; Shaw et al., 1998; Biron et al., 1999). The changes of NK cells may be measurable in peripheral blood, tumor tissues and lymph nodes.

STATUS OF BLOOD NK CELLS IN CANCER PATIENTS

Experimental studies in rodents have provided compelling evidence that anticancer activities of peripheral blood NK cells mediate elimination of bloodborne metastases and consequently prevent cancer spreading and development of distant metastases (Trinchieri, 1989; Vujanovic et al., 1996a). These findings have resulted in the notion that numbers and functions of NK cells in peripheral blood might positively correlate with the host resistance to development of metastases and therefore may serve as prognostic markers. The notion has been extensively tested in patients with various cancer types.

The number of peripheral blood NK cells as a single parameter has been correlated with cancer prognosis in a few studies. In these studies, NK cells have been defined as $CD56^+CD3^-$ lymphocytes and enumerated in Ficoll gradient-purified peripheral blood mononuclear cell (PBMNC) populations, using fluorochrome-conjugated specific antibodies and two-color flow cytometry analysis (Zhou and Jiang, 1994; Soygur et al., 1999; Sephton et al., 2000; Marana et al., 2000). Although limited, these studies have shown that NK cell numbers in peripheral blood may positively correlate with cancer prognosis (Zhou and Jiang, 1994; Soygur et al., 1999; Sephton et al., 2000; Marana et al., 2000). Thus, in patients with metastatic breast carcinoma, it was determined that a decreased NK cell count coincided with flattened diurnal cortisol rhythm and both correlated with early mortality (Sephton et al., 2000). Patients with invasive bladder transitional cell carcinoma showed significantly lower percentages of NK cells in peripheral blood than normal individuals and those patients who responded to chemotherapy had significantly higher levels of NK cells then those who did not respond (Soygur et al., 1999). Patients with esophageal carcinoma in stages II, III and IV of the disease had significantly decreased numbers of NK cells. The numbers of circulating NK cells increased after radical operation of the patients, but did not reach normal levels. Those patients who developed tumor recurrence or metastases had a fall in NK cell number, which was evident 2–8 months before clinical diagnosis of the relapse (Zhou and Jiang, 1994). In patients with cervical carcinoma who had a good clinical response to chemotherapy, the numbers of NK cells in peripheral blood were higher before the treatment, in comparison with the patients with a poor clinical response (Marana et al., 2000).

Contrary to the limited quantitative studies, numerous studies have correlated functions of peripheral blood NK cells with cancer prognosis. The most frequently tested function of NK cells in these studies has been the perforin/granzyme-mediated spontaneous lysis of K562 myeloid leukemia target cells (Pross et al., 1981; Whiteside et al., 1990). In these assays, target cells are labeled with the radioactive isotope chromium-51 (sodium chromate-51, ^{51}Cr) and mixed with whole peripheral blood lymphocytes as effector cells in various effector:target (E:T) ratios. The effector cell–target cell mixtures are briefly centrifuged, to make contacts between effector and target cells and incubated at 37°C, for 4 h, to allow direct recognition of target cells by and triggering of cytolytic activity in NK cells via engagement of KARs with corresponding cell membrane-bound ligands expressed on target cells. The triggering process is followed by a localized secretion of cytolytic granules and release of perforin/granzymes by NK cells at the contact point between NK cell and tumor cell, insertion of perforin and formation of pores in target cell membrane, entering of granzymes into and further damage of target cells, calcium and water influx into target cells, swelling of target cells, cell membrane disruption and release of the ^{51}Cr labeled cytoplasmic content by target cells (Vujanovic, 2001).

To examine the apoptotic tumoricidal mechanism of peripheral blood NK cells mediated by TNF family ligands, we have recently selected and utilized perforin/granzyme resistant tumor cell lines as target cells and applied apoptotic cytotoxicity assays such as 1 h [^{3}H]thymidine release, 1–24 h MTT, 1–4 h TUNEL assays and 4–24 h microcytotoxicity assays (Vujanovic, 2001; Wahlberg et al., 2001).

To evaluate NK cells further functionally, cytoplasmic levels of the cytolytic molecules perforin and granulysin (Kishi et al., 2002) and the signaling molecule ζ chain (Kuss et al., 1999) have been evaluated by flow cytometry assays. In addition, the expression of IL-18R and responsiveness of peripheral blood NK cells to IL-18 by production of IFN-γ, using RT-PCR and ELISA, respectively, have been examined (Kobashi et al., 2001; Lee et al., 2001).

By applying these assays, multiple studies have consistently shown that peripheral blood NK cell activities positively correlate with cancer prognosis. Thus, breast carcinoma patients with low peripheral blood NK cytolytic activity after therapy more frequently, and in a shorter period of time developed metastases than those with normal NK activity (Pross and Lotzova, 1993). In addition, stress levels in breast carcinoma patients and daughters of these patients negatively correlated with NK cytolytic activity, cytolytic response of NK cells to IFN-γ, in vitro secretion of IFN-γ and/or prognosis (Andersen et al., 1998; Tahir et al., 2001; Cohen et al., 2002). Our

Table 34.1 Malignancies in which prognosis positively correlates with number and function of NK cells

Breast carcinoma
Squamous cell carcinoma of head and neck
Esophageal carcinoma
Lung adenocarcinoma
Lung squamous cell carcinoma
Gastric carcinoma
Colorectal carcinoma
Pancreatic carcinoma
Ovarian carcinoma
Cervical carcinoma
Prostate carcinoma
Bladder carcinoma
Hodgkin's disease
Lymphoma and leukemia

studies indicated that the assessment of TNF family ligand-mediated apoptotic mechanism might be more sensitive and more reliable in the examination of breast carcinoma-related NK cell dysfunction than the assessment of perforin/granzyme-mediated necrotic pathway (Wahlberg et al., 2001). In lung carcinoma patients with distant metastases, NK cytolytic activity was found to be lower than in patients without metastases (Nakamura et al., 2000). Similarly, lung carcinoma patients who died from the cancer during the course of radiotherapy had lower NK activity prior to therapy than patients who remained disease-free during this therapy (Ogata et al., 1989). In patients with squamous cell carcinoma of head and neck (SCCHN), NK cytolytic activity before therapy was found to correlate inversely with development of regional and distant metastases and disease-related death (Schantz and Ordonez, 1991; Gonzalez et al., 1998), but directly correlated with disease-free survival (Schantz et al., 1986). Our studies suggested that in patients with SCCHN, similar to patients with breast carcinoma, the NK assays of TNF family ligand-mediated apoptotic mechanism more sensitively detect cancer-related NK cell dysfunction than the NK assays of perforin/granzyme-mediated necrotic pathway (unpublished data). In addition, patients with SCCHN showed a decreased expression of ζ chain in peripheral blood NK cells and T cells and the lowest expression of ζ chain was found in patients who had cancer recurrence or developed secondary primary cancers within 2 years (Kuss et al., 1999). Gastric carcinoma patients who showed increased NK cytolytic activity before surgical treatment had longer survival than those patients who had decreased NK activity (Akiyoshi et al., 1990; Takeuchi et al., 2001). In addition, the patients with low NK activity had large advanced tumors and regional lymph node metastases (Nio et al., 1991). In patients with colorectal carcinoma, NK cytolytic activity increased following radical surgical treatment (Tartter et al., 1986). In contrast, when the patients had cancer recurrences within 2 years of the treatment, their NK activity was found to be suppressed before and after this therapy (Tartter et al., 1987). Patients with cervical carcinoma who had good clinical responses and good prognosis exhibited NK cytolytic activity significantly higher before and after chemotherapy than patients with poor clinical responses and poor prognosis. In addition, in vitro IL-12 stimulation of peripheral blood mononuclear cells after chemotherapy selectively induced increases in NK cytolytic activity only in patients with good clinical responses (Marana et al., 2000). Importantly, both E6 and E7 oncoproteins of human papillomavirus 16, which has been implicated in the etiology of human cervical carcinoma, inhibited IL-18-induced IFN-γ production in NK cells by competing for IL-18R α-chain (Lee et al., 2001), indicating potential mechanism of cancer-mediated suppression of NK cells in these patients. Patients with advanced pancreatic and esophageal carcinomas showed a marked impairment of NK activity, in contrast to the patients with the localized diseases (Aparicio-Pages et al., 1991). In patients with ovarian carcinoma, low NK activity prior to treatment correlated with the progression of disease after treatment (Garzetti et al., 1993). Patients with atypical prostate or prostate carcinoma in the progressive stage D2 showed a pronounced impairment of NK activity (Tarle et al., 1993). Prostate carcinoma patients also exhibited a decreased expression of ζ chain in peripheral blood NK cells and T cells (Healy et al., 1998). In addition, in patients with advanced prostate carcinoma, blood NKT cells and NK cells were found impaired in production of IFN-γ (Tahir et al., 2001). Patients with active stages III and IV of Hodgkin's disease, either untreated or during treatment, exhibited significantly decreased NK activity in comparison to normal controls and NK activity positively correlated with the response to treatment (Frydecka, 1985). In patients with various progressive cancers, NK cells showed significant decrease in expression of granulysin and IL-18R and in secretion of IFN-γ in response to IL-18 (Kobashi et al., 2001; Kishi et al., 2002). In contrast, tumor-free patients showed normal levels of granulysin (Kobashi et al., 2001). Importantly, recent studies have shown that epithelial tumor cells spontaneously produce a soluble form of MICA ligand by the proteolytic activity of cell membrane metaloproteases and that soluble MICA is present at high levels in the sera of patients with gastrointestinal malignancies, but not in the sera of healthy individuals (Groh et al., 2002; Gleimer and Parham, 2003). In addition, binding of MICA or MICB to NKG2D receptor induced endocytosis and degradation of the receptor, causing a marked reduction of NKG2D expression on both tumor-infiltrating and peripheral blood NK cells and T cells and consequently their severe functional impairment in patients with cancer (Groh et al., 2002; Gleimer and Parham, 2003). This form of NK cell and T cell silencing might be an important mechanism of tumor immune evasion and a significant correlate of cancer prognosis.

TUMOR-INFILTRATING NK CELLS (TINK)

TINK are potentially directly able to kill tumor cells, secrete cytotoxic/cytostatic cytokines (e.g. IFN-γ, IFN-α and TNF), arm other tumor-infiltrating immune cells (e.g. macrophages) and thus mediate elimination or growth inhibition of cancer cells and blood neovasculature cells in tumor tissues. Consequently, TINK may control tumor growth. In humans, NK cells have been consistently found to infiltrate tumors, although in relatively low numbers (Harabuchi et al., 1985; Vujanovic et al., 1996a; Li et al., 2003). The majority of TINK has been found scattered in tumor stroma and mostly distributed around the cancer cell micronodules, where most of tumor infiltrating lymphocytes (TILs) and newly forming tumor blood vessels are located (Okamoto et al., 1987; Ogawa et al., 1988). The characteristic distribution of TINK and their relatively low numbers in tumors suggest that their major antitumor activities might be mediated via secreted cytokines, arming of other TILs, direct killing of potentially metastatic tumor cells which enter into tumor stroma, generation of cellular tumor antigens for the priming of specific antitumor immunity, providing help to tumor-infiltrating DC in induction of adaptive antitumor immunity and/or control of neovasculature development; but not via direct destruction of the majority of cancer cells located in cancer cell micronodules. The potential antitumor activities of TINK and related control of tumor growth and cancer prognosis might be directly dependent on the number of TINK/area of the tumor stromal tissue. These possibilities have been recently assessed by in situ immunohistochemical investigations of TINK. In these studies, TINK are typically specifically labeled in tumor tissue sections with anti-CD57 monoclonal antibody and counted in arbitrarily defined areas of tumor tissue sections (e.g. 0.5–1.0 cm^2/section), using a semiautomated quantitative light microscopy analysis (Coca et al., 1997; Villegas et al., 2002). Several of these studies have resulted in highly significant findings (Coca et al., 1997; Ishigami et al., 2000a, b; Takanami et al., 2001; Villegas et al., 2002). In patients with lung adenocarcinoma, it was found that tumor infiltrating CD57$^+$ cells ranged from 3 to 257/mm^2 (mean = 32.0) of tumor tissue sections and their higher numbers (>32/mm^2 of tumor tissue section) correlated with a longer survival, while their lower numbers (<32/mm^2 of tumor tissue section) correlated with a shorter survival. That was observed in both stage I of the disease and overall groups (Takanami et al., 2001). Similar findings were obtained in patients with lung squamous cell carcinoma (Villegas et al., 2002), colorectal carcinoma (Coca et al., 1997) and gastric carcinoma (Ishigami et al., 2000a, b). Lung squamous cell carcinoma patients were shown to have 1–25 (mean = 6.74) TINK/0.173 mm^2 of tumor tissue section and a significantly better survival if 5 or more TINK/field infiltrated the tumor tissue. In contrast, the risk of death was 2.40 fold higher if less than 5 TINK/microscopic field of tumor tissue section were present (Villegas et al., 2002). Patients with colorectal carcinoma 5 years after radical surgical treatment, especially those having TNM stage III of the disease with a little or moderate NK cell infiltration of tumors, had significantly shorter survival rates and disease-free survival than the patients with abundant NK cell infiltration of tumors. The degree of NK cell infiltration was defined as little (<50 NK cells/50 microscopic fields of tumor sections), moderate (50–150 NK cells/50 microscopic fields) and abundant (>150 NK cells/50 microscopic fields). Multivariate analysis using the Cox regression model identified two significant prognostic parameters: number of involved lymph nodes and NK cell infiltration. A combined analyses of these parameters determined two groups of patients in each stage of the disease: those with high levels of NK cell infiltration and better prognosis, and those with low/moderate levels of NK cell infiltration and worse prognosis (Coca

et al., 1997). In patients with gastric carcinoma, higher levels of TINK (>25 NK cells/25 microscopic fields) correlated with a less advanced and less invasive gastric carcinoma and lower lymphatic invasion and fewer metastases in the lymph nodes. More importantly, the patients with high levels of TINK had a significantly better prognosis than the patients with low levels of TINK. Similar correlations were established with tumor-infiltrating S-100 protein-expressing cells (presumably DC). In addition, combinational analysis of the numbers of TINK, lymphocytes and DC in tumors and lymph node metastases showed that these parameters had independent prognostic values (Ishigami et al., 2000a,b).

NK CELLS IN TUMOR-DRAINING LYMPH NODES

NK cells resident in tumor-draining (regional) lymph nodes may mediate in the microenvironment elimination of micrometastases and control development of metastatic foci by direct killing of tumor cells. They may also participate in preferential induction and regulation of tumor-specific Th1 type adaptive immune responses and induction of antitumor CTLs via secretion of IFN-γ and TNF. Therefore, NK cells in tumor-draining lymph nodes might significantly contribute to host antitumor resistance and might have an important prognostic value. Indeed, several published studies support this possibility. Lymph node NK cells have been assessed both quantitatively, following their immunohistochemical staining with anti-CD57 mAb, and functionally, using 4 h ^{51}Cr release cytotoxicity assays against K562 cell targets. It was determined that patients with various cancers, who exhibited in regional lymph nodes hyperplasias of B cell follicles with high contents of NK cells and T cells, had a favorable prognosis (Tsyplakov and Petrov, 1997). Similarly, node-negative gastric carcinoma patients with decreased numbers of NK cells in regional lymph nodes more frequently exhibited cancer recurrence than patients with normal numbers of NK cells in the microenvironment (Ishigami et al., 2000c). In addition, in SCCHN patients, regional lymph nodes with micrometastases exhibited significantly diminished NK activity, in comparison to uninvolved or control nodes (Mickel et al., 1988).

CONCLUSIONS AND PERSPECTIVES

The studies reviewed here on the number and function of NK cells in peripheral blood, tumor tissues and tumor-draining lymph nodes of cancer patients provide evidence that NK cells sensitively recognize and characteristically respond to cancer and that these responses may serve as reliable markers of host resistance/susceptibility to cancer and cancer prognosis. The available data also indicate that NK cells infiltrating tumor tissues and lymph nodes might be more reliable predictors of cancer outcome than blood NK cells. Therefore, future studies should be more focused on tumor- and lymph node-infiltrating NK cells. Previous studies have examined morphometrically NK cells in these tissues by employing anti-CD57 antibody as a single marker and have neither discriminated NK cells and NKT cells, two phenotypically and functionally distinct anti-tumor immune effector cell subpopulations expressing CD57, nor investigated their distinct functions. Combined morphometric and functional differential investigations of NK and NKT cells in tumor tissues and tumor-draining lymph nodes are likely to increase the precision and reliability of NK cell-based cancer staging and prognostic studies. Therefore, future efforts should be directed to differential numerical analyses of NK cells and NKT cells using two-color immunohistochemistry with anti-CD57 (or anti-CD56) and anti-CD3 antibodies. In parallel, novel functional parameters of NK cells should be evaluated, including NK cell receptors (KIRs and KARs) and their ligands (MHC class I molecules, MICA and MICB), cytolytic mediators (TNF family ligands, perforin, granzymes and granulysin), cytokine receptors (IL-18R, IL-12R, IL-2R, IL15R, IFN-αR and IFN-γR), receptor signaling pathways, apoptotic tumoricidal activity and spontaneous and induced secretion of Th1 or Th2 cytokines. In addition, to obtain more clinically valuable data, more sensitive, more automated and higher throughput new technologies, including novel flow cytometry and cytotoxicity assays, confocal microscopy quantitative imaging analyses, real-time RT-PCR, LUMINEX, Cellomics, Genomics and Proteomics, should be applied. Thus improved future studies of NK cells in cancer patients will provide novel important information and will critically increase our understanding of the complex interactions between NK cells and cancer in humans and will define highly sensitive, precise and reliable clinically relevant assays for effective cancer staging and cancer prognostic.

ACKNOWLEDGEMENTS

This work was supported by National Institute of Health Grant 1-P60 DE13059 and National Institute of Health Grant RO1 DE14775.

REFERENCES

Andersen, B.L., Farrar, W.B., Golden-Kreutz, D. et al. (1998). Stress and immune responses after surgical treatment for regional breast cancer. J Natl Cancer Inst 90, 30–36.

Akiyoshi, T., Koba, F., Arinaga, S. and Ueo, H. (1990). Preoperative cell-mediated immune function and the prognosis of patients with gastric carcinoma. J Surg Oncol 45, 137–142.

Aparicio-Pages, M.N., Verspaget, H.W., Pena, A.S. and Lamers, C.B. (1991). Natural killer cell activity in patients with adenocarcinoma in the upper gastrointestinal tract. J Clin Lab Immuno 35, 27–32.

Biron, C.A., Nguyen, K.B., Pien, C.G., Cousens, L.P. and Salazar-Mather, T.P. (1999). Natural killer cells in antiviral defense: function and regulation by innate cytokines. Annu Rev Immunol 17, 189–220.

Coca, S., Perez-Piquera, J., Martinez, D. et al. (1997). The prognostic significance of intratumoral natural killer cells in patients with colorectal carcinoma. Cancer 79, 2320–2328.

Cohen, M., Kline, E., Kuten, A., Fried, G., Zinder, O. and Pollack, S. (2002). Increased emotional distress in daughters of breast cancer patients is associated with decreased natural cytotoxic activity, elevated levels of stress hormones and decreased secretion of Th1 cytokines. Internat J Cancer 100, 347–354.

Cooper, M.A., Fehniger, T.A. and Caligiuri, M.A. (2001). The biology of human natural killer-cell subsets. Trends Immunol 2, 633–640.

Ferlazzo, G., Tsang, M.L., Moretta, L., Melioli, G., Steinman, R.M. and Munz, C. (2002). Human dendritic cells activate resting natural killer (NK) cells and are recognized via the NKp30 receptor by activated NK cells. J Exp Med 195, 343–351.

Fernandez, N.C., Lozier, A., Flament, C. et al. (1999). Dendritic cells directly trigger NK cell functions: Cross-talk relevant in innate anti-tumor immune responses in vivo. Nat Med 5, 405–411.

Frydecka, I. (1985). Natural killer cell activity during the course of disease in patients with Hodgkin's disease. Cancer 56, 2799–2803.

Garzetti, G.G., Cignitti, M., Ciavattini, A., Fabris, N. and Romanini, C. (1993). Natural killer cell activity and progression-free survival in ovarian cancer. Gynecol Obstet Invest 35, 118–120.

Gerosa, F., Baldani-Guerra, B., Nisii, C., Marchesini, V., Carra, G. and Trinchieri, G. (2002). Reciprocal activating interaction between natural killer cells and dendritic cells. J Exp Med 195, 327–333.

Gleimer, M. and Parham, P. (2003). Stress management: MHC class I and class I-like molecules as reporters of cellular stress. Immunity 19, 469–477.

Gonzalez, F.M., Vargas, J.A., Lopez-Cortijo, C. et al. (1998). Prognostic significance of natural killer cell activity in patients with laryngeal carcinoma. Arch Otolaryngol Head Neck Surg 124, 852–856.

Groh, V., Wu, J., Yee, C. and Spies, T. (2002). Tumor-derived soluble MIC ligands impair expression of NKG2D and T cell activation. Nature 419, 734–738.

Harabuchi, Y., Yamanaka, N. and Kataura, A. (1985). Identification of lymphocyte subsets and natural killer cells in head and neck cancers. An immunohistological study using monoclonal antibodies. Arch Oto-Rhino-Laryngol 242, 89–97.

Healy, C.G., Simons, J.W., Carducci, M.A. et al. (1998). Impaired expression and function of signal-transducing zeta chain in peripheral T cells and natural killer cells in patients with prostate cancer. Cytometry 32, 109–119.

Ishigami, S., Natsugoe, S., Tokuda, K. et al. (2000a). Prognostic value of intratumoral natural killer cells in gastric carcinoma. Cancer 88, 577–583.

Ishigami, S., Natsugoe, S., Tokuda, K. et al. (2000b). Clinical impact of intratumoral natural killer cell and dendritic cell infiltration in gastric cancer. Cancer Lett 159, 103–108.

Ishigami, S., Natsugoe, S., Hokita, S. et al. (2000c). Intranodal antitumor immunocyte infiltration in node-negative gastric cancers. Clin Cancer Res 6, 2611–2617.

Kashii, Y., Giorda, R., Herberman, R.B., Whiteside, T.L. and Vujanovic, N.L. (1999). Constitutive expression and role of the tumor necrosis factor family ligands in apoptotic killing by human natural killer cells. J Immunol *163*, 5358–5366.

Kishi, A., Takamori, Y., Ogawa, K. et al. (2002). Differential expression of granulysin and perforin by NK cells in cancer patients and correlation of impaired granulysin expression with progression of cancer. Cancer Immunol Immunother *50*, 604–614.

Kobashi, K., Iwagaki, H., Yoshino, T. et al. (2001). Down-regulation of IL-18 receptor in cancer patients: its clinical significance. Anticancer Res *21*, 3285–3293.

Kos, F.J. and Engleman, E.G. (1995). Requirement for natural killer cells in the induction of cytotoxic T cells. J Immunol *155*, 578–584.

Kos, F.J. and Engleman, E.G. (1996). Role of natural killer cells in the generation of influenza virus-specific cytotoxic T cells. Cell Immunol *173*, 1–6.

Kuss, I., Saito, T., Johnson, J.T. and Whiteside, T.L. (1999). Clinical significance of decreased zeta chain expression in peripheral blood lymphocytes of patients with head and neck cancer. Clin Cancer Res *5*, 329–334.

Lanier, L.L. (1998). NK cell receptors. Annu Rev Immunol *16*, 359–393.

Lanier, L.L. and Phillips, J.H. (1992). Natural killer cells. Curr Opin Immunol *4*, 38–42.

Lee, S.-J., Cho, Y.-S., Cho, M.-C. et al. (2001). Both E6 and E7 oncoproteins of human papillomavirus 16 inhibit IL-18-induced IFN-γ production in human peripheral blood mononuclear and NK cells. J Immunol *167*, 497–504.

Li, S., Makarenkova, V.P., Tjandrawan, T. et al. (2003). A novel N-CAM epitope defines precursors of human adherent NK cells. J Leuk Biol in press.

Lu, G., Janjic, B.M., Janjic, J., Whiteside, T.L., Storkus, W.J. and Vujanovic, N.L. (2002). Innate direct anticancer effector function of human immature dendritic cells. II. Role of TNF, LT-α1β2, Fas ligand and TRAIL. J Immunol *168*, 1831–1839.

Marana, H.R.C., de Silva, J.S. and de Andrade, J.M. (2000). NK cell activity in the presence of IL-12 is a prognostic assay to neoadjuvant chemotherapy of cervical cancer. Gynecol Oncol *78*, 318–323.

Mickel, R.A., Kessler, D.J., Taylor, J.M. and Lichtenstein, A. (1988). Natural killer cell cytotoxicity in the peripheral blood, cervical lymph nodes, and tumor of head and neck cancer patients. Cancer Res *48*, 5017–5022.

Moretta, A., Biassoni, R., Bottino, C., Mingari, M.C. and Moretta, L. (2000). Natural cytotoxicity receptors that trigger human NK-cell-mediated cytolysis. Immunol Today *21*, 228–234.

Moretta, A. (2002). Natural killer cells and dendritic cells: rendezvous in abused tissues. Nat Rev Immunol *2*, 957–964.

Nakamura, H., Kawasaki, N., Hagiwara, M., Saito, M., Konaka, C. and Kato, H. (2000). Cellular immunologic parameters related to age, gender, and stage in lung cancer patients. Lung Cancer *28*, 139–145.

Naruke, T., Goya, T., Tsuchiya, R. and Suematsu, K. (1998). Prognosis and survival in resected lung carcinoma based on the new internal staging system. J Thorac Cardiovasc Surg *96*, 440–447.

Nio, Y., Shiraishi, T., Imai, S. et al. (1991) The clinical status and histopathological factors affecting natural killer cells of peripheral blood lymphocytes in patients with gastric cancer. J Clin Lab Immunol *35*, 97–108.

Ogata, H., Miyoshi, T., Itami, J. et al. (1989). A clinical study of a multiregression analysis on the NK activity and related clinical

factors in patients with lung cancer. Jap J Cancer Clin *35*, 554–559.

Ogawa, Y., Maeda, T., Inomata, T. et al. (1988). Immuno-histochemical study of cancer tissues. 1. Special reference to Leu-11b positive lymphocytes (NK cells). J Jap Soc Cancer *23*, 1236–1242.

Okamoto, Y., Sano, T., Okamura, S., Ueki, M. and Sugimoto, O. (1987). An immunohistochemical study with monoclonal antibodies on lymphocytes infiltrating in cervical cancer. Acta Obstet Gynecol Jap *39*, 925–932.

Oliva, A., Kinter, A.L., Vaccareza, M. et al. (1998). Natural killer cells from human immunodeficiency virus (HIV)-infected individuals are an important source of CC-chemokines and suppress HIV-I entry and replication in vitro. J Clin Invest *102*, 223–231.

Peritt, D., Robertson, S., Gri, G., Showe, L., Aste-Amezaga, M. and Trinchieri, G. (1998). Differentiation of human NK cells into NK1 and NK2 subsets. J Immunol *161*, 5821–5824.

Peron, J.-M., Esch, C., Subbotin, V.M., Maliszewski, C., Lotze, M.T. and Shurin, M.R. (1998). Flt3-ligand administration inhibits liver metastases: Role of NK cells. J Immunol *161*, 6164–6170.

Piccioli, D., Sbrana, S., Melandri, E. and Valiante, N.M. (2002). Contact-dependent stimulation and inhibition of dendritic cells by natural killer cells. J Exp Med *195*, 335–341.

Pross, H.F., Baines, M.G., Rubin, P., Shagge, P. and Patterson, M.S. (1981). Spontaneous human lymphocyte mediated cytotoxicity against tumor target cells. IX. The quantitation of natural killer cell activity. J Clin Immunol *1*, 51–63.

Pross, H.F. and Lotzova, E. (1993). Role of natural killer cells in cancer. Nat Immun *12*, 279–292.

Robertson, M.J. and Ritz, J. (1990). Biology and clinical relevance of human NK cells. Blood *76*, 2421–1990.

Ruggeri, L., Capanni, M., Urbani, E. et al. (2002). Effectiveness of donor natural killer cell alloreactivity in mismatched hematopoietic transplants. Science *295*, 2097–2100.

Schantz, S.P. and Ordonez, N.G. (1991). Quantitation of natural killer cell function and risk of metastatic poorly differentiated head and neck cancer. Nat Immun Cell Growth Reg *10*, 278–288.

Schantz, S.P., Shillitoe, E.J., Brown, B. and Campbell, B. (1986). Natural killer cell activity and head and neck cancer: a clinical assessment. J Natl Cancer Inst *77*, 869–875.

Sephton, S.E., Sapolsky, R.M., Kraemer, H.C. and Spiegel, D. (2000). Diurnal cortisol rhythm as a predictor of breast cancer survival. J Natl Cancer Inst *92*, 994–1000.

Shaw, S.G., Maung, A.A., Steptoe, R.J., Thomson, A.W. and Vujanovic, N.L. (1998). Expansion of functional natural killer cells in multiple tissue compartments of mice treated with Flt3-ligand: Implication for anti-cancer and anti-viral therapy. J Immunol *161*, 2817–2824.

Soygur, T., Beduk, Y., Baltaci, S., Yaman, O. and Tokgoz, G. (1999). The prognostic value of peripheral blood lymphocyte subsets in patients with bladder carcinoma treated using neoadjuvant M-VEC chemotherapy. BJU Internatl *84*, 1069–1072.

Sulica, A., Morel, P., Mates, D. and Herberman, R.B. (2001). Ig-binding receptors on human NK cells as effector and regulatory surface molecules. Internatl Rev Immunol *20*, 371–414.

Tahir, S.M., Cheng, O., Shaulov, A. et al. (2001). Loss of IFN-gamma production by invariant NK T cells in advanced cancer. J Immunol *167*, 4046–4050.

Takanami, I., Takeuchi, K. and Giga, M. (2001). The prognostic value of natural killer cell infiltration in resected pulmonary adenocarcinoma. J Thorac Cardiovasc Surg 121, 1058–1063.

Takeuchi, H., Machara, Y., Tokunaga, E., Koga, T., Kakeji, Y. and Sugimachi, K. (2001). Prognostic significance of natural killer cell activity in patients with gastric carcinoma: a multivariate analysis. Am J Gastroenterol 96, 574–578.

Tarle, M., Kovacic, K. and Kastelan, M. (1993). Correlation of cell proliferation marker (TPS), natural killer (NK) activity and tumor load serotest (PSA) in untreated and treated prostatic tumors. Anticancer Res 13, 215–218.

Tartter, P.I., Martinelli, G., Steinberg, B. and Barron, D. (1986). Changes in peripheral T cell subsets and natural-killer cytotoxicity in relation to colorectal cancer. Cancer Detect Prevent 9, 359–364.

Tartter, P.I., Steinberg, B., Barron, D.M. and Martinelli, G. (1987). The prognostic significance of natural killer cytotoxicity in patients with colorectal cancer. Arch Surg 122, 1264–1268.

Trinchieri, G. (1989). Biology of natural killer cells. Adv Immunol 47, 187–376.

Tsyplakov, D.E. and Petrov, S.V. (1997). Hyperplastic follicular response of the regional lymph nodes in cancer: immunohistochemistry, ultrastructure, prognostic importance. Ark Patol 59, 55–60.

Villegas, F.R., Coca. S., Villarubia, V.G. et al. (2002). Prognostic significance of tumor infiltrating natural killer cells subset CD57 in patients with squamous cell lung cancer. Lung Cancer 35, 23–28.

Vitolo, D., Vujanovic, N.L., Rabinowich, H., Schlesinger, M., Herberman, R.B. and Whiteside, T.L. (1993). Rapid interleukin 2-induced adherence of human natural killer (NK) cells. Expression of mRNA for cytokines and IL-2 receptors in adherent NK cells. J Immunol 151, 1926–1937.

Vivier, E. and Biron, C.A. (2002). A pathogen receptor on natural killer cells. Science 296, 1248–1249.

Vujanovic, N.L., Basse, P., Herberman, R.B. and Whiteside, T.L. (1996a). Antitumor functions of natural killer cells and control of metastases. METHODES 9, 394–408.

Vujanovic, N.L., Nagashima S., Herberman, R.B. and Whiteside, T.L. (1996b). Non-secretory apoptotic killing by human natural killer cells. J Immunol 157, 1117–1126.

Vujanovic, N.L. (2001). Role of TNF family ligands in antitumor activity of natural killer cells. Intern Rev Immunol 20, 407–429.

Wahlberg B.J., Burholt, D.R., Kornblith, P. et al. (2001). Measurement of NK activity by the microcytotoxicity assay (MCA): A new application for an old assay. J Immunol Methods 253, 69–81.

Whiteside, T.L., Bryant, J., Day, R. and Herberman, R.B. (1990). Natural killer cytotoxicity in diagnosis of immune dysfunction: criteria for a reproducible assay. J Clin Lab Anal 4, 102–214.

Whiteside, T.L. and Rabinowich, H. (1998). The role of Fas/FasL in immunosuppression induced by human tumors. Cancer Immunol Immunother 46, 175–184.

Yokoyama, W.M. and Plougastel, B.F.M. (2003). Immune functions encoded by the natural killer gene complex. Nat Rev 3, 304–316.

Zhou, J.H. and Jiang, Y.G. (1994). Pre- and postoperative NK cell number and plasma levels of TNF and PGE2 in patients with esophageal carcinoma and their clinical significance. Chinese J Oncol 16, 132–136.

Section V

Provocative assays *in vivo*

Delayed Type Hypersensitivity Responses

William J. Burlingham[1], Ewa Jankowska-Gan[1], Anne M. VanBuskirk[2], Ronald P. Pelletier[3] and Charles G. Orosz[3]

[1]*Department of Surgery, University of Wisconsin, Madison, WI;* [2]*Department of Surgical Oncology,* [3]*Department of Surgery/Transplant, The Ohio State University College of Medicine, Columbus, OH, USA*

> If we value the pursuit of knowledge, we must be free to follow wherever the search may lead us.
>
> Adlai Stevenson Jr 1900–1965

INTRODUCTION

Many tests have been designed to monitor T cell behavior and function in humans and experimental animals. Most of these are performed *in vitro*. Since *in vitro* tests remove T cells from the constraints imposed by living tissues, interpretation of these tests should be made with some degree of caution. However, there are tests of T cell behavior that can be performed *in vivo*, one of which is type IV, or delayed type hypersensitivity (DTH) reactions. Although this test was first performed by Koch to monitor immune responses to an infectious agent, most individuals are familiar with DTH reactivity as the clinical test for reactivity to allergens including pollens or dander. Allergic individuals will generate localized redness and swelling within 24–48 h of the subcutaneous deposition of a previously experienced allergen. In such responses, macrophages are recruited by tissue damage products (presumably hyaluronan, HMGB1, uric acid, ATP or HSP70) to the injection site, where they acquire, process and present allergen components to similarly recruited memory T cells. Upon antigen recognition, the memory T cells produce gamma interferon, which promotes a cytokine cascade that activates local vascular endothelial cells. This promotes the rapid recruitment of neutrophils and subsequently additional macrophages and T cells. This leukocyte infiltrating process disturbs local tissue architecture. It also induces vasodilatation (redness) and edema (swelling) that is characteristic of cutaneous DTH responses. It is the area of redness and sometimes the degree of swelling that can be measured to provide an index of DTH reactivity.

As a rule, DTH responses require prior immunologic sensitization to a specific antigen and thus are categorized as recall, or memory T cell responses. As such, they cannot be used to measure the potential to respond to an antigen that has not yet been encountered by a given individual. Rather, they can identify specific antigens to which the individual has already made an immune response and they provide an index of the current T cell reactivity to specific recall antigens. Clinically, the DTH response has been utilized to identify pathogens with which the patient has been previously infected, e.g. *Mycobacterium tuberculosis*. Specifically a purified protein derivative (PPD), usually used at intermediate strength, is applied to assess evidence of prior exposure to the organism. Typically used for an assessment of global immune responses, frequent tests include tetanus toxoid, Diphtheria toxoid, group C *Streptococcus*, tuberculin from *M. tuberculosis* and *M. bovis*, *Candida*, *Trichophyton* and *Proteus* and a glycerin control (Pasteur Merieux Connaught, Swiftwater, PA). DTH reactivity is typically suppressed in the setting of several tumors, including Hodgkin's disease and other hematologic malignancies, malnutrition, during high dose IL-2 administration (Wiebke et al., 1988) and chronic stress/viral infections.

Measuring Immunity, edited by Michael T. Lotze and Angus W. Thomson
ISBN 0-12-455900-X, London

By extension, the DTH assay can be used to provide an index of T cell-mediated immunity to a wide variety of antigens derived from environmental elements (pollens, etc.), infectious agents, tumors or allografts. In addition, DTH responses can be used to confirm successful vaccination, or to determine the degree of residual immunocompetence after injury or immunosuppressive therapy. In the setting of childhood immunodeficiencies or HIV associated acquired immunodeficiency (AIDS), it can be used serially to assess immune reactivity (see Chapter 55). As described in detail below, illustrating many of the principles of the assay, DTH responses can also be used to determine the nature of the T cell responses made by an individual to a particular antigen, for example, to graft alloantigens.

TRANSVIVO DTH

By the late 1990s, it had become clear that mice which would normally reject cardiac allografts within 7–10 days could be made to accept the allografts after transient treatment with any of several therapeutic agents, including antibodies that bound to the T cell receptor (Pearson et al., 1992), antibodies and agents that bound to co-stimulator molecules (Baliga et al., 1994; Hancock et al., 1996) and antibodies that bound to endothelial cells (Orosz et al., 1993). This raised questions about the immunobiology associated with the development of the acceptor versus rejector phenotype in transplant recipients. One difference that became apparent was that allograft rejector mice display donor-reactive delayed type hypersensitivity (DTH) responses, whereas allograft acceptor mice do not (VanBuskirk et al., 1998). Mice can be tested for DTH reactivity in two ways:

1 the direct DTH assay wherein sensitized mice are injected subcutaneously in the pinnae or footpads with challenge antigen, or
2 the transfer DTH assay wherein splenocytes from sensitized mice are injected subcutaneously into the pinnae or footpads of naive mice along with challenge antigen.

In either case, subsequent swelling that can be measured with a micrometer within 24 h indicates an immune response to the challenge antigen. DTH responses are informative because they are recall responses, i.e. T cell responses that develop only after a prior sensitizing event. Thus, DTH responses in allograft recipients demonstrate that recipient T cells have previously recognized and responded immunologically to graft alloantigens.

However, it soon became apparent that allograft acceptance is a more complicated issue. Investigators reported that allograft acceptance could be transferred from mouse to mouse with splenic T cells (Graca et al., 2000), suggesting that immune regulation rather than non-sensitization, anergy or clonal deletion, was responsible for allograft acceptance. Furthermore, allograft acceptor mice that had

been sensitized to a third party antigen, like tetanus toxoid, prior to transplantation, lost the ability to mount tetanus-reactive DTH responses when the tetanus antigen was mixed with donor alloantigens at the time of DTH challenge. Thus, DTH responses in allograft acceptor mice demonstrate the property of linked suppression described by Waldmann (Wise et al., 1998). It was then demonstrated that allograft acceptor mice recovered the ability to mount donor-reactive DTH responses when antibodies that neutralized TGFβ or IL10 were provided at the DTH challenge site (Bickerstaff et al., 2000). This explained the phenomenon of linked suppression. Apparently, T cells of allograft acceptor mice, in contrast to allograft rejector mice, respond to donor alloantigen challenge by producing little of the pro-inflammatory cytokine interferon gamma (IFN). Instead, they produce the immunosuppressive cytokines transforming growth factor beta (TGFβ) and interleukin-10 (IL10) (Xia et al., 2001). Once produced, TGFβ and IL10 block local DTH responses indiscriminately, so the induction of TGFβ/IL10 by donor alloantigens at the DTH site blocks both the alloreactive DTH response and the DTH response to the co-localized tetanus antigens.

The clinical implications of these studies are readily apparent. DTH assays could be used to determine if transplant patients had developed the pro-inflammatory or anti-inflammatory form of T cell allosensitization to donor alloantigens. At the time, no other clinical tests could do this. Historically, the clinical test for cellular alloimmunity was the mixed lymphocyte response (MLR). While the MLR readily detects alloreactive T cells, it indiscriminately measures the responses of donor-reactive T cells that have responded to alloantigens along with those that have not. Thus, the MLR provides an index of total alloreactivity, rather than an index of prior allosensitization. However, clinical assays of donor-reactive DTH activity in transplant patients are complicated by the risk of allosensitization and rejection presented by subcutaneous deposition of donor alloantigens.

To circumvent this, the *transvivo DTH assay* was developed. This test is essentially a transfer DTH assay, in which human peripheral blood mononuclear cells are placed subcutaneously into the pinnae or footpads of naive mice along with challenge alloantigen (Carrodeguas et al., 1999). Measurable DTH-like swelling occurs within 24 h if MHC-matched human T cells and human APC are both available at the DTH site and the human PBMC donor had been pre-sensitized to the challenge antigen. The transvivo DTH responses are induced only by the human PBMC, since the murine lymphocytes are not pre-sensitized to either the DTH challenge antigens or to human leukocyte antigens and the human DTH responses are driven only by the challenge antigens, provided that the human PBMCs are not pre-sensitized to any murine antigens. A positive donor-reactive DTH response in the transvivo DTH assay reflects the fact that the transplant patient has developed a pro-inflammatory immune disposition toward graft alloantigens.

The principle of linked suppression can be employed in the transvivo DTH assay to detect the development of anti-inflammatory allosensitization mediated by donor-reactive immune regulation. According to this principle, DTH responses to third party antigens are lost when the antigen is co-localized with donor alloantigens that induce regulatory T cell responses. Most adult patients are environmentally pre-sensitized to Epstein-Barr virus (EBV) and respond strongly to EBV antigen in the transvivo DTH assay. PBMC from transplant patients can be challenged with EBV antigen, with donor alloantigen and with a combination of both. This protocol provides a highly informative analytic system. First, the DTH response to EBV provides an internal positive control for recall responses by PBMC from immunosuppressed patients. Second, three definitive patterns of DTH responses are possible:

1 DTH-positive for donor antigen, DTH-positive for EBV, DTH-positive for the antigen mixture, reflecting a pro-inflammatory allosensitization to donor alloantigens
2 DTH-negative for donor alloantigen, DTH-positive for EBV antigen and DTH-positive for the antigen mixture, reflecting a lack of prior sensitization to donor alloantigens
3 DTH-negative for donor alloantigen, DTH-positive for EBV antigen and DTH-negative for the antigen mixture, reflecting an anti-inflammatory allosensitization to donor alloantigens.

This analytic system has been successfully tested in the clinical setting (VanBuskirk et al., 2000).

Technical design and execution of the transvivo DTH assay

The transvivo DTH assay was originally designed to measure a transplant patient's immune responses to graft antigens under physiologic conditions, but without putting the patient at increased risk for sensitization to their transplanted organ. It is also useful for detecting immune responses to any recall antigen, such as tetanus toxoid (TT) or Epstein Barr virus (EBV) antigens. In general, the transvivo DTH assay detects memory responses to antigens presented via the indirect pathway of antigen presentation. Specifically, it detects the inflammatory response that is engendered by specific human memory T cells interacting with human antigen presenting cells (APC) in the presence of a recall antigen. This antigen is presented to the T cells by the APC and subsequent activation of both the T cell and APC causes edema and leukocytic infiltration into the injection site. It is this edema and infiltration that is measured in the transvivo DTH assay.

The minimal requirements for successful implementation of the transvivo DTH assay are human peripheral blood mononuclear cells (PBMC), a recall antigen or alloantigen and a severe combined immunodeficient

(SCID) mouse. SCID mice are the mouse type of choice, rather than immunocompetent mice, to avoid any xeno-reactivity to mouse IgG and to prevent any complicating factors of mouse lymphocytes responding to the human PBMC. However, immunocompetent mice have been used successfully to detect graft-reactive and recall antigen reactive immune responses when no xeno-reactivity is present. PBMC with or without antigen are injected into the pre-measured hind footpads or pinnae of a mouse and swelling is measured after 18 h. This time is sufficient to induce swelling that is dependent upon human recall responses, but not sufficient to detect primary human anti-mouse responses. SCID mice are used rather than immunocompetent mice to avoid any reactivity to mouse IgG that may be present in the patient's serum. To measure net antigen-induced swelling, the 18 h swelling elicited by the injection of PBMC alone is subtracted from the swelling elicited by the injection of PBMC plus antigen. Either pinnae or footpads can be used as the injection site, although each has its own advantages and disadvantages. The advantage to using the ear pinnae is that the measurement is very quick and simple. However, the volume of cells + antigen that can be injected is limited, the injection is technically more difficult and the risk of hematoma is present if the injection breaks one of the many blood vessels in the pinnae. In addition, the pinnae have an impressive network of dendritic cells, which could influence the swelling responses. The advantage of the footpad is that they are easily injected with larger volumes of cells. However, the disadvantage is that measurement of the footpad takes a considerably longer period of time compared to ear measurement.

The following is the technical protocol for the transvivo DTH assay:

Reagents

Phosphate-buffered saline, pH 7.4 (PBS)
Sterile, anticoagulated blood
Ficoll-Hypaque solution to remove red blood cells
Recall antigen

EBV lysate (8 µg/injection, Viral Antigens, Inc.)
TT (25LF/injection, Wyeth)

Alloantigen (10 µg/ injection)
Protease inhibitor (PMSF) at 1 M

Materials/supplies

50 ml sterile centrifuge tubes
10 ml, 5 ml, 1 ml pipets and pipettor
1.5 ml eppendorf-type centrifuge tubes
100 µl, 10 µl pipetman with sterile tips
hemocytometer and trypan blue
full size centrifuge and microfuge
2 ml insulin syringes (27-ga needle)
Vibracell sonicator (2 mm probe)

Spring-loaded, dial face calipers (Swiss Precision
   Instruments)
SCID mice
Inhalant anesthesia (isoflurane)

Preparation of alloantigen

Isolate donor PBMC from blood and wash three times in
PBS. Resuspend PBMC to 1.2×10^8 cells/ml (4 million
cells per 30 μl). Add 1 μM PMSF to the mixture. Sonicate
using five-to-six 1-second pulses with a probe sonicator.
Be careful to keep the material cold and avoid excessive
bubbles. Check for disruption of >90 per cent of the cells
using a hemocytometer. When the cells are disrupted,
centrifuge the mixture at 14000 rpm at 4°C for 20 min.
Carefully siphon off the supernatant and determine protein
concentration. Use 8 μg/injection.

Preparation of leukocytes and injection mixture

Separate PBMC from red blood cells using ficoll hypaque
(Histopaque) solution according to standard methods.
Wash the PBMC three times with PBS to remove hypaque
and contaminating platelets. It is important to remove the
platelets, otherwise there will be increased background
swelling. Resuspend the PBMC in PBS at a concentration
of 8 million PBMC/ml. Separate PBMC into two aliquots;
one for PBMC alone and one for PBMC + antigen. Place
the cells into microfuge tubes and pulse spin to pellet the
PBMC. Suction off the supernatant. To each tube, add
5 μl of PBS. To the PBMC + antigen tube 10 μg of EBV
lysate. Add the same volume of PBS to the PBL alone.
Then add sufficient PBS to bring both tubes to 25 μl.
Gently resuspend the cells using a pipetman and tip and
inject.

Injection of footpads

Anesthetize mouse with isoflurane. Measure rear footpad
thickness with dial gauge calipers. Carefully inject one
footpad with PBMC alone and the other footpad with
PBMC + antigen. Make sure there is no leakage.

Injection of pinnae

Anesthetize mouse with isoflurane. Measure ear pinnae
with dial gauge calipers, avoiding cartilage. Carefully inject
one ear pinna with PBMC, the other with PBMC + antigen,
avoiding rupturing any blood vessels. Make sure there is
no leakage.

Measurement

Eighteen hours after injection, anesthetize mouse with
isoflurane and measure footpad (or ear) swelling. Subtract
the pre-injection measurement from the post-injection

measurement to obtain the increase in swelling. The net
increase can then be determined by subtracting the
swelling obtained from PBL alone from the swelling
obtained from PBL + antigen. After subtracting the
swelling of PBMC alone, net swelling $<10 \times 10^{-4}$ inches
is considered negative, $10–20 \times 10^{-4}$ inches is a weakly
positive result, $25–35 \times 10^{-4}$ inches is a moderately positive result and an increase of over 40×10^{-4} inches is
considered a strongly positive result.

USE OF THE TRANSVIVO DTH ASSAY FOR DETECTION OF DONOR ANTIGEN-DRIVEN IMMUNE REGULATION

The transvivo DTH assay can be adapted to detect antigen-
driven downregulation of DTH responses, also called linked
recognition. This adaptation takes advantage of the fact
that a downregulated response to donor antigens is an
active process that can inhibit a parallel response to an
unrelated antigen if both antigens are present at the same
site. In human DTH responses, donor antigen-driven down-
regulation can be mediated by TGFβ, IL-10 or both
cytokines (VanBuskirk et al., 2000). In this adaptation of the
transvivo DTH assay, the swelling responses elicited by
PBMC + recall antigen are compared to the responses
elicited by PBMC alone, by PBMC + donor antigen and by
PBMC + recall antigen + donor antigen. If linked recognition is present, a weak or negative response will be elicited
by PBMC + donor antigen and a strong response elicited
by PBMC + recall antigen. However, the response to recall
antigen will be significantly dampened when donor antigen
is also present in the injection mixture. The responses to the
different injection mixtures and their interpretations are
shown in Table 35.1.

Confounding elements of the assay

During the course of developing the transvivo DTH assay, it
became clear that several conditions can affect this assay,
including the length of time between blood collection
and assay, platelet contamination of the PBMC, RBC
contamination of the PBMC and donor sensitization to
mice or mouse IgG.

Table 35.1 Transvivo DTH assay adapted to detect donor
antigen-driven regulation

Immune status	PBMC alone	PBMC + Recall antigen	PBMC + Donor antigens	PBMC + Recall antigen + Donor antigens
Naive	−	+	−	+
Sensitized	−	+	+	+
Regulated	−	+	−	−

Length of time between blood collection and assay performance

The most consistent results are routinely obtained when PBMC are isolated from freshly drawn blood. However, that is not always feasible. We have observed that when the time between blood collection and assay performance increases, the functionality of the cells decreases. For example, when freshly drawn blood is compared with 24-h blood or 48-h blood, the PBMC from freshly drawn blood are quite active in the transvivo DTH assay. However, PBMC from blood drawn greater than 24 h before is not functional in this assay. As an alternative, PBMC can be isolated from freshly drawn blood and cryopreserved in 90 per cent FBS/10 per cent DMSO, without loss of function in the transvivo DTH assay. However, substantial loss of viable cells due to freeze/thawing can be problematic.

Platelet contamination of PBMC

Variable numbers of platelets are present in PBMC preparations from different donors. This is dependent upon the donors, but also on how the PBMC were isolated. Contamination of the PBMC with 2×10^7 platelets per injection resulted in high background swelling (Carrodeguas et al., 1999). To avoid this problem, the PBMC can be washed with PBS until the platelet count has been reduced to a level of less than 1×10^7 per injection.

RBC contamination of PBMC

Occasionally, RBC can contaminate the PBMC preparations and these RBC can also contribute to high background swelling. Visual inspection of the PBMC will determine if RBC are present. If so, they can be removed by lysis with ammonium chloride buffer. However, if ammonium chloride buffer is used, it is imperative that the resultant PBMC preparation be washed at least three times to remove any residual lysis buffer. If the buffer is not removed completely, the PBMC can become activated, resulting in high background swelling. This is typically a problem with blood that is not freshly drawn, but it can occur with patient blood samples that are freshly drawn, as well.

Donor sensitization to mice or to mouse IgG

Occasionally, PBMC are obtained from individuals who are sensitized to mice or to mouse IgG. If an individual has a history of allergic reactions to mice, their PBMC may promote a strong swelling response when they are injected into mice, even in the absence of co-injected, exogenous antigen. Furthermore, some transplant patients are sensitized to mouse IgG due to prior treatment with murine-derived therapeutic agents, such as OKT3, a mouse IgG directed against human CD3+ cells. These patients may

have developed an immune response to mouse IgG that sometimes, but not always, includes the development of antibodies to mouse IgG. For these patients, interpretable transvivo DTH responses can be elicited if SCID mice are used for the transvivo DTH assay, since SCID mice lack IgG. In general, we recommend the use of SCID mice for detection of regulated DTH responses in transplant patients. However, SCID mice are much more expensive than normal, naive mice and this needs to be considered for high volume testing.

CLINICAL STUDIES WITH THE TRANSVIVO DTH ASSAY (OHIO STATE UNIVERSITY)

The transvivo DTH assay has been in use for the past several years at the Ohio State University (OSU) as one of the clinical assays used to monitor donor-specific immune behavior following kidney or simultaneous kidney/pancreas transplantation. Patients were routinely tested at 6 months and then annually following transplantation. They were also tested during any hospital readmissions. The transvivo DTH assay conditions at OSU involved the injection of 7×10^6 fresh human peripheral blood mononuclear cells (PBMC) into the pinnae of normal C57Bl/6 mice. To date the OSU transplant program has tested 467 patients at least once post-transplant for the presence of donor-reactive DTH reactivity and 445 of these patients were also tested for regulated, donor-reactive DTH reactivity. These two types of DTH reactivities are referred to as the 'pro-inflammatory' and 'anti-inflammatory' DTH phenotypes, respectively. In addition, a subset of 147 patients was also tested for donor-reactive DTH phenotype immediately prior to transplantation. It should be noted that these two DTH phenotypes are not mutually exclusive. In general, it appears that the two phenotypes are mediated by two interacting lymphocyte subpopulations and that the overall immune response represents the proportional contributions of these two subpopulations. When one or the other dominates, their phenotype is uniquely expressed. However, when neither subpopulation dominates, the phenotype reflects the relative contributions of both. Thus, a partially regulated individual can express both a weak pro-inflammatory DTH response and a weak anti-inflammatory DTH response during transvivo DTH testing.

A critical factor for this clinical trial of transvivo DTH is the reproducibility/stability of this assay. The assay requires a substantial number of PBMC (about 35 million), so patient PBMC are often limiting. For this reason, repetitive testing of patient samples has not been feasible. However, eight patients have had separate blood samples obtained less than 2 weeks apart (1–13 days) which were tested in the transvivo DTH assay. In six out of eight patients (75 per cent), the two test results were concordant for pro-inflammatory donor-reactive DTH phenotype. For the remaining two patients, an initial pro-inflammatory phenotype was lost. Ten of these patients were also tested for anti-inflammatory donor-reactive DTH phenotype. In four out of eight patients (50 per cent) the two test results were concordant. In three of the four discordant cases, an initial anti-inflammatory donor phenotype was lost.

Pre-transplant DTH reactivity

Immediately prior to transplantation, pro-inflammatory donor-reactive DTH reactivity was detected in 37 per cent (55/147) of tested transplant recipients. Thus, a surprisingly large number of the patients, more than one-third, were DTH-reactive to donor alloantigens prior to transplantation. This is even more interesting, considering that all of these patients were donor cross-match negative. This is the first suggestion that cellular (DTH) and humoral (IgG) alloimmunity correlate poorly (see below). Seventy-four of these 147 patients were re-tested at some point post-transplant. There was only 46 per cent concordance (34/74) with the pre-transplant DTH phenotype. Most of the discordant patients (70 per cent) were not donor-reactive before transplantation, but developed donor-reactive DTH responses after transplant. However, the remaining 12/40 discordant patients displayed pro-inflammatory, donor-reactive DTH activity prior to transplant, but lost it by the time they were tested post-transplant. This represents 22 per cent of the patients who were DTH-reactive pre-transplant. This is the first indication that DTH phenotype is not stable in transplant patients.

Immediately prior to transplantation, anti-inflammatory donor-reactive DTH reactivity was detected in 20 per cent (24/122) of tested transplant recipients. Thus, in pre-transplant testing for donor-reactivity, the pro-inflammatory DTH phenotype is about twice as common as the anti-inflammatory phenotype. Twelve of the patients with the pre-transplant anti-inflammatory DTH phenotype were retested post-transplant, of whom most (11) had lost the anti-inflammatory DTH phenotype. This, again, indicates that DTH phenotype is not stable in transplant patients. In general, it is not uncommon for transplant recipients to display pro-inflammatory or anti-inflammatory DTH reactivity toward donor alloantigens as they undergo transplantation. Apparently the pre-transplant DTH phenotype is relatively unstable. Further, it does not appear to influence post-transplant outcome. Pre-transplant detection of either donor-reactive DTH phenotype did not correlate statistically with any of the measured post-transplant outcomes, including the incidence of acute rejection, chronic allograft nephropathy, graft loss or patient death. For example, one-year graft survival was 94 per cent in DTH-negative patients, 95 per cent in patients with the pro-inflammatory DTH phenotype and 96 per cent in patients with the anti-inflammatory DTH phenotype. This is the first indication that DTH phenotype may not predict clinical outcome in transplant patients.

Post-transplant DTH reactivity – the pro-inflammatory phenotype

For this analysis, the results of DTH testing performed within the first post-transplant year ($n = 235$ patients) were analyzed separately from the results of testing performed beyond the first year ($n = 291$ patients). A total of 59 patients had testing performed during both of these periods. Additionally, of the 235 patients tested within the first post-transplant year, 78 had additional, serial tests performed within the first year. Of the 291 patients tested beyond the first post-transplant year, 80 had subsequent serial testing.

The first post-transplant year

When tested at some point within the first year post-transplant, 47 per cent (111/235) of tested patients displayed pro-inflammatory DTH responses toward donor alloantigens. Thus, almost half of the transplant patients appear to undergo DTH-detectable cellular allosensitization to donor alloantigens within the first year post-transplant. This is much higher than the number of patients who undergo humoral allosensitization. Only about 19 per cent of this patient population (45/235) produced alloreactive IgG, as detected by Flow PRA analysis. This, again, illustrates the poor correlation between cellular and humoral alloimmunity in transplant patients. Of the 78 patients who were serially tested within the first year post-transplant, 28 per cent ($n = 22$) maintained the pro-inflammatory DTH phenotype, while 18 per cent ($n = 14$) lost it. Further, 22 per cent ($n = 17$) acquired the pro-inflammatory DTH phenotype, while 32 per cent ($n = 25$) never displayed it. Thus, the post-transplant pro-inflammatory DTH phenotype of individual patients is relatively unstable within the first year post-transplant, with 40 per cent of patients changing their phenotype during this period.

Beyond the first post-transplant year

When tested at some point after the first year post-transplant, 49 per cent ($n = 143$) of tested patients displayed pro-inflammatory DTH responses toward donor alloantigens. This is similar to the frequency of reactivity observed during the first year post-transplant, so the overall incidence of the pro-inflammatory DTH phenotype within the transplant population appears to be generally stable. For the 80 patients who were serially tested after the first year, 31 per cent ($n = 25$) maintained the pro-inflammatory DTH phenotype, while 10 per cent ($n = 8$) lost it. Further, 29 per cent ($n = 23$) acquired the pro-inflammatory DTH phenotype, while 30 per cent ($n = 24$) never displayed it. Thus, the pro-inflammatory DTH phenotype of individual patients remains relatively unstable after the first year post-transplant, with 40 per cent of the patients changing their phenotype during this period.

Clinical impact

Since acute rejection is a cell-mediated immune response and pro-inflammatory DTH reactivity reflects cellular allosensitization toward graft alloantigens, it is intuitively obvious that patients who display donor-reactive DTH responses would be at increased risk for pathologic developments at the graft site. Thus, it is somewhat surprising that no statistically significant correlation has been observed between the expression of the pro-inflammatory DTH phenotype and the incidence of acute rejection, chronic allograft nephropathy, organ loss or patient death among patients who were tested for pro-inflammatory DTH phenotype either within or after the first year post-transplant. It should be noted that this outcome may be unique to the analytic and therapeutic conditions employed at OSU (center effect). At the very least, it suggests that good clinical immunosuppression does not necessarily block cellular allosensitization, as it has been thought to do. Instead, it appears to block the pathologic consequences of that allosensitization.

Post-transplant DTH reactivity – the anti-inflammatory phenotype

For this analysis, the results of DTH testing performed within the first post-transplant year ($n = 220$ patients) were analyzed separately from the results of testing performed beyond the first year ($n = 300$ patients). A total of 75 patients had testing performed during both of these periods. Additionally, of the 220 patients tested within the first post-transplant year, 71 had additional, serial tests performed within the first year. Of the 300 patients tested beyond the first post-transplant year, 75 had subsequent serial testing.

The first post-transplant year

When tested sometime within the first year post-transplant, 23 per cent ($n = 50$) of tested patients displayed the anti-inflammatory DTH phenotype toward donor alloantigens. Thus, about a quarter of the transplant patients appear to undergo DTH-detectable anti-inflammatory cellular allosensitization to donor alloantigens within the first year post-transplant. This is about half as many patients as those who undergo pro-inflammatory allosensitization within the same period. Overall, almost two-thirds of transplant patients display some form of DTH-detectable cellular allosensitization within a year of transplantation, despite the use of immunosuppressive agents that effectively minimize acute allograft rejection. Of the 71 patients who were serially tested within the first year, 4 per cent ($n = 3$) maintained the anti-inflammatory DTH phenotype, while 17 per cent ($n = 12$) lost it. Further, 25 per cent ($n = 18$) acquired the anti-inflammatory DTH phenotype, while 54 per cent ($n = 38$) never displayed it. Thus, the anti-inflammatory DTH phenotype of individual patients, like

the pro-inflammatory DTH phenotype, is relatively unstable within the first year post-transplant, with 42 per cent of patients changing their phenotype during this period.

Beyond the first post-transplant year

When tested at some point after the first year post-transplant, 22 per cent ($n = 65$) of tested patients displayed anti-inflammatory DTH responses toward donor alloantigens. This is similar to the frequency of reactivity observed during the first year post-transplant, so the overall incidence of the anti-inflammatory DTH phenotype within the transplant population appears to be generally stable. For the 75 patients who were serially tested after the first year, 7 per cent ($n = 5$) maintained the anti-inflammatory DTH phenotype, while 16 per cent ($n = 12$) lost it. Further, 16 per cent ($n = 12$) acquired the anti-inflammatory DTH phenotype, while 61 per cent ($n = 46$) never displayed it. Thus, the anti-inflammatory DTH phenotype of individual patients, like the pro-inflammatory DTH phenotype, remains relatively unstable after the first year post-transplant, with 32 per cent of patients changing their phenotype during this period.

Clinical impact

Since anti-inflammatory DTH reactivity reflects an inhibitory predisposition towards donor-reactive cell-mediated immunity, it might be expected that patients who display such DTH responses would be at decreased risk for pathologic developments at the graft site. Thus, it is somewhat surprising that no statistically significant correlation has been observed between the expression of the anti-inflammatory DTH phenotype and the incidence of acute rejection, chronic allograft nephropathy, organ loss or patient death among patients who were tested for anti-inflammatory DTH phenotype either within or after the first year post-transplant. Again, it should be noted that this outcome may be unique to the analytic and therapeutic conditions employed at OSU (center effect). This observation suggests that good clinical immunosuppression may not only block the pathologic consequences of pro-inflammatory cellular allosensitization, but also the beneficial consequences of anti-inflammatory cellular allosensitization.

RELATIONSHIP OF CELLULAR AND HUMORAL ALLOIMMUNITY IN TRANSPLANT PATIENTS

In addition to testing these transplant recipients for anti-donor pro- and anti-inflammatory DTH, their sera were also evaluated for the presence of alloantibodies by flow bead PRA analysis. No significant correlation was found between the presence of alloantibodies and presence of either the pro-inflammatory or the anti-inflammatory DTH phenotype. Detectable alloantibodies were produced by only 26 per cent of patients who displayed the pro-inflammatory DTH phenotype and 31 per cent of those who displayed the anti-inflammatory DTH phenotype. Furthermore, 39 per cent of alloantibody-positive patients displayed neither type of DTH reactivity. This indicates that the presence of detectable circulating alloantibodies correlates poorly with cellular allosensitization and that monitoring alloantibodies severely underestimates the percentage of patients who have become cellularly allosensitized. Nevertheless, the display of alloantibodies by transplant recipients clearly reflects an increased risk for pathologic developments in the allograft (Pelletier et al., 2002a), while their DTH status does not (Pelletier et al., 2002b).

CLINICAL AND PRE-CLINICAL STUDIES WITH THE TRANSVIVO DTH ASSAY: THE UNIVERSITY OF WISCONSIN EXPERIENCE

Investigators at the University of Wisconsin (UW) have used the transvivo DTH assay as an index of cell-mediated immunity in patients after organ transplantation. DTH analysis can readily detect donor antigen-linked suppression, whereas traditional assays such as mixed lymphocyte culture (MLC) and cytotoxic T lymphocyte (CTL) tests have failed to do so (Geissler et al., 2001). They adopted this assay not only to determine the incidence of post-transplant donor-reactive T cell sensitization, but more importantly to detect donor-specific human T regulatory cells, since their ultimate goal is the replacement of immunosuppression (IS) drug therapy by immunologic tolerance. Their transvivo DTH assay conditions involved the injection of 7×10^6 fresh or 9×10^6 frozen human peripheral blood mononuclear cells (PBMC) into the footpads of CB17 SCID mice.

DTH reactivity in tolerant patients

The organ allograft recipient who has stopped taking immunosuppressive drugs, yet retains good allograft function for long periods of time offers a unique opportunity to explore the mechanisms of peripheral tolerance (Uehling et al., 1976; Kusaka et al., 2000). Investigators at the University of Wisconsin Transplant Center have identified four patients (three kidney and one liver) who have accepted a transplanted organ for >3 years after discontinuing immunosuppression. At the time of DTH testing, two kidney patients (6.5 and 33 years post-transplant) and one liver patient (5 years post-transplant) had good graft function. The fourth, a recipient of a kidney transplant from his mother, retained excellent allograft function for 7 years after discontinuing his medication at year 2 and then lost renal function due to acute and chronic rejection at year 10, at which time fresh and frozen samples of PBMC were tested in DTH.

PBMC from all three allograft acceptors were found to exhibit a regulated response to donor antigens characterized by weak anti-donor DTH, strong recall antigen DTH

and a suppressed DTH to recall antigen when co-localized with donor antigen at the challenge site (VanBuskirk et al., 2000). In contrast, the allograft rejector showed a vigorous anti-donor DTH. To evaluate further the phenomenon of donor antigen-linked suppression, they tested patients with good graft function who were still taking maintenance immunosuppressive (IS) drug therapy (VanBuskirk et al., 2000; Geissler et al., 2001). Interestingly, the regulated phenotype was observed in some, but not all kidney and liver transplant patients still receiving IS drugs. Therefore, the term 'regulator' may be used to characterize patients who may still be taking IS drugs but whose PBMC exhibit the same features of immune regulation found in cases of long-term allograft acceptance. The relevance of regulator status to the need of an individual transplant patient for IS drugs remains to be determined.

In summary, the phenomenon of donor antigen-linked DTH suppression is characteristic of, but may not necessarily be limited to transplant recipients who accept their graft without immunosuppressive therapy. Therefore, assessment of donor reactive DTH responses and donor antigen-linked suppression may prove valuable in characterizing the evolving relationship between a recipient and their graft. Specifically, the transvivo DTH assay may help to identify patients who could benefit from IS reduction trials.

Lessons from individual patients

The establishment of a regulated DTH response to the transplant donor alloantigens appears to depend upon an equilibrium between effector (IFNγ-producing) and regulator (TGFβ, IL-10-producing) T cells, resulting in a net response that is low (Cai, et al., 2004). Neutralizing TGFβ or IL-10 reverses linked suppression and restores a strong anti-donor DTH response (VanBuskirk et al., 2000). Responses to recall antigens such as TT or EBV remain relatively constant and thus are used as a positive control. Donor-reactive DTH response is therefore a dynamic process that could change over time, especially during the loss of peripheral tolerance and the onset of graft rejection (Burlingham et al., 2000). The investigators studied the breakdown of tolerance in a patient who received a kidney transplant 10 years earlier from his mother and who had been off IS drugs for 7 years. The clinical course of the patient between years 8.8 and 10.5 post-transplant showed that the breakdown of tolerance to donor antigen was correlated with the recovery of anti-donor DTH response from an unresponsive state. At the pre-rejection time point, year 8.8, there was no detectable DTH response to donor alloantigen above the background level (i.e. the response to donor antigen = response to PBS alone). Beginning at year 9.2 there was a noticeable rise in the level of donor reactivity in DTH with a peak response at time point 9.7. A gradual recovery of anti-donor DTH response between years 9 and 10 closely paralleled the change in clinical status from tolerant to rejector. At the end of year 8 and the beginning of year 9 post-transplant, the renal function of the patient was stable with a serum creatinine of 2.0 mg/dl. A biopsy performed at year 9 revealed large lymphoid aggregates but no tubulitis or evidence of acute rejection. Ten months later the patient's creatinine had risen above 3.4 mg/dl, which prompted a biopsy at year 9.7 that revealed extensive tubulitis, cellular rejection and glomerular sclerosis. Besides anti-donor DTH reactivity, donor-specific antibody was detected in patient serum between year 10 and 10.7 post-transplantation; interestingly, both antibody and DTH responses were specific for maternal donor HLA class II/DR, rather than HLA-A, B alloantigens (Burlingham et al., 2000). These results provided the first hint that HLA-DR differences may be more immunogenic and less tolerogenic than HLA-class I, as had previously been observed in DTH studies of recombinant inbred mice (Smith and Miller, 1979).

A second patient, studied 6 years after liver transplantation and more than 3 years after discontinuing IS therapy, was evaluated for DTH reactivity at four different time points (5.3, 5.4, 5.7 and 5.9 years) during the transplant course. When the study began at year 5.3 post-transplant, the patient PBMC showed a low DTH response to donor antigen (Δ 15 over background PBS response) and a very strong regulation effect: Δ 40 versus TT, and Δ 0 versus dAg+TT. The extent of linked suppression may be a calculated as 100 per cent based on the following formula:

$$\text{Per cent Suppression} = 1 - \frac{\text{co-injection of recall Ag+ dAg}}{\text{recall Ag}} \times 100\%$$

where recall Ag+dAg is the net swelling response to the combination of recall and donor antigen, recall Ag the response to TT (in this example) or EBV alone. At time points 5.4, 5.7 and 5.9 post-transplant, patient PBMC exhibited an increased DTH response to donor antigen (Δ 30, 58, and 40 over background) with a simultaneous decrease in the extent of linked suppression (96 per cent, 54 per cent and 63 per cent, respectively). A biopsy taken during this time was negative for rejection, but laboratory results did show an elevation in liver enzymes. The patient died 1 year later due to acute liver failure. The investigators were unable to obtain sequential blood samples for DTH testing during this critical period.

Another patient, 4 years post liver transplant and still taking prednisone and FK506, showed a different clinical pattern. At the time of initial DTH testing, the patient was diagnosed with excellent graft function; however, the DTH results displayed a very strong donor-reactive response (Δ 45) and a non-regulator phenotype (Δ 45 versus TT; Δ 45 versus dAg+TT). The patient lost graft function 1.5 years later as a result of late hepatic artery thrombosis, considered a form of chronic rejection (Geissler et al., 2001).

A similar situation was observed in a patient who was 8 years post heart transplant and 2 years free of IS therapy. The recipient was referred to the laboratory as a potentially tolerant patient. Results from the DTH assay indicated that the patient was sensitized to the donor antigen (Δ 47.5) and was a non-regulator (Δ 35 versus EBV, Δ 47.5 versus dAg+EBV; 0 per cent suppression). A biopsy performed at the same time point revealed grade 3A rejection and decreased cardiac function (40 per cent ejection fraction). The patient refused IS medication and died 2 months later.

The loss of peripheral DTH regulation does not always result in graft rejection. A patient who withdrew himself from immunosuppression 1.5 years after receiving a cadaver donor kidney and who for 5 years maintained excellent kidney graft function, was studied in detail. Initial tests at 5–6 years post transplant with patient PBMC showed a consistently low DTH response to donor type/soluble HLA-B*1501 antigen. This regulated donor-reactive DTH response began as early as year 3 (based on studies of cryopreserved PBMC) and continued through year 7.2 post-transplant. It was correlated with excellent renal function as defined by serum creatinine of 1.3 mg/dl. A second leukophoresis was obtained from the patient at time point 7.6 years post-transplant to further our efforts in understanding the mechanism of tolerance. At this time, renal function was still excellent (serum creatinine = 1.4 mg/dl) but an increase was observed in the response of patient PBMC to donor HLA-B*1501. Specifically, the net DTH response to allopeptide p37 (which corresponded to the immunodominant polymorphic region of the heavy chain of HLA-B*1501) doubled, from Δ 20 to Δ 40.5 indicating that the patient had lost the ability to regulate his DTH response to a donor class I antigen. Since that time the DTH response to donor antigen HLA-B*1501 as well as p37 peptide, has remained high. A similarly high response was seen to soluble HLA-B44, another donor HLA-B antigen. Although renal function remains stable (current serum creatinine = 1.3 mg/dl), the patient is being closely monitored at regular clinical visits for any signs that may indicate a change in transplant status. An important aspect of this study was that CD4+CD25+ T cells from the regulated time period were able fully to restore a regulated DTH response to donor alloantigen by the year 7.6 PBMC. This meant that the long period of regulated DTH (years 3.0–7.2 post-transplant) was the result of the activity of a donor antigen-specific, CD4+CD25+ T regulatory cells. Thus, DTH may be an excellent way to detect the presence of such T cells in PBMC (Lee, manuscript submitted).

Primate studies with the transvivo DTH assay

In collaboration with Dr Stuart Knechtle, the investigators undertook a DTH study of 13 Rhesus monkeys that were given a kidney allograft along with transient (<200 days) IS therapy. Donor-reactive DTH responses were found to be strongly correlated with clinical status. For example, 6/6 Rhesus monkeys with metastable tolerance to the renal allograft showed strong linked suppression (>60 per cent) and weak anti-donor DTH, while 7/7 monkeys with rejection were DTH sensitized to donor alloantigens, as indicated by anti-donor DTH response equal to the response to a positive control (TT) recall antigen (Torrealba, et al., 2004). All regulator monkeys showed a strong anti-donor DTH response (similar to recall antigen response) when TGFβ, but not IL-10, was neutralized by antibody in the footpad injection site. One monkey followed over a 10-month period after discontinuing IS showed an initially regulated DTH response to donor, then progressively lost DTH regulation concomitant with loss of renal function and acute rejection, similar to the patient case described above (Burlingham et al., 2000). The loss of renal function also correlated with the disappearance from the graft interstitium of CD4+ T cells that stained positively for latent TGFβ. The latter may be the *local* arm of the regulated DTH response. Indeed, the investigators have found a TGFβ-dependent, regulated DTH response in leukocytes harvested by collagenase digestion from monkey, which accepted allograft kidney (Burlingham, unpublished observations). In addition, they were able to identify CD4+ CD25+ T cells expressing TGFβ within the allograft during graft acceptance (Torrealba, et al., 2004).

What drives regulation in graft acceptors? Donor HLA class I and class II antigens

Initial studies established that a single donor antigen was sufficient to trigger linked suppression. Specifically, a single donor-mismatched HLA class I antigen (HLA-B62) when co-injected with a recall antigen in the footpad of a SCID mouse could trigger DTH regulation, whereas a self-HLA class I antigen (HLA-A2) could not (VanBuskirk et al., 2000). In addition, rejection of a kidney allograft from the mother was correlated with DTH versus donor HLA-DR but not with DTH to donor A, B antigens (Burlingham et al., 2000). To determine if DTH regulated responses are biased to recognition of donor HLA- class I, HLA specificity analysis of donor antigen-linked suppression was performed on four highly mismatched liver transplant recipients who demonstrated donor antigen-regulated DTH responses. EBV-transformed LCL expressing single HLA antigens and soluble purified HLA were used as sources of donor type antigen. All purified HLA were tested at a dose of 50 ng per injection. The results clearly showed that a single donor HLA class I-A or -B triggered partial to complete suppression of DTH response to a recall antigen, while donor type HLA-DR antigen consistently failed to induce linked suppression (Jankowska-Gan et al., 2002).

In order to determine fully if the lack of regulation by donor HLA-DR in comparison to HLA-A or -B was dose dependent, HLA-DR and HLA-B were tested over a wide range (0.5–500 ng) of doses in two patients. The dose response of HLA-B8 versus HLA-DR17 (dAg for one patient) and HLA-B7 versus HLA-DR7 (dAg for second patient) revealed that donor type HLA-DR, regardless of concentration, were not capable of triggering linked suppression, whereas a dose of donor HLA-B as low as 5 ng

per injection was sufficient in each case to trigger linked suppression and 50 ng were sufficient to cause >80 per cent suppression.

These data were interesting since it suggested the possibility that class I but not class II-derived allopeptides trigger regulatory T cell responses. However, further analysis of one of the liver transplant recipients demonstrated that soluble HLA-DQ as well as allopeptides derived from the DQA chain polymorphic region, could also trigger DTH linked suppression. This indicates that at least some HLA-class II antigens may trigger the regulator T cells in allograft acceptors.

Minor H antigens

In addition to class I HLA-A and -B antigens, it is also clear that certain minor H antigens can activate regulation of DTH in transplant patients. Initial studies (VanBuskirk et al., 2000) identified an HLA-identical kidney recipient that exhibited donor antigen-linked suppression to EBV and TT recall antigens. Currently, the patient is 36 years post-transplant and remains one of the earliest documented cases of successful cessation of immunosuppression (Uehling et al., 1976). Using PCR techniques, the investigators identified a minor H antigen, HA-1, that differed between the recipient and her donor (both HLA-A2+). The recipient was typed as HA-1 R/R, while the donor was typed as HA-1H/H. A single nonamer peptide, HA-1H, at concentration of 1 μg per injection was sufficient to trigger linked suppression. Interestingly, HA-1 antigen expression is known to be restricted to cells of hematopoietic origin. Therefore, the finding that a single donor type minor H peptide expressed only by donor leukocytes can trigger regulation of DTH in a long-term allograft acceptor suggests that microchimerism may continue to drive immune regulation long after organ transplantation. Interestingly, the minor antigen-specific T reg cells were CD8+, not CD4+, as had been observed previously (Cai, et al., 2004).

Immune regulation and graft survival in kidney transplant recipients may both be enhanced by HLA-DR sharing

Because the patients showing DTH regulation and kidney allograft acceptance were closely matched for HLA-DR/DQ or were HLA identical (Cai, et al., 2004), a retrospective study was performed to determine the influence of HLA matching on DTH regulation, acute rejection and graft survival in primary cadaveric kidney transplant recipients (from 1993 to 2001) and LRD kidney transplant recipients (from 1978 to 2001). HLA-DR matching in cadaver recipients ($n = 849$) was significantly correlated with freedom from acute rejection episodes ($P = 0.0001$) as well as graft survival ($P = 0.0001$). In addition, 29 cadaveric and 33 living related renal transplant recipients with stable renal function (creatinine = 1.8 mg/dl) were tested using the transvivo DTH assay. Within the cadaveric population, nine (31 per cent) patients exhibited a regulated phenotype, 15 (52 per cent) a non-regulated phenotype and five (17 per cent) were sensitized to donor antigen. Living related donor (LRD) transplant recipients had a stronger tendency toward DTH regulation when compared to cadaver recipients ($P = 0.002$). In the 1-haplotype LRD group ($n = 27$), 18 (67 per cent) patients were determined to be regulators, nine (33 per cent) were non-regulators and none were sensitized to their donor. In the smaller LRD HLA-identical cohort, all of the patients ($n = 6$) tested positive for DTH regulation in response to donor minor H antigens. Statistical analysis of the cadaver group data revealed that HLA-DR matching significantly correlated with development of immune regulation ($P = 0.046$). Of the total number of nine regulators in the cadaver donor RTx group, six had a 2 DR antigen match, two had a 1 DR match and only one had a 0 antigen match. Overall, the results of DTH analysis were correlated with the beneficial effect of HLA-DR matching on long-term outcome: those patients with highest incidence of DTH regulation to donor antigens (2 DR-matched) were the same ones enjoying the best graft survival at 7 years post-transplant (Rodriges, et al., 2004).

At the present time a UW-sponsored, randomized clinical trial is underway to evaluate the use of the DTH assay to predict risk of rejection in conjunction with steroid withdrawal. This trial will enroll 75 kidney transplant recipients age 55 or greater maintained on MMF as a part of trial therapy regimen since the time of transplant. Fifty subjects will be withdrawn from steroids over a 3-month period, 25 control subjects will be maintained on current therapy. As of this writing seven patients have been enrolled in the trial. The DTH results will be analyzed before and after steroid withdrawal to determine its predictive value.

CONCLUSIONS

The transvivo DTH assay represents an interesting tool with which to monitor the in vivo disposition of T cells from a given individual toward specific antigens. It is valuable for two reasons. It not only monitors only recall T cell responses, but it can detect both pro-inflammatory and anti-inflammatory T cell responses. This allows its use for the determination of whether and how a given individual has recognized and responded to a specific set of antigens. While straightforward in theory and design, the execution of the transvivo DTH assay is complicated by some technical issues that remain to be resolved. In this regard, the clinical application of the transvivo DTH assay represents a work in progress. The first sets of clinical studies with the transvivo DTH assay have been encouraging. The OSU experience demonstrates that the assay can be used routinely to monitor graft-reactive DTH responses in transplant patients. Surprisingly, this study was unable to show statistical correlations between DTH results and various parameters of clinical outcome. Nevertheless, the UW experience

has shown that the transvivo DTH assay can be very informative in studies on the behavior of donor-reactive T cells from tolerant transplant patients. It is hoped that other investigators will utilize the transvivo DTH assay in additional clinical trials. This would confirm or contest existing data, help to fine-tune the assay and add to the growing body of information about transvivo DTH reactivity in humans.

ACKNOWLEDGEMENTS

The UW authors would like to acknowledge the contributions of Daniel Rodriguez, Junglim Lee, Junchao Cai, Masaki Katayama and Jose Torrealba to the development of our understanding of the regulated DTH response in transplant recipients. The OSU authors would like to acknowledge the physicians and medical staff, who made the clinical trial possible and Jacob Jansen, who performed most of the DTH analyses.

REFERENCES

Baliga, P., Chavin, K.D., Qin, L. et al. (1994). CTLA4Ig prolongs allograft survival while suppressing cell-mediated immunity. Transplantation 58, 1082–1090.

Bickerstaff, A.A., VanBuskirk, A.M., Wakely, E. and Orosz, C.G. (2000). Transforming growth factor-β and interleukin-10 subvert alloreactive delayed type hypersensitivity in cardiac allograft acceptor mice. Transplantation 69, 1517–1520.

Burlingham, W.J., Jankowska-Gan, E., VanBuskirk, A., Orosz, C.G., Lee, J.H. and Kusaka, S. (2000). Loss of tolerance to a maternal kidney transplant is selective for HLA class II: evidence from trans-vivo DTH and alloantibody analysis. Hum Immunol 61, 1395–1402.

Cai, J., Lee, J., Jankowska-Gan, E. et al. (2004). Minor H antigen HA-I-specific regulator and effector CD8+T cells, and HA-1 microchimerism, in allogroft tollerance J Exp Med 199, 1017–1023.

Carrodeguas, L., Orosz, C.G., Waldman, W.J., Sedmak, D.D., Adams, P.W. and VanBuskirk, A.M. (1999). Trans vivo analysis of human delayed-type hypersensitivity reactivity. Hum Immunol 60, 640–651.

Geissler, F., Jankowska-Gan, E., DeVito-Haynes, L.D. et al. (2001). Human liver allograft acceptance and the 'tolerance assay': in vitro anti-donor T cell assays show hyporeactivity to donor cells, but unlike DTH, fail to detect linked suppression. Transplantation 72, 571–580.

Graca, L., Honey, K., Adams, E., Cobbold, S.P. and Waldmann, H. (2000). Cutting edge: anti-CD154 therapeutic antibodies induce infectious transplantation tolerance. J Immunol 165, 4783–4786.

Hancock, W.W., Sayegh, M.H., Zheng, X.-G., Peach, R., Linsley, P.S. and Turka, L.A. (1996). Costimulatory function and expression of CD40 ligand, CD80, and CD86 in vascularized murine cardiac allograft rejection. Proc Natl Acad Sci USA 93, 13967–13972.

Jankowska-Gan, E., Rhein, T., Haynes, L.D. et al. (2002). Human liver allograft acceptance and the 'tolerance assay'. II. Donor HLA-A, -B but not DR antigens are able to trigger regulation of DTH. Hum Immunol 63, 862–870.

Kusaka, S., Grailer, A.P., Fechner, J.H. Jr et al. (2000). Clonotype analysis of human alloreactive T cells: a novel approach to studying peripheral tolerance in a transplant recipient. J Immunol *164*, 2240–2247.

Orosz, C.G., Ohye, R.G., Pelletier, R.P. et al. (1993). Treatment with anti-vascular cell adhesion molecule 1 monoclonal antibody induces long-term murine cardiac allograft acceptance. Transplantation *56*, 453–460.

Pearson, T.C., Madsen, J.C., Larsen, C.P., Morris, P.J. and Wood, K.J. (1992). Induction of transplantation tolerance in adults using donor antigen and anti-CD4 monoclonal antibody. Transplantation *54*, 475–483.

Pelletier, R.P., Hennessy, P.K., Adams, P.W., VanBuskirk, A.M., Ferguson, R.M. and Orosz, C.G. (2002a). Clinical significance of MHC-reactive alloantibodies that develop after kidney or kidney-pancreas transplantation. Am J Transplant *2*, 134–141.

Pelletier, R.P., Hennessy, P.K., Adams, P.W. and Orosz, C.G. (2002b). High incidence of donor-reactive delayed-type hypersensitivity reactivity in transplant patients. Am J Transplant *2*, 926–933.

Rodriguez, D.S., Jankowska-Gan, E., Haynes, L.D. et al. (2004). Immune regulation and graft survival in kidney transplant recipients are both enhanced by human leukocyte antigen matching. Am J Transplant *4*, 537–543.

Smith, F.I. and Miller, J.F. (1979). Delayed-type hypersensitivity to allogeneic cells in mice. III. Sensitivity to cell-surface antigens coded by the major histocompatibility complex and by other genes. J Exp Med *150*, 965–976.

Torrealba, J.R., Katayama, M., Fechner, J.H. Jr. et al. (2004). Metastable tolerance to rhesus monkey renal transplants is correlated with allograft TGF-B1-CD4+T regulatory cell infiltrates. J Immunol *172*, 5753–5764.

Uehling, D.T., Hussey, J.L., Weinstein, A.B., Wank, R. and Bach, F.H. (1976). Cessation of immunosuppression after renal transplantation. Surgery *79*, 278–282.

VanBuskirk, A.M., Wakely, M.E., Sirak, J.H. and Orosz, C.G. (1998). Patterns of allosensitization in allograft recipients: Long-term cardiac allograft acceptance is associated with active alloantibody production in conjunction with active inhibition of alloreactive delayed-type hypersensitivity. Transplantation *65*, 1115–1123.

VanBuskirk, A.M., Burlingham, W.J., Jankowska-Gan, E. et al. (2000). Human allograft acceptance is associated with immune regulation. J Clin Invest *106*, 145–155.

Wiebke, E.A., Rosenberg, S.A. and Lotze, M.T. (1988). Acute immunologic effects of IL-2 in cancer patients: Decreased delayed type hypersensitivity response and decreased proliferative response to soluble antigens. J Clin Oncol *6*, 1440–1449.

Wise, M.P., Bemelman, F., Cobbold, S.P. and Waldmann, H. (1998). Cutting Edge: Linked suppression of skin graft rejection can operate through indirect recognition. J Immunol *161*, 5813–5816.

Xia, D., Sanders, A., Shah, M., Bickerstaff, A. and Orosz, C. (2001). Real-time polymerase chain reaction analysis reveals an evolution of cytokine mRNA production in allograft acceptor mice. Transplantation *72*, 907–914.

Rebuck Windows: Granulocyte Function

Chapter 36

Daniel R. Ambruso

Department of Pediatrics, University of Colorado School of Medicine, Denver, CO, USA

Diapedesis and accumulation of white corpuscles in inflammatory diseases must be regarded as modes of defense against microorganisms, the leukocytes in this struggle devouring and destroying the parasites.

I. Metchnikov, 1968

INTRODUCTION

The inflammatory response is the summation of a complex series of events in which vascular endothelial and other mesenchymal or parenchymal cells, plasma protein systems and leukocytes respond to infection or injury in the tissues (Vaporciyan and Ward, 1995). The coordinated reaction to the noxious event focuses a large number of mechanisms which abolish the microbe or injurious agent and initiate healing. Despite its beneficial effects, excessive inflammation has the potential for tissue damage and destruction (Vaporciyan and Ward, 1995). Unregulated, inflammatory processes play a significant role in many diseases.

The cardinal signs of inflammation were noted by the Roman, Celsius, as redness and swelling with heat and pain (Majino, 1975). These physical findings are largely initiated by changes in local hemodynamics and vascular permeability followed by accumulation of leukocytes at the site. Phagocytic cells, neutrophils and monocytes play a critical role as effectors of inflammation. As recognized and described by Metchnikov in the nineteenth century, these cells create an important first line of host defense through their ability to emigrate to sites of microbial invasion or to the presence of substances and by a variety of mechanisms eliminate them or neutralize their noxious effects.

In this chapter, a review of humoral mediators and phagocyte function will be presented and these will be correlated with *in vitro* and *in vivo* measures of the response of these inflammatory constituents in an effort to define a crucial part of the immune response.

HUMORAL MEDIATORS OF INFLAMMATION

The release of humoral mediators is important for initiation and orderly progression of the inflammatory response. These compounds produced from several sources include substances released from microbes (e.g. endotoxin or formulated peptides), plasma proteins (e.g. coagulation factors, kinins, vasoactive amines and constituents of complement system) and active agents produced by a variety of cell types including endothelial cells, other mesenchymal cells and leukocytes (lipids, cytokines and chemokines) (Dinarello and Moldawer, 2000). These systems or mediators are summarized in Table 36.1 which describes their source and target(s) or action(s).

IL-1 and TNF are the central pro-inflammatory cytokines which are responsible for the major signs and symptoms including cachexia, fever, muscle breakdown, other non-immune effects and induction and release of other

Measuring Immunity, edited by Michael T. Lotze and Angus W. Thomson
ISBN 0-12-455900-X, London

Table 36.1 Inflammatory mediators

Mediator/system	Source	Target/action
Lipids		
PAF	Leukocytes (myeloid cells and monocytes), endothelial cells	Vascular permeability and cell activation (neutrophils, eosinophils, platelets)
LTB$_4$	Neutrophils, monocytes	Vascular permeability, neutrophil, monocyte activation
Cytokines		
IL-1	Multiple cells including monocytes and macrophages	Multiple biologic activities in various organs mediating effects of inflammation, production of other cytokines (e.g. IL-6)
TNF	Multiple cell types	Multiple biologic activities like IL-1, fever, increase acute phase proteins, activation and priming, endothelium and neutrophils
IL-6	Lymphocytes, monocytes, epithelial and endothelial cells, mesenchymal cells	Release of acute phase reactants, proliferation and activation of a variety of cells
INF-γ	Leukocytes	Enhances responses of leukocytes to inflammatory stimuli
Chemokines (CXC)		
IL-8	Monocytes, neutrophils, endothelial and other cells	Priming and activation of neutrophils and basophils
GROα,β,γ	Monocytes, endothelial cells and others	Neutrophil chemotaxis and activation
NAP-2	Platelets	Activation of neutrophils
Chemokines (CC)		
MCP-1	Monocytes, endothelial and others	Degranulation of basophils, activation of monocytes
RANTES	Monocytes and eosinophils	Chemotactic for eosinophils, basophils, monocytes, lymphocytes
Eotaxin	Monocytes, eosinophils and others	Eosinophils, basophils, lymphocytes
Complement		
C3a	Activation of complement system, plasma proteins	Increases capillary permeability
C5a	Activation of complement system, plasma proteins	Chemotactic for neutrophils and monocytes
C3b (iC3b)	Activation of complement system, plasma proteins	Opsonin for phagocytosis
C5b-9	Activation of complement system, plasma proteins	Cytolytic activity
Kinins		
Bradykinin and kallikrein	Plasma proteins	Pain, vascular permeability, vasodilatation
Vasoactive amines		
Serotonin, histamine	Platelets, mast cells, basophils	Vascular permeability and cell activation
Coagulation		
Plasma clotting factors	Plasma proteins	Chemotaxis, vascular permeability, complement activation

cytokines such as INF-γ, IL-6 (Dinarello and Wolff, 1993; Hill, 1993; Strieter and Kunkel, 1994). These cytokines enhance endothelial adhesion, leukocyte functional responsiveness and production of chemokines which have the dual role of chemoattractants luring phagocytes to the inflammatory site as well as activating other aspects of cell function (Oppenheim et al., 1991; Dinarello, 1996). Balancing these substances are the anti-inflammatory cytokines, IL-4, IL-10 and TGF-β which dampen the acute inflammatory response (Kulkarni et al., 1993; Moore et al., 1993).

Vasodilatation and enhanced vascular permeability are key events in the development of the inflammatory response (Vaporciyan and Ward, 1995; Gabay and Kushner, 1999). Lipid metabolites such as platelet activating factor (PAF) and leukotrienes (e.g. LTB$_4$) produced by leukocytes, endothelial cells and mast cells as well as vasoactive amines released by mast cells, basophils and platelets induce both events (Serhan, 1994; Prescott et al., 2000). Activation of complement with release of potent anaphylatoxins, activation of coagulation and concomitant generation of bradykinin and kallekriens also have potent effects on the local vascular bed (Sharma, 1992; Vaporciyan and Ward, 1995). Vasodilatation may also be triggered by local release of nitric oxide from a variety of cells including endothelial and smooth muscle cells, monocytes and macrophages (Lowenstein and Snyder, 1992; Nathan, 1992). The change in vascular integrity results in leakage of complement proteins and antibodies which induce movement of cells into the area and prompt their phagocytic function (1990). Many of the agents noted above have a chemotactic activity supporting the cellular phase of acute inflammation.

A powerful group of compounds generated during acute inflammation are the chemokines. Named for their dual activities as chemotaxins and cytokines, chemokines contain heparin binding domains which allow interactions between proteoglycans on endothelial cells and subendothelial matrix (Baggiolini, 1998). These molecules also interact with neutrophils, monocytes and specific populations of lymphocytes and support emigration of these cells into the site of inflammation. The chemokines fall into two groups, based on conserved pairs of cysteine residues and whether they contain an intervening amino acid (CXC) or not (CC) (Zlotnik and Yoshie, 2000). Included in the former are IL-8, GROα,β,γ and NAP-2. Generated by a variety of cell types (see Table 36.1), these compounds are strong chemoattractants and activate other functions of neutrophils (Baggiolini et al., 1989; Walz and Baggiolini, 1990). The CC chemokines, which include MCP-1, Rantes and eotaxin, are released from a wide variety of cells and are chemotactic for monocytes, basophils, eosinophils and subclasses of lymphocytes (Schall et al., 1990; Rollins et al., 1991).

Humoral factors of inflammation induce chemotactic activity in their cellular targets and activation of other cell functions through binding to specific surface receptors (Murphy, 1994; Locati and Murphy, 1999). Although there may be some overlap in the ability to interact with more than one receptor (e.g. a chemokine may bind more than one receptor and chemokine receptors may interact with more than one molecule), interaction of humoral substances with their cognate receptors leads to an orderly sequence of emigration of phagocytes to the site of the microbial invasion or noxious substances.

THE PHAGOCYTE AND THE INFLAMMATORY RESPONSE

An adequate pool of functional phagocytes provides the host with a first line of defense against microbial invasion. The predominant cell of the acute inflammatory response is the neutrophil (PMN) or granulocyte. The function of this cell relies upon integration of extracellular signals through receptor linked intracellular signaling pathways. This leads to an orderly sequence of adhesion to and movement through the endothelial surface, emigration to the site of inflammation and ingestion or destruction of the inciting agent through the focus of a variety of oxygen dependent or independent mechanisms (Figure 36.1).

Neutrophil function

The first step in PMN function is adherence to the endothelium adjacent to the area of infection. This requires expression of adhesion molecules (Table 36.2) and their interaction with complementary molecules on the endothelial surface (Harlan et al., 1992). Loose adhesion which mediates neutrophil rolling along post-capillary venules requires L-selectin and the sialyl-Lewis X (Sle^x) interacting with endothelial E-selectin and P-selectin (Foxall et al., 1992; Kansas et al., 1993). Tight adherence of neutrophils is effected through the interaction of neutrophil β-2 integrins, CD11b/CD18 with ICAM-1 and/or ICAM-2 (Springer, 1990). The neutrophil contains a large supply of CD11b/CD18 in specific granule membranes which become expressed with secretion occurring during adherence. Qualitative changes which increase the affinity of CD11b/CD18 to its ligands also occur during this process (Zimmerman et al., 1992). By these mechanisms, then, neutrophils are recruited from the laminar flow of blood to roll along the endothelial surface. Subsequently, with tight adherence and spreading, the cells begin their transmigration through the endothelial barrier.

Once the neutrophil is past the endothelial barrier, it encounters gradients of a variety of molecules released

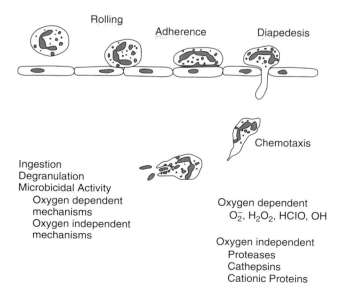

Figure 36.1 Neutrophil function. Taken from Peterson, V.M. and Ambruso, D.R. (1994). Phagocyte production and function following burn injury. Austin: RG Landes Company, p. 61.

Table 36.2 Leukocyte and endothelial adhesion molecules and their proposed roles in host defense and inflammation

Leukocyte associated	Endothelial associated	Function

Selectins
 L selectin
  (neutrophils, monocytes,
  lymphocytes)
	Selectins
	 P-selectin (stimulated endothelium)
	 E-selectin
	  (stimulated endothelium,
	  activated platelets)
		Neutrophil rolling, lymphocyte homing
		Inflammation, hemostasis
		Ligands for all are sialyated, fucosylated
		  carbohydrates

β_2 integrins
 CD11a/CD18
  (all leukocytes)
	Intracellular adhesion molecules (ICAM)
	 ICAM-1
	  (endothelium, also monocytes and
	  lymphocytes)
		Neutrophil and monocyte
		Adherence, diapedesis
		Chemotaxis

CD11b/CD18
  (neutrophils, monocytes,
  macrophages, some lymphocytes)
 CD11c/CD18 (ligand C3bi)
  (macrophages, monocytes,
  neutrophils, activated lymphocytes)
	ICAM-2
	  (endothelium, some lymphocytes)
		Inflammation, immune responsiveness

CD11d/CD18
  (macrophages, monocytes,
  neutrophils, T lymphocytes)
	ICAM-3
	  (lymphocytes, monocytes, neutrophils)	

β_1 integrins
 VLA-4 (very late activated antigen)
  (lymphocytes, eosinophils,
  monocytes)
	VCAM-1
	  (vascular cell adhesion molecule)
		Leukocyte homing, inflammatory response

Adapted from Peterson, V.M. and Ambruso, D.R. (1994). Phagocyte production and function following burn injury. Austin: RG Landes Company, p. 68.

by microbes and inflammatory, parenchymal and mesenchymal cells (Ambruso, 1994). Neutrophils move up the concentration gradient. The most potent *in vivo* chemoattractants include the complement fragment, C5a, N-formyl oligopeptides (e.g. fMLP) and lipid compounds (e.g. PAF), cytokines and chemokines (Bokoch, 1995). Most of the relevant stimuli have receptors which can initiate directed migration (Bokoch, 1995).

During movement, the cell transforms its spherical shape to a linear form extending organelle poor pseudopods (Ambruso, 1994). The cell may change directions by reorienting existing pseudopods or extending new ones. Uropods in the posterior portion of the neutrophil anchor the cell during movement. Movement requires a microtubular system, a cortical actin network cycling actin between monomeric and polymeric pools and cross-link polymers into three-dimensional networks and actin binding proteins (Bokoch, 1995).

Once at the site of infection or inflammation, neutrophils begin to ingest the offending microorganisms. The first step, opsonization, coats the microbe with specific proteins usually IgG or complement (C3) (Ambruso, 1994; Dinauer, 2003). Ingestion is initiated by the interaction between these ligands attached to the microbe and specific receptors on the neutrophil. The most important phagocytic receptors are the Fc and C3bi receptors (Berger et al., 1984; Unkeless, 1989; Huizinga et al., 1990). Neutrophils express three types of Fc receptors: FcRI, FcRII and FcγRIII, which bind different forms of IgG. Initiation of phagocytosis may require the proximity of two or more receptors occupied by the specific ligand.

The interactions between combinations of receptors may stimulate other functions besides phagocytosis. FcRI and FcRII activate the NADPH oxidase, while FcRII and FcRIII stimulate exocytosis (Huizinga et al., 1990). The C3bi receptor mediates adhesion, recognizes C3bi coated particles and initiates phagocytosis and the respiratory burst (Berger et al., 1984).

Activation of phagocytosis through receptor ligand interactions and subsequent signal transduction results in changes in membrane fluidity, reorganization of the cortical actin cytoskeleton and formation of phagocytic pseudopods which extend around the ingested microbe (Ambruso, 1994; Dinauer, 2003). The pseudopods are rich in actin and actin-associated proteins. These proteins form and remodel a three-dimensional network which promotes the formation of the phagocytic vacuole. As the extending pseudopods encompass the microbe, the plasma membrane at the advancing ends fuses to complete the phagosome.

Stimulation of the neutrophil by phagocytosis or exposure to a soluble stimulus leads to the consumption of oxygen and production of O_2^-. This reaction is under control of the NADPH oxidase which contains several components, including the cytochrome b_{558}, a heterodimer composed of the p22 phox and gp91 phox and proteins designated as p47 phox, p67 phox and p40 phox, the low molecular weight GTP binding protein, Rac2 (Ambruso and Johnston, 1998). In resting neutrophils, some components reside in the cytosol (Rac2, p47 phox, p67 phox, p40 phox), while cytochrome b_{558} is membrane-associated (plasma membrane and specific granules)

(Ambruso et al., 1990; Clark et al., 1990). With activation of the neutrophil, p47 phox, p67 phox and Rac2 translocate to the plasma membrane (Ambruso et al., 1990; Clark et al., 1990; Quinn et al., 1993). Secretion of specific granules increases the plasma membrane associated cytochrome b$_{558}$ (Ambruso et al., 1990). During activation of the oxidase, these components undergo processing (e.g. phosphorylation of p47 phox) or interact to form complexes (e.g. p67 phox with Rac, p47 phox and p40 phox), subsequently finding their way to the plasma membrane (Rotrosen and Leto, 1990; Park et al., 1992; Nisimoto et al., 1997). These processes are not completely understood but, as membrane and cytosol associated components are assembled, activity of the oxidase is expressed.

Specific and azurophilic granules contain a variety of degradative and directly bactericidal compounds (Borregaard and Cowland, 1997). Fusion of specific and azurophilic granules with release of toxic oxygen metabolites and granule contents into the phagolysosome is critical to the destruction of the microorganism (Ambruso, 1994; Dinauer, 2003). As with motility and ingestion, degranulation requires that microtubular system, cortical actin cytoskeleton and Ca^{++} dependent proteins which promote membrane fusion, must all be intact.

Signal transduction

The classic view of signal transduction in neutrophils is centered around the pathways described with chemoattractant receptors such as those described for fMLP. Linked to heterotrimeric G-proteins, these pathways affect functional activity through activation of phospholipase C, phosphoinositide metabolism, changes in cytosolic calcium, activation of protein kinase C and subsequent protein phosphorylation (Bokoch, 1995). However, recent data have implicated a number of other signaling pathways and mechanisms including activation of tyrosine kinases, inhibition of phosphatases, other kinases such as PI-3 kinases and GTPases belonging to the Ras superfamily (Bokoch, 1995).

Ras GTPases can be broken into five subfamilies (Bokoch, 1995). Neutrophils contain GTPases that fit into many of these subfamilies but those belonging to the Rho subfamily play a dominant role in neutrophil function. The Rho GTPases, including Rho, Rac and Cdc42, play critical roles in actin reorganization, integrin complex formation, cell adhesion, gene transcription, cell cycle progression and cell proliferation (Nobes and Hall, 1995; Ridley, 1996; Hall, 1998). Each appears to have a distinct function. For example, in fibroblasts, activation of Rho results in actin assembly, stress fiber formation and production of adhesion complexes (Hall, 1998). Cdc42 appears more related to formation of spike-like filopodra, while Rac activity appears to be associated with broad lamellipodia. There is cross-talk or interaction between these members (Allen et al., 1997; Cox et al., 1997). In fibroblasts, activation

of Cdc42 can lead to activation of Rac and, subsequently, Rho (Kjoller and Hall, 1999). Rac has been implicated in Ras associated transformation (Rebollo and Martinez, 1999).

Activation of Rho GTPases is regulated by binding of guanine nucleotides

Regulatory proteins control the cycling between the GDP-bound or inactive and the GTP-bound or active states (Bourne et al., 1991; Hotchin and Hall, 1996; Mackay and Hall, 1998; Ambruso et al., 2000). Guanine nucleotide exchange factors (GEFs) facilitate exchange of GTP for GDP on the guanine nucleotide binding site leading to activation of the GTPase. Hydrolysis of GTP occurs quite rapidly through the interaction with guanine nucleotide activating proteins (GAPs). Guanine nucleotide dissociation inhibitors (GDIs) prevent the activation of these GTPases by inhibiting transfer of guanine nucleotides to the active site. The targets of activated Rac have not been completely determined. In the active state, Rac binds and activates a kinase p21 activated kinase (PAK) (Geijsen et al., 1999). Subsequent activation pathways may also include activation of p42/44 MAP kinase, p38 MAP kinase and c-Jun kinase (Coso et al., 1995; Hill et al., 1995; Minden et al., 1995; Borregaard and Cowland, 1997; Van Aelst and D'Souza-Schorey, 1997).

In neutrophils, Rho GTPases are critical to shape change, adherence, chemotaxis, ingestion and NADPH oxidase activity (el Benna et al., 1994; Borregaard and Cowland, 1997; Glogauer et al., 2000). These cells contain Rho A, Rac1 and Rac2 and Cdc42. Although these GTPases may exhibit specific functions or activities, there is some overlap. For example, Rac2 and Cdc42 affect actin nucleation, activate MAP kinase cascades (p38 MAPK and c-Jun) and bind PAK at a common motif (Coso et al., 1995; Hill et al., 1995; Minden et al., 1995; Borregaard and Cowland, 1997; Van Aelst and D'Souza-Schorey, 1997; Glogauer et al., 2000). Rac1 and Rac2 contain 92 per cent identity (Didsbury et al., 1989). Rac1 has a ubiquitous distribution whereas Rac2 appears in myeloid cells (Heyworth et al., 1994). Although Rac2 is the specific GTPase for the NADPH oxidase, Rac1 can activate this enzyme complex. The physiologic roles for these proteins are not well defined and it is unclear if the overlapping functions represent a dual dependency or dual requirement.

EVALUATION OF INFLAMMATORY MECHANISMS

Investigation of inflammatory mechanisms may be organized according to determination of humoral constituents or cellular function (Table 36.3). Studies of humoral constituents depend on the model identified and materials available. Quantitation of cytokines, growth factors, lipids, complement and coagulation components may be completed by a number of sensitive techniques including

Table 36.3 Evaluation of neutrophil function

Function	Screening studies	Detailed studies
Adherence	<ul><li>Adherence of monocytes and neutrophils from anticoagulated whole blood to nylon or glass wool</li><li>Adherence of isolated cells to plastic or glass</li></ul>	<ul><li>Adherence of isolated neutrophils to protein coated surfaces, cultured endothelial cells; pretreatment of either cell type with cytokines, inhibitors or antibodies to cell surface adhesion molecules; evaluate/monitor endothelial and/or phagocyte contribution to adherence</li><li>Aggregation: evaluation of light transmission after an agonist; evaluates homotypic adhesion</li><li>Immunofluorescence staining of cells with labeled antibodies for various cell surface adhesive antigens in resting state or after stimulation with various agents</li><li>Direct evaluation, rolling, adherence</li></ul>
Chemotaxis	<ul><li>Gross and microscopic examination of infected sites for presence of phagocytes</li><li>Evaluation of total complement system activity and generation of C5a. Measurement of cytokines or chemokines from blood, or fluid isolated from specific sites or from cells</li><li>Rebuck skin window</li><li>Directed or random migration with Boyden chamber or agarose assays using C5a, fMLP or other chemokines or chemoattractants</li></ul>	<ul><li>Modified systems based on double well diffusion with endothelial cells alone or in combination with subendothelial barrier</li><li>Fluorescent assays documenting actin assembly</li><li>Immunofluorescent evaluation of receptors and cell surface constituents</li><li>Direct measurement of actin, actin binding proteins and other proteins involved in motility</li></ul>
Ingestion	<ul><li>Serum opsonizing activity and screening studies of complement (see above)</li><li>Direct observation of tissues or blood smears</li><li>Microscopic observations of neutrophils or monocytes in bactericidal activity assay: quantify number of bacteria ingested per cell or percentage of cells which have ingested bacteria</li><li>Oil red O dye ingestion</li></ul>	<ul><li>Ingestion of radiolabeled microorganisms or other particulate stimulae</li><li>Direct evaluation of Fc, fMLP, C3b receptors with immunofluorescent or radiolabeled ligands</li><li>Direct measurement of O_2 consumption, O_2 production, generation of H_2O_2, other toxic oxygen metabolites, HMP shunt activity or chemiluminescence</li></ul>
Killing/degranulation	<ul><li>Bactericidal or candidicidal activity: direct measurement of viable microbes over time</li><li>NBT dye reduction (histochemical)</li><li>Dihydrorhodamine oxidation (flow cytometry)</li></ul>	<ul><li>Measurement of oxidase activity in plasma membrane from activated cells</li><li>Measurement of oxidase activity in SDS cell-free system to evaluate cytosol and membrane contributions</li><li>Quantitation of oxidase components by activity, Western blot assay with specific antibodies and spectral analysis (cytochrome b_{558})</li><li>Total content of various granule constituents (e.g. lysozyme, myeloperoxidase, lactoferrin, elastase, β-glucororidase)</li><li>Release of granule constituents in response to various stimuli</li><li>Direct evaluation of receptors required for activation of respiratory burst (fMLP, Fc, etc.)</li><li>Cytocydal effects of activated leukocytes on endothelial or cultured cells</li></ul>
Signal transduction	—	<ul><li>Changes in cytosolic Ca^{2+} concentration after stimulation</li><li>Levels of inositide phosphates</li><li>Activity of phospholipase A, C and D</li><li>Protein phosphorylation (serine/threonine and tyrosine)</li><li>Quantitation and activation of specific signal molecules or pathways (e.g. small GTPases, Rho, Rac; p38, p42/44 MAPK; PKC, etc.)</li></ul>
Miscellaneous biochemical	—	<ul><li>Levels of superoxide dismutase, catalase</li><li>Activity of glutathione system</li><li>Activity of glycolytic pathway</li></ul>

Adapted from Peterson, V.M., and Ambruso, D.R. (1994). Phagocyte production and function following burn injury. Austin: RG Landes Company, p. 68.

ELISA, flow cytometric and other approaches (de Jager et al., 2003; Kellar and Douglass, 2003). Measurement of levels in blood, tissue, inflammatory fluids as well as cell lysates can be completed. Assays can also be performed on purified cell populations incubated under a variety of stimulatory conditions with cell, tissue, organ or whole animal systems. Because structure, sequence and genetic information is available for most if not all of the biologically active compounds, gene expression can be determined as well. This is not only true for the biologically active molecules but also for their cognate receptors. A profile of gene expression, intracellular and extracellular levels can be obtained in a variety of models. Furthermore, knockout animals with specific deficiency of protein or receptor are available to confirm the significance of a specific compound or receptor.

IN VIVO STUDIES OF INFLAMMATION: THE REBUCK WINDOW

In 1955, the Rebuck skin window was introduced to study the kinetics of the cellular phase of inflammation (Rebuck, 1983). Utilizing adherence of leukocytes to sterile glass coverslips applied to superficially abraded areas of skin, direct visualization of leukocytes moving into the site may be completed over time. These studies provide insight into the sequential emigration of cells into an area of inflammation. Because this method is qualitative and detects only adherent cells, additional approaches have been developed using blisters or skin chambers (Boggs et al., 1964; Mass et al., 1975). These techniques have been used to determine abnormalities in phagocyte migration in a variety of congenital and acquired disorders of phagocyte function including specific granule deficiency, hyper IgE syndrome, Becket's syndrome, leukocyte adhesion deficiency, the newborn, burn patients, cancer patients, neutropenias and others (McCabe et al., 1973; Miler et al., 1979; Deinard et al., 1980; Gallin et al., 1982; Israel et al., 1982; Soderberg-Warner et al., 1983; Djawari et al., 1985; Zimmerli & Gallin, 1987; Bedlow et al., 1998). The major drawback to these studies is the semi-quantitative nature of the data obtained and incomplete agreement among the various in vivo assays and in vitro motility assays.

Similar information may be obtained from a variety of animal models and human disease by evaluation of the morphologic features of leukocytes in peripheral blood and inflammatory sites. The relative absence of a cell type suggests decreased production or an inability to emigrate into the area. The presence of antibodies specific for well-defined leukocyte antigens may aid in the identification of specific subpopulations of leukocytes. Abnormalities may compel a more thorough investigation of adherence, motility and emigration. The presence of appropriate numbers and types of cells as an appropriate response may suggest an inability of mechanisms meant to destroy microbes or toxic substances. An excessive number of cells could suggest failure of programmed cell death. All of these processes may be further evaluated with cell based in vitro assays.

IN VITRO ASSAYS OF CELL FUNCTION

Specific activities of neutrophils, monocytes or other cell types can be assessed by in vitro functional or biochemical analysis of cells isolated and/or purified from the site of inflammation or the peripheral blood (see Table 36.3). These can be organized according to the functional characteristics of phagocytic cells including adherence, chemotaxis, ingestion and killing or degranulation (Ambruso, 1994). A summary of commonly used measures of phagocyte function is provided in Table 36.3. The biochemical processes or pathways supporting the functional activities may be investigated including analysis of the receptors and associated signaling pathways. This will provide a profile of the biologic mechanisms critical to the inflammatory response.

SUMMARY

The process of inflammation is complicated and includes the generation of multiple humoral mediators as well as the response to a variety of leukocytes, most significantly, the phagocytic cells including neutrophils and monocytes. In vitro and in vivo assessment of these mechanisms will help elucidate the critical physiologic and biochemical events of this process. Understanding inflammation will clarify mechanisms associated with disease states and suggest therapeutic strategies to improve the body's ability to defend itself from microbes or noxious substances.

REFERENCES

Allen, W.E., Jones, G.E., Pollard, J.W. and Ridley, A.J. (1997). Rho, Rac and Cdc42 regulate actin organization and cell adhesion in macrophages. J Cell Sci 110, 707–720.

Ambruso, D.R. (1994). Phagocyte function. In Phagocyte production and function following burn injury, Peterson, V.A. and Ambruso, D.R., ed. Austin, TX: R.G. Landes Company, pp. 60–92.

Ambruso, D.R., Bolscher, B.G., Stokman, P.M., Verhoeven, A.J. and Roos, D. (1990). Assembly and activation of the NADPH:O2 oxidoreductase in human neutrophils after stimulation with phorbol myristate acetate. J Biol Chem 265, 924–930.

Ambruso, D.R. and Johnston, R.B. (1998). Chronic granulomatous disease of childhood. In Kendig's disorders of the respiratory tract in children, Chernick, V. and Boat, T.F., eds. Phildelphia, PA: W.B. Saunders Company, pp. 1107–1117.

Ambruso, D.R., Knall, C., Abell, A.N. et al. (2000). Human neutrophil immunodeficiency syndrome is associated with an inhibitory Rac2 mutation. Proc Natl Acad Sci USA 97, 4654–4659.

Baggiolini, M. (1998). Chemokines and leukocyte traffic. Nature 392, 565–568.

Baggiolini, M., Walz, A. and Kunkel, S.L. (1989). Neutrophil-activating peptide-1/interleukin 8, a novel cytokine that activates neutrophils. J Clin Invest 84, 1045–1049.

Bedlow, A.J., Davies, E.G., Moss, A.L., Rebuck, N., Finn, A. and Marsden, R.A. (1998). Pyoderma gangrenosum in a child with congenital partial deficiency of leucocyte adherence glycoproteins. Br J Dermatol 139, 1064–1067.

Berger, M., O'Shea, J., Cross, A.S. et al. (1984). Human neutrophils increase expression of C3bi as well as C3b receptors upon activation. J Clin Invest 74, 1566–1571.

Boggs, D.R., Athens, J.W., Cartwright, G.E. and Wintrobe, M.M. (1964). The effect of adrenal glucocorticosteroids upon the cellular composition of inflammatory exudates. Am J Pathol 44, 763–773.

Bokoch, G.M. (1995). Chemoattractant signaling and leukocyte activation. Blood 86, 1649–1660.

Borregaard, N. and Cowland, J.B. (1997). Granules of the human neutrophilic polymorphonuclear leukocyte. Blood 89, 3503–3521.

Bourne, H.R., Sanders, D.A. and McCormick, F. (1991). The GTPase superfamily: conserved structure and molecular mechanism. Nature 349, 117–127.

Clark, R.A., Volpp, B.D., Leidal, K.G. and Nauseef, W.M. (1990). Two cytosolic components of the human neutrophil respiratory burst oxidase translocate to the plasma membrane during cell activation. J Clin Invest 85, 714–721.

Coso, O.A., Chiariello, M., Yu, J.C. et al. (1995). The small GTP-binding proteins Rac1 and Cdc42 regulate the activity of the JNK/SAPK signaling pathway. Cell 81, 1137–1146.

Cox, D., Chang, P., Zhang, Q., Reddy, P.G., Bokoch, G.M. and Greenberg, S. (1997). Requirements for both Rac1 and Cdc42 in membrane ruffling and phagocytosis in leukocytes. J Exp Med 186, 1487–1494.

de Jager, W., te, V.H., Prakken, B.J., Kuis, W. and Rijkers, G.T. (2003). Simultaneous detection of 15 human cytokines in a single sample of stimulated peripheral blood mononuclear cells. Clin Diagn Lab Immunol 10, 133–139.

Deinard, A.S., Geehan, G., Page, A.R. and Holmes, B. (1980). Function studies of monocytes from patients with cyclic neutropenia. Am J Pediatr Hematol Oncol 2, 201–206.

Didsbury, J., Weber, R.F., Bokoch, G.M., Evans, T. and Snyderman, R. (1989). rac, a novel ras-related family of proteins that are botulinum toxin substrates. J Biol Chem 264, 16378–16382.

Dinarello, C.A. (1996). Cytokines as mediators in the pathogenesis of septic shock. Curr Top Microbiol Immunol 216, 133–165.

Dinarello, C.A. and Moldawer, L.L. (2000). Proinflammatory and anti-inflammatory cytokines in rheumatoid arthritis: a primer for clinicians. Thousand Oaks, CA: Amgen, Inc.

Dinarello, C.A. and Wolff, S.M. (1993). The role of interleukin-1 in disease. N Engl J Med 328, 106–113.

Dinauer, M.C. (2003). The phagocyte system and disorders of granuloparesis and granulocyte function. In Nathan and Oski's Hematology of Infancy and Childhood, 6th edn, Nathan, D.G., Orkin, S.H., Ginsburg, D. and Look, A.T., eds. Philadelphia, PA: W.B. Saunders, pp. 938–945.

Djawari, D., Hornstein, O.P. and Luckner, L. (1985). Skin window examination according to Rebuck and cutaneous pathergy tests in patients with Behcet's disease. Dermatologica 170, 265–270.

el Benna, J., Ruedi, J.M. and Babior, B.M. (1994). Cytosolic guanine nucleotide-binding protein Rac2 operates in vivo as a component of the neutrophil respiratory burst oxidase. Transfer of Rac2 and the cytosolic oxidase components p47phox and p67phox to the submembranous actin cytoskeleton during oxidase activation. J Biol Chem 269, 6729–6734.

Foxall, C., Watson, S.R., Dowbenko, D. et al. (1992). The three members of the selectin receptor family recognize a common carbohydrate epitope, the sialyl Lewis(x) oligosaccharide. J Cell Biol 117, 895–902.

Gabay, C. and Kushner, I. (1999). Acute-phase proteins and other systemic responses to inflammation. N Engl J Med 340, 448–454.

Gallin, J.I., Fletcher, M.P., Seligmann, B.E., Hoffstein, S., Cehrs, K. and Mounessa, N. (1982). Human neutrophil-specific granule deficiency: a model to assess the role of neutrophil-specific granules in the evolution of the inflammatory response. Blood 59, 1317–1329.

Geijsen, N., van Delft, S., Raaijmakers, J.A. et al. (1999). Regulation of p21rac activation in human neutrophils. Blood 94, 1121–1130.

Glogauer, M., Hartwig, J. and Stossel, T. (2000). Two pathways through Cdc42 couple the N-formyl receptor to actin nucleation in permeabilized human neutrophils. J Cell Biol 150, 785–796.

Hall, A. (1998). Rho GTPases and the actin cytoskeleton. Science 279, 509–514.

Harlan, J.M., Winn, R.K., Vedder, N.B., Doershick, C.M. and Rice, C.L. (1992). In vivo models of leukocyte adherence. In Adhesion: its role in inflammatory diseases, Harlan, J.M. and Liu, E., eds. New York: W.H.Freeman Company, pp. 151–182.

Heyworth, P.G., Bohl, B.P., Bokoch, G.M. and Curnutte, J.T. (1994). Rac translocates independently of the neutrophil NADPH oxidase components p47phox and p67phox. Evidence for its interaction with flavocytochrome b558. J Biol Chem 269, 30749–30752.

Hill, C.S., Wynne, J. and Treisman, R. (1995). The Rho family GTPases RhoA, Rac1, and CDC42Hs regulate transcriptional activation by SRF. Cell 81, 1159–1170.

Hill, H.R. (1993). Modulation of host defenses with interferon-gamma in pediatrics. J Infect Dis 167 Suppl 1. S23–S28.

Hotchin, N.A. and Hall, A. (1996). Regulation of the actin cytoskeleton, integrins and cell growth by the Rho family of small GTPases. Cancer Surv 27, 311–322.

Huizinga, T.W., Roos, D. and dem Borne, A.E. (1990). Neutrophil Fc-gamma receptors: a two-way bridge in the immune system. Blood 75, 1211–1214.

Israel, L., Samak, R., Edelstein, R., Amouroux, J., Battesti, J.P. and de Saint, F.G. (1982). In vivo nonspecific macrophage chemotaxis in cancer patients and its correlation with extent of disease, regional lymph node status, and disease-free survival. Cancer Res 42, 2489–2494.

Kansas, G.S., Ley, K., Munro, J.M. and Tedder, T.F. (1993). Regulation of leukocyte rolling and adhesion to high endothelial venules through the cytoplasmic domain of L-selectin. J Exp Med 177, 833–838.

Kellar, K.L. and Douglass, J.P. (2003). Multiplexed microsphere-based flow cytometric immunoassays for human cytokines. J Immunol Methods 279, 277–285.

Kjoller, L. and Hall, A. (1999). Signaling to Rho GTPases. Exp Cell Res *253*, 166–179.

Kulkarni, A.B., Huh, C.G., Becker, D. et al. (1993). Transforming growth factor beta 1 null mutation in mice causes excessive inflammatory response and early death. Proc Natl Acad Sci USA *90*, 770–774.

Locati, M. and Murphy, P.M. (1999). Chemokines and chemokine receptors: biology and clinical relevance in inflammation and AIDS. Annu Rev Med *50*, 425–440.

Lowenstein, C.J. and Snyder, S.H. (1992). Nitric oxide, a novel biologic messenger. Cell *70*, 705–707.

Mackay, D.J. and Hall, A. (1998). Rho GTPases. J Biol Chem *273*, 20685–20688.

Majino, G. (1975). The healing hand: man and wound in the ancient world. Cambridge, MA: Harvard University Press.

Mass, M.F., Dean, P.B., Weston, W.L. and Humbert, J.R. (1975). Leukocyte migration in vivo: a new method of study. J Lab Clin Med *86*, 1040–1046.

McCabe, W.P., Rebuck, J.W., Kelly, A.P. Jr and Ditmars, D.M. Jr (1973). Leukocytic response as a monitor of immunodepression in burn patients. Arch Surg *106*, 155–159.

Metchnikov, I. (1968). Immunity in infective disease. In Comparative pathology of inflammation, Starling F.A. and Starling, E.H., eds. New York: Dover, p. 244.

Miler, I., Holub, M., Vondracek, J., Jouja, V. and Hromadkova, L. (1979). Skin-window study on the migration of leukocytes of newborns and infants. Folia Microbiol (Praha) *24*, 408–414.

Minden, A., Lin, A., Claret, F.X., Abo, A. and Karin, M. (1995). Selective activation of the JNK signaling cascade and c-Jun transcriptional activity by the small GTPases Rac and Cdc42Hs. Cell *81*, 1147–1157.

Moore, K.W., O'Garra, A., de Waal, M.R., Vieira, P. and Mosmann, T.R. (1993). Interleukin-10. Annu Rev Immunol *11*, 165–190.

Murphy, P.M. (1994). The molecular biology of leukocyte chemoattractant receptors. Annu Rev Immunol *12*, 593–633.

Nathan, C. (1992). Nitric oxide as a secretory product of mammalian cells. FASEB J *6*, 3051–3064.

Nisimoto, Y., Freeman, J.L., Motalebi, S.A., Hirshberg, M. and Lambeth, J.D. (1997). Rac binding to p67(phox). Structural basis for interactions of the Rac1 effector region and insert region with components of the respiratory burst oxidase. J Biol Chem *272*, 18834–18841.

Nobes, C.D. and Hall, A. (1995). Rho, rac, and cdc42 GTPases regulate the assembly of multimolecular focal complexes associated with actin stress fibers, lamellipodia, and filopodia. Cell *81*, 53–62.

Oppenheim, J.J., Zachariae, C.O., Mukaida, N. and Matsushima, K. (1991). Properties of the novel proinflammatory supergene 'intercrine' cytokine family. Annu Rev Immunol *9*, 617–648.

Park, J.W., Ma, M., Ruedi, J.M., Smith, R.M. and Babior, B.M. (1992). The cytosolic components of the respiratory burst oxidase exist as a M(r) approximately 240 000 complex that acquires a membrane-binding site during activation of the oxidase in a cell-free system. J Biol Chem *267*, 17327–17332.

Peterson, V.M. and Ambruso, D.R. (1994). Phagocyte production and function following burn injury. Austin: RG Landes Company.

Prescott, S.M., Zimmerman, G.A., Stafforini, D.M. and McIntyre, T.M. (2000). Platelet-activating factor and related lipid mediators. Annu Rev Biochem *69*, 419–445.

Quinn, M.T., Evans, T., Loetterle, L.R., Jesaitis, A.J. and Bokoch, G.M. (1993). Translocation of Rac correlates with NADPH oxidase activation. Evidence for equimolar translocation of oxidase components. J Biol Chem *268*, 20983–20987.

Rebollo, A. and Martinez, A. (1999). Ras proteins: recent advances and new functions. Blood *94*, 2971–2980.

Rebuck, J.W. (1983). The skin window as a monitor of leukocytic functions in contact activation factor deficiencies in man. Am J Clin Pathol *79*, 405–413.

Ridley, A.J. (1996). Rho: theme and variations. Curr Biol *6*, 1256–1264.

Rollins, B.J., Walz, A. and Baggiolini, M. (1991). Recombinant human MCP-1/JE induces chemotaxis, calcium flux, and the respiratory burst in human monocytes. Blood *78*, 1112–1116.

Rotrosen, D. and Leto, T.L. (1990). Phosphorylation of neutrophil 47-kDa cytosolic oxidase factor. Translocation to membrane is associated with distinct phosphorylation events. J Biol Chem *265*, 19910–19915.

Rubin, E. and Faber, J.L. (eds) (1990). Essential pathology. Philadelphia, PA: Lippincott.

Schall, T.J., Bacon, K., Toy, K.J. and Goeddel, D.V. (1990). Selective attraction of monocytes and T lymphocytes of the memory phenotype by cytokine RANTES. Nature *347*, 669–671.

Serhan, C.N. (1994). Eicosanoids in leukocyte function. Curr Opin Hematol *1*, 69–77.

Sharma, J.N. (1992). Involvement of the kinin-forming system in the physiopathology of rheumatoid inflammation. Agents Actions Suppl 38, 343–361.

Soderberg-Warner, M., Rice-Mendoza, C.A., Mendoza, G.R. and Stiehm, E.R. (1983). Neutrophil and T lymphocyte characteristics of two patients with hyper-IgE syndrome. Pediatr Res *17*, 820–824.

Springer, T.A. (1990). Adhesion receptors of the immune system. Nature *346*, 425–434.

Strieter, R.M. and Kunkel, S.L. (1994). Acute lung injury: the role of cytokines in the elicitation of neutrophils. J Invest Med *42*, 640–651.

Unkeless, J.C. (1989). Function and heterogeneity of human Fc receptors for immunoglobulin G. J Clin Invest *83*, 355–361.

Van Aelst, L. and D'Souza-Schorey, C. (1997). Rho GTPases and signaling networks. Genes Dev *11*, 2295–2322.

Vaporciyan, A.A. and Ward, P.A. (1995). The inflammatory response. In Williams Hematology, Beutler, E., Lichtman, M.A., Coller, B.S. and Kipps, T.J., eds. New York: McGraw Hill, Inc., pp. 48–57.

Walz, A. and Baggiolini, M. (1990). Generation of the neutrophil-activating peptide NAP-2 from platelet basic protein or connective tissue-activating peptide III through monocyte proteases. J Exp Med *171*, 449–454.

Zimmerli, W. and Gallin, J.I. (1987). Monocytes accumulate on Rebuck skin window coverslips but not in skin chamber fluid. A comparative evaluation of two in vivo migration models. J Immunol Methods *96*, 11–17.

Zimmerman, G.A., Prescott, S.M. and McIntyre, T.M. (1992). Endothelial cell interactions with granulocytes: tethering and signaling molecules. Immunol Today *13*, 93–100.

Zlotnik, A. and Yoshie, O. (2000). Chemokines: a new classification system and their role in immunity. Immunity *12*, 121–127.

The Vascular and Coagulation Systems

Chapter 37

Franklin A. Bontempo

University of Pittsburgh School of Medicine, Pittsburgh, PA, USA

There's a good time coming, boys! A good time coming.
Charles Mackay, The Good Time Coming

INTRODUCTION

The vascular system, while not particularly associated with immunogenicity, is the conduit for the mediators of immunity and is a common site of immunologic attack. The vascular system includes the vessel wall, the endothelium and the vascular contents including the white blood cells, red blood cells (RBCs), platelets, macrophages, complement, cytokines, immunoglobulins, coagulation mediators and other plasma proteins. It consists of the arteries, arterioles, capillaries, veins, venous sinuses and venules with fenestrations allowing the passage of polymorphonuclear leukocytes and lymphocytes to sites of disease and with the capability of modulation of capacitance through vasoconstriction and dilatation. In the steady state approximately 79 per cent of the blood volume is contained in the systemic circulation with 59 per cent in the veins, 15 per cent in the arteries and only 5 per cent in the capillaries; 12 per cent is contained in the pulmonary vessels and the remaining 9 per cent is contained in the heart (Guyton, 1971).

Despite this, the cross-sectional areas of the various vessels, if summed, are as follows:

Aorta	2.5 cm^2
Small arteries	20 cm^2
Arterioles	40 cm^2
Capillaries	2500 cm^2
Venules	250 cm^2
Small veins	80 cm^2
Venae cavae	8 cm^2

with the large cross-sectional area of the capillaries allowing for the exchange of nutrients with the tissues.

THE COAGULATION SYSTEM

The coagulation system consists of three lines of defense in the maintenance of the integrity of the vascular system: the vessel wall, the platelets and the coagulation factors. The vessel wall plays an important role in the integrity of the vasculature because of its collagen-containing basement membrane which, when breached, functions as an activator of platelets. In addition, the vascular wall endothelial cells produce and/or contain the coagulation proteins prostacyclin, plasminogen activator, plasminogen activator inhibitor-1, thrombomodulin, tissue factor pathway inhibitor and von Willebrand's factor and exert an important regulatory function on the clotting cascade external to the liver, which is the site of production of most clotting proteins. The clotting cascade functions to form a stable fibrin clot after activation at several possible points which enables it to maintain the integrity of a vessel wall if breached and platelet interaction with the clotting cascade enhances the clotting function. Both the platelets and the clotting cascade may be a site of immunologic

Measuring Immunity, edited by Michael T. Lotze and Angus W. Thomson
ISBN 0-12-455900-X, London

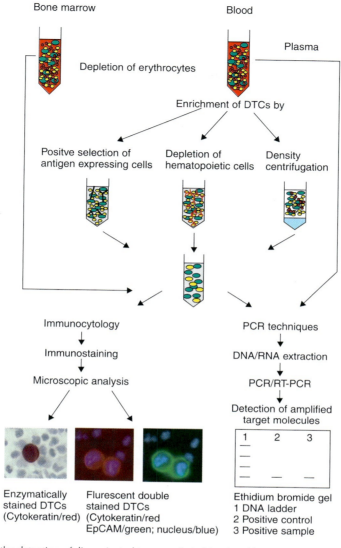

Bone marrow

Blood

Plasma

Depletion of erythrocytes

Enrichment of DTCs by

Positve selection of antigen expressing cells

Depletion of hematopoietic cells

Density centrifugation

Immunocytology

PCR techniques

Immunostaining

DNA/RNA extraction

Microscopic analysis

PCR/RT-PCR

Detection of amplified target molecules

Enzymatically stained DTCs (Cytokeratin/red)

Flurescent double stained DTCs (Cytokeratin/red EpCAM/green; nucleus/blue)

Ethidium bromide gel
1 DNA ladder
2 Positive control
3 Positive sample

Figure 26.1 Illustration of methods for the detection of disseminated tumor cells in blood and bone marrow.

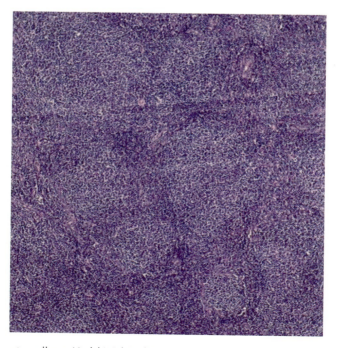

Figure 41.2 H&E section of a follicular center cell non-Hodgkin's lymphoma.

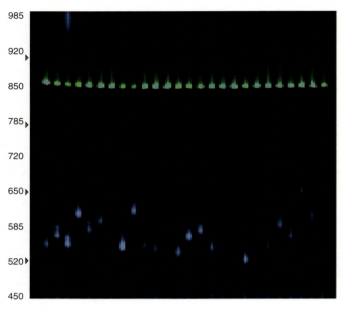

Figure 43.2 Photograph of the computer screen displaying a gel of peripheral blood lymphocytes from a type 1 diabetic child subjected to TCR Vβ-specific amplification. The fluorescent blue PCR products corresponding to Vβ gene families 1-24 were electrophoresed on a 16-cm, 5 per cent polyacrylamide non-denaturing gel for 1 h on an ABI 377 DNA Sequencer and automatically analyzed by GeneScan software. As internal control, a portion of the Cα region of the TCR is also amplified by using primers labeled with a different dye (6-TET), which originate green bands. The relative abundance of T cells carrying each Vβ chain transcript is estimated by calculating a ratio of Vβ fluorescent and Cα fluorescent areas for each Vβ gene family.

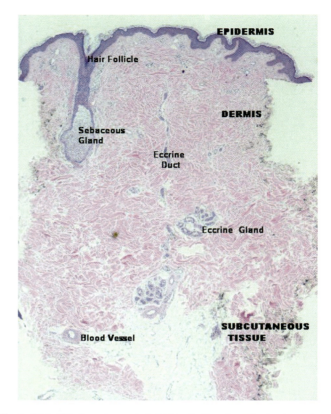

Figure 53.1 Skin is composed of epidermis, dermis and subcutaneous tissue. (Courtesy of Drs P.M. Manolson and T.L. Barrett, Johns Hopkins.)

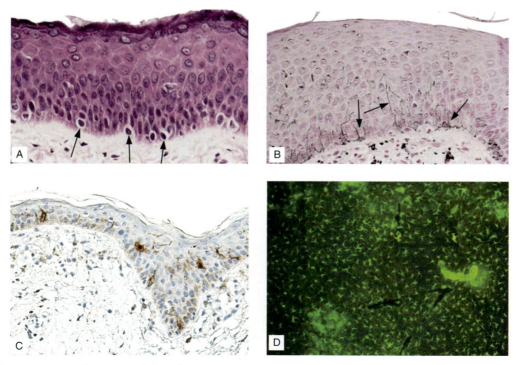

Figure 53.2 (A) Melanocytes (arrowed). (C) Langerhans cells express CD1a protein. (D) Immunofluorescence staining for HLA-DR in an epidermal sheet. (Courtesy of Drs P.M. Manolson and T.L. Barrett, Johns Hopkins (A–C) and N. Romani, University of Innsbruck, Austria (D).)

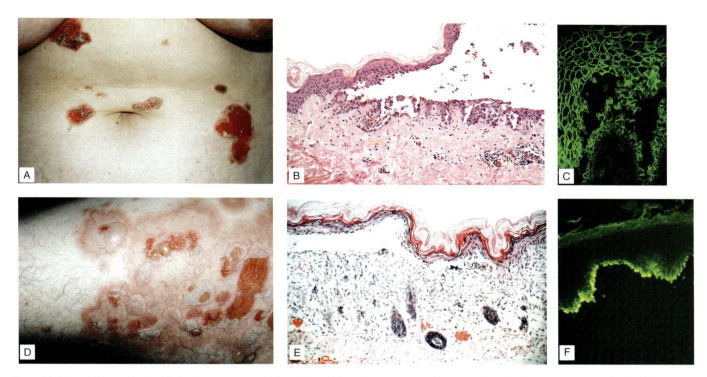

Figure 53.3 Pemphigus vulgaris. (A) Bullae occur intraepidermally and therefore rupture easily, leaving denuded erosions. (B) Suprabasilar blistering. (C) Direct immunofluorescence demonstrates IgG in the intracellular regions of the epidermis. Bullous pemphigoid. (D) Bullae occur on erythematous patches and urticarial plaques. (E) Subepidermal blistering. (F) Direct immunofluorescence staining shows linear deposit of IgG and complement at the dermal-epidermal junction. (Courtesy of Dr G.J. Anhalt, Johns Hopkins.)

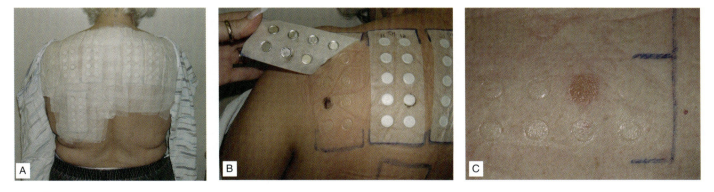

Figure 53.4 Patch testing. (A) Test materials are applied to the skin under occlusive patches. (B) that are removed after 48 h. (C) +2 reaction.

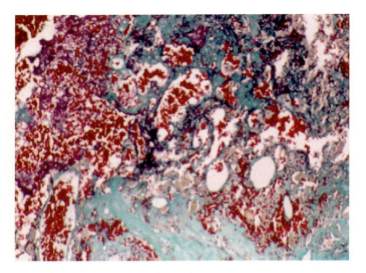

Figure 54.1 Unstable carotid plaque.

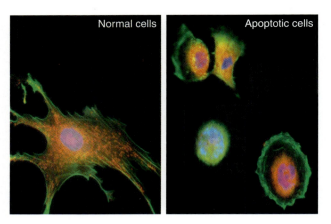

Figure 58.5 Multiple apoptosis analysis. F-actin appears in green, nuclei in blue and mitochondria in red.

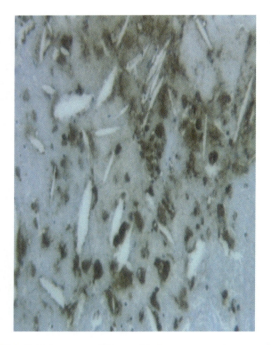

Figure 54.2 Cells in an unstable carotid plaque: macrophages and T lymphocytes.

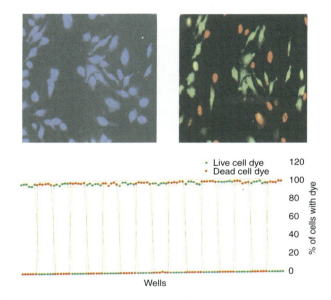

Figure 58.6 Cell viability assay by ArrayScan II.

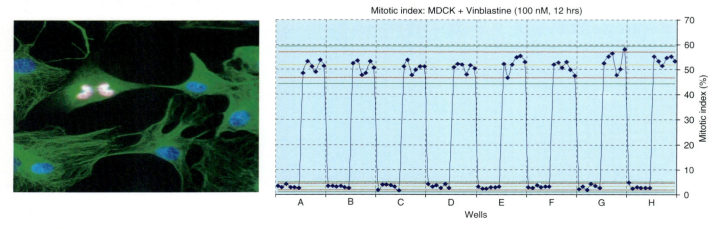

Figure 58.7 Mitotic index to quantify curacin A antimitotic effect.

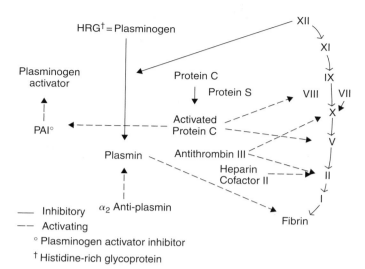

HRG† = Plasminogen

Plasminogen activator

PAI°

Plasmin

α₂ Anti-plasmin

Protein C

Protein S

Activated Protein C

Antithrombin III

Heparin Cofactor II

XII

XI

IX

VIII   VII

X

V

II

I

Fibrin

—— Inhibitory

-- Activating

° Plasminogen activator inhibitor

† Histidine-rich glycoprotein

Figure 37.1 Coagulation cascade. The role of inhibitory and activating molecules in the coagulation cascade is shown. Multiple steps are susceptible to inhibition or enhancement in the setting of both acute and chronic inflammation.

attack. A basic schematic diagram of the clotting cascade and fibrinolytic system is shown in Figure 37.1 with factor II being thrombin and factor I being fibrinogen.

TESTING OF THE VASCULAR AND COAGULATION SYSTEMS

Measurements of immunity involving the vascular and coagulation systems may be either direct or indirect. Direct tests measure immunologic markers such as immunoglobulins or antigenic proteins but many indirect tests measure the residual effects of immunologic attack on the vascular or coagulation systems with markers, which are not specifically immunologic in themselves. Some of the testing useful in analysis of the vascular and coagulation systems is similar to that used in clinical rheumatologic disorders in general which is covered in greater detail elsewhere in this volume. Testing in this section will focus on that which is particularly useful in immunologic disorders of the vascular and coagulation systems.

Testing for immunity to platelets and capillaries

Bleeding and closure times

The bleeding time is a general measure of the clotting function of all three major parts of the clotting system and may also be affected by damage or dysfunction of the microvasculature, however, it is primarily a measure of platelet function. If platelet function is normal, it begins to become prolonged when the platelet count falls to 50 000–75 000 due to the inability of that lowered number of platelets to maintain adequate hemostasis in response

to trauma. At levels <10 000, petechiae may occur due to passage of red blood cells into the skin near the capillary walls. If platelet function is abnormal, bleeding times may be prolonged at any platelet number. Historically, bleeding times have been devised on ear lobes, the skin of the index finger and the skin of the forearm, with the latter having the widest acceptance because of its better reproducibility due to the use of a spring-loaded lancet making a standardized 5 mm long, 1 mm deep cut in the skin. The skin is wiped clear and filter paper is used to dab the site every 30 seconds until bleeding is stopped. The number of dabs is then divided by two to determine the number of minutes of the bleeding time. Bleeding times have limitations in that their reproducibility is sometimes variable due to cutting of variable-sized capillaries, the effect of various skin disorders, age-related differences in skin thickness and the experience of the technician. Their utility is also limited by the need for a technician to be available on demand and to present at the bedside or clinic.

Because of these limitations, bleeding times are beginning to be replaced in some centers by the closure time (Kundu et al, 1995), which is essentially an automated bleeding time done in the laboratory. In the closure time whole blood is passed through a standardized capillary tube and platelets are stimulated by both collagen/epinephrine and collagen/ADP and the number of seconds required to clot the capillary tube is measured with each in an attempt to mimic what is measured by the bleeding time in the skin. Differences in closure time with one stimulant versus the another may have an advantage in determining if a platelet defect is due to aspirin or non-steroidal anti-inflammatory drugs and may more specifically identify defects due to other disorders compared with the bleeding time. Because a standardized *in vitro* system is used with the closure time, its reproducibility is probably better than the bleeding time.

Bleeding or closure times may have utility in measuring immunity in immune thrombocytopenic purpura, where they may be prolonged with a falling platelet count or occasionally in patients with immune-mediated capillary dysfunction. They are unlikely to be diagnostic in either of these types of disorders but may be beneficial in determining the overall platelet function and the need to transfuse with platelets in order to keep either time in the normal range.

Heparin-induced thrombocytopenia testing

Heparin-induced thrombocytopenia (HIT) (Warkentin et al, 2001) is an immune-mediated cause of thrombocytopenia which occurs in up to 4–5 per cent of patients who receive standard unfractionated heparin and probably 1–2 per cent of patients who receive low molecular weight heparins. Typically, thrombocytopenia in the first 10–14 (Kunicki et al, 1987) after the first dose of heparin may be the only manifestation but up to 50 per cent of patients may develop serious thrombotic complications, which may be life threatening. Recognition of HIT is important to prevent the latter from occurring by discontinuing heparin and/or switching to an alternate anticoagulant. In the HIT syndrome, patients develop antibodies against the heparin-platelet factor 4 complex on the surface of the platelet which leads to cross-linking of platelets and a cycle of platelet activation which leads to thrombosis. While clinical recognition of HIT is of primary importance, laboratory testing usually serves at least an adjunctive role in making the diagnosis.

Tests that are used for making a diagnosis of HIT include:

1 Heparin platelet antibody by aggregation method. This test measures the presence of antibodies against the heparin-platelet factor 4 complex on the surface of the platelet after exposure to unfractionated or low-molecular weight heparins. Testing is done in a platelet aggregometer and measures platelet aggregation in response to the addition of heparin which is not normally an aggregating agent. The clinical utility of this test is limited by the relatively low sensitivity of most formulations of this test for the presence of HIT.
2 Platelet factor 4 enzyme immunoassay. Several variations of antigenic assays intended to measure binding of specific antibody to the platelet factor 4–heparin complex exist. These may be solid phase or fluid phase but the target antigen for both is the platelet factor 4 heparin complex. These antigenic assays tend to have a lower specificity but a higher sensitivity than the HIT tests by the aggregation method, i.e. there may be a high false positive rate. Some laboratories recommend using both an antigenic test along with an aggregation test on patients with suspected HIT due to the high clinical significance of a correct diagnosis, particularly with the availablility of newer anticoagulants for treatment of HIT or when urgent cardiac bypass is being considered.
3 Serotonin release assay. The serotonin release assay quantitates the release of ^{14}C-radiolabeled serotonin from the dense granules of activated platelets in patients with HIT. Studies suggest that the serotonin release assay has the highest sensitivity and specificity for making a diagnosis of HIT but this assay has had limited availability in the USA because of the requirement for radiolabeling and because it is labor intensive, costly and difficult to perform on demand for a disorder where a rapid diagnosis is often essential.

Strong controversy Kottke-Marchant et al (2003) exists regarding the relative accuracy of a laboratory compared with a clinical diagnosis of HIT but the need for a correct diagnosis remains important due to the serious clinical consequences from this disorder. In addition, accuracy in the diagnosis of HIT is the source of a high degree of anxiety among clinicians due to the frequent occurrence of legal actions related to its recognition and management.

PI^{A1} antibody

In the USA, 98 per cent of the population expresses the PI^{A1} antigen (Kunicki et al, 1987) on the surface of platelets with a slightly higher incidence in African-Americans compared with Caucasians. Standard serologic typing of platelets for this antibody may be beneficial in thrombocytopenia patients in specific clinical situations. In particular, in pregnant mothers who are PI^{A1} negative with fathers who are PI^{A1} positive, the syndrome of neonatal alloimmune thrombocytopenic purpura (NATP) may occur, which is an incompatibility analogous in platelets to the mechanism of Rh incompatibility and hemolysis of the RBCs. Babies with NATP, often first born, develop thrombocytopenia <50 000 in the neonatal period due to placental transmission of maternal alloantibodies against PI^{A1}. This syndrome is associated with more hemorrhagic complications in infants than are seen in infants born to mothers with idiopathic thrombocytopenic purpura (ITP). Subsequent pregnancies with the same parents may have similar risks to the first. Accurate identification is beneficial since the usual treatment of the thrombocytopenic infant with NATP is to raise the infant's platelet count by transfusing the mother's PI^{A1} negative platelets into the neonate until the alloantibodies have fallen in titer, which commonly occurs during the first 1–2 weeks of life at which time the thrombocytopenia usually resolves.

A second use of the PI^{A1} antibody is in occasional, mostly PI^{A1} negative patients, more commonly women, who develop thrombocytopenia approximately 1 week after transfusion of RBCs or plasma due to the rare and poorly understood syndrome (Nijjar et al, 1987 and Mueller-Eckhard et al, 1991) of post-transfusion purpura (PTP). These patients are also most commonly, but not exclusively, positive for the PI^{A1} antibodies. The pathogenesis of this syndrome is obscure but seems to be that transfused PI^{A1} antibodies cause platelet destruction and thrombocytopenia in the PI^{A1} negative recipient. The enigma is why antibodies should attack platelets which do not express the targeted antigen on the platelet surface. Patients with PTP may have prolonged and severe periods of bleeding which may be fatal, thrombocytopenia may persist for up to 6 months and anti-PI^{A1} antibodies may persist for as long as a year after diagnosis. The standard therapy is treatment with intravenous immunoglobulin, which is associated with a high response rate.

Platelet associated immunoglobulin G or M testing

The platelet associated IgG or IgM (PAIgG or PAIgM) tests are a group of different tests, which attempt to quantitate various antibodies on the surface of platelets to aid in the diagnosis of ITP. These tests use antigen capture techniques to detect antibodies on the surface of patient platelets or normal platelets exposed to the patient's plasma. While newer formulations of this test are an improvement over those developed previously, antibodies are not found in many patients with ITP and false positives tend to occur in numerous disorders. As a result many find their utility limited for making a diagnosis of ITP.

Testing for immunity of red blood cells

Direct antiglobulin test

The direct antiglobulin (Walker, 1990) test (DAT, direct Coombs' test) detects the presence of IgG or complement on the surface of the red blood cell (RBC) membrane. This is done by adding antiserum containing antibodies to complement and IgG to a patient's washed RBCs and evaluating for agglutination caused by bridging of previously sensitized red cell membranes. This test is useful in making a diagnosis of autoimmune hemolytic anemia, drug-induced hemolysis, hemolytic disease of the newborn and transfusion reactions.

Indirect antiglobulin test

The indirect antiglobulin (Walker, 1990) test (IAT, indirect Coombs' test) enables the detection of autoantibodies in patient's serum. Normal RBCs are incubated with a patient's serum after which the RBCs are washed and antiserum as used in the DAT is added and the sample is read for the presence of agglutination also as in the DAT. The IAT may be useful in autoimmune hemolysis but may also recognize alloantibodies in serum from alloimmunization due to previous transfusion or maternal/fetal incompatibility.

Testing for immunity in the clotting cascade

Lupus anticoagulant testing

Lupus anticoagulants (LACs) are a heterogeneous group of antiphospholipid antibodies which may occur in 2–4 per cent of the US population and may be related to infection, malignancy, autoimmune disorders, thrombocytopenia, miscarriage and thrombosis. There is no single test which defines the presence of a lupus anticoagulant and consensus on what testing should be used for making a diagnosis does not exist. The general guidelines for making a diagnosis of a lupus anticoagulant are to demonstrate interference in the clotting cascade and further to demonstrate that the interference is phospholipid dependent. All testing essentially aims to manipulate phospholipid in the test system to demonstrate the presence of antibody against it or to measure directly specific antiphospholipid antibody immunologic types, which are numerous and vary in clinical significance. Specific tests (Triplett, 1990) which are frequently used include:

1 Activated partial thromboplastin time (APTT) mix. The phospholipid based activator of the APTT may be inhibited by the presence of an LAC causing persistent prolongation of the APTT after mixing with normal plasma. Unfortunately only about 60 per cent of patients with LACs have a both a prolonged APTT and APTT mix making the APTT mix unsuitable as a screening test.

2 Russell viper venom time. The Russell viper venom time (RVVT) uses a snake venom reagent which is also phospholipid based to stimulate the clotting cascade at the level of factor X. Failure to correct the RVVT with the addition of normal plasma is also suggestive of an LAC. A disadvantage of the RVVT is that it is probably less specific for the presence of an LAC than other tests and tends to be falsely positive in patients taking warfarin.

3 Hexagonal phase phospholipid neutralization. The hexagonal phase phospholipid neutralization tests for the ability of a highly specific type of phospholipid to cause correction of a long APTT when added to plasma from a patient suspected of having a lupus anticoagulant. The advantage of this test is its high specificity but its relatively low specificity for LACs (about 25 per cent) makes it unsuitable as a sole definitive test.

4 Tissue thromboplastin inhibition index (TTI). The tissue thromboplastin inhibition index tests for inhibition of the prothrombin time (PT) assay with increasing dilution of an activator of the PT in a patient with a suspected LAC compared to a control plasma. Exaggeration of the effect of dilution on the PT is suspicious for a lupus anticoagulant. Because of its dependence on a normal initial it is invalid in patients taking warfarin or with some other reason for a prolonged PT.

5 Anticardiolipin antibody. A direct measure of a specific type of antibody which may be IgG, IgA or IgM, thought to be associated with a higher incidence of thrombosis, particularly with the IgG type. The presence of an LAC or specific antiphospholipid antibody may have implications for the duration of anticoagulant therapy in a patient with a thrombotic event, may be a causative factor for thrombosis, miscarriage, stroke, or unexplained thrombocytopenia and may be related to the presence of an underlying autoimmune disorder.

Anti-factor VIII antibody

Both autoantibodies and alloantibodies may occur against the factor VIII molecule, which is the specific factor against which there are more antibodies than any other in the clotting cascade. Specific testing and titering of an anti-factor VIII antibody, measured in Bethesda units, may provide an answer for the cause of a low factor VIII level in a patient without a previous bleeding history in the case of an acquired autoantibody against factor VIII. Alloantibodies against factor VIII may occur in patients with hemophilia A who develop an immune response against transfused factor VIII which was previously given for bleeding. A rapid and specific diagnosis of an acquired antibody against factor VIII is necessary to prevent possible life-threatening hemorrhage which may develop in patients with these antibodies and the height of the antibody titer may have an impact on the type of therapy used in treating them. Unrecognized alloantibodies against factor VIII in hemophiliacs may lead to the failure of clotting factor concentrates to provide their expected clinical benefit after a clotting factor transfusion is used to stop bleeding or prevent bleeding at surgery.

Factor X

The factor X level may occasionally be depressed due to binding by amyloid protein in patients with amyloidosis who form specific types of amyloid protein (Choufani et al, 2001). The amyloid-protein complexes are subsequently removed from the circulation and the factor X level falls. This may help in the unrecognized diagnosis of amyloidosis and the low factor X level in this disorder may lead to hemorrhage, which may be treated by splenectomy.

Protein S

Acquired deficiencies of the natural anticoagulant protein S have been noted to occur transiently due to formation of autoantibodies in children with varicella infection and have been associated with thromboembolic disease (Pashankar et al, 1996). Prophylactic anticoagulation may therefore be beneficial in young patients who develop antibodies to protein S.

Factor II

Antibodies against factor II in the clotting cascade can occasionally be seen in patients with lupus anticoagulants (Baca et al, 2002), depressing the prothrombin (factor II) level and giving rise to the unusual occurrence of a lupus anticoagulant which presents with bleeding manifestations rather than the more commonly seen thrombotic manifestations. Bleeding in this situation may need to be treated with plasma, plasma concentrates or danazol.

Testing for immunity in the vascular system

von Willebrand's antigen

von Willebrand's antigen is produced by the vascular endothelial cell and is a common acute phase reactant. While highly non-specific, von Willebrand's antigen is elevated in vasculitis (Nusinow et al, 1984 and Woolf et al, 1987) and attempts have been made to use it as a measure of immune vascular damage in a variety of rheumatologic disorders where vasculitis may accompany the disease (Belch et al,1987).

Cryoglobulins

Cryoglobulins are immunoglobulins which are capable of reversibly precipitating in the cold; they may exist as monoclonal (type I) cryoglobulins or mixed (type II) cyroglobulins, with the latter consisting of more than one immunoglobulin class. Testing for cryoglobulins can be difficult since specimens may need to be collected in pre-warmed syringes. Cryoglobulinemia may be seen in a number of autoimmune, infectious and malignant processes and may sometimes be associated with a mild vasculitis caused by complemented-mediated inflammation, which may be treated with plasmapheresis. Particular disorders which may be associated with cryoglobulinemia include hepatitis C, multiple myeloma, macroglobulinemia, systemic lupus erythematosus, rheumatoid arthritis, infectious mononucleosis, polyarteritis nodosa and Sjogren's syndrome (Schumacher 1993).

REFERENCES

Baca, V., Montiel, G., Meillon, L. et al. (2002). Diagnosis of lupus anticoagulant in the lupus anticoagulant-hypoprothrombinemia syndrome: report of two cases and review of the literature. Am J Hematol 71, 200–207.

Belch, J.J., Zoma, A.A., Richards, I.M., McLaughlin, K., Forbes, C.D. and Sturrock, R.D. (1987). Vascular damage and factor-VIII-related antigen in the rheumatic diseases. Rheumatol Int 7, 107–111.

Choufani, E.B., Sanchorawala, V., Ernst, T. et al. (2001). Acquired factor X deficiency in patients with amyloid light-chain amyloidosis: incidence, bleeding manifestations, and response to high-dose chemotherapy. Blood 97, 1885–1887.

Guyton, A.C. (1971). Textbook of Medical Physiology, 4th edn. Philadelphia: W.B. Saunders.

Kottke-Marchant, K. and Bontempo, F.A. (2003). A positive in vitro assay is required to diagnose heparin-induced thrombocytopenia. Med Clin North Am 87, 1215–1224.

Kundu, S.K., Heilman, E.J., Sio, R., Garcia, C., Davidson, R. and Ostgaard, R.A. (1995). Description of an in vitro platelet function analyzer – PFA-100. Semin Thromb Hemost 21 Suppl 2, 106–112.

Kunicki, T.J., Furihata, K., Bull, B. and Nugent, D.J. (1987). The immunogenicity of platelet membrane glycoproteins. Transf Med Rev 1, 21–33.

Mueller-Eckhard, C., Kroll, H., Kiefel, V. et al. (1991). Post-transfusion purpura. In Platelet Immunology: Fundamental and Clinical Aspects, Kaplan-Gouet, C., Schlegel, N., Salmon, C.H. and McGregor, J., eds. London: ColloqueINSERM/John Libbey Eurotext.

Nijjar, T.S., Bonacosa, I.A. and Israels, L.G. (1987). Severe acute thrombocytopenia following infusion of plasma containing anti-Pl[A1]. Am J Hematol 25, 219–221.

Nusinow, S.R., Federici, A.B., Zimmerman, T.S. and Curd, J.G. (1984). Increased von Willebrand factor antigen in the plasma of patients with vasculitis. Arthritis Rheum 27, 1405–1410.

Pashankar, D., Robinson, A. and Tait, R.C. (1996). Protein S deficiency after varicella. J Pediatr 129, 315–316.

Schumacher, H.R. (ed.) (1993). Primer on the Rheumatic Diseases, 10th edn. Atlanta, Georgia: The Arthritis Foundation.

Triplett, D.A. (1990). Laboratory diagnosis of lupus anticoagulants. Semin Thromb Hemost 16, 182–192.

Walker, R.H. (ed.) (1990). Technical Manual, 10th edn. Arlington, VA: American Association of Blood Banks.

Warkentin, T.E. and Greinacher, A. (eds) (2001). Heparin-induced Thrombocytopenia, 2nd edn. New York: Marcel Dekker.

Woolf, A.D., Wakerley, G., Wallington, T.B., Scott, D.G. and Dieppe, P.A. (1987). Factor VIII related antigen in the assessment of vasculitis. Ann Rheum Dis 46, 441–447.

Sentinel Node Assays

Galina V. Yamshchikov and Craig L. Slingluff, Jr
Department of Surgery, University of Virginia, Charlottesville, VA, USA

Happy families are all alike; every unhappy family is unhappy in its own way.

Leo Nikolaevic Tolstoi, *Anna Karenina* (1875)

INTRODUCTION

Unfortunately, therapeutic cancer vaccines have not yet been as successful as prophylactic bacterial or viral vaccines. This may be attributed to numerous factors including the presence of cancer-associated immune dysfunction and pre-existing tolerance to cancer antigens. To improve cancer vaccine strategies, it is necessary to dissect the response to cancer vaccines so that obstacles to successful immune therapy can be identified and addressed. The induction of effective tumor immunity by cancer vaccines depends on multiple sequential events:

1 antigen delivery to antigen-presenting cells
2 maturation of the dendritic cells involving delivery of additional environmental signals driving intensity (Signal 2), nature of the pathogen (Signal 3) and location of the 'danger signal'
3 migration of appropriately polarized and instructed antigen-laden dendritic cells to the draining nodes
4 antigen presentation to circulating T cells that enter the nodes through the high endothelial venules
5 selection and expansion of antigen-reactive T cells in the nodes
6 dissemination of the responding T cells systemically to tumor deposits

7 induction of tumor cell apoptosis by activated tumor-reactive T cells.

The dissection of immune responses could help to identify the limitations in the process of tumor vaccination and eventually increase the efficiency of vaccination against cancer.

Development of immune responses requires interaction between antigen-presenting cells and lymphocytes. Dendritic cells (DCs) are considered the critical antigen-presenting cells *in vivo* (Schuler et al., 1997; Banchereau and Steinman, 1998; Mellman and Steinman. 2001). Immature DCs, such as Langerhans cells, take up antigens in the periphery, process them and present antigenic peptides in a complex with MHC molecules. Following recruitment and activation by endogenous or exogenous 'danger' signals, DC take up antigen and mature subsequent to exposure to inflammatory cytokines, characterized by increased surface expression of MHC and co-stimulatory molecules (Steinman et al., 1999). Maturation of DCs is also accompanied by a rapid coordinated switch in the chemokine receptors expressed on the cell surface. While immature DCs express CCR1, CCR2, CCR5 and CXCR1 receptors associated with retention at inflammatory sites, maturation results in an upregulation of CCR7 that drives the migration of DCs to lymph nodes (Sallusto et al., 1998; Marzo et al., 1999). The process of DC migration to the lymph nodes from a site of immunization has been extensively studied using animal models (Macatonia et al., 1987; Richters et al., 1996; Dieu et al., 1998; MartIn-Fontecha et al., 2003). Animal studies also suggest that

Measuring Immunity, edited by Michael T. Lotze and Angus W. Thomson
ISBN 0-12-455900-X, London

the route of immunization controls the distribution of DC, as well as memory and effector T cells (Mullins et al., 2003).

The encounter of antigen-specific T lymphocytes and DCs presenting relevant antigen are rare events. Naive T lymphocytes constantly circulate through the body, entering lymphoid tissues due to expression of specific adhesion molecules (Campbell and Butcher, 2000). Recent studies provide insights into spatial and temporal aspects of DC–T cell interactions within draining lymph nodes using dynamic imaging methods (Delon et al., 2002; Stoll et al., 2002; Bajenoff et al., 2003). This initial antigen recognition along with appropriate co-stimulation induces clonal expansion of antigen-specific T cells followed by differentiation and migration to sites of inflammation or other lymphoid system compartments (Rosato et al., 1996; Miller et al., 2002; Bajenoff and Guerder, 2003; MartIn-Fontecha et al., 2003).

MONITORING IMMUNE RESPONSES IN THE BLOOD MAY NOT REFLECT VACCINE IMMUNOGENICITY

The primary site of the immune response to cutaneous antigen exposure is the lymph node draining the site of vaccination; similarly, immune responses to tumor occur in lymph nodes draining sites of cutaneous tumors such as melanoma (Marzo et al., 1999; Mullins et al., 2003). Lymph nodes draining tumor deposits as well as tumor-involved nodes resected from cancer patients are an excellent source of tumor specific CTL lines (Cox et al., 1994; Yamshchikov et al., 2001a; Seiter et al., 2002). Because of the central role of draining lymph nodes in the immune response to cutaneous antigen exposure, it is critical for tumor vaccines to induce immune responses in the lymph nodes draining the vaccine site, from which those antigen-specific CTL may subsequently enter the circulation and traffic to sites of tumor. Thus, an important first endpoint for tumor vaccines is the immune response generated in the vaccine-draining lymph nodes. It is not clear that measuring T cell responses in the blood alone is an adequate method for characterizing immunologic responses to vaccines in cancer patients.

However, most cancer vaccine trials are evaluated for immunogenicity only in peripheral blood lymphocytes. Paradoxically, in some studies, T cell responses do not correlate well with clinical tumor regressions. In one study, vaccination with a modified gp100 peptide led to detectable CTL responses in the peripheral blood in over 90 per cent of patients, but no clinical tumor regressions (Rosenberg et al., 1998). In another arm of that study, in which patients were vaccinated and received high-dose IL-2, there were objective clinical tumor regressions in 41 per cent of patients, but T cell responses were observed in only a small minority of patients (Rosenberg et al., 1998). It has been postulated that this may be due

to alterations of T cell trafficking by interleukin-2 (Rosenberg et al., 1999), but this hypothesis could not be tested because T cell responses in the trials were assessed only in the blood and not in other compartments.

Vaccines may fail because of poor immunogenicity. In fact, T cell responses to some melanoma vaccines have been difficult to detect, despite observed regressions of metastatic tumor deposits. In one study, patients were vaccinated with a MAGE-A3 peptide and regressions of one or more metastatic tumor deposits were observed in 25 per cent of patients, but T cell responses were not detectable in the blood in the original analyses. Subsequent analysis with very rigorous single-cell measures has demonstrated T cells reactive to this peptide in two responding patients, but the frequency of responding T cells is far below the level expected for a therapeutic CTL response (Coulie et al., 2001). The biologic relevance of these responses remains uncertain.

A vaccine must be immunogenic to have a therapeutic effect; so the finding of a clinical benefit in the absence of clear evidence of immunogenicity may be attributable to random fluctuations in tumor size independent of vaccine effect. Alternatively, it may represent a vaccine effect that occurs but is not detectable in the peripheral blood. A T cell response to vaccination may be difficult to detect in the peripheral blood because of dilution, depletion by trafficking to tumor deposits, or peripheral depletion due to other causes. However, if the vaccine is immunogenic, the T cell response should be detectable in the node(s) draining the vaccine site and evaluation of T cell responses in that node would permit a more sensitive measure of immunogenicity than evaluation of T cell responses in the blood alone.

SENTINEL IMMUNIZED NODE BIOPSY

Sentinel lymph node biopsy has become a widespread practice that is commonly used to detect occult tumor metastases in clinical oncology (Barranger and Darai, 2003; Edge et al., 2003; Evans et al., 2003). This approach defines the dominant lymph nodes draining a cutaneous tumor site by intradermal injection of a blue dye or a radioactive colloid suspension (e.g. Tc99 sulfur colloid) at the skin site to be mapped. The dye or colloid enters lymphatic channels and accumulates in draining lymph nodes. Then, excisional biopsy is performed of the node(s) identified by those methods. The same procedure has been adapted for use in identifying lymph nodes draining the sites of cutaneous vaccination, which we call a sentinel immunized node (SIN) biopsy (Yamshchikov et al., 2001b; Ayyoub et al., 2003).

The methodology for evaluation of the draining nodes is based on published murine experience with Langerhans cell migration after cutaneous antigen exposure (Macatonia et al., 1987; Richters et al., 1996). These and other studies define the optimal time for identifying immune responses in the node to be about a week after vaccination (Macatonia et al., 1987; Rosato et al., 1996).

Evaluation of immune responses in lymph nodes draining vaccination sites was introduced in the regular clinical trials assessments at the University of Virginia (UVA) (Yamshchikov et al., 2001b). Feasibility and limitations of SIN biopsy as an outpatient procedure were evaluated in four clinical trials at UVA where 119 SIN procedures were attempted or planned. Among these, 116 SIN biopsies (97 per cent) were completed in 113 patients. Three patients underwent SIN biopsy twice because of sequential enrollment in two of these trials. In three cases (3 per cent), SIN biopsy was aborted or failed for reasons detailed in Table 38.1. Only one patient out of 120 declined the procedure.

Patients were injected intradermally one week (6–9 days) after the third vaccine with approximately 0.5 mCi technetium-99 sulfur colloid, distributed at multiple injection sites at the periphery of the vaccine-site inflammatory reaction. Lymphoscintigraphy was performed and the patient was brought to the outpatient Cancer Center clinic for excisional biopsy of the dominant sentinel node identified by this radiocolloid lymphatic mapping. The SIN location was identified by transcutaneous evaluation of gamma counts using a standard hand-held gamma probe (C-trak, Care Wise Medical Products Corp., Morgan Hill, CA). In those cases where more than one hot spot node was identified by lymphoscintigraphy and the gamma probe, the hottest node closest to the vaccine injection site was selected. Because this was a research procedure, no attempt was made to remove all hot nodes, but only to remove a representative hot spot node. In one case, the only sentinel node was in the iliac chain. In the interest of avoiding patient morbidity, that node was not removed for this research study. Typical radiocolloid SIN mapping is shown in Figure 38.1.

The procedure can be performed in an outpatient clinic procedure room as we have done at the University of Virginia (Yamshchikov et al., 2001b). The procedure is performed as follows:

1 A minor procedure tray was used, containing suture scissors, Metzenbaum scissors, Adson forceps, one other pair of forceps, several Crile clamps, a scalpel, a needle driver and two shallow phrenic retractors.

2 Infiltration of skin and subcutaneous tissue with approximately 20 ml of 1 per cent lidocaine with epinephrine and bicarbonate as local anesthetic.
3 The location of the sentinel immunized node was identified by use of a gamma probe.
4 A 2–3 cm incision was made in skin overlying the node and the node was removed using standard surgical techniques, ligating vascular pedicles to the node with 3-0 silk ligatures.
5 Electrocautery was not needed and not used. Occasionally a suture was used for hemostasis.
6 The incisions were closed with a layer of running 3-0 polyglactin suture (Polysorb, US Surgical) in the subcutaneous tissue and another layer of running deep dermal suture, plus a 4-0 Polysorb subcuticular stitch. Benzoin and steristrips were applied.
7 Each node, at the time of surgical resection, was measured in three dimensions (excluding surrounding adipose tissue) and these values were used to calculate a crude volume, as a product of the three dimensions.
8 A central slice was cut from each SIN after it was removed and was submitted in formalin for formal histologic review, to rule out the presence of metastatic melanoma and for immunohistochemical stains and microscopic histologic evaluation.
9 The remainder of each SIN was processed to a single cell suspension by mechanical dissociation under sterile conditions in the Tissue Procurement Facility. The resulting lymphocyte suspensions were viably cryopreserved in 90 per cent human AB serum (Sigma, St Louis, MO) and 10 per cent DMSO (Sigma) and stored in liquid nitrogen.

Table 38.1 Success and limitations of SIN biopsy; experience at the Human Immune Therapy Center at the University of Virginia

Total number of SIN biopsy procedures attempted or planned	119
Number of SIN biopsy procedures failed or aborted	3
too deep for removal in clinic – morbidly obese	1
failed due to prior SIN biopsy that took the same node	1
aborted – drainage to iliac node, not attempted	1
Total number of SIN biopsy procedures completed	116
Number of patients with one successful SIN biopsy	110
Number of patients with two successful SIN biopsies[a]	3

[a] Due to sequential enrollment into two of the trials. (From Annals of Surgical Oncology.)

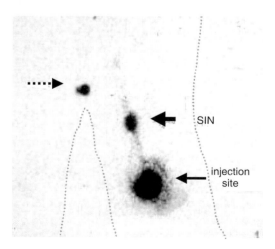

Figure 38.1 Identification of the lymph node in the groin, which drains a cutaneous vaccine site in the thigh by Tc99-sulfur colloid and excision guided by a gamma probe. Technetium-labeled sulfur colloid was injected intradermally around the vaccine injection site reaction in the left thigh. The resulting gamma camera scan demonstrates the radioactivity at the injection site, the lymphatic channel draining toward the sentinel immunized node and the hot spot representing the location of the SIN in the left groin. The location of the symphysis pubis was identified with a radioactive marker (dotted arrow). The body contours are marked with dotted gray lines.

Table 38.2 Sentinel immunized nodes and random nodes compared clinically

		Gamma counts (10 s)	LN volume (mm³)	Number of cells (millions)
SIN	Mean	7598	1422	111
n = 122	Median	3792	1080	65
	(Range)	(327–50 387)	(196–4590)	(3–692)
Random nodes	Mean	50	494	33
n = 10	Median	29	212	18
	(Range)	(1–222)	(125–2080)	(4–124)

These data represent the recorded data for maximal gamma counts (n = 106), LN volume (n = 107) and cell counts (n = 122) for SIN samples, as well as maximal gamma counts (n = 8), LN volume (n = 8) and cell counts (n = 10) for random node samples. (From Annals of Surgical Oncology.)

The yield of cells for immunologic studies averaged approximately 100 million per node. For one of the clinical trials at the University of Virginia (UVA-Mel36) and as described (Ayyoub et al., 2003), patients consented to a removal of a non-radioactive node in addition to a sentinel immunized node, when such a random node (RN) could be identified and removed without enlarging the incision and without substantial additional dissection. At UVA, this was feasible in a minority of cases. In a few other cases, a non-sentinel node was removed incidentally, because it was attached to the SIN. The gamma counts and crude lymph node volume were measured for each of these nodes and were compared to the corresponding values for the SINs in all 116 cases. In addition, the total number of mononuclear cells obtained from each node was recorded. Clinical comparison between sentinel immunized nodes and random nodes is presented in Table 38.2.

The mean age of patients at the time of the procedure was 55 years (range 25–82). On lymphoscintigraphy, the number of hot spots visualized ranged from 1 to 6 (mean 1.88, median 2). A total of 122 sentinel immunized nodes were removed (mean 1.05/patient procedure, median 1, range 1–2). The vast majority of SIN biopsies were performed on inguinal nodes (97 per cent, see Figure 38.1), but three were left axillary node biopsies in patients who had previously had bilateral inguinal node dissections or biopsies. Among those with inguinal SIN biopsies, 43 (37 per cent) were performed on the right and 70 (60 per cent) were performed on the left. Patients tolerated all of these procedures well under local anesthesia.

The SIN were evaluated on hematoxylin and eosin (H&E) sections by a surgical pathologist. None contained metastatic melanoma, nor did any of the random nodes contain evidence of melanoma. The nodes were evaluated further by immunohistochemical stains for dendritic cell infiltrates using S100, CD23 and CD1a antibodies and some were evaluated for CD4+ T cells and CD8+ T cells. S100+ cells routinely stained very strongly and were clustered in the paracortical areas (Figure 38.2). CD1a+ cells were more lightly stained and routinely were fewer in number, but in the same general distribution as the S100+ cells (not shown). CD23 stains DCs and B cells, and prominent cell clusters in the paracortical areas were

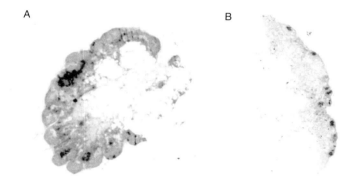

Figure 38.2 Immunohistochemical identification and quantification of S100+ dendritic cells in sentinel immunized nodes. A central slice of each immunized node was preserved in formalin and evaluated by immunohistochemical stains for S100+ dendritic cells. The proportion of the cross-sectional area occupied by DC ranged from about 2 to 20 per cent. Examples are shown for patient VMM226 with 6.6 per cent of the node containing S100+ dendritic cells and for VMM193 with 2.7 per cent of the node containing S100+ dendritic cells. Histologically, node A had reactive features, whereas node B did not have reactive features.

observed in most SIN (not shown). It was possible to measure the extent of DC infiltration of nodes by the use of image analysis software, dividing the cross-sectional area of S100+ cells by the total cross-sectional area of the node (excluding the fatty hilum); these values varied widely from 1.7 to 19.6 per cent in 13 patients evaluated in UVA-Mel31. Examples of staining are shown in Figure 38.2.

EVALUATION OF IMMUNE RESPONSES IN LYMPH NODES DRAINING THE VACCINATION SITE

As expected, evaluations of tumor-specific responses in the lymph nodes draining the vaccination site provided more sensitive measures of vaccine immunogenicity (Yamshchikov et al., 2001b). Several studies incorporated this novel technology in the trial design, where evaluation of immune responses in the lymph node draining vaccination site were performed in parallel with responses in the blood (Ayyoub et al., 2003; Slingluff et al., 2003b). Here we describe the experience accumulated at the Human Immune Therapy Center of the University of Virginia. All patients on trials UVA-Mel31 and Mel36 and half of patients on Mel39 received a vaccine comprising four melanoma peptides (100 µg each of the HLA-A1-restricted peptide tyrosinase$_{240-251S}$ (DAEKSDICTDEY), the HLA-A2-restricted peptides tyrosinase$_{368-376D}$ (YMDG-TMSQV) and gp100$_{280-288}$ (YLEPGPVTA), the HLA-A3-restricted peptide gp100$_{17-25}$ (ALLAVGATK) and 190 µg of the HLA-DR-restricted tetanus helper peptide AQYIKAN-SKFIGITEL. In addition, half of patients on UVA-Mel39 were vaccinated with a mixture of 12 peptides, including the four incorporated in the earlier trials, plus eight

others. All peptides used for immunizations are listed in Table 38.3.

Along with the SIN, peripheral blood lymphocytes were also collected from all patients before initiation of the vaccine regimen, each week prior to each vaccine, on the day of the SIN biopsy and in follow-up after completion of the vaccines. Lymphocyte samples from these dates and also from the SIN were thawed and evaluated simultaneously for T cell responses to multiple defined peptide antigens. As we have previously reported, T cell responses in the SIN could be detected by tetramer analyses directly *ex vivo* (Figure 38.3), by intracellular IFNγ release

Table 38.3 Peptides used in vaccines

Allele	Sequence	Epitope	Reference
HLA-A1	DAEKSDICTDEY	Tyrosinase$_{(240-251)}$[a]	(Kittlesen et al., 1998)
	SSDYVIPIGTY	Tyrosinase$_{(146-156)}$	(Kawakami et al., 1998)
	EADPTGHSY	MAGE-A1$_{(161-169)}$	(Traversari et al., 1992)
	EVDPIGHLY	MAGE-A3$_{(168-176)}$	(Gaugler et al., 1994)
HLA-A2	YMDGTMSQV	Tyrosinase$_{(368-376)}$[b]	(Skipper et al., 1996a)
	IMDQVPFSV	gp100$_{(209-217)}$[c]	(Parkhurst et al., 1996)
	YLEPGPVTA	gp100$_{(280-288)}$	(Cox et al., 1994)
	GLYDGMEHL	MAGE-A10$_{(254-262)}$	(Huang et al., 1999)
HLA-A3	ALLAVGATK	gp100$_{(17-25)}$	(Skipper et al., 1996b)
	LIYRRRLMK	gp100$_{(614-622)}$	(Kawakami et al., 1998)
	SLFRAVITK	MAGE-A1$_{(96-104)}$	(Chaux et al., 1999)
	ASGPGGGAPR	NY-ESO-1$_{(53-62)}$	(Wang et al., 1998)

[a] substitution of S for C at residue 244
[b] post-translational change of N to D at residue 370
[c] 209–2M, substitution of M for T at position 210.

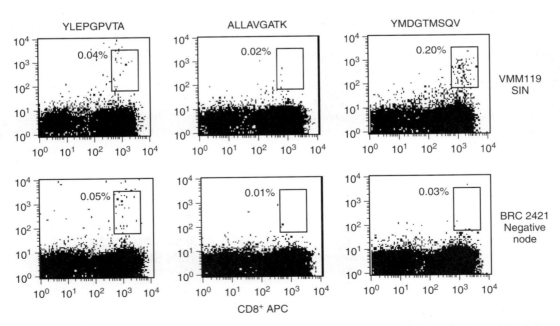

Figure 38.3 Cryopreserved cells from the SIN of patient VMM119 and from a tumor negative lymph node (BRC2421, HLA-A2) of a breast cancer patient were thawed and enriched for CD8$^+$ cells. Cells were triple-stained with the tetramers, anti-CD8 antibody and anti-TCR-γ/β-1 antibody. We used FACScan with CELLQuest software to enumerate tetramer$^+$ CD8$^+$ cells. The population of tetramer$^+$ CD8$^+$ cells is designated with a small rectangle on each plot. The percentage of CD8$^+$ cells that are tetramer$^+$ is shown. The difference between SIN and negative node binding corresponds to 0.17 per cent of CD8$^+$ lymphocytes bearing TCR specific for YMDGTMSQV peptide, and the absence of CD8$^+$ cells with YLEPGPVTA specific TCR. (From Yamshchikov et al., 2001b.)

(Figure 38.4), by bulk cytokine release assay followed by ELISA on cell supernatants (not shown) and by ELIspot assay (Figure 38.5). We also found that peptide-reactive CTL detected in the SIN are capable of recognizing and lysing tumor cells naturally expressing the corresponding peptides from gp100 and tyrosinase (Figure 38.6).

The primary measure of T cell responses in the clinical trials was the ELIspot assay, in which the numbers of T cells secreting IFNγ in response to each tested peptide were enumerated. The samples were sensitized once *in vitro* with a mixture of the peptides, then cultured 14 days in RPMI 1640 containing 10 per cent human AB serum and low-dose IL-2. These cell populations were then evaluated by ELIspot assay as previously described (Slingluff, 2003). Briefly, lymphocytes were plated at 10 000– 150 000 cells per well in 96 well plates with equal numbers of antigen-presenting cells (C1R-A1, C1R-A2, T2 or C1R-A3) pulsed with 10 μg/ml of each peptide and washed after

2 h. Negative controls were lymphocytes tested with antigen-presenting cells alone or pulsed with an irrelevant peptide from HIV or malarial proteins (Johnson et al., 1991; Blum-Tirouvanziam et al., 1995). As a positive control the responder T cells were stimulated with PMA (1 ng/ml, Sigma) and ionomycin (1 μM, Sigma).

These assays were performed over several years and there were some improvements in the assay systems over time. Specifically, the earlier studies were done on plastic plates (Immulon 2 flat bottom plates, Dynatech, Chantilly, VA), but more recent ELIspot assays used filter-bottom MultiScreen plates (Millipore, Bedford, MA). Also, spots in early assays were read visually with a binocular microscope; more recently, an automated ELIspot plate reader (Biosys-Bioreader-3000, Karben, Germany) was used to count spots for all assays.

Criteria used for defining a positive response were consistent throughout the study. Results are reported as

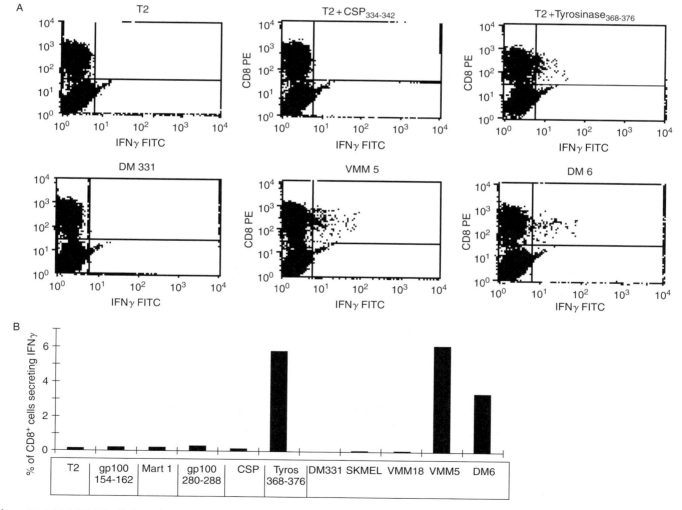

Figure 38.4 VMM204 T cells from the SIN were sensitized once *in vitro* with the four immunizing peptides and then expanded with anti-CD3 antibody. They were added to T2 cells pulsed with one of five peptides or to one of 5 different tumor cells. The number of CD8+ cells secreting IFNγ was determined by FACS after staining for CD8 and intracellular staining for IFNγ. In (A), raw FACS data are shown for six different stimulators. In (B), results represent the percentage of CD8+ cells secreting IFNγ as measured in this assay. (From Yamshchikov et al., 2001b.)

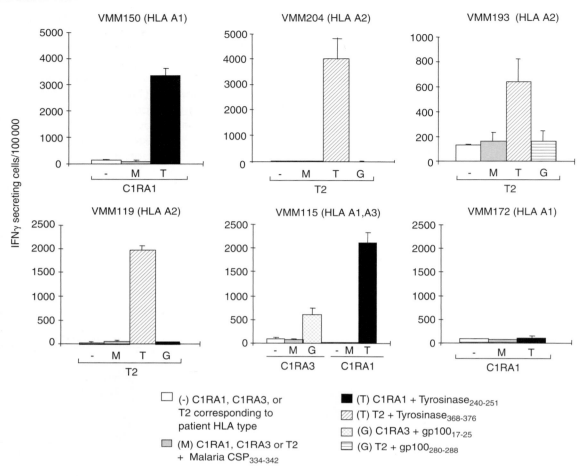

Figure 38.5 Mononuclear cells from the SIN of five patients were cryopreserved at the time of resection. These cryopreserved cells were thawed and sensitized with the mixture of four immunizing peptides, cultured 14 days, then evaluated in an ELIspot assay for reactivity to the immunizing peptides pulsed on C1RA1, T2 or C1RA3. Negative controls include C1RA1, T2 or C1RA3 alone or pulsed with the irrelevant peptide YLKKIKNSL (CSP$_{334-342}$). Error bars represent 1 standard deviation. Mononuclear cells from the SIN of patient VMM172, receiving a different vaccine, were similarly stimulated and evaluated. The x-axis labels represent the target cells (C1RA1, T2 or C1RA3) and the peptide pulsed on that target cell (- for no peptide, **M** for irrelevant malaria peptide, **G** for gp100 peptide, **T** for tyrosinase peptide). (From Yamshchikov et al., 2001b.)

the number of peptide-reactive T cells per 10^5 cells. The response to peptide is considered positive if the following criteria are met:

1. The ratio of the post-vaccine T cell response to peptide ($T_{exp\ post}$) divided by the highest T cell response to the negative controls ($T_{con\ post}$) is at least 2 ($R_{exp\ post}$).
2. The actual number of spots counted for an experimental peptide ($T_{exp\ post}$) is at least 30 (spots per 10^5 cells) greater than the number of spots counted for a negative control ($T_{con\ post}$). (Note: The threshold for the number of spots over background (30) represents 30 spots per 100 000 lymphocytes, of which approximately 20 per cent are CD8 cells. Thus, 30 spots per 100 000 lymphocytes represent approximately 30 spots per 20 000 CD8+ cells (0.15 per cent).)
3. The number of spots counted for an experimental peptide ($T_{exp\ post}$) minus 1 SD is greater than the number of spots counted for the highest negative control ($T_{con\ post}$)

plus 1 SD. Depending upon patient allele type, each patient may generate a T cell response against more than one of the synthetic peptides.

4. For evaluation of PBL, responses are positive if there is at least a doubling of the response after vaccination ($R_{exp\ post} > 2 \times R_{exp\ pre}$) compared to the prevaccine value and if all three of the criteria above are also met.

Evaluation of random nodes, when available, also served as negative controls for the SIN values.

Data on the immune responses detected in the PBL and SIN are being reported in detail separately for each of the four studies (Slingluff et al., 2003b and manuscripts in preparation). Combined summary data from Mel31 and Mel36 ($n = 60$) are shown in Figure 38.6. Evaluation of the SIN alone detected T cell responses 46 per cent more often than in PBL (57 per cent versus 39 per cent); combined evaluation of the SIN and the PBL detected immunogenicity 62 per cent more often than in PBL alone

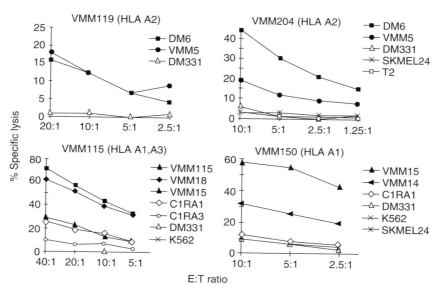

Figure 38.6 T cells from the SIN of patients VMM119 and VMM204 were stimulated once *in vitro* with the four immunizing melanoma peptides at 40 μg/ml, then expanded with anti-CD3 antibodies at 14 days. The T cells from VMM115 and VMM150 were stimulated once with the peptides, then restimulated once with the peptides pulsed on autologous irradiated PBL, prior to anti-CD3 expansion. These cultured T cells were then assayed for cytotoxicity against several melanoma- and non-melanoma target cells in 4-h chromium release assays. DM6 (■) and VMM5 (●) are HLA-A2+, tyrosinase+, gp100+. VMM15 (▲) and VMM14 (◄) are HLA-A1+, tyrosinase+. VMM18 (◆) is HLA-A3+, tyrosinase+, gp100+. VMM115 (■) is an autologous tumor line from the VMM115 nodal metastases, which is HLA-A1+, HLA-A3+, tyrosinase+, gp100+. Negative control melanoma cells include DM331 (△) and SkMel24 (*), which are both HLA-A1+A2+ and are tyrosinase and gp100 negative. Non-melanoma targets include C1R-A1 (◇), C1R-A3 (○), T2 (□), and K562 (×). They are all negative for tyrosinase and gp100 and they express HLA-A1, -A3, -A2, or no class I MHC, respectively. (From Yamshchikov et al., 2001b.)

(63 per cent versus 39 per cent). Thus, 35–40 per cent of T cell responses would have been missed if only the PBL were evaluated. The biologic relevance of responses detected in the SIN but not in the PBL can be debated, but since the SIN is believed to represent the site at which an immune response to cutaneous antigen occurs, the presence of an immune response in the SIN is evidence of immunogenicity of the vaccine, whereas the measure of the response in the peripheral blood may be considered a composite measure of immunogenicity of the vaccine, dissemination of the response, persistence of memory responses and success or failure of circulating T cells to traffic to tumor or to be sequestered in other secondary lymphoid organs. In patients with measurable metastatic disease, it seems likely that an effective vaccine will generate T cells in the SIN that disseminate into the circulation and then are depleted from the circulation by trafficking to tumor deposits. Thus, it may be desirable to observe high responses in the SIN and in tumor deposits, but low or absent responses in the circulation, as we have observed in the patient whose data are shown in Figure 38.7 (Yamshchikov et al., 2001b).

For those four patients from whom a SIN and a random node were prospectively collected in accord with the protocol, T cell responses were measured in parallel using lymphocytes from the SIN and from the random node after one *in vitro* sensitization with a mixture of four melanoma peptides from gp100 and tyrosinase (DAEKSDICTDEY, YLEPGPVTA, YMDGTMSQV, ALLAVGATK). These data are presented in Figure 38.8. Responses were observed in three of the four patients and in all three of those patients, there was a response in the SIN, but not in the random nodes. These responses were observed to two different peptides, with values 12–41-fold the background reactivity.

These data document the uniqueness of the SIN as the primary site of immune response to a cutaneous melanoma vaccination which can provide information not available from PBL or random nodes. Evaluation of the SIN plus PBL permits a more sensitive measure of T cell immunogenicity than evaluation of PBL alone.

Ayyoub et al. (2003) reached similar conclusions about the importance of SIN analysis for evaluation of vaccine immunogenicity in their studies. They used sensitive tetramer technology for enumeration of MART-1 specific T cells. It was confirmed by phenotyping analysis that peptide-specific T cells in the SIN had a memory phenotype and expressed the CCR7 receptor that is characteristic for T cells residing in lymph nodes. However, this group found much smaller differences between the SIN and RN in their studies with RN being positive for peptide-specific T cells. A possible reason for the discrepancy between the results may be the different timing in the SIN excisions. In their vaccination protocol, the SIN was resected at 2–4 weeks post immunization, when induced

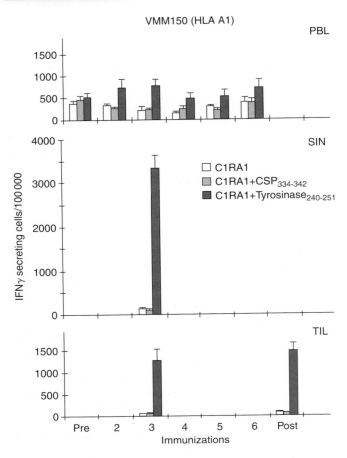

VMM150 (HLA A1)

PBL

SIN

☐ C1RA1
☐ C1RA1+CSP₃₃₄₋₃₄₂
■ C1RA1+Tyrosinase₂₄₀₋₂₅₁

TIL

Figure 38.7 Mononuclear cells from peripheral blood (PBL), from two metastatic tumor deposits (TIL) and from the SIN of patient VMM150 were cryopreserved at the time of collection. These cells were thawed and sensitized with the mixture of the four immunizing peptides in parallel cultures. After 14 days they were evaluated in an ELIspot assay for reactivity to the immunizing peptide tyrosinase₂₄₀₋₂₅₁S pulsed on C1RA1. Negative controls include C1RA1 alone or pulsed with the irrelevant malaria peptide CSP₃₃₄₋₃₄₂. (From Yamshchikov et al., 2001b).

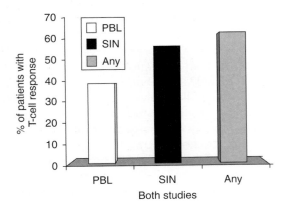

Figure 38.8 Patients on the two vaccine trials Mel31 and Mel36, using the four melanoma peptide vaccine preparation, were evaluated for evidence of T cell response in the PBL and in the SIN. The proportion of patients with T cell responses to at least one peptide in the PBL, in the SIN, or in either are presented as summary data from both trials combined (n = 60).

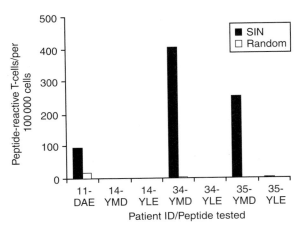

Figure 38.9 T cell response in SIN is specific and is not evident in a random node from the same basin (Mel36). Lymphocytes from a sentinel immunized node and from a random, non-radioactive node were sensitized *in vitro* once with the four melanoma peptide mixture, then assayed by ELIspot assay for reactivity to each of the peptides relevant for the patients' HLA type. Patients 11, 14, 34 and 35 were studied. Patient 11 is HLA-A1+ and reactivity was tested to the tyrosinase DAEKSDICTDEY. The other three patients are HLA-A2+ and reactivity was tested to the gp100 and tyrosinase peptides YLEPGPVTA and YMDGTMSQV. The reactivity from the SIN is shown in the solid black bars. Reactivity from the random nodes is shown in the white empty bars. Reactivity was negative for patient 14 and reactivity to YLEPGPVTA was negative in all three cases evaluated.

T cells could have already migrated out of the SIN to other lymphoid compartments or tumor sites and therefore no statistical difference was found between T cell measurements for SIN and RN. All evaluations of SINs at the University of Virginia clinical trials were done a week after the third vaccine and in this case SIN demonstrated superior readouts of peptide-specific T cells in comparison to PBL and RN, which were still found negative or low positive. There is a great deal more to learn about the optimal methods for identifying immune responses and characterizing those that are most reflective of protective immunity. Variables include the compartment being studied, the timing of the evaluation and the precise method used for analysis.

CONCLUSIONS

1 The sentinel immunized node is a primary site of cellular immune responses to cutaneous vaccination, but optimal detection of responses in that node may be time-dependent.

2 T cell responses to tumor vaccines may be more readily detectable in the sentinel immunized node than in the peripheral blood.

3 Cells from the SIN can be evaluated by flow cytometry or immunohistochemically for expression of activation markers on dendritic cells or T cells.

4 Evaluation of T cell dissemination from the SIN to the periphery may aid in understanding failures or successes of tumor vaccines.

5 Sentinel immunized nodes may be useful in characterizing immune responses to cancer vaccines and in optimizing them.

Areas of future investigation should include:

1 Dissection of the immune responses based on compartment including the blood, the vaccine-draining nodes and the sites of metastatic tumor. This may help to define if either the responses in the blood or the SIN can predict the extent of T cell targeting to tumor deposits. We would expect that additional tumor-cell-dependent variables may augment or interfere with the ability of antigen-specific T cells to infiltrate tumor deposits or to survive in that environment.

2 Characterization of antigen-specific T cells in the SIN and the peripheral blood for activation status and Tc1/Tc2 or Th1/Th2 bias, to determine if these can predict clinical tumor regression or protection from tumor progression.

3 Development of new techniques for measurement of antigen-specific T cell responses using small numbers of cells to permit such evaluations by fine needle aspiration biopsy of the SIN and/or tumor.

4 Characterization of the time course of immune response development and regulation of immune responses in the SIN and characterization of regulatory T cell infiltration in the SIN over time.

5 Evaluation of DC in the SIN of responders and non-responders, to determine if pre-existing or vaccine-induced changes in DC bias towards an immunogenic or tolerogenic phenotype.

It is increasingly evident that tumors evolve in immunocompetent hosts because of their ability to evade immune-mediated destruction, such that human cancers have generally undergone some form of immune escape and/or immune editing (Shankaran et al., 2001). Thus, it would be surprising if simply increasing the numbers of antigen-specific T cells would induce dramatic tumor regressions in most patients. On the other hand, some dramatic tumor regressions have been observed in small numbers of patients on experimental vaccine trials (Nestle, 1998; Slingluff, 2003), suggesting that immune-mediated protection can be achieved in optimal circumstances. To extend such results to a larger proportion of patients will require a stepwise approach to dissect the components of the immune response to cancer antigens and component mechanisms of immune escape by tumor cells. Evaluation of T cells, dendritic cells and tumor cells in multiple compartments during the course of vaccination is a step toward this kind of knowledge about the physiology and pathophysiology of the immune response to cancer.

REFERENCES

Ayyoub, M., Zippelius, A., Pittet, M. J. et al. (2003). Activation of human melanoma reactive CD8+ T cells by vaccination with an immunogenic peptide analog derived from Melan-A/melanoma antigen recognized by T cells-1. Clin Cancer Res 9, 669–677.

Bajenoff, M., Granjeaud, S., Guerder, S. et al. (2003). The strategy of T cell antigen-presenting cell encounter in antigen-draining lymph nodes revealed by imaging of initial T cell activation. J Exp Med 198, 715–724.

Bajenoff, M. and Guerder, S. (2003). Homing to nonlymphoid tissues is not necessary for effector Th1 cell differentiation. J Immunol 171, 6355–6362.

Banchereau, J. and Steinman, R. M. (1998). Dendritic cells and the control of immunity. Nature 392, 245–252.

Barranger, E. and Darai, E. (2003). Sentinel lymph nodes. Cancer 98, 2524–2525; author reply 2525–2526.

Blum-Tirouvanziam, U., Servis, C., Habluetzel, A. et al. (1995). Localization of HLA-A2.1-restricted T cell epitopes in the circumsporozoite protein of Plasmodium falciparum. J Immunol 154, 3922–3931.

Campbell, J. J. and Butcher, E. C. (2000). Chemokines in tissue-specific and microenvironment-specific lymphocyte homing. Curr Opin Immunol 12, 336–341.

Chaux, P., Luiten, R., Demotte, N. et al. (1999). Identification of five MAGE-A1 epitopes recognized by cytolytic T lymphocytes obtained by in vitro stimulation with dendritic cells transduced with MAGE-A1. J Immunol 163, 2928–2936.

Coulie, P. G., Karanikas, V., Colau, D. et al. (2001). A monoclonal cytolytic T-lymphocyte response observed in a melanoma patient vaccinated with a tumor-specific antigenic peptide encoded by gene MAGE-3. Proc Natl Acad Sci USA 98, 10290–10295.

Cox, A. L., Skipper, J., Chen, Y. et al. (1994). Identification of a peptide recognized by five melanoma-specific human cytotoxic T cell lines. Science 264, 716–719.

Delon, J., Stoll, S. and Germain, R. N. (2002). Imaging of T-cell interactions with antigen presenting cells in culture and in intact lymphoid tissue. Immunol Rev 189, 51–63.

Dieu, M. C., Vanbervliet, B., Vicari, A. et al. (1998). Selective recruitment of immature and mature dendritic cells by distinct chemokines expressed in different anatomic sites. J Exp Med 188, 373–386.

Edge, S. B., Niland, J. C., Bookman, M. A. et al. (2003). Emergence of sentinel node biopsy in breast cancer as standard-of-care in academic comprehensive cancer centers. J Natl Cancer Inst 95, 1514–1521.

Evans, H. L., Krag, D. N., Teates, C. D. et al. (2003). Lymphoscintigraphy and sentinel node biopsy accurately stage melanoma in patients presenting after wide local excision. Ann Surg Oncol 10, 416–425.

Gaugler, B., Van den Eynde, B., van der Bruggen, P. et al. (1994). Human gene MAGE-3 codes for an antigen recognized on a melanoma by autologous cytolytic T lymphocytes. J Exp Med 179, 921–930.

Huang, L. Q., Brasseur, F., Serrano, A. et al. (1999). Cytolytic T lymphocytes recognize an antigen encoded by MAGE-A10 on a human melanoma. J Immunol 162, 6849–6854.

Johnson, R. P., Trocha, A., Yang, L. et al. (1991). HIV-1 gag-specific cytotoxic T lymphocytes recognize multiple highly conserved epitopes. Fine specificity of the gag-specific response defined by using unstimulated peripheral blood mononuclear cells and cloned effector cells. J Immunol 147, 1512–1521.

Kawakami, Y., Robbins, P. F., Wang, X. et al. (1998). Identification of new melanoma epitopes on melanosomal proteins recognized by tumor infiltrating T lymphocytes restricted by HLA-A1, -A2, and -A3 alleles. J Immunol 161, 6985–6992.

Kittlesen, D. J., Thompson, L. W., Gulden, P.H. et al. (1998). Human melanoma patients recognize an HLA-A1-restricted CTL epitope from tyrosinase containing two cysteine residues: implications for tumor vaccine development. J Immunol 160, 2099–2106.

Macatonia, S. E., Knight, S. C., Edwards, A. J. et al. (1987). Localization of antigen on lymph node dendritic cells after exposure to the contact sensitizer fluorescein isothiocyanate. Functional and morphological studies. J Exp Med 166, 1654–1667.

Martln-Fontecha, A., Sebastiani, S., Hopken, U. E. et al. (2003). Regulation of dendritic cell migration to the draining lymph node: impact on T lymphocyte traffic and priming. J Exp Med 198, 615–621.

Marzo, A. L., Lake, R. A., Lo, D. et al. (1999). Tumor antigens are constitutively presented in the draining lymph nodes. J Immunol 162, 5838–5845.

Mellman, I. and Steinman, R. M. (2001). Dendritic cells: specialized and regulated antigen processing machines. Cell 106, 255–258.

Miller, M. J., Wei, S. H., Parker, I. et al. (2002). Two-photon imaging of lymphocyte motility and antigen response in intact lymph node. Science 296, 1869–1873.

Mullins, D. W., Sheasley, S. L., Ream, R. M. et al. (2003). Route of immunization with peptide-pulsed dendritic cells controls the distribution of memory and effector T cells in lymphoid tissues and determines the pattern of regional tumor control. J Exp Med 198, 1023–1034.

Parkhurst, M. R., Salgaller, M. L., Southwood, S. et al. (1996). Improved induction of melanoma-reactive CTL with peptides from the melanoma antigen gp100 modified at HLA-A*0201-binding residues. J Immunol 157, 2539–2548.

Richters, C. D., van Pelt, A. M., van Geldrop, E. et al. (1996). Migration of rat skin dendritic cells. J Leukoc Biol 60, 317–322.

Rosato, A., Zambon, A., Macino, B. et al. (1996). Anti-L-selectin monoclonal antibody treatment in mice enhances tumor growth by preventing CTL sensitization in peripheral lymph nodes draining the tumor area. Int J Cancer 65, 847–851.

Rosenberg, S. A., Yang, J. C., Schwartzentruber, D. J. et al. (1998). Immunologic and therapeutic evaluation of a synthetic peptide vaccine for the treatment of patients with metastatic melanoma. Nat Med 4, 321–327.

Rosenberg, S. A., Yang, J. C., Schwartzentruber, D. J. et al. (1999). Impact of cytokine administration on the generation of antitumor reactivity in patients with metastatic melanoma receiving a peptide vaccine. J Immunol 163, 1690–1695.

Sallusto, F., Schaerli, P., Loetscher, P. et al. (1998). Rapid and coordinated switch in chemokine receptor expression during dendritic cell maturation. Eur J Immunol 28, 2760–2769.

Schuler, G., Thurner, B. and Romani, N. (1997). Dendritic cells: from ignored cells to major players in T-cell-mediated immunity. Int Arch Allergy Immunol 112, 317–322.

Seiter, S., Monsurro, V., Nielsen, M. B. et al. (2002). Frequency of MART-1/MelanA and gp100/PMel17-specific T cells in tumor metastases and cultured tumor-infiltrating lymphocytes. J Immunother 25, 252–263.

Shankaran, V., Ikeda, H., Bruce, A. T. et al. (2001). IFNgamma and lymphocytes prevent primary tumour development and shape tumour immunogenicity. Nature 410, 1107–1111.

Skipper, J. C., Hendrickson, R. C., Gulden, P. H. et al. (1996a). An HLA-A2-restricted tyrosinase antigen on melanoma cells results from posttranslational modification and suggests a novel pathway for processing of membrane proteins. J Exp Med 183, 527–534.

Skipper, J. C., Kittlesen, D. J., Hendrickson, R. C. et al. (1996b). Shared epitopes for HLA-A3-restricted melanoma-reactive human CTL include a naturally processed epitope from Pmel-17/gp100. J Immunol 157, 5027–5033.

Slingluff, C.L., Gina, J., Petroni, R. et al. (2003a). Immunologic and clinical outcomes of vaccination with a multi-epitope melanoma peptide vaccine plus low-dose IL-2 administered either concurrently or on a delayed schedule. Submitted for publication.

Slingluff, C. L., Jr, Petroni, G. R., Yamshchikov, G. Y. et al. (2003b). Clinical and immunologic results of a randomized phase II trial of vaccination using four melanoma peptides either administered in granulocyte-macrophage colony-stimulating factor in adjuvant or pulsed on dendritic cells. J Clin Oncol 21, 4016–4026.

Steinman, R. M., Inaba, K., Turley, S. et al. (1999). Antigen capture, processing, and presentation by dendritic cells: recent cell biological studies. Hum Immunol 60, 562–567.

Stoll, S., Delon, J., Brotz, T. M. et al. (2002). Dynamic imaging of T cell-dendritic cell interactions in lymph nodes. Science 296, 1873–1876.

Traversari, C., van der Bruggen, P., Luescher, I. F. et al. (1992). A nonapeptide encoded by human gene MAGE-1 is recognized on HLA-A1 by cytolytic T lymphocytes directed against tumor antigen MZ2-E. J Exp Med 176, 1453–1457.

Wang, R. F., Johnston, S. L., Southwood, S. et al. (1998). Recognition of an antigenic peptide derived from tyrosinase-related protein-2 by CTL in the context of HLA-A31 and -A33. J Immunol 160, 890–897.

Yamshchikov, G., Thompson, L., Ross, W. G. et al. (2001a). Analysis of a natural immune response against tumor antigens in a melanoma survivor: lessons applicable to clinical trial evaluations. Clin Cancer Res 7, 909s–916s.

Yamshchikov, G. V., Barnd, D. L., Eastham, S. et al. (2001b). Evaluation of peptide vaccine immunogenicity in draining lymph nodes and peripheral blood of melanoma patients. Int J Cancer 92, 703–711.

Imaging Inflammation

Chapter 39

N. Scott Mason, Brian J. Lopresti and Chester A. Mathis

Department of Radiology, University of Pittsburgh, Pittsburgh, PA, USA

The morbid process designated by the term inflammation, being one to which every organ and probably every tissue of the body is liable, and comprehending as it does in its progress and consequences by far the greatest number of ills to which flesh is heir, possesses a deeper interest for the physician or surgeon than any other material subject which could be named.

Joseph Lister, 1858

INTRODUCTION

A non-invasive method that would allow reliable and accurate visualization of subacute, acute and chronic inflammation and infection would benefit the diagnosis and the delineation of infection/inflammatory processes in the clinical setting. While magnetic resonance imaging and computed tomography are able to localize relatively small focal abnormalities, these imaging modalities are based primarily upon the detection of anatomical changes. As such, these techniques are of limited utility in the early stages of infective or inflammatory processes and do not allow for the discrimination of active processes from anatomical changes resulting from a treated process or after surgery. The development of a variety of radiopharmaceuticals (both in traditional nuclear medicine and in positron emission tomography) for use in non-invasive imaging of infective/inflammatory processes, both peripherally and centrally, reflects the significant scientific interest in this area. The utility of

non-invasive radiopharmaceutical methods is based upon the specific accumulation of the radiotracer in an infective/inflammatory process as a result of local perturbation of the physiologic condition. In order for a radiopharmaceutical to be useful it should:

1 demonstrate fairly rapid accumulation and retention in foci of interest
2 not accumulate in non-affected areas
3 clear rapidly from non-affected background areas
4 not produce side effects
5 provide the clinician with information regarding the localization, severity and extent of the disease process.

In this chapter, we attempt to provide a general overview of the radiopharmaceuticals available for the non-invasive monitoring of systemic inflammation (and infection) as well as discuss in more detail the application of these radiotracer techniques in monitoring neuroinflammation.

Tissues will invariably react to injurious events with an inflammatory response. The cascade of cellular signaling events that follows the presence of a foreign entity or tissue degradation ultimately leads to a local response through the recruitment of white blood cells (leukocytes) from the blood. White blood cells are classified into two main groups: granulocytes and agranulocytes (lymphoid cells). Granulocytes (whose name is based upon the presence of granules in the cell cytoplasm) include neutrophils, eosinophils and basophils. Granulocytes also possess a multi-lobed nucleus and as a result are also called

Measuring Immunity, edited by Michael T. Lotze and Angus W. Thomson
ISBN 0-12-455900-X, London

polymorphonuclear leukocytes or 'polys'. Neutrophils are primarily active in the process of bacterial phagocytosis. These cells do not possess the ability to regenerate lysosomes involved in the digestion of microbes and die after the phagocytosis of only a few microbes. Eosinophils attack parasites and aid in the removal of antigen–antibody complexes. The primary function of basophils is the secretion of anticoagulant and vasodilatory substances that mediate the hypersensitivity (inflammation) reaction.

Agranulocytes (lymphocytes and monocytes) have neither granules in their cytoplasm nor multi-lobular nuclei. These cells are also referred to as mononuclear leukocytes. Lymphocytes are present not only in the peripheral blood supply, but also in lymphoid organs and tissues including the thymus, bone marrow, spleen and lymphoid nodules. The lymphocytes are the main constituents of the immune system. Monocytes are the precursors of macrophages that exist in the peripheral blood supply for 24–36 h. In the presence of an inflammation site, monocytes are responsible for not only phagocytotic activity but also play a secretory role. A variety of molecules serve as components of these cellular signaling events including substance P, interleukin-1 (IL-1), tumor necrosis factor-α (TNF-α), intercellular adhesion molecule-1 (ICAM-1, found on endothelial cells) and complementary adhesion molecules located on leukocytes (leukocyte function associated antigen-1 (LFA-1))

EDEMA IMAGING

[Ga-67]citrate has been used for over 30 years for imaging infection and inflammation. Gallium acts as an iron analog *in vivo*, binding to transferrin. The [Ga-67] citrate/transferrin complex most likely is delivered to the site of inflammation as a result of locally increased vascular permeability (Tsan, 1985). The exact mechanism of retention of Ga-67 citrate/transferrin is not known; however, there is evidence from *in vitro* models suggesting a role of siderophores released by microorganisms or the involvement of lactoferrin present in leukocytes (Weiner, 1990).

[Ga-67]citrate is limited in its clinical application by several shortcomings. While this agent demonstrates good sensitivity for a variety of pathological conditions including both acute and chronic infections, inflammation and several skeletal disorders, Ga-67 demonstrates low specificity. This low specificity is a result of several factors including a non-specific mechanism of uptake, the route of biological elimination (intestinal tract), as well as accumulation of the radiotracer in other processes (malignant tissue and bone repair and modeling) (Perkins, 1981; Bekerman et al., 1984; Seabold et al., 1989). Additional disadvantages include the long physical and biological half-lives which, in combination with the high energy gamma rays associated with the decay process, lead to relatively high radiation exposures for the subject (ICRP, 1987). Furthermore, delayed imaging

of up to 72 h is often required to obtain optimal imaging information.

These drawbacks, along with the development of newer radiolabeled tracers (including labeled leukocytes), have limited the use of Ga-67 imaging. However, [Ga-67]citrate imaging is still viewed as useful in the diagnosis of vertebral osteomyelitis (Hadjipavlou et al., 1998; Seabold et al., 1989; Turpin and Lambert, 2001) as well as studies in patients with fever of unknown origin (FUO) (Peters, 1999). In addition, in immunocompromised patients, Ga-67 imaging is the procedure of choice for the detection of lymph node irregularities and lung infections as this method does not require the handling of blood or blood products (Wassie et al., 1994).

IgG

Non-specific human polyclonal immunoglobulin(s) (hIgG) labeled with either In-111 or Tc-99m have been proposed as imaging agents for the detection of both subacute and acute infection and inflammation. The specific uptake and accumulation of these agents in inflammatory/infectious foci is thought to be a result of extravasation and locally increased vascular permeability (Morrel et al., 1990; Fischman et al., 1992). Both In-111 and Tc-99m labeled hIgGs demonstrate physiologic uptake in normal liver and spleen as well as a relatively slow clearance from the blood pool. There are also differences in the *in vivo* distribution that depend upon the radionuclide. The In-111 labeled agent demonstrates higher uptake in the liver compared to the Tc-99m labeled agent; however, the Tc-99m labeled agent shows higher uptake in the kidneys, urinary tract and bowel compared to the In-111 labeled compound (Goh et al., 1990). These agents have demonstrated utility in applications associated with bone and joint imaging (Oyen et al., 1992; Nijhof et al., 1997) and pulmonary infection/inflammation imaging (Buscombe et al., 1993). Currently, the primary clinical application of radiolabeled IgG is in subjects with rheumatoid arthritis. In general, the Tc-99m labeled agent has advantages when compared to the In-111 labeled agent in terms of dosimetry issues, imaging properties and availability of the radionuclide.

AVIDIN/BIOTIN

Another non-specific infection/inflammation imaging agent is based upon the high affinity interaction of biotin for avidin (protein contained in the eggs of avians and reptiles). The In-111 labeled biotin/avidin system utilizes the non-specific uptake and accumulation of avidin in inflammation/infection foci as a surrogate target. Following sufficient time to allow for the localization of the avidin, In-111 biotin is administered. While free In-111 biotin shows little uptake in normal tissues and clears rapidly through the urinary tract, the high affinity binding interaction of In-111 biotin with avidin leads to significant accumulation in inflammation/infection foci with relatively good target to background ratios *in vivo* (Rusckowski et al., 1992). The avidin/biotin system has also been utilized with Tc-99m (Tc-99m biotin-PEG liposomes) (Laverman et al., 2000) and F-18 (Shoup et al., 1994) in animal models of infection and inflammation. The In-111 system has been used in humans in osteomyelitis (Lazzeri et al., 1999) as well as for the detection of vascular infections in prosthetic vascular grafts (Samuel et al., 1996).

CELL IMAGING

Radiolabeled leukocytes

Radiolabeling leukocytes with either In-111 or Tc-99m represents a more specific method of detecting inflammation/infection based upon the role of leukocyte migration in the inflammatory process. Radiolabeling cell populations can be accomplished either by a direct or indirect labeling approach. In the direct approach, leukocytes are isolated from the individual's (or a donor's) blood, radiolabeled and then readministered to the individual. While the procedure is relatively simple, it takes several hours to perform and requires the handling of blood and/or blood products that could lead to the transmission of blood-borne pathogens. Radiolabeled leukocytes are initially localized in the lungs following intravenous administration, but subsequently clear quickly from this organ. A significant fraction of the radioactivity (most likely associated with cells damaged during the labeling process) accumulates in the spleen, while labeled leukocytes migrate to the site of inflammation. One proposed mechanism of uptake for radiolabeled leukocytes is based upon the increase of cellular adhesion molecules found on the vascular endothelium. Following this initial event, the radiolabeled leukocytes diffuse through the vascular endothelium and basal membrane finally to localize by chemotaxis at the inflammatory foci.

The most common method of direct labeling for leukocytes uses an oxinate chelator to carry the In-111 into the cell (Segal et al., 1976; Thakur et al., 1977a,b). In a similar fashion, a lipophilic chelation agent (hexamethylpropylene amineoxime [HMPAO]) has been used to label white blood cells with Tc-99m (McAfee and Thakur, 1976a,b; Peters et al., 1986; Peters, 1994). As a result of the lower radiation dose and more favorable imaging characteristics of Tc-99m labeled white blood cells, Tc-99m labeled leukocytes have, for the most part, replaced In-111 labeled preparations. However, the product resultant from the HMPAO labeling procedure is not as stable *in vivo* as the In-111 oxime product. Upon intravenous administration white blood cells labeled with Tc-99m HMPAO release radioactivity at a rate of approximately 7 per cent per hour (Becker et al., 1988). This 'free' radioactivity is eliminated at early time points through the kidneys and bladder and at later time points leads to increased radioactivity in the gall bladder and bowel. As a result, In-111 labeled white blood cells are the preferred agent for the evaluation of kidney, bladder and gall bladder infections (Peters, 1994). Labeled white blood cell preparations are also used for the detection of skeletal infections (Krznaric et al., 1996; Liberatore et al., 2000) and for post-procedure evaluations of individuals who have received vascular grafts or orthopedic prostheses (Becker et al., 1987; Liberatore et al., 1998; Larikka et al., 2001).

Indirect labelling of cells

Other attempts to develop radiolabeled imaging agents for the non-invasive evaluation of inflammatory/infective processes are based on the labeling of agents that demonstrate specificity for any of the myriad receptors and surface antigens found on the surface of the various cell types involved in the body's inflammatory response. These include monoclonal antibody and antibody fragment-based radiolabeled agents, labeled cytokines for various cell surface receptors, labeled peptides and other chemical entities that demonstrate specificity for specific receptor subtypes (i.e. peripheral benzodiazepine receptor (PBR)) found on macrophages and activated microglia. The utility of these agents may be based upon the active recruitment of a particular cell type to the site of inflammation or the upregulation of a particular receptor/surface antigen in response to the inflammatory process.

Monoclonal antibodies

A variety of approaches have been utilized to label white blood cells *in vivo*. One method involves the use of radiolabeled monoclonal antibodies (MAbs) for surface antigens/receptors of granulocytes. A variety of monoclonal antibodies specific for antigens found on granulocytes have been developed and several have been evaluated for imaging inflammatory/infection foci. Among these are: anti NCA-95 (non-specific cross-reacting antigen 95) immunoglobulin G (BW250/183) (Becker et al., 1990, 1992) and anti CD15 IgM (a stage specific embryonic antigen, LeuTech®, Palatin Technologies, Princeton, NJ) (Thakur et al., 1996; Kipper et al., 2000).

In general, there are inherent disadvantages and limitations to the use of MAbs. The high molecular weight of these entities may limit delivery of the agents to the inflammatory sites of interest. In addition, the biological half-life of these compounds is generally long as these compounds are metabolized in the liver rather than the more rapid elimination through the urinary tract. The most serious potential limitation is the possible production of human antimouse antibodies (HAMA) following the administration of these agents. HAMA response may lead to altered biodistribution and pharmacokinetics of these agents, or allergic reactions. A HAMA response also increases the risk of an immune response following subsequent injections. Further, the administration of these radiolabeled MAbs may lead to transient neutropenia.

While these MAbs were designed to bind to specific antigens on the cell surfaces of leukocytes, it soon became apparent that labeled MAbs did not demonstrate an *in vivo* distribution that was similar to the distribution observed in *ex vivo* labeled studies. Subsequent studies have demonstrated that as little as 10 per cent (BW250/183) (Becker et al., 1989) and possibly as much as 50 per cent (CD15-IgM) (Thakur et al., 1996; Mozley et al., 1999) of the radioactivity was actually associated with granulocytes. It is now thought that these radiolabeled MAb agents localize at the site of inflammation in much the same manner as the non-specific edema agents discussed earlier; i.e. through extravasation resultant from enhanced vascular permeability in the area of the inflammatory/infection foci.

Even with this lack of true specificity and the problems inherent with the use of MAbs in general, these compounds have demonstrated some utility in a variety of clinical settings. Tc-99m labeled BW250/183 has been used in the evaluation of inflammatory bowel disease (Mahida et al., 1992), foot infections in diabetic patients (Dominguez-Gadea et al., 1993) and in the evaluation of suspected bone infections (Peltier et al., 1993).

As a result of the limitations associated with MAbs, the utility of radiolabeled antibody fragments (Fab' or F(ab')$_2$) has been examined. The utilization of antibody fragments in diagnostic applications might alleviate many of the drawbacks associated with MAbs. As expected, antibody fragments demonstrate rapid blood clearance and a significantly lower immunogenic response when compared to monoclonal antibodies. One such antigranulocyte antibody fragment (Fab'-anti NCA-90) labeled with Tc-99m (Tc-99m-labeled sulesomab, Leukoscan®) has demonstrated little immunogenic (HAMA) response and infection/inflammation localization results were comparable to those obtained with leukocytes labeled by the direct method (Becker et al., 1994; Stokkel et al., 2002). Leukoscan® has also been used for the localization of osteomyelitis (Harwood et al., 1999) and in the detection of appendicitis (Barron et al., 1999).

Cytokines

Another approach to the development of radiolabeled agents for inflammatory/infection imaging is based on the wide variety of proteins and glycoproteins with high affinity for specific membrane receptors found on cells involved in the inflammatory response (granulocytes, macrophages, leukocytes, etc.). As a class these compounds (cytokines) are involved in a variety of homeostatic functions with respect to immunity, inflammation and hematopoiesis and are produced *de novo* in response to an immune stimulus. A single cytokine may act on several different cell types and the same cytokine may be secreted by different cell types. The site of action of the cytokine may be on the cell from which it was originally secreted, on nearby cells, or on cells that are some distance removed from the original secreting cell. In general, cytokines possess several characteristics which lend themselves to the development of inflammation imaging agents (Signore et al., 2003a,b). These compounds are generally of low molecular weight (15–25 kD), demonstrate rapid plasma clearance, possess a short biologic half-life and bind to specific receptor sites with high affinity.

Interleukin-1 (IL-1)α and IL-1β are inflammatory cytokines that bind with high affinity to receptors that are primarily on the surfaces of granulocytes, monocytes and lymphocytes (Lowenthal and MacDonald, 1986; Dinarello, 1991). IL-1α and IL-1β have been radiolabeled with I-123 and have demonstrated specific uptake in focal *S. aureus* infections in both mice and rabbits (van der Laken et al., 1995, 1997, 1998a). However adverse biologic effects were associated with IL-1 administration, even at doses as low as 10 ng/kg, which made these radiolabeled cytokines unsuitable for clinical use.

Further work was aimed at the development of a radiolabeled analog of the naturally occurring IL-1 receptor antagonist (IL-1Ra). This antagonist demonstrated none of the adverse effects associated with IL-1 administration in humans, even at doses up to 10 mg/kg (Granowitz et al., 1992). The radiolabeled compound demonstrated selective retention in mouse and rabbit models of inflammation (van der Laken et al., 1996, 1998a). Subsequently, [I-123]IL-1Ra was used in the imaging of rheumatoid arthritis in a small group of patients. While the radiolabeled compound demonstrated the ability to delineate inflamed joints, the compound also demonstrated significant non-specific accumulation in the intestinal tract (Barrera et al., 2000).

Another leukocyte cytokine, interleukin-8 (IL-8) has been utilized as a lead in the development of imaging agents for inflammation. IL-8 is a chemotactic cytokine (CXC subfamily) and is involved in the recruitment and activation of neutrophils to inflammatory foci. High concentrations of IL-8 resulting from recruitment of neutrophils have been found in a variety of inflammatory diseases including rheumatoid arthritis (Endo et al., 1991) and colitis (Izzo et al., 1992). IL-8 has been labeled with I-123 and the resultant compound localized to inflammatory foci in animal models of inflammation/infection (Hay et al., 1997; van der Laken et al., 1998b). Interestingly, the biodistribution of [I-123]IL-8 *in vivo* varies depending upon the oxidative method (Bolton-Hunter reagent versus Iodogen method) used in the radiosynthesis (van der Laken et al., 2000). The development of a Tc-99m labeled IL-8 analog using hydrazinonicotinamide (HYNIC) as a chelation agent was viewed as an improvement over the iodinated derivatives based upon the higher specific activity obtained in the technetium preparations as compared to the iodinated analogs (Rennen et al., 2000, 2001). [Tc-99m]IL-8 yielded higher specific uptake in animal models of inflammation as compared to the radioiodinated derivative (0.33 per cent ID/g versus 0.057 per cent ID/g) (Gratz et al., 2001; Rennen et al., 2001). However, concerns regarding a drop in peripheral leukocyte counts and leukocytosis following the administration of these IL-8 derivatives were found to be drawbacks that limited the clinical utility of these compounds in humans (Rennen et al., 2000, 2001).

Platelet factor 4 (PF4), another member of the CXC subfamily of cytokines, binds to the same receptors as IL-8 and has been used as a lead compound in the development of a potential inflammation imaging agent. A synthetic peptide P483H (Diatide, Inc. (now Diatide Research Laboratories a Division of Berlex Laboratories)) which included the heparin-binding portion of PF4 as well as a lysine-rich sequence (to promote clearance through the kidneys) has been labeled with Tc-99m. The radiolabeled compound has demonstrated the ability to accumulate in inflammatory foci in humans without some of the adverse effects associated with radiolabeled IL-8 agents (Moyer et al., 1996). However, there is some evidence that the radionuclide is released from the agent *in vivo* evidenced by high lung and thyroid uptake (Palestro et al., 2001).

Peptides

Another target area for the development of inflammation/infection imaging utilizes the variety of peptides for specific receptors found on white blood cells. Formyl-Met-Leu-Phe is one such peptide that acts as a chemotactic peptide released by bacteria. The peptide binds with high affinity to receptors on granulocytes and monocytes. This particular peptide was radiolabeled in the early 1980s and evaluated as a potential imaging agent (McAfee et al., 1984). In general this class of agents demonstrated unsuitable *in vivo* biodistribution (significant non-specific accumulation in spleen, liver, kidney and intestinal tract) as well as undesirable biological activity (granulocytopenia) (Fischman et al., 1993; Pollak et al., 1996).

Tuftsin (Thr-Lys-Pro-Arg) is another chemotactic peptide that promotes phagocytosis of neutrophils, monocytes and macrophages by means of a receptor-mediated process. Another peptide (Thr-Lys-Pro-Pro-Arg) has demonstrated higher affinity for the tuftsin receptor than native tuftsin and is the basis for a Tc-99m labeled imaging agent for inflammation (RP-128, Resolution Pharmaceuticals with rights sold to Bracco, Inc.) (Caveliers et al., 2001). A few small studies with RP-128 have been reported (Paul et al., 2000; Caveliers et al., 2001). While RP-128 demonstrates low background activity, fast renal clearance and no adverse biologic effect, the sensitivity and specificity (73 per cent and 64 per cent) are not favorable when compared to other imaging agents for inflammation such as radiolabeled immunoglobulins.

In-111 Octreotide (Octreoscan®) is a radiolabeled somatostatin analog that has been used primarily for imaging of neuroendocrine tumors (Kwekkeboom et al., 2000; Kwekkeboom and Krenning, 2002; van der Lely et al., 2003). Octreoscan® is a diethylenetriamine pentaacetic acid (DTPA) modified derivative that chelates In-111 effectively. The eight amino acid peptide octreotide demonstrated a longer biological half-life than somatostatin itself. Octreoscan® became the first peptide-based diagnostic agent approved by the Food and Drug Administration.

The primary clinical applications of Octreoscan® are based upon the presence of increased numbers of somatostatin receptors (SSR) in tumors of neuroendocrine origin. While five SSR subtypes are known, octreotide binds with high affinity to only two of these receptor subtypes (SSR-2 and SSR-5) (Breeman et al., 1998). The presence of SSR-2 on activated lymphocytes has been used to rationalize the utilization of Octreoscan® in chronic inflammatory disease/infections. A number of studies have been performed to determine the efficacy of Octreoscan® in imaging chronic infections where lymphocytes predominate with varied results (Kwekkeboom et al., 1998; Weinmann et al., 2000; Lebtahi et al., 2001).

FDG

[F-18]Fluorodeoxyglucose (FDG) is a radiopharmaceutical that provides an *in vivo* index of glucose metabolism and has become the standard clinical radiopharmaceutical for positron emission tomography (PET), a technique that provides improvements in resolution and sensitivity over single photon methods. In addition, PET provides the ability to quantify the amount of radioactivity present in a given area of interest in the acquired image. The primary clinical application of FDG-PET has been in the area of oncology where the techniques have demonstrated utility in the differentiation of malignant versus benign tumors, the evaluation of treatment efficacy in cancer patients and the determination of tumor stage (Delbecke, 1999; Ak et al., 2000). The biochemical basis for FDG uptake in malignant processes is the increase in glucose metabolism normally found in tumor cells as compared to normal cells. Granulocytes and macrophages normally present in infective/inflammatory processes also demonstrate increased glucose metabolism relative to normal cells and it is this feature that allows FDG imaging to be useful in these processes. FDG-PET has been used non-invasively to image a wide variety of infective processes, including bacterial and fungal infections as well as bone and soft tissue infective processes (O'Doherty et al., 1997; Sugawara et al., 1998; Kalicke et al., 2000; Stumpe et al., 2000; Vanquickenborne et al., 2003; Bleeker-Rovers et al., 2004). FDG-PET has demonstrated particular utility in the differentiation of osteomyelitis and infective processes involving soft tissue surrounding bone (Guhlmann et al., 1998; Kalicke et al., 2000; Zhuang et al., 2000). The sensitivity and specificity of FDG-PET in these narrow applications exceeds 90 per cent. However, there is still significant debate regarding the utility and cost effectiveness of FDG-PET imaging in these applications (Buscombe and Signore, 2003; Oyen and Mansi, 2003). One drawback to this application is the obvious inability to distinguish between neoplastic lesions and infective/inflammation processes as both yield increases in FDG uptake based upon increases in glucose metabolism (Shreve et al., 1999). One possible solution to the differentiation of inflammatory processes versus neoplastic lesions is based upon differences in uptake demonstrated at early and later time points during the biodistribution of FDG. These studies (both animal and clinical) suggest that FDG will continue to accumulate in neoplastic lesions over time while accumulation will peak at approximately 1 h post-injection in inflammatory processes and then continue to decrease (Zhuang et al., 2001).

Apoptosis

A variety of diseases including cancer, neurodegenerative diseases, infectious diseases and organ and bone marrow transplant rejection involve apoptosis or programmed cell death (Thompson, 1995). Normally phosphatidylserine is confined to the inner leaflet portion of the plasma membrane lipid bilayer. However, it is externalized to the outer leaflet of the plasma membrane during apoptosis (Martin et al., 1995). Annexin-V is an endogenous human protein that binds with nanomolar affinity to phosphatidylserine present on the outer surface of apoptotic cells. This protein has been radiolabeled with a variety of radioisotopes in efforts to develop radiotracers to image apoptosis. [Tc-99m] annexin V has been utilized in several animal model studies and in human studies to examine acute myocardial infarction (Blankenberg et al., 1998; Hofstra et al., 2000; Ogura et al., 2000). Efforts directed at the development of positron-labeled annexin derivatives have also been undertaken. A F-18 labeled derivative utilizing a N-succinimidyl-[F-18]fluorobenzoate as the labeling synthon has been compared to the [Tc-99m]annexin in an animal model of myocardial ischemia (Murakami et al., 2003). While the two tracers demonstrated roughly the same uptake in infarct areas compared to non-infarct areas (approximately threefold), the fluorine-18 labeled compound demonstrated lower uptake in liver, spleen and kidney in normal animals compared to the Tc-99m derivative. Annexin V has also been labeled with iodine-124 both through a direct iodination of the protein and through the use of a radiolabeled synthon (N-succinimidyl iodobenzoate). In animal studies both tracers showed significant uptake in the kidneys and bladder. The direct iodination product also demonstrated significant thyroid uptake, presumably due to in vivo deiodination (Collingridge et al., 2003; Glaser et al., 2003).

In contrast to subacute and acute inflammatory processes, chronic inflammation is characterized by an *in situ* clonal expansion of infiltrating lymphocytes as opposed to the migration of these cells from the peripheral blood supply. A complicating factor in the use of labeled lymphocytes is their sensitivity to radiation damage resulting from labeling procedures utilizing In-111 (Signore et al., 1983). While lymphocyte labeling methods utilizing [Tc-99m]HMPAO have not demonstrated the same propensity for cellular damage (Jaakkola et al., 1998), the lack of recruitment from the peripheral blood supply limits their use.

Monocytes labeled with Tc-99m and In-111 have also been used to image chronic inflammation (Weinberg et al., 1986; Grimm et al., 1995). While the same limitations discussed for lymphocytes (radiation sensitivity and lack of recruitment from peripheral blood supply) apply, an additional limitation with respect to labeled monocytes is the low number of monocytes (2–8 per cent or 200–600 monocytes/ml of blood) normally present. The low number of monocytes not only makes the isolation and labeling of these cells difficult, but also limits the sensitivity of the method.

There are several cytokines that have been radiolabeled and evaluated as *in vivo* imaging agents for chronic inflammation. Interleukin-2 (IL-2) is a single chain glycoprotein consisting of 133 amino acids (Morgan et al., 1976). Following specific antigen stimulation, IL-2 is secreted *in vivo* by T lymphocytes (designated as T lymphocytes based upon the fact that while their precursor cells are produced in the bone marrow, these cells leave the bone marrow and mature in the thymus). Under normal physiologic conditions the expression of IL-2 receptors in lymphoid tissues and on the surface of peripherally localized blood lymphocytes is extremely low (Robb et al., 1984; Semenzato et al., 1992). IL-2 expression is greatly increased in target organs following *in vivo* activation; however, the presence of IL-2 on the surface of peripherally localized T lymphocytes remains very low, even during inflammatory/pathological processes. As a consequence, there are low levels of background radioactivity associated with circulating lymphocytes. IL-2 has been radiolabeled with several radionuclides including S-35, I-125, I-123, I-131 and Tc-99m and evaluated in a variety of animal models (Koths and Halenbech, 1985; Robb et al., 1985; Signore et al., 1987; Chianelli et al., 1997). In humans, studies utilizing IL-2 radiolabeled with either I-123 or Tc-99m have been performed to evaluate the utility of these radiolabeled agents in a variety of disease pathologies including inflammatory bowel diseases (Crohn's disease) and insulin-dependent diabetes. In a small group of patients suffering from Crohn's disease, [I-123]IL-2 uptake was shown not only to differentiate active/inactive disease from control subjects, but also demonstrated a positive correlation between the number of regions of interest denoted as 'positive' and the time to disease relapse (Signore et al., 2000a,b).

One critical area of concern with respect to inflammation imaging is the discrimination between sterile inflammation and bacterial infection. Several different radiotracers have been evaluated for their potential to differentiate between

Table 39.1 Radiopharmaceuticals for inflammation/infection

Inflammatory process	Radiopharmaceuticals
Various infections (bacterial, viral, fungal)	^{99m}Tc-Ciprofloxacin, ^{99m}Tc-Fluconazole
Edema (extravasal leakage)	^{111}In/^{99m}Tc-human polyclonal immunoglobulin, Avidin/^{111}In-biotin, ^{67}Ga-citrate
Infiltrating cells	^{111}In/^{99m}Tc-white blood cells, MAbs, cytokines (IL-1, IL-6, IL-8), chemotactic peptides, ^{18}F-FDG
Cell death (apoptosis)	^{99m}Tc/^{18}F-Annexin V derivatives
Chronic inflammation	^{111}In/^{99m}Tc-lymphocytes and monocytes, cytolines (IL-2), peptides (^{111}In-octreotide, RP-128)

a sterile inflammatory process and inflammation resulting from a bacterial infection. One such agent is a [Tc-99m]-labeled fluoroquinolone ([Tc-99m]ciprofloxacin or Infecton™) (Gabay and Kushner, 1999), which has been used in imaging studies for a variety of infectious diseases (Vinjamuri et al., 1996; Britton et al., 1997, 2002; Hall et al., 1998; Yapar et al., 2001). Since ciprofloxin only binds to the DNA gyrase present in dividing bacteria, it allows for the differentiation of sterile and bacterial processes. The radiolabeled compound is primarily eliminated through the kidneys with low bowel and bone marrow accumulation (De Winter et al., 2001).

The peripheral benzodiazepine receptor

Benzodiazepines are a class of drugs widely prescribed for their anxiolytic, anticonvulsant, hypnotic and sedative effects. The activity of benzodiazepines is mediated in the central nervous system by the central benzodiazepine receptor (CBR), which constitutes part of a 5-subunit macromolecular receptor complex that includes a post-synaptic GABA$_A$ receptor and a chloride channel (Braestrup and Squires, 1977; DeLorey and Olsen, 1992). A second class of benzodiazepine receptor, pharmacologically distinct from the CBR, was first identified in non-neuronal peripheral tissues such as the kidney (Braestrup and Squires, 1977). These binding sites have come to be known as peripheral benzodiazepine receptors (PBR) as a result of the relative abundance of these receptors in peripheral tissues (Hertz, 1993). PBR receptor densities are highest in the adrenal glands, though abundant concentrations have been shown to exist in other peripheral tissues such as the kidneys, heart, testes, ovaries, uterus (Awad and Gavish, 1987; Kurumaji and Toru, 1996) and hematogenous cells (Canat et al., 1993; Maeda et al., 1998; Lockhart et al., 2003). Low concentrations of PBR sites have also been identified in non-neuronal brain tissue.

The PBR is an 18-kDa subunit of a hetero-oligomeric complex with three known subunits. The PBR also includes a 32-kDa voltage dependent anion channel and a 30-kDa adenine nucleotide translocase. This complex has been localized to the outer and inner mitochondrial

membrane (Anholt et al., 1986; Mukherjee and Das, 1989; Papadopoulos et al., 1994), though non-mitochondrial PBR sites have been observed in heart, liver and testes (as reviewed by Gavish et al., 1999). PBR sites are also located on the plasma membrane of mature human erythrocytes, which lack mitochondria altogether (Olson et al., 1988).

The cellular source of PBR expression is heterogeneous, though most are closely associated with steroidogenic tissue in the adrenal cortex (Benavides et al., 1983a; De Souza et al., 1985), testicular Leydig cells (Garnier et al., 1993), uterine epithelium (Fares et al., 1988; Verma and Snyder, 1989), acinar cells in the mammary glands (Tong et al., 1991), and ovaries (Toranzo et al., 1994). PBR sites are abundant in many types of blood cells, particularly granulocytes (polymorphonuclear cells), monocytes and lymphocytes (Canat et al., 1993; Maeda et al., 1998). In normal brain, low concentrations of PBR sites are known to exist in the parenchyma, ependyma and choroid plexus (Benavides et al., 1983b) with even lower concentrations in cortex (Benavides et al., 1988). While the cellular source of PBR expression in normal brain has been the subject of some debate, a growing body of evidence implicates microglia, the brain's intrinsic macrophages, as the principal component of brain PBR expression (Dubois et al., 1988; Myers et al., 1991a,b; Stephenson et al., 1995; Banati et al., 1997; Wilms et al., 2003), rather than reactive astrocytes also known to express PBR sites (Hertz, 1993; Itzhak et al., 1993).

While a complete understanding of its physiologic function remains to be elucidated, the PBR has been implicated in a variety of biological processes including the regulation of transmembrane cholesterol transport in steroidogenesis (Hall, 1991; Culty et al., 1999), immunomodulation (Ruff et al., 1985; Zavala, 1997), cellular respiration (Hirsch et al., 1989), acute and chronic stress (Novas et al., 1987; Karp et al., 1989; Drugan and Holmes, 1991), apoptosis (Hirsch et al., 1998; Bono et al., 1999), secretion of cytokines (Zavala et al., 1990; Taupin et al., 1993), heme biosynthesis (Taketani et al., 1994), chemotaxis (Ruff et al., 1985) and in cellular proliferation (Black et al., 1994). These and other putative physiologic roles for the PBR are the subject of a comprehensive review (Gavish et al., 1999). As a result of the variety of physiologic roles attributed to the PBR, there has been considerable interest in the role of the PBR in inflammatory processes. This is particularly true with regard to inflammatory processes that primarily affect the CNS.

Injury of the mammalian brain often results in a permanent functional impairment, which may be the result of a singular traumatic or biochemical insult (e.g. ischemic stroke and mechanical percussion) or a protracted process of chronic inflammation (e.g. multiple sclerosis) or neurodegeneration (e.g. Alzheimer's disease). In any case, the brain's reduced capacity to recover function after injury is largely due to the fact that the neuron is post-mitotic and therefore unable to regenerate damaged neural tissue by proliferative processes. Collateral or secondary degeneration, which involves the spread of damage to neurons that were spared direct injury, may amplify the functional deficit. For this reason, it is imperative that the brain has effective and responsive mechanisms for combating pathologic insults and protecting intact neurons from secondary degeneration.

Inflammation of the CNS can be mediated by microglia, macrophages from the periphery that infiltrate brain, or a combination of these elements. Microglia are distributed throughout the CNS and are the brain's intrinsic macrophage and immune response effector. Under normal circumstances, microglia are dormant and remain isolated from other cells. In response to neuronal injury, microglia can transform themselves into a form which is morphologically and functionally analogous to macrophages in the peripheral immune system. This process of microglial activation has been associated with an upregulation of cell-surface receptors and ion channels as well as the secretion of a plurality of proinflammatory cytokines and growth factors involved in cell signaling, including interleukin-1 (IL-1), IL-3, IL-5, IL-6, tumor necrosis factor-α (TNF-α), nerve growth factor (NGF), brain-derived neurotrophic factor (BDNF), transforming growth factor-beta 1 (TGF-β1) neurotrophin-3 (NT-3) and NT-4/5 (Thoenen and Barde, 1980; Giulian et al., 1988; Hama et al., 1989; Kamegai et al., 1990; Merrill, 1992; Sawada et al., 1993; Heese et al., 1998; Gavish et al., 1999; Batchelor et al., 2000; Shaffer et al., 2003). These cytokines and growth factors stimulate mitotic proliferation of microglia (Vaca and Wendt, 1992; Chirumamilla et al., 2002), recruitment of reactive astrocytes (Penkowa et al., 1999) and neuronal sprouting (Batchelor et al., 2000). Importantly, in the activated state microglia express PBR sites which, in contrast, are comparatively absent from dormant microglia (Banati et al., 2000). Once activated, microglia migrate to the damaged neural tissue where they proliferate and participate in the inflammatory response. In instances where the pathological event or disease results in blood–brain barrier disruption, microglial activation may involve the recruitment of mononuclear phagocytes from the peripheral immune system that infiltrate brain, as is the case in traumatic-ischemic brain injury (Myers et al., 1991a). A more detailed survey of the role of microglia in disease can be found in one of many comprehensive reviews of the subject (Perry et al., 1993; Kreutzberg, 1996; Gavish et al., 1999; Streit et al., 1999; Banati, 2002, 2003).

Microglia are an attractive cellular target for the development of molecular imaging probes that could potentially provide non-invasive *in vivo* measures of the inflammatory response to pathologic insult of the CNS for several reasons. First, activated microglia are relatively absent from healthy brain tissue and therefore constitutive PBR expression is low. This is an important characteristic as it provides a low background against which to measure increased PBR expression on activated microglia. In addition, activated microglia concentrate in areas where neuronal injury is present and are relatively absent elsewhere, though considerable evidence shows that microglial

activation may also extend to areas which are projected to from the sites of direct injury (Banati et al., 1997; Cicchetti et al., 2002). It is this spatial localization of microglia to areas of active neuronal injury that provides the most convincing rationale for the development of non-invasive imaging agents to detect microglial activation.

R-[N-methyl-¹¹C]PK11195 and R,S-[N-methyl-¹¹C]PK11195

The isoquinoline carboxamide derivative 1-(2-chlorophenyl)-N-methyl-N-(1-methylpropyl)-3-isoquinolinecarboxamide (PK11195) is a potent and selective PBR antagonist with well characterized pharmacology (Benavides et al., 1983b, 1988; Le Fur et al., 1983a,b; Camsonne et al., 1984). Racemic [N-methyl-¹¹C]PK11195 was shown to be rapidly and highly extracted from blood into brain and, in the absence of pathology, distribute in a uniform manner across brain tissue (Price et al., 1990; Cremer et al., 1992). In saturation binding experiments where baboons were administered a pharmacologic dose (1 mg/kg) of unlabeled PK11195 prior to PET imaging, a consistent two- to threefold increase in peak brain radioactivity concentrations (from 0.005–0.008 per cent ID/ml to 0.012–0.03 per cent ID/ml) were observed compared to control animals. One possible explanation for this increase is that the blockade of abundant PBR sites in peripheral tissues inhibits some degree of systemic binding of R,S-[N-methyl-¹¹C]PK11195, resulting in higher plasma concentrations of free R,S-[N-methyl-¹¹C]PK11195 and subsequent increased availability to the brain. Similarly, when a displacing dose (1 mg/kg) of unlabeled PK11195 was administered 8 minutes after the bolus injection of R,S-[N-methyl-¹¹C]PK11195 in normal baboons, a rapid rise in cortical radioactivity concentration was observed followed by a transient period of accelerated washout lasting ~8 minutes and a return to control clearance rates (Petit-Taboue et al., 1991). The displacement of bound R,S-[N-methyl-¹¹C]PK11195 from peripheral PBR sites results in a transient increase in free radiotracer concentration in plasma and increased availability to the brain in a manner consistent with the saturation binding studies discussed previously.

While the PK11195 racemate was first radiolabeled with carbon-11 as a potential agent for imaging PBR expression in the human myocardium, the R-enantiomer (R-[N-methyl-¹¹C]PK11195) has been shown to have higher affinity for PBR than the racemic mixture and might allow improved detection of specific binding (Shah et al., 1994). For this reason, the use of the single enantiomer precursor is now favored over use of the racemate.

[C-11]PK11195 is, to date, the most widely used PET imaging agent for the PBR, in part the result of the lack of suitable alternatives. This radiotracer has been employed successfully to detect inflammatory pathology in human imaging studies of multiple sclerosis (MS), Alzheimer's disease (AD), glioma and glioblastoma, ischemic stroke, Rasmussen's encephalitis, herpes encephalitis, cerebral vasculitis, multiple system atrophy (MSA) and peripheral nerve damage (Table 39.2). Additional preclinical studies in animal models of disease indicate other potential applications that may be translated to the clinic in the future, such as neuroAIDS (Venneti et al., 2004) and chronic obstructive pulmonary disease (Jones et al., 2003). However, certain methodological considerations preclude the use of [C-11]PK11195 for quantitative assessment of microglial activation in the CNS. The first of these considerations is one of specificity. While it has been demonstrated that microglia are the predominant source of [C-11]PK11195 binding in the intact brain (Banati et al., 1997), there is evidence to show that in certain conditions recruitment of peripheral immune cells into brain may also occur (Raivich et al., 1998; Flugel et al., 2001). Monocytes and lymphocytes from the periphery express PBR sites and once they have infiltrated brain are indistinguishable from activated microglia. In the case where the disease pathology involves disruption of the blood–brain barrier, infiltrating peripheral macrophages may be a considerable cellular source of PBR expression (Myers et al., 1991a; Nesbit et al., 1991; Williams et al., 2001) that is indistinguishable from activated microglia using [C-11]PK11195 and non-invasive imaging.

One of the advantages of positron emission tomography is the ability to extract quantifiable information from the studies. This ability is predicated upon accurate determination of the amount of radiopharmaceutical present during the course of the study. A variety of biomathematical modeling techniques, such as compartmental analysis, are often employed to make quantitative estimates of specific radiotracer binding in PET imaging experiments. These methods rely on the accurate description of radiotracer input function to brain, requiring discrete sampling of arterial blood and determination of radiolabeled plasma metabolites. It has been reported that the unstable behavior of [C-11]PK11195 in plasma complicates input function determination and is not conducive to accurate estimates of *in vivo* radiotracer specific binding (Banati et al., 2000). Recently, it has been shown that base-promoted dechlorination of PK11195 precursor during the radiosynthetic procedure may result in a radiolabeled impurity with similar chromatographic properties as authentic [C-11]PK11195. Adjustments to the radiosynthetic procedure can be implemented which inhibit the dechlorination side-chain reaction and may make arterial input function determination more reliable (Cleij et al., 2003).

Table 39.2 Synopsis of [C-11]PK11195 findings in inflammatory pathologies

Affliction	Effect on [C-11]PK11195 binding	Reference
Glioma	Increase in 8 of 10 patients	(Junck et al., 1989)
Glioblastoma	Twofold higher in tumor, 30 per cent displaceable	(Pappata et al., 1991)
Ischemic stroke	2.5-fold higher in afflicted hemisphere	(Ramsay et al., 1992)
Ischemic stroke	20–50 per cent increase in afflicted hemisphere	(Gerhard et al., 2000)
Ischemic stroke	Increase in ipsilateral thalamus	(Pappata et al., 2000)
AD	No increase detected	(Groom et al., 1995)
AD	Increase in entorhinal, temporoparietal and cingulated cortex	(Cagnin et al., 2001a)
MS	Increase in sites of active MS lesions	(Vowinckel et al., 1997)
MS	Increase in sites of active MS lesions	(Banati et al., 2000)
MS	15–30 per cent increase in two patients	(Debruyne et al., 2002)
Rasmussen's encephalitis	18–28 per cent increase in affected hemisphere	(Banati et al., 1999)
Cerebral vasculitis	Increased binding in occipital and temporal lobes of affected side	(Goerres et al., 2001)
Herpes encephalitis	Increase in focal lesion site and distal projections	(Cagnin et al., 2001b)
Peripheral nerve injury	Increase in thalamus following limb denervation	(Banati et al., 2001)
Multiple system atrophy	Increase in dorsolateral prefrontal cortex, caudate, putamen, thalamus and substantia nigra	(Gerhard et al., 2003)

The problems associated with rigorous quantitation of the amount of circulating [C-11]PK11195 has led investigators to utilize semiquantitative methods of data analysis or methods which employ tissue-based input, such as the simplified reference tissue model (SRTM: Lammertsma and Hume, 1996; Gunn et al., 1997), for the analysis of [C-11]PK11195 human PET studies. A complication of tissue-based input methods of analysis, such as SRTM, is that they require that a region of interest devoid of specific binding be defined (reference region) on the PET image. In the presence of inflammatory pathology, it is well established that activated microglia are found not only in the foci of the lesion but also along neural pathways that project from the injured neurons to other brain regions (Banati et al., 2000; Cagnin et al., 2001b; Cicchetti et al., 2002). Furthermore, diseases with multifocal or diffuse pathology may be characterized by ubiquitous microglial activation or the lack of a predictable anatomical pattern of inflammatory response, thereby rendering the consistent definition of a reference region very difficult, if not impossible. Nevertheless, these approaches (Gunn et al., 1997) have been utilized in the analysis of [C-11]PK11195 binding in a variety of studies including multiple sclerosis (Banati et al., 2000).

[C-11]DAA1106 and fluorinated analogues

N-(2,5-dimethoxybenzyl)-N-(5-fluoro-2-phenoxyphenyl) acetamide (DAA1106) is a novel ligand with sub-nanomolar affinity and excellent selectivity for the PBR. *In vitro* autoradiography of rat brain demonstrated a regional distribution of [H-3]DAA1106 consistent with the known distribution of PBR receptors (Benavides et al., 1983b), with highest binding in olfactory bulb and choroid plexus and moderate binding in cerebellum (Chaki et al., 1999).

Zhang et al. (2003a) reported the labelling of DAA1106 with carbon-11 by methylation of the corresponding desmethyl precursor (DAA1123; Okubo et al., 2004) with high end-of-synthesis radiochemical yield (72 ± 16 per cent) and specific activity (90–156 GBq/μmol). Co-injection of mice with [C-11]DAA1106 and a blocking dose (1 mg/kg) of either unlabeled DAA1106 or PK11195 resulted in a significant reduction of radioactivity throughout the brain that was greatest in the olfactory bulb (14 per cent of control) and cerebellum (16 per cent of control), with moderate reductions in other cortical and subcortical structures (20–54 per cent of control; Zhang et al., 2003a). These results suggest that a dominant portion of brain radioactivity following the injection of [C-11]DAA1106 is specifically bound to constitutive PBR receptors in brain.

Two analogs of DAA1106 labeled with the longer lived positron-emitting radioisotope fluorine-18 have been developed as putative imaging agents for the PBR (Zhang et al., 2003b). Preliminary studies of these analogs, a fluoromethyl derivative (N-5-fluoro-2-phenoxyphenyl)-N-(2-[F-18]fluoromethyl-5-methoxybenzyl)acetamide ([F-18]FMDAA1106) and a fluoroethyl derivative (N-5-fluoro- 2-phenoxyphenyl)-N-(2-[F-18]fluoroethyl-5-methoxybenzyl) acetamide ([F-18]FEDAA1106) indicate that they possess similar binding characteristics and brain distributions to that observed using [C-11]DAA1106 (Zhang et al., 2003a,b). While [C-11]DAA1106 and its radiofluorinated analogues are still novel and largely uncharacterized, the *in vivo* and *in vitro* properties of these ligands in rodent and monkey brain warrant further study and potential development for human PET imaging.

CONCLUSION

Overall the area of non-invasive imaging of inflammation has routinely relied upon relatively non-specific radiotracers, such as gallium citrate and radiolabeled white blood cells for the majority of clinical applications. A multitude of efforts at more specific agents based upon a variety of cellular and chemical entities, including cell specific antibodies, cytokines and chemotactic peptides have led to a variety of interesting compounds which all possess some of the attributes of the 'ideal' inflammation tracer discussed at the outset. Nevertheless, none of these agents has completely replaced the routine application of the standard radiopharmaceuticals ([Ga-67]citrate and labeled white blood cells) in the field. The development of PET radiotracers for inflammation imaging, especially neuroinflammation, presents an interesting direction that may take advantage of the increase in resolution and the quantification aspects inherent with PET to lead to advances in this area. However, there is still significant work to be done in the area of radiotracer synthesis and validation for these applications. While the application of PBR ligands in this area has shown some early promise, there is still much work to be done in order to demonstrate the routine clinical utility of this application. In addition, other interesting areas of radiotracer development are essentially unexplored. The potential utility of radiotracers for the cyclo-oxygenase system, especially COX-2 remains a wide open area of investigation. There have been no convincing demonstrations of specific radiotracers for the COX-2 system to date, even though the involvement of this system in inflammation is well established.

REFERENCES

Ak, I., Stokkel, M.P. and Pauwels, E.K. (2000). Positron emission tomography with 2-[18F]fluoro-2-deoxy-D-glucose in oncology. Part II. The clinical value in detecting and staging primary tumours. J Cancer Res Clin Oncol 126, 560–574.

Anholt, R.R., Pederson, P.L., DeSouza, E.B. and Snyder, S.H. (1986). The peripheral-type benzodiazepine receptor. Localization to the mitochondrial outer membrane. J Biol Chem 261, 776–783.

Awad, M. and Gavish, M. (1987). Binding of [H-3]Ro 5-4864 and [H-3]PK11195 to cerebral cortex and peripheral tissues of various species: Species differences and heterogeneity in peripheral benzodiazepine binding sites. J Neurochem 49, 1407–1414.

Banati, R.B., Myers, R. and Kreutzberg, G.W. (1997). PK ('peripheral benzodiazepine')-binding sites in the CNS indicate early and discrete brain lesions: microautoradiographic detection of [3H]PK11195 binding to activated microglia. J Neurocytol 26, 77–82.

Banati, R.B., Goerres, G.W., Myers, R. et al. (1999). [11C](R)-PK11195 positron emission tomography imaging of activated microglia in vivo in Rasmussen's encephalitis. Neurology 53, 2199–2203.

Banati, R.B., Newcombe, J., Gunn, R.N. et al. (2000). The peripheral benzodiazepine binding site in the brain in multiple sclerosis: quantitative in vivo imaging of microglia as a measure of disease activity. Brain 123, 2321–2337.

Banati, R.B., Cagnin, A., Brooks, D.J. et al. (2001). Long-term trans-synaptic glial responses in the human thalamus after peripheral nerve injury. Neuroreport 12, 3439–3442.

Banati, R.B. (2002). Visualising microglial activation in vivo. Glia 40, 206–217.

Banati, R.B. (2003). Neuropathological imaging: in vivo detection of glial activation as a measure of disease and adaptive change in the brain. Br Med Bull 65, 121–131.

Barrera, P., van der Laken, C.J., Boerman, O.C. et al. (2000). Radiolabeled interleukin-1 receptor antagonist for detection of synovitis in patients with rheumatoid arthritis. Rheumatology (Oxford) 39, 870–874.

Barron, B., Hanna, C., Passalaqua, A.M., Lamki, L., Wegener, W.A. and Goldenberg, D.M. (1999). Rapid diagnostic imaging of acute, nonclassic appendicitis by leukoscintigraphy with sulesomab, a technetium 99m-labeled antigranulocyte antibody Fab' fragment. LeukoScan Appendicitis Clinical Trial Group. Surgery 125, 288–296.

Batchelor, P.E., Liberatore, G.T., Porritt, M.J., Donnan, G.A. and Howells, D.W. (2000). Inhibition of brain-derived neurotrophic factor and glial cell line-derived neurotrophic factor expression reduces dopaminergic sprouting in the injured striatum. Eur J Neurosci 12, 3462–3468.

Becker, W., Dusel, W., Berger, P. and Spiegel, W. (1987). The 111In-granulocyte scan in prosthetic vascular graft infections: imaging technique and results. Eur J Nucl Med 13, 225–229.

Becker, W., Schomann, E., Fischbach, W., Borner, W. and Gruner, K.R. (1988). Comparison of 99Tcm-HMPAO and 111In-oxine labeled granulocytes in man: first clinical results. Nucl Med Commun 9, 435–447.

Becker, W., Borst, U., Fischbach, W., Pasurka, B., Schafer, R. and Borner, W. (1989). Kinetic data of in-vivo labeled granulocytes in humans with a murine Tc-99m-labeled monoclonal antibody. Eur J Nucl Med 15, 361–366.

Becker, W., Marienhagen, J., Ordnung, D. and Wolf, F. (1990). Kinetic of Tc-99m-anti-NCA-95-Moab in vitro labeled granulocytes in comparison to in-vivo Moab-labeled and In-111-oxine-labeled granulocytes. Prog Clin Biol Res 355, 151–158.

Becker, W., Bair, J., Behr, T. et al. (1994). Detection of soft-tissue infections and osteomyelitis using a technetium-99m-labeled anti-granulocyte monoclonal antibody fragment. J Nucl Med 35, 1436–1443.

Becker, W.S., Saptogino, A. and Wolf, F.G. (1992). The single late 99Tcm granulocyte antibody scan in inflammatory diseases. Nucl Med Commun 13, 186–192.

Bekerman, C., Hoffer, P.B. and Bitran, J.D. (1984). The role of gallium-67 in the clinical evaluation of cancer. Semin Nucl Med 14, 296–323.

Benavides, J., Malgouris, C., Imbault, F. et al. (1983a). 'Peripheral type' benzodiazepine binding sites in rat adrenals: binding studies with [3H]PK 11195 and autoradiographic localization. Arch Int Pharmacodyn Ther 266, 38–49.

Benavides, J., Quarteronet, D., Imbault, F. et al. (1983b). Labelling of 'peripheral-type' benzodiazepine binding sites in the rat brain by using [3H]PK 11195, an isoquinoline carboxamide derivative: kinetic studies and autoradiographic localization. J Neurochem 41, 1744–1750.

Benavides, J., Cornu, P., Dennis, T. et al. (1988). Imaging of human brain lesions with an omega 3 site radioligand. Ann Neurol 24, 708–712.

Black, K.L., Shiraishi, T., Ikezak, K., Tabuchi, K. and Becker, D.P. (1994). Peripheral benzodiazepine stimulates secretion of growth hormone and mitochondrial proliferation in pituitary tumour GH3 cells. Neurol Res 16, 74–80.

Blankenberg, F.G., Katsikis, P.D., Tait, J.F. et al. (1998). In vivo detection and imaging of phosphatidylserine expression during programmed cell death. Proc Natl Acad Sci USA 95, 6349–6354.

Bleeker-Rovers, C.P., De Kleijn, E.M., Corstens, F.H., Van Der Meer, J.W. and Oyen, W.J. (2004). Clinical value of FDG PET in patients with fever of unknown origin and patients suspected of focal infection or inflammation. Eur J Nucl Med Mol Imaging 31, 29–37.

Bono, F., Lamarche, I., Prabonnaud, V., Le Fur, G. and Herbert, F.M. (1999). Peripheral benzodiazepine receptor agonists exhibit potent antiapoptotic activities.

Braestrup, C. and Squires, R.F. (1977). Specific benzodiazepine receptors in rat brain characterized by high-affinity [H-3]diazepam binding. Proc Natl Acad Sci USA 74, 3805–3809.

Breeman, W.A., van Hagen, P.M., Kwekkeboom, D.J., Visser, T.J. and Krenning, E.P. (1998). Somatostatin receptor scintigraphy using [111In-DTPA0]RC-160 in humans: a comparison with [111In-DTPA0]octreotide. Eur J Nucl Med 25, 182–186.

Britton, K.E., Vinjamuri, S., Hall, A.V. et al. (1997). Clinical evaluation of technetium-99m infecton for the localisation of bacterial infection. Eur J Nucl Med 24, 553–556.

Britton, K.E., Wareham, D.W., Das, S.S. et al. (2002). Imaging bacterial infection with (99m)Tc-ciprofloxacin (Infection). J Clin Pathol 55, 817–823.

Buscombe, J. and Signore, A. (2003). FDG-PET in infectious and inflammatory disease. Eur J Nucl Med Mol Imaging 30, 1571–1573.

Buscombe, J.R., Oyen, W.J., Grant, A. et al. (1993). Indium-111-labeled polyclonal human immunoglobulin: identifying focal infection in patients positive for human immunodeficiency virus. J Nucl Med 34, 1621–1625.

Cagnin, A., Brooks, D.J., Kennedy, A.M. et al. (2001a). In-vivo measurement of activated microglia in dementia. Lancet 358, 461–467.

Cagnin, A., Myers, R., Gunn, R.N. et al. (2001b). In vivo visualization of activated glia by [11C] (R)-PK11195-PET following herpes encephalitis reveals projected neuronal damage beyond the primary focal lesion. Brain 124, 2014–2027.

Camsonne, R., Crouzel, C., Comar, D. et al. (1984). Synthesis of N-(methyl-1 propyl), chloro-2-phenyl-1 isoquinoline carboxamide-2 (PK11195): a new ligand for peripheral benzodiazepine receptors. J Labeled Comp Radiopharm 21, 985–991.

Canat, X., Carayon, P., Bouaboula, M. et al. (1993). Distribution profile and properties of peripheral-type benzodiazepine receptors on human hemopoietic cells. Life Sci 52, 107–118.

Caveliers, V., Goodbody, A.E., Tran, L.L., Peers, S.H., Thornback, J.R. and Bossuyt, A. (2001). Evaluation of 99mTc-RP128 as a potential inflammation imaging agent: human dosimetry and first clinical results. J Nucl Med 42, 154–161.

Chaki, S., Funakoshi, T., Yoshikawa, R. et al. (1999). Binding characteristics of [3H]DAA1106, a novel and selective ligand for peripheral benzodiazepine receptors. Eur J Pharmacol 371, 197–204.

Chianelli, M., Signore, A., Fritzberg, A.R. and Mather, S.J. (1997). The development of technetium-99m-labeled interleukin-2: a new radiopharmaceutical for the in vivo detection of mononuclear cell infiltrates in immune-mediated diseases. Nucl Med Biol 24, 579–586.

Chirumamilla, S., Sun, D., Bullock, M.R. and Colello, R.J. (2002). Traumatic brain injury induced cell proliferation in the adult mammalian central nervous system. J Neurotrauma 19, 693–703.

Cicchetti, F., Brownell, A.L., Williams, K., Chen, Y.I., Livni, E. and Isacson, O. (2002). Neuroinflammation of the nigrostriatal pathway during progressive 6-OHDA dopamine degeneration in rats monitored by immunohistochemistry and PET imaging. Eur J Neurosci 15, 991–998.

Cleij, M.C., Aigbirhio, F.I., Baron, J.C. and Clark, J.C. (2003). Base-promoted dechlorination of (R)-[C-11]PK11195. J Labeled Comp Radiopharm (Suppl.1), S88.

Collingridge, D.R., Glaser, M., Osman, S. et al. (2003). In vitro selectivity, in vivo biodistribution and tumour uptake of annexin V radiolabeled with a positron emitting radioisotope. Br J Cancer 89, 1327–1333.

Cremer, J.E., Hume, S.P., Cullen, B.M. et al. (1992). The distribution of radioactivity in brains of rats given [N-methyl-11C]PK 11195 in vivo after induction of a cortical ischaemic lesion. Int J Rad Appl Instrum B 19, 159–166.

Culty, M., Li, H., Boujrad, N. et al. (1999). In vitro studies on the role of the peripheral-type benzodiazepine receptor in steroidogenesis. J Steroid Biochem Mol Biol 69, 123–130.

De Souza, E.B., Anholt, R.R., Murphy, K.M., Snyder, S.H. and Kuhar, M.J. (1985). Peripheral-type benzodiazepine receptors in endocrine organs: autoradiographic localization in rat pituitary, adrenal, and testis. Endocrinology 116, 567–573.

De Winter, F., Van de Wiele, C., Dumont, F. et al. (2001). Biodistribution and dosimetry of 99mTc-ciprofloxacin, a promising agent for the diagnosis of bacterial infection. Eur J Nucl Med 28, 570–574.

Debruyne, J.C., Van Laere, K.J., Versijpt, J. et al. (2002). Semiquantification of the peripheral-type benzodiazepine ligand [11C]PK11195 in normal human brain and application in multiple sclerosis patients. Acta Neurol Belg 102, 127–135.

Delbecke, D. (1999). Oncological applications of FDG PET imaging: brain tumors, colorectal cancer, lymphoma and melanoma. J Nucl Med 40, 591–603.

DeLorey, T.M. and Olsen, R.W. (1992). Gamma-aminobutryic acid A receptor structure and function. J Biol Chem 267, 16747–16750.

Dinarello, C.A. (1991). Interleukin-1 and interleukin-1 antagonism. Blood 77, 1627–1652.

Dominguez-Gadea, L., Martin-Curto, L.M., de la Calle, H. and Crespo, A. (1993). Diabetic foot infections: scintigraphic evaluation with 99Tcm-labeled anti-granulocyte antibodies. Nucl Med Commun 14, 212–218.

Drugan, R.C. and Holmes, P.V. (1991). Central and peripheral benzodiazepine receptors: involvement in an organism's response to physical and psychological stress. Neurosci Biobehav Rev 15, 277–298.

Dubois, A., Benavides, J., Peny, B. et al. (1988). Imaging of primary and remote ischaemic and excitotoxic brain lesions. An autoradiographic study of peripheral type benzodiazepine binding sites in the rat and cat. Brain Res 445, 77–90.

Endo, H., Akahoshi, T., Takagishi, K., Kashiwazaki, S. and Matsushima, K. (1991). Elevation of interleukin-8 (IL-8) levels in joint fluids of patients with rheumatoid arthritis and the induction by IL-8 of leukocyte infiltration and synovitis in rabbit joints. Lymphokine Cytokine Res 10, 245–252.

Fares, F., Bar-Ami, S., Brandes, J.M. and Gavish, M. (1988). Changes in the density of peripheral benzodiazepine binding sites in genital organs of the female rat during the oestrous cycle. J Reprod Fertil 83, 619–625.

Fischman, A.J., Fucello, A.J., Pellegrino-Gensey, J.L. et al. (1992). Effect of carbohydrate modification on the localization of human polyclonal IgG at focal sites of bacterial infection. J Nucl Med 33, 1378–1382.

Fischman, A.J., Rauh, D., Solomon, H. et al. (1993). In vivo bioactivity and biodistribution of chemotactic peptide analogs in nonhuman primates. J Nucl Med 34, 2130–2134.

Flugel, A., Matsumuro, K., Neumann, H. et al. (2001). Anti-inflammatory activity of nerve growth factor in experimental autoimmune encephalomyelitis: inhibition of monocyte transendothelial migration. Eur J Immunol 31, 11–22.

Gabay, C. and Kushner, I. (1999). Acute-phase proteins and other systemic responses to inflammation. N Engl J Med 340, 448–454.

Garnier, M., Boujrad, N., Oke, B.O. et al. (1993). Diazepam binding inhibitor is a paracrine/autocrine regulator of Leydig cell proliferation and steroidogenesis: action via peripheral-type benzodiazepine receptor and independent mechanisms. Endocrinology 132, 444–458.

Gavish, M., Bachman, I., Shoukrun, R. et al. (1999). Enigma of the peripheral benzodiazepine receptor. Pharmacol Rev 51, 629–650.

Gerhard, A., Neumaier, B., Elitok, E. et al. (2000). In vivo imaging of activated microglia using [11C]PK11195 and positron emission tomography in patients after ischemic stroke. Neuroreport 11, 2957–2960.

Gerhard, A., Banati, R.B., Goerres, G.W. et al. (2003). [11C](R)-PK11195 PET imaging of microglial activation in multiple system atrophy. Neurology 61, 686–689.

Giulian, D., Young, D.G., Woodward, J., Brown, D.C. and Lachman, L.B. (1988). Interleukin-1 is an astroglial growth factor in the developing brain. J Neurosci 8, 709–714.

Glaser, M., Collingridge, D.R., Aboagye, E.O. et al. (2003). Iodine-124 labeled annexin-V as a potential radiotracer to study apoptosis using positron emission tomography. Appl Radiat Isot 58, 55–62.

Goerres, G.W., Revesz, T., Duncan, J. and Banati, R.B. (2001). Imaging cerebral vasculitis in refractory epilepsy using [(11)C](R)-PK11195 positron emission tomography. AJR Am J Roentgenol 176, 1016–1018.

Goh, A.S., Aw, S.E., Sundram, F.X., Ang, E.S., Goh, S.K. and Leong, K.H. (1990). Imaging of focal inflammation with 99Tcm-labeled human polyclonal immunoglobulin G. Nucl Med Commun 11, 843–856.

Granowitz, E.V., Porat, R., Mier, J.W. et al. (1992). Pharmacokinetics, safety and immunomodulatory effects of human recombinant interleukin-1 receptor antagonist in healthy humans. Cytokine 4, 353–360.

Gratz, S., Rennen, H.J., Boerman, O.C., Oyen, W.J. and Corstens, F.H. (2001). Rapid imaging of experimental colitis with (99m)Tc-interleukin-8 in rabbits. J Nucl Med 42, 917–923.

Grimm, M.C., Pullman, W.E., Bennett, G.M., Sullivan, P.J., Pavli, P. and Doe, W.F. (1995). Direct evidence of monocyte recruitment to inflammatory bowel disease mucosa. J Gastroenterol Hepatol 10, 387–395.

Groom, G.N., Junck, L., Foster, N.L., Frey, K.A. and Kuhl, D.E. (1995). PET of peripheral benzodiazepine binding sites in the microgliosis of Alzheimer's disease. J Nucl Med 36, 2207–2210.

Guhlmann, A., Brecht-Krauss, D., Suger, G. et al. (1998). Fluorine-18-FDG PET and technetium-99m antigranulocyte antibody scintigraphy in chronic osteomyelitis. J Nucl Med 39, 2145–2152.

Gunn, R.N., Lammertsma, A.A., Hume, S.P. and Cunningham, V.J. (1997). Parametric imaging of ligand-receptor binding in PET using a simplified reference region model. Neuroimage 6, 279–287.

Hadjipavlou, A.G., Cesani-Vazquez, F., Villaneuva-Meyer, J. et al. (1998). The effectiveness of gallium citrate Ga 67 radionuclide imaging in vertebral osteomyelitis revisited. Am J Orthop 27, 179–183.

Hall, A.V., Solanki, K.K., Vinjamuri, S., Britton, K.E. and Das, S.S. (1998). Evaluation of the efficacy of 99mTc-Infecton, a novel agent for detecting sites of infection. J Clin Pathol 51, 215–219.

Hall, P.F. (1991). The role of diazepam binding inhibitor in the regulation of steroidogenesis. Neuropharmacology 30, 1411–1416.

Hama, T., Miyamoto, M., Tsukui, H., Nishio, C. and Hatanaka, H. (1989). Interleukin-6 as a neurotrophic factor for promoting the survival of cultured basal forebrain cholinergic neurons from postnatal rats. Neurosci Lett 104, 340–344.

Harwood, S.J., Valdivia, S., Hung, G.L. and Quenzer, R.W. (1999). Use of Sulesomab, a radiolabeled antibody fragment, to detect osteomyelitis in diabetic patients with foot ulcers by leukoscintigraphy. Clin Infect Dis 28, 1200–1205.

Hay, R.V., Skinner, R.S., Newman, O.C. et al. (1997). Scintigraphy of acute inflammatory lesions in rats with radiolabeled recombinant human interleukin-8. Nucl Med Commun 18, 367–378.

Heese, K., Hock, C. and Otten, U. (1998). Inflammatory signals induce neurotrophin expression in human microglial cells. J Neurochem 70, 699–707.

Hertz, L. (1993). Binding characteristics of the receptor and coupling to transport proteins. In Peripheral benzodiazepine receptors, Giessen-Crouse, E., ed. London: Academic Press, pp. 27–51.

Hirsch, J.D., Beyer, C.F., Malkowitz, L., Loullis, C.C. and Blume, A.J. (1989). Characterization of ligand binding to mitochondrial benzodiazepine receptors. Mol Pharmacol 35, 164–172.

Hirsch, T., Decaudin, D., Susin, S.A. et al. (1998). PK11195, a ligand of the mitochondrial benzodiazepine receptor, facilitates the induction of apoptosis and reverses Bcl-2-mediated cytoprotection. Exp Cell Res 241, 426–434.

Hofstra, L., Liem, I.H., Dumont, E.A. et al. (2000). Visualisation of cell death in vivo in patients with acute myocardial infarction. Lancet 356, 209–212.

ICRP (1987). Radiation dose to patients from Radiopharmaceuticals: Gallium citrate, International Commision on Radiation Protection. 18, 141–143.

Itzhak, Y., Baker, L. and Norenberg, M.D. (1993). Characterization of the peripheral-type benzodiazepine receptors in cultured astrocytes: evidence for multiplicity. Glia 9, 211–218.

Izzo, R.S., Witkon, K., Chen, A.I., Hadjiyane, C., Weinstein, M.I. and Pellecchia, C. (1992). Interleukin-8 and neutrophil markers in colonic mucosa from patients with ulcerative colitis. Am J Gastroenterol 87, 1447–1452.

Jaakkola, K., Knuuti, J., Soderlund, K., Saraste, A., Jalkanen, S. and Voipio-Pulkki, L.M. (1998). Labelling lymphocytes with technetium99m-hexamethyl propyleneamine oxime for scintigraphy: an improved labelling procedure. J Immunol Methods 214, 187–197.

Jones, H.A., Marino, P.S., Shakur, B.H. and Morrell, N.W. (2003). In vivo assessment of lung inflammatory cell activity in patients with COPD and asthma. Eur Respir J 21, 567–573.

Junck, L., Olson, J.M., Ciliax, B.J. et al. (1989). PET imaging of human gliomas with ligands for the peripheral benzodiazepine binding site. Ann Neurol 26, 752–758.

Kalicke, T., Schmitz, A., Risse, J.H. et al. (2000). Fluorine-18 fluorodeoxyglucose PET in infectious bone diseases: results of histologically confirmed cases. Eur J Nucl Med 27, 524–528.

Kamegai, M., Niijima, K., Kunishita, T. et al. (1990). Interleukin 3 as a trophic factor for central cholinergic neurons in vitro and in vivo. Neuron 4, 429–436.

Karp, L., Weizman, A., Tyano, S. and Gavish, M. (1989). Examination stress, platelet peripheral benzodiazepine binding sites, and plasma hormone levels. Life Sci 44, 1077–1082.

Kipper, S.L., Rypins, E.B., Evans, D.G., Thakur, M.L., Smith, T.D. and Rhodes, B. (2000). Neutrophil-specific 99mTc-labeled anti-CD15 monoclonal antibody imaging for diagnosis of equivocal appendicitis. J Nucl Med 41, 449–455.

Koths, K. and Halenbech, R. (1985). Pharmacokinetic studies on 35S-labeled recombinant interleukin-2 in mice. In Cellular and molecular biology of lymphokines. London: Academic Press, 779–783.

Kreutzberg, G.W. (1996). Microglia: a sensor for pathological events in the CNS. Trends Neurosci 19, 312–318.

Krznaric, E., Roo, M.D., Verbruggen, A., Stuyck, J. and Mortelmans, L. (1996). Chronic osteomyelitis: diagnosis with technetium-99m-d, l-hexamethylpropylene amine oxime labeled leucocytes. Eur J Nucl Med 23, 792–797.

Kurumaji, A. and Toru, M. (1996). Postnatal development of peripheral-type benzodiazepine receptors in rat brain and peripheral tissues. Develop Brain Res 97, 148–151.

Kwekkeboom, D., Krenning, E.P. and de Jong, M. (2000). Peptide receptor imaging and therapy. J Nucl Med 41, 1704–1713.

Kwekkeboom, D.J., Krenning, E.P., Kho, G.S., Breeman, W.A. and Van Hagen, P.M. (1998). Somatostatin receptor imaging in patients with sarcoidosis. Eur J Nucl Med 25, 1284–1292.

Kwekkeboom, D.J. and Krenning, E.P. (2002). Somatostatin receptor imaging. Semin Nucl Med 32, 84–91.

Lammertsma, A.A. and Hume, S.P. (1996). Simplified reference tissue model for PET receptor studies. Neuroimage 4, 153–158.

Larikka, M.J., Ahonen, A.K., Junila, J.A., Niemela, O., Hamalainen, M.M. and Syrjala, H.P. (2001). Extended combined 99mTc-white blood cell and bone imaging improves the diagnostic accuracy in the detection of hip replacement infections. Eur J Nucl Med 28, 288–293.

Laverman, P., Zalipsky, S., Oyen, W.J. et al. (2000). Improved imaging of infections by avidin-induced clearance of 99mTc-biotin-PEG liposomes. J Nucl Med 41, 912–918.

Lazzeri, E., Manca, M., Molea, N. et al. (1999). Clinical validation of the avidin/indium-111 biotin approach for imaging infection/inflammation in orthopaedic patients. Eur J Nucl Med 26, 606–614.

Le Fur, G., Guilloux, F., Rufat, P. et al. (1983a). Peripheral benzodiazepine binding sites: effect of PK 11195, 1-(2-chlorophenyl)-N-methyl-(1-methylpropyl)-3 isoquinolinecarboxamide. II. In vivo studies. Life Sci 32, 1849–1856.

Le Fur, G., Perrier, M.L., Vaucher, N. et al. (1983b). Peripheral benzodiazepine binding sites: effect of PK 11195, 1-(2-chlorophenyl)-N-methyl-N-(1-methylpropyl)-3-isoquinolinecarboxamide. I. In vitro studies. Life Sci 32, 1839–1847.

Lebtahi, R., Crestani, B., Belmatoug, N. et al. (2001). Somatostatin receptor scintigraphy and gallium scintigraphy in patients with sarcoidosis. J Nucl Med 42, 21–26.

Liberatore, M., Iurilli, A.P., Ponzo, F. et al. (1998). Clinical usefulness of technetium-99m-HMPAO-labeled leukocyte scan in prosthetic vascular graft infection. J Nucl Med 39, 875–879.

Liberatore, M., Fiore, V., D'Agostini, A. et al. (2000). Sternal wound infection revisited. Eur J Nucl Med 27, 660–667.

Lockhart, A., Davis, B., Matthews, J.C. et al. (2003). The peripheral benzodiazepine receptor ligand PK11195 binds with high affinity to the acute phase reactant alpha1-acid glycoprotein: implications for the use of the ligand as a CNS inflammatory marker. Nucl Med Biol 30, 199–206.

Lowenthal, J.W. and MacDonald, H.R. (1986). Binding and internalization of interleukin 1 by T cells. Direct evidence for high- and low-affinity classes of interleukin 1 receptor. J Exp Med 164, 1060–1074.

Maeda, S., Miyawaki, T., Nakanishi, T., Takigawa, M. and Shimada, M. (1998). Peripheral type benzodiazepine receptor in T lymphocyte rich preparation. Life Sci 63, 1423–1430.

Mahida, Y.R., Perkins, A.C., Frier, M., Wastie, M.L. and Hawkey, C.J. (1992). Monoclonal antigranulocyte antibody imaging in inflammatory bowel disease: a preliminary report. Nucl Med Commun 13, 330–335.

Martin, S.J., Reutelingsperger, C.P., McGahon, A.J. et al. (1995). Early redistribution of plasma membrane phosphatidylserine is a general feature of apoptosis regardless of the initiating stimulus: inhibition by overexpression of Bcl-2 and Abl. J Exp Med 182, 1545–1556.

McAfee, J.G. and Thakur, M.L. (1976a). Survey of radioactive agents for in vitro labeling of phagocytic leukocytes. II. Particles. J Nucl Med 17, 488–492.

McAfee, J.G. and Thakur, M.L. (1976b). Survey of radioactive agents for in vitro labeling of phagocytic leukocytes. I. Soluble agents. J Nucl Med 17, 480–487.

McAfee, J.G., Subramanian, G. and Gagne, G. (1984). Technique of leukocyte harvesting and labeling: problems and perspectives. Semin Nucl Med 14, 83–106.

Merrill, J.E. (1992). Tumor necrosis factor alpha, interleukin 1 and related cytokines in brain development: normal and pathological. Dev Neurosci 14, 1–10.

Morgan, D.A., Ruscetti, F.W. and Gallo, R. (1976). Selective in vitro growth of T lymphocytes from normal human bone marrows. Science 193, 1007–1008.

Morrel, E.M., Tompkins, R.G., Fischman, A.J., Wilkinson, R.A. and Yarmush, M.L. (1990). Imaging infections with antibodies. A quantitative autoradiographic analysis. J Immunol Methods 130, 39–48.

Moyer, B.R., Vallabhajosula, S., Lister-James, J. et al. (1996). Technetium-99m-white blood cell-specific imaging agent developed from platelet factor 4 to detect infection. J Nucl Med 37, 673–679.

Mozley, P.D., Thakur, M.L., Alavi, A. et al. (1999). Effects of a 99mTc-labeled murine immunoglobulin M antibody to CD15 antigens on human granulocyte membranes in healthy volunteers. J Nucl Med 40, 2107–2114.

Mukherjee, S. and Das, S.K. (1989). Subcellular localization of 'peripheral type' benzodiazepine receptors for [H-3]Ro5-4864 in guinea pig lung: localization to the mitochondrial inner membrane. J Biol Chem 164, 16713–16718.

Murakami, Y., Takamatsu, H., Taki, J. et al. (2003). 18F-labeled annexin V: a PET tracer for apoptosis imaging. Eur J Nucl Med Mol Imaging.

Myers, R., Manjil, L.G., Cullen, B.M., Price, G.W., Frackowiak, R.S. and Cremer, J.E. (1991a). Macrophage and astrocyte populations in relation to [3H]PK 11195 binding in rat cerebral cortex following a local ischaemic lesion. J Cereb Blood Flow Metab 11, 314–322.

Myers, R., Manjil, L.G., Frackowiak, R.S. and Cremer, J.E. (1991b). [3H]PK 11195 and the localisation of secondary thalamic lesions following focal ischaemia in rat motor cortex. Neurosci Lett 133, 20–24.

Nesbit, G.M., Forbes, G.S., Scheithauer, B.W., Okazaki, H. and Rodriguez, M. (1991). Multiple sclerosis: histopathologic and MR and/or CT correlation in 37 cases at biopsy and three cases at autopsy. Radiology 180, 467–474.

Nijhof, M.W., Oyen, W.J., van Kampen, A., Claessens, R.A., van der Meer, J.W. and Corstens, F.H. (1997). Evaluation of infections of the locomotor system with indium-111-labeled human IgG scintigraphy. J Nucl Med 38, 1300–1305.

Novas, M.L., Medina, J.H., Calvo, D. and De Robertis, E. (1987). Increase of peripheral type benzodiazepine binding sites in kidney and olfactory bulb in acutely stressed rats. Eur J Pharmacol 135, 243–246.

O'Doherty, M.J., Barrington, S.F., Campbell, M., Lowe, J. and Bradbeer, C.S. (1997). PET scanning and the human immunodeficiency virus-positive patient. J Nucl Med 38, 1575–1583.

Ogura, Y., Krams, S.M., Martinez, O.M. et al. (2000). Radiolabeled annexin V imaging: diagnosis of allograft rejection in an experimental rodent model of liver transplantation. Radiology 214, 795–800.

Okubo, T., Yoshikawa, R., Chaki, S., Okuyama, S. and Nakazato, A. (2004). Design, synthesis and structure-affinity relationships of aryloxyanilide derivatives as novel peripheral benzodiazepine receptor ligands. Bioorg Med Chem 12, 423–438.

Olson, J.M., Ciliax, B.J., Mancini, W.R. and Young, A.B. (1988). Presence of peripheral-type benzodiazepine binding sites on human erythrocyte membranes. Eur J Pharmacol 152, 47–53.

Oyen, W.J., Claessens, R.A., van der Meer, J.W., Rubin, R.H., Strauss, H.W. and Corstens, F.H. (1992). Indium-111-labeled human nonspecific immunoglobulin G: a new radiopharmaceutical for imaging infectious and inflammatory foci. Clin Infect Dis 14, 1110–1118.

Oyen, W.J. and Mansi, L. (2003). FDG-PET in infectious and inflammatory disease. Eur J Nucl Med Mol Imaging 30, 1568–1570.

Palestro, C.J., Weiland, F.L., Seabold, J.E. et al. (2001). Localizing infection with a technetium-99m-labeled peptide: initial results. Nucl Med Commun 22, 695–701.

Papadopoulos, V., Boujrad, N., Ikonomovic, M.D., Ferrara, O. and Vidic, B. (1994). Topography of the Leydig cell mitochondrial peripheral-type benzodiazepine receptor. Mol Cell Endocrinol 104, R5–R9.

Pappata, S., Cornu, P., Samson, Y. et al. (1991). PET study of carbon-11-PK 11195 binding to peripheral type benzodiazepine sites in glioblastoma: a case report. J Nucl Med 32, 1608–1610.

Pappata, S., Levasseur, M., Gunn, R.N. et al. (2000). Thalamic microglial activation in ischemic stroke detected in vivo by PET and [11C]PK11195. Neurology 55, 1052–1054.

Paul, C., Peers, S.H., Woodhouse, L.E., Thornback, J.R., Goodbody, A.E. and Bolton, C. (2000). The detection and quantitation of inflammation in the central nervous system during experimental allergic encephalomyelitis using the radiopharmaceutical 99mTc-RP128. J Neurosci Methods 98, 83–90.

Peltier, P., Potel, G., Lovat, E., Baron, D. and Chatal, J.F. (1993). Detection of lung and bone infection with anti-granulocyte monoclonal antibody BW 250/183 radiolabeled with 99Tcm. Nucl Med Commun 14, 766–774.

Penkowa, M., Moos, T., Carrasco, J. et al. (1999). Strongly compromised inflammatory response to brain injury in interleukin-6-deficient mice. Glia 25, 343–357.

Perkins, P.J. (1981). Early gallium-67 abdominal imaging: pitfalls due to bowel activity. Am J Roentgenol 136, 1016–1017.

Perry, V.H., Andersson, P.B. and Gordon, S. (1993). Macrophages and inflammation in the central nervous system. Trends Neurosci 16, 268–273.

Peters, A.M., Danpure, H.J., Osman, S. et al. (1986). Clinical experience with 99mTc-hexamethylpropylene-amineoxime for labelling leucocytes and imaging inflammation. Lancet 2, 946–949.

Peters, A.M. (1994). The utility of [99mTc]HMPAO-leukocytes for imaging infection. Semin Nucl Med 24, 110–127.

Peters, A.M. (1999). Nuclear medicine imaging in fever of unknown origin. Q J Nucl Med 43, 61–73.

Petit-Taboue, M.C., Baron, J.C., Barre, L. et al. (1991). Brain kinetics and specific binding of [11C]PK 11195 to omega 3 sites in baboons: positron emission tomography study. Eur J Pharmacol 200, 347–351.

Pollak, A., Goodbody, A.E., Ballinger, J.R. et al. (1996). Imaging inflammation with 99Tcm-labeled chemotactic peptides: analogues with reduced neutropenia. Nucl Med Commun 17, 132–139.

Price, G.W., Ahier, R.G., Hume, S.P. et al. (1990). In vivo binding to peripheral benzodiazepine binding sites in lesioned rat brain: comparison between [3H]PK11195 and [18F]PK14105 as markers for neuronal damage. J Neurochem 55, 175–185.

Raivich, G., Jones, L.L., Kloss, C.U., Werner, A., Neumann, H. and Kreutzberg, G.W. (1998). Immune surveillance in the injured nervous system: T-lymphocytes invade the axotomized mouse facial motor nucleus and aggregate around sites of neuronal degeneration. J Neurosci 18, 5804–5816.

Ramsay, S.C., Weiller, C., Myers, R. et al. (1992). Monitoring by PET of macrophage accumulation in brain after ischaemic stroke. Lancet 339, 1054–1055.

Rennen, H.J., Boerman, O.C., Koenders, E.B., Oyen, W.J. and Corstens, F.H. (2000). Labeling proteins with Tc-99m via hydrazinonicotinamide (HYNIC): optimization of the conjugation reaction. Nucl Med Biol 27, 599–604.

Rennen, H.J., Boerman, O.C., Oyen, W.J., van der Meer, J.W. and Corstens, F.H. (2001). Specific and rapid scintigraphic detection of infection with 99mTc-labeled interleukin-8. J Nucl Med 42, 117–123.

Robb, R.J., Greene, W.C. and Rusk, C.M. (1984). Low and high affinity receptors for IL-2. J Exp Med 160, 1126–1146.

Robb, R.J., Mayer, P.C. and Garlick, R. (1985). Retention of biological activity following radioiodination of human interleukin-2: comparison with biosynthetically labeled growth factor in receptor binding assay. J Immunol Methods 81, 15–30.

Ruff, M.R., Pert, C.B., Weber, R.J., Wahl, L.M., Wahl, S.M. and Paul, S.M. (1985). Benzodiazepine receptor-mediated chemotaxis of human monocytes. Science 229, 1281–1283.

Rusckowski, M., Fritz, B. and Hnatowich, D.J. (1992). Localization of infection using streptavidin and biotin: an alternative to nonspecific polyclonal immunoglobulin. J Nucl Med 33, 1810–1815.

Samuel, A., Paganelli, G., Chiesa, R. et al. (1996). Detection of prosthetic vascular graft infection using avidin/indium-111-biotin scintigraphy. J Nucl Med 37, 55–61.

Sawada, M., Suzumura, A., Itoh, Y. and Marunochi, T. (1993). Production of interleukin-5 by mouse astrocytes and microglia in culture. Neurosci Lett 155, 175–178.

Seabold, J.E., Nepola, J.V., Conrad, G.R. et al. (1989). Detection of osteomyelitis at fracture nonunion sites: comparison of two scintigraphic methods. Am J Roentgenol 152, 1021–1027.

Segal, A.W., Arnot, R.N., Thakur, M.L. and Lavender, J.P. (1976). Indium-111-labeled leucocytes for localisation of abscesses. Lancet 2, 1056–1058.

Semenzato, G., Zambello, R. and Pizzolo, G. (1992). Interleukin-2 receptor expression in health and disease. In Interleukin-2, Balkwill, F., ed. Oxford: Blackwell Scientific Publications, 78–105.

Shaffer, L.L., McNulty, J.A. and Young, M.R. (2003). Brain activation of monocyte-lineage cells: involvement of interleukin-6. Neuroimmunomodulation 10, 295–304.

Shah, F., Hume, S.P., Pike, V.W., Ashworth, S. and McDermott, J. (1994). Synthesis of the enantiomers of [N-methyl-11C]PK 11195 and comparison of their behaviours as radioligands for PK binding sites in rats. Nucl Med Biol 21, 573–581.

Shoup, T.M., Fischman, A.J., Jaywook, S., Babich, J.W., Strauss, H.W. and Elmaleh, D.R. (1994). Synthesis of fluorine-18-labeled biotin derivatives: biodistribution and infection localization. J Nucl Med 35, 1685–1690.

Shreve, P.D., Anzai, Y. and Wahl, R.L. (1999). Pitfalls in oncologic diagnosis with FDG PET imaging: Physiologic and benign variants. Radiographics 19, 61–77.

Signore, A., Beales, P., Sensi, M., Zuccarini, O. and Pozzilli, P. (1983). Labelling of lymphocytes with indium 111 oxine: effect on cell surface phenotype and antibody-dependent cellular cytotoxicity. Immunol Lett 6, 151–154.

Signore, A., Parman, A., Pozzilli, P., Andreani, D. and Beverley, P.C. (1987). Detection of activated lymphocytes in endocrine pancreas of BB/W rats by injection of 123I-interleukin-2: an early sign of type 1 diabetes. Lancet 2, 537–540.

Signore, A., Chianelli, M., Annovazzi, A. et al. (2000a). 123I-interleukin-2 scintigraphy for in vivo assessment of intestinal mononuclear cell infiltration in Crohn's disease. J Nucl Med 41, 242–249.

Signore, A., Procaccini, E., Annovazzi, A., Chianelli, M., van der Laken, C. and Mire-Sluis, A. (2000b). The developing role of cytokines for imaging inflammation and infection. Cytokine 12, 1445–1454.

Signore, A., Chianelli, M., Bei, R., Oyen, W. and Modesti, A. (2003a). Targeting cytokine/chemokine receptors: a challenge for molecular nuclear medicine. Eur J Nucl Med Mol Imaging 30, 149–156.

Signore, A., Picarelli, A., Annovazzi, A. et al. (2003b). 123I-Interleukin-2: biochemical characterization and in vivo use for imaging autoimmune diseases. Nucl Med Commun 24, 305–316.

Stephenson, D.T., Schober, D.A., Smalstig, E.B., Mincy, R.E., Gehlert, D.R. and Clemens, J.A. (1995). Peripheral benzodiazepine receptors are colocalized with activated microglia following transient global forebrain ischemia in the rat. J Neurosci 15, 5263–5274.

Stokkel, M.P., Reigman, H.E. and Pauwels, E.K. (2002). Scintigraphic head-to-head comparison between 99mTc-WBCs and 99mTc-LeukoScan in the evaluation of inflammatory bowel disease: a pilot study. Eur J Nucl Med Mol Imaging 29, 251–254.

Streit, W.J., Walter, S.A. and Pennell, N.A. (1999). Reactive microgliosis. Prog Neurobiol 57, 563–581.

Stumpe, K.D., Dazzi, H., Schaffner, A. and von Schulthess, G.K. (2000). Infection imaging using whole-body FDG-PET. Eur J Nucl Med 27, 822–832.

Sugawara, Y., Braun, D.K., Kison, P.V., Russo, J.E., Zasadny, K.R. and Wahl, R.L. (1998). Rapid detection of human infections with fluorine-18 fluorodeoxyglucose and positron emission tomography: preliminary results. Eur J Nucl Med 25, 1238–1243.

Taketani, S., Kohno, H., Okuda, M., Furukawa, T. and Tokunaga, R. (1994). Induction of peripheral-type benzodiazepine receptors during differentiation of mouse erythroleukemia cells. A possible involvement of these receptors in heme biosynthesis. J Biol Chem 269, 7527–7531.

Taupin, V., Toulmond, S., Serrano, A., Benavides, J. and Zavala, F. (1993). Increase in IL-6, IL-1 and TNF levels in rat brain following traumatic lesion. Influence of pre- and post-traumatic treatment with Ro5 4864, a peripheral-type (p site) benzodiazepine ligand. J Neuroimmunol 42, 177–185.

Thakur, M.L., Coleman, R.E. and Welch, M.J. (1977a). Indium-111-labeled leukocytes for the localization of abscesses: preparation, analysis, tissue distribution, and comparison with gallium-67 citrate in dogs. J Lab Clin Med 89, 217–228.

Thakur, M.L., Lavender, J.P., Arnot, R.N., Silvester, D.J. and Segal, A.W. (1977b). Indium-111-labeled autologous leukocytes in man. J Nucl Med 18, 1014–1021.

Thakur, M.L., Marcus, C.S., Henneman, P. et al. (1996). Imaging inflammatory diseases with neutrophil-specific technetium-99m-labeled monoclonal antibody anti-SSEA-1. J Nucl Med 37, 1789–1795.

Thoenen, H. and Barde, Y.A. (1980). Physiology of nerve growth factor. Physiol Rev 60, 1284–1335.

Thompson, C.B. (1995). Apoptosis in the pathogenesis and treatment of disease. Science 267, 1456–1462.

Tong, Y., Rheaume, E., Simard, J. and Pelletier, G. (1991). Localization of peripheral benzodiazepine binding sites and diazepam-binding inhibitor (DBI) mRNA in mammary glands and dimethylbenz(a)antracene (DMBA)-induced mammary tumors in the rat. Regul Pept 33, 263–273.

Toranzo, D., Tong, Y., Tonon, M.C., Vaudry, H. and Pelletier, G. (1994). Localization of diazepam-binding inhibitor and peripheral type benzodiazepine binding sites in the rat ovary. Anat Embryol (Berl) 190, 383–388.

Tsan, M.F. (1985). Mechanism of gallium-67 accumulation in inflammatory lesions. J Nucl Med 26, 88–92.

Turpin, S. and Lambert, R. (2001). Role of scintigraphy in musculoskeletal and spinal infections. Radiol Clin North Am 39, 169–189.

Vaca, K. and Wendt, E. (1992). Divergent effects of astroglial and microglial secretions on neuron growth and survival. Exp Neurol 118, 62–72.

van der Laken, C.J., Boerman, O.C., Oyen, W.J. et al. (1995). Specific targeting of infectious foci with radioiodinated human recombinant interleukin-1 in an experimental model. Eur J Nucl Med 22, 1249–1255.

van der Laken, C.J., Boerman, O.C., Oyen, W.J. et al. (1996). Different behaviour of radioiodinated human recombinant interleukin-1 and its receptor antagonist in an animal model of infection. Eur J Nucl Med 23, 1531–1535.

van der Laken, C.J., Boerman, O.C., Oyen, W.J. et al. (1997). Preferential localization of systemically administered radiolabeled interleukin 1alpha in experimental inflammation in mice by binding to the type II receptor. J Clin Invest 100, 2970–2976.

van der Laken, C.J., Boerman, O.C., Oyen, W.J., van de Ven, M.T., van der Meer, J.W. and Corstens, F.H. (1998a). Imaging of infection in rabbits with radioiodinated interleukin-1 (alpha and beta), its receptor antagonist and a chemotactic peptide: a comparative study. Eur J Nucl Med 25, 347–352.

van der Laken, C.J., Boerman, O.C., Oyen, W.J., Van de Ven, M.T., Ven der Meer, J.W. and Corstens, F.H. (1998b). The kinetics of radiolabeled interleukin-8 in infection and sterile inflammation. Nucl Med Commun 19, 271–281.

van der Laken, C.J., Boerman, O.C., Oyen, W.J., van de Ven, M.T., van der Meer, J.W. and Corstens, F.H. (2000). Radiolabeled interleukin-8: specific scintigraphic detection of infection within a few hours. J Nucl Med 41, 463–469.

van der Lely, A.J., de Herder, W.W., Krenning, E.P. and Kwekkeboom, D.J. (2003). Octreoscan radioreceptor imaging. Endocrine 20, 307–311.

Vanquickenborne, B., Maes, A., Nuyts, J. et al. (2003). The value of (18)FDG-PET for the detection of infected hip prosthesis. Eur J Nucl Med Mol Imaging.

Venneti, S., Lopresti, B.J., Wang, G. et al. (2004). PET imaging of brain macrophages using the peripheral benzodiazepine receptor in a macaque model of NeuroAIDS. J Clin Invest 113.

Verma, A. and Snyder, S.H. (1989). Peripheral type benzodiazepine receptors. Annu Rev Pharmacol Toxicol 29, 307–322.

Vinjamuri, S., Hall, A.V., Solanki, K.K. et al. (1996). Comparison of 99mTc infecton imaging with radiolabeled white-cell imaging in the evaluation of bacterial infection. Lancet 347, 233–235.

Vowinckel, E., Reutens, D., Becher, B. et al. (1997). PK11195 binding to the peripheral benzodiazepine receptor as a marker of microglia activation in multiple sclerosis and experimental autoimmune encephalomyelitis. J Neurosci Res 50, 345–353.

Wassie, E., Buscombe, J.R., Miller, R.F. and Ell, P.J. (1994). 67Ga scintigraphy in HIV antibody positive patients; a review of its clinical usefulness. Br J Radiol 67, 349–352.

Weinberg, J.B., Blinder, R.A. and Coleman, R.E. (1986). In vitro function of indium-111 oxine-labeled human monocytes. J Immunol Methods 95, 9–14.

Weiner, R. (1990). The role of transferrin and other receptors in the mechanism of 67Ga localization. Int J Rad Appl Instrum B 17, 141–149.

Weinmann, P., Crestani, B., Tazi, A. et al. (2000). 111In-pentetreotide scintigraphy in patients with Langerhans' cell histiocytosis. J Nucl Med 41, 1808–1812.

Williams, K.C., Corey, S., Westmoreland, S.V. et al. (2001). Perivascular macrophages are the primary cell type productively infected by simian immunodeficiency virus in the brains of macaques: implications for the neuropathogenesis of AIDS. J Exp Med 193, 905–915.

Wilms, H., Claasen, J., Rohl, C., Sievers, J., Deuschl, G. and Lucius, R. (2003). Involvement of benzodiazepine receptors in neuroinflammatory and neurodegenerative diseases: evidence from activated microglial cells in vitro. Neurobiol Dis *14*, 417–424.

Yapar, Z., Kibar, M., Yapar, A.F., Togrul, E., Kayaselcuk, U. and Sarpel, Y. (2001). The efficacy of technetium-99m ciprofloxacin (Infecton) imaging in suspected orthopaedic infection: a comparison with sequential bone/gallium imaging. Eur J Nucl Med *28*, 822–830.

Zavala, F., Taupin, V. and Descamps-Latscha, B. (1990). In vivo treatment with benzodiazepines inhibits murine phagocyte oxidative metabolism and production of interleukin 1, tumor necrosis factor and interleukin-6. J Pharmacol Exp Ther *255*, 442–450.

Zavala, F. (1997). Benzodiazepines, anxiety and immunity. Pharmacol Ther *5*, 199–216.

Zhang, M.R., Kida, T., Noguchi, J. et al. (2003a). [(11)C]DAA1106: radiosynthesis and in vivo binding to peripheral benzodiazepine receptors in mouse brain. Nucl Med Biol *30*, 513–519.

Zhang, M.R., Maeda, J., Furutsuka, K. et al. (2003b). [18F]FMDAA1106 and [18F]FEDAA1106: two positron-emitter labeled ligands for peripheral benzodiazepine receptor (PBR). Bioorg Med Chem Lett *13*, 201–204.

Zhuang, H., Duarte, P.S., Pourdeh, M., Shnier, D. and Alavi, A. (2000). Exclusion of chronic osteomyelitis with F-18 fluorodeoxyglucose positron emission tomographic imaging. Clin Nucl Med *25*, 281–284.

Zhuang, H., Pourdehnad, M., Lambright, E.S. et al. (2001). Dual time point 18F-FDG PET imaging for differentiating malignant from inflammatory processes. J Nucl Med *42*, 1412–1417.

Section VI

Assays in Acute and Chronic Diseases

Cancer – Solid Tumors

Chapter 40

Mary L. Disis and the Immunologic Monitoring Consortium

Tumor Vaccine Group, University of Washington, Seattle, WA, USA

> The great tragedy of science – the slaying of a beautiful hypothesis by an ugly fact.
>
> Thomas Huxley

INTRODUCTION

Recent advances in molecular biology and basic immunology have resulted in the development of highly quantitative assays to measure tumor-specific T cell immunity. The definition of specific tumor antigens and a more detailed understanding of T cell-antigen recognition and the character of peptides presented in the major histocompatibitiy complex (MHC) have resulted in the development of novel methods to quantitate the human T cell response to cancer. As compared to older methods of immune response analysis such as delayed type hypersensitivity (DTH) response, chromium release assays (^{51}Cr) and tritiated thymidine incorporation, new immunologic monitoring techniques are, in general, more robust and reproducible (Table 40.1).

Currently there are no standard methods of assessing immunity after an immunotherapeutic intervention. The ideal immunologic assay would be one whose detection of immunity correlated with a clinical response and could be adapted to wide scale clinical use. The amount of clinical material that can be obtained on individual cancer patients would limit the choice of assay used (Table 40.2). Currently, clinical trials of immunotherapeutics should be designed to incorporate validation of any particular

biomarker into the statistical assessment correlating laboratory results with clinical outcome. As we wait and see whether any particular assay will be predictive of clinical outcome, many immunologic monitoring methods have proven to be of utility as a measure of potency. Vaccines designed to elicit a specific immune response, e.g. to class I peptides or a Th1 response, can be analyzed exquisitely to determine whether immunization resulted in the desired outcome. In addition, reproducible immunologic monitoring methods have allowed comparison of different vaccine strategies as well as the identification and characterization of baseline immunity in cancer patients.

Evaluation of cytokine production or expression after antigenic stimulation via ELISPOT or cytokine flow cytometry (CFC) and assessment of a clonal T cell response in terms of measuring T cell binding to particular

Table 40.1 Comparison of assay characteristics

Feature	ELISPOT	CFC	MHC tetramer
Limit of detection	1:100 000	1:20 000	1:20 000
Assay time (h)	24–48	8	2
Requires *in vitro* stimulation	Limited to prolonged	Limited	No
Functional readout	Yes	Yes	No
Non-MHC restricted	Yes	Yes	No
Easily automated	No	Yes	Yes
T cell subset response	After a pre-selection step	Yes	Yes

Measuring Immunity, edited by Michael T. Lotze and Angus W. Thomson
ISBN 0-12-455900-X, London

Table 40.2 Cellular requirements for common assays per a single antigen and control

Assay type	Amount of PBMC needed
LDA	50×10^6
ELISPOT	10×10^6
Flow based assays (CFC, tetramer)	1×10^6

MHC-peptide complexes have become standard immunologic tools for measuring human tumor-specific T cell immunity. The studies described below are representative examples of the types of analysis that can be performed evaluating and characterizing tumor specific immunity in patients with solid tumors.

ASSESSMENT OF CELLULAR IMMUNITY BASED ON ANTIGEN SPECIFIC CYTOKINE PRODUCTION

Antigen specific immune responses are largely regulated by secretion of cytokines whose function is to govern the growth and differentiation of T cell populations. Secretion of cytokines by T cells responding to a specific antigen has become a common measure of a functional immune response. Although the measurement of cytokine production by T cells using ELISA methodologies is not quantitative, measurement of cytokines offers a detailed characterization of the function of the T cell and the phenotype of the immune environment generated after antigen recognition. Evaluation of cytokine production by an individual T cell can be assessed using either ELISPOT or CFC. Thus, these assays are a highly quantitative measure of potentially functional T cells.

ELISPOT

Cytokine release assays have been modified to provide a quantitative measure of precursor frequency. Recently, enzyme-linked immunosorbent-spot (ELISPOT) has been used to characterize cytokine release at the single cell level (Scheibenbogen et al., 1997, 2003; Schmittel et al., 1997; Vaquerano et al., 1998). ELISPOT is a sensitive T cell quantitation method and can detect specific precursors at 1:100 000. Indeed, ELISPOT is being increasingly used as a tool for monitoring immunologic responses to cancer vaccines (Wang and Rosenberg, 1999; Asai et al., 2000; Meidenbauer et al., 2000). The methods individual laboratories employ for ELISPOT vary greatly (Asai et al., 2000). Standardization of technique and definition of the sensitivity and range of the assay are needed to develop ELISPOT as a clinical tool.

ELISPOT analysis has been used by several investigators to define and characterize baseline T cell immunity to specific tumor antigens in a variety of solid tumor patient populations. Tatsumi et al. (2002) used interferon (IFN)-gamma and interleukin (IL)-5 ELISPOT assays on fractionated T cell populations to examine the magnitude of Th1 and Th2 responses to HLA-DRB1*0401 epitopes of MAGE-6. They demonstrated that patients with active melanoma or renal cell carcinoma displayed a strongly polarized Th2-type reactivity to these peptides, while normal donors and patients who were disease-free following therapeutic intervention exhibited either a weak mixed Th1/Th2-type or strongly polarized Th1-type response to the same epitopes. It should be emphasized that these polarized CD4+ responses are specific for these specific epitopes and do not represent a general tendency of the donor or patient to respond in a generically Th2-biased or Th1-biased fashion. Mitogen treatment of peripheral blood mononuclear cells (PBMC) stimulated IFN-gamma and IL-5 responses that were indistinguishable between the patients with active melanoma or renal cell carcinoma and normal donors and patients who were disease-free. While the numbers of patients in the study were relatively small, the results do imply that a Th2-type dominated CD4+ response against the MAGE-6 epitopes may correlate with active disease status. Investigators are extending these studies to determine the prognostic significance of Th1-type and Th2-type balance. Studies of baseline immunity to tumor antigens may also indicate differences in immune responses to the same antigens between tumor types. Investigators evaluated T cell responses against Ep-CAM, HER-2/neu and CEA in patients with breast and colorectal cancer by IFN-gamma ELISPOT. Although influenza specific responses were similar in both populations, tumor antigen specific T cell immunity could only be detected in the colorectal cancer patients (Nagorsen et al., 2003).

ELISPOT has also been used to assess the potency of a particular vaccine approach. Vaccine studies comparing vaccination strategies and adjuvants have utilized ELISPOT to determine which approach to be superior. One study evaluated DNA plasmid, peptide and modified vaccinia Ankara virus (MVA) combinations in their ability to elicit influenza specific responses in mice (Woodberry et al., 2003). Investigators demonstrated while DNA/MVA combinations could enhance IFN-gamma secretion by CD8+ T cells, protection against infection was not enhanced. Studies such as this, in preclinical models, will influence the design of human vaccine trials. Vaccine comparative evaluations are already ongoing in humans. For example, investigators vaccinated melanoma patients with tyrosinase peptides in granulocyte macrophage colony stimulating factor (GM-CSF), keyhole limpit hemocyanin (KLH), or both (Scheibenbogen et al., 2003). Using IFN-gamma ELISPOT as a biomarker, they determined that the use of both adjuvants resulted in the generation of immunity in a larger number of patients than either adjuvant alone.

Finally, human clinical trials of cancer vaccines suggest that a positive ELISPOT response may correlate with improved clinical outcome after vaccination. Evidence of a correlation between immunologic responses defined by the ELISPOT assay and clinical response has been reported in a recent study in melanoma patients testing tumor derived heat shock protein gp96-peptide complexes (Belli et al., 2002). Notably, this group measured responses using freshly isolated PBMC without any *in vitro* culture step and used a stringent definition of a positive ELISPOT (Keilholz et al., 2002). The study showed a strong correlation ($P < 0.01$) between T cell responses measured by IFN-gamma ELISPOT and patient clinical responses in 23 patients. This is, to date, the largest study showing a correlation between ELISPOT and clinical outcome and underscores the need for further studies to determine if the IFN-gamma ELISPOT assay is a correlate of *in vivo* tumor rejection. Furthermore, it is important to note that the PBMC samples in this study did not undergo *in vitro* stimulation. The ability to detect tumor specific immunity without an *in vitro* stimulation step may indicate a more robust immune response generated after vaccination.

ELISPOT is a highly sensitive method for detecting tumor specific T cell responses in patients undergoing experimental immunotherapy for solid tumors. However, there is considerable methodologic variation between individual laboratories at present. This variability makes it difficult to compare responses induced by different vaccines at different clinical centers. The acceptance of clearly defined protocols for the ELISPOT assay and validated measures of what represents an immunologic response will allow ELISPOT to be compared to clinical response in the large patient numbers needed to determine if it can be a surrogate marker for clinically relevant levels of vaccination.

Cytokine flow cytometry (CFC)

CFC is a relatively new method of quantifying antigen-specific T cells (Waldrop et al., 1997; Suni et al., 1998). Immune effector cells are identified by virtue of their cytokine production upon short-term *in vitro* incubation with antigen (e.g. virus, protein, or peptide(s)). Either all or the terminal portion of the incubation is done in the presence of a secretion inhibitor such as brefeldin A, which allows the detection of cytokines intracellularly. The short-term incubation, often 6 h, avoids the confounding effects of cell proliferation and/or apoptosis and thus allows for accurate quantitation of the frequency of responsive T cells in peripheral blood (Maecker et al., 2000). The cells are fixed, permeabilized and stained for surface and intracellular epitopes and analyzed by flow cytometry (Maecker, 2003).

CFC has an advantage over ELISPOT in that the assay can simultaneously analyze multiple T cell subsets responding to a specific antigen. CFC has been used to analyze T cell frequencies in a large number of infectious disease settings, including HIV (Maecker and Maino, 2003),

CMV (Maecker et al., 2000) and other viral and bacterial systems. The data from viral systems, especially CMV, have demonstrated that an unexpectedly large proportion of the CD4+ and CD8+ T cell repertoire of seropositive individuals can be devoted to this response (Bitmansour et al., 2001; Dunn et al., 2002). This may be due in part to the biology of the virus, including its presence in the blood and lymphatic system and its ability periodically to reactivate and thereby boost immune responses. In part because of concerns about the sensitivity of CFC in detecting responses to non-viral antigens, its use in monitoring cancer responses has been more limited. However, CFC has been used in detecting responses to tumor antigens in both mouse and human systems.

CFC assays in mouse models were pioneered by work on viral infections, including LCMV (Murali-Krishna et al., 1998; Varga and Welsh, 1998; Whitmire et al., 1998; Hassett et al., 2000; De Boer et al., 2001; Homann et al., 2001; Slifka and Whitton, 2001). Studies of vaccination for the intracellular parasite *Leishmania major* also used CFC to demonstrate the requirement for sustained IL-12 production in maintaining antigen-specific IFN gamma-producing T cells (Gurunathan et al., 1998, 2000; Stobie et al., 2000; Mendez et al., 2001). Similar correlation of IFN gamma CFC with protection was shown in a *Listeria monocytogenes* vaccination model (Leavey and Tarleton, 2003). These studies were important in establishing the concept of CFC as a surrogate marker for vaccine-induced protection from disease.

Turning to virus-induced tumor systems, CFC was used to track the CD8+ T cell response to polyoma virus in neonatal and adult mice (Lukacher et al., 1999; Moser et al., 2001). These studies observed that IFN gamma-producing CD8+ T cells developed in both tumor-resistant and susceptible mice, but that the responses in susceptible mice lacked cytotoxic potential as measured by ^{51}Cr release (Moser et al., 2001).

Investigators also noted that tetramer and CFC assays correlated well, except during acute viremia, when T cell receptor (TCR) down-modulation appeared to cause underestimation of the number of specific T cells by tetramer assays (Moser et al., 2001). These studies helped to validate CFC methodology against tetramer staining and demonstrated that high levels of specific T cells could be detected by CFC for a viral tumor antigen. They also suggested the possibility that IFN-gamma CFC alone might not predict protection from disease, but that other effector functions, like cytotoxicity, might be important. Studies of non-viral tumor models soon began to use CFC to assess immunity. One study used DNA fusion constructs of fragment C of tetanus toxin and a peptide from CEA to vaccinate mice (Rice et al., 2001). The vaccine responses were then quantitated by cytotoxic T cell (CTL) assay and by IFN-gamma CFC. Dramatic responses could be demonstrated using both assays and results corresponded to protection from challenge with a fragment C-expressing tumor.

One of the earliest studies to use CFC in a human tumor system analyzed the responses of cloned melanoma-specific T cells (Fonteneau et al., 1997). Investigators used peptide titration to demonstrate that antigen density affected not only the fraction of cells that responded, but also the effector functions induced. In terms of cytokines, IFN-gamma and tumor necrosis factor (TNF)-alpha production required 10- to 100-fold less antigen than did IL-2 and GM-CSF production. More recently, CFC has been used to study ex vivo responses to human cancer vaccines. Brossart et al. showed that MUC1 or HER-2/neu peptide-pulsed dendritic cell vaccination could induce CFC responses of 0.5–2 per cent of CD8 T cells after three injections of patients with breast and ovarian cancer (Brossart et al., 2000). These responses were also detectable by CTL assays. CFC responses to MUC1, a tumor-associated mucin, have also been reported in another study of various solid tumor patients and shown to increase with MUC1 vaccination (Karanikas et al., 2000). The responses ranged as high as 2.7 per cent. CFC responses have frequently been measured in melanoma, a relatively antigenic tumor for which CTL targets have been well defined. In fact, Lee et al. have shown that melanoma patients may have circulating T cells, detected by tetramer assays, specific for MART-1 or tyrosinase, in the absence of any vaccination (Lee et al., 1999b). In at least one such case, these cells appeared to be anergic as measured by lack of cytokine production in a CFC assay.

CFC responses have also been detected following vaccination of melanoma patients (Lee et al., 1999a; Nielsen et al., 2000; Smith et al., 2003; Whiteside et al., 2003). Interestingly, the magnitude or activation status of the melanoma-specific CD8+ cells does not appear to correlate with clinical response (Lee et al., 1999a; Nielsen et al., 2000). However, the ability to induce responses by peptide vaccination of up to 3.5 per cent of CD8+ T cells demonstrates that vaccine-elicited tumor responses can be readily detectable by CFC (Smith et al., 2003). Interestingly, at least one patient immunized with gp100 peptide appeared to develop a population of peptide-specific cells that lacked IFN-gamma production (Smith et al., 2003), suggesting that a vaccine-induced response can be susceptible to anergy induction. Finally, comparison of tetramer, CFC and ELISPOT responses to a melanoma vaccine showed that the highest number of peptide-specific CD8+ T cells were detected by tetramer, followed by CFC and then ELISPOT assays (Whiteside et al., 2003). One concept for tumor evasion of host immune responses involves the polarization of T cells towards a Th2 phenotype (Hu et al., 1998). CFC data using Th2 cytokines in human systems is largely lacking; however, one report examining tumor-infiltrating lymphocytes in human cervical cancer found a disproportionate number of IL-5-producing CD8+ and non-CD8+ T cells (Sheu et al., 2001) in response to mitogen stimulation. Thus, further studies designed to measure tumor-specific

Th2 cells in untreated as well as vaccinated tumor patients are suggested.

From the above studies, it is clear that T cell responses to solid tumor antigens can be detected by CFC. In fact, even relatively simple vaccination strategies such as peptide-in-adjuvant can induce readily detectable levels of IFN-gamma-producing T cells. However, it is also possible to detect anergic T cells either in untreated or vaccinated tumor patients by a combination of tetramer and CFC assays. Furthermore, the presence of an IFN-gamma CFC response may be necessary but not sufficient to predict protection from tumor progression. Production of other cytokines, proliferative and cytotoxic capacity and other phenotypic measures may also be important in predicting outcome.

ASSESSMENT OF CELLULAR IMMUNITY BASED ON DIRECT ENUMERATION OF T CELLS SPECIFIC FOR A PARTICULAR PEPTIDE-MHC COMPLEX

One of the most widely used methods to evaluate T cell responses to tumor antigens is the MHC tetramer assay. MHC tetramers are complexes of four MHC molecules associated with a specific antigenic peptide and a fluorochrome (Altman et al., 1996). MHC tetramer specificity is conveyed at the level of both the MHC and the antigen. Tetramer allows direct ex vivo enumeration of antigen-specific CD8+ T cells by flow cytometry (Ogg et al., 1998; Romero et al., 1998). Tetramer binding to T cells ex vivo can be detected with high sensitivity and the lower detection limit reaches 0.01 per cent in peripheral blood lymphocytes in whole blood assays (Klenerman et al., 2002).

The majority of the clinical studies using tetramers have focused on assessing responses to immunotherapy in melanoma patients. A number of antigens expressed on melanoma cells have been discovered (Boon and Old, 1997). More importantly, specific amino acid peptide sequences from melanoma-associated antigens have been identified to bind MHC class I molecules, especially HLA-A2, and to form epitopes recognizable by specific TCRs on CD8+ CTL. To date, tetramer-positive lymphocytes have been detected in patient samples for most of these antigens including melanocyte/melanoma differentiation antigens MelanA/Mart-1, tyrosinase and gp100; as well as cancer-testis antigens NY-ESO-1 and CAMEL (Rimoldi et al., 2000; Dutoit et al., 2001; Oertli et al., 2002; Weber et al., 2003). Several clinical trials of cancer vaccines targeting melanoma have focused on vaccination with CD8+ epitopes derived from tumor antigens, therefore, the enumeration of T cells specific for those peptide-MHC complexes by MHC tetramer evaluation is a rational choice for a biomarker of the immune response.

In studies to quantitate and characterize immune responses induced by vaccination, Valmori et al. (2002) demonstrated that immunization of melanoma patients with Melan-A peptides selected high-avidity T cell clones exhibiting increased tumor reactivity. The number of circulating Melan-A tetramer+ CD8+ T cells increased after vaccination and remained at a stable level of 1.1–2.3 per cent of total circulating CD8+ T cells. MHC tetramers can be used to discern the structural avidity of antigen specific T cells as well (Bullock et al., 2001). Investigators vaccinated human class I transgenic mice with melanoma peptides altered to improve class I binding. Analysis of CD8+ antigen specific T cells derived from these animals demonstrated that functional avidity assessed by cytokine secretion did not necessarily correlate to structural avidity as assessed by tetramer analysis (Bullock et al., 2001). Thus, tetramers can be used not only to enumerate antigen specific T cells but also to define T cell-MHC binding characteristics. In a vaccination study by Coulie et al. (2001), the authors observed a monoclonal 100-fold expansion of MAGE-3-specific CD8+ T cells in a melanoma patient immunized with a MAGE-3 peptide presented by HLA-A1. In this study, the same patient also exhibited a partial rejection of a large metastasis after vaccination. Tetramers have been used to enumerate antigen-specific CD8+ T cells ex vivo, not only in peripheral blood, but also in metastatic lymph nodes and tumor infiltrating lymphocytes (TIL). Investigators using Melan-A/MART-1 tetramer staining demonstrated relatively high levels of specific CD8+ T cells in TIL as well as in metastatic lymph nodes, but not in normal lymph nodes (Romero et al., 1998). This observation indicates that Melan-A/MART-1-specific CD8+ T cells accumulated at sites where tumor-associated antigens were present. In evaluation of melanoma immunity it was also demonstrated that using tetramers to evaluate the tumor specific immune response enumerated all antigen specific T cells including those that may not effect an anti-tumor function (Lee et al., 1999b).

The limited tetramer literature in cancers other than melanoma includes studies in squamous cell carcinoma of the head and neck (SCCHN), synovial sarcoma, colon and lung cancers. In SCCHN, Hoffmann et al. (2002) used tetramers to enumerate the frequency of $p53_{264-272}$ peptide-specific CD8+ T cells in patients' blood. They found, contrary to expectations, high frequencies of specific CD8+ cells in blood of patients whose tumors had normal p53 expression, but low frequencies of peptide-specific CD8+ T in patients whose tumors accumulated p53. Based on these data, the authors speculated that patients who had an elevated p53 expression in their tumors and a low frequency of $p53_{264-272}$ specific T cells will not benefit from the $p53_{264-272}$ vaccine. Indeed, these patients may benefit from vaccines consisting of other p53 epitopes. One study used tetramers to detect immunity to synovial sarcoma. Sato et al. (2002) found increased frequencies of circulating CTL in patients who had pulmonary metastasis, as compared to patients without metastasis. The tetramers used in this study contained peptides derived from SYT-SSX, which is a chimeric fusion gene product

resulting from tumor-specific chromosomal translocation. This gene product has been considered to play a key role in the genesis (Barr, 1998) of synovial sarcomas, as well as to serve as an immune target. In advanced colon and lung cancer, Fong et al. (2001) observed a correlation of clinical response with the expansion of tetramer+ CD8+ T cells in two of 12 vaccinated patients. Patients in this study were vaccinated with autologous dendritic cells loaded with peptide derived from CEA. The resultant tetramer+ T cells, which were found to expand upon vaccination, were also shown to recognize tumor cells expressing endogenous CEA.

In addition to their use in monitoring T cell responses in patients, MHC class I tetramers can be used as a tool for the isolation of tumor-specific CD8+ T cells from a heterologous population of cells such as PBMC, tumor-infiltrating lymphocytes or cultured cells (Yee et al., 1999). The isolated tumor-specific T cells can then be activated to expand ex vivo to transfer to cancer patients as a way of adoptive immunotherapy. Tetramers are also of value in tracking adoptively transferred T cells to define any correlations between their number, activity or distribution and disease progression (Dudley et al., 2002).

Thus, MHC tetramers can serve as an assay to monitor immunity present de novo in patients with solid tumor malignancy, to assess the effects of active immunization and even to isolate T cells for further expansion and immunotherapy. Studies are ongoing to determine whether MHC tetramers can also predict the functional avidity of the tumor specific T cell response.

ADDITIONAL PARAMETERS OF IMMUNITY THAT MAY PREDICT CLINICAL RESPONSE

While the assays described above are all quantitative measuring the magnitude of the induced tumor specific immune response, there are other parameters induced by immunotherapy that may also predict functional tumor specific immunity. For example, the functional avidity of a T cell population may predict the ability of T cells to bind to and lyse tumors in vivo. Furthermore, if T cells cannot migrate to the site of antigen bearing tumor once they are activated, then there would be little chance of the generation of a functional anti-tumor response. Moreover, vaccination with a single antigen could result in the development of a broadening of the immune response, i.e. epitope spreading. Any of these additional parameters has characteristics which could predict an anti-tumor effect.

Investigators vaccinated patients with an MCH class I peptide specific for a well-defined tumor antigen, NY-ESO (Dutoit et al., 2002). Active immunization of peptide in GM-CSF was able to elicit a peptide-specific T cell response as measured by MHC tetramer assay. However, only the minority of p157-165 peptide-specific T cells were of high enough avidity to recognize the naturally processed NY-ESO protein in HLA-matched tumor cells. The majority of p157-165 specific CD8+ T cells were of low functional avidity and did not respond to tumor cells *in vitro*. In this trial, the sole measurement of peptide-specific CD8+ T cells would not have revealed the potential functional diversity of the epitope specific T cell population elicited (Dutoit et al., 2002).

When evaluating immunotherapies such as adoptive T cell transfer, it is critical to be able to determine whether the infused T cells actually 'home' to the site of tumor. Immunologic monitoring may also include some aspect of evaluation of T cell migration *in vivo*. One technique used is to label T cells with reagents such as indium-111 to assess distribution after infusion. A recent study evaluated the *in vivo* migration of T cells specific for Melan-A expanded *ex vivo* and infused into patients with advanced stage melanoma (Meidenbauer et al., 2003). Indium-111 labeling of the Melan-A specific CTL demonstrated localization of the infused tumor antigen specific T cells to metastatic sites within 24 h after injection.

A phenomenon that is being increasingly reported after active tumor antigen specific immunization is the broadening of the immune response via epitope or determinant spreading. Epitope spreading was first described in autoimmune disease (Lehmann et al., 1992) and has been associated with both MHC class I- and MHC class II-restricted responses (Vanderlugt and Miller, 1996; el-Shami et al., 1999). Epitope spreading represents the generation of an immune response to a particular portion of an immunogenic protein and then the natural spread of that immunity to other areas of the protein or even to other antigens present in the environment. Theoretically, a broadening of the immune response may represent endogenous processing of antigen at sites of inflammation initiated by a specific T cell response or 'driver clone' (Sercarz, 2000). That is, the initial immune response can create a microenvironment at the site of the tumor that enhances endogenous immune effector cells present locally. These immune cells, e.g. APC and T cells, may begin to respond more effectively to tumor antigen that is present in the body. Several cancer vaccines studies have reported epitope spreading developing after active immunization. One such trial immunizing patients with Th epitopes derived from HER-2/neu demonstrated that intramolecular epitope spreading within HER-2/neu predicted the patients whose T cells could recognize endogenously processed antigen after peptide immunization (Disis et al., 2002). Another vaccine trial immunizing breast and ovarian cancer patients with autologous DC pulsed with MUC-1 or HER-2/neu peptides also resulted in epitope spreading (Brossart et al., 2000). In this trial 10 patients were immunized. Half the patients developed CD8+ T cell precursors to their immunizing peptides. Moreover, some patients developed new immunity to other tumor antigens expressed in their cancers such as CEA and MAGE-3. Epitope spreading has also been induced after immunization with a prostate cancer and melanoma specific vaccine (Cavacini et al., 2002; Weber et al., 2003). Epitope spreading has been related to the tissue destruction induced in autoimmune disease. It remains to be determined whether a similar phenomenon in cancer specific immunity will be associated with an anti-tumor response (Vanderlugt and Miller, 2002).

CONCLUSIONS

Highly quantitative measures of T cell immunity to tumor antigens have revolutionized our approach to the clinical application of immune based therapies and even the baseline assessment of tumor specific immunity. ELISPOT, CFC and MHC tetramer assays are reproducible and can be performed in most immunologic laboratories. These methods of analysis are allowing a more detailed evaluation of the immune response to cancer as well as facilitating prioritization of a variety of immunotherapeutic approaches. Which monitoring method, if any, will predict a clinical response is still an open experimental question.

ACKNOWLEDGEMENTS

The authors in the Immunologic Monitoring Consortium are Holden T. Maeker, Timothy M. Clay, H. Kim Lyerly and Jennie C.C. Chang.

This work was supported for MLD, JCCC, HTM, TMC and HKL by NIH NCI grant U54CA090818. We thank Ms Chalie Livingston for assistance in manuscript preparation.

REFERENCES

Altman, J. D., Moss, P. A. H., Goulder, P. J. R. et al. (1996). Phenotypic analysis of antigen-specific T lymphocytes. Science 274, 94–96.

Asai, T., Storkus, W. J. and Whiteside, T. L. (2000). Evaluation of the modified ELISPOT assay for gamma interferon production in cancer patients receiving antitumor vaccines. Clin Diagn Lab Immunol 7, 145–154.

Barr, F. G. (1998). Translocations, cancer and the puzzle of specificity. Nat Genet 19, 121–124.

Belli, F., Testori, A., Rivoltini, L. et al. (2002). Vaccination of metastatic melanoma patients with autologous tumor-derived heat shock protein gp96-peptide complexes: clinical and immunologic findings. J Clin Oncol 20, 4169–4180.

Bitmansour, A. D., Waldrop, S. L., Pitcher, C. J. et al. (2001). Clonotypic structure of the human CD4(+) memory T cell response to cytomegalovirus. J Immunol 167, 1151–1163.

Boon, T. and Old, L. J. (1997). Cancer tumor antigens. Curr Opin Immunol 9, 681–683.

Brossart, P., Wirths, S., Stuhler, G., Reichardt, V. L., Kanz, L. and Brugger, W. (2000). Induction of cytotoxic T-lymphocyte responses *in vivo* after vaccinations with peptide-pulsed dendritic cells. Blood 96, 3102–3108.

Bullock, T. N., Mullins, D. W., Colella, T. A. and Engelhard, V. H. (2001). Manipulation of avidity to improve effectiveness of adoptively transferred CD8(+) T cells for melanoma immunotherapy in human MHC class I-transgenic mice. J Immunol 167, 5824–5831.

Cavacini, L. A., Duval, M., Eder, J. P. and Posner, M. R. (2002). Evidence of determinant spreading in the antibody responses to prostate cell surface antigens in patients immunized with prostate-specific antigen. Clin Cancer Res 8, 368–373.

Coulie, P. G., Karanikas, V., Colau, D. et al. (2001). A monoclonal cytolytic T-lymphocyte response observed in a melanoma patient vaccinated with a tumor-specific antigenic peptide encoded by gene MAGE-3. Proc Natl Acad Sci USA 98, 10290–10295.

De Boer, R. J., Oprea, M., Antia, R., Murali-Krishna, K., Ahmed, R. and Perelson, A. S. (2001). Recruitment times, proliferation, and apoptosis rates during the cd8(+) t-cell response to lymphocytic choriomeningitis virus. J Virol 75, 10663–10669.

Disis, M. L., Gooley, T. A., Rinn, K. et al. (2002). Generation of T-cell immunity to the HER-2/neu protein after active immunization with HER-2/neu peptide-based vaccines. J Clin Oncol 20, 2624–2632.

Dudley, M. E., Wunderlich, J. R., Robbins, P. F. et al. (2002). Cancer regression and autoimmunity in patients after clonal repopulation with antitumor lymphocytes. Science, 298, 850–854.

Dunn, H. S., Haney, D. J., Ghanekar, S. A., Stepick-Biek, P., Lewis, D. B. and Maecker, H. T. (2002). Dynamics of CD4 and CD8 T cell responses to cytomegalovirus in healthy human donors. J Infect Dis 186, 15–22.

Dutoit, V., Rubio-Godoy, V., Dietrich, P. Y. et al. (2001). Heterogeneous T-cell response to MAGE-A10(254-262): high avidity-specific cytolytic T lymphocytes show superior antitumor activity. Cancer Res 61, 5850–5856.

Dutoit, V., Taub, R. N., Papadopoulos, K. P. et al. (2002). Multi epitope CD8(+) T cell response to a NY-ESO-1 peptide vaccine results in imprecise tumor targeting. J Clin Invest 110, 1813–1822.

el-Shami, K., Tirosh, B., Bar-Haim, E. et al. (1999). MHC class I-restricted epitope spreading in the context of tumor rejection following vaccination with a single immunodominant CTL epitope. Eur J Immunol 29, 3295–3301.

Fong, L., Hou, Y., Rivas, A. et al. (2001). Altered peptide ligand vaccination with Flt3 ligand expanded dendritic cells for tumor immunotherapy. Proc Natl Acad Sci USA 98, 8809–8814.

Fonteneau, J. F., Le Drean, E., Le Guiner, S., Gervois, N., Diez, E. and Jotereau, F. (1997). Heterogeneity of biologic responses of melanoma-specific CTL. J Immunol 159, 2831–2839.

Gurunathan, S., Prussin, C., Sacks, D. L. and Seder, R. A. (1998). Vaccine requirements for sustained cellular immunity to an intracellular parasitic infection. Nat Med 4, 1409–1415.

Gurunathan, S., Stobie, L., Prussin, C. et al. (2000). Requirements for the maintenance of Th1 immunity in vivo following DNA vaccination: a potential immunoregulatory role for CD8+ T cells. J Immunol 165, 915–924.

Hassett, D. E., Slifka, M. K., Zhang, J. and Whitton, J. L. (2000). Direct ex vivo kinetic and phenotypic analyses of CD8(+) T-cell responses induced by DNA immunization. J Virol 74, 8286–8291.

Hoffmann, T. K., Donnenberg, A. D., Finkelstein, S. D. et al. (2002). Frequencies of tetramer+ T cells specific for the wild-type sequence p53(264-272) peptide in the circulation of patients with head and neck cancer. Cancer Res 62, 3521–3529.

Homann, D., Teyton, L. and Oldstone, M. B. (2001). Differential regulation of antiviral T-cell immunity results in stable CD8+ but declining CD4+ T-cell memory. Nat Med 7, 913–919.

Hu, H. M., Urba, W. J. and Fox, B. A. (1998). Gene-modified tumor vaccine with therapeutic potential shifts tumor-specific T cell response from a type 2 to a type 1 cytokine profile. J Immunol 161, 3033–3041.

Karanikas, V., Lodding, J., Maino, V. C. and McKenzie, I. F. (2000). Flow cytometric measurement of intracellular cytokines detects immune responses in MUC1 immunotherapy. Clin Cancer Res 6, 829–837.

Keilholz, U., Weber, J., Finke, J. H. et al. (2002). Immunologic monitoring of cancer vaccine therapy: results of a workshop sponsored by the Society for Biological Therapy. J Immunother 25, 97–138.

Klenerman, P., Cerundolo, V. and Dunbar, P. R. (2002). Tracking T cells with tetramers: new tales from new tools. Nat Rev Immunol 2, 263–272.

Leavey, J. K. and Tarleton, R. L. (2003). Cutting edge: dysfunctional CD8+ T cells reside in nonlymphoid tissues during chronic Trypanosoma cruzi infection. J Immunol 170, 2264–2268.

Lee, K. H., Wang, E., Nielsen, M. B. et al. (1999a). Increased vaccine-specific T cell frequency after peptide-based vaccination correlates with increased susceptibility to in vitro stimulation but does not lead to tumor regression. J Immunol 163, 6292–6300.

Lee, P. P., Yee, C., Savage, P. A. et al. (1999b). Characterization of circulating T cells specific for tumor-associated antigens in melanoma patients. Nat Med 5, 677–685.

Lehmann, P. V., Forsthuber, T., Miller, A. and Sercarz, E. E. (1992). Spreading of T-cell autoimmunity to cryptic determinants of an autoantigen. Nature 358, 155–157.

Lukacher, A. E., Moser, J. M., Hadley, A. and Altman, J. D. (1999). Visualization of polyoma virus-specific CD8+ T cells in vivo during infection and tumor rejection. J Immunol 161, 3369–3378.

Maecker, H. T. (2003). Cytokine flow cytometry. In Flow Cytometry Protocols, T.S. Hawley, ed. Humana Press, pp. in press.

Maecker, H. T. and Maino, V. C. (2003). T cell immunity to HIV: defining parameters of protection. Curr HIV Res 1, 249–259.

Maecker, H. T., Maino, V. C. and Picker, L. J. (2000). Immunofluorescence analysis of T-cell responses in health and disease. J Clin Immunol 20, 391–399.

Meidenbauer, N., Harris, D. T., Spitler, L. E. and Whiteside, T. L. (2000). Generation of PSA-reactive effector cells after vaccination with a PSA-based vaccine in patients with prostate cancer. Prostate 43, 88–100.

Meidenbauer, N., Marienhagen, J., Laumer, M. et al. (2003). Survival and tumor localization of adoptively transferred Melan-A- specific T cells in melanoma patients. J Immunol 170, 2161–2169.

Mendez, S., Gurunathan, S., Kamhawi, S. et al. (2001). The potency and durability of DNA- and protein-based vaccines against Leishmania major evaluated using low-dose, intradermal challenge. J Immunol 166, 5122–5128.

Moser, J. M., Altman, J. D. and Lukacher, A. E. (2001). Antiviral CD8+ T cell responses in neonatal mice: susceptibility to polyoma virus-induced tumors is associated with lack of cytotoxic function by viral antigen-specific T cells. J Exp Med 193, 595–606.

Murali-Krishna, K., Altman, J. D., Suresh, M. et al. (1998). Counting antigen-specific CD8 T cells: a reevaluation of bystander activation during viral infection. Immunity 8, 177–187.

Nagorsen, D., Scheibenbogen, C., Schaller, G. et al. (2003). Differences in T-cell immunity toward tumor-associated antigens in colorectal cancer and breast cancer patients. Int J Cancer 105, 221–225.

Nielsen, M. B., Monsurro, V., Migueles, S. A. et al. (2000). Status of activation of circulating vaccine-elicited CD8+ T cells. J Immunol 165, 2287–2296.

Oertli, D., Marti, W. R., Zajac, P. et al. (2002). Rapid induction of specific cytotoxic T lymphocytes against melanoma-associated antigens by a recombinant vaccinia virus vector expressing multiple immunodominant epitopes and costimulatory molecules in vivo. Hum Gene Ther 13, 569–575.

Ogg, G. S., Jin, X., Bonhoeffer, S. et al. (1998). Quantitation of HIV-1-specific cytotoxic T lymphocytes and plasma load of viral RNA. Science 279, 2103–2106.

Rice, J., Elliott, T., Buchan, S. and Stevenson, F. K. (2001). DNA fusion vaccine designed to induce cytotoxic T cell responses against defined peptide motifs: implications for cancer vaccines. J Immunol 167, 1558–1565.

Rimoldi, D., Rubio-Godoy, V., Dutoit, V. et al. (2000). Efficient simultaneous presentation of NY-ESO-1/LAGE-1 primary and nonprimary open reading frame-derived CTL epitopes in melanoma. J Immunol 165, 7253–7261.

Romero, P., Dunbar, P. R., Valmori, D. et al. (1998). Ex vivo staining of metastatic lymph nodes by class I major histocompatibility complex tetramers reveals high numbers of antigen-experienced tumor-specific cytolytic T lymphocytes. J Exp Med 188, 1641–1650.

Sato, Y., Nabeta, Y., Tsukahara, T. et al. (2002). Detection and induction of CTLs specific for SYT-SSX-derived peptides in HLA-A24(+) patients with synovial sarcoma. J Immunol 169, 1611–1618.

Scheibenbogen, C., Lee, K. H., Mayer, S. et al. (1997). A sensitive ELISPOT assay for detection of CD8+ T lymphocytes specific for HLA class I-binding peptide epitopes derived from influenza proteins in the blood of healthy donors and melanoma patients. Clin Cancer Res 3, 221–226.

Scheibenbogen, C., Schadendorf, D., Bechrakis, N. E. et al. (2003). Effects of granulocyte-macrophage colony-stimulating factor and foreign helper protein as immunologic adjuvants on the T-cell response to vaccination with tyrosinase peptides. Int J Cancer 104, 188–194.

Schmittel, A., Keilholz, U. and Scheibenbogen, C. (1997). Evaluation of the interferon-gamma ELISPOT-assay for quantification of peptide specific T lymphocytes from peripheral blood. 210, 167–174.

Sercarz, E. E. (2000). Driver clones and determinant spreading. J Autoimmun 14, 275–277.

Sheu, B. C., Lin, R. H., Lien, H. C., Ho, H. N., Hsu, S. M. and Huang, S. C. (2001). Predominant Th2/Tc2 polarity of tumor-infiltrating lymphocytes in human cervical cancer. J Immunol 167, 2972–2978.

Slifka, M. K. and Whitton, J. L. (2001). Functional avidity maturation of CD8(+) T cells without selection of higher affinity TCR. Nat Immunol 2, 711–717.

Smith, J. W., 2nd, Walker, E. B., Fox, B. A. et al. (2003). Adjuvant immunization of HLA-A2-positive melanoma patients with a modified gp100 peptide induces peptide-specific CD8+ T-cell responses. J Clin Oncol 21, 1562–1573.

Stobie, L., Gurunathan, S., Prussin, C. et al. (2000). The role of antigen and IL-12 in sustaining Th1 memory cells in vivo: IL-12 is required to maintain memory/effector Th1 cells sufficient to mediate protection to an infectious parasite challenge. Proc Natl Acad Sci USA 97, 8427–8432.

Suni, M. A., Picker, L. J. and Maino, V. C. (1998). Detection of antigen-specific T cell cytokine expression in whole blood by flow cytometry. J Immunol Methods 212, 89–98.

Tatsumi, T., Kierstead, L. S., Ranieri, E. et al. (2002). Disease-associated bias in T helper type 1 (Th1)/Th2 CD4(+) T cell responses against MAGE-6 in HLA-DRB10401(+) patients with renal cell carcinoma or melanoma. J Exp Med 196, 619–628.

Valmori, D., Dutoit, V., Schnuriger, V. et al. (2002). Vaccination with a Melan-A peptide selects an oligoclonal T cell population with increased functional avidity and tumor reactivity. J Immunol 168, 4231–4240.

Vanderlugt, C. J. and Miller, S. D. (1996). Epitope spreading. Curr Opin Immunol 8, 831–836.

Vanderlugt, C. L. and Miller, S. D. (2002). Epitope spreading in immune-mediated diseases: implications for immunotherapy. Nat Rev Immunol 2, 85–95.

Vaquerano, J. E., Peng, M., Chang, J. W., Zhou, Y. M. and Leong, S. P. (1998). Digital quantification of the enzyme-linked immunospot (ELISPOT). Biotechniques 25, 830–834, 836.

Varga, S. M. and Welsh, R. M. (1998). Detection of a high frequency of virus-specific CD4+ T cells during acute infection with lymphocytic choriomeningitis virus. J Immunol 161, 3215–3218.

Waldrop, S. L., Pitcher, C. J., Peterson, D. M., Maino, V. C. and Picker, L. J. (1997). Determination of antigen-specific memory/effector CD4+ T cell frequencies by flow cytometry: evidence for a novel, antigen-specific homeostatic mechanism in HIV-associated immunodeficiency. J Clin Invest 99, 1739–1750.

Wang, R. F. and Rosenberg, S. A. (1999). Human tumor antigens for cancer vaccine development. 170, 85–100.

Weber, J., Sondak, V. K., Scotland, R. et al. (2003). Granulocyte-macrophage-colony-stimulating factor added to a multipeptide vaccine for resected Stage II melanoma. Cancer 97, 186–200.

Whiteside, T. L., Zhao, Y., Tsukishiro, T., Elder, E. M., Gooding, W. and Baar, J. (2003). Enzyme-linked immunospot, cytokine flow cytometry, and tetramers in the detection of T-cell responses to a dendritic cell-based multipeptide vaccine in patients with melanoma. Clin Cancer Res 9, 641–649.

Whitmire, J. K., Asano, M. S., Murali-Krishna, K., Suresh, M. and Ahmed, R. (1998). Long-term CD4 Th1 and Th2 memory following acute lymphocytic choriomeningitis virus infection. J Virol 72, 8281–8288.

Woodberry, T., Gardner, J., Elliott, S. L. et al. (2003). Prime boost vaccination strategies: CD8 T cell numbers, protection, and Th1 bias. J Immunol 170, 2599–2604.

Yee, C., Savage, P. A., Lee, P. P., Davis, M. M. and Greenberg, P. D. (1999). Isolation of high avidity melanoma-reactive CTL from heterogeneous populations using peptide-MHC tetramers. J Immunol 162, 2227–2234.

Cancer – Hematologic Disorders

Chapter
41

Edward D. Ball and Peter R. Holman

Blood and Marrow Transplantation Program and Division, University of California, San Diego, CA, USA

To be conscious that you are ignorant is a great step to knowledge.

Benjamin Disraeli (1804–1881)

INTRODUCTION

Advances in the treatment of hematological malignancy have been steady and impressive. Most exciting is the fact that the majority of advances are being made through better understanding of the molecular pathogenesis of the diseases, thus allowing more rationally targeted therapy as reported by Gilliland (2002). For example, the treatment of chronic myeloid leukemia (CML) has been revolutionized by the advent of the small molecule inhibitor of the abl tyrosine kinase, STI571, now known as imatinib (Gleevec). Hematologic and cytogenetic remissions are now routinely being achieved with this oral and easily tolerated drug. However, this is by far an uncommon situation, a disease with a consistent molecular target that is central to the pathogenesis of the disorder. That is, the activated kinase induced by the translocation is responsible for the excessive proliferation of CML cells; blocking the kinase reverses its activity and quells the disease. B lymphoproliferative diseases such as non-Hodgkin's lymphoma (NHL) and multiple myeloma also express a consistent but patient-specific target, the specific idiotype of the monoclonal immunoglobulin expressed or secreted by the malignant cells. This surface expressed idiotypic protein can be used to create patient-specific vaccines for active immunotherapy. Cells of the various hematological neoplasms also express surface antigens characteristic of their lineage. Antigens such as CD20 or CD52 can be targeted 'passively' with monoclonal antibodies (mAb) directed to the relevant antigen with therapeutic effects.

All of the approaches to immunotherapy to date are either imperfect or experimental and need to withstand rigorous clinical testing. Progress will come from improved understanding of the basic biology of cancer and the immune system's reaction to altered normal tissues.

One of the more fundamental obstacles to advances in the treatment of the diseases of the hematopoietic system is the paucity of known and validated targets for novel therapies. Most malignant cells are phenotypically indistinguishable from their corresponding normal tissues. For example, cells from patients with acute myeloid leukemia (AML) express a variety of cell surface antigens such as CD33, CD64 and CD34, all expressed on normal hematopoietic cells. Leukemia stem cells may be distinguished from normal hematopoietic stem cells since they tend to be CD90$^-$ CD117$^-$ and CD123$^+$. In contrast, normal stem cells are CD90$^+$, CD117$^+$ and CD123$^-$. However, it is preferable to target antigens that are truly unique to the leukemia cell and not found on normal tissues. AML-specific antigens may exist. Candidates include FLT-3, WT-1, proteinase 3 and possibly a number of neoantigens created as a result of chromosomal translocations that occur with some frequency, but with considerable diversity, in AML (Elisseeva et al., 2002). For example, FLT-3 is a

Measuring Immunity, edited by Michael T. Lotze and Angus W. Thomson
ISBN 0-12-455900-X, London

cell surface receptor for FLT-ligand that is mutated in up to 30 per cent of AML patients, possibly creating unique peptides for presentation through HLA molecules. As more is learned about AML-associated peptide antigens, specific vaccine protocols will be possible using pulsed dendritic cells or a peptide plus adjuvant strategy.

This chapter will discuss the aspects of immune monitoring that apply to this group of malignant disorders of the hematopoietic system. We will focus on AML and non-Hodgkin's lymphoma, two diseases that have tumor-specific markers that have been targeted for immuno-therapy.

ACUTE MYELOID LEUKEMIA

AML is a clonal proliferation of an aberrant hematopoietic myeloid stem cell that fails to differentiate, thus leading to an accumulation of immature cells, blasts and bone marrow failure. AML is a heterogeneous disease at every level examined. Morphology, cell surface antigen expression and cytogenetics vary considerably among patients, though some common findings do exist. Specific mutations occur in many known genes including FLT-3, p53 and ras. Chromosomal translocations result in the creation of fusion proteins that may represent neoantigens recognizable to the immune system.

Treatment of AML requires the use of potent myelo-suppressive chemotherapeutic agents that selectively cause cytoreduction of malignant cells compared to normal bone marrow cells. Allogeneic bone marrow transplantation is often used in order to allow a donor versus

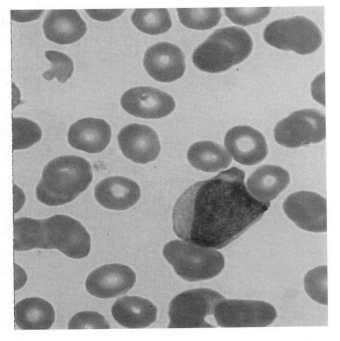

Figure 41.1 Peripheral blood smear showing a blast cell from a patient with AML.

leukemia (GVL) cell reaction to contribute to ongoing immunosurveillance (Horowitz et al., 1990). The target antigens of the GVL effect are not well-characterized but include polymorphic minor histocompatibility antigens (Falkenburg et al., 1997, 2000). Other immunological approaches are under study such as the use of adoptive transfer of cytotoxic T lymphocytes or the use of selected cytokines.

AML cells commonly contain chromosomal translocations leading to the creation of fusion proteins. A prototypical example is promyelocytic leukemia (FABM3 AML) wherein there is a translocation involving chromosomes 15 and 17. This translocation t(15;17) results in the juxtaposition of the PML and RARA genes which encode a fusion protein referred to as PML-RAR-α. This fusion protein is unique to the leukemia and possibly contains amino acid sequences that are immunogenic. An interesting mouse model has recently been reported that shows the potential power of vaccination with the PML-RAR-α fusion protein. The APL transgenic mouse bearing the human PML-RARA oncogene offers an excellent model for the human disease (Brown et al., 1997). Padua et al. (2003) created a DNA vaccine by fusing the human PML-RARA oncogene to tetanus fragment C. The investigators vaccinated syngeneic murine recipients with this DNA vaccine before challenging the mice with APL transgenic mouse splenocytes. Vaccination protected these normal syngeneic mice from developing leukemia. This DNA vaccine induced a humoral and cellular immune response against the leukemia cells of tumor-bearing mice. Further, they performed studies to mimic clinical disease by establishing leukemia in mice and then inducing immunity through vaccination. This study showed improved survival in cohorts of mice treated with DNA plus ATRA. The mechanism of the therapeutic effect was both humoral and cellular. Using ELISA, sustained antibody production was noted in mice treated with ATRA alone as well as with ATRA plus vaccine. Natural killer cell populations were increased in both treated and untreated mice. It was impossible to detect significant cytotoxic T cell responses to mouse APL spleen cells. The cellular immune response was primarily seen in CD4+ B lymphocytes. No autoimmune effects were seen through this experiment that breaks tolerance to PML-RARA alpha. This study provides very useful lessons for the possible treatment of human disease. Though human APL responds very well to chemotherapy and ATRA, some patients do relapse, indicating in some the continued presence of disease. There are a number of other AML-associated translocations that could be targeted for this approach.

Overcoming tolerance to normal or mutated antigens offers an approach to immunotherapy for AML. Candidate peptides that are presented in class I HLA can be identified. They can be presented to dendritic or other antigen-presenting cells to create cell vaccines for *in vivo* therapeutics. In AML the search for relevant peptides has led to WT-1, proteinase 3 peptides representing translocations such as t (15;17). Molldrum et al. (2002) immunized patients with AML with a peptide from proteinase 3 with a GM-CSF adjuvant. The protein, proteinase 3 has been found to be over-expressed in AML and chronic myeloid leukemia (CML) cells. A nine amino acid peptide sequence derived from proteinase 3 termed PR1, that can only be recognized by T lymphocytes through the histocompatibility molecule, HLA-A2, can induce T cell immunity to proteinase 3. A phase 1 vaccine study examined the effects of PR1 on nine patients (three with CML, three with AML and three with myelodysplastic syndrome; all of whom had proteinase 3 in their abnormal cells). The patients were monitored for immune responses including the generation of peptide-specific CTL and tetramer sort-purified cells. PR1-specific CTL were identified, as were tetramer-sorted PR1-CTL that were able to lyse AML cells. One patient who had relapsed after allogeneic stem cell transplant for APL with the t (15;17) had a cytogenetic and molecular response to vaccination. Donor-derived PR1-CTL could be demonstrated. All three patients at the highest dose level of the peptide vaccine achieved complete remission. Two patients with relapsed AML prior to vaccination attained cytogenetic remissions and remain in continuous complete remission. Several patients had mild cutaneous reactions to the vaccine. These remarkable findings show that vaccination with a peptide can induce remission in an AML patient and encourage further development of tumor vaccines for this disease as well as other tumor vaccines.

Clinical trials of immunotherapy in AML are likely to employ mAb, cytokines, immunomodulatory small molecules and cells such as CTLs and dendritic cells either alone or combined with peptide vaccinations. Outcomes of such therapy will be measured by effects on leukemia cells in the circulation and the bone marrow. Morphological examination is standard. In addition, performance of cytogenetic analysis, FISH and PCR for specific informative markers may be useful in determining the efficacy of such therapy. Biological effects of such therapies will be monitored by effects on T cells such as expansion of selected clones of T cells. This can be done by the method of TCR spectrotyping wherein the TCR beta unit gene utilization is measured by PCR. Specific peptide-specific T cells can be measured by tetramer binding. T cell reactivity or activation can be measured by ELISPOT assays or by intracellular cytokine assays (by flow cytometry). Humoral responses to malignant cells may be measured by flow cytometry testing the reactivity of sera from patients with autologous blasts.

Zhong et al. (2002) described a method of generating large numbers of CTL reactive against AML cells. Evidence from allogeneic hematopoietic stem cell transplantation indicates that there can be an immune response against leukemia-associated antigens in patients with both acute and chronic myeloid leukemia (AML, CML). However, an autologous anti-tumor cell response is either actively suppressed or non-evident due to replacement of the lymphohematopoietic space with rapidly growing malignant cells. We have shown that specific anti-AML T cells can be generated and expanded from primary cultures of mononuclear cells from all newly diagnosed patients with AML using a novel method of sequential modulation of growth factors (SMGF). The purpose of the culture is to induce greater degrees of antigen presentation than previously described methods by inducing dendritic cell differentiation of the AML blast cells in the presence of autologous lymphocytes. The sensitized anti-AML lymphocytes are then expanded through the use of growth factors and co-stimulatory molecule ligation. The unique feature of the SMGF protocol is that larger numbers (10^9–10^{10}) of CD8+ T cells that are myeloid leukemia-specific can be generated compared with currently available protocols. Moreover, there is selective use of T cell receptor Vβ regions in these expanded cells. The number and function of CTLs is augmented in these cultures when the anti-CTLA-4 mAb (MDX-010) is included to block the negative proliferative signal of CTLA-4 after binding to CD80/86. Clinical trials of adoptive T cell therapy in patients with AML are planned. Peripheral blood cells will be obtained from patients with AML at first diagnosis or relapse. Mononuclear cells (MNC) containing AML blasts and normal T cells will be separated from red blood cells and granulocytes. The MNC fraction will be cultured in GM-CSF and IL-4 to induce dendritic cell differentiation in the AML blast cells. IL-2 will then be added to initiate T cell proliferation in the presence of the differentiated AML cells possessing augmented antigen-presenting activity. Finally, anti-CD3 (OKT-3) and anti-CTLA-4 mAb (MDX-010) will be added to expand the numbers of T cells. The cells will be tested *in vitro* for their ability to kill autologous AML cells. The first study will test safety by using graded numbers of T cells in cohorts of patients. When safety is established and the best dose of T cells is determined, a second study will test for efficacy of the infusions in a larger number of patients. *In vitro* assays designed to determine the mechanism of action of the T cell killing will be incorporated into the clinical protocol. These will include cytotoxicity assays to monitor AML reactivity of T cells. The cytotoxicity of the anti-AML CTL obtained in SMGF cultures will be analyzed in standard 4-h ^{51}Cr release assays against autologous AML blasts, autologous

Table 41.1 Assays employed to monitor immunotherapy

CTL activity
ELISPOT
Tetramers
PCR for detection of residual disease
Spectrotyping (TCR repertoire)
Flow cytometry for intracellular cytokines
Antibody responses to TAA

remission PHA blasts or bone marrow (BM) cells and AML cell lines. TCR Vβ repertoire analysis will be performed on the expanded T cells and on peripheral blood cells collected pre-infusion (baseline) and on days 7, 14, 21, 28 and 160 after the infusion. The TCR Vβ repertoire will be measured pre-culture, at day 8 in culture and post-culture prior to infusion for alterations in the expressed T cell Vα and Vβ genes consistent with a cellular immune response to AML cells. To extend these studies, CD4+ or CD8+ T cells will be purified with anti-CD4 or CD8 mAb and magnetic beads. The CD4+ or CD8+ TCR repertoire will be analyzed at day 0, day 8 and day 35 of SMGF culture. The AML-specific cytotoxicity of the specific T cell clones from the SMGF culture will be obtained using the limiting dilution technique, or will be examined in effector cell blocking experiments in CTL assay with specific anti-Vβ mAb. The best AML cytotoxic clones can then be selected for studies of AML-specific antigens recognized by particular clones. In addition, an analysis of the frequency of anti-leukemia T cells pre- and post- culture by ELISPOT will be performed. The ELISPOT technique is a sensitive method that can measure cytokine release from a single cell, allowing for direct calculation of the frequency of antigen-specific CD8+ T cells and/or Th1 type CD4+ T cells that secrete a specific cytokine in response to tumor-associated antigens. ELISPOT assays have the sensitivity to detect and measure the number of antigen-specific T cells among blood lymphocytes, without previously having to expand the T cells *ex vivo*. ELISPOT will be performed for pre- and post-SMGF cultures of AML patient cells to determine the frequency of specific T cell activation testing both Th1 and Th2 responses (IFN-γ, IL-5). ELISPOT will also be performed on PB cells from patients in the clinical trial at the same time points as the TCR Vβ analysis (days 7, 14, 21, 28 and 160) after CTL infusion.

NON-HODGKIN'S LYMPHOMA

Standard approaches to the treatment of hematological malignancy have included chemotherapy and radiation. In some relatively aggressive lymphoid malignancies, such therapy can be curative but in the more slowly growing lymphoproliferative disorders, such as indolent lymphoma and chronic lymphocytic leukemia (CLL), cure with these modalities is exceedingly rare. In recent years, immunological approaches to the treatment of these diseases have emerged as a promising therapeutic option. Such treatments have been administered either alone or in combination with chemotherapy or radiation therapy. Immune therapeutic approaches have emerged as a result of dramatic advances in the understanding of the molecular alterations associated with neoplasia. They include identification of cell surface proteins that can be targeted by therapeutic antibodies and vaccination with idiotype, a lymphoma specific protein, two of the most thoroughly evaluated newer modalities in this arena. Currently, these approaches and others are either in common clinical use or are in late stage clinical trial development.

These newer immunological approaches present many novel challenges in terms of the conduct of clinical trials and the evaluation of treatment efficacy (Simon et al., 2001). Whereas mAb appropriately continue to be evaluated via traditional clinical trial paradigms, vaccine approaches historically have been associated with few serious adverse effects. Therefore, subsequent phase I trials, in which an agent's toxicity profile is initially evaluated, may be unnecessary. Also, as phase I trials generally have enrolled patients with more heavily pretreated and advanced disease, this patient population is less likely to have an intact immune response system capable of benefiting from such therapy. Many of these newer immunological approaches could be taken, with appropriate caution, directly to phase II or phase III studies for maximum efficiency in translating such approaches to the clinic.

Lymphomas are particularly well suited to immunologically targeted approaches. The affected cells are generally readily available, and have an assortment of potential protein targets on the cell surface including immunoglobulin idiotype (Id), which can function as a specific clonal protein tumor marker. Lymphomas are broadly classified into two groups, non-Hodgkin's lymphoma (NHL) and Hodgkin's disease (HD). In HD, the malignant cell is the Reed-Sternberg (R-S) cell, which tends to be distributed only sparsely in involved tissues. Surrounding the malignant cells is a prominent polyclonal inflammatory cell infiltrate. Immunoglobulin gene rearrangement studies have demonstrated the R-S cell to be of B cell origin (Kanzler et al., 1996). The development of immune based therapies for Hodgkin's disease (apart from allogeneic transplantation) has lagged behind that for NHL. However, given the recent greater understanding of the role of the Epstein-Barr virus (EBV) in the pathogenesis of Hodgkin's disease, immune therapeutic approaches are anticipated in the near future. The expression of viral antigens such as Epstein-Barr nuclear antigen-1 (EBNA-1), latent membrane protein 1 (LMP-1) and latent membrane protein 2 (LMP-2) in R-S cells and the elucidation of the resulting immune response may allow *ex vivo* expansion of antigen specific T cells with therapeutic benefit in EBV-positive HD.

The NHL are broadly classified into B cell and T cell derived tumors. Clonal surface immunoglobulin idiotype is uniformly expressed by the majority of B cell lymphomas. T cell lymphomas similarly express a clonal T cell receptor. These surface molecules allow interaction of lymphocytes with antigen presenting cells (APC). Numerous other molecules are also displayed on the lymphocyte cell surface. One such important molecule is CD20, which appears to be involved in B cell regulation, B cell growth and transmembrane calcium flux (Riley and Sliwkowski, 2000). CD22 is another B cell surface molecule which is also the target of immune therapy currently being evaluated in clinical trials (Coleman et al., 2003). It is expressed in 60–80 per cent of B cell malignancies (Cesano et al.,

Figure 41.2 H&E section of a follicular center cell non-Hodgkin's lymphoma. **See colour plate 41.2.**

2003) and appears to be involved in cellular homing, adhesion and regulation of B cell activation. In murine knock-out studies when CD22 is absent, cells are more susceptible to apoptotic signals (Nitschke et al., 1997). CD52 is another target on both normal and malignant B cells. Alemtuzumab (Campath-1H, Ilex Pharmaceuticals, San Antonio, TX) is a humanized mAb that is FDA approved for use in patients with CLL. HLA-DR, CD80 and CD30 are additional targets of immunotherapeutic approaches. To date, most passive immune based treatment approaches have used mAb for targeting such cell surface structures.

In contrast, active immune therapy approaches are designed to utilize *in vivo* immune effector mechanisms as the primary therapeutic modality. The best studied and most promising example of this approach for NHL is idiotype vaccination. This involves administering idiotype combined with a hapten and administered in association with adjuvant. The idiotype is the clonal hypervariable region of the corresponding heavy and light chains. The most commonly used adjuvant is the immunostimulatory myeloid growth factor, GM-CSF. Idiotype protein is generated either through gene capture methodology or via hybridoma technology starting with a lymph node biopsy specimen. The idiotype protein is a relatively weak antigen, thus, it is linked to a hapten, most commonly Keyhole Limpet Hemocyanin (KLH). Phase III randomized clinical trials are currently evaluating the efficacy of such an approach. Animal studies (Campbell et al., 1988, 1990) have demonstrated the ability of such vaccines to protect against tumor challenge and also to induce responses against established tumors. Further, the NCI described 20

patients receiving idiotype vaccine conjugated to KLH and administered with GM-CSF (Bendandi et al., 1999). All patients were previously untreated and in a clinical complete remission (CR) after receiving chemotherapy. Of these 20 patients, 11 had an informative translocation (Bcl-2/IgH) detectable by PCR both prior to treatment and after completing chemotherapy, despite being in a clinical CR. Eight of 11 patients converted to PCR negativity after vaccination. These eight patients had sustained molecular remissions.

Clinical trials evaluating mAb therapies in NHL have relied on objective measurements of evaluable tumors to determine efficacy. More recently, such agents have been evaluated in maintenance therapy regimens. The primary endpoint in such trials has been response duration as seen in two recent reports (Hainsworth, 2002; Hainsworth et al., 2003), but molecular monitoring of the bcl-2 gene rearrangement has also been performed (Martinelli et al., 2003). Relying on radiological measurements of tumor size or waiting for clinical evidence of disease recurrence is cumbersome and inefficient when evaluating many immune mediated therapies such as idiotype vaccination. Such treatments are patient specific and components of the strategy such as the dose or schedule of vaccine, the specific hapten or adjuvant used often need to be adjusted as the design is refined. Using traditional endpoints would therefore make such approaches prohibitively burdensome. This demonstrates the need for the development and standardization of surrogate outcome measurements. While a number of assays are available to evaluate an immune response to specific interventions, to date there has been no standardization. Ultimately, any useful surrogate assay has to correlate with the important clinical endpoints of response, freedom from disease progression and survival. Additionally, finding surrogate evidence of a tumor specific immune response *per se* is often insufficient evidence of therapeutic efficacy as the local tumor microenvironment may actually be inhibitory to peripherally detected immune effector cells. Given the heterogeneity of the immune response, it is also frequently unclear what aspect of the measured immune response is clinically important. In NHL and a number of other malignancies, it appears that measurement of the cellular immune response is more likely to correlate with clinical outcome. The importance of measuring antibody or NK cell responses to idiotype vaccination is less clear.

IMMUNOLOGIC MONITORING ASSAYS

Assays reported as potentially useful surrogate markers for immunotherapeutic studies can be *in vivo* tests such as delayed type hypersensitivity (DTH). *In vitro* studies include both phenotypic (quantitative) and functional assays. No one test has proven to be ideal.

DTH testing has been commonly used in clinical trials. Antigen is injected directly or loaded onto APC into the dermis and after 48–72 h the diameter of erythema or induration is measured. This response is mediated by CD4+ T cells which, on interaction with antigen, release cytokines resulting in an inflammatory reaction. Concern about this test as a useful surrogate includes the specificity of the response. For example, DTH responses have occurred with both peptide loaded DCs and control DCs (Thurner et al., 1999) and responses to GM-CSF have also been reported (McNeel et al., 1999). The optimal dose and timing of antigen administration relative to vaccination is also unclear. Due to small numbers of patients enrolled in most trials, it is difficult to draw firm conclusions regarding the relationship of the DTH response to clinical outcomes in any specific malignancy. Control antigen administered along with tumor specific antigen would also help to determine the ability of patients to respond to antigen at all. Due to such concerns, DTH has been infrequently used in idiotype vaccine trials in NHL.

A more commonly used *in vitro* assay in NHL has been the lymphocyte proliferation assay. This test is also usually a measure of CD4+ T helper cells. Samples are obtained from the peripheral blood following which the lymphocyte population is separated, usually using Ficoll Hypaque density gradient centrifugation. The cells are then incubated with antigen (with or without APC) or control at varying concentrations for a defined period following which [^{3}H] thymidine is added. The amount of [^{3}H] thymidine incorporated into DNA is then measured as a function of DNA synthesis and antigen specific cell proliferation. The ratio of antigen specific proliferation to control proliferation determines the stimulation index. A positive response is usually indicated by the incorporation of at least two times the control. A major concern regarding this assay relates to the lack of demonstrated clinical correlation. In an idiotype vaccine study of 41 patients with NHL, cellular proliferative responses were evaluated (Hsu et al., 1997). An antigen specific cellular proliferative response was only identified in seven patients whereas responses to KLH occurred in 39. Antigen specific humoral immune responses were identified in 17 patients. Although there appeared to be a correlation between any immune response and clinical outcome, the small number of antigen specific cellular responses seen precluded any such conclusion. It has yet to be demonstrated that the presence and magnitude of a cellular proliferative response directly correlates with anti-tumor efficacy.

Cytotoxicity assays have been commonly used in immunotherapy studies. Such assays are designed as an *in vitro* measure of tumor specific CD8+ T cells. The degree to which this reflects *in vivo* tumor killing ability however remains unclear. Assays are performed by measuring the release of chromium or indium from target cells following incubation with peripheral blood lymphocytes. The lymphocytes generally require a number of stimulation rounds prior to performing the assay as it is relatively insensitive. These manipulations may result in skewing of the responding population away from the *in vivo* composition. The antigen chosen for stimulation and the concentration used are also important. When an autologous tumor is not available, alternative targets such as irradiated HLA matched allogeneic tumor or antigen loaded DC are used. A specific target has the potential to produce a false negative cytotoxicity result or one that does not correlate with *in vivo* responses. Furthermore, due to local inhibitory tumor induced changes, a positive cytotoxicity assay may not reflect *in vivo* tumor cell killing. Such changes include local tumor downregulation of HLA class I molecules, resulting in deficient antigen presentation to CD8+ T cells. Some tumors also produce gangliosides which can suppress NF-κB, important in the T cell response to certain malignancies (Uzzo et al., 1999).

In the NCI idiotype vaccine study of Bendandi et al. (1999), specific lysis of autologous follicular lymphoma targets was evaluated. Malignant lymphocytes were first stimulated by co-culture with CD40L-transfected fibroblasts before irradiation. After being labeled with indium, they were used as stimulators for culture with pre- and post-vaccination PBMC. Obviously, such conditions may not accurately reflect the *in vivo* conditions.

Cytokine release is another frequently used assay of *in vivo* cytotoxicity. This is also a functional assay. Secreted cytokines can be detected either by ELISA or by ELISPOT. Alternatively, intracellular cytokines can be detected by multiparameter flow cytometry. In the ELISA assay, cytokines including IFN-γ, TNF-α and IL-2 can be measured in the supernatant following incubation of PBMC with tumor target tissue. The supernatant is then added to microtiter plates coated with specific antibody to the cytokine of interest. Once again, the major criticism of this assay is that this *in vitro* system is artificial, not necessarily reflecting the ability of identified cells to respond to relevant antigens *in vivo*.

In the ELISPOT assay used to detect antigen specific T cells, a 96-well plate is coated with antibody to the cytokine to be detected. Lymphocytes in the form of purified populations of CD4+ or CD8+ cells or unseparated PBMC are then added along with stimulating antigen. Antigen specific T cells release cytokine that binds to the antibody coating the wells. A detection antibody along with its chromogenic substrate is then added and each cell is identified as an individual spot. Studies in melanoma have suggested that IFN-γ release as detected in an ELISPOT assay correlated with clinical outcome following vaccination (Reynolds et al., 1997). This assay has also been utilized in multiple myeloma patients following vaccination with idiotype (Osterborg et al., 1998).

Intracellular cytokine monitoring can be performed to evaluate T cell activation in peripheral blood or tissues including lymph nodes. Following activation of the responding cells *in vitro* with relevant antigen, further cytokine secretion is blocked. The cell population is next fixed and permeabilized and fluorochrome labeled anti-cytokine antibodies are used for detection in a flow cytometry assay. This is a sensitive assay, able to detect relatively low frequencies of stimulated cells and the pattern of cytokine expression detected allows for evaluation of the type of response, either Th1 or Th2. This assay has been utilized in a number of clinical studies in cancer patients including multiple myeloma patients following vaccination with immunoglobulin idiotype (Maecker et al., 2001), although definitive correlation with clinical outcome requires further validation. This is the assay we are currently using to evaluate antigen specific T cell proliferative responses in an ongoing clinical trial evaluating immunoglobulin idiotype protein conjugated to KLH and administered with GM-CSF. The setting is post-autologous stem cell transplantation for indolent lymphoma, mantle cell lymphoma or transformed NHL. Starting 3 months post-transplant, a series of monthly vaccinations is administered. In this setting, the likelihood of minimal residual disease is maximized, a setting shown to be associated with an increased likelihood of developing an antigen specific response following vaccination. Another important aspect of this trial is determining whether post-transplant, patients can develop antigen specific immune responses. Mackall et al. (1996) have demonstrated in a murine model that the recovering T cell repertoire can undergo skewing upon exposure to antigen in the post-transplant setting. Although the clinical trial is in an early stage, five of the initial six patients have developed idiotype specific immune responses early after the initiation of vaccination as demonstrated by detection of intracellular cytokine (Holman et al., 2003).

PCR evaluation of the third complementarity determining region (CDR3) of the TCR can help to identify a skewed population of T cells following vaccination. The CDR3 encodes the highly polymorphic antigen recognition site of the TCR and when restricted, indicates a skewed T cell population. Its correlation with clinical outcomes has not been documented.

For a test to be a useful surrogate marker of clinical outcome following any form of immunotherapy, it should ideally be simple to perform, have a high degree of correlation between laboratories and be meaningful in terms of predicting outcome. Current methodologies evaluate either phenotypic or functional changes usually occurring in response to ex vivo antigenic stimulation. These manipulations, performed to enhance the sensitivity or specificity of the assay can alter the cell population of interest resulting in a distortion of the true in vivo state. Also, the mechanism of tumor cell killing following immunotherapy continues to be unraveled. Whether cell killing occurs as a result of cytokine mediated mechanisms or apoptosis via Fas or the perforin/granzyme pathway will have relevance to the utility of assays involving cytokine release. Ultimately, efficient evaluation of vaccines and other immunotherapies will require the use of relevant assays that reliably predict clinical outcome.

FUTURE PROSPECTS

The future of immunotherapy for diseases of the hematopoietic cell system depends on continued advances in the understanding of the immune response to tumor-associated antigens (TAA), elucidation of the molecular nature of TAA and means of augmenting the immune response to TAA through the use of cellular and molecular vaccines, cytokines and stem cell transplants. It should be considered in future trials that immunotherapy alone will probably not be curative for the majority of patients, since TAA will not likely be expressed on every cell of a patient's

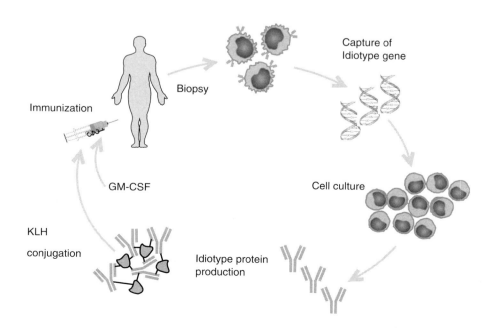

Figure 41.3 Schema of an idiotypic vaccine clinical trial.

tumor, thus predicting escape of these antigen-negative variants. Targeting multiple TAA may help overcome this obstacle, since it is more likely to kill more cancer cells the more antigens are targeted. In addition, augmentation of the innate immune system may help by complementing the antigen-specific responses.

ACKNOWLEDGEMENTS

The authors gratefully acknowledge Dr Elizabeth Broome of UCSD for providing the photomicrographs.

REFERENCES

Bendandi, M, Gocke, C. D. Kobrin, C. B. et al. (1999). Complete molecular remissions induced by patient-specific vaccination plus granulocyte-monocyte colony-stimulating factor against lymphoma. Nat Med 5, 1171–1177.

Brown, D., Kogan, S., Lagasse, E. et al. (1997). A PMLRAR alpha transgene initiates murine acute promyelocytic leukemia. Proc Natl Acad Sci USA 94, 2551–2556.

Campbell, M. J., Esserman, L. and Levy, R. (1988). Immunotherapy of established murine B cell lymphoma. Combination of idiotype immunization and cyclophosphamide. J Immunol 141, 3227–3233.

Campbell, M. J., Esserman, L. and Byars, N. E. (1990). Idiotype vaccination against murine B cell lymphoma. Humoral and cellular requirements for the full expression of antitumor immunity. J Immunol 145, 1029–1036.

Cesano, A., Gayko, U., Brannan, J. et al. (2002). Differential expression of CD22 in indolent and aggressive non-Hodgkin's lymphoma (NHL): Implications for Targeted Immunotherapy. Blood 100(11), 1358, 350a.

Coleman, M., Goldenberg, D. M., Siegel, A. B. et al., (2003). Epratuzumab: targeting B-cell malignancies through CD22. Clin Cancer Res 9, 3991S–3994S.

Elisseeva, O. A., Oka, Y., Tsuboi, A. et al. (2002). Humoral immune responses against Wilms tumor gene WT1 product in patients with hematopoietic malignancies. Blood 99, 3272–3279.

Falkenburg, J. H., Smit, W. M. and Willemze, R. (1997). Cytotoxic T-lymphocyte (CTL) responses against acute or chronic myeloid leukemia. Immunol Rev 157, 223–230.

Falkenburg, J. H., van de Corput, L., Marijt, E. W. et al. (2003). Minor histocompatibility antigens in human stem cell transplantation. Exp Hematol 31, 743–751.

Gilliland, D. G. (2002). Molecular genetics of human leukemias: new insights into therapy. Semin Hematol 39 Suppl 3, 6–11.

Hainsworth, J. D., Litchy, S., Burris, H. A. III et al. (2003). Single-agent Rituximab as first-line and maintenance treatment for patients with chronic lymphocytic leukemia or small lymphocytic lymphoma: a phase II trial of the Minnie Pearl Cancer Research Network. J Clin Oncol 21, 1746–1751.

Hainsworth, J. D. (2002). Rituximab as first-line and maintenance therapy for patients with indolent non-Hodgkin's lymphoma. J Clin Oncol 20, 4261–4267.

Holman, P., Medina, B., Corringham, S. et al. (2003). Early and robust immune responses to idiotype (Id) vaccination occur in mantle cell lymphoma (MCL) and indolent lymphoma (IL) patients following autologous stem cell transplantation (ASCT). Blood 11, 899a.

Horowitz, M. M., Gale, R. P., Sondel, P. M. et al. (1990). Graft-versus-leukemia reactions after bone marrow transplantation. Blood 75, 555–562.

Hsu, F. J., Caspar, C. B., Czerwinski, D. et al. (1997). Tumor-specific idiotype vaccines in the treatment of patients with B-cell lymphoma: long-term results of a clinical trial. Blood 89, 3129–3135.

Kanzler, H., Kuppers, R., Hansmann, M. L. et al. (1996). Hodgkin and Reed-Sternberg cells in Hodgkin's disease represent the outgrowth of a dominant tumor clone derived from (crippled) germinal center B cells. J Exp Med 184, 1495–1505.

Mackall, C. L., Bare, C. V., Granger, L. A. et al. (1996). Thymic-independent T cell regeneration occurs via antigen-driven expansion of peripheral T cells resulting in a repertoire that is limited in diversity and prone to skewing. J Immunol 156, 4609–4916.

Maecker, H. T., Auffermann-Gretzinger, S., Nomura, L. E. et al. (2001). Detection of CD4 T-cell responses to a tumor vaccine by cytokine flow cytometry. Clin Cancer Res 7 Suppl, 902s–908s.

Martinelli, G., Laszlo, D., Bertolini, F. et al. (2003). Chlorambucil in combination with induction and maintenance rituximab is feasible and active in indolent non-Hodgkin's lymphoma. B J Haematol 123, 271–277.

McNeel, D. G., Schiffman, K. and Disis, M. L. (1999). Immunization with recombinant human granulocyte-macrophage colony-stimulating factor as a vaccine adjuvant elicits both a cellular and humoral response to recombinant human granulocyte-macrophage colony-stimulating factor. Blood 93, 2653–2659.

Molldrem, J. J., Kant, S., Lu, S. et al. (2002). Peptide vaccination with PR1 elicits active T cell immunity that induces cytogenetic remission in acute myelogenous leukemia. Blood 100, 6a.

Nitschke, L., Carsetti, R., Ocker, B. et al. (1997). CD22 is a negative regulator of B-cell receptor signalling. Curr Biol 7, 133–143.

Osterborg, A., Yi, Q., Henriksson, L. et al. (1998). Idiotype immunization combined with granulocyte-macrophage colony-stimulating factor in myeloma patients induced type I, major histocompatibility complex-restricted, CD8- and CD4-specific T-cell responses. Blood 91, 2459–2466.

Padua, R. A., Larghero, J., Robin, M. et al. (2003). PML-RARA-targeted DNA vaccine induces protective immunity in a mouse model of leukemia. Nat Med 9, 1413–1417.

Reynolds, S. R., Oratz, R., Shapiro, R. L. et al. (1997). Stimulation of CD8+ T cell responses to MAGE-3 and Melan A/MART-1 by immunization to a polyvalent melanoma vaccine. Int J Cancer 72, 972–976.

Riley, J. and Sliwkowski, M. X. (2000). CD20: a gene in search of a function. Semin Oncol 27 Suppl 12, 17–24.

Simon, R. M., Steinberg, S. M., Hamilton, M. et al. (2001). Clinical Trial Designs for the E Clinical Development of Therapeutic Cancer Vaccines. J Clin Oncol. 19(6), 1848–1854.

Thurner, B., Haendle, I. Roder, C. et al. (1999). Vaccination with mage-3A1 peptide-pulsed mature, monocyte-derived dendritic cells expands specific cytotoxic T cells and induces regression of some metastases in advanced stage IV melanoma. J Exp Med 190, 1669–1678.

Uzzo, R. G., Rayman, P., Kolenko, V. et al. (1999). Mechanisms of apoptosis in T cells from patients with renal cell carcinoma. Clin Cancer Res 5, 1219–1229.

Zhong, R. K., Rassenti, L. Z., Kipps, T. J. et al. (2002). Sequential modulation of growth factors: a novel strategy for adoptive immunotherapy of acute myeloid leukemia. Biol Blood Marrow Transplant 8, 557–568.

Autoimmunity – Rheumatoid Arthritis

Chapter 42

Peter C. Taylor

The Kennedy Institute of Rheumatology Division, Faculty of Medicine, Imperial College London, London, UK

Perfect activity leaves no tracks behind it . . .

Lao Tzu, Chapter 27, Tao Te Ching, ~3000 BC

INTRODUCTION

The clinical presentation of rheumatoid arthritis (RA) is heterogeneous with a wide spectrum of age of onset, degree of joint involvement and severity. Up to 90 per cent of patients with aggressive synovitis have radiological evidence of bone erosion within 2 years of diagnosis, despite treatment (Sharp et al., 1991). Early identification of patients with RA and, in particular, those likely to assume a more rapidly destructive form of disease, is important because of the considerable evidence that is now available for the benefit of early, aggressive intervention with disease modifying agents (Boers et al., 1997; Mottonen et al., 1999, 2002). Preservation of joint integrity is closely associated with maintenance of functional capability. This realization has prompted the investigation and measurement of numerous biologic 'markers' in blood and joint fluids that may serve as indicators of prognosis and the response to therapy. Although some of the markers under consideration are accessible in routine practice, many are in the stage of experimental evaluation and require access to specialized technology and customized reagents.

Rheumatoid factors, autoantibodies that react with the Fc portion of IgG, can have diagnostic and prognostic value in the assessment of RA and have been on the rheumatologic stage for over 60 years. However, as we

shall see, numerous other markers have been investigated, although few are in routine clinical practice.

PRINCIPLES BEHIND MEASUREMENT OF BIOLOGIC 'MARKERS'

Although the cause of RA remains unknown, advances in molecular technology have facilitated identification of cell subsets and cytokines contributing to the inflammatory and destructive components of the disease. However, these advances have been based on studies of synovial tissue from rheumatoid joints. Such tissue is not readily accessible in routine clinical practice or even in the context of clinical trials. The majority of biologic markers of potential value in the diagnosis and assessment of outcome in RA are measured in peripheral blood or urine. Although, in general, cytokines and immune cell subsets within the peripheral blood compartment are not measured clinically they are considered to be important in the pathogenesis of RA. Serum cytokine measurements and peripheral blood cellular enumeration and phenotyping are discussed elsewhere in this volume.

The biologic markers of potential value in the diagnosis and assessment of outcome in RA to be discussed in this chapter can be considered in four categories (Table 42.1).

These are:

1 Immunologic abnormalities such as rheumatoid factors.
2 Genetic factors such as HLA class II and the 'shared epitope'.

Measuring Immunity, edited by Michael T. Lotze and Angus W. Thomson
ISBN 0-12-455900-X, London

Table 42.1 Biologic markers of rheumatoid arthritis

Immunological abnormalities		Rheumatoid factor
		Anti-citrunillated peptides
		Anti-A2/RA33
		Agalactosyl IgG
		Anti-p68 (BiP)
Genetic		HLA DRβ1
		Sulfoxidation status
		Matrix metalloproteinase genotype
Acute phase response		ESR, CRP, SAA
		IL-6
Tissue specific		
	Synovium	Hyaluronan
	Cartilage	Aggrecan epitopes, COMP
	Bone	Bone sialoprotein
		Pyridinoline cross-links
		Collagen type 1 fragments
	Vascular	VEGF

3 The acute phase response elicited by hepatocytes as part of the inflammatory process.
4 Macromolecules specific for joint associated tissues that are released into synovial fluid, the circulation or excreted in the urine as part of degenerative and repair processes.

MEASUREMENT OF BIOLOGIC 'MARKERS'

The only biomarkers currently in routine clinical use for the purpose of following RA disease activity are ESR and CRP, measures of acute phase response. The ESR is a measurement of the distance in millimeters that red blood cells fall within a specified tube (westergen or Wintrobe) over 1 h. The ESR is an indirect measurement of alterations in acute phase reactants and quantitative immunoglobulins, discussed further below in the section entitled acute phase reactants. CRP is a pentameric protein comprised of five identical, non-covalently bound subunits, arranged in cyclic symmetry in a single plane. Unlike the ESR, CRP can be measured using stored serum samples and is independent of the hemoglobin concentration. CRP can be measured by ELISA, radioimmunodiffusion or nephelometry.

In terms of RA diagnosis, rheumatoid factors (discussed in the section entitled immunological abnormalities) remain the sole serological measure included in the widely used American College of Rheumatology classification criteria for RA (Arnett et al., 1988). However, there is currently increasing interest in the measurement of antibodies to cyclic citrullinated peptides (anti-CCP) as a more specific marker of RA, as discussed in detail in the section entitled immunological abnormalities. Importantly, new studies using a scoring system that includes measurement of anti-CCP antibodies together with rheumatoid factor, duration of symptoms, arthritis in

three or more joint groups and metatarsophalangeal tenderness show an ability to differentiate persistent arthritis from self-limiting disease and erosive arthritis from persistent, non-erosive arthritis with better discrimination than the American College of Rheumatology classification criteria for RA (Visser et al., 2002).

Practical considerations in the measurement of rheumatoid factors are detailed in Section II (Serologic assays) of this handbook. In brief, IgM rheumatoid factor is the only one routinely measured by clinical laboratories. A titer of ≥1:160 is usually considered significant if measured by the widely used latex agglutination technique utilizing latex particles coated with human IgG. More recently, many laboratories have begun using nephelometry and enzyme-linked immunosorbent assay (ELISA) techniques to measure IgM rheumatoid factor. However, a study of the performance of commercially available ELISA test kits for rheumatoid factor measurement found large variations among kits in the ability to detect rheumatoid factor (Bas et al., 2002).

Antibodies to citrullinated peptides were initially measured in research laboratories by indirect immunofluorescence and immunoblotting. More recently, to overcome the technical difficulties and expense of the assays and to enhance the detection limits, ELISAs have been developed for antifilaggrin antibodies. The antigens used in these ELISAs have been recombinant rat or human filaggrin deaminated in vivo (Nogueira et al., 2001; Vincent et al., 2002), filaggrin extracted from human epidermis (Nogueira et al., 2001) and a synthetic cyclic citrullinated peptide (CCP) derived from human filaggrin (Bizzaro et al., 2001; Nogueira et al., 2001; Bas et al., 2002; Vincent et al., 2002). An ELISA using CCP as the antigen is now available commercially although not yet widespread in routine clinical usage.

Other biomarkers discussed in this chapter have been used as research tools in attempts to delineate their value as markers of prognosis, markers to monitor response to therapy or surrogate markers of a biological process.

MARKERS UNDER INVESTIGATION IN THE DIAGNOSIS AND ASSESSMENT OF OUTCOME IN RHEUMATOID ARTHRITIS

Immunologic abnormalities

Several immunologic abnormalities, particularly autoantibodies, are associated with the presence of rheumatoid arthritis.

Rheumatoid factors

Rheumatoid factors (RF) are autoantibodies directed against the Fc portion of IgG. They may be of any immunoglobulin class although only those of IgM class are in routine use. They are found in 75–80 per cent of RA patients at some time during the course of their disease.

Rheumatoid patients with a positive rheumatoid factor test are designated as having 'seropositive' RA.

The disease specificity of RF for rheumatic diseases is dependent on the concentration (titer) designated as being of likely clinical significance. The specificity of RF for RA is considerably higher at elevated titers, although this is at the expense of sensitivity. Thus, in the context of a chronic polyarthritis, high titer IgM RF is relatively specific for the diagnosis of RA and remains the sole serologic criterion widely used in classification criteria for RA (Arnett et al., 1988). It has little predictive value in the general population, however, since the overall disease prevalence is relatively low.

RF also occur in other diseases, for example, some connective tissue diseases, such as systemic lupus erythematosus (SLE) and primary Sjogren's syndrome. In addition, RF may be measured in patients with certain infections, such as malaria and rubella and following vaccinations.

Interestingly, RF are not detected in most experimental models of RA. Only MRL/lpr mice, a strain characterized phenotypically by a lupus-like disease, including anti-dsDNA and anti-Sm antibodies express RF (Table 42.2). However, these mice present with overlapping disease features including arthritis that may become erosive (Koopman and Gay, 1988).

Rheumatoid factor may have some prognostic value with regard to disease manifestations and activity as well as the severity of structural damage to joints as assessed by radiology. Seropositive disease, especially when the RF titer is high, is often associated with more rapid and severe progression of radiological joint destruction and functional loss (Listing et al., 2000; Combe et al., 2001; Drossaers-Bakker et al., 2002). Furthermore, among patients meeting classification criteria for RA, extra-articular manifestations occur more commonly in those seropositive for RF than those who are seronegative (Jacoby et al., 1973; Masi et al., 1976; Alarcon et al., 1982; Egeland and Munthe, 1983; Westedt et al., 1985; Aho et al., 1993a). Rheumatoid nodules, one of the commonest extra-articular manifestations of RA and vasculitis occur almost exclusively in seropositive patients (Sharp et al., 1964; Masi et al., 1976; Alarcon et al., 1982; Westedt et al., 1985; Aho et al., 1993a) and are associated with increased mortality (Erhardt et al., 1989). For example, in a retrospective case control study of 135 women with early RA, patients with persistently positive RF had more erosions, nodules, extra-articular disease, functional disability

and disease activity than seronegative, or intermittently seronegative individuals over a mean period of 6 years of follow up (Van Zeben et al., 1992).

In a study of seropositive RA patients attending specialist clinics the rate of formation of new erosions correlated with the RF titer (Sievers, 1965). However, this observation was not confirmed in a study of a community-based cohort of patients with recent-onset arthritis over 8 years of follow up (Aho et al., 1989). In part these differences reflect the heterogeneous nature of the RA phenotype but interpretation may also be confounded by differences in pharmacological intervention.

Intriguingly, the presence of RF may antedate the clinical manifestations of RA. A study of a large cohort of healthy individuals from Finland found that nine of 129 subjects with positive RF subsequently developed seropositive RA over a 10-year investigation period, as compared to only 12 of 7000 subjects with negative tests (Aho et al., 1991). These findings imply that the presence of a positive RF in a healthy individual is associated with a relative risk of approximately 40 for the development of RA. Despite this striking observation, in the same study, 120 of 129 patients with positive RF did not develop RA over 10 years of observation. Therefore the RF test lacks predictive value for development of clinical disease.

Although RF titers in individual RA patients at any given time-point in the course of the disease are not considered to be an accurate reflection of disease activity, it is interesting to note that in a placebo-controlled study of the anti-TNF agent infliximab, RF titers fell significantly in the infliximab group without change in the placebo group (Maini et al., 1999).

Antibodies to citrullinated antigens

Unlike other autoimmune rheumatic diseases such as SLE or Sjogren's syndrome, the autoantigens in rheumatoid arthritis have been particularly elusive. The search for novel antigens has been driven by the need to identify molecules that could initiate or maintain autoimmunity in RA and for diagnostic assays for the disease beyond rheumatoid factors. Among numerous autoantigens that have been proposed, autoantibodies directed against three in particular have stood the test of time and reproducibility in independent laboratories: the antiperinuclear factor (APF), anti-rat esophageal keratin antibodies (AKA) and the anti-Sa antibodies (Aho et al., 1994; Hayem et al., 1999).

It has recently emerged that all three antigens share a common feature, namely that they are citrullinated. Citrullination involves the removal of side amino groups from the highly basic arginine residues by the action of the enzyme peptidylarginine deiminase converting them to the neutral citrulline. This process fundamentally changes the charge and hence the antigenicity of the protein. Peptidylarginine deiminase is widely distributed in tissues including placenta, keratinocytes, polymorphonuclear leukocytes, HL-60 cells and *Porphyromonas gingivalis*, a

Table 42.2 Autoantibodies in murine models of arthritis

Model	Rheumatoid factor	Anti-citrulline	Anti-RA33
Collagen-induced arthritis	No	No	No
MRL/lpr mice	Yes	Unknown	Yes
Pristane-induced arthritis	No	Unknown	Yes
TNF transgenic mice	No	No	Yes

well-established cause of a mild chronic gingivitis in humans. The target antigen for the APF has now been identified as citrullinated fillagrin (Schellekens et al., 1998), probably caused by infection of buccal epithelial cells (used as the substrate) with *P. gingivalis*. The target antigen for rat esophageal keratin is citrullinated keratin (Van Venrooij and Pruijn, 2000), or a keratin like molecule and that for the Sa antigen, originally identified in placenta, is citrullinated vimentin (Menard et al., 2000). Recently other citrullinated molecules have also been proposed, including citrullinated fibrin (Masson-Bessiere et al., 2001), as a possible target antigen in RA. Peptides derived from citrullinated fillagrin are now used in commercially available kits (Kroot et al., 2000) and may well have a future role in the diagnosis and predicting prognosis in RA. Thus it seems that the important autoantigens in RA are likely to have undergone the post-translational modification of citrullination before they react with autoantibodies.

The diagnostic sensitivity and specificity of APF, AKA and anti-Sa antibodies vary depending on the methods of detection used (Table 42.3). APF detected by means of indirect immunofluorescence using buccal epithelium has a reported specificity for RA of 73–99 per cent (Nienhuis and Mandema, 1964; Vivino and Maul, 1990) and a sensitivity of 49–87 per cent (Nienhuis and Mandema, 1964; Janssens et al., 1988). For AKA, detected by the use of rat esophagus as a substrate (Young et al., 1979), the reported specificity for RA generally exceeds 90 per cent with a sensitivity between 40 and 60 per cent (Hoet et al., 1991). An immunoblotting method for the detection of AKA, using three protein antigens extracted from rat esophagus epithelium and separated by non-denaturing polyacrylamide gel electrophoresis, found that AKA had a sensitivity for RA of 43 to 50 per cent and a specificity of 99 per cent (Gomes-Daudrix et al., 1994). The intensity of labeling of the three rat esophagus protein antigens and that of human epidermal filaggrin when RA sera are tested by immunoblotting, correlates with the APF titers of the sera (Sebbag et al., 1995).

Table 42.3 Novel autoantibodies in rheumatoid arthritis

Antibody	Antigen	Sensitivity (%)	Specificity (%)	Reference
Antikeratin	Filaggrin	40–60	92–99	Young et al., 1979 Gomes-Daudrix et al., 1994
	Anti-citrullinated peptides	76	96	Schellekens et al., 1998
Anti-Sa	Vimentin	42	98	Masson-Bessiere et al., 2001 Hayem et al., 1999
Anti-RA33	HnRNP-A2	40	90	Hassfeld et al., 1995
Anti-p68 (BiP)	BiP	68	96	Blass et al., 2001

ELISA assays based upon either filaggrin derived from human skin or synthetic peptides have high specificity and sensitivity for RA (Palosuo et al., 1998; Schellekens et al., 1998) (see Table 42.3). An ELISA assay consisting of several citrulline-containing peptide variants reportedly has a sensitivity and specificity of 76 and 96 per cent for RA, respectively (Schellekens et al., 1998) (see Table 42.3). This test may ultimately prove useful in the differential diagnosis of early stage RA, particularly in the ability to distinguish RA from primary Sjogren's syndrome or SLE. The assay is not currently in wide clinical use.

The combination of testing for AKA and RF (by both IgM ELISA and latex methods) may be of value in patients with undiagnosed polyarthritis. This was illustrated in a study of 270 patients with early arthritis who were initially tested, then followed for up to 2 years. The most common final diagnoses were RA, spondyloarthropathy and undifferentiated arthritis in 94, 56, and 61 patients, respectively (Saraux et al., 2002). The sensitivity and specificity of the three tests in combination for an eventual diagnosis of RA were 75 and 82 per cent, respectively, if at least one test was positive. If all three tests were positive the sensitivity was 33 per cent, specificity was 99 per cent and positive predictive value 97 per cent. The findings of this study are highly relevant to routine clinical practice where it is often difficult to establish a definitive diagnosis of RA in patients presenting with an inflammatory arthropathy but not yet fulfilling classification criteria (Arnett et al., 1988) and there is now considerable evidence that suppression of synovitis at the earliest stages of disease leads to significantly improved outcomes.

The prognostic significance of AKA and APF has been studied in three cohorts of early RA with follow ups of 3 and 8 years respectively (von Essen et al., 1993; Kurki et al., 1997; Combe et al., 2001). All patients with detectable AKA developed at least some erosions by the end of the 8-year follow up (Kurki et al., 1997). One cohort with recent onset RA was followed by the same investigators; the initial presence of AKA was associated with active and treatment resistant disease at up to 3 years but did not predict radiologic progression (Paimela et al., 2001). Others have reported similar findings (Combe et al., 2001). Furthermore, among patients with chronic erosive RA, APF and AKA do not define any subgroup with a particularly aggressive course.

As in the case of RF, the presence of AKA, APF or anti-filaggrin antibodies may antedate clinical RA (Kurki et al., 1992; Aho et al., 1993b, 2000). In addition, detection of either AKA or APF in a healthy individual with a positive sensitized sheep red blood cell agglutination test further increases the relative risk of developing RF-positive RA by a factor of five (Aho et al., 1993b). However, a significant number of antibody positive patients do not develop disease. As an example, in the study just quoted, 12 of 70 RF positive patients who did not develop RA tested positive for either AKA, APF or both antibodies (Aho et al., 1993b).

Positive RF, AKA or APF tests prior to clinical disease may also indicate that initiation of disease antedates symptoms by many years. This possibility has profound implications for epidemiologic studies seeking an initiating cause of RA.

Anti-p68 (BiP) antibodies

The autoantigen named BiP is a ubiquitously expressed 68 kDa glycoprotein that serves as a chaperone in the endoplasmic reticulum and binds to immunoglobulin heavy chains. Increased T cell proliferative responses against BiP have been noted in patients with RA and antibodies directed against the protein may be a marker for the disease. In a study of 400 patients with RA, 200 patients with other rheumatic diseases and healthy donors, the reported specificity of anti-BiP antibodies for RA is 96 per cent with a sensitivity of 68 per cent (Blass et al., 2001).

Anti-RA33 antibodies

Anti-A2/anti-RA33 antibodies are directed to the heterogeneous nuclear ribonucleoprotein A2 (hnRNP-A2), a nuclear protein that is involved in mRNA splicing and transport (Hassfeld et al., 1993). The antibodies occur in approximately one-third of RA patients but can also be detected in 20–30 per cent of patients with SLE and in up to 40 per cent of patients with the rare overlap syndrome mixed connective tissue disease (MCTD). Thus the sensitivity of anti-A2/anti-RA33 autoantibodies for RA is low (at around ~40 per cent). Nevertheless, in a representative cohort of patients with various rheumatic diseases including autoimmune and non-autoimmune arthritides, the specificity of anti-A2/anti-RA33 antibodies for RA was approximately 90 per cent (Hassfeld et al., 1995) (see Table 42.3). However, if a diagnosis of SLE and MCTD (or MCTD alone) is excluded or in the absence of autoantibodies associated with SLE (such as anti-DNA, anti-Sm and anti-U1 RNP antibodies), the specificity of anti-RA33 antibodies for RA can be as high as 96 per cent (Hassfeld et al., 1995).

Anti-RA33 antibodies are associated with prominent arthritis in patients with MCTD and SLE (Isenberg et al., 1994), suggesting a relationship of this antibody to autoimmune inflammatory joint disease in general. Furthermore, it has been postulated that anti-RA33 antibodies are an early and stable marker of RA on the basis of observations in a cohort of patients with various rheumatic diseases where all of seven anti-RA33 positive patients initially presenting with an undifferentiated arthritis went on to meet classification criteria for RA within 3 years (Hassfeld et al., 1993). However, the presence of anti-RA33 antibodies is not associated with an increased risk of progressive radiographic joint damage (Combe et al., 2001).

Gal 0 glycoforms

RA is associated with a marked increase in IgG lacking galactose (designated as Gal 0 glycoforms) and terminating in N-acetyl glucosamine in the Fc region (Parekh et al., 1985). In vitro, agalactosyl immunoglobulins (Gal 0 IgG) activate complement by means of a mannose-binding protein dependent pathway (Malhotra et al., 1995). Gal 0 levels correlate with disease severity in RA and revert to normal during the course of pregnancy-induced remissions (Rook et al., 1991). More rapid radiographic progression of RA has been associated with low serum levels of mannose-binding lectin, which is determined genetically (Graudal et al., 2000; Ip et al., 2000). Furthermore, the finding of mannose-binding protein and enrichment of Gal 0 IgG in RA synovial fluids has prompted the suggestion that these events are of pathologic significance in the joint destruction of RA.

Gal 0 IgG and RF were measured at presentation and at a 2-year follow up, in a prospective study of 60 British patients with a history of synovitis of less than 1 year's duration (Young et al., 1991). Over the study period, 39 patients developed RA as defined by the ACR classification criteria. The initial Gal 0 IgG correctly predicted the development of RA, or otherwise, in 47 of the 60 patients. The combination of Gal 0 IgG and RF status gave a test with 90 per cent sensitivity, 95 per cent specificity and 94 per cent predictive value.

Cell surface expression of CD40 ligand

The CD40 ligand (CD154) is expressed on activated T cells and underlies many interactions between these and other haematopoietic cells. Enhanced surface expression of the CD40 ligand on circulating T cells is associated with more active disease in RA (Berner et al., 2000).

Antibodies to alpha-enolase and calpastatin

Antibodies to alpha-enolase and calpastatin have been reported in patients in the early phase of RA, often in the absence of RF (Vittecoq et al., 2001; Saulot et al., 2002). However, because of the low prevalence of these antibodies in RA patients it is unlikely that they will be clinically useful diagnostic markers. For example, among 255 patients with early arthritis, elevated serum levels of antibodies to an enzyme in the glycolytic pathway, alpha-enolase, were found in 25 per cent of those who were later determined to have rheumatoid arthritis (Saulot et al., 2002). One-half of those with RA and anti-enolase antibodies did not have serum rheumatoid factor or antifilaggrin antibodies. Among 40 patients whose arthritis remained undifferentiated after 1 year of observation, 10 per cent had antibodies to alpha-enolase.

Genetic factors

The risk of developing RA is associated with carriage of particular HLA alleles. A patient's HLA DR type and other genetic factors may also play a role in determining the severity of disease. More severe forms of RA are significantly associated with genotypes that contain the Dw4/Dw14 and Dw4/DR1 alleles (Lanchbury et al., 1991; van Zeben et al., 1991; Wordsworth et al., 1992) and almost all patients with Felty's syndrome have the Dw4 subtype (Lanchbury et al., 1991). The immunogenetics of the immune response is discussed in detail in Section I of this book.

Shared epitope

RA is positively associated with certain HLA DR alleles (particularly HLA DR4) encoding a conserved amino acid sequence in the third hypervariable region of the DRβ1 chain termed the 'shared epitope'. The 'shared epitope' is present in 80–90 per cent of patients with established disease and has been extensively studied (Gregersen et al., 1987; Wordsworth et al., 1989; Gorman and Criswell, 2002). Numerous studies have demonstrated an association between the presence of the shared epitope and poor radiological outcome (van der Heijde, et al., 1992; Constantin et al., 2002a,b; Massardo et al., 2002). However, other investigators have failed to confirm this association, for example in a clinic-based study from Argentina (Citera et al., 2001) and the Norfolk Arthritis Registry study (Bukhari et al., 2002) reporting on a large inception cohort in the UK. Such apparent discrepancies may be explained on the basis of interaction between genetic and other variables as suggested by a study reporting an association between carriage of the shared epitope and more severe bone damage in patients seronegative for rheumatoid factor but not in seropositive patients (Mattey et al., 2001). Furthermore, the variable effects of therapeutic intervention may confound the interpretation of such studies. For example, in a reanalysis of data from two prior prospective treatment studies, the shared epitope was associated with accelerated radiographic destruction in patient groups receiving a less aggressive treatment regimen but the association was not observed in patients receiving disease-modifying anti-rheumatic drugs at an early stage after disease onset or in those treated with a more aggressive, combination therapy regimen (Lard et al., 2002).

Matrix metalloproteinase genotype

Matrix metalloproteinases degrade collagen and contribute to cartilage and bone destruction in RA. These molecules are discussed further below in the section entitled Tissue-specific markers. Carriage of a polymorphism in the promoter region of the gene for matrix metalloproteinase 3 (MMP-3) is reported to be associated with more severe disease. In a study of 103 patients with early RA, homozygous carriage of a particular polymorphism in the promoter region of the MMP-3 gene (6A/6A) was associated with the presence of more severe joint damage at first presentation and higher subsequent rate of progression of structural damage to joints as

compared with patients carrying one or more alleles of a different type (5A) (Constantin et al., 2002b).

Sulfoxidation status

The inherited ability to oxidize the sulfur compound S-carboxy-methyl-L-cysteine varies widely among individuals. The prevalence of individuals with poor sulfoxidation status is increased in patients with established RA (Emery et al., 1992) and, in early RA, defective sulfoxidation status correlates strongly with persistent clinical disease. In 54 patients with recent onset symmetrical polyarthritis, the S-oxidation capacity was evaluated and the clinical course was monitored over 4 years. At 4 years, 74 per cent of patients with a diagnosis of RA were poor S-oxidizers compared to 31 per cent of those who were asymptomatic (Emery et al., 1992).

Acute phase response

Acute phase reactants are a heterogeneous group of proteins synthesized by hepatocytes in response to inflammation under the regulation of cytokines signaling via the gp130 receptor, in particular, the pro-inflammatory cytokine interleukin-6 (IL-6) (Gauldie et al., 1987). CRP is the most commonly measured acute phase protein and becomes elevated in serum within 4 h of tissue injury with peak concentrations between 24 and 72 h after an acute insult. The ESR is an indirect measurement of alterations in acute phase reactants and quantitative immunoglobulins. It is affected by multiple variables and as such, is somewhat imprecise. Nevertheless, it is inexpensive and very easy to measure, hence its widespread use in clinical practice and clinical trials. It rises more slowly after the onset of inflammation than CRP and tends to remain elevated for longer, decreasing by about 50 per cent a week once inflammation subsides. In the context of active RA, ESR and CRP tend to be elevated in parallel.

C reactive protein and ESR

At the present time, the most widely accepted methods of assessing RA disease activity and response to therapy involve clinical assessment of the numbers of swollen and tender joints and laboratory measures of the inflammatory burden in the form of ESR and CRP. Using these parameters a total disease activity score can be formulated (Prevoo et al., 1995). For many years in routine clinical assessment ESR and CRP have been considered the most objective measures of disease activity in RA.

Anti-TNF therapy is accompanied by a rapid reduction in clinical measures of disease activity and serum concentrations of CRP strongly suggesting that the clinical and biological responses are linked. Published studies using these agents in therapy for RA demonstrate that the magnitude of improvement in tender joint counts, swollen joint counts and CRP is about 60–70 per cent from baseline (Maini et al., 1999; Weinblatt et al., 1999; Lipsky et al., 2000).

Structural damage to joints, as assessed by plain radiology, is significantly more likely to progress when either of these measures of acute phase response is elevated. This observation holds good irrespective of the presence or absence of RF and irrespective of therapeutic intervention with conventional disease-modifying anti-rheumatic drugs (Amos et al., 1977; Combe et al., 2001). The relationship between the rate of advance in radiological damage to joints and acute phase markers is more pronounced when both ESR and CRP are elevated than when CRP concentrations alone are raised (Davis et al., 1990).

As will be apparent from the discussion so far, in cohort studies, a number of measures have been defined that are indicative of progressive joint damage with the passage of time. By combining ESR, CRP or disease activity score at presentation with other poor prognostic factors such as positive DR4 and RF status, the absence or progression of radiographic joint damage over 2 years of follow up was correctly predicted in 83 per cent of a group of 147 patients (van der Heijde et al., 1992).

There has been considerable interest in the relationship between the rate of structural damage to joints and the cumulative inflammatory burden in RA. This has been investigated by measuring time-integrated values of acute phase markers. In a study of 110 patients with early RA with symptom duration of less than 1 year, a highly significant correlation between radiological progression and cumulative CRP production was noted (van Leeuwen et al., 1993). However, there was a wide variation in the relationship between the magnitude of radiographic change and cumulative CRP, particularly in those with low CRP levels. HLA DR4, positive RF, gender or age could not account for this inter-individual variability. Therefore, as is the case for other markers of poor prognosis, on an individual patient basis serial measurements of modestly elevated acute phase proteins lack the predictive accuracy reliably to inform treatment decisions.

Interleukin-6

IL-6 regulates the production of acute phase proteins by hepatocytes (Gauldie et al., 1987) and activates osteoclasts to absorb bone (Tamura et al., 1993). Inflamed synovium is thought to be the principal source of plasma IL-6 in RA since IL-6 is often detected in high concentration in the synovial fluid. Therefore it was reasoned that plasma IL-6 concentrations might reflect joint inflammation better than acute phase protein levels. However, in a small cohort of patients with early RA, there was no relationship between radiological progression and time integrated values of plasma IL-6 concentration despite a significant correlation between IL-6 and the acute phase measures (van Leeuwen et al., 1995). Such apparent discrepancies may be due to a known diurnal variation in concentrations of this cytokine.

The rapid reductions in CRP following infliximab therapy are accompanied by changes in IL-6 (Elliott et al., 1994; Charles et al., 1999) providing formal proof that TNFα regulates other pro-inflammatory cytokines.

Tissue-specific markers

A number of biochemical markers of joint damage have been described in RA. They are predominantly derived from a single tissue such as cartilage, bone or synovium, and may be detected in joint fluids, serum or urine. These molecules may be synthetic or degradative, their presence in body fluids arising as a consequence of metabolism of the tissue of origin. However, in general, joint fluids are not readily available in comparison to serum or urine. At present there is limited information regarding the usefulness of tissue-specific markers as measures of disease activity or response to therapy in RA. Assays for measurement of these markers are not routinely available and their usage has largely been restricted to research studies. However, it is emerging that some tissue-specific markers may have prognostic value.

Synovium-specific markers

The synovium is thought to be the dominant source of matrix metalloproteinase 3 (MMP-3), an enzyme that is essential to the fragmentation of collagen matrix. Elevated serum levels are reported to correlate with severity of radiographic joint damage in some studies (Yamanaka et al., 2000), although no such relationship was observed in others (Roux-Lombard et al., 2001). However, serum pro-MMP-3 concentrations closely correlated at all time points with CRP levels in serum sampled at multiple time points over a 5-year study period (Roux-Lombard et al., 2001).

The anti-TNF therapy infliximab results in significant arrest of structural damage to joints in RA patients (Taylor, 2001). In keeping with this finding, there is marked reduction in circulating concentrations of precursor MMP-1 and MMP-3 (Brennan et al., 1997). However, in serial synovial biopsies taken at baseline and 8 weeks after etanercept, another anti-TNF therapy, no significant change was observed in synovial tissue expression of MMP (Catrina et al., 2002). Similarly, serum levels of osteoprotegerin (OPG) and soluble receptor activator of nuclear factor kappa B ligand (sRANKL), both of which are elevated in rheumatoid compared to normal sera, are normalized following infliximab therapy without influencing the OPG:sRANKL ratio (Ziolkowska et al., 2002).

Hyaluronan, another marker that may be predominantly released from the synovium, is strikingly elevated in the serum of patients with RA (Engstrom-Laurent and Hallgren, 1985; Poole et al., 1990). Hyaluronan is produced by synovial lining cells in rheumatoid joints but not by lining cells from normal joints (Dahl and Husby, 1985). In RA, serum hyaluronan concentrations correlate with disease activity despite a short half-life of 15 minutes or less (Poole et al., 1990) and prospective studies suggest that in early RA serum hyaluronan may reflect ongoing joint destruction and even predict subsequent joint damage (Paimela et al., 1991). However, these findings must be interpreted with caution as elevated serum levels of hyaluronan may vary with physical activity independently of the magnitude of synovitis (Manicourt et al., 1999).

Cartilage-specific markers

Markers of cartilage metabolism such as cartilage oligomeric matrix protein (COMP), a member of the thrombospondin protein family, may have some prognostic value in patients with RA. In early RA patients, elevated serum COMP levels are reported to be predictive of severe disease characterized by subsequent large and small joint destruction (Forslind et al., 1992; Mansson et al., 1995). In another 5-year prospective study of early RA patients, COMP tended to correlate with radiological joint damage score at the start but thereafter did not reflect the destructive aspect of disease or the inflammatory component as judged by CRP concentrations (Roux-Lombard et al., 2001).

Treatment of RA with TNF blockade results in a significant, sustained reduction in serum COMP (den Broeder, et al., 2002; Crnkic et al., 2003). Of interest, reductions in COMP are reported even in patients failing to achieve clinical parameters of modest response (Crnkic et al., 2003). This is in keeping with studies demonstrating joint protection in the majority of patients receiving anti-TNF therapies, even those failing to achieve modest clinical responses (Lipsky et al., 2000).

Increased serum concentrations of COMP in RA patients have been reported to be indicative of the rapid development of hip joint destruction (Mansson et al., 1995). Serum levels of a putative marker of cartilage aggrecan synthesis were also measured in these patients. The marker, epitope 846, is located on the chondroitin sulfate rich area of the aggrecan molecule and may be a marker of favorable prognosis. Epitope 846 levels were elevated in those patients with slow joint destruction, as compared with a group matched for age, gender and disease duration but with more destructive joint disease (Mansson et al., 1995). These data are suggestive of ongoing cartilage reparative processes in the group with a more benign course.

There is reported to be an association between the aggrecan content of synovial fluid obtained from knee joints and the severity of knee and hip joint destruction in RA (Mansson et al., 1997). The chondroitin sulfate rich region of aggrecan is most abundantly detected in synovial fluids recovered from joints with little radiological evidence of destruction, whereas the hyaluronan binding region of core protein is released in more severely damaged joints (Saxne and Heinegard, 1992).

Measurement of cross-linked c-terminal peptides from type II collagen in urine may provide some prognostic information. A correlation between the excretion of these peptides and radiographic progression over 4 years was noted in a prospective study of 110 patients with early RA (Garnero et al., 2002).

Bone-specific markers

As in the case of cartilage-specific markers, several bone-derived molecules have been investigated as potential markers of prognosis and therapeutic efficacy with respect to joint protection. However, the specificity of bone-specific markers may be confounded by concurrent osteoporosis.

Pyridinoline cross-links measured in urine are a marker of bone degradation. Urinary concentrations of this marker correlate with disease activity in RA and diminish after treatment with pulsed glucocorticoids and disease modifying antirheumatic drugs (Kollerup et al., 1994; Dolan et al., 2002).

Bone sialoprotein is an osteoblast-derived protein preferentially expressed in juxta-articular bone. Bone sialoprotein levels in synovial fluid correlate with knee joint destruction in both RA and osteoarthritis (Saxne et al., 1995). Bone sialoprotein levels are also reported to be elevated in RA serum, but in contrast to synovial fluid, serum concentrations do not correlate with joint destruction.

Another bone marker is a type I collagen degradation product, cross-linked carboxyterminal telopeptides of type I collagen (ICTP). ICTP can be measured by immunoassays in serum and synovial fluids. In a 3-year prospective study of 66 patients with early RA, at baseline 51 per cent had elevated serum ICTP concentrations compared to healthy controls (Paimela et al., 1994). Throughout the follow-up period, serum ICTP levels correlated with inflammatory parameters. Furthermore, ICTP concentrations correlated with the rate of radiological destruction. There was a stronger relationship between baseline ICTP levels than the other variables of disease activity with the rate of progression of joint erosions. The findings were independently confirmed in another cohort of 110 early RA patients (Garnero et al., 2002). Collectively, these data suggest a potential role for measurement of serum ICTP as a prognostic marker for joint damage in early RA. Synovial fluid ICTP concentrations are reported to correlate better with assessment of knee joint destruction than serum levels (Aman et al., 1999). However, such markers of bone turnover remain a research tool and have not found a role in the routine management of RA patients.

Vascular markers

Vascular endothelial growth factor (VEGF) is the most endothelial cell specific growth factor characterized to date (Brown et al., 1997; Neufeld et al., 1999). It also induces vascular permeability (Ferrara, 1995). VEGF concentrations are elevated in RA patients as compared to healthy controls and to patients with osteoarthritis (Harada et al., 1998; Nagashima, et al., 2000; Ballara, et al., 2001). Furthermore, in patients with early RA, there is a significant correlation between serum VEGF levels at presentation and the rate of radiological joint destruction over the subsequent year (Ballara et al., 2001). Serum VEGF concentrations fall rapidly, but do not normalize, after treatment with anti-TNF agents (Paleolog et al., 1998).

FUTURE PROSPECTS

Evaluation of disease activity in RA is essential both for routine clinical management and in RA clinical trials. Disease activity in RA joints is conventionally assessed clinically, in the form of numbers of tender and swollen joints in combination with routine laboratory measures of surrogate markers of inflammation in blood samples such as C-reactive protein (CRP) and erythrocyte sedimentation rate (ESR). In cohort studies, a number of poor prognostic factors have been defined that are indicative of progressive joint damage with the passage of time. These include high titer rheumatoid factor, possession of the shared epitope, high numbers of joints involved at baseline, high disability at baseline and persistently elevated acute phase reactants. In particular, time-integrated values of acute phase reactants correlate well with the rate of progression of joint damage, as assessed radiologically. However, on an individual patient basis these markers lack the predictive accuracy reliably to inform treatment decisions. As yet, of the various biomarkers discussed in this chapter, none have been unequivocally shown to surpass the prognostic potential of ESR and CRP. Therefore, for the foreseeable future it is likely that ESR and CRP will remain the most valuable laboratory surrogate markers of disease activity.

It is likely that antibodies to citrullinated peptides will be used increasingly in routine clinical practice as a new classification criterion for diagnosis of RA in the early phase of disease. Furthermore, research into the role of citrullinated antigens in RA may give important insights into the etiopathogenesis of this disease.

In recent years, clinical trials of biologic therapies directed against cytokine targets, in particular TNFα, have demonstrated significant arrest of structural damage to joints as assessed by plain radiography. However, radiography is a relatively insensitive tool and it is not possible reliably to determine structural change in less than 6–12 months. Therefore, there has been considerable interest in the measurement of serum and urine markers of cartilage metabolism before and after therapeutic intervention with a view to determining the potential of these markers as indicators of therapeutic efficacy with respect to joint protection. Tissue-specific markers of the type discussed in this chapter hold considerable promise as a means to cut short the time necessary to

determine disease-modifying efficacy of test compounds in clinical trials. However, much research is yet to be done on existing and new biomarkers in order to give sufficiently accurate information regarding the rate of joint destruction to permit reliably informed treatment decisions in a routine clinic setting.

REFERENCES

Aho, K., Tuomi, T., Palosuo, T. et al. (1989). Is seropositive rheumatoid arthritis becoming less severe? Clin Exp Rheumatol 7, 287–290.

Aho, K., Heliovaara, M., Maatela, J. et al. (1991). Rheumatoid factors antedating clinical rheumatoid arthritis. J Rheumatol 18, 1282–1284.

Aho, K., Steiner, G., Kurki, P. et al. (1993a). Anti-RA 33 as a marker of rheumatoid arthritis in a Finnish population. Clin Exp Rheumatol 11, 645–647.

Aho, K., von Essen, R., Kurki, P. et al. (1993b). Antikeratin antibody and the perinuclear factor as markers for subclinical rheumatoid disease process. J Rheumatol 20, 1278–1281.

Aho, K., Palusuo, T. and Kurki, P. (1994). Marker antibodies of rheumatoid arthritis: diagnostic and pathogenetic implications. Semin Arthritis Rheum 23, 379–387.

Aho, K., Palosuo, T., Heliovaara, M. et al. (2000). Antifilaggrin antibodies within 'normal' range predict rheumatoid arthritis in a linear fashion. J Rheumatol 27, 2743–2746.

Alarcon, G.S., Koopman, W.J., Acton, R.T. et al. (1982). Seronegative rheumatoid arthritis. A distinct immunogenetic disease? Arthritis Rheum 25, 502–507.

Aman, S., Risteli, J., Luukkainen, R. et al. (1999). The value of synovial fluid analysis in the assessment of knee joint destruction in arthritis in a three year follow up study. Ann Rheum Dis 58, 559–562.

Amos, R.S., Constable, T.J., Crockson, R.A. et al. (1977). Rheumatoid arthritis: relation of C-reactive protein and erythrocyte sedimentation rates to radiographic changes. Br Med J 1, 195–197.

Arnett, F.C., Edworthy, S.M., Bloch, D.A. et al. (1988). The American Rheumatism Association 1987 revised criteria for classification of rheumatoid arthritis. Arthritis Rheum 31, 315–324.

Ballara, S., Taylor, P.C., Reusch, P. et al. (2001). Raised serum vascular endothelial growth factor levels are associated with destructive change in inflammatory arthritis. Arthritis Rheum 44, 2055–2064.

Bas, S., Perneger, T.V., Kunzle, E. et al. (2002). Comparative study of different enzyme immunoassays for measurement of IgM and IgA rheumatoid factors. Ann Rheum Dis 61, 505–510.

Berner, B., Wolf, G., Hummel, K.M. et al. (2000). Increased expression of CD40 ligand (CD154) on CD4+ T cells as a marker of disease activity in rheumatoid arthritis. Ann Rheum Dis 59, 190–195.

Bizzaro, N., Mazzanti, G., Tonutti, E. et al. (2001). Diagnostic accuracy of the anti-citrulline antibody assay for rheumatoid arthritis. Clin Chem 47, 1089–1093.

Blass, S., Union, A., Raymackers, J. et al. (2001). The stress protein BiP is overexpressed and is a major B and T cell target in rheumatoid arthritis. Arthritis Rheum 44, 761–771.

Boers, M., Verhoeven, A.C., Markusse, H.M. et al. (1997). Randomised comparison of combined step-down prednisolone, methotrexate and sulphasalazine with sulphasalazine alone in early rheumatoid arthritis. Lancet 350, 309–318.

Brennan, F.M., Browne, K.A., Green, P.A. et al. (1997). Reduction of serum matrix metalloproteinase 1 and matrix metalloproteinase 3 in rheumatoid arthritis patients following anti-tumour necrosis factor-alpha (cA2) therapy. Br J Rheumatol 36, 643–650.

Brown, L.F., Detmar, M., Claffey, K. et al. (1997). Vascular permeability factor/vascular endothelial growth factor: a multifunctional angiogenic cytokine. EXS 79, 233–269.

Bukhari, M., Lunt, M., Harrison, B.J. et al. (2002). Rheumatoid factor is the major predictor of increasing severity of radiographic erosions in rheumatoid arthritis: results from the Norfolk Arthritis Register Study, a large inception cohort. Arthritis Rheum 46, 906–912.

Catrina, A.I., Lampa, J., Ernestam, S. et al. (2002). Anti-tumour necrosis factor (TNF)-alpha therapy (etanercept) down-regulates serum matrix metalloproteinase (MMP)-3 and MMP-1 in rheumatid arthritis. Rheumatology 41, 484–489.

Charles, P., Elliott, M.J., Davis, D. et al. (1999). Regulation of cytokines, cytokine inhibitors, and acute-phase proteins following anti-TNF-alpha therapy in rheumatoid arthritis. J Immunol 163, 1521–1528.

Citera, G., Padulo, L.A., Fernandez, G. et al. (2001). Influence of HLA-DR alleles on rheumatoid arthritis: susceptibility and severity in Argentine patients. J Rheumatol 28, 1486–1491.

Combe, B., Dougados, M., Goupille, P. et al. (2001). Prognostic factors for radiographic damage in early rheumatoid arthritis: a multiparameter prospective study. Arthritis Rheum 44, 1736–1743.

Constantin, A., Lauwers-Cances, V., Navaux, F. et al. (2002a). Collagenase-1 (MMP-1) and HLA-DRB1 gene polymorphisms in rheumatoid arthritis: a prospective longitudinal study. J Rheumatol 29, 15–20.

Constantin, A., Lauwers-Cances, V., Navaux, F. et al. (2002b). Stromelysin 1 (matrix metalloproteinase 3) and HLA-DRB1 gene polymorphisms: Association with severity and progression of rheumatoid arthritis in a prospective study. Arthritis Rheum 46, 1754–1762.

Crnkic, M., Mansson, B., Larsson, L. et al. (2003). Serum cartilage oligomeric protein (COMP) decreases in rheumatoid arthritis patients treated with infliximab or etanercept. Arthritis Res Ther 5, R181–R185.

Dahl, I.M.S. and Husby, G. (1985). Hyaluronic acid production in vitro by synovial lining cells from normal and rheumatoid joints. Ann Rheum Dis 44, 647–657.

Davis, M.J., Dawes, P.T., Fowler, P.D. et al. (1990). Comparison and evaluation of a disease activity index for use in patients with rheumatoid arthritis. Br J Rheumatol 29, 111–115.

den Broeder, A.A., Joosten, L.A., Saxne, T. et al. (2002). Long term anti-tumour necrosis factor alpha monotherapy in rheumatoid arthritis: effect on radiological course and prognostic value of markers of cartilage turnover and endothelial activation. Ann Rheum Dis, 61, 311–318.

Dolan, A.L., Moniz, C., Abraha, H. et al. (2002). Does active treatment of rheumatoid arthritis limit disease-associated bone loss? Rheumatology (Oxford) 41, 1047–1051.

Drossaers-Bakker, K.W., Zwinderman, A.H., Vlieland, T.P. et al. (2002). Long-term outcome in rheumatoid arthritis: a simple algorithm of baseline parameters can predict radiographic damage, disability, and disease course at 12-year follow up. Arthritis Rheum 47, 383–390.

Egeland, T. and Munthe, E. (1983). The role of the laboratory in rheumatology. Rheumatoid factors. Clin Rheum Dis 9, 135–160.

Elliott, M.J., Maini, R.N., Feldmann, M. et al. (1994). Randomised double-blind comparison of chimeric monoclonal antibody to tumour necrosis factor alpha (cA2) versus placebo in rheumatoid arthritis. Lancet 344, 1105–1110.

Emery, P., Bradley, H., Arthur, V. et al. (1992). Genetic factors influencing the outcome of early arthritis: The role of sulphoxidation status. Br J Rheumatol 31, 449–551.

Engstrom-Laurent, A. and Hallgren, R. (1985). Circulating hyaluronate in rheumatoid arthritis: Relationship to inflammatory activity and the effect of corticosteroid therapy. Ann Rheum Dis 44, 83–88.

Erhardt, C.C., Mumford, P.A., Venables, P.J.W. et al. (1989). Factors predicting a poor life prognosis in rheumatoid arthritis: An eight year prospective study. Ann Rheum Dis 48, 7–13.

Ferrara, N. (1995). The role of vascular endothelial growth factor in pathological angiogenesis. Breast Cancer Res Treat 36, 127–137.

Forslind, K., Eberhardt, K., Jonsson, A. et al. (1992). Increased serum concentration of cartilage oligomeric matrix protein. A prognostic marker in early rheumatoid arthritis. Br J Rheumatol 31, 593–598.

Garnero, P., Landewe, R., Boers et al. (2002). Association of baseline levels of markers of bone and cartilage degradation with long-term progression of joint damage in patients with early rheumatoid arthritis: the COBRA study. Arthritis Rheum 46, 2847–2856.

Gauldie, J., Richards, C., Harnish, D. et al. (1987). Interferon b2/B-cell stimulatory factor type 2 shares identity with monocyte-derived hepatocyte-stimulating factor and regulates the major acute phase protein response in liver cells. Proc Natl Acad Sci USA 84, 7251–7259.

Gomes-Daudrix, V., Sebbag, M., Girbal, C. et al. (1994). Immunoblotting detection of so-called 'antikeratin antibodies': A new assay for the diagnosis of rheumatid arthritis. Ann Rheum Dis 53, 735–742.

Gorman, J.D. and Criswell, L.A. (2002). The shared epitope and severity of rheumatoid arthritis. Rheum Dis Clin North Am 28, 59–78.

Graudal, N.A., Madsen, H.O., Tarp, U. et al. (2000). The association of variant mannose-binding lectin genotypes with radiographic outcome in rheumatoid arthritis. Arthritis Rheum 43, 515–521.

Gregersen, P.K., Silver, J. and Winchester, R.J. (1987). The shared epitope hypothesis. An approach to understanding the molecular genetics of susceptibility to rheumatoid arthritis. Arthritis Rheum 30, 1205–1213.

Harada, M., Mitsuyama, K., Yoshida, H. et al. (1998). Vascular endothelial growth factor in patients with rheumatoid arthritis. Scand J Rheumatol 27, 377–380.

Hassfeld, W., Steiner, G., Grainger, W. et al. (1993). Autoantibody to the nuclear antigen RA33: A marker for early rheumatoid arthritis. Br J Rheumatol 32, 199–203.

Hassfeld, W., Steiner, G., Studnicka-Benke, A. et al. (1995). Autoimmune response to the spliceosome: an immunological link between rheumatoid arthritis, mixed connective tissue disease, and systemic lupus erythematosus. Arthritis Rheum 38, 777–785.

Hayem, G., Chazerain, P., Combe, B. et al. (1999). Anti-Sa antibody is an accurate diagnostic and prognostic marker in adult rheumatoid arthritis. J Rheumatol 2, 7–13.

Hoet, R.M.A., Boerbooms, A., Arends, M. et al. (1991). Antiperinuclear factor, a marker antibody for rheumatoid arthritis: colocalisation of the perinuclear factor and profilaggrin. Ann Rheum Dis 50, 611–618.

Ip, W.K., Lau, Y.L., Chan, S.Y. et al. (2000). Mannose-binding lectin and rheumatoid arthritis in Southern Chinese. Arthritis Rheum 43, 1679–1687.

Isenberg, D.A., Steiner, G. and Smolen, J.S. (1994). Clinical utility and serological connections of anti-RA33 antibodies in systemic lupus erythematosus. J Rheumatol 21, 1260–1263

Jacoby, R.K., Jayson, M.I. and Cosh, J.A. (1973). Onset, early stages, and prognosis of rheumatoid arthritis: a clinical study of 100 patients with 11-year follow-up. Br Med J 2, 96–100.

Janssens, X., Veys, E.M., Verbruggen, G. et al. (1988). The diagnostic significance of the antiperinuclear factor for rheumatoid arthritis. J Rheumatol 15, 1346–1350.

Kollerup, G., Hanswsen, M. and Horslev-Peterson, K. (1994). Urinary hydroxypridinium cross-links of collagen in rheumatoid arthritis, relation to disease activity and effects of methyl prednisolone. Br J Rheumatol 33, 816–820.

Koopman, W.J. and Gay, S. (1988). The MRL-lpr/lpr mouse. A model for the study of rheumatoid arthritis. Scand J Rheumatol 75, 284–289.

Kroot, E.J., de Jong, B.A., van Leeuwen, M.A. et al. (2000). The prognostic value of anti-cyclic citrullinated peptide antibody in patients with recent-onset rheumatoid arthritis. Arthritis Rheum 43, 1831–1835.

Kurki, P., Aho, K., Palosuo, T. et al. (1992). Immunopathology of rheumatoid arthritis: antikeratin antibodies precede the clinical disease. Arthritis Rheum 35, 914–917.

Kurki, P., von Essen, R., Kaarela, K. et al. (1997). Antibody to stratum corneum (antikeratin antibody) and antiperinuclear factor: Markers for progressive rheumatoid arthritis. Scand J Rheumatol 26, 346–349.

Lanchbury, J.S., Jaeger, E.E., Sansom, D.M. et al. (1991). Strong primary selection for the Dw4 subtype of DR4 accounts for the HLA-DQw7 association with Felty's syndrome. Hum Immunol 32, 56–64.

Lard, L.R., Boers, M., Verhoeven, A. et al. (2002). Early and aggressive treatment of rheumatoid arthritis patients affects the association of HLA class II antigens with progression of joint damage. Arthritis Rheum 46, 899–905.

Lipsky, P.E., van der Heidje, D.M., St Clair, E.W. et al. (2000). Infliximab and methotrexate in the treatment of rheumatoid arthritis. N Engl J Med 343, 1594–1602.

Listing, J., Rau, R., Muller, B. et al. (2000). HLA-DRB1 genes, rheumatoid factor, and elevated C-reactive protein: independent risk factors of radiographic progression in early rheumatoid arthritis. Berlin Collaborating Rheumatological Study Group. J Rheumatol 27, 2100–2109.

Maini, R.N., St Clair, E. W., Breedveld, F. et al. (1999). Infliximab (chimeric anti-tumour necrosis factor a monoclonal antibody) versus placebo in rheumatoid arthritis patients receiving concomitant methotrexate: a randomised phase III trial. Lancet 354, 1932–1939.

Malhotra, R., Wormald, M.R., Rudd, P.M. et al. (1995). Glycosylation changes of IgG associated with rheumatoid arthritis can activate complement via the mannose-binding protein. Nat Med 1, 237–243.

Mansson, B., Carey, D., Alini, M. et al. (1995). Cartilage and bone metabolism in rheumatoid arthritis. Differences between rapid and slow progression of disease identified by serum markers of cartilage metabolism. J Clin Invest 95, 1071–1077.

Mansson, B., Geborek, P. and Saxne, T. (1997). Cartilage and bone macromolecules in knee joint synovial fluid in rheumatoid arthritis: relation to development of knee or hip joint destruction. Ann Rheum Dis 56, 91–96

Masi, A.T., Maldonado-Cocco, J.A., Kaplan, S.B. et al. (1976). Prospective study of the early course of rheumatoid arthritis in young adults: comparison of patients with and without rheumatoid factor positivity at entry and identification of variables correlating with outcome. Semin Arthritis Rheum 4, 299–326.

Massardo, L., Gareca, N., Cartes, M.A. et al. (2002). The presence of the HLA-DRB1 shared epitope correlates with erosive disease in Chilean patients with rheumatoid arthritis. Rheumatology (Oxford) 41, 153–156.

Masson-Bessiere, C., Sebbag, M., Girbal-Neuhauser, E. et al. (2001). The major synovial targets of the rheumatoid arthritis-specific antifilaggrin autoantibodies are deiminated forms of the alpha- and beta-chains of fibrin. J Immunol 166, 4177–4184.

Mattey, D.L., Hassell, A.B., Dawes, P.T. et al. (2001). Independent association of rheumatoid factor and the HLA-DRB1 shared epitope with radiographic outcome in rheumatoid arthritis. Arthritis Rheum 44, 1529–1533.

Menard, H.A., Lapointe, E., Rochdi, M.D. et al. (2000). Insights into rheumatoid arthritis derived from the Sa immune system. Arthritis Res 2, 429–432.

Mottonen, T., Hannonen, P., Leirisalo-Repo, M. et al. (1999). Comparison of combination therapy with single-drug therapy in early rheumatoid arthritis: a randomised trial. FIN-RACo trial group. Lancet 353, 1568–1573.

Mottonen, T., Hannonen, P., Korpela, M. et al. (2002). Delay to institution of therapy and induction of remission using single-drug or combination-disease-modifying antirheumatic drug therapy in early rheumatoid arthritis. Arthritis Rheum 46, 894–898.

Nagashima, M., Wauke, K., Hirano, D. et al. (2000). Effects of combinations of anti-rheumatic drugs on the production of vascular endothelial growth factor and basic fibroblast growth factor in cultured synoviocytes and patients with rheumatoid arthritis. Rheumatology (Oxford) 39, 1255–1262.

Neufeld, G., Cohen, T., Gengrinovitch, S. et al. (1999). Vascular endothelial growth factor (VEGF) and its receptors. FASEB J 13, 9–22.

Nienhuis, R.L.F and Mandema, F. (1964). A new serum factor in patients with rheumatoid arthritis: The antiperinuclear factor. Ann Rheum Dis 23, 302.

Nogueira, L., Sebbag, M., Vincent, C. et al. (2001). Performance of two ELISAs for antifilaggrin autoantibodies, using either affinity purified or deiminated recombinant human filaggrin, in the diagnosis of rheumatoid arthritis. Ann Rheum Dis 60, 882–887.

Paimela, L., Heiskanen, A., Kurki, P. et al. (1991). Serum hyaluronate levels as a predictor of radiographic progression in early rheumatoid arthritis. Arthritis Rheum 34, 815–821.

Paimela, L., Leirisalo-Repo, M., Risteli, L. et al. (1994). Type I collagen degradation product in serum of patients with early rheumatoid arthritis: relationship to disease activity and radiological progression in a three year follow-up. Br J Rheumatol 33, 1012–1016.

Paimela, L., Palosuo, T., Aho, K. et al. (2001). Association of autoantibodies to filaggrin with an active disease in early rheumatoid arthritis. Ann Rheum Dis 60, 32–35.

Paleolog, E.M., Young, S., Stark, A.C. et al. (1998). Modulation of angiogenic vascular endothelial growth factor by tumor necrosis factor alpha and interleukin-1 in rheumatoid arthritis. Arthritis Rheum 41, 1258–1265.

Palosuo, T., Lukka, M., Alenius, H. et al. (1998). Purification of filaggrin from human epidermis and measurement of antifilaggrin autoantibodies in sera from patients with rheumatoid arthritis by an enzyme-linked immunosorbent assay. Int Arch Allergy Immunol 115, 294–302.

Parekh, R.B., Dwek, R.A., Sutton, B.J. et al. (1985). Association of rheumatoid arthritis and primary osteoarthritis with changes in the glycosylation pattern of total serum IgG. Nature 316, 452–457.

Poole, A.R., Witter, J., Roberts, N. et al. (1990). Inflammation and cartilage metabolism in rheumatoid arthritis. Studies of the blood markers hyaluronic acid, orosomucoid and keratan sulfate. Arthritis Rheum 33, 790–799.

Prevoo, M.L., van 't Hof, M.A., Kuper, H.H. et al. (1995). Modified disease activity scores that include twenty-eight-joint counts. Development and validation in a prospective longitudinal study of patients with rheumatoid arthritis. Arthritis Rheum 38, 44–48.

Rook, G.A., Steele, J., Brealey, R. et al. (1991). Changes in IgG glycoform levels are associated with remission of arthritis during pregnancy. J Autoimmun 4, 779–794.

Roux-Lombard, P., Eberhardt, K., Saxne, T. et al. (2001). Cytokines, metalloproteinases, their inhibitors and cartilage oligomeric matrix protein: relationship to radiological progression and inflammation in early rheumatoid arthritis. A prospective 5-year study. Rheumatology (Oxford) 40, 544–551.

Saraux, A., Berthelot, J.M., Charles, G. et al. (2002). Value of laboratory tests in early prediction of rheumatoid arthritis. Arthritis Rheum 47, 155–165.

Saulot, V., Vittecoq, O., Charlionet, R. et al. (2002). Presence of autoantibodies to the glycolytic enzyme alpha-enolase in sera from patients with early rheumatoid arthritis. Arthritis Rheum 46, 1196–1201.

Saxne, T. and Heinegard, D. (1992). Synovial fluid analysis of two groups of proteoglycan epitopes distinguishes early and late cartilage lesions. Arthritis Rheum 35, 385–390.

Saxne, T., Zunino, L. and Heinegard, D. (1995). Increased release of bone sialoprotein into synovial fluid reflects tissue destruction in rheumatoid arthritis. Arthritis Rheum 38, 82–90.

Schellekens, G.A., de Jong, B.A., van den Hoogen, F.H. et al. (1998). Citrulline is an essential constituent of antigenic determinants recognized by rheumatoid arthritis-specific autoantibodies. J Clin Invest 101, 273–281.

Sebbag, M., Simon, M., Vincent, C. et al. (1995). The antiperinuclear factor and the so-called antikeratin antibodies are the same rheumatoid arthritis-specific autoantibodies. J Clin Invest 95, 2672–2679.

Sharp, J.T., Calkins, E., Cohen A. et al. (1964). Observations on the clinical, chemical and serological manifestations of rheumatoid arthritis based on the course of 154 cases. Medicine 43, 41.

Sharp, J.T., Wolfe, F., Mitchell, D.M. et al. (1991). The progression of erosion and joint space narrowing scores in rheumatoid arthritis during the first twenty-five years of disease. Arthritis Rheum 34, 660–668.

Sievers, K. (1965). The rheumatoid factor in definite rheumatoid arthritis. An analysis of 1279 adult patients with a follow-up study. Acta Rheumatol Scand 11, 1.

Tamura, T., Udagawa, N., Takahashi, N. et al. (1993). Soluble interleukin-6 receptor triggers osteoclast formation by interleukin-6. Proc Natl Acad Sci USA 90, 11924–11928.

Taylor, P.C. (2001). Anti-TNF therapies. Curr Opin Rheumatol 13, 164–169.

van der Heijde, D.M., van Riel, P.L., van Leeuween, M. et al. (1992). Prognostic factors for radiographic damage and physical disability in early rheumatoid arthritis. A prospective follow-up study of 147 patients. Br J Rheumatol 31, 519–525.

van Leeuwen, M.A., van Rijswijk, M.H., van der Heijde, D.M. et al. (1993). The acute phase response in relation to radiographic progression in early rheumatoid arthritis: a prospective study during the first three years of the disease. Br J Rheumatol 32 Suppl 3, 9–13.

van Leeuwen, M.A., Westra, J., Limburg, P.C. et al. (1995). Clinical significance of interleukin-6 measurement in early rheumatoid arthritis: relation with laboratory and clinical variables and radiological progression in a three year prospective study. Ann Rheum Dis 54, 674–677.

Van Venrooij, W.J. and Pruijn, G.J. (2000). Citrullination: a small change for a protein with great consequences for rheumatoid arthritis. Arthritis Res 2, 249–251.

van Zeben, D., Hazes, J.M., Zwiderman, A.H. et al. (1991). Association of HLA-DR4 with a more progressive disease course in patients with rheumatoid arthritis. Arthritis Rheum 34, 822–830.

Van Zeben, D., Hazes, J.M.W., Zwinderman, A.H.D. et al. (1992). Clinical significance of rheumatoid factors in early rheumatoid arthritis: results of a follow-up study. Ann Rheum Dis 51, 1029–1035.

Vincent, C., Nogueira, L., Sebbag, M. et al. (2002). Detection of antibodies to disseminated recombinant rat filaggrin by enzyme-linked immunosorbent assay: a highly effective test for the diagnosis of rheumatoid arthritis. Arthritis Rheum 46, 2051–2058.

Visser, H., le Cessie, S., Vos, K. et al. (2002). How to diagnose rheumatoid arthritis early: a prediction model for persistent (erosive) arthritis. Arthritis Rheum 46, 357–365.

Vittecoq, O., Salle, V., Jouen-Beades, F. et al. (2001). Autoantibodies to the 27 C-terminal amino acids of calpastatin are detected in a restricted set of connective tissue diseases and may be useful for diagnosis of rheumatoid arthritis in community cases of very early arthritis. Rheumatology (Oxford) 40, 1126–1134.

Vivino, F.B. and Maul, G.G. (1990). Histological and electron microscopic characterization of the antiperinuclear factor antigen. Arthritis Rheum 33, 960–969.

von Essen, R., Kurki, P., Isomaki, P. et al. (1993). Prospect for an additional laboratory criterion for rheumatoid arthritis. Scand J Rheumatol 22, 267–272.

Weinblatt, M.E., Kremer, J.M., Bankhurst, A.D. et al. (1999). A trial of etanercept, a recombinant tumor necrosis factor receptor:Fc fusion protein, in patients with rheumatoid arthritis receiving methotrexate. N Engl J Med *340*, 253–259.

Westedt, M.L., Herbrink, P., Molenaar, J.L. et al. (1985). Rheumatoid factors in rheumatoid arthritis and vasculitis. Rheumatol Int *5*, 209–214.

Wordsworth, B.P., Lanchbury, J.S., Sakkas, L.I. et al. (1989). HLA-DR4 subtype frequencies in rheumatoid arthritis indicate that DRB1 is the major susceptibility locus within the class II region. Proc Natl Acad Sci USA *86*, 10049–10053.

Wordsworth, P., Pile, K.D., Buckley, J.D. et al. (1992). HLA heterozygosity contributes to susceptibility to rheumatoid arthritis. Am J Hum Genet *51*, 585–591.

Yamanaka, H., Matsuda, Y., Tanaka, M. et al. (2000). Serum matrix metalloproteinase 3 as a predictor of the degree of joint destruction during the six months after measurement, in patients with early rheumatoid arthritis. Arthritis Rheum *43*, 852–858.

Young, A., Sumar, N., Bodman, K. et al. (1991). Agalactosyl IgG: an aid to differential diagnosis in early synovitis. Arthritis Rheum *34*, 1425–1429.

Young, B.J.J., Mallya, R.K., Leslie, R.D.G. et al. (1979). Anti-keratin antibodies in rheumatoid arthritis. Br Med J *2*, 97–99.

Ziolkowska, M., Kurowska, M., Radzikowska, A. et al. (2002). High levels of osteoprotegerin and soluble receptor activator of nuclear factor kappa B ligand in serum of rheumatoid arthritis patients and their normalisation after anti-tumor necrosis factor alpha treatment. Arthritis Rheum *46*, 1744–1753.

Autoimmunity – Type 1 Diabetes

Chapter 43

Patrizia Luppi and Massimo Trucco

Division of Immunogenetics, Department of Pediatrics, Rangos Research Center, Children's Hospital of Pittsburgh, University of Pittsburgh School of Medicine, Pittsburgh, PA, USA

Kilimanjaro is a snow covered mountain 19 710 feet high, and it is said to be the highest mountain in Africa. Its western summit is called the Masai 'Ngàje Ngài', the House of God. Close to the western summit there is the dried and frozen carcass of a leopard. No one has explained what the leopard was seeking at that altitude.

Ernest Hemingway, The Snows Of Kiliminjaro

AUTOIMMUNITY: GENERAL CONCEPTS

Thousands and thousands of immature T cells are generated every day by our bone marrow. They carry different T cell receptors (TCRs) as a result of the random association of numerous variable and constant segments constituting the functional TCR molecule (Pietropaolo and Trucco, 2000). These cells, each carrying one of the more than 10^9 possible different TCR molecules, travel via the blood vessels eventually reaching the thymus. Here, on the basis of their affinity for self-antigenic epitopes and the major histocompatiblity complex (MHC) molecules that, at the surface of the antigen-presenting cells (APCs), accommodate them in their groove, receive a positive or negative signal. The positive signal brings the T cells to final maturation; the negative signal blocks them in the thymus where they finally die.

Generally, T cells that are negatively selected in the thymus represent autoreactive elements which are potentially dangerous as they could attack targets harboring tissue-specific self-antigens. The physical conformation of the alleles of the MHC class II molecule is one of the most influential variables in this sophisticated selection process, together with the quantity and quality of the antigenic peptides derived from self-proteins. The death of the anti-self or autoreactive T cell clones (i.e. clonal deletion) provides immunologic tolerance (i.e. central tolerance) against self-structures, while preserving an efficient patrolling by T cells for non-self structures carried by foreign invaders that need eventually to be eliminated (Pietropaolo and Trucco, 2000).

Like everything in nature, there are exceptions. Due to the combination of different factors negatively influencing the peptide/MHC/TCR molecular relationship, in fact, some possibly autoreactive T cell clones manage to pass the thymus censorship and proceed untouched into the periphery.

Once in circulation, these T cells remain quiescent until some event, promoted by the environment, activates them. Activated T cells proliferate and specifically attack those target cells carrying self-antigens, eventually leading to target cell destruction. This immune attack against self-structures is conventionally defined as 'autoimmunity'. In this context, when the recognized self-antigen(s) is specifically expressed by the insulin secreting β-cells of the endocrine pancreas, the autoimmune process leads to β-cell destruction and eventually to type 1 diabetes. Moreover, when β-cells are destroyed, they expose to the immune system previously hidden or cryptic self-antigens of whom it was until then not aware, i.e. 'ignorant'. The newly presented self-antigens amplify the initial immune

Measuring Immunity, edited by Michael T. Lotze and Angus W. Thomson
ISBN 0-12-455900-X, London

response by activating a B lymphocyte reaction resulting in the production of antibodies. Since these antibodies are specifically reacting against structures of the self they are called 'autoantibodies'.

The best evidence of the role played by the T cells in the pathogenesis of type 1 diabetes is the histological picture defined as 'insulitis', a term referring to the inflammatory invasion of the islets of Langerhans, the agglomerate of cells constituting the endocrine pancreas, by mononuclear cells (Trucco and Dorman, 1989). Besides the insulin-producing β-cells, the islets of Langerhans include α-cells producing glucagon and δ-cells secreting somatostatin. Another type of pancreatic cell produces an array of polypeptides, whose function is not yet fully understood. In a normal pancreas, we can count close to half a million islets (Bottino et al., 2002).

Evidence for the requirement of an environmental agent necessary to activate the autoimmune reaction against β-cells is offered by the concordance of the disease in monozygotic twins, a coincidence that actually does not reach 50 per cent (Olmos et al., 1988; Lo et al., 1991). This finding indicates that a considerable 'environmental' factor participates in the pathogenesis of the disease. In fact, infections caused by a few different viruses have been found to be temporally associated with the onset of the disease. Coxsackie, mumps and rubella virus infections are the most frequently reported in conjunction with diabetes onset (Hyoty et al., 1995; Luppi et al., 2000).

TYPE 1 DIABETES

Type 1 diabetes is an autoimmune disease most frequently affecting children, characterized by infiltrating mononuclear cells in the islets of Langerhans (i.e. insulitis) and selective destruction of the insulin-producing β-cells. As a consequence, the maintenance of normal blood glucose levels is severely impaired and the patient becomes dependent on daily injections of exogenous insulin to correct hyperglycemia. It is not known what is the length of time required for the autoimmune process to complete destruction of the β-cells. The general view considers that this process may occur over a prolonged period of time (Eisenbarth, 1986). During the majority of this time the disease is clinically silent, but the appearance of polyuria, polydipsia and weight loss, especially in subjects of pubertal age, represents subtle but very characteristic symptoms prodromic of the clinical onset of type 1 diabetes. These are the symptoms that should attract the attention of parents and physicians. In the majority of cases, however, the diagnosis of type 1 diabetes is made only when acute ketoacidosis complicates the patient's clinical conditions. When appearing in younger children (<5 years of age), type 1 diabetes is particularly severe. A more aggressive and rapid process of β-cell destruction than in teenagers seems to take place here (Komulainen et al., 1999).

Despite many years of intensive studies, the precise autoantigen(s) and mechanism(s) triggering the autoimmune β-cell-specific attack still remain undetermined. One of the limitations in the study of the etiopathogenesis of type 1 diabetes is the fact that it is not possible to monitor properly the kinetics of β-cell destruction in humans. In fact, human specimens from diseased pancreata cannot be obtained at different time-points during the course of the disease. Moreover, with the scientific knowledge available, it is not yet possible to predict with absolute approximation who or when an individual will develop the disease. However, in individuals defined as genetically 'at risk' because of their histocompatibility or human leukocyte antigen (HLA) make-up (Trucco, 1992), indirect, yet reliable, evidence of autoimmunity is provided by the detectable presence of high titers of serum autoantibodies (Bottazzo et al., 1974; Lipton et al., 1992; Verge et al., 1996) and of T cell sensitization (Brooks-Worrell et al., 1996) to a vast array of islet-cell antigens even at early, still asymptomatic, stages of the disease.

Additional immunologic abnormalities have been recently identified in the peripheral circulation of pre-diabetic individuals. These immunologic features are novel, potential markers that, in association with the disease-associated HLA alleles and the presence of autoantibodies, allow a more refined characterization of individuals at risk for diabetes. Early identification of individuals at risk for diabetes will, in turn, permit prompt treatment once effective and safe strategies of intervention become available to block the autoimmune damage of the β-cells (Herold et al., 2002).

Hereafter, we will describe the canonical assays and techniques available to date to approach the study of the autoimmune phenomenon in type 1 diabetic patients.

Determining the genetic background: HLA typing

Nucleotide polymorphisms at certain HLA loci correlate with susceptibility to a variety of autoimmune diseases (Friday et al., 1999). Genetic studies of diabetics and their immediate family members have provided critical information, identifying genetic markers for diabetes (Davies et al., 1994) with specific polymorphism of the HLA-DQB1 locus being the strongest indicator of type 1 diabetes mellitus susceptibility (Trucco, 1992).

Methods for screening the highly polymorphic HLA loci for alleles associated with disease are important for risk evaluation of genetically susceptible individuals. HLA-DQB1 alleles containing a polymorphism encoding the presence of a neutral amino acid residue (e.g. alanine, valine or serine) at amino acid 57 represent the most sensitive, single susceptibility marker, while an aspartate at the same position (Asp-57) confers resistance (Todd et al., 1987; Morel et al., 1988; McDevitt, 2001). However, sequence data, including those of the DQ and DRB alleles, result in haplotype information that can be used to interpret better the degrees of association and susceptibility of various genotypes for type 1 diabetes. These are among the same HLA markers required to be matched between donor and recipient for successful kidney (Hsia et al., 1993; Tong et al., 1993) and bone marrow transplantation (Hurley et al., 2000; Rosner et al., 2000).

Originally HLA typing was performed using sera from polygravidae immunized against the alleles of the father expressed by the cells of the fetus, or from individuals who received multiple, HLA-unmatched blood transfusions, able to kill antigen-positive, donor lymphocytes isolated from venous blood (Rosner et al., 2000).

More recently the advent of molecular biology transformed the HLA typing approach and antibody-mediated cytotoxicity was substituted with genomic DNA probing using libraries of oligonucleotides recognizing the majorities of the HLA alleles at the various loci (Rudert and Trucco, 1989, 1992; Trucco and Ball, 1989; Trucco et al., 1989; Faas et al., 1996; Hurley et al., 2000). Advances in DNA sequencing technology via automated acquisition and analysis are important additions to the screening and characterization of genetic markers. Again, more recently, pyrosequencing methodology offered an improvement to data acquisition, analysis and allelic identification, including the advantages of real time data output, resistance to sequencing artifacts associated with analysis by gel electrophoresis, no need of DNA fluorescent labeling and compatibility with 96- and 384-well microplate formats (Ringquist et al., 2002).

Pyrosequencing was originally designed for expressed sequence tag (EST) sequencing in which short (roughly 10 nucleotide) stretches of DNA are analyzed. The pyrosequencing method, reviewed by Ronaghi (2001), is a four-enzyme process combining the activities of DNA polymerase, ATP sulfurylase, luciferase and apyrase. Briefly, the method can be described in four steps:

1 hybridization of sequencing primer to a single stranded DNA template
2 incorporation of a complementary nucleotide and release of pyrophosphate
3 use of ATP sulfurylase to convert pyrophosphate and exogenous adenosine 5' phosphosulfate into ATP, followed by conversion into light via the activity of luciferase
4 degradation of unincorporated dNTP by means of apyrase.

Sequencing continues by reiteration of steps 2 through 4 using the next dNTP to be tested for incorporation into the nascent nucleotide chain. The data output is represented graphically by a 'pyrogram' consisting of a plot of time versus intensity of light produced (Ronaghi et al., 1996). Generation of light represents incorporation of a particular nucleotide.

An important advantage of pyrosequencing over other sequencing technologies is that nucleotides are tested individually for incorporation into nascent DNA. The result is that mixed populations of DNA expected from heterozygous individuals are sequenced independently, allowing the resolution of allelic combinations which are impossible to distinguish by conventional sequencing approaches (Alexander et al., 2002).

Pyrosequencing can easily complete a 70 nucleotide read length of each sample in a 96-well sample tray within an hour, potentially yielding 768 sequence reactions in an 8-h shift or as many as 3072 when performed in a 384-well format, sufficient to sequence fully the polymorphic region at one HLA class II locus from roughly 768 individuals. Its accuracy and throughput make pyrosequence-based typing (PSBT) an important addition to the methods available for identification of these markers in genetic studies and genotyping donors for transplant recipient matching (Ringquist et al., 2002). We have expanded on our previous work, developing PSBT for the identification of HLA-DQB1 alleles in clinical samples (Ringquist et al., 2002), by tackling the genotyping of the complex multi-loci HLA-DRB system (Alexander et al., 2002). As illustrated in Figure 43.1, HLA-DRB genes have been successfully analyzed by pyrosequencing. Comparison of pyrograms obtained from cloned DNA and cell line genomic DNA has indicated, for HLA-DRB alleles DRB1*1302 and DRB3*0301, that genomic DNA can be analyzed. Analysis of the pyrograms indicated that DRB1*1302 specific nucleotide dispensations occurred at events A2, G5, A17, A36, A41, C46, A54, G59 and C60, while DRB3*0301 associated events were at dispensations C10, G12, C43, G45, A47 and C56. Pyrosequencing of HLA-DRB, while matching the expected sequence for these alleles, yielded readily interpreted pyrosequence data whether originating from cloned stocks or from genomic DNA.

Determining the immunological β-cell damage: the cellular role

Evidence in mice and humans has clearly demonstrated the central role played by T cells in β-cell destruction (Wicker et al., 1986; Conrad et al., 1994; Delovitch and Singh, 1997). These T cells are autoreactive in as much as they destroy targets harboring unique β-cell antigens and, in fact, circulating T cells responding to the islet/brain specific self-antigen glutamic acid decarboxylase (GAD) or insulin have been demonstrated in type 1 diabetic patients (Tisch et al., 1993). This finding demonstrates a failure in the mechanism(s) devoted to the maintenance of the state of immune tolerance or hyporesponsiveness towards self-antigens, a condition that is fundamental to prevention of autoimmunity. Additionally, a subset of CD4$^+$ T cells, constituting 5–10 per cent of peripheral CD4$^+$ T cells in healthy mice and humans, express the interleukin-2 receptor-α chain, CD25 and are thought to perform the specialized role of peripheral regulation of both the adaptive (i.e. T cells) and the innate (i.e. dendritic cells) immune system (Sakaguchi et al., 2001) normally preventing the negative consequences

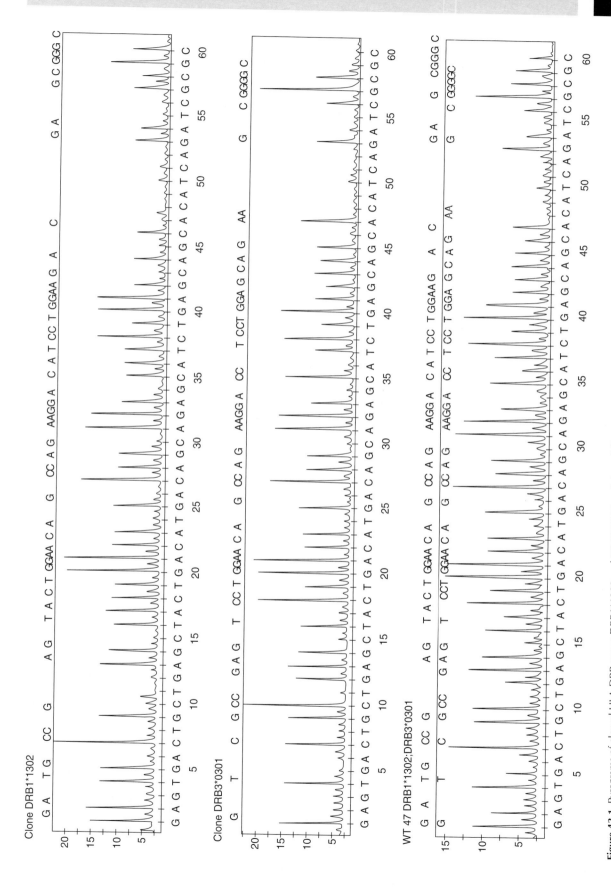

Figure 43.1 Pyrograms of cloned HLA-DRB genes DRB1*1302 and DRB3*0301 and the cell line WT47 HLA-DRB1*1302;DRB3*0301 genomic DNA. Samples were prepared for pyrosequencing from cloned DNA (top and middle panels) or from genomic DNA purified from the HLA containing cell line WT47 (bottom panel). The nucleotide sequence for the HLA-DRB alleles for each sample is indicated. Read lengths were at least 50 nucleotides.

of an incomplete thymic selection. In particular, these regulatory CD4$^+$CD25$^+$ T cells have been shown to be crucially important in the maintenance of tolerance to self-antigens in rodent models of autoimmune diabetes (Salomon et al., 2000; Stephens and Mason, 2000). Their removal by neonatal thymectomy or their functional inactivation by mutation in the gene Foxp3, which is important for their development and function, causes spontaneous development of a rapidly fatal lymphoproliferative disease which includes autoimmune polyendocrinopathy, early-onset type 1 diabetes, autoimmune entheropathy, hemolytic anemia and orchitis (Chatila et al., 2000; Brunkow et al., 2001; Sakaguchi et al., 2001).

Defects in CD4$^+$CD25$^+$ frequency and/or in their function have also been suggested to underlie immune dysregulation and development of type 1 diabetes in humans as well (Chatila et al., 2000; Kukreja et al., 2002). The study of CD4$^+$CD25$^+$ T cells and their importance in the regulation of immune responses represents a very exciting area of research and future studies will definitively clarify their role in modulating immune system function in diabetic patients as well as in other patients with autoimmune diseases.

Recognition of an antigen by a T cell involves interaction with the MHC/peptide complex on an APC through the TCR. The specificity of the interaction is determined by the TCR on the T cell. The TCR is composed of an α and a β chain divided into a variable region that recognizes antigens and a constant region that anchors the TCR to the cell membrane. As with immunoglobulin molecules, the TCR gets diversity from genomic DNA rearrangements of multiple segments, such as variable (V), diversity (D) and joining (J) regions. After the process of rearrangement, each T lymphocyte expresses a clonally unique TCR (Pietropaolo and Trucco, 2000). Current models of T cell activation assume that successful T cell activation occurs if recognition of the MHC/peptide complex via TCR (signal 1) is accompanied by a co-stimulatory signal (signal 2). The presence of signal 1 in the absence of signal 2 is either ignored or is tolerizing. Co-stimulatory signals include cell surface antigens, cytokines and other secreted molecules (Trucco et al., 2002).

The possibility of analyzing the TCR repertoire of the T cells accumulating in a tissue targeted by an autoimmune response is extremely important as it provides information on the phenotype of T cells engaged in that immune response against a putative self-antigen. This is particularly true for type 1 diabetes, in which the identification of the T cells infiltrating the pancreatic islets of Langherhans at different time-points during diabetes development would not only be useful but necessary to gain a better definition of the unique T cell subsets that initiate β-cell destruction. Our laboratory had the opportunity to perform such a study in two typical cases of type 1 diabetes complicated with ketoacidosis (Conrad et al., 1994). This was possible because severe neurological complications had rendered the patients unresponsive to further medical management and upon their arrival at Children's Hospital of Pittsburgh they were already brain-dead. Analysis of the TCR repertoire of the T cells infiltrating their pancreatic islets showed presence of an exceptionally high frequency (>30 per cent) of T cells carrying the Vβ7 gene family, thus indicating the presence of a specific antigen present on the islets, able to stimulate the recruitment of a selected subset of T cells from the peripheral blood. While the nature of this islet-cell specific antigen is still not known, additional studies from our group have suggested that this subpopulation of T cells can be activated by a virus (Luppi et al., 2000, 2003a).

Although the possibility of analyzing T cells from the pancreatic material of diabetic patients is critical for unraveling many aspects of the complex pathogenesis of type 1 diabetes in humans, it represented a rare, anecdotal, event. Researchers who are interested in investigating T cell phenotype and function in diabetic patients can only have access to the circulating lymphocytes that can be easily isolated from the peripheral blood of the affected individuals by using a density gradient.

The study of the circulating immune cells from diabetic patients is extremely valuable as it might represent a direct means to ascertain the presence of subsets of T cells important in disease pathogenesis eventually infiltrating the pancreatic islets of Langherhans. Furthermore, it would provide a tool for monitoring disease progression and the design of T cell directed intervention regimens. This has been demonstrated by the results of recent investigations performed on circulating T cells from diabetic patients at the onset of the disease in which we detected a high frequency of T cells expressing the TCR Vβ7 region (Luppi et al., 2000). The highest frequency of Vβ7$^+$ T cells was detected in the peripheral blood of very young children (Luppi et al., 2003b). Furthermore, a longitudinal study on the cases, who presented with the clinical onset of the disease while under our clinical monitoring (i.e. converters), demonstrated that a high frequency of circulating Vβ7 T cells had already been present for years, suggesting an on-going infiltration of T cells, sharing a TCR with similar characteristics (i.e. Vβ7), within the islets (Luppi et al., 2000).

The analysis of the TCR of the T cells infiltrating the pancreatic islets of the two diabetic children described above and of circulating lymphocytes in diabetic converters was performed by using a polymerase chain reaction (PCR)-based strategy using cDNA generated from reverse transcribed mRNA extracted from either the purified islets or from ficoll-isolated peripheral blood mononuclear cells (PBMC). This technique allows the semi-quantitative characterization of the TCR variable gene usage by using sequence-specific oligonucleotide primer panels. A system with fluorescence-tagged primers, which are specific for each of the known TCR V-region families, is routinely used by our laboratory to generate PCR products that can easily be detected and quantitated using a fluorescence detection system of the ABI

377 DNA Sequencer (PE Biosystems, Foster City, CA). Specifically, we are using a 3'-oligonucleotide specific for the constant region of the TCR that is labeled with 6-carboxyfluorescein (6-FAM, PE Biosystems) paired with a panel of 5'-oligonucleotides specific for each single V gene family or subfamily of the TCR α or β chain (Luppi et al., 2000). The amplified products are then resolved in a 5 per cent polyacrylamide non-denaturing gel on ABI 377 DNA Sequencer and each fluorescent band, corresponding to a V region of the TCR α or β chain, is analyzed with GeneScan software (PE Biosystems) which allows quantitation of fluorescence peak heights and areas corresponding to each band (Figure 43.2).

This strategy has advantages in its ease of use, although it is time consuming as it is based on a high number of individual reactions, each employing a different sequence-specific primer. In fact, the study of the TCR-Vα and -Vβ gene segment usage requires individual amplification of at least 29 TCR-Vα and 26 TCR-Vβ cDNA families and subfamilies. Moreover, the need to run polyacrylamide gels to resolve TCR-amplified products for each individual to be tested limits its suitability for routine clinical analysis. To overcome this problem, we set out to quantitate the TCR-amplified fluorescent products on an ABI Prism 3100 Genetic Analyzer (PE Biosystems), which is based on a capillary system for detection of the

fluorescent PCR products and does not require gels to be run. Furthermore, this system allows the analysis of TCR repertoire from multiple patients in the same run, thus opening the possibility to be employed for TCR analysis in a clinical setting.

Another analysis that is easily performed on the ABI Prism 3100 Genetic Analyzer is the study of the size distribution of the TCR-βchain, referred to as Complementarity Determining Region 3 (CDR3) size imaging or CDR3 size-pattern analysis. This analysis provides information regarding the complexity of the TCR repertoire in each sample. Since the CDR3 region of the β-chain is the non-germline-encoded distribution hypervariable region (inclusive of the Variable, Diversity and Joining segments) thought to carry the specificity for antigen recognition by T cells (Jorgensen et al., 1992), an irregular distribution of CDR3 sizes can reveal evidence of an antigen-driven clonal (or oligoclonal) expansion (Pannetier et al., 1995). To obtain the CDR3 size-pattern analysis, the fluorescence-amplified PCR products corresponding to each TCR-Vβ region are run on the ABI 3100 Genetic Analyzer and displayed as peaks, which are then qualitatively analyzed by using Genescan software. The interpretation of the CDR3 spectratype profile is based on the observation of, generally, an average of eight discrete bands, each spaced by three nucleotides for each Vβ family. Each band intensity (i.e. peak) represents the abundance of the clones of T cells with a certain CDR3 length. The definition of clonal, oligoclonal or polyclonal CDR3 profiles is based on the size distribution, pattern and number of peaks in each spectratype (Manfras et al., 1997).

Another technique to study TCR usage on circulating T lymphocytes is the detection of TCR phenotypes at the cell surface by using V region-specific monoclonal antibodies (mAb) and flow cytometry. The multiparameter analysis in flow cytometry permits the simultaneous detection of additional surface and cytoplasmic antigens on the same cells, which allows a clear and complete analysis of the cell subset under examination. For example, by using mAb against the CD4 and the CD8 T cell surface antigens it is possible to evaluate frequency of each of these subsets of T cells in the peripheral blood of diabetic patients. By combining use of mAb against a panel of leukocyte-specific adhesion molecules (CD62L, CD54, CD11a, CD49d) and activation markers (i.e. CD69, CD71) it is then possible to study the expression of these molecules on the surface of the selected CD4+ and CD8+ T lymphocytes (Luppi et al., 2002). The major problem of the flow cytometry approach in studying TCR repertoire usage is that the panel of mAb available for TCR analysis is incomplete. Secondly, no information about the non-germline-encoded hypervariable CDR3 region can be obtained because clonotypic reagents are not available for routine use.

Adhesion molecules have an important role in mediating leukocyte responses to inflammatory stimuli and in binding of cells to each other or to the extracellular

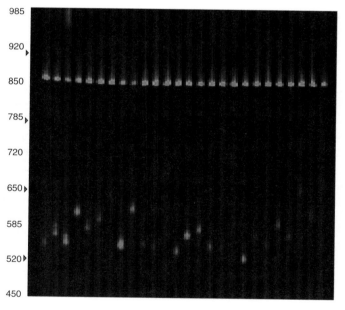

Figure 43.2 Photograph of the computer screen displaying a gel of peripheral blood lymphocytes from a type 1 diabetic child subjected to TCR Vβ-specific amplification. The fluorescent blue PCR products corresponding to Vβ gene families 1–24 were electrophoresed on a 16-cm, 5 per cent polyacrylamide non-denaturing gel for 1 h on an ABI 377 DNA Sequencer and automatically analyzed by GeneScan software. As internal control, a portion of the Cα region of the TCR is also amplified by using primers labeled with a different dye (6-TET), which originate green bands. The relative abundance of T cells carrying each Vβ chain transcript is estimated by calculating a ratio of Vβ fluorescent and Cα fluorescent areas for each Vβ gene family. **See colour plate 43.2.**

matrix. In an immune response, for example, interaction of intercellular adhesion molecule-I (ICAM-I; CD54) on APC with its ligand, lymphocyte function-associated antigen-1 (LFA-1; CD11a), on T cells helps T cells to activate, thus allowing migration of activated T cells from the circulation to the sites of inflammation. L-selectin (CD62L) expressed on lymphocytes, is another adhesion molecule modulated during cellular activation allowing lymphocyte rolling and adhesion to endothelial cells. Both L-selectin and ICAM-I are shed from the cell membrane and are found in the circulation in soluble form. A recent investigation on a large group of subjects at high risk of developing type 1 diabetes showed increased concentrations of soluble adhesion molecules in highest risk relatives (Toivonen et al., 2001). Furthermore, there appears to be an inverse correlation between age of the high-risk subjects and the levels of both ICAM-I and L-selectin. Similar results were also reported by another group who studied patients with type 1 diabetes (Dogruel et al., 2001). Overall, these studies suggest that adhesion molecules could be considered markers of progressive β-cell destruction (Toivonen et al., 2001). The source of the circulating soluble adhesion molecules could be both endothelial and immune cells. We are routinely performing this type of analysis in leukocytes of type 1 diabetic patients by using whole blood from diabetic individuals in a four-color flow cytometry analysis (Luppi et al., 2002, 2003b). This means that we are able to detect up to four different surface antigen molecules on the surface of each cell, thus allowing the possibility to investigate in detail the phenotype of the T cells. Within the T lymphocytes, we are particularly focusing on the investigation of adhesion molecule expression on the Vβ7+ T cell subpopulation as these are the subset of T cells that seem to play an important pathogenic role in β-cell destruction (Figure 43.3). As leukocyte activation is characterized by changes in expression of adhesion molecules present on resting immune cells or by the expression of new molecules on the cell surface, the use of a whole blood flow-cytometry technique (Luppi et al., 2002, 2003b) will avoid any non-specific activation of lymphocytes that could result from the isolation procedure. Moreover, the use of whole blood allows the analysis of the cell phenotype by using small amounts of blood (50–100 μl of blood), which is a limiting factor when working with children of a young age.

Determining the immunologic β-cell damage: the humoral role

Uncertainty exists regarding the role played by autoantibodies in type 1 diabetes pathogenesis, although they are considered to be the best markers of the ongoing autoimmune process. In fact, although there is not direct participation of autoantibodies in the initial immune-mediated attack to β-cells, autoantibodies specific for a number of islet-cell autoantigens are present in the sera of subjects defined genetically at-risk for the disease

during the long, prodromal period, before symptoms arise (Pietropaolo and Eisenbarth, 2001).

The progress made in the field of immunology of diabetes in the past decade, supports the optimistic intent to be able in the near future to predict more accurately the timing of the onset of overt type 1 diabetes. New therapeutic strategies, such as a variety of immunomodulation as well as gene and cell therapeutic approaches can also be developed (Trucco et al., 2002).

Autoantibodies are some of the most potent risk determinants for autoimmune diseases with relative risk exceeding 100 (Pietropaolo and Eisenbarth, 2001). The quintessential model for the application of autoantibody markers in the prediction of a selective immune-mediated tissue damage is type 1 diabetes. Several recent studies have suggested that using a combination of humoral immunological markers detecting autoantibodies to glutamic acid decarboxylase, 65 isoform (GAD65), the neuroendocrine antigen IA-2 and insulin gives a higher predictive value for type 1 diabetes and great sensitivity without significant loss of specificity (Bingley et al., 1994; Verge et al., 1996; Pietropaolo et al., 1998). An increasing number of studies have shown that multiple autoantibodies to islet antigens conferred a cumulative risk of developing diabetes of nearly 90 per cent during follow-up (Bingley et al., 1994; Verge et al., 1996; Maclaren et al., 1999). With this degree of predictability, a strategy can be devised, whereby individuals with high genetic risk of developing type 1 diabetes can be identified even several years prior to the onset of the overt disease. These are very important prerequisites for designing effective intervention strategies for the prevention of type 1 diabetes.

GAD65 autoantibodies are detected in triplicate after immunoprecipitation of serum with the *in vitro* transcribed/translated recombinant ^{35}S-[Met]-labeled recombinant human GAD65, as originally described by Grubin et al. (1994). The assay is performed in 96-well filtration plates with autoantibody-bound ^{35}S-[Met]-GAD65 that is precipitated with Protein A Sepharose. The results are expressed as an index: index = sample cpm − negative control cpm/positive control cpm − negative control cpm (Pietropaolo et al., 2002). The cut-off point for the assay is established as the 99th percentile of the autoantibody index calculated using a sufficiently high number of control subjects.

IA-2 autoantibodies are detected using a similar technique as for detecting GAD65. The assay is performed in 96-well filtration plates with autoantibody-bound ^{35}S-[Met]-IA-2 that is precipitated with Protein A Sepharose. Here again, the results are expressed as the index plus the coefficient of variation (CV). Our CV for both GAD65 and IA-2 antibody assays was previously reported (Pietropaolo et al., 1998). Proficiency workshops results, organized by the University of Florida in Gainesville (1995, 1996 and 1997) and the Diabetes Autoantibody Standardization Program (DASP, 2000, 2002), organized by WHO, are summarized

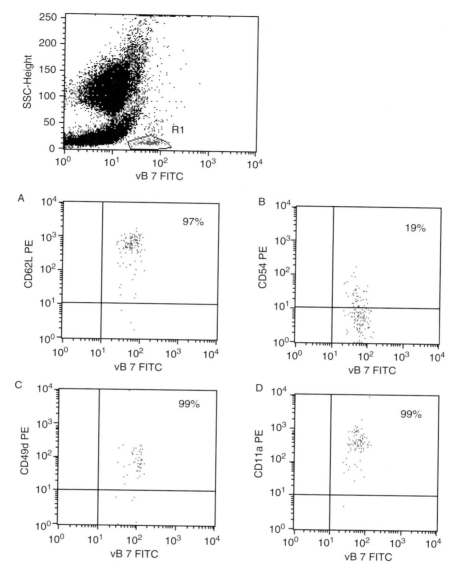

Figure 43.3 Flow cytometry analysis of adhesion molecules expression on Vβ7⁺ T lymphocytes in a diabetic patient; 50 μl of whole heparinized blood was stained with directly conjugated anti-human monoclonal antibodies (mAb) against the Vβ chain of the TCR and to a panel of adhesion molecules and run on a FACSCalibur machine (Becton Dickinson, San Jose, CA). The analysis of the expression of adhesion molecules on the surface of the circulating Vβ7⁺ T cells was made first by setting a specific gate for the Vβ7⁺ T cell subset based on dot-plot graphs of side-scatter (SSC) versus the cells positive for the Vβ7⁺ mAb (R1 on top dot-plot graph). Dot-plot graphs of Vβ7⁺ T cells versus the positive cells for mAb to CD62L (A), CD54 (B), CD49d (C) and CD11a (D) were then drawn. The frequency of Vβ7⁺T cells positive for the different adhesion molecules tested is reported.

as follows: 76–100 per cent sensitivity, 90–100 per cent specificity (100 per cent specificity 3 times) and 100 per cent validity for GAD autoantibodies.

For the insulin autoantibody (IAA) radioimmunoassay, serum samples are incubated with ¹²⁵I-labeled insulin, as described by Williams et al. (1997). Three quality controls are generally included in each assay:

1 sera obtained from long-standing insulin treated patients (positive control)
2 IAA positive first degree relative of type 1 diabetic patients (medium control)
3 serum from a healthy volunteer (negative control).

A standard curve is generated for each assay. The cut-off point is here established as the 99th percentile and in our more recent studies was set at 0.16 units. For IAA the inter-assay CV was 19.4 per cent ($n = 15$), whereas the intra-assay CV was 8.0 per cent ($n = 15$). Insulin autoantibodies gave 16 per cent sensitivity and 100 per cent specificity, which was averaged in recent DASP workshops.

Enterovirus detection

Exposure to viral infections has been recognized as one of the most important events able to accelerate the autoimmune process of β-cell destruction (Luppi et al., 2000;

Serreze et al., 2000). In particular, infections caused by enterovirus (EV) have been found associated with diabetes onset in humans since 1979 (Yoon et al., 1979). Therefore, the analysis of the presence of an acute or chronic EV infection in children could be extremely important for the identification of the individuals who will eventually progress to the clinical onset, among those genetically at-risk for the development of diabetes. We started routinely to analyze serum samples from different individuals for the presence of enterovirus EV RNA and anti-EV antibodies (Luppi et al., 2000). Detection of EV-RNA is done by an RT-PCR method which is generally carried out from coded samples (Lonnrot et al., 1999). This RT-PCR method amplifies a genome sequence of the highly conserved 5′ non-coding region of all EV serotypes and RT-PCR products are identified by a lanthanide chelate labeled EV specific probe in a liquid phase hybridization assay. The detection limit of this assay is 0.015 fg of viral RNA. The IgG and IgA class antibodies to coxsackievirus B4 (CVB4) antigen and to a synthetic EV peptide are routinely analyzed using an enzyme immunoassay (EIA) method (Hyoty et al., 1995; Juhela et al., 1999) and IgM class antibodies using a heavy chain capture EIA using a panel of three EV antigens (CVB3, echovirus 11, and CVA16) (Juhela et al., 1999). These antibody assays were designed to detect antibodies to several EV serotypes. Virus antigens are also heat-treated at +56 °C for 15 minutes to expose antigenic determinants which are cross-reactive between different EV serotypes. The antibody results are expressed as enzyme immunoassay units (EIU) which show the relative antibody activity of the sample compared to positive and negative control sera included in each test and which are therefore comparable between different test runs. All serum samples are tested in triplicate. Samples are considered seropositive if EIU > 15. Diagnosis of acute infection during the follow up in the converters is based on the presence of twofold or greater increase in the concentration of IgA and/or IgG and/or detection of IgM in amounts exceeding previously defined cut-off limits and/or presence of EV-RNA in serum (Hyoty et al., 1995; Luppi et al., 2000).

CONCLUDING REMARKS

We actually know then 'what the leopard was seeking at that altitude . . .' or why T cells are aiming at the thymus. The task for us scientists is now that of finding appropriate means to force the diabetogenic T cells that escaped thymic negative selection, to remain in a state of hyporesponsiveness so to reconstitute, for example, an efficient peripheral tolerance against the β-cell specific structures. Once a correct way to re-establish tolerance is found, efficient ways to treat diabetes will easily be found, as well.

ACKNOWLEDGEMENTS

The authors want to thank Dr Massimo Pietropaolo for allowing them to include in this chapter his procedures to determine properly autoantibody titers in the sera of our patients and Dr Steven Ringquist for volunteering the description of his pyrosequencer approach to HLA molecular typing.

REFERENCES

Alexander, A., Nichol, L., Ringquist, S., Styche, A., Rudert, W. and Trucco, M. (2002). Pyrosequencing sheds light on HLA genotyping. Hum Immunol 63 Suppl, S95.

Bingley, P.J., Christie, M.R., Bonifacio, E. et al. (1994). Combined analysis of autoantibodies improves prediction of IDDM in islet cell antibody-positive relatives. Diabetes 43, 1304–1310.

Bottazzo, G.F., Florin-Christensen, A. and Doniach, D. (1974). Islet-cell antibodies in diabetes mellitus with autoimmune polyendocrine deficiencies. Lancet 2, 1279–1282.

Bottino, R., Balamurugan, A.N., Giannoukakis, N. and Trucco. M. (2002). Islet/pancreas transplantation: challenges for pediatrics. Pediatr Diabetes 3, 210–223.

Brooks-Worrell, B.M., Starkebaum, G.A., Greenbaum, C. and Palmer, J.P. (1996). Peripheral blood mononuclear cells of insulin-dependent diabetic patients respond to multiple islet cell proteins. J Immunol 157, 5668–5674.

Brunkow, M.E., Jeffery, E.W., Hjerrild, K.A. et al. (2001). Disruption of a new forkead/winged-helix protein, scurfin, results in the fatal lymphoproliferative disorder of the scurfy mouse. Nat Genet 27, 68–73.

Chatila, T.A., Blaeser, F., Ho, N. et al. (2000). JM2, encoding a fork head-related protein, is mutated in X-linked autoimmunity-allergic disregulation syndrome. J Clin Invest 106, R75–81.

Conrad, B., Weidmann, E., Trucco, G. et al. (1994). Evidence for superantigen involvement in insulin-dependent diabetes mellitus etiology. Nature 371, 351–355.

Davies, J.L., Kawaguchi, Y., Bennett, S.T. et al. (1994). A genome-wide search for human type 1 diabetes susceptibility genes. Nature 371, 130–136.

Delovitch, T.L. and Singh, B. (1997). The nonobese diabetic mouse as a model of autoimmune diabetes: immune dysregulation gets the NOD. Immunity 7, 727–738.

Dogruel, N., Kirel, B., Akgun Y. and Us, T. (2001). Serum soluble endothelial-cell specific adhesion molecules in children with insulin-dependent diabetes mellitus. J Pediatr Endocrinol Metab 14, 287–293.

Eisenbarth, G.S. (1986) Type I diabetes mellitus: a chronic autoimmune disease. N Engl J Med 314, 1360–1368.

Faas, S.J., Menon, R., Braun, E.R., Rudert, W.A. and Trucco, M. (1996). Sequence-specific priming and exonuclease-released fluorescence detection of HLA-DQB1 alleles. Tissue Antigens 48, 97–112.

Friday, R.P., Trucco, M. and Pietropaolo, M. (1999). Genetics of Type 1 diabetes mellitus. Diabetes Nutr Metab 12, 3–26.

Grubin, C.E., Daniels, T., Toivola, B. et al. (1994). A novel radiobinding assay to determine diagnostic accuracy of isoform-specific glutamic acid decarboxylase antibodies in childhood IDDM. Diabetologia 37, 344–350.

Herold, K.C., Hagopian, W., Auger, J.A. et al. (2002). Anti-CD3 monoclonal antibody in new-onset type 1 diabetes mellitus. N Engl J Med 346, 1692–1698.

Hsia, S., Tong, J.Y., Parris, G.L. et al. (1993). Molecular compatibility and renal graft survival – the HLA DRB1 genotyping. Transplantation 55, 395–399.

Hurley, C.K., Maiers, M., Ng, J. et al. (2000). Large-scale DNA-based typing of HLA-A and HLA-B at low resolution is highly accurate specific and reliable. Tissue Antigens 55, 352–358.

Hyoty, H., Hiltunen, M., Knip, M. et al. (1995). A prospective study of the role of Coxsackie B and other enterovirus infections in the pathogenesis of IDDM. Diabetes 44, 652–657.

Jorgensen, J.L., Esser, U., Fazekas de St Groth, B., Reay, P.A. and Davis, M.M. (1992). Mapping T-cell receptor-peptide contacts by variant peptide immunization of single-chain transgenics. Nature 355, 224–230.

Juhela, S., Hyöty, H., Hinkkanen, A. et al. (1999). T cell responses to enterovirus antigens and to β-cell autoantigens in unaffected children positive for IDDM-associated autoantibodies. J Autoimm 12, 269–278.

Komulainen, J., Kulmala, P., Savola, K. et al. (1999). Clinical, autoimmune, and genetic characteristics of very young children with type 1 diabetes. Childhood Diabetes in Finland (DiMe) Study Group. Diabetes Care 22, 1950–1955.

Kukreja, A., Cost, G., Marker, J. et al. (2002). Multiple immnoregulatory defects in type-1 diabetes. J Clin Invest 109, 131–140.

Lipton, R.B., Kocova, M., LaPorte, R.E. et al. (1992). Autoimmunity and genetics contribute to the risk of insulin-dependent diabetes mellitus in families: islet cell antibodies and HLA DQ heterodimers. Am J Epidemiol 136, 503–512.

Lo, S.S., Tun, R.Y.M., Hawa, H. and Leslie, R.D.G. (1991). Studies of diabetic twins. Diab Metab Rev 7, 223–238.

Lonnrot, M., Sjoroos, M., Salminen, K., Maaronen, M., Hyypia, T. and Hyoty, H. (1999). Diagnosis of entero- and rhinovirus infections by RT-PCR and time-resolved fluorometry with lanthanide chelate labelled probes. J Med Virol 59, 378–384.

Luppi,P., Zanone, M.M., Hyoty, H. et al. (2000). Restricted TCR Vβ gene usage and enterovirus infections in Type 1 diabetes: a pilot study. Diabetologia 43, 1484–1497.

Luppi, P., Haluszcazk, C., Trucco, M. and DeLoia, J.A. (2002). Normal pregnancy is associated with peripheral leukocyte activation. Am J Reproductive Immunol 47, 72–81.

Luppi, P., Rudert, W.A., Licata, A. et al. (2003a). Expansion of specific $\alpha\beta^+$ T cell subsets in the myocardium of patients with myocarditis and idiopathic dilated cardiomyopathy associated with Coxsackievirus B infection. Human Immunol 64, 194–210.

Luppi, P., Betters, D., Tse, T., Becker, D. and Trucco, M. (2003b). Children with early-onset type 1 diabetes show selective activation of T cells in the peripheral blood. Submitted.

Maclaren, N., Lan, M., Coutant, R. et al. (1999). Only multiple autoantibodies to islet cells (ICA), insulin, GAD65, IA-2 and IA-2α predict immune-mediated (Type 1) diabetes in relatives. J Autoimmun 12, 279–287.

Manfras, B.J., Rudert, W.A., Trucco, M. and Boehm, B.O. (1997). Analysis of the alpha/beta T-cell receptor repertoire by competitive and quantitative family-specific PCR with exogenous standards and high resolution fluorescence based CDR3 size imaging. J Immunol Methods 210, 235–249.

McDevitt, H. (2001). Closing in on type 1 diabetes. N Engl J Med 345, 1060–1061.

Morel, P.A., Dorman, J.S., Todd, J.A., McDevitt, H.O. and Trucco, M. (1988). Aspartic acid at position 57 of the HLA-DQ beta chain protects against type I diabetes: a family study. Proc Natl Acad Sci USA 85, 8111–8115.

Olmos, P., A'Hern, R., Heaton, D.A. et al. (1988). Significance of the concordance rate for type 1 (insulin-dependent) diabetes in identical twins. Diabetologia 31, 747–750.

Pannetier, C., Even, J. and Kourilsky, P. (1995). T-cell repertoire diversity and clonal expansions in normal and clinical samples. Immunol Today 16, 176–181.

Pietropaolo, M. and Eisenbarth, G.S. (2001). Autoantibodies in human diabetes. Curr Dir Autoimmun 4, 252–282.

Pietropaolo, M. and Trucco, M. (2000). Major histocompatibility locus and other genes that determine the risk of development of type 1 diabetes mellitus. In Diabetes Mellitus: a Fundamental and Clinical Text, 2nd edn, LeRoith, D., Taylor, S.I. and Olefsky, J.M. eds. Philadelphia: Lippincott Williams and Wilkins, pp. 399–410.

Pietropaolo, M., Becker, D.J., LaPorte, R.E. et al. (2002). Progression to insulin-requiring diabetes in seronegative prediabetic subjects: the role of two HLA-DQ high risk haplotypes. Diabetologia 45, 66–76.

Pietropaolo, M., Peakman, M., Pietropaolo, S.L. et al. (1998). Combined analysis of GAD65 and ICA512(IA-2) autoantibodies in organ and non-organ specific autoimmune diseases confers high specificity for insulin-dependent diabetes mellitus. J Autoimmun 11, 1–10.

Ringquist, S., Alexander, A.M., Rudert, W.A., Styche, A. and Trucco, M. (2002). Pyrosequence based typing of alleles of the HLA-DQB1 gene. BioTechniques 33, 166–175.

Ronaghi, M. (2001). Pyrosequencing sheds light on DNA sequencing. Genome Research 11, 3–11.

Ronaghi, M., Karamohamed, S., Pettersson, B., Uhlen, M., Nyzen, P. (1996). Real-time DNA sequencing using detection of pyrophosphate release. Annal Biochem 242, 84–89.

Rosner, G., Martell, B.S. and Trucco, M. (2000). Histocompatibility. In Hematopoietic Stem Cell Therapy, Ball, E.D., Lister, J. and Law, P., eds. Philadelphia: Churchill Linvingstone, pp. 233–251.

Rudert, W.A. and Trucco, M. (1989). A rapid test for IDDM susceptibility detection. Pharmacy Times October, 38–43.

Rudert, W.A. and Trucco, M. (1992). Rapid detection of sequence variations using polymers of specific oligonucleotides. Nucl Acid Res 5, 1146.

Sakaguchi, S., Sakaguchi, N., Shimizu, J. et al. (2001). Immunologic tolerance maintained by CD25+ CD4+ regulatory T cells: their common role in controlling autoimmunity, tumor immunity, and transplantation tolerance. Immunol Rev 182, 18–32.

Salomon, B., Lenschow, D.J., Rhee, L. et al. (2000). B7/CD28 costimulation is essential for the homeostasis of the CD4+ CD25+ immunoregulatory T cells that control autoimmune diabetes. Immunity 12, 431–440.

Serreze, D.V., Ottendorfer, E.W., Ellis, T.M., Gauntt, C.J. and Atkinson, M.A. (2000). Acceleration of type 1 diabetes by a coxsackievirus infection requires a preexisting critical mass of auto reactive T-cells in pancreatic islets. Diabetes 49, 708–711.

Stephens, L.A. and Mason, D. (2000). CD25 is a marker for CD4+ thymocytes that prevent autoimmune diabetes in rats, but peripheral T cells with this function are found in both CD25+ and CD25− subpopulations. J Immunol 165, 3105–3110.

Tisch, R., Yang, X.D., Singer, S.M., Liblau, R.S., Fugger, L. and McDevitt, H.O. (1993). Immune response to glutamic acid decarboxylase correlates with insulitis in non-obese diabetic mice. Nature 366, 72–75.

Todd, J.A., Bell, J.I. and McDevitt, H.O. (1987). HLA-DQ beta gene contributes to susceptibility and resistance to insulin-dependent diabetes mellitus. Nature 329, 599–604.

Toivonen, A., Kulmala, P., Savola, K., Akerblom, H.K. and Knip, M., The Childhood Diabetes in Finland. (2001). Soluble adhesion molecules in preclinical type 1 daibetes. The Childhood Diabetes in Finland Study Group. Pediatr Res *49*, 24–29.

Tong, J.Y., Hsia, S., Parris, G.L. et al. (1993). Molecular compatibility and renal graft survival – the HLA DQB1 genotyping. Transplantation *55*, 390–395.

Trucco, M. (1992) To be or not to be Asp 57, that is the question. Diabetes Care *15*, 705–715.

Trucco, M. and Ball, E. (1989). RFLP analysis of DQ-beta chain gene: Workshop report. In Histocompatibility Testing 1987 *1*, 860.

Trucco, M. and Dorman, J. (1989). Immunogenetics of insulin-dependent diabetes mellitus in humans. CRC Crit Rev Immunol *9*, 201–245.

Trucco, G., Fritsch, R., Giorda, R. and Trucco, M. (1989). Rapid detection of IDDM susceptibility, using amino acid 57 of the HLA-DQ beta chain as a marker. Diabetes *38*, 1617–1622.

Trucco, M., Robbins, P.D., Thomson, A.W. and Giannoukakis, N. (2002). Gene therapy strategies to prevent autoimmune disorders. Curr Gene Ther *2*, 341–354.

Verge, C.F., Gianani, R., Kawasaki, E. et al. (1996). Prediction of type I diabetes in first-degree relatives using a combination of insulin, GAD, and ICA512bdc/IA-2 autoantibodies. Diabetes *45*, 926–933.

Wicker, L.S., Miller, B.J. and Mullen, Y. (1986). Transfer of autoimmune diabetes mellitus with splenocytes from nonobese diabetic (NOD) mice. Diabetes *35*, 855–860.

Williams, A.J.K., Bingley, P.J., Bonifacio, E., Palmer, J.P. and Gale, E.A.M. (1997). A novel micro-assay for insulin autoantibodies. J Autoimmun *10*, 473–478.

Yoon, J.W., Austin, M., Onodera, T. and Notkins, A.L. (1979). Virus-induced diabetes mellitus: isolation of a virus from the pancreas of a child with diabetic ketoacidosis. New Engl J Med *300*, 1173–1179.

Autoimmunity – Systemic Lupus Erythematosus

Chapter 44

Sharon Chambers and David A. Isenberg
Centre for Rheumatology, University College London, London, UK

Even the finest weapons are instruments of great evil.

Lao Tzu, Chinese Philosopher

SLE 3

Systemic lupus erythematosus (SLE) is a classic autoimmune rheumatic disease characterized by a wide variety of clinical features and a broad selection of antinuclear and other antibodies. The hallmark of the disease is widespread inflammation, which may affect virtually any organ of the body. The propensity of the disease to involve multiple organs/systems requires a multidisciplinary approach to its management.

There is some debate, but the term lupus (Latin for wolf) may first have been used by the thirteenth century physician Rogerius who likened the erythematous, erosive facial lesions of the disease to those produced by the bite of a wolf.

In 1948, Hargraves and colleagues described the LE cell phenomenon. Observing this in cells in the bone marrow of patients with systemic lupus, they described the phagocytosis of free nuclear material by mature polymorphonuclear leukocytes. The LE cell phenomenon was the specific test for the diagnosis of SLE and led to the search for other immunological markers.

In 1957 Friou and colleagues used indirect immunofluorescence to demonstrate antinuclear antibodies in the blood of patients with SLE. Since then, some 40–50 cellular targets for antibodies, many directed against nuclear components, have been demonstrated.

Some of these antibodies are disease specific, e.g. anti dsDNA and anti-Sm antibodies. Others including anti Ro/La may be found in other autoimmune diseases, e.g. Sjogren's syndrome.

EPIDEMIOLOGY

SLE is found worldwide. It is 10–20 times more common in females than males, with a distinct predominance of the disease among Afro-Caribbeans and probably Chinese and Hispanics. The majority of women develop the disease in the childbearing years. Only 10–15 per cent develop the disease after age 50 and in this latter group the female:male ratio approaches 4:1.

The genetic contribution to the etiology of SLE is indicated by studies of twin concordance, which show an increased prevalence in monozygotic twins (24 per cent) compared to dizygotic twins (2 per cent) (Deapen et al., 1992).

CLINICAL FEATURES

The many clinical features of SLE and cumulative frequencies are documented in Table 44.1.

Measuring Immunity, edited by Michael T. Lotze and Angus W. Thomson
ISBN 0-12-455900-X, London

Table 44.1 Clinical features of SLE cohort attending UCH/The Middlesex SLE clinic 1978–2002 ($n = 300$)

Organ involvement	No.	% of total
Alopecia	51	17
Oral ulcers	84	28
Joints	290	97
Jaccoud's	7	
Erosive	15	
Serositis	153	51
Kidney	100	33
CNS	70	23
Lung	7	2
Hemolytic anemia	16	5
Thrombocytopenia	52	17
Sjogren's syndrome	36	12
Antiphospholipid antibody syndrome	25	8

CNS, central nervous system.

Non-specific features

Fatigue, anorexia, lymphadenopathy and weight loss occur in many patients with SLE and often serve as useful indicators of disease activity.

Musculoskeletal

The musculoskeletal involvement usually takes the form of polyarticular, symmetrical episodic arthralgia. Overt arthritis and bone erosions/deformities rarely occur. There is minimal cellular inflammation in the synovial membrane of lupus joints with only occasional hematoxylin bodies (tissue equivalent of LE cells) and non-specific vasculitis and perivasculitis demonstrated histologically.

A small subset of lupus patients have an erosive arthropathy (approx 5 per cent) that seems to be an overlap with rheumatoid arthritis.

Tenosynovitis is more evident in SLE and may give rise to tendon rupture or joint deformities without bone destruction.

Myalgia may occur in up to 50 per cent of patients and is thought to be secondary to adjacent joint inflammation. A vacuolar myopathy has been described in lupus. This is characterized by the presence of plump, swollen sarcolemmal nuclei with other prominent vacuolated nuclei centrally located within the muscle fiber. A true accompanying myositis is uncommon (<5 per cent). Treatment with corticosteroids and other antimalarials may also cause a myopathy.

Cutaneous involvement

The classic malar 'butterfly' rash is found in only one-third of patients with the disease. It presents as an erythematous, elevated lesion on the bridge of the nose and cheeks, sparing the nasolabial fold. On direct immunofluorescence immune deposits and complement at the dermal–epidermal junction may be seen. The rash tends to be precipitated and exacerbated by sun-exposure and may last from days to weeks. It has been postulated that sunlight damages chromatin which then acts as a substrate for autoantibody production leading to a local inflammatory reaction. Some studies have shown that UV irradiation of keratinocytes *in vitro* induces release of dermal and epidermal cytokines and increases the expression of cell adhesion molecules such as ICAM-1 which, *in vivo*, may lead to vascular activation culminating in the photosensitive lupus syndromes (Norris, 1993). More recent work has linked UV light to an increase in apoptosis (see later).

Subacute cutaneous lupus

The lesions of subacute cutaneous lupus erythematosus (SCLE) are non-fixed and non-scarring. They occur on sun-exposed skin as erythematous papules or small scaly plaques, which may merge and form annular lesions. SCLE may be accompanied by the presence of anti-Ro antibodies in sera and in the lesion.

Other skin lesions of SLE include discoid lesions, various photosensitive skin rashes, splinter hemorrhages, buccal and nasal ulceration, angioneurotic edema and vasculitis of the digits.

Renal disease

Renal complications are a major cause of morbidity in lupus patients. The World Health Organization (WHO) has subdivided renal lupus into six major categories according to biopsy-derived information.

    I   = normal appearance
    II = mesangial disease
    III = focal segmental glomerulonephritis
    IV = diffuse proliferative glomerulonephritis
    V   = membranous
    VI = glomerulosclerosis.

Histologically, the range of glomerular changes include swelling and proliferation of mesangial, endothelial and parietal epithelial cells, with infiltration by monocytes and polymorphonuclear leukocytes. In addition, immune complexes, foci of necrosis and hematoxylin bodies can be identified in the glomeruli of lupus patients.

The WHO classification has been widely adopted worldwide. Some centers also use disease activity and damage scores when reporting biopsy results and, although not universally accepted, many clinicians have found this practice useful in predicting the outcome and planning treatment interventions. The WHO classification however does not consider tubulointerstitial disease and makes no allowance for varying degrees of severity within individual categories. Neither does it recognize the recently described overlap of lupus nephritis and the multiple small thrombi associated with the antiphospholipid antibodies.

The decision on the timing and value of the renal biopsy is still controversial. Goulet et al. (1993) used regression tree techniques to show that combinations of serum creatinine, 24-h urine protein levels, nephrotic syndrome and duration of prior renal disease provide accurate prognostic information about lupus nephritis without recourse to biopsy.

McLaughlin et al. (1994) in a long-term follow-up study of 123 SLE patients who had a renal biopsy between 1970 and 1984 showed that the biopsy was helpful in assessing prognosis in patients with normal serum creatinine. In those with elevated serum creatinine, the biopsy did not contribute additional information about the risk of dying.

More recently, Godfrey et al. (2002) showed that the EDTA-GFR is a better predictor of renal involvement than either serum creatinine concentration or creatinine clearance calculated by the Cockcroft-Gault formula. They concluded that a normal serum creatinine concentration does not exclude the possibility of significant renal involvement including WHO classes III, IV and V and therefore should not be used to determine the indication for renal biopsy.

We recommend that patients should therefore have regular urinalysis for protein and red cell casts as well as serum urea and creatinine estimations. Those with significant hematuria/proteinuria and diminished glomerular filtration rates should be considered for a renal biopsy.

AUTOANTIBODIES IN SLE

A major feature of SLE is its apparent diversity of autoantibodies. The cumulative frequency of these antibodies and their clinical associations are indicated in Table 44.2.

Arbuckle et al. (2003) demonstrated that many of these autoantibodies may present many years before the clinical diagnosis of SLE.

Some of these antibodies are strongly associated with particular disease features as indicated in Table 44.2.

Antinuclear antibodies

These heterogeneous antibodies belong primarily to the IgG1 and IgG3 immunoglobulin subclasses and are directed against components of the nucleus.

Antinuclear antibodies (ANA) are not specific for SLE and may be found in other conditions such as Sjogren's syndrome, polymyositis and scleroderma and in 10 per cent of normal individuals.

ANA may be detected by enzyme immunoassay or more commonly by indirect immunofluorescence using tissue culture cells such as human epithelioid cells (Hep 2 cells) or frozen sections of rodent liver or kidney as substrate.

The pattern of nuclear fluorescence has been used to indicate the specificity of antibody present. The homogeneous pattern is common in SLE and may be due to anti-dsDNA or anti-histone antibodies. Anti-histone may be

Table 44.2

Antibody specificity	Literature	Disease association
ANA	>90	
dsDNA	40–90	Renal/cardiovascular-respiratory
ssDNA	up to 70	
Histone	30–80	
Sm	5–30	
RNP	20–35	
Ro	30–40	Photosensitive rashes/subacute cutaneous lupus
La	10–15	Coincident Sjogren's syndrome
Cardiolipin	20–50	Thrombosis/fetal loss/thrombocytopenia
LAC	20–50	Thrombosis/fetal loss/thrombocytopenia
Fc IgG (RF)	25	
hsp90	5–50	
hsp70	5–40	
Thyroid Ags	up to 35	
C1q	20–45	Renal
Antiribosomal P	approx 15	CNS lupus (controversial!)
Anti glutamate receptor	NWE	CNS lupus
Anti-ASE-1	NWE	Serositis

The 'Literature' column refers to an approximate range derived from several published studies. LAC = lupus anticoagulant; G = IgG; Ags = antigens; NWE = not well established.

associated with drug-induced lupus. Speckled staining is often found in Sjogren's syndrome and is associated with anti-Sm, -Ro, -La or anti-RNP antibodies. The nucleolar pattern has been weakly associated with scleroderma, although anti-SCl-70 and centromere antibodies are much more specific tests.

DNA antibodies

DNA antibodies were first described in 1957. Since then, the dsDNA–binding test has remained the single most important laboratory test for the diagnosis of SLE.

Several studies demonstrate that in many, though not all patients, the levels of anti-dsDNA correlate well with the occurrence and severity of renal disease and the response to treatment.

Swaak et al. (1979) contrasted 51 patients with SLE and 660 patients who had autoimmune conditions. Fifty of the sera from the lupus patients contained anti-dsDNA antibodies in contrast to just one of the control sera. Furthermore, in many patients with renal exacerbations of their lupus, a sharp fall in the anti-dsDNA level was usually preceded by a rise suggesting that the antibodies were being deposited in an organ such as the kidney.

Bootsma et al. (1995) in a rather controversial paper proposed that a rise in anti-dsDNA antibody levels could be used to predict and avoid a clinical relapse by treating these patients with high levels of prednisolone (30 mg/day). The relapse rate compared with the control group treated with more conventional therapy was significantly lower.

Antibodies to extractable nuclear antigens

Extractable nuclear antigens (ENA) are ribonucleoproteins (protein antigens not containing DNA) that are extractable from cell nuclei using phosphate buffered saline. These ENA are Ro (SS-A), La (SS-B), Sm and RNP.

Sm is a 95 kDa protein that exists as a nuclear protein-RNA complex as part of the ribonucleoprotein (RNP) antigen. Sm and RNP both function to splice transcriptional mRNA. Antibodies to Sm are virtually diagnostic of SLE, but like anti-RNP do not have a strong association with any particular disease feature. Anti-Sm and anti-U1 RNP are more frequently associated with Afro-Caribbeans than Caucasians (Isenberg et al., 1997). Antibodies to U1 RNP are usually associated with mild disease, a lower incidence of renal involvement and the MHC haplotype DR4.

Antibodies to ribosomal P protein

The ribosomal P proteins: P0, P1 and P2 are acidic phosphoproteins required for protein synthesis and ribosome-associated GTPase activity. These antibodies produce a fine granular cytoplasmic immunofluorescence on human epithelial substrate. These antibodies appear relatively specific for lupus (Yasuma et al., 1990). Claims have been made suggesting an association of autoantibodies to ribosomal P proteins in SLE patients with cerebral involvement and lupus psychosis (Bonfa et al., 1987). This has generated much controversy (reviewed by Teh and Isenberg, 1994). Not all lupus patients with neuropsychiatric involvement will be positive for ribosome P antibodies and many patients with anti-ribosomal part bodies will not have CNS disease. At present there appears to be little value in routinely measuring anti-ribosomal antibodies in the management of patients with neuropsychiatric lupus.

Anti ASE-1 antibodies

Anti-bodies against the ASE-1 antigen (anti-sense to ErCC-1) interfere with critical DNA repair and are strongly correlated with serositis (Edworthy et al., 2002).

Other autoantibodies

Anti-platelet, anti-erythrocyte and lymphocytotoxic antibodies have been identified in lupus. They are associated with thrombocytopenia, Coombs' positive hemolytic anemia and lymphopenia, respectively.

Antibodies to RNA are found in SLE in a higher incidence than in patients with other autoimmune disease. They appear to have relatively little clinical significance in lupus.

Antibodies to C1q may be elevated in SLE and are indicative of proliferative glomerulonephritis. Recent evidence suggests that the measurement of antiC1q, anti-DNA and anticardiolipin antibodies is highly specific for glomerulonephritis in lupus patients (Siegert et al., 1999; Loizou et al., 2000).

ABNORMALITIES AND DYSREGULATION AT THE CELLULAR LEVEL

Numerous abnormalities of cellular function, cytokine regulation and apoptosis contribute to the immunopathogenesis of SLE.

A wide array of functional and quantitative defects is seen among cells of the immune system – T and B lymphocytes, natural killer cells and antigen-presenting cells.

Various authors describe increased numbers of hyperactive B cells expressing elevated levels of CD86 with coexistent T cell lymphocytopenia. The increase in activated B cells contributes to the hypergammaglobulinemia associated with reactivity to self-antigens. On circulating B cells, receptors for the cytokine IL-2 are increased while the CR-1 (receptor for C3b) expression is decreased.

The role of heat shock proteins (hsp) is also under scrutiny. These are proteins produced by cells in response to stress including viral infection and heat shock. They are concerned with the folding and unfolding of proteins and the intracellular trafficking of protein necessary for proper antigen presentation.

There is increased cytoplasmic and surface expression of heat shock protein 90 on B cells and CD4$^+$ T cells compared with normal cells (Twomey et al., 1996). The potential importance of hsp90 in at least a subset of patients is emphasized by observations in MRL/lpr mice, which confirm that hsp90 was elevated in the splenocytes of these animals when compared with the MRL$^{+/+}$ and BALB/c controls and that this increased expression preceded the onset of the disease. In addition, antibodies to hsp90 were detected in these mice shortly before the development of antibodies to double-stranded DNA.

Increased DNA mutations on T cells have been identified in both human and murine models of lupus. The mutations are believed to cause T cell death and the release of DNA by necrosis leading to the production of anti-DNA antibodies.

The role of T cell antibodies in the lack of suppression of hyperactive B cells has been explored. Indeed the titers of such antibodies have been reported to show a correlation with disease activity (Yamada et al., 1993).

Other studies show a reduction in CD4$^+$ cells bearing the CD45R$^+$ phenotype. This population of cells helps to induce suppression by signaling CD8 T cells. The reduction in this subset may explain the failure of T cells to suppress the hyperactive B cells. Anti-T-cell autoantibodies may be responsible for the depletion of this particular subset. CD45 autoantibodies mediate neutralization of activated T cells from lupus patients through anergy or apoptosis (Mamoune et al., 2000).

Subtle biochemical deficiencies including the T cell CAMP pathway as well as abnormal capping of cell surface protein (CD4 and CD8) and decreased cAMP production leading to inability to switch phenotype and suppress activity have been proposed.

CYTOKINES

Some other biomarkers have been recognized including cytokine levels. Cytokines in lupus can be classified according to whether they are pro- or anti-inflammatory. It is likely that this balance of opposing cytokines and their inhibitory receptors not only determines disease severity but also the particular organ involvement.

One report suggests that interleukin-6 (IL-6) is increased in the cerebrospinal fluid (CSF) of patients with CNS involvement in SLE but not in patients with SLE who lack neurological symptoms. Similarly, TGFβ has been implicated in preventing renal disease and decreased levels are also found in renal disease.

The characterization of different subsets of T helper (Th) cells is directly related to their cytokine profiles. Th1 cells support cell-mediated immunity while Th2 cells provide B cell help and also suppress cell-mediated immunity. The balance between cytokines from Th1 and those from Th2 cells is thus critical in determining the outcome of the immune response and any imbalance could have profound pathological effects.

It appears that Th2 cells predominate in SLE resulting in too much help for B cells and overproduction of antibodies. In support for this concept, increased levels of IL-10 have been found in lupus patients and this cytokine suppresses Th1 cells and thus impairs cell-mediated immunity. In mice continuous administration of anti-IL-10 delays the onset of the disease.

Tumour necrosis factor (TNFα) is produced by T (Th1) and B lymphocytes, natural killer cells and mononuclear phagocytic cells. TNFβ, originally called lymphotoxin, is produced by activated lymphocytes. The genes for TNFα and TNFβ are closely linked and located within the major histocompatibility complex (MHC). *In vitro* TNFα production by mitogen-activated peripheral blood lymphocytes varies according to the HLA class II haplotype of the donor. Elevated production is found in DR3 and DR4 subjects, whereas low production is found in DR2 and DQw1postive donors. The DR2, DQw1 genotype in lupus patients is associated with lupus nephritis. DR3+ lupus patients are not predisposed to lupus nephritis and have elevated levels of TNFα production. The DR4 haplotype is associated with high TNFα inducibility and negatively correlated with lupus nephritis (Jacob et al., 1990a).

Both macrophage and natural killer (NK) cell-mediated cytotoxicity are frequently impaired in lupus patients. Interferon-γ (IFN-γ) induced enhancement of both types of cytotoxicity is also impaired despite normal levels of IFN-γ production by lupus Th1 cells. SLE NK cells fail to release soluble factors required for killing. Recombinant interferon-γ (rIFN-γ) has been used to induce remission in patients with RA but exacerbated disease in both lupus patients (Machold and Smolen, 1990) and lupus-prone strains of mice (Jacob et al., 1990b).

Accessory cells in lupus may produce insufficient amounts of IL-1 to provide the necessary activation signal for T cells. This effect cannot be overcome *in vitro* by addition of exogenous IL-1, suggesting a defect may exist at the level of the IL-1 receptor on T cells. Alternatively, the defect could exist at a distal point in some biochemical pathway.

Both CD4+ and CD8+ T cells produce either normal or decreased amounts of IL-2 in response to exogenous antigens, mitogens and allo- and autoantigens. Reduced IL-2 generation would have a profound effect on T cell responses. This impairment is not reversed by the addition of exogenous IL-2. However, *in vitro* treatment of SLE accessory cells with IFN-γ plus the addition of IL-2 has been shown to restore T cell proliferation and the expression of T suppressor activity.

APOPTOSIS

Apoptosis is the normal method of cell death in multicellular organs. The process involves DNA fragmentation, condensation of chromatin, membrane blebbing and externalization of phosphatidylserine.

Apoptosis appears to have dual role in lupus pathogenesis. First, this process is an important mechanism for deletion of autoreactive lymphocytes and secondly, apoptosis results in the availability of autoantigens which can be presented to the immune system.

Normally apoptotic cells are rapidly cleared by macrophages, but recent evidence has demonstrated that there is a profound defect in this clearance pathway in lupus patients. When macrophages from a subgroup of SLE patients were differentiated *in vitro*, they displayed markedly impaired phagocytosis of apoptotic cells leading to the accumulation of secondary necrotic cells (Herrmann et al., 1998). These and other data have led to the notion that SLE may be a disease of 'waste disposal'.

Genetic studies of murine models suggest the role of defective apoptosis in lupus pathogenesis. Mice that have had the DNAse 1 gene deleted show symptoms of lupus including the presence of antinuclear antibodies and an immune complex positive nephritis (Napirei et al., 2000). DNAse 1 is a nuclease responsible for the removal of DNA from nuclear antigens of spent cells at the sites of rapid cell turnover.

Similar lupus-type phenotypes arise in mice lacking C1q or serum amyloid P, molecules which are involved in the clearance of immune complexes and apoptotic material.

The importance of removing apoptotic cells is explained by the appearance of a variety of nuclear autoantigens which are sequestered in blebs on the surface of apoptotic cells and may become accessible for dendritic cells (Andrade et al., 2000).

The Fas or Fas ligand does not seem to be involved in immune dysregulation in human lupus. In contrast, the MRL *lpr* and MRL *gld* mouse models of lupus have single point mutations in either Fas (CD95) or the Fas ligand. This abnormality results in failure of self-reactive T cells to undergo apoptosis in the thymus and may account for the accumulation of double negative T cells (CD4-CD8), which infiltrate many tissues in these mice. These mice develop massive lymphoproliferation and autoimmune nephritis.

There has been little strong evidence that patients with SLE have any mutations of the genes for Fas or the Fas ligand. Only one patient with SLE who has a mutation in the Fas ligand has been described (Wu et al., 1998).

The Bcl-2 proto-oncogene exerts a regulatory function during development and maintenance of adult tissue by preventing apoptosis in specific cell types. It is involved in T cell development and thymic selection and is found in long-lived B lymphocytes within the follicular mantle zone. Elevated Bcl-2 levels have been found in lymphocytes derived from some lupus patients and a number of cytokines (IL-2, IL-4, IL-7 and IL-15) can increase this expression and prevent cellular apoptosis preferentially in lupus patients (Graninger et al., 2002).

ANIMAL MODELS OF SLE

Both spontaneous and experimental murine models of SLE have been used to glean information on the cytokine and cellular abnormalities that may contribute to the pathogenesis of SLE in humans.

The 'older' mouse models of lupus are summarized in Table 44.3. These include the New Zealand Black (NZB)

mice which develop hemolytic anemia and chronic glomerulonephritis. The mice produce IgM antinuclear antibodies, but do not secrete IgG antibodies. When mated with the phenotypically normal New Zealand White (NZW), an F1 hybrid (B/W F1) is produced. The hybrid develops a chronic obliterative glomerulonephritis and also high levels of antinuclear antibodies and cationic IgG anti-dsDNA in the serum. Granular deposits of IgG and complement are observed in the renal mesangium and anti-ds DNA has been eluted from the kidneys.

One of the main cellular defects accounting for this clinical picture is B cell hyperactivity. These B cells have increased responses to T cell derived B cell growth factors including interleukin-5 (IL-5) and have increased mRNA for c-myc, an oncogene expressed in activated and proliferating cells. Excessive T cell help, impaired T cell mediated suppression or both may contribute to B cell hyperactivity in B/W F1 mice. The IgG isotype of the pathogenic antinuclear antibodies suggests that T cell help has been necessary for the production of these autoantibodies. Evidence in support of this is the amelioration of the disease severity in B/W F1 mice by treatment with anti-CD4 monoclonal antibodies reactive with Th cells. Evidence of impaired T suppressor mechanism after the onset of autoimmunity includes decreased IgG anti-DNA antibody secretion by B/W F1 splenocytes cultured with young, but not old, B/W F1 T cells with suppressor phenotype.

Table 44.3 Features of lupus-prone mouse strains

Strain	50% survival time	Major clinical features	Major immunological features
NZB	18 months	Hemolytic anemia, glomerulonephritis, lymphomas	Anti-erythrocyte antibodies IgM hyperproduction Generalized lymphocyte dysfunction
(NZBxNZW)F$_1$	7–8 months	Severe immune complex nephritis	Anti-nuclear and anti-DNA autoantibodies Generalized lymphocyte dysfunction
MRL/*lprl/lpr*	2–4 months	Lymphoproliferation immune complex nephritis, rheumatoid arthritis, vasculitis	Anti-nuclear antibodies and rheumatoid factors Proliferation of Ly1 cells, generalized lymphocyte dysfunction
MRL$^{+/+}$	18 months	As for MRL/*lpr* but less severe	As for MRL/*lpr*
BXSB	2–4 months	Hemolytic anemia, lymphadenopathy, glomerulonephritis	Anti-DNA, NTA and erythrocyte antibodies Thymic atrophy occurs early
Moth-eaten	1 month	Hair loss, glomerulonephritis, infections	Anti-DNA, NTA and erythrocyte antibodies Immunosuppression
Palmerston-North	11 months	Polyarteritis nodosa, immune complex nephritis	Anti-DNA autoantibodies, B cell hyperactivity
Swan	18 months	Mild glomerulonephritis	Anti-DNA autoantibodies, early thymic atrophy
(SWRxNZB)F$_1$	4–8 months	Severe glomerulonephritis	Anti-DNA, anti-nucleosome antibodies

NTA = natural thymocytotoxic antibody.

Abnormalities of the thymic epithelial cells as well as accelerated thymic atrophy have been described in NZB and B/W F1 mice. No global abnormalities in the generation of self-tolerance by the B/W F1 thymus have been detected. Data demonstrating that B/W F1 athymic mice do not develop kidney disease while those mice engrafted with a thymus do develop autoimmune disease support the requirement for T cells in the development of the full blown lupus-like disease.

The MRL/*lpr* mouse and the moth-eaten mouse have a single gene defect, the absence of fas and protein tyrosine phosphatase SHP-1, respectively, which significantly accelerates disease in a specific susceptible genetic background.

The Yaa (Y-chromosome-linked-autoimmune acceleration) gene accelerates disease in MRL$^{+/+}$ mice. These mice have increased levels of gp70-anti-gp70 immune complexes but no increase in the levels of circulating antibodies to DNA. Disease expression may be controlled by a least four genes, three of which have been mapped to chromosomes 7 and 17.

TREATMENT

There is no cure for SLE. The goals of treatment are therefore to control troublesome symptoms and suppress disease activity. Conventional treatment for lupus using the four main groups of drugs and the situations in which they are most useful are outlined in Table 44.4.

Antimalarials

Hydroxychloroquine is the antimalarial of choice. Many patients with fatigue, arthralgia and/or cutaneous SLE respond well to this drug, but a minority may require treatment with a combination of hydroxychloroquine and quinacrine or with more potent agents such as dapsone or possibly thalidomide.

Corticosteroids

Corticosteroids are useful in moderate doses up to 30 mg/day in severe arthritis, pericarditis or pleuritis. They are used at higher doses in the treatment of autoimmune hemolytic anemia, nephritis and thrombocytopenia.

Steroids may also be given as slow intravenous infusions in high doses, e.g. 1 g on 3 successive days to control severe symptoms.

It is advisable that all patients requiring 7.5 mg prednisolone/day or more be given calcium and vitamin D supplements to reduce the risk of corticosteroid-induced osteoporosis. Bisphosphonates such as alendronate and risedronate may also be offered. Bone densitometry should be done every 2 years in those on regular steroid to monitor bone loss.

Cytotoxic drugs

The main cytotxic drugs in use are cyclophosphamide, azathioprine, and mycophenolate mofetil.

The group from the National Institutes of Health at Bethesda has argued that intravenous boluses of cyclophosphamide, monthly for 6 months and subsequently every 3 months for 2 years in combination with monthly methylprednisolone therapy for 1 year is the treatment of choice in patients with severe renal involvement (Boumpas et al., 1992, 1993; Gourley et al., 1996). The problems of side effects with cyclophosphamide have made us more wary about its routine use, though this drug remains the treatment of choice for patients with serious renal and cerebral disease.

In common with many European groups, we use steroids and maintenance azathioprine in the first instance for patients with mild/moderately active renal disease.

Azathioprine may also be used as a steroid-sparing agent in cases where it proves difficult to reduce the dose of oral steroid without causing a flare of symptoms. Some data suggest that methotrexate may be used for mildly active disease and as a 'steroid sparer' (Carneiro and Sato, 1999) and to treat antimalarial resistant lupus arthritis.

A combination of mycophenolate mofetil and prednisolone has been compared with prednisolone and oral cyclophosphamide in the treatment of renal SLE (Chan et al., 2000). Both regimens were equally effective but mycophenolate had fewer major side effects.

We are now entering a new and exciting era in the treatment of SLE. Many new ideas about treatment are being translated from laboratory bench to the clinic. These include LJP 394, anticytokine, antiCD40 ligand, leflunomide, B cell depletion, anti BLys, anti-IFN-γ.

Table 44.4 Drug therapy in systemic lupus

	NSAID	Antimalarial	Corticosteroids	Cytotoxic agents
Malaise	+	+	+	−
Fever	+	−	+	−
Serositis	+	−	+	−
Arthralgia	+	+	+	−
Arthritis	+	+	+	+
Myalgia	+	+	+	−
Myositis	−	−	+	+
Malar/discoid rash	−	+	+	−
Pneumonitis	−	−	+	+
Carditis	−	−	+	+
Vasculitis	−	−	+	+
CNS disease	−	−		?
Renal	−	−	+	+
Hemolytic anemia	−	−	+	+
Thrombocytopenia	−	−	+	+
Raynaud's	−	−	?	?
Alopecia	−	−	?	?

Note: + = usually beneficial; − = not beneficial; ? = dubious/controversial.
*Widely prescribed but doubts remain that steroids are beneficial in many cases.

LJP 394

This drug has been developed specifically to inactivate B cells which produce anti-dsDNA antibodies. The drug consists of four oligonucleotides, each 20 bases in length which are attached to an inert scaffold. When these nucleotides bind surface Ig anti-dsDNA molecules on B cells, they can cross-link those molecules. This leads to anergy or deletion of the B cells rather than activation because the drug molecule does not carry any T cell epitopes and cannot recruit T cell help.

Alarcon-Segovia et al. (2003) demonstrated that treatment with LJP 394 in patients with high-affinity antibodies to its DNA epitope prolonged the time to renal flare, decreased the number of renal flares and required fewer treatments with high-dose corticosteroid compared to placebo.

Anti CD40

CD154 (CD40 ligand) is expressed as a cytokine, but also as a transmembrane protein on the surface of activated CD4 T lymphocytes. It interacts with its receptor, CD40, on B cells and promotes B cell growth, differentiation and antibody isotype class switching. It also primes dendritic cells to stimulate IL-12 production and indirectly enhances T cell dependent antibody responses.

Murine models of SLE demonstrate an overexpression of CD154 on T cells. Blockade of the CD154–CD40 interaction in mice with lupus has been shown to delay and decrease the incidence of glomerulonephritis. In humans, overexpression of CD154 on CD4 T cells also occurs in SLE. Monoclonal antibodies to CD40L have been used to treat patients with lupus and in at least one study were found to be safe and well tolerated (Davis et al., 2001). Another study reported an increased risk of thrombotic events.

Anti-cytokine therapy (anti BLyS)

B cell activating factor, also known as BLyS, has been highlighted in recent studies as a regulator of B cell activation and differentiation. High levels of BLyS have been found in lupus prone mice. Blocking the interaction between BLyS and its receptor TACI-Ig in female 21-week-old B/W mice markedly delayed the onset of proteinuria in these mice and resulted in increased survival. Trials using monoclonal anti-BLys antibodies in humans are now ongoing.

Anti-cytokine therapy (anti-IL-10)

IL-10 levels are elevated in the blood of lupus patients. Monoclonal anti-IL-10 antibodies have been used to treat six patients with SLE for 21 days each (Llorente et al., 2000). These patients reported improvements of the skin and joints which persisted for up to 6 months in the majority of cases.

Leflunomide

Leflunomide inhibits the pyrimidine synthesis pathway, thus blocking RNA and DNA synthesis in T and B cells and inhibiting proliferation of these cells. The first studies of this drug in the treatment of SLE have appeared (e.g. Remer et al., 2001). It appears to be safe and efficacious in short-term studies.

DISEASE MONITORING

In order to assess the totality of the effects of lupus on a patient, it is necessary to use tools which distinguish activity (ongoing inflammation), damage (permanent change) and patient perception.

The lupus community has been at the forefront of attempts to produce valid and reliable tools whose ultimate goal has been to help provide measures for assessing the efficacy of therapeutic agents. The history/derivation of these indices is recorded elsewhere (Isenberg and Ramsey-Goldman, 1999).

In 1984, the British Isles Lupus Assessment Group (BILAG) was formed. The group developed the BILAG index of SLE disease activity. The scoring system identifies features attributable to active lupus present within the last 4 weeks. It is based on the 'physician's intention to treat' provided this index proves to be reliable, comprehensive, sensitive to change and requiring only basic hematology and biochemistry indices. It utilizes 86 items which are divided into eight systems with a graded score for each system. The systems are general, mucocutaneous, neurological, musculoskeletal, cardiorespiratory, vasculitis, renal and hematological. The index allows for indication of features which are improving, the same, worse or new.

In the new computerized BLIPS (British Lupus Integrated Program) version, several amendments have been made to the activity index (Isenberg and Gordon, 2000).

The Systemic Lupus International Cooperating Clinics and American College of Rheumatology (SLICC/ACR) damage index is used to assess chronic damage. This index outlines non-reversible changes occurring since onset of lupus, changes which are not related to active inflammation and are present for at least 6 months. Clinical assessment, urinalysis and x-rays are used to assess damage. The SF (short form) 36 questionnaire is widely used to assess patients' perception of disease in patients with SLE.

CONCLUSION

The mortality of lupus has improved from a 5-year survival of less than 50 per cent to a 15-year survival of 80 per cent (Pistiner et al., 1991). Much remains to be done, however, as even in our own cohort of nearly 400 patients at the Centre for Rheumatology, we have found that some teenage patients with lupus have succumbed to SLE and the average age of death of the first 50 patients in our cohort who have died is 51 years (Isenberg, personal observation). Moss et al. (2002) noted that for the same cohort of patients, followed up between 1978 and 2002, malignancy, infection and vascular disease were the most common causes of death, although 40 per cent of early deaths were due to SLE-related renal disease. There was a fourfold increased risk of death in the cohort of patients with SLE compared with the general population.

We therefore seek more specific treatments with reduced side effects to help improve mortality and morbidity rates.

REFERENCES

Alarcon-Segovia, D., Tumlin, J., Furie, R. et al. (2003). LPJ 394 for the prevention of renal flare in patients with systemic lupus erythematosus. Arthritis Rheum 48, 442–454.

Andrade, F., Casciola-Rosen, L. and Rosen, A. (2000). Apoptosis in systemic lupus erythematosus. Clinical implications. Rheum Dis Clin N Am 26, 215–227.

Arbuckle, M.R., McClain, M.T., Rubertone, M.V. et al. (2003). Development of autoantibodies before the clinical onset of systemic lupus erythematosus. N Engl J Med 349, 1526–1533.

Bonfa, E., Golombek, S.J., Kaufman L.D. et al. (1987). Association between lupus psychosis and anti-ribosomal P protein antibodies. N Engl J Med 317, 265–271.

Bootsma, H., Spronk, P. and Derksen, R. (1995). Prevention of relapses in systemic lupus erythematosus. Lancet 345, 1595–1599.

Boumpas, D.T., Austin, H.A., Vaughan E.M. et al. (1992). Controlled trial of methylprednisolone versus two regimens of pulse cyclophosphamide in severe lupus nephritis. Lancet 340, 741–745.

Boumpas, D., Austin. H.A., Vaughan, E.M., Yarboro, C.H., Klippel, J.H. and Balow J.E. (1993). Risk for sustained amenorrhoea in patients with systemic lupus erythematosus receiving intermittent pulse cyclophosphamide therapy. Ann Intern Med 119, 366–369.

Carnerio, J.R.M. and Sato, E.M. (1999). Double blind randomised, placebo controlled clinical trial of methotrexate in systemic lupus erythematosus. J Rheumatol 26, 1275–1279.

Chan, T. M., Li, F.K., Tang, C.S. et al. (2000). Efficacy of mycophenolate mofetil in patients with diffuse proliferative lupus nephritis. N Engl J Med 343, 1156–1162.

Davis, J.C. Jr, Torortis, M.C., Rosenberg, J., Skelnar, T.A. and Wolfsy, D. (2001). Phase 1 clinical trial of a monoclonal antibody against CD40 ligand (IDEC-131) in patients with systemic lupus erythematosus. J Rheumatol 28, 95–101.

Deapen, D., Escalante, A. and Weinrib, L. (1992). A revised estimate of twin concordance in systemic lupus erythematosus. Arthritis Rheum 35, 311–318.

Edworthy, S., Fritzler, M., Whitehead, C., Martin, L. and Rattner, J.B. (2000). ASE-1: an autoantigen in systemic lupus erythematosus. Lupus 9, 681–687.

Godfrey, T., Cuadrado, M.J., Fofi, C. et al. (2001). Chromium-51 ethylenediamine tetraacetic acid glomerular filtration rate: a better predictor than glomerular filtration rate calculated by the Cockcroft-Gault formula for renal involvement in systemic lupus erythematosus patients. Rheumatology 40, 324–328.

Goulet, J.R., Mackenzie, T., Lewinton, C., Hayslett, J.P., Campi, A. and Esdaille, J.M. (1993). The long term prognosis of lupus nephritis: the impact of disease activity. J Rheumatol 20, 59–65.

Gourley, M.F., Austin, H.A., Scott, D. et al. (1996). Methylprednisolone and cyclophosphamide, alone or in combination in patients with lupus nephritis. Ann Intern Med 125, 549–557.

Graninger, W.B., Steiner, C.W., Graninger M.T., Aringer, M. and Smolen, J.S. (2000). Cytokine regulation of apoptosis and Bcl-2 expression in lymphocytes of patients with systemic lupus erythematosus. Cell Death Different 7, 966–972.

Herrmann, M., Voll, R. E., Zoller, O.M., Hagenhofer, M., Ponner, B. B. and Kalden, J.R. (1998). Impaired phagocytosis of apoptotic cell material by monocyte-derived macrophages from patients with systemic lupus erythematosus. Arthritis Rheum 41, 1241–1250.

Isenberg, D.A. and Ramsey-Goldman, R. (1999). Assessing patients with lupus: towards a drug responder index. Rheumatology 38, 1045–1049.

Isenberg, D.A. and Gordon, C. (2000). From Bilag to Blips – disease activity assessment in lupus past, present and future. Lupus 9, 651–654.

Jacob, C.O., Fronek, Z., Lewis, G.D., Koo, M., Hansen, J.A. and McDevitt, H.O. (1990a). Heritable major histocompatibility complex class II-associated differences in relevance to genetic predisposition to systemic lupus erythematosus. Proc Natl Acad Sci USA 87, 1233–1237.

Jacob, C.O., Van der Meide, P. H. and McDevitt, H.O. (1990b). In vivo treatment of (NZB X NZW) F1 lupus-like nephritis with monoclonal antibody to γ interferon. J Exp Med 166, 798–803.

Llorente, L., Richaud-Patin, Y. Garcia-Padilla, C. et al. (2000). Clinical and biologic effects of anti-interleukin-10 monoclonal antibody administration in systemic lupus erythematosus. Arthritis Rheum 43, 1790–1800.

Loizou, S., Samarkos, M., Norsworthy, P.J., Cazabon, J.K., Walport, M.J. and Davies, K.A. (2000). Significance of anti-cardiolipin and anti-beta(2) glycoprotein antibodies in lupus nephritis. Rheumatology (Oxford) 39, 962–968.

Machold, K.P. and Smolen, J.S. (1990). Interferon-γ induced exacerbation of systemic lupus erythematosus. J Rheumatol 17, 831–832.

Mamoune, A., Kerdreux, S., Durand, V. et al. (2000). CD45 autoantibodies mediate neutralization of activated T cells from lupus patients through anergy or apoptosis. Lupus 9, 622–631.

McLaughlin, J.R., Bombardier, C., Farewell, V.T., Gladman, D.A., and Urowitz, M.B. (1994). Kidney biopsy in systemic lupus erythematosus. III. Survival analysis, controlling for clinical and laboratory variables. Arthritis Rheum 4, 559–567.

Moss, K.E., Ioannou, Y., Sultan, S.M., Haq, I. and Isenberg, D.A (2002). Outcome of a cohort of 300 patients with systemic lupus erythematosus attending a dedicated clinic for over two decades. Ann Rheum Dis 61, 409–413.

Napirei, M., Karsunky, H., Zevnik, B., Stephan, H., Mannherz, H.G. and Moroy, T. (2002). Features of systemic lupus erythematosus in Dnase-1 deficient mice. Nat Genet 25, 177–181.

Norris, D.A. (1993). Pathomechanisms of photosensitive lupus erythematosus (review). J Invest Dermatol *100*, 58S–68S.

Pistiner, M., Wallace, D.J., Nessim, S., Metzger, A. L. and Klinenberg, J. R. (1992). Lupus erythematosus in the 1980s: a survey of 570 patients. Semin Arthritis Rheum *21*, 358–363.

Remer, C. F., Wiseman, M.H. and Wallace, D.J. (2001). Benefits of Leflunomide in systemic lupus erythematosus: a pilot observational study. Lupus *10*, 480–483.

Siegert, C.E., Kazatchkine, M.D., Sjoholm, A., Wurznerr Loos, M. and Daha, M.R. (1999). Autoantibodies against C1q view on clinical relevance and pathogenic role. Clin Exp Immunol *116*, 4–8.

Swaak, A.J.G., Aarden, L.A. and Statius van Eps, L.W. (1979). Anti dsDNA and complement profiles as prognostic guides in systemic lupus erythematosus. Arthritis Rheum *22*, 226–235.

Teh, L.S. and Isenberg, D.A. (1994). Antiribosomal P protein antibodies in systemic lupus erythematosus. A reappraisal. Arthritis Rheum *37*, 307–315.

Twomey, B.N., Dhillon, V.B., Latchman, D.S. et al. (1996). Lupus and heat shock proteins. In Stress Proteins in Medicine, Van Eden, W. and Young, D.B., eds. New York: Marcel Dekker Inc., pp. 345–357.

Wu, J., Wilson, J., He, J., Xiang, L., Schur, P.H. and Mountz, J.D. (1996). Fas ligand mutation in a patient with systemic lupus erythematosus and lymphoproliferative disease. J Clin Invest *98*, 1107–1113.

Yamada, A., Minota, S., Nojima, Y. and Yazaki, Y. (1993). Changes in subset specificity of anti-T cell autoantibodies in systemic lupus erythematosus. Autoimmunity *14*, 269–273.

Yasuma, M., Takasaki, Y., Marsumoto, K. et al. (1990). Clinical significance of IgG anti-Sm antibodies in patients with systemic lupus erythematosus. J Rheumatol *17*, 469–475.

Autoimmunity – Multiple Sclerosis

Chapter 45

Beau M. Ances[1], Nancy J. Newman[2] and Laura J. Balcer[1]

[1] Department of Neurology, Hospital of the University of Pennsylvania, Philadelphia, PA; [2] Department of Neurology, Emory School of Medicine, Emory University, Atlanta, GA, USA

Dreams are nothing but incoherent ideas, occasioned by partial or imperfect sleep.

Benjamin Rush (1746–1813)

EPIDEMIOLOGY

MS is a common cause of neurological disability in middle-aged adults. This disease affects over one million people worldwide and is very common within the USA (Minden et al., 1993; Pugliatti et al., 2002; O'Connor et al., 2002). Age, sex, race, geographical latitude, genetics and environmental exposure are risk factors for developing MS.

The median age of onset of MS is approximately 24 years of age (Minden et al., 1993) with a female to male ratio of two to one (O'Connor et al., 2002). The mean age of death of MS patients is 58 years old, compared to the general national average in the USA of 72 years old (Minden et al., 1993). Within the USA, MS is observed more often in Caucasians compared to African-Americans (Minden et al., 1993). However, the typical clinical course is more severe within African-Americans who are affected (Pugliatti et al., 2002). In regard to geographical patterns, a higher incidence of MS occurs when moving either more north or south of the equator, especially in countries with colder climates (Pugliatti et al., 2002). This latitude effect is also present within the USA as the incidence of MS is highest within the upper Midwest and Northeast compared to the South (Minden et al., 1993).

Family studies have shown that genetic factors contribute to MS (Sadovnick, 2002; Herrera and Ebers, 2003; Kenealy et al., 2003; Willer et al., 2003). The risk for developing MS within dizygotic twins is the same as for other siblings (3–5 per cent). However, the risk for monozygotic twins is greater than 30 per cent (O'Connor et al., 2002; Willer et al., 2003). A greater than 10-fold increased risk of developing MS exists within individuals having certain human leukocyte antigens (HLA) genotypes (O'Connor et al., 2002; Sadovnick, 2002; Herrera and Ebers , 2003; Kenealy et al., 2003). The major predisposing associated haplotype is HLA-DR2 in cellular typing nomenclature (DR15,DQ6 by serology and DRB5*0101-DQA1*0102-DQB1*0602 by sequence-based terminology) (Haegert and Francis, 1993; Hillert, 1994). Even though an association between HLA class II DRB1*15 and DRB1*17 alleles and MS has been seen in individuals of northern European and Mediterranean descent, the presence of these haplotypes does not preclude the development of MS (Sadovnick, 2002; Herrera and Ebers, 2003; Kenealy et al., 2003). Genetic interactions may also occur between certain haplotypes and certain T cell receptors, immunoglobulins and tumor necrosis factors which may lead to an increased chance of developing MS (O'Connor et al., 2002; Alizadeh et al., 2003).

Not only genetic but also one or more exogenous or environmental factors may influence the development of MS (O'Connor et al., 2002). Although twin studies have provided strong evidence for genetic factors in the development of MS, the concordance rate for monozygotic twins has never been demonstrated to be greater than 40 per cent (Compston and Ebers, 1990; Sadovnick, 2002;

Measuring Immunity, edited by Michael T. Lotze and Angus W. Thomson
ISBN 0-12-455900-X, London

Willer et al., 2003). Thus, at least 60 per cent of persons with an identical twin who has MS will not develop the disease.

Certain foods, toxins, psychological stress, anesthesia, surgery and physical trauma have been implicated in the development of MS (O'Connor et al., 2002). However, no direct causal relationships have been proven to date. Overall, it is believed that both genetic and environmental factors are responsible for the subsequent development of MS within a susceptible individual (O'Connor et al., 2002). The resulting disability that results from MS leads to a major burden not only to the affected individual but also to the health care system and society (Whetten-Goldstein et al., 1998).

PATHOPHYSIOLOGY

Loss of myelin due to inflammation with limited subsequent remyelination are the two cardinal features of MS (Noseworthy et al., 2000). Breakdown of the blood–brain barrier is typically observed with early inflammatory changes (Smith et al., 1993). Immunocytochemical studies of active MS lesions have shown damage to vascular walls with intramural deposition of complement on smooth muscle components as well as protein-rich leakage (Noseworthy et al., 2000). These abnormalities can occur within hours to days of an acute attack and slowly resolve over subsequent weeks to months (Poser, 1986).

Typical pathological findings seen in MS are plaques containing inflammatory cells scattered throughout the affected parenchyma and arranged in cuffs around blood vessels (Figure 45.1). Inflammatory cells that are stimulated during an acute flare include macrophages, lymphocytes, large mononuclear cells and plasma cells (Prineas and Wright, 1978; Tourbah et al., 1993). In MS macrophages are immunologically active and can stimulate T cells leading to the subsequent production of large quantities of cytokines and inflammatory mediators (Hafler and Weiner, 1995; Hohlfeld et al., 1995; Martin and McFarland, 1995;

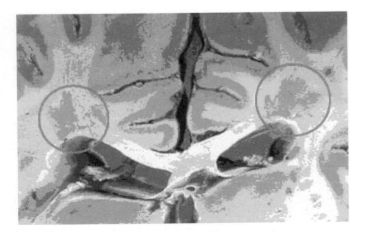

Figure 45.1 Circles surround perventricular plaques seen on pathology.

O'Connor et al., 2000). These cytokines can be either pro- or anti-inflammatory in nature (Hafler and Weiner, 1995) with a T cell either stimulatory or inhibitory depending on surrounding environment factors (Hafler and Weiner, 1995; McFarland, 1995; Hohlfeld, 1997).

Axonal loss has also shown to be a key factor in the pathogenesis of MS and is responsible for part of the irreversible clinical impairment and disability (O'Connor et al., 2002). Axonal loss could stem from:

1 direct autoimmune attack against axons
2 a 'bystander injury' due to exposure of axons to immune attack following demyelination
3 degeneration of axons as a result of chronic demyelination
4 primary degeneration of axons, stimulating a secondary inflammatory response (Trapp et al., 1999; Lassmann, 2003).

The importance of these potential associated mechanisms remains to be determined.

ETIOLOGY

The exact etiology of MS remains unknown, but it is believed that this disease most likely results from a viral infection. These organisms can induce disturbances within a previously competent or compromised immune system (Allen and Brankin, 1993; Cook et al., 1995; O'Connor et al., 2002). MS may either be due to infection by viruses that directly induce neurological dysfunction from the onset or result from reactivation later in life. A number of organisms or their nucleic acids have been observed within the CSF or brain parenchyma of patients with MS (Booss and Kim, 1990; O'Connor et al., 2002). These organisms include mycoplasma (Cevassut, 1930), protozoa (Bequignon, 1956), spirochetes (Ichelson, 1957), as well as a number of both DNA and RNA viruses, such as herpes simplex viruses types 1, 2 and 6 (Sanders et al., 1996), rabies virus (Bychkova, 1964), parainfluenza virus type I (ter Meulen et al., 1972), coronavirus (Talbot et al., 1996), canine distemper virus (Rohowsky-Kochan et al., 1995), measles virus (Haase et al., 1981), human immunodeficiency virus type 1 (HIV-1) (Berger et al., 1989) and human T lymphotrophic virus type I (HTLV-I) (Salmi et al., 1983; Greenberg et al., 1989). However, none of the above organisms have been successfully isolated from large groups of clinically definite MS patients. Furthermore, within MS patients infected with these organisms, levels did not correlate with disease activity (O'Connor et al., 2002).

Despite the lack of definitive evidence of a viral source for MS, it is commonly believed that one or more viruses may be responsible for the development of MS within certain genetically susceptible individuals (Allen and Brankin, 1993; Cook et al., 1995). One hypothesis for the mechanism in which viruses cause MS has been proposed which involves both direct and indirect pathways (Clausen, 2003). Viruses could directly damage and lead to functional alterations within oligodendrocytes, resulting in demyelination. Because a single oligodendrocyte can send processes to many neighboring axons, impairment can cause demyelination within a large volume of brain tissue (Silberberg, 1986). Viral invasion may also directly damage endothelial cells within blood vessels and lead to a disruption of the blood–brain barrier. This may subsequently allow for indirect mechanisms in which immunocompetent or activated T lymphocytes can gain entry into the CNS. Demyelination could develop due to the release of cytokines from these activated cells (Poser, 1986; Noseworthy et al., 2000).

Another theory has suggested that viral infection leads to demyelination due to repeated constant exposure of certain antigens to the immune system (Clausen, 2003). An inappropriate immune sensitivity results with antibodies cross-reacting against the oligodendrocyte and/or vascular endothelial cells (Allen and Brankin, 1993; Cook et al., 1995). Alternatively, viral infection might cause a disorder of immunoregulation and secondary demyelination (Salonen et al., 1982). Myelin may not be the primary focus of attack but instead may be an 'innocent bystander' with the large-scale destruction that occurs resulting from the interaction of the immune system and reactivated viral infection (Silberberg, 1986; Clausen, 2003).

CLINICAL MANIFESTATIONS

There are no clinical findings that are unique to MS (Kurtzke, 1983; Lisak, 2004). Symptoms and signs that result from MS can include neurological, neuro-ophthalmologic and psychiatric features.

Neurological signs and symptoms

Neurological signs and symptoms of MS are caused primarily by both demyelination and axonal loss that can occur within the cerebral hemispheres, cerebellum, brain stem and spinal cord. Demyelination and destruction of axons produce a variety of somatosensory, motor, cerebellar symptoms and signs (Miller, 1990; Matthews et al., 1991; Kinkel and Rudick, 2002; Lisak, 2004).

Sensory symptoms are the most common clinical manifestations of MS and present as the initial manifestation of the disease in over 70 per cent of MS patients (Kurtzke, 1970; McAlpine, 1972). The anatomic distribution of sensory symptoms often does not correspond to a recognized dermatome, peripheral nerve or homuncular pattern. Some patients may complain of numbness, whereas others are bothered by sensations of tingling, burning or tightness.

Up to 40 per cent of cases of MS will initially present with motor symptoms and signs (Mueller, 1949; Miller,

1990; Matthews et al., 1991; Kinkel and Rudick, 2002; Lisak, 2004). Patients with motor dysfunction may complain of heaviness, stiffness and/or pain in one or more extremities. Typically these symptoms are present in the legs more often than within the arms. Spasticity can also develop and often produces significant discomfort or frank pain (Hooge and Redekop, 1992, 1993).

Cerebellar symptoms and signs can sometimes be seen on initial presentation but typically occur in patients with well-established MS. Cerebellar signs usually manifest as gait ataxia, limb dysmetria and intention tremor (Kurtzke, 1970; McAlpine, 1972). Many patients develop a non-specific impairment of articulation leading to a speech disturbance called 'scanning speech'.

A Lhermitte's sign, sudden electric-like sensations that radiate down the spine or extremities upon neck flexion, can also be observed. This sign results from a demyelinating lesion in the cervical spinal cord. However, it is not pathognomonic for MS and can be observed within patients with cervical pathology, neck trauma, radiation myelopathy and subacute combined degeneration of the spinal cord (Matthews et al., 1991).

Fatigue can also be seen within MS patients and is usually present in greater than 80 per cent of individuals eventually diagnosed with MS (Tartaglia et al., 2004; Racke and Hawker, 2004; Fisk et al., 1994; Vercoulen et al., 1996; Kinkel and Rudick, 2002; Lisak, 2004). This symptom is particularly bothersome for those with mild to moderate disease. Many patients will complain of a complete lack of motivation. These symptoms can be so severe that they are unable to carry out even the most simple activities of daily living (Miller, 1990; Kinkel and Rudick, 2002). Typically these patients experience fatigue in the setting of motor difficulties (Vercoulen et al., 1996).

Neuro-ophthalmologic manifestations

Optic neuritis (ON) may be the initial presentation of MS (Leibowitz and Alter, 1968; Kuroiwa and Shibasaki, 1973; McDonald and Barnes, 1992). ON usually presents as acute or subacute unilateral eye pain (about 2/3 of the time) accentuated by retro-orbital pain with eye movements. A variable degree of visual loss within the central vision can be observed (Leibowitz and Alter, 1968; Kuroiwa and Shibasaki, 1973). Often the patient with ON will complain of a loss of color vision (red desaturation). Physical examination can reveal a relative afferent pupillary defect. Most often the lesion in ON is retrobulbar with the fundoscopic examination normal during the acute stages (Nordmann et al., 1987). Later, as the disease progresses, the optic disc can become pale as a result of axonal loss and resultant gliosis with temporal pallor present. Typically acute ON will get worse over a time period of several days to 2 weeks, with subsequent visual recovery slowly occurring over 2–4 weeks (Beck et al., 1994). Improvement from ON can continue to progress for up to 1 year after the initial onset of visual symptoms (Beck et al., 1993c).

The Optic Neuritis Treatment Trial (ONTT) was a multicenter trial that attempted to assess the benefit of treatment with corticosteroids on visual recovery in acute optic neuritis (Optic Neuritis Study Group, 1991, 2004; Beck et al., 1993a; Jacobs et al., 2000; Liu, 2000; CHAMPS Study Group, 2001). The ONTT enrolled 457 patients, aged 18–46 years, with acute unilateral optic neuritis. Patients in the ONTT were randomized to one of three treatment protocols:

1 oral prednisone (1 mg/kg/day) for 14 days with a 4-day taper
2 intravenous (IV) methylprednisolone sodium succinate (250 mg every 6 h for 3 days) followed by a course of oral prednisone (1 mg/kg/day) for 11 days with a 4-day taper
3 oral placebo for 14 days (Beck et al., 1992; Trobe et al., 1996).

The major findings of the ONTT were:

1 IV methylprednisolone hastened the recovery of visual function in acute optic neuritis, but had no long-term benefits in visual outcome at either 6 months or at 10 years when compared to placebo or oral prednisone. This medication was most beneficial if given within the first 15 days of presentation
2 treatment with oral prednisone alone was associated with an increased rate of recurrent optic neuritis in not only the affected eye but the contralateral eye as well at both 6 months and at 10 years
3 monosymptomatic patients in the IV methylprednisolone group had a reduced rate for the subsequent development of MS during the first 2 years of follow up, but this benefit was not observed beyond 2 years (Optic Neuritis Study Group, 1991, 2004).

These results suggest that no effective treatment exists for preventing patients who develop acute ON from subsequently developing long-term visual disability (Söderström, 2001; Biousse and Newman, 2002; Foroozan et al., 2002).

The average interval from initial presentation of ON symptoms until subsequent development of MS can vary but typically occurs within 5–7 years (Optic Neuritis Study Group, 1991, 2004). Brain MRI is a powerful technique for predicting subsequent events in MS patients with acute ON (Optic Neuritis Study Group, 1991, 2004; Beck et al., 1993b). The presence of even a single characteristic brain MRI lesion at the time of acute ON is associated with a significantly increased risk (Optic Neuritis Study Group, 2004). More than one lesion on MRI does not substantially increase this risk. Patients with no lesions on MRI and with atypical ON have a very low risk of developing MS.

Internuclear ophthalmoplegia (INO) refers to abnormal horizontal ocular movements with loss or delayed adduction and horizontal nystagmus of the abducting eye due to a lesion in the medial longitudinal fasciculus on the side of diminished adduction (Reulen et al., 1983; Müri and Meienberg, 1985; Gass and Hennerici, 1997). The adduction weakness may be manifest as:

1 complete inability to adduct the eye beyond the midline
2 a mild limitation of adduction associated with decreased velocity of adduction or
3 a mild decrease in the velocity of adducting saccades without any limitation of adduction (Meienberg et al., 1986).

Patients with a unilateral INO can also have a skew deviation with the higher eye on the side of the lesion (Thömke et al., 1992).

Psychiatric manifestations

Neuropsychiatric manifestations may appear at any time of the disease and commonly precede definitive neurological manifestations by months to years (Schiffer and Babigian, 1984; Herndon, 1990; Hutchinson et al., 1993). Overall, cognitive changes can be observed in almost 50 per cent of MS patients (Patti et al., 2003; Benedict et al., 2004). Symptoms tend to progress as the disease worsens (Hutchinson et al., 1993). The most common neuropsychiatric signs and symptoms are disturbances in cognition especially within recent memory, information processing, abstraction and conceptual reasoning (Herndon, 1990; Miller, 1990; Ron and Feinstein, 1992; Benedict et al., 2000; Patti et al., 2003; Lisak, 2004).

Depression can also be a common finding in MS patients with up to 75 per cent experiencing some form of depression during their illness (Schiffer and Babigian, 1984; Kinkel and Rudick, 2002; Patti et al., 2003; Lisak, 2004). The degree of depression can range from mild to severe (Patti et al., 2003; Lisak, 2004) and typically develops after other clinical manifestations. This progression suggests that depression may result within individuals from a greater understanding and knowledge of their disease process rather than due to a direct reaction to the illness. Depression may be quite difficult to identify in some patients, as symptoms can overlap with other disease features, including fatigue, diminished attention and concentration and pain (Kinkel and Rudick, 2002).

GUIDES TO THE DIAGNOSIS OF MS

MS is clinically diagnosed with additional support coming from neuroimaging and paraclinical sources, such as cerebral spinal fluid and evoked potentials. A detailed clinical history requires documentation of at least two discrete episodes within time affecting the CNS (Poser et al., 1983). The McDonald criteria have been developed to assist in the diagnosis of MS. Based on the extent to which the diagnostic criteria are fulfilled for a particular clinical presentation, patients can be categorized as 'MS' (diagnostic criteria fulfilled), 'possible MS' (criteria not completely met – patient at risk but diagnostic evaluation is equivocal) or 'not MS' (criteria fully explored and not met) (McDonald, et al., 2001). The McDonald criteria have successfully been shown to accurately diagnose MS in patients with recent onset of a clinically isolated syndrome. At least two studies have evaluated the sensitivity and specificity of these criteria. One study prospectively evaluated 50 patients at 3 months, 1 year and 3 years of follow up and demonstrated a sensitivity and specificity of 83 per cent (McDonald, et al., 2001). A second study analyzed 139 patients using a retrospective analysis found similar results (Dalton et al., 2004).

The diagnosis of MS is assisted by neuroimaging findings that show evidence of dissemination of lesions within time and space. MRI is particularly sensitive for detecting lesions in the brain stem, cerebellum and spinal cord (Cutler et al., 1986; Ormerod et al., 1986; Grossman and McGowan, 1998; Fazekas et al., 1999; Arnold and Matthews, 2002; Bot et al., 2004) (Figure 45.2). Gadolinium (Gad) can be injected and assists in the diagnosis of newly active plaques. Gad enhancement diminishes or disappears after treatment with corticosteroids due to restoration of the blood–brain barrier. Lesions that are more suggestive of MS include those that are 6 mm or more in diameter, ovoid, abutting the lateral ventricles and infratentorial (Arnold and Matthews, 2002). Usually lesions will be observed within the periventricular region, corpus callosum, centrum semiovale and, to a lesser extent, within deeper white matter structures and the basal ganglia. Lesions seen on MRI in MS patients often will fluctuate over time (Grossman and McGowan, 1998; Arnold and Matthews, 2002) with some lesions disappearing, some reappearing, some enlarging, some decreasing and some remaining unchanged (Grossman and

McGowan, 1998; Arnold and Matthews, 2002). However, the extent of MRI abnormalities may not correlate with the degree of clinical disability.

Despite these advances in neuroimaging, lesions that are observed may not always be MS (Arnold and Matthews, 2002). Healthy patients over 50 years of age can have similar lesions due to atherosclerotic and hypertensive cerebrovascular disease, CNS vasculitis, migraine, sarcoidosis, venous angiomas and both primary and metastatic brain tumors (Paty, 1990; Boppana and Zagzag, 1993; Arnold and Matthews, 2002). Therefore neuroimaging findings alone cannot be used in the diagnosis of MS.

In addition to demyelinating lesion burden and activity, neuronal and axonal loss are likely to have a crucial role in the development of neurological and visual impairment in MS (Raine and Cross, 1989; Ferguson et al., 1997). Proton MR spectroscopy (MRS) can also provide information on phospholipid metabolism as well as other metabolic components, such as N-acetyl aspartate (NAA) (an exclusively neuronal marker), creatine phosphate (Cr) (a marker of energy metabolism), choline (a cell membrane component), and lactic acid (LA) (Larsson et al., 1991; DeStefano et al., 1995; Kimura et al., 1996; Matthews et al., 1996). Acute MS lesions can have a decrease in NAA and an increase in LA. Chronic MS brains have a reduced amount of NAA as well as a reduced NAA/Cr ratio due to loss of neurons or axons (DeStefano et al., 1995).

Cerebrospinal fluid analysis

Examination of CSF can also assists in the diagnosis of MS (McDonald et al., 2001). Typically glucose and protein levels in the cerebrospinal fluid (CSF) are normal in MS. A few mononuclear cells per cubic millimeter may also be observed. Often a significant elevation of the CSF immunoglobulin level relative to other protein components is present. This immunoglobulin increase is predominantly IgG with an excess primarily in lambda and kappa light chains (Whitaker et al., 1990; Fukazawa et al., 1993). The IgG level may be expressed as a percentage of total protein (normal < 11 per cent), as a percentage of albumin (normal < 27 per cent) or by the use of the IgG index (normal value < 0.66) (Whitaker et al., 1990). CSF IgG production abnormalities, as measured by the IgG index, are found in more than 75 per cent of clinically definite MS patients (Miller et al., 1983; Zeman et al., 1993, 1996; Lowenthal and Karcher, 1994). An elevation in oligoclonal bands can also be observed and is seen in more than 80 per cent of patients with clinically definite MS (Zeman et al., 1993, 1996). More recently, the presence of serum anti-myelin basic protein (MBP) antibodies can predict progression to MS after a clinically isolated event. MBP is one of the major components of myelin and is normally negligible in the CSF. During an acute MS flare it rises and falls quickly (Warren and Catz, 2003).

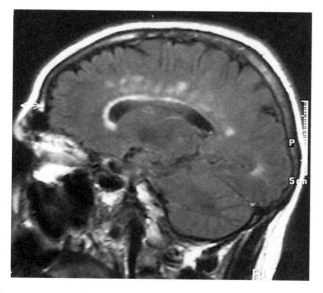

Figure 45.2 MRI of patient showing multiple demyelinating plaques.

Visually evoked potentials (VEPs)

VEPs are electric potentials or voltages evoked by brief sensory stimuli. These signals are delayed, attenuated or absent within regions of demyelination. An abnormal VEP is seen in 85 per cent of clinically definite MS cases (Brooks and Chiappa, 1982). However, almost any pathophysiologic process that damages the optic nerve can affect VEP results (Asselman et al., 1975; Wilson, 1978). In addition, even though VEPs are considered an 'objective' test and are used in the McDonald criteria they may be affected by the patient's age, attention and concentration (Regan, 1972; Regan et al., 1977; Hawkes and Stow, 1981).

TREATMENT

Although some patients with MS have an illness that is slowly progressive from onset (primary progressive MS, or PPMS) and others have an acute, rapidly progressive disease (acute MS), most cases of MS begin with a relapsing-remitting course (RRMS). While not all patients with RRMS develop a progressive course, secondary progressive MS (SPMS) is a long-term sequela of RRMS for many patients (Lublin et al., 1996). While patients with RRMS have clearly defined relapses with a lack of disease progression during inter-relapse intervals, SPMS is characterized by disease progression and worsening of neurologic baseline following an initially relapsing-remitting course. Treatments must therefore be targeted not only toward reducing inflammatory responses and numbers of exacerbations in patients with MS, but ideally should minimize disease progression and axonal loss (Noseworthy et al., 2000; O'Connor, 2002).

Corticosteroids are often used in acute attacks. Treatment usually consists of a short course of IV methylprednisolone, 500 to 1000 mg daily for 3–5 days, with or without a taper. As demonstrated by the ONTT, oral steroid therapy alone should probably not be offered to patients with acute optic neuritis. Patients treated with oral prednisone alone are more likely to suffer recurrent episodes of optic neuritis than those treated with methylprednisolone followed by oral prednisone taper (Optic Neuritis Study Group, 1991, 2004).

Treatment for RRMS consists of starting disease modifying medications, including the interferons or glatiramer acetate. These medications can lead to a decrease in the frequency of relapses and reduce disability in patients with RRMS.

Interferon-beta-1b (Betaseron)

This drug is a cytokine that modulates immune responsiveness, although its precise mechanism of action in MS is unknown. Interferon-beta-1b is administered every other day subcutaneously by self-injection (Arnason, 1993). The efficacy of interferon-beta-1b was demonstrated in a double blind, placebo-controlled trial of patients with RRMS who were randomly assigned to either interferon-beta-1b or placebo (Paty and Li, 1993). After 2 years, the exacerbation rate was significantly lower for patients receiving interferon-beta-1b compared to placebo. The INCOMIN study (independent comparison of interferons) compared interferon-beta-1b (Betaseron) with intramuscular interferon-beta-1a (Avonex) in 188 patients with relapsing-remitting MS and found the former to be more effective on both clinical and MRI outcomes. Over a 2-year period, patients had more relapse free periods as well as developing fewer new MRI lesions on interferon-beta-1b compared to those assigned to interferon-beta-1a (Durelli et al., 2002).

Interferon-beta-1a (Avonex)

Like interferon-beta-1b this drug is a cytokine that modulates immune responsiveness. Interferon-beta-1a is given by weekly intramuscular injections. The efficacy of interferon-beta-1a in patients with RRMS was demonstrated in a randomized, double blind study comparing interferon-beta-1a to placebo (Jacobs et al., 1996). Over a 2-year period, patients treated with interferon-beta-1a had a reduction in the annual exacerbation rate, a decrease in MRI lesion volume burden and less disability compared to patients receiving placebo. In a subsequent study, the Controlled High-Risk Avonex MS Prevention Study (CHAMPS), patients newly diagnosed with MS (those who suffered a first acute clinical demyelinating event and who also had evidence of prior subclinical demyelination on brain MRI) were treated with either Avonex or placebo after initial treatment with corticosteroid therapy. Treatment with Avonex led to a significantly lower probability of developing clinically definitive MS during the subsequent 3 years of follow up compared to patients who were treated with corticosteroids followed by placebo (Jacobs et al., 2000; Galetta, 2001; CHAMPS Study Group, 2002). An extension study of the CHAMPS with all patients on active interferon beta-1a therapy, the Controlled High-Risk Avonex MS Prevention Surveillance (CHAMPIONS) has provided additional data in support of early use of Avonex for the treatment of MS (Kinkel et al., 2003).

Interferon-beta-1a at higher doses (Rebif) has also been shown to be beneficial in RRMS. This medication is given subcutaneously three times a week. The efficacy of interferon-beta-1a was shown through the Prevention of Relapses and Disability by Interferon-beta-1a Subcutaneously in Multiple Sclerosis (PRISMS) study. In this study RRMS patients were given placebo or Rebif three times per week for 2 years. Treatment with Rebif also led to a significant reduction in the MRI lesion burden. Approval for Rebif in the USA arose from results from the EVIDENCE trial in which Rebif was compared directly to Avonex (PRISMS Study Group, 1998). Relapse rate was less frequent and the mean number of active MRI lesions was lower for patients on Rebif compared to those on Avonex.

The main side effects of interferons are flu-like symptoms and depression that tend to diminish with time. Periodic laboratory evaluations including liver enzymes, complete white blood cell counts and thyroid function tests should be performed every 3–6 months. All of the interferons are capable of stimulating the production of neutralizing antibodies that can limit the efficacy of these agents (Sorensen et al., 2003). The risk of antibody formation over 18 months of treatment is highest with Betaseron, intermediate with Rebif and lowest with Avonex (Bertolotto et al., 2003).

Glatiramer acetate (Copaxone)

Glatiramer acetate (Copaxone), a daily subcutaneous injectable synthetic polymer, has been shown to have some positive effects in a small double-blind trial of RRMS (Bornstein et al., 1987). Studies have shown a lower relapse rate and a significant reduction in the number of new T2 lesions compared to placebo. Side effects can include local injection site reactions and transient systemic post-injection reactions such as chest pain, flushing, dyspnea, palpitations and/or anxiety. No laboratory monitoring is necessary and no neutralizing antibodies have been detected.

There are now a number of medications approved by the US Food and Drug Administration for the treatment of RRMS. There are no clear guidelines, nor is there strong evidence for choosing one drug versus another (Galetta et al., 2002). After making a diagnosis of MS the patient should be started on one of the medications listed above. MS patients should be notified that these therapies primarily slow the disease course but are not a cure. These drugs are typically continued indefinitely unless side effects are intolerable or the patient begins to fail in terms of response, after which use of another agent can be considered.

ACKNOWLEDGEMENTS

This chapter was revised from Multiple Sclerosis and Related Demyelinating Diseases by Nancy J. Newman and Laura J. Balcer in Walsh and Hoyt's Clinical Neuro-ophthalmology (2004).

REFERENCES

Alizadeh, M., Babron, M.C., Birebent, B. et al. (2003). Genetic interaction of CTLA-4 with HLA-DR15 in multiple sclerosis patients. Ann Neurol 54,119–122.
Allen, I.V. and Brankin, B. (1993). Pathogenesis of multiple sclerosis – the immune diathesis and the role of viruses. J Neuropathol Exp Neurol 52, 95–105.
Arnason, B.G. (1993). Interferon beta in multiple sclerosis (editorial; comment). Neurology 43, 641–643.
Arnold, D.L. and Matthews, P.M. (2002). MRI in the diagnosis and management of multiple sclerosis. Neurology 58, S23–S31.
Asselman, P., Chadwick, D.W. and Marsden, C.D. (1975). Visual evoked responses in the diagnosis and management of patients suspected of multiple sclerosis. Brain 98, 261–282.
Beck, R.W., Cleary, P.A., Anderson, M.M, Jr et al. (1992). A randomized, controlled trial of corticosteroids in the treatment of acute optic neuritis. N Engl J Med 326, 581–588.
Beck, R.W., Cleary, P.A., Trobe, J.D. et al. (1993a). The effect of corticosteroids for acute optic neuritis on the subsequent development of multiple sclerosis. N Engl J Med 329, 1764–1769.
Beck, R.W., Arrington, J., Murtagh, F.R. et al. and The Optic Neuritis Study Group (1993b). Brain magnetic resonance imaging in acute optic neuritis: Experience of The Optic Neuritis Study Group. Arch Ophthalmol 50, 841–846.
Beck, R.W., Cleary, P.A. and The Optic Neuritis Study Group. (1993c). Optic Neuritis Treatment Trial. One-year follow-up results. Arch Ophthalmol 111, 773–775.
Beck, R.W., Cleary, P.A., Backlund, J.C. et al. (1994). The course of visual recovery after optic neuritis: experience of the Optic Neuritis Treatment Trial. Ophthalmology 101, 1771–1778.
Benedict, R.H.B., Weinstock-Guttman, B., Fishman, I. et al. (2004). Prediction of neuropsychological impairment in multiple sclerosis: comparison of conventional magnetic resonance imaging measures of atrophy and lesion burden. Arch Neurol 61, 226–230.
Bequignon, R. (1956). De l'étiologie de la sclérose en plaques. CR Acad Sci 242, 1380–1382.
Berger, J.R., Sheremata, W.A., Resnick, L. et al. (1989). Multiple sclerosis-like illness occurring with human immunodeficiency virus infection. Neurology 39, 324–329.
Bertolotto, A., Gilli, F., Sala, A. et al. (2003). Persistent neutralizing antibodies abolish the interferon beta bioavailability in MS patients. Neurology 60, 634–639.
Biousse, V. and Newman, N.J. (2002). Optic neuritis. In Conn's Current Therapy. Philadelphia: W. B. Saunders, pp. 943–945.
Booss, J. and Kim, J.H. (1990). Evidence for a viral etiology of multiple sclerosis. In Handbook of Multiple Sclerosis, Cook, S.D., ed. New York: Marcel Dekker, pp. 41–62.
Boppana, M. and Zagzag, D. (1993). Central nervous system demyelination presenting as a mass lesion: A diagnostic challenge. Ann Neurol 34, 312.
Bornstein, M.B., Miller, A., Slagle, S. et al. (1987). A pilot trial of Cop 1 in exacerbating-remitting multiple sclerosis. N Engl J Med 317, 408–414.
Bot, J.C.J., Barkhof, F., Polman, C.H. et al. (2004). Spinal cord abnormalities in recently diagnosed MS patients: added value of spinal MRI examination. Neurology 62, 226–233.
Brooks, E.B. and Chiappa, K.H. (1982). A comparison of clinical neuro-ophthalmological findings and pattern shift evoked potentials in multiple sclerosis. In Clinical Applications of Evoked Potentials in Neurology, Courjan, J.J., Mauguiere, F. and Revol, M., eds. New York: Raven Press, pp. 435–437.
Bychkova, E.N. (1964). Viruses isolated from patients with encephalomyelitis and multiple sclerosis. Communication I: pathogenic and antigenic properties. Vopr Virusol 9, 173–176.
CHAMPS Study Group. (2001). Interferon β-1a for optic neuritis patients at high risk for multiple sclerosis. Am J Ophthalmol 132, 463–471.
CHAMPS Study Group. (2002). Baseline MRI characteristics of patients at high risk for multiple sclerosis: results from the CHAMPS trial. Multiple Sclerosis 8, 330–338.

Chevassut, K. (1930). The aetiology of disseminated sclerosis. Lancet 1, 552–560.

Clausen, J. (2003). Endogenous retroviruses and MS: using ERV's as disease markers. Int MS J 10, 20–21.

Compston, A. and Ebers, G.C. (1990). The genetics of multiple sclerosis. In Handbook of Multiple Sclerosis. Cook, S.D., ed. New York: Marcel Dekker, pp. 25–40.

Cook, S.D., Bansil, S., Boos, J. et al. (1995). Total lymphoid irradiation (TLI) and low-dose prednisone (LDP) in progressive multiple sclerosis (PMS). Neurology 45, A417.

Cutler, J.R., Aminoff, M.J. and Brant-Zawadzki M. (1986). Evaluation of patients with multiple sclerosis by evoked potentials and magnetic resonance imaging: A comparative study. Ann Neurol 20, 645–648.

Dalton, C.M., Brex, P.A., Miszkiel, K.A. et al. (2002). Application of the new McDonald Criteria to patients with clinically isolated syndromes suggestive of multiple sclerosis. Ann Neurol 52, 47–53.

DeStefano, N., Matthews, P., Antel, J. et al. (1995). Chemical pathology of acute demyelinating lesions and its correlation with disability. Ann Neurol 38, 901–909.

Durelli, L., Verdun, E., Barbero, P. et al., Independent Comparison of Interferon (INCOMIN) Trial Study Group (2002). Every-other-day interferon beta-1b versus once-weekly interferon beta-1a for multiple sclerosis: results of a 2-year prospective randomised multicentre study (INCOMIN). Lancet 359, 1453–1460.

Fazekas, F., Barkhof, F., Filippi, M. et al. (1998). The contribution of magnetic resonance imaging to the diagnosis of multiple sclerosis. Neurology 53, 448–456.

Ferguson, B., Matyszak, M.K., Esiri, M.M. and Perry V.H. (1997). Axonal damage in acute multiple sclerosis lesions. Brain 120, 393–399.

Fisk, J.D., Pontefract, A., Ritvo, P.G. et al. (1994). The impact of fatigue on patients with multiple sclerosis. Can J Neurol Sci 21, 9–14.

Foroozan, R., Buono, L.M., Savino, P.J. et al. (2002). Acute demyelinating optic neuritis. Curr Opin Ophthalmol 13, 375–380.

Fukazawa, T., Moriwaka, F., Sugiyama, K. et al. (1993). Cerebrospinal fluid IgG profiles and multiple sclerosis in Japan. Acta Neurol Scand 88, 178–183.

Galetta, S.L. (2001). The Controlled High-Risk Avonex Multiple Sclerosis Trial (CHAMPS Study). J Neuro-Ophthalmol 21, 292–295.

Galetta, S.L., Markowitz, C. and Lee, A.G. (2002). Immunomodulatory agents for the treatment of relapsing multiple sclerosis: a systematic review. Arch Intern Med 162, 2161–2169.

Gass, A. and Hennerici, M.G. (1997). Bilateral internuclear ophthalmoplegia in multiple sclerosis. J Neurol Neurosurg Psychiatr 63, 564.

Greenberg, S.J., Ehrlich, G.D., Abbott, M.A. et al. (1989). Detection of sequences homologous to retroviral DNA in multiple sclerosis by gene amplification. Proc Natl Acad Sci USA 86, 2878–2882.

Grossman, R.I. and McGowan, J.C. (1998). Perspectives on multiple sclerosis. Am J Neurol Radiol 19, 1251–1265.

Haase, A.T., Ventrua, P., Gibbs, C.J. Jr et al. (1981). Measles virus nucleotide sequences: Detection by hybridization in situ. Science 212, 672–674.

Haegert, D.G. and Francis, G.S. (1993). HLA-DQ polymorphisms do not explain HLA class II associations with multiple sclerosis in two Canadian groups. Neurology 43, 1207–1210.

Hafler, D.A. and Weiner, H.L. (1995). Immunologic mechanisms and therapy in multiple sclerosis. Immunol Rev 144, 75–105.

Hawkes, C.H. and Stow, B. (1981). Pupil size and the pattern evoked visual response. J Neurol Neurosurg Psychiatr 44, 90–91.

Herndon, R.M. (1990). Cognitive deficits and emotional dysfunction in multiple sclerosis. Arch Neurol 47,18.

Herrera, B.M. and Ebers, G.C. (2003). Progress in deciphering the genetics of multiple sclerosis. Curr Opin Neurol 16, 253–258.

Hillert, J. (1994). Human leukocyte antigen studies in multiple sclerosis. Ann Neurol 36, S15–S17.

Hohlfeld, R. (1997). Biotechnological agents for the immunotherapy of multiple sclerosis: Principles, problems and perspectives. Brain 120, 865–916.

Hohlfeld, R., Meinl, E., Weber, F. et al. (1995). The role of autoimmune T-lymphocytes in the pathogenesis of multiple sclerosis. Neurology 45, S33-S38.

Hooge, J.P. and Redekop, W.K. (1992). Multiple sclerosis with very late onset. Neurology 42, 1907–1910.

Hooge, J.P. and Redekop, W.K. (1993). Late-onset MS. Neurology 43, 1629.

Hutchinson, M., Stack, J. and Buckley, P. (1993). Bipolar affective disorder prior to the onset of multiple sclerosis. Acta Neurol Scand 88, 388–393.

Ichelson, R.R. (1957). Cultivation of spirochaetes from spinal fluids with multiple sclerosis cases and negative controls. Proc Soc Exp Biol Med 95, 57–58.

Jacobs, L.D., Cookfair, D.L., Rudick, R.A. et al. (1996). Intramuscular interferon beta-1a for disease progression in relapsing multiple sclerosis. The Multiple Sclerosis Collaborative Research Group (MSCRG). Ann Neurol 39, 285–294.

Jacobs, L.D., Beck, R.W., Simon, J.H. et al. (2000). Intramuscular interferon beta-1a therapy initiated during a first demyelinating event in multiple sclerosis. N Engl J Med 343, 898–904.

Kenealy, S.J., Pericak-Vance, M.A. and Haines, J.L. (2003). The genetic epidemiology of multiple sclerosis. J Neuroimmunol 143, 7–12.

Kimura, H., Grossman, R.I., Lenkinski, R.E. et al. (1996). Proton MR spectroscopy and magnetization transfer ratio in multiple sclerosis: correlative findings of active versus irreversible plaque disease. Am J Neurol Radiol 17, 1539–1547.

Kinkel, R.P. and Rudick, R.A. (2002). Multiple sclerosis. In Conn's Current Therapy, Rakel, R.E. and Bope, E.T., eds. Philadelphia: W.B. Saunders, pp. 922–937.

Kinkel, R.P. and the CHAMPIONS Study Group. (2003). Initial results of the CHAMPIONS study, an open-label 5-year extension of the CHAMPS study. Presented at the 19th Congress of the European Committee for Treatment and Research in Multiple Sclerosis (ECTRIMS), September 17–20, 2003, Milan, Italy.

Kuroiwa, Y. and Shibasaki, H. (1973). Clinical studies of multiple sclerosis in Japan. I. A current appraisal of 83 cases. Neurology 23, 609–617.

Kurtzke, J.F. (1970). Clinical manifestations of multiple sclerosis. In Handbook of Clinical Neurology, Vol 9, Vinken, P.J. and Bruyn, G.W., eds. Amsterdam: North-Holland, pp. 161–216.

Kurtzke, J.F. (1983). Epidemiology of multiple sclerosis. In Multiple Sclerosis, Hallpike, J.F., Adams, C.W.M. and Toutellotte, W.W., eds. Baltimore: Williams & Wilkins, pp. 47–96.

Larsson, H.B., Christiansen, P., Jensen, M. et al. (1991). Localized in vivo proton spectroscopy in the brain of patients with multiple sclerosis. Magn Reson Med 22, 23–31.

Lassmann, H. (2003). Axonal injury in multiple sclerosis: renewed interest in axonal destruction in MS (editorial). J Neurol Neurosurg Psychiatr 74, 695–697.

Leibowitz, U. and Alter, M. (1968). Optic nerve involvement and diplopia as initial manifestations of multiple sclerosis. Acta Neurol Scand 44, 70–80.

Lisak, R.P. (2004). Multiple sclerosis. In Conn's Current Therapy, Rakel, R.E. and Bope, E.T., eds. Philadelphia: W.B. Saunders, pp. 973–981.

Liu, G.T. (2000). Visual loss: optic neuropathies. In Neuro-Ophthalmology: Diagnosis and Management, Liu, G.T., Volpe, N.J. and Galetta, S. Philadelphia: W.B. Saunders, pp. 103–187.

Lowenthal, A. and Karcher, D. (1994). Cerebrospinal fluid in multiple sclerosis. Clin Neurosci 2, 211–214.

Lublin, F.D., Reingold, S.C. for the National Multiple Sclerosis Society (USA) Advisory Committee on Clinical Trials of New Agents in Multiple Sclerosis. (1996). Defining the clinical course of multiple sclerosis: results of an international survey. Neurology 46, 907–911.

McAlpine, D. (1972). Symptoms and signs. In Multiple Sclerosis: A Reappraisal, 2nd edn, McAlpine, D., Lumsden, C.E. and Acheson, E., eds. Baltimore: Williams & Wilkins, pp. 132–196.

McDonald, W.I. and Barnes, D. (1992). The ocular manifestations of multiple sclerosis. 1. Abnormalities of the afferent visual system. J Neurol Neurosurg Psychiatr 55, 747–752.

McDonald, W.I., Compston, A. and Edan, G. (2001). Recommended diagnostic criteria for multiple sclerosis: guidelines from the International Panel on the Diagnosis of Multiple Sclerosis. Ann Neurol 50, 121–127.

McFarland, H/F. (1995). The multiple sclerosis lesion. Ann Neurol 37, 419–421.

Martin, R. and McFarland, H.F. (1995). Immunological aspects of experimental allergic encephalomyelitis and multiple sclerosis. Crit Rev Clin Lab Sci 32, 121–182.

Matthews, P.M., Grancis, G., Antel, J. et al. (1991). Proton magnetic resonance spectroscopy for metabolic characterization of plaques in multiple sclerosis. Neurology 41, 1251–1256.

Matthews, P.M., Pioro, E., Narayanan, S. et al. (1996). Assessment of lesion pathology in multiple sclerosis using quantitative MRI morphometry and magnetic resonance spectroscopy. Brain 119, 715–722.

Meienberg, O., Müri, R. and Rabineau, P.A. (1986). Clinical and oculographic examinations of saccadic eye movements in the diagnosis of multiple sclerosis. Arch Neurol 43, 438–443.

Miller, A.E. (1990). Clinical features. In Handbook of Multiple Sclerosis, Cook, S.D., ed. New York: Marcel Dekker, pp. 169–186.

Miller, J.R., Burke, A.M. and Bever, C.T. (1983). Occurrence of oligoclonal bands in multiple sclerosis and other CNS diseases. Ann Neurol 13, 53–58.

Minden, S.L., Marder, W.D., Harrold, L.N. and Dor, A. (1993). Multiple Sclerosis: a statistical portrait. A compendium of data on demographics, disability, and health services utilization in the United States. Cambridge, MA: Abt Associates.

Mueller, R. (1949). Studies on disseminated sclerosis with special reference to symptomatology, course and prognosis. Acta Med Scand 133 Suppl 222, 1–214.

Müri, R.M. and Meienberg, O. (1985). The clinical spectrum of internuclear ophthalmoplegia in multiple sclerosis. Arch Neurol 42, 851–855.

Nordmann, J.P., Saraux, H. and Roullet, E. (1987). Contrast sensitivity in multiple sclerosis: a study in 35 patients with and without optic neuritis. Ophthalmologica 195, 199–204.

Noseworthy, J.H., Lucchinetti, C., Rodriguez, M. et al. (2000). Multiple sclerosis. N Engl J Med 343, 938–952.

O'Connor, P. on behalf of The Canadian Multiple Sclerosis Working Group. (2002). Key issues in the diagnosis and treatment of multiple sclerosis. Neurology 59, S1–S33.

Optic Neuritis Study Group. (1991). The clinical profile of optic neuritis: experience of the Optic Neuritis Treatment Trial. Arch Ophthalmol 109, 1673–1678.

Optic Neuritis Study Group. (2004). Visual function more than 10 years after optic neuritis: experience of the Optic Neuritis Treatment Trial. Am J Ophthalmol 137, 77–83.

Ormerod, I.E.C., Bronstein, A., Rudge, P. et al. (1986). Magnetic resonance imaging in clinically isolated lesions of the brain stem. J Neurol Neurosurg Psychiatr 49, 737–743.

Patti, F., Cacopardo, M., Palermo, F. et al. (2003). Health-related quality of life and depression in an Italian sample of multiple sclerosis patients. J Neurol Sci 211, 55–62.

Paty, D.W. (1990). Neuroimaging in multiple sclerosis. In Handbook of Multiple Sclerosis, Cook, S.D., ed. New York: Marcel Dekker, pp. 291–316.

Paty, D.W. and Li, D.K. (1993). Interferon beta-1b is effective in relapsing-remitting multiple sclerosis. I. Clinical results of a multicenter, randomized, double-blind, placebo-controlled trial. The IFNB Multiple Sclerosis Study Group. Neurology 43, 662–667.

Poser, C.M. (1986). Pathogenesis of multiple sclerosis: A critical reappraisal. Acta Neuropathol 71, 1–10.

Poser, C.M., Paty, D.W., Scheinberg, L. et al. (1983). New diagnostic criteria for multiple sclerosis: guidelines for research protocols. Ann Neurol 13, 227–231.

Prineas, J.W. and Wright, R.G. (1978). Macrophages, lymphocytes, and plasma cells in the perivascular compartment in chronic multiple sclerosis. Lab Invest 38, 409–421.

PRISMS Study Group. (1998). Randomised double-blind placebo-controlled study of interferon beta-1a in relapsing/remitting multiple sclerosis. PRISMS (Prevention of Relapses and Disability by Interferon beta-1a Subcutaneously in Multiple Sclerosis) Study Group. Lancet 352, 1498–1504.

Pugliatti, M., Sotgiu, S. and Rosati, G. (2002). The worldwide prevalence of multiple sclerosis. Clin Neurol Neurosurg 104, 182–191.

Raine, C.S. and Cross, A.H. (1989). Axonal dystrophy as a consequence of long-term demyelination. Lab Invest 60, 714–725.

Regan, D. (1972). Evoked Potentials in Psychology, Sensory Physiology and Clinical Medicine. London: Chapman and Hall, Ltd.

Regan, D., Murray, T.J. and Silver, R. (1977). Effect of body temperature on visual evoked potential delay and visual perception in multiple sclerosis. J Neurol Neurosurg Psychiatr 40, 1083–1091.

Reulen, J.P.H., Sanders, E.A.C.M. and Hogenuis, L.A.H. (1983). Eye movement disorders in multiple sclerosis and optic neuritis. Brain 106, 121–140.

Rohowsky-Kochan, C., Dowling, P.C. and Cook, S.D. (1995). Canine distemper virus-specific antibodies in multiple sclerosis. Neurology 45, 1554–1560.

Ron, M.A. and Feinstein, A. (1992). Multiple sclerosis and the mind. J Neurol Neurosurg Psychiatr 55, 1–3.

Sadovnick, A.D. (2002). The genetics of multiple sclerosis. Clin Neurol Neurosurg 104, 199–202.

Salmi, A., Reunanen, M., Ilonen, J. et al. (1983). Intrathecal antibody synthesis to virus antigens in multiple sclerosis. Clin Exp Immunol 52, 241–249.

Salonen, R., Ilonen, J., Reunanen, M. et al. (1982). PPD-, PWM-, and PHA-induced interferon in stable multiple sclerosis: Association with HLA-Dw2 antigen and clinical variables. Ann Neurol *11*, 279–284.

Sanders, V.J., Waddell, A.E., Felisan, S.L. et al. (1996). Herpes simplex virus in postmortem multiple sclerosis brain tissue. Arch Neurol *53*, 125–133.

Schiffer, R.B. and Babigian, H.M. (1984). Behavioral disorders in multiple sclerosis, temporal lobe epilepsy, and amyotrophic lateral sclerosis. Arch Neurol *41*, 1067–1069.

Silberberg, D.H. (1986). Pathogenesis of demyelination. In Multiple Sclerosis, McDonald, W.I. and Silberberg, D.H., eds. London: Butterworths, pp. 99–111.

Smith, M.E., Stone, L.A., Albert, P.S. et al. (1993). Clinical worsening in multiple sclerosis is associated with increased frequency and area of gadopentetate dimeglumine-enhancing magnetic resonance imaging lesions. Ann Neurol *33*, 480–489.

Söderström, M. (2001). Optic neuritis and multiple sclerosis. Acta Ophthalmol Scand *79*, 223–227.

Sorensen, P.S., Ross, C. and Clemmesen, K.M. Danish Multiple Sclerosis Study Group. (2003). Clinical importance of neutralising antibodies against interferon beta in patients with relapsing-remitting multiple sclerosis. Lancet *362*, 1184–1191.

Talbot, P.J., Paquette, J.S., Ciurli, C. et al. (1996). Myelin basic protein and human coronavirus 229E cross-reactive T cells in multiple sclerosis. Ann Neurol *39*, 233–240.

Tartaglia, M.C., Narayanan, S., Francis, S.J. et al. (2004). The relationship between diffuse axonal damage and fatigue in multiple sclerosis. Arch Neurol *61*, 201–207.

ter Meulen, V., Koprowski, H., Iwasaki, Y. et al. (1972). Fusion of cultured multiple-sclerosis brain cells with indicator cells: Presence of nucleocapsids and virion with isolation of parainfluenza-type virus. Lancet *1*, 1–5.

Thömke, F., Hopf, H.C. and Breen, L.A. (1992). Slowed abduction saccades in bilateral internuclear ophthalmoplegia. Neuro-Ophthalmology *12*, 241–246.

Tourbah, A., Fontaine, B. and Lyon-Caen, O. (1993). Immunologie de la sclerose en plaques: Donneés recentes et perspectives therapeutiques. Rev Neurol *149*, 373–384.

Trapp, B.D., Ransohoff, R.M., Fisher, E. and Rudick, R.A. (1999). Neurodegeneration in multiple sclerosis: relationship to neurological disability. Neuroscientist *5*, 48–57.

Trobe, J.D., Beck, R.W., Moke, P.S. et al. (1996). Contrast sensitivity and other vision tests in the Optic Neuritis Treatment Trial. Am J Ophthalmol *121*, 547–553.

Vercoulen, J.H.M.M., Hommes, O.R., Swanink, C.M.A. et al. (1996). The measurement of fatigue in patients with multiple sclerosis. A multidimensional comparison with patients with chronic fatigue syndrome and healthy subjects. Arch Neurol *53*, 642–649.

Warren, K.G. and Catz, I. (1985). The relationship between levels of cerebrospinal fluid myelin basic protein and IgG measurements in patients with multiple sclerosis. Ann Neurol.

Whetten-Goldstein, K., Sloan, F.A., Goldstein, L.B. and Kulas, E.D. (1998). A comprehensive assessment of the cost of multiple sclerosis in the United States. Multiple Sclerosis *4*, 419–425.

Whitaker, J.N., Benveniste, E.N. and Zhou, S-r. (1990). Cerebrospinal fluid. In Handbook of Multiple Sclerosis, Cook, S.D., ed. New York: Marcel Dekker, pp. 251–270.

Willer, C.J., Dyment, D.A., Risch, N.J. et al. (2003). Twin concordance and sibling recurrence rates in Multiple Sclerosis. Proc Natl Acad Sci USA *100*, 12877–12882.

Wilson, H.B. (1978). Visual-evoked response differentiation of ischemic optic neuritis from the optic neuritis of multiple sclerosis. Am J Ophthalmol *86*, 530–535.

Zeman, A., McLean, B., Keir, G. et al. (1993). The significance of serum oligoclonal bands in neurological diseases. J Neurol Neurosurg Psychiatr *56*, 32–35.

Zeman, A., Kidd, D., McLean, B.N. et al. (1996). A study of oligoclonal band negative multiple sclerosis. J Neurol Neurosurg Psychiatr *60*, 27–30.

Autoimmunity – Inflammatory Bowel Disease

Chapter
46

Scott E. Plevy and Miguel Reguiero

*Division of Gastroenterology, Hepatology and Nutrition,
Inflammatory Bowel Disease Center, Pittsburgh, PA, USA*

My bowels, my bowels! I am pained at my very heart; my heart maketh a noise in me; I cannot hold my peace.

Jeremiah 4:19

INTRODUCTION

The idiopathic inflammatory bowel diseases (IBDs), Crohn's disease (CD) and ulcerative colitis (UC), are characterized by chronic, intermittent inflammation of the gastrointestinal tract. Ulcerative colitis (UC) and Crohn's disease (CD) describe clinical entities based on definitions established eight decades ago and revised remarkably little since (Crohn et al., 1932; Kirsner, 1988). These clinical definitions are utilized to predict natural history as well as medical and surgical outcomes. The distinction between CD and UC is based largely on the distribution of inflammation. The inflammation in UC invariably involves the distal rectum and extends proximally through the colon in a symmetric, continuous manner. Inflammatory changes affect only the innermost layers of the colonic wall. In contrast, the inflammation of CD can affect any portion of the gastrointestinal tract, with involvement of the terminal ileum being most common. Inflammation in CD is often patchy and discontinuous in nature. It can also involve all layers of the bowel wall, leading to inflammatory complications unique to CD, such as fistula formation, abscess and perforation. In 5–10 per cent of patients, categorization is not certain based on these definitions, leading to the clinical entity of 'indeterminate' colitis (Ceboes and De Hertogh, 2003).

The highest incidence and prevalence rates for IBD have been reported in studies from Northern European countries and North America (Langholz et al., 1991; Shivanda et al., 1996; Loftus et al., 2000). Recently this concept of geographic distribution of IBD has been altered by the increase in reports of CD and UC from continental Europe, the Pacific Rim, the Middle East, Africa and Latin America (Rozen et al., 1979; Higashi et al., 1988; Timmer et al., 1999). The prevalence of CD and UC in North America ranges from 26.0 to 198.5 cases per 100 000 persons and 37.5 to 229 cases, respectively (Calkins, 1994). The incidence rates for CD and UC in North America range from 3.1 to 14.6 cases per 100 000 persons and 2.2 to 14.3 cases per 100 000, respectively (Loftus, 2004). UC and CD occur in infancy and childhood, but the incidence of either disorder is low in individuals younger than 10 years of age (Calkins et al., 1984). Both forms of IBD occur most frequently in persons between the ages of 15 and 30 years (Calkins et al., 1984; Calkins, 1994). In general, the gender distribution between UC and CD is equivalent, but in regions with a high incidence of IBD, a slight female predominance for CD and male predominance in UC have been reported (Trallori et al., 1996; Yapp et al., 2000). Although the incidence of UC has remained relatively constant in populations, the incidence of CD appears to be increasing at a dramatic level (Kugathasan et al., 2003).

The differential diagnosis of IBD is extensive. As will be discussed, immunogenetic testing has been purported to help distinguish among diagnostic possibilities. The

Measuring Immunity, edited by Michael T. Lotze and Angus W. Thomson
ISBN 0-12-455900-X, London

differential diagnosis of IBD includes infectious entero-colitides, ischemic colitis, microscopic colitis, collagenous colitis, celiac disease and functional disorders of the GI tract that are not associated with inflammatory responses, termed irritable bowel syndrome (IBS). Also, drug-related inflammatory conditions of the GI tract can mimic or exacerbate IBD, for example, non-steroidal anti-inflammatory drug-induced mucosal injury. Furthermore, the distinction between CD and UC in patients with colonic inflammation is clinically important as it guides medical therapy and, most significantly, surgical options for UC provide more definitive long-term solutions than those for CD.

Characterization of immunogenetic profiles within the IBDs has led to initial descriptions of clinically relevant subgroups and raises the possibility that immunogenetic testing of patients with IBD may lead to better diagnosis and the more rational use of medical and surgical interventions. This chapter will review recent work that begins to define subgroups within the IBDs based on immunologic and genetic markers. For detailed reviews of the clinical history of these disorders, the reader is referred to other sources (Kirsner, 1988; Podolsky, 2002).

GENETIC MARKERS AND CLINICAL STRATIFICATION OF IBD

The single, strongest risk factor for development of IBD, independent of type, is a family member with the disease (Andres and Friedman, 1999). Farmer (1986) observed a 40 per cent frequency of IBD in first-degree family members. A subsequent investigation documented a 10-fold increase in an individual's risk of IBD for those with a first-degree relative afflicted with either CD or UC (Orholm et al., 1991). Although some studies have shown a greater occurrence of familial CD than UC (Orholm et al., 1991; Peeters et al., 1996), other data indicate that the relative risk of familial disease is similar for both forms of IBD and that these disorders are genetically related, sharing some but not all genetic loci (Ahmad et al., 2001).

The increased rate of IBD observed in twins, especially monozygotic twins, provides further evidence of genetic involvement in IBD. Twin studies have shown significantly higher concordance rates in monozygotic twins compared with dizygotic twins for both UC and CD (Tysk et al., 1988; Thompson et al., 1996; Orholm et al., 2000). Among Danish twins with UC, probandwise concordance rates were 18 per cent and 58 per cent for UC and CD among monozygotic pairs, respectively and 4.5 per cent and 0 among dizygotic pairs, respectively (Orholm et al., 2000). In British twin pairs, Thompson et al. (1996) reported that the relative risk of a monozygotic twin developing IBD was 3.49 versus that of a dizygotic twin. These findings confirm a genetic etiology in IBD, but the lack of 100 per cent concordance in monozygotic twins suggests that non-genetic factors, e.g. environmental interactions, also play a role.

Findings of genome-wide searches have begun to elucidate the genetic predisposition in IBD. Several genetic loci have been identified that convey susceptibility to IBD in general (Satsangi et al., 1996); other genes appear to influence the specific characteristics (e.g. location, extent, severity and course) of the disease that develops in susceptible individuals (Ahmad et al., 2001). Satsangi et al. (1996) found evidence of susceptibility to UC and CD on chromosomes 3, 7 and 12. The strongest linkage was found on chromosome 12, which conveyed a 2.0 relative risk of disease development in siblings. Several groups have also reported a link between chromosome 16 (labeled *IBD1*) and IBD susceptibility (Ahmad et al., 1996; Hugot and Thomas, 1998). *IBD1* contributes an inherited risk of 1.3 for CD development (Hugot and Thomas, 1998). Recently, mutations in the *NOD2* gene were discovered within the CD-linked *IBD1* locus (Hugot et al., 2001; Ogura et al., 2001a). The *NOD2* gene encodes for an intracellular protein expressed in monocytes, dendritic cells (Ogura et al., 2001b) and intestinal epithelial Paneth cells (Lala et al., 2003; Ogura et al., 2003). *NOD2* activation enables the activation of nuclear factor kappa B in response to bacterial peptidoglycan component, muramyl dipeptide (Inohara et al., 2003). Although the functional significance of a defect in the *NOD2* gene is not yet clear, a working hypothesis is that it leads to disruption of the innate immune response to enteric bacteria. This may lead to defective killing of intracellular bacteria by macrophages and dendritic cells with persistent innate and adaptive immune responses stimulated through other pathways. *NOD2* gene mutations are estimated to occur in approximately 25 per cent of patients with CD.

Chromosome 6 (*IBD3*) may also influence CD and UC development. This chromosome encodes the genes for the human leukocyte antigen (HLA) classes I and II

Table 46.1 Epidemiologic and clinical characteristics of CD and UC

Characteristic	Finding
Geographic distribution	Northern Europe and North America
Prevalence (per 100 000 persons in North America)	CD: 26–198.5 UC: 37.5–229
Incidence (per 100 000 persons in North America)	CD: 3.1–14.6 UC: 2.2–14.3
Age of onset (years)	15–30
Gender distribution	Equivalent in males and females (slight female predominance in CD)
Symptoms	Similar for colonic CD and UC
Disease course	Chronic remitting and relapsing course
Extraintestinal manifestations	Similar arthritic, ocular and dermatologic complications in CD and UC Primary sclerosing cholangitis and ankylosing spondylitis more common in UC
Cancer risk	Similar for colonic CD and UC
Mortality	Similar for both UC and CD

molecules. The association between the HLA region on chromosome 6 and the risk of IBD is estimated at 64–100 per cent for UC and 10–33 per cent for CD (Ahmad et al., 2001). Specifically, a positive association has been observed between *DR2, DRB1*1502* and *DRB1*103* in UC and *DR7* and *DQ4* in CD (Stokkers et al., 1999). Given the different allele associations in UC and CD, these genes probably do not convey susceptibility to the disease but possibly modify the IBD phenotype, allowing for the different presentations of the diseases. Another hypothesis is that HLA associations are markers for closely linked susceptibility genes that have yet to be identified. The TNF genes are located within the HLA region on chromosome 6. In CD, dramatic and prolonged clinical responses to a single infusion of anti-TNF monoclonal antibody (infliximab, Centocor, Malvern, PA) demonstrate that TNF is a key mediator in mucosal inflammation (Targan et al., 1997). Genetic polymorphisms within the TNF locus have been associated with CD (Plevy et al., 1997) and correlated with functional differences in TNF production (Hajeer and Hutchinson, 2001).

A recent study has demonstrated an intriguing association between IBD and the X chromosome. Confirming epidemiological observations (i.e. high incidence of IBD and Turner's syndrome, the higher incidence of CD in females versus males and greater number of affected mother and child pairs than father and child pairs), Vermeire et al. (2001) found evidence suggestive of X-chromosome susceptibility in 79 affected sibling pairs. The peak linkage was documented in the pericentromeric region which is also the location of immunoregulatory genes. This region is also the site of translocation between chromosome 1 and the X chromosome, predisposing an individual to renal cell carcinoma, a cancer that may occur with increased frequency in a subset of UC patients (Vermeire et al., 2001).

DISTINCT CLINICAL SUBGROUPS OF IBD PATIENTS DEFINED BY GENETIC MARKERS

Of great interest clinically, there is concordance for anatomic site and clinical type of Crohn's disease within families. In 60 families, clinical site (small bowel, ileum, right colon, left colon and perianal region) and clinical type of disease (inflammatory, stricturing and fistulizing) were evaluated. An 86 per cent concordance for site and an 82 per cent concordance for type of disease were found (Bayless et al., 1996). Thus, different clinical subtypes of CD run in families, demonstrating how genetics influences expression of disease. Furthermore, age at diagnosis correlated with anatomic site and clinical type of disease. CD has a bimodal age distribution with peaks at 20 and 40 years. Younger age at diagnosis (<20 years) was associated with a family history of CD, stricturing disease and a higher frequency of surgery. Older age at diagnosis (>40 years) was associated with the presence of

colonic disease and the inflammatory subtype. Thus, patients with a family history of CD have a distinct clinical phenotype, with earlier onset and more aggressive disease (Bayless et al., 1996).

Recently, genetic markers have provided valuable information about clinical heterogeneity within IBD. Ultimately, for this research to impact clinical practice, these markers should help guide medical or surgical therapy of IBD patients.

An interesting candidate gene in IBD is the interleukin-1 receptor antagonist (IL-1ra) gene. IL-1 is a pro-inflammatory cytokine and IL-1ra downregulates inflammatory responses by blocking the effects of IL-1. In IBD patients, there is decreased intestinal IL-1ra expression (Casini-Raggi et al., 1995). A genetic association with a specific IL-1ra polymorphism has been described in UC (Papo et al., 1999; Tountas et al., 1999). This allele was associated with total colonic inflammation, a more severe form of disease (Roussomoustakaki et al., 1997). Thus, disease severity may be modulated by functional differences in IL-1ra production which, in turn, is determined by genetic factors (Tountas et al., 1999; Carter et al., 2004).

HLA alleles may also define clinically useful subgroups of IBD patients. In 99 UC patients undergoing total protocolectomy, 14.3 per cent versus 3.2 per cent of non-IBD controls possessed the rare HLA DRB1*0103 allele. This allele is associated with extensive disease and extraintestinal manifestations such as oral aphthous ulcers, arthritis and uveitis (Roussomoustakaki et al., 1997). Potentially, this allele can be used to identify UC patients who may develop aggressive disease early in their disease course.

Abdominal colectomy and mucosal proctectomy with IPAA has become the surgical treatment of choice for most patients with ulcerative colitis. The most frequent complication following IPAA is idiopathic inflammation of the ileal pouch commonly known as pouchitis. From a large study at the Mayo Clinic, the cumulative risk for the first episode of pouchitis at 1, 5 and 10 years after IPAA is 15 per cent, 36 per cent and 46 per cent, respectively (Penna et al., 1996). Pouchitis appears to be a unique form of recurrent IBD specific to the ileal reservoir. The occurrence of pouchitis in UC but not in familial adenomatous polyposis patients (Salemans et al., 1992) and evidence of an aberrant immunologic response in pouchitis with increased inflammatory cytokine production (Gionchetti et al., 1994), suggest an immunogenetic etiology. In fact, IL-1 receptor antagonist and lymphotoxin genetic polymorphisms have been correlated with the incidence and severity of pouchitis (Brett et al., 1996; Facklis et al., 1999; Aisenberg et al., 2004). Within the UC population, a CD-associated TNF microsatellite haplotype marker also correlated with treatment-refractory UC patients before colectomy (Facklis et al., 1999).

Since its first description, the NOD2 genotype has been strongly associated with a specific clinical phenotype. Studies from different patient populations correlate

NOD2 mutations with the presence of ileal fibrostenotic disease (Abreu et al., 2002; Cuthbert et al., 2002; Hampe et al., 2002; Lesage et al., 2002). In a study on 163 patients with CD, the early development of stricturing or perforating disease 5 years after diagnosis was influenced by the disease location, the clinical activity and the smoking habits, but not by the NOD2 genotype (Louis et al., 2002). Thus NOD2 may confer genetic predisposition to CD, but environmental factors influence the disease course and aggressiveness.

As other genes are described, other clinical correlations will be made. For example, a recent study showed that the CD associated susceptibility haplotype on chromosome 5q31 correlates with perianal CD (Armuzzi et al., 2003).

INFECTIOUS AND ENVIRONMENTAL TRIGGERS OF MUCOSAL INFLAMMATION

In individuals predisposed to develop IBD, as determined by the presence of genetic factors, some initiating event appears to trigger the inappropriate immune response. The specific triggering event has yet to be determined, but potential antigens and microbial factors have been extensively studied. Specifically, onset of disease has been associated with foreign travel, enteric infections and perinatal viral infections (Sartor, 1995; Papadakis and Targan, 1999). Additionally, patients with CD have increased concentrations of Eubacteria, Peptostreptococcus, Coprococcus and Bacteroides in their feces as well as elevated serum antibodies against these organisms (Sartor, 1995). Abnormal bacterial byproducts such as hydrogen sulfide are also found in patients with UC, leading to decreased epithelial cell butyrate metabolism and subsequent tissue injury (Sartor, 1995).

CD and UC, when active, lead to a significant decrease in aerobic bacteria and Lactobacillus, suggesting that intestinal flora changes may be involved in the development or promotion of inflammation (Fiocchi, 1998). The triggering infection or antigen is only one step in the development of IBD, as many implicated microbial triggers are not detectable years after disease onset and antibiotics are not consistently effective in disease treatment (Sartor, 1995).

The importance of the bacterial flora in the initiation and perpetuation of IBD is most clearly demonstrated by studies in mouse models of IBD. Colitis prone, germ-free derived mice do not develop IBD until recolonized with constituents of the normal enteric microflora (Sartor, 1996). In some animal models, a single bacterial strain can induce colitis. However, the same strain in a different animal model may have no effect on the development of colitis (Rath et al., 1996, 1999, 2001). For example, the addition of Bacteroides vulgatus to a group of five bacteria isolated from CD patients induced colitis in HLA-B27 transgenic rats (Rath et al., 1996), but did not induce disease in germ-free derived interleukin-10 deficient mice

(Sellon et al., 1998). Furthermore, IL-10 deficient mice monoassociated with Streptococcus faecalis develop colitis (Sellon et al., 1998). Additionally, IL-10 deficient mice develop colitis when Helicobacter species are introduced (Kullberg et al., 2001). Furthermore, preliminary work has demonstrated that in germ-free derived IL-10 deficient mice, there is an association between specific bacteria and disease location and severity (Mow et al., 2004). Taken as a whole, these animal model studies can be interpreted as having two important meanings in the context of the human IBDs. First, the loss of immunologic tolerance to the normal intestinal microflora is not global, rather it appears that specific bacteria and therefore specific bacterial antigens are recognized. In support of this theory, in another mouse model of IBD, the C3H/HeJBir mouse, serological B cell and T cell reactivity occurs in response to a limited repertoire among the enormous enteric microbial load of antigens (Brandwein et al., 1997; Cong et al., 1998). Interestingly, in the TNBS model of induced murine colitis, mucosal T cells lose tolerance to enteric bacterial antigen preparations, but tolerance can be restored by IL-10 and anti-IL-12 (Duchmann et al., 1996). Likewise, bacterial antigen specific T regulatory cells can inhibit the adoptive transfer of colitis by pathogenic antigen specific T cells from C3H/HeJBir mice (Cong et al., 2002). Thus, these studies suggest that immunologic interventions in IBD can potentially restore tolerance to the enteric flora. In summary, the genetic composition of the host as well as specific microbial determinants may influence the concomitant immune response and therefore the clinical phenotype of disease.

The role of bacterial antigens in human IBD has been suggested through several observations. In CD, some patients clinically improve upon alteration of the enteric bacterial flora by antibiotics (Prantera et al., 1996, 1998). Studies have demonstrated that reintroduction of the diverted fecal stream into a segment of bowel can reactivate CD in that segment (Rutgeerts et al., 1991). Through characterization of serological B cell and mucosal T cell responses, it has been proposed that patients with IBD specifically lose tolerance to their own bacterial populations. Furthermore, probiotic bacteria, normal constituents of the enteric flora, have been demonstrated in small clinical trials to have anti-inflammatory effects in IBD (Gionchetti et al., 2000, 2003; Mimura et al., 2004). Although the exact mechanisms of action are unclear, some hypotheses include alteration of the bacterial flora with increased ratios of probiotic to aerobic adherent bacteria (Madsen et al., 1999, 2001), direct effects on intestinal epithelial cell permeability preventing translocation of bacteria and bacterial products (Madsen et al., 2001) and direct anti-inflammatory effects demonstrated by alterations in cytokine and growth factor production (Lammers et al., 2002; Schultz et al., 2002). Enteric helminths – evolutionarily, normal constituents of the enteric flora, but greatly diminished in carriage in industrialized countries (Elliott et al., 2000) – may have similar ameliorative effects in intestinal inflammation in mice (Khan et al., 2002; Elliott et al., 2003) and humans (Summers et al., 2003). In a landmark mechanistic study, Duchmann et al. (1995) demonstrated that in human lamina propria mononuclear cells (LPMC), tolerance selectively exists to intestinal flora from autologous but not heterologous intestine and that this tolerance is broken in LPMC from IBD patients. Finally, an interesting observation highlights the essential link between human genetics and the enteric microbial flora in IBD. A study of CD patients, their first degree relatives and healthy unrelated controls demonstrated that the flora of CD patients contained more anaerobic gram-positive coccoid rods and gram-negative rods than that of healthy subjects and this abnormality was also observed in nine of 26 (34 per cent) of first degree relatives (Van de Merwe et al., 1988).

These observations have led to the hypothesis that specific microbes are directly involved in the pathogenesis of IBD, particularly CD, as an infectious pathogenic agent. Many specific organisms have been proposed to contribute directly to the development of CD, including *Mycobacteria, Listeria* and measles virus, however, the detection of immune responses to antigens from these microbes has been variable and not reproducible among studies. No organism studied to date fulfills Koch's postulates, although Koch's postulates may not apply to the model of IBD. For example, bacteria that are part of the normal flora or common in the environment may become pathogenic in certain situations. First, bacteria from the normal flora may acquire extra virulence factors; second, harmless bacteria can cause disease if they gain access to deep tissue; and thirdly, in immunocompromised patients, components of the normal flora can cause disease. Also, not all of those infected or colonized by pathogenic bacteria will develop disease. Subclinical infection may be more common. Finally, to fulfill Koch's postulates, bacteria need to be culturable *in vitro* and transfer disease to an animal model. Given the enormous complexity of the commensal enteric microbial flora, most of which remain to be identified, some bacteria are not culturable *in vitro* and there may not be a suitable animal model of infection. Perhaps the organism that has attracted the most attention as a pathogenic agent in CD has been *Mycobacterium avium*, subspecies *paratuberculosis* (MAP), a ubiquitous environmental mycobacterial species that has been detected in water supplies, meat and dairy products. As with other mycobacterial infections, it is likely that host genetic determinants will predict outcome to infection. *Mycobacterium avium* subspecies *paratuberculosis* causes a disease in cattle and sheep known as Johne's disease (Hulten et al., 2000a), characterized by transmural intestinal inflammation similar in some, but not all aspects, to CD (Van Kruinningen, 1999). MAP specific immune responses (Wayne et al., 1992; Peetermans et al., 1995; Walmsley et al., 1996; Cohavy et al., 1999; Olsen et al., 2001) as well as MAP detection in intestinal tissue in

Crohn's patients (McFadden et al., 1987, 1992; Gitnick et al., 1989; Peetermans et al., 1995) have been reported; however, data from studies are not consistent (Kobayashi et al., 1988; Ibbotson et al., 1992; Stainsby et al., 1993; Rowbotham et al., 1995; Dumonceau et al., 1996). Large clinical trials performed with anti-mycobacterial therapy in CD have been negative (Prantera et al., 1994; Thomas et al., 1998). However, proponents of this theory would argue that anti-mycobacterial agents used were not highly active against MAP, mandating the need for newer, large placebo controlled trials with active antibiotics (Hulten et al., 2000b). Large scale epidemiologic studies to detect immune responses and the presence of particular environmental and commensal microorganisms will be necessary to clarify whether a specific microbial species may have a direct pathogenic role in IBD. If a single organism is found, this does not exclude the possibility, even the likelihood, that an infectious agent would only explain the presence of IBD in a subset of genetically predisposed patients.

IBD-SPECIFIC SEROLOGICAL MARKERS

Several serum immune markers have been well characterized in subgroups of patients with IBD over the past two decades. The common theme among these many markers is that they represent antibodies that are reactive with constituents of the enteric bacterial flora. Some of these markers have been purported to help distinguish the clinical diagnosis of IBD from other inflammatory and non-inflammatory conditions of the GI tract, to help distinguish between CD and UC and that these markers may be able to define clinically important subgroups within CD and UC. The two serological tests that are the most widely studied are anti-neutrophil cytoplasmic antibody with a perinuclear staining pattern (pANCA) and anti-*Saccharomyces cerevisiae* antibody (ASCA).

The incidence of serum pANCA in UC patients has been reported to be between 50 and 80 per cent (Papadakis and Targan, 1999; Landers et al., 2002). As ANCA is the best-characterized serological marker in IBD, it will be discussed in detail. The antigens used to detect ASCA in IBD patients are oligomannoside epitopes derived from yeast and this serum antibody may be a marker of immunoreactivity against enteric microbial products. ASCA is expressed in sera in up to 70 per cent of CD patients (Papadakis and Targan, 1999; Landers et al., 2002).

Two new serological tests have been recently demonstrated in IBD patients. OmpC is an outer membrane porin purified from *E. coli*. Initially, human sera from UC patients demonstrated elevated IgG anti-OmpC compared to healthy controls (Cohavy et al., 2000). Subsequently, in patients with CD, IgA responses to OmpC were found in 55 per cent of patients (Landers et al., 2002; Mow et al., 2004). Similarly, the *Pseudomonas fluorescens* I2 antigen was recently detected inside macrophages isolated from the intestinal mucosa of CD patients (Sutton et al., 2000; Dalwadi et al., 2001; Weo et al., 2002). Serum reactivity to this antigen, measured by IgA, is detected far more frequently in CD patients compared to UC patients and other patients with inflammatory conditions (Sutton et al., 2000; Landers et al., 2002; Mow et al., 2004). As will be discussed, serum reactivity to pANCA, ASCA, OmpC and I2 may discern clinically important subgroups of IBD patients.

Serum ANCAs are antibodies directed against intracellular components of neutrophils. ANCA is best known as a marker for inflammatory vasculitides such as Wegener's granulomatosis (Gross and Csernok, 1995; Gross et al., 1995). The main neutrophilic antigen associated with vasculitis has been identified as a cytoplasmic serine proteinase (Jennette et al., 1990). Immunostaining of neutrophils for ANCA with antibodies to proteinase-3 results in a cytoplasmic fluorescent pattern (cANCA) (Jennette et al., 1990). Perinuclear anti-neutrophilic cytoplasmic antibody (pANCA) staining is also observed. This phenomenon occurs after alcohol fixation of substrate cells, as positively charged protein molecules are soluble in alcohol. Cytoplasmic granules redistribute around the nuclei, resulting in a pANCA pattern for antibodies against elastase, lactoferrin, cathepsin G and myeloperoxidase (Falk et al., 1990).

pANCA was subsequently associated with IBD (Saxon et al., 1990; Vasiliauskas et al., 1996; Dubinsky et al., 2001). The incidence of serum pANCA in UC patients has been reported to be between 50 and 80 per cent (Saxon et al., 1990; Ruemmele et al., 1998; Dubinsky et al., 2001; Sandborn et al., 2001a). pANCA production occurs in B cells located in the colonic mucosa (Targan et al., 1995a). It therefore appears that mucosal antigens lead to local production of pANCA. The ANCA that has been reported in UC appears to differ in immunoglobulin class and IgG subclasses from ANCAs detected in the vasculitic diseases (Muller-Ladner et al., 1996). pANCAs have been detected in the serum of patients with autoimmune hepatitis, primary sclerosing cholangitis and other autoimmune liver diseases. This staining pattern has been seen in greater than 90 per cent of sera from patients with type 1 autoimmune hepatitis (Hardarson et al., 1993; Mulder et al., 1993; Targan et al., 1995b; Schwarze et al., 2003) and up to 70 per cent of patients with primary sclerosing cholangitis (Hardarson et al., 1993; Mulder et al., 1993; Terjung et al., 1998; Angulo et al., 2000; Schwarze et al., 2003).

Another distinction between the pANCA in UC from that in vasculitis is that the UC pANCA is actually nuclear in location. Confocal and electron microscopy demonstrated that the UC associated pANCA was localized primarily over chromatin concentrated toward the periphery of the nuclei (Billing et al., 1995). There may be multiple antigens recognized by this pANCA, including histone H1 (Eggena et al., 2000), high mobility group (HMG) nuclear

protein 1 and 2 (Sobajima et al., 1998, 1999) and a 50 kD nuclear envelope protein (Terjung et al., 2000). Interestingly, pANCA that reacts with HMG proteins has been reported in 90 per cent of patients with autoimmune hepatitis (Sobajima et al., 1999). A similar frequency of patients with autoimmune hepatitis and primary sclerosing cholangitis has a serum pANCA that reacts with the 50 kD nuclear envelope protein (Terjung et al., 2000). However, there is a difference between the pANCAs seen in UC from the pANCAs seen in inflammatory liver diseases. After treatment with the enzyme DNAse I, the majority of autoimmune hepatitis and PSC patients show a pANCA that recognizes cytoplasmic constituents. In IBD, after treatment with DNAse I, the pANCA staining pattern is lost. In approximately 70 per cent of the cases of UC, there is complete loss of antigen recognition, while in 30 per cent of cases there is conversion to cytoplasmic staining (Vidrich et al., 1995).

The question persists whether pANCA recognizes components of the enteric microflora or may in fact recognize a putative autoantigen. These processes are not necessarily mutually exclusive because recognition of a bacterial antigen can lead to a process of molecular mimicry. Human pANCA monoclonal antibodies isolated from B cells obtained from UC patients recognize histone H1 (Eggena et al., 2000). Subsequently, a novel mycobacterial histone H1 homolog (HupB) was described as an antigenic target of pANCA as well as a target for serum IgA isolated from patients with CD (Cohavy et al., 1999). Thus, pANCA likely recognizes components of the enteric flora, but through molecular mimicry, may also represent a true autoantibody.

Other putative autoantibodies have been described in the sera of IBD patients. Several groups have described the presence of anti-colon antibodies in IBD. Antibodies to at least three colon antigens have been identified. The first antibody described recognized a lipopolysaccharide antigen extractable from colonic tissue (Arashi et al., 1995). These antibodies are present in both CD and UC and also occur in a variety of non-intestinal and intestinal inflammatory diseases. A second anti-colon antibody was identified by elution of IgG antibodies from surgically resected UC intestinal tissue (Fiocchi et al., 1989). This antibody has been determined to be specific for UC as opposed to CD and other inflammatory or non-inflammatory controls. The antigen has been identified as a tropomyosin, an actin binding protein found in most cells (Onuma et al., 2000; Taniguchi et al., 2001). These antibodies are synthesized by lamina propria B cells, and epithelial deposits of IgG1 and an activated complement appear to co-localize with a 40 kD protein in UC specimens (Biancone et al., 1995). Lamina propria B cells producing IgG and IgA were subsequently determined to be reactive against the tropomyosin isoform tropomyosin-5 (Geng et al., 1998; Taniguchi et al., 2001). Another anti-colon antibody has been described against various epithelial cell associated antigens (Fiocchi et al., 1989).

These were demonstrable in 70 per cent of patients with IBD as opposed to 8 per cent of controls. Approximately half of healthy relatives of IBD patients were found to have a similar circulating antibody. Other p and cANCAs to lactoferrin, cathepsin G and bactericidal/permeability-increasing protein have been described in IBD patients (Skogh and Peen, 1993; Broekroelofs et al., 1994; Kossa et al., 1995; Walmsley et al., 1997; Sugi et al., 1999), but lack of reproducibility between studies makes interpretation of these results difficult. Finally, lymphocytoxic IgMs have been reported in 20 to 40 per cent of IBD patients (Korsmeyer et al., 1974; Henderson et al., 1976).

CLINICAL SIGNIFICANCE OF SEROLOGICAL MARKERS

pANCA and ASCA have gained familiarity with clinicians because of their diagnostic potential and specificity in IBD (Targan et al., 1999; Rutgeerts and Vermeire, 2000; Reumaux et al., 2003). ASCA, a CD specific antibody, is present in 55–65 per cent of CD patients. It is important to note that the prevalence of ASCA in UC is 5–20 per cent. Conversely, pANCA, a UC specific antibody, is present in 50–65 per cent of UC patients and 10–25 per cent of CD patients (Targan et al., 1999; Rutgeerts and Vermeire, 2000; Reumaux et al., 2003). Differences in ANCA and ASCA prevalence between studies may reflect different and heterogeneous patient groups, but the methodology to detect ANCA and ASCA – sensitivity, specificity and even the actual antigen detected – varies between studies (Sandborn et al., 2001). Both of these antibodies are present at very low frequency in patients without IBD. When interpreting clinical studies on serologic markers in IBD, it is important to note that most studies (exceptions will be noted) are retrospective. In these studies, the gold standard is clinical, endoscopic, radiographic and histopathologic diagnosis of CD and UC.

Although the specificity of these markers for UC and CD is high, their sensitivity is considerably lower, making them less useful as diagnostic tests. In a study by Annese et al. (2001), ASCA was detected in the serum of 34 of 96 patients with sporadic CD (35 per cent) and 11 of 97 patients with sporadic UC (12 per cent). This marker was significantly more common in patients with familial CD (55 per cent) and familial UC (25 per cent) and was detected in 25 per cent of unaffected relatives. Similarly, ANCA has been widely reported in greater than 10 per cent of CD patients (Paoadakis and Targan, 1999). Vasiliauskas et al. (1996) found that 55 per cent of the CD population displayed serum ANCA levels, including 53 per cent with cytoplasmic ANCA (cANCA) and 47 per cent with pANCA. The patients positive for pANCA were characterized as having left-sided colitis with symptoms of rectal bleeding, mucous discharge and urgency, i.e. 'UC-like inflammation'.

UC patients positive for pANCA often have aggressive, treatment-resistant, left-sided disease and require surgery early in the disease course (Sandborn et al., 1996; Vasiliauskas et al., 1996). Patients with treatment-resistant left-sided UC are pANCA+ over 90 per cent of the time. pANCA is also associated with chronic pouchitis in UC following ileal-pouch anal anastomosis (IPAA) (Sandborn et al., 1995; Facklis et al., 1999). Although the etiology of pouchitis is unknown, it may represent a form of recurrent UC in the pouch and its manifestation exclusively in UC patients demonstrates an underlying immunoregulatory disturbance. In patients with UC and familial adenomatous polyposis (FAP) who had undergone total colectomy with IPAA, 100 per cent of patients with chronic pouchitis and UC were pANCA positive, versus 50 per cent with UC and no pouchitis and 0 per cent with FAP and no pouchitis (Fonkalsrud, 1996; Hurst et al., 1996; Barton et al., 2001). Furthermore, preoperative high levels of pANCA (not ASCA) correlated with chronic pouchitis following ileal pouch/anal anastomosis in a small but prospective analysis (Fleshner et al., 2001).

These findings suggest that ASCA and ANCA in UC and CD may define clinically useful immunologic subgroups. The combination of serologic markers, i.e. ANCA-positive and ASCA-negative for UC or ANCA-negative and ASCA-positive for CD, may have particular predictive value (Fonkalsrud, 1996; Hurst et al., 1996; Ruemmele et al., 1998; Barton et al., 2001; Sandborn et al., 2001a; Peeters et al., 2001). In three large retrospective studies, the specificity of these markers to distinguish CD from UC is 92–98 per cent (Ruemmele et al., 1998; Quinton et al., 1998; Peeters et al., 2001). However, sensitivities are low: 44–57 per cent. Therefore, half of patients cannot be classified by this analysis, which significantly limits clinical utility. In children with an uncertain diagnosis of IBD incorporation of sequential non-invasive testing into a diagnostic strategy may avoid costly evaluations and facilitate clinical decision making. One hundred and twenty-eight children received in parallel a complete clinical and endoscopic work-up for IBD and serologic testing with ASCA and ANCA. Sequential testing, using a sensitive ASCA/ANCA assay was followed, if positive, by more specific ASCA and pANCA reducing false-positive diagnoses by 81 per cent. Only four of 128 patients would have received unnecessary colonoscopy for definitive diagnosis (Dubinsky et al., 2001).

In the 5–10 per cent of patients who defy categorization as CD or UC, the term indeterminate colitis has been adopted. A pivotal prospective study evaluated ASCA and pANCA in patients with indeterminate colitis (Joossens et al., 2002). This analysis followed 97 patients with clinically and endoscopically defined indeterminate colitis prospectively for 6 years. Their initial serum antibody characterization demonstrated that 48 per cent of the population was ASCA−/pANCA−, 27 per cent were ASCA+/pANCA−, 21 per cent were ASCA−/pANCA+ and 4 per cent were ASCA+/pANCA+. Over the 6 years of prospective follow up, 17 of 97 patients were diagnosed with CD, 66 of the 97 patients remained indeterminate and 14 patients of the 97 declared as UC. Eight of 17 CD patients were ASCA+/pANCA−. In patients who remained indeterminate, 16 of 66 were ASCA+/pANCA− and in UC, two of 14 were ASCA+/pANCA−. Therefore, ASCA is a marker for the development of CD. In pANCA+/ASCA− indeterminate patients, four developed CD, nine remained indeterminate and 7 (50 per cent) were diagnosed with UC. In patients with CD who were pANCA+, a 'UC-like' phenotype was described. The most striking finding is that in patients who remained indeterminate, 40 of 66 remained ASCA−/pANCA−. Therefore, the major conclusion is that indeterminate colitis may represent a distinct form of IBD based on the lack of IBD associated antibodies. ASCA+/pANCA− is predictive of CD, pANCA+/ASCA− is predictive of UC or UC-like CD. Unfortunately, these two CD groups cannot be distinguished prospectively. ASCA/pANCA− patients are likely to remain indeterminate with 6 years of follow up.

Recent work has characterized clinical subgroups of CD patients using ANCA, ASCA, OmpC and I2 serologic responses. In sera from 330 Crohn's patients, ASCA was detected in 56 per cent of patients, 55 per cent were reactive to OmpC, 50 per cent had I2 immunoreactivity and 23 per cent were pANCA positive (Landers et al., 2002). Eighty-five per cent responded to at least one antigen; only 4 per cent responded to all four (Landers et al., 2002). The level of response was stable over time and with change in disease activity. Cluster analysis of these antibody responses described four groups: ASCA, OmpC/I2, pANCA or no/low response (Landers et al., 2002). This study concluded that rather than a global loss of tolerance, there seem to be patient subsets with differing responses to selected microbial and potential autoantigens.

Subesquently, anti-I2 was independently associated with fibrostenosis and small bowel surgery, anti-Omp C with internal perforating behavior and ASCA with small bowel disease, fibrostenosis and small bowel surgery (Mow et al., 2004). Taken together, these results suggest that antibody responses to I2, OmpC and ASCA are associated with complicated small bowel Crohn's disease. The more antibody responses against different antigens present, the more likely that the patient will have a severe disease course (Mow et al., 2004). Patients expressing reactivity to all three markers (ASCA, I2 and anti-OmpC) were more likely to have fibrostenotic disease (72 per cent), internal perforating disease (58.7 per cent) and small bowel surgery (72 per cent), compared with the patients without reactivity (23 per cent, 27.9 per cent and 23 per cent respectively). The presence of all three markers (ASCA, I2 and anti-OmpC) carried an 8.6-fold increased risk for small bowel surgery, compared with patients without reactivity (Mow et al., 2004).

Although selective loss of tolerance to microbial antigens has begun to define clinically important subgroups of CD patients, the clinical value of these serodiagnostic tests is a matter of debate and large prospective analyses are mandated to determine whether these markers do in fact predict natural history and ultimately guide clinical decisions.

CORRELATION OF GENETIC MARKERS WITH SERUM ANTIBODIES IN IBD: DEFINING DISTINCT CLINICAL PHENOTYPES

As pANCA is present in 15–18 per cent of unaffected family members of UC patients, it may be a marker of genetic susceptibility (Yang, 1995). In the UC population, pANCA was associated with a specific HLA class II allele (DR2), while in pANCA negative UC, a different HLA association was found (HLA DR4) (Yang et al., 1993). In CD, pANCA expression was correlated with the presence of a polymorphism in the gene for the intracellular adhesion molecule-1 (ICAM-1) (Yang et al., 1995), an important surface protein involved in cell adhesion in the immune system. Thus, pANCA expression in both UC and CD defines subgroups of patients with unique genetic associations.

Patients with antibody responses toward microbial antigens (ASCA, I2, OmpC) have a high frequency of clinical complications regardless of NOD2 genotype (Mow et al., 2004). NOD2 variants were not associated with complicated small bowel surgery, indicating that disease behavior and severe course are more closely associated with immune responses toward microbial antigens than is the NOD2 genotype. Therefore, NOD2 can be seen as a marker for Crohn's disease susceptibility, whereas microbial antibody responses are indicators of disease course and severity. Confirming this conclusion, in another study of 163 patients with CD, the early development of stricturing or perforating disease after diagnosis was influenced by disease location, clinical activity and smoking habits, but not by the NOD2 genotype (Louis et al., 2003).

IMMUNE SYSTEM DYSREGULATION

Inappropriate immune responses evident in both UC and CD include alterations in the intestinal mucosal barrier and amplification of inflammation through the activation of lymphocytes and macrophages. In an exaggerated response to antigen, T cells are activated in UC and CD, leading to cytokine overproduction. Schreiber et al. (1991) documented increased expression of lymphocyte activation antigens on the cell surface of B cells, T cells, CD4+ T cells and CD8+ T cells found in the intestines of both UC and CD patients.

Although both forms of IBD are associated with T cell activation, CD and UC have traditionally been distinguished by distinct patterns of helper T cell dysfunction. Lamina propria cells of patients with CD have been shown to overproduce cytokines typically associated with a helper T cell 1 (Th1) response, such as IL-12 and interferon gamma (Fuss et al., 1996; Monteleone et al., 1997). In contrast, in patients with UC, a cytokine profile compatible with a helper T cell 2 (Th2) response has been observed, with increased production of IL-5, although not the major Th2 cytokine IL-4 (Mullin et al., 1992; Fuss et al., 1996). Discovery of murine models of mucosal inflammation resembling human IBD has been espoused as further evidence that Th1 and Th2 pathways predominate in CD and UC, respectively. However, because findings on the production of immunoregulatory cytokines in human IBD have been inconsistent and tremendous overlap consistently described between individual patients, the distinction from CD and UC by the production of Th1 and Th2 cytokines respectively is a vast oversimplification of a complicated question. Two caveats to this immunologic generalization are particularly pertinent to human IBD. First, mucosal cytokine patterns depend on when in the course of disease they are analyzed. Th1 cytokines have been detected in chronic, late-stage CD. However, in early ileal CD lesions seen in the postoperative setting, a Th2 cytokine pattern has been described (Desreumaux et al., 1997). Secondly, when cytokine production is systematically analyzed in mucosal tissue, there are heterogeneous cytokine responses among patients with both CD and UC (Andus et al., 1993; Plevy et al., 1997).

Additional research is needed to determine whether these T cell pathways differentiate the immunopathogenesis of CD and UC. Important regulatory T cell subsets have recently been described in the intestinal mucosa, which likely have a primary role in inhibiting inflammatory responses. T regulatory-1 (Tr1) cells make large amounts of IL-10 and some IFN-γ, while Th3 cells produce TGFβ (Smith et al., 2000). TGFβ producing T cells likely mediate the phenomenon of oral tolerance, which is a state of immune unresponsiveness to intestinal luminal antigens. For example, lymphocytes from mice do not proliferate when stimulated with antigens from their own enteric flora, but proliferate when stimulated with flora from other mice. Furthermore, mice (and, as discussed, people) with Th1-mediated IBD lose this tolerance to their own enteric flora, demonstrating the importance of regulatory T cell subsets in maintaining intestinal homeostasis (Duchmann et al., 1997). Most likely, cytokine profiles and elucidation of T cell subsets will be useful to determine subgroups within CD and UC rather than to distinguish one entity from the other.

TNF is a pro-inflammatory mediator secreted by mucosal macrophages and T cells and has been shown to play an integral role in the pathogenesis of IBD. Several studies have documented significant increases in TNF in the colonic mucosa of individuals with UC and CD compared with normal controls (MacDonald et al., 1990; Murch et al., 1993; Reinecker et al., 1993; Breese et al., 1994) and stool samples of patients with active UC and CD (Braegger et al., 1992).

High concentrations of mucosal IL-2 and IL-2 receptors have also been observed in both UC and CD (Kusugami et al., 1989). Moreover, patients with UC and CD have demonstrated impaired activity of IL-1 receptor antagonist

(RA). Decreased IL-1RA levels are associated with unopposed IL-1 secretion. Cominelli (1994) documented the ratio of intestinal IL-RA to IL-1 to be 5.6 ± 1.8 and 6.3 ± 1.5 in CD and UC patients, respectively, versus 24.8 ± 6.5 in normal controls ($P < 0.02$ control versus UC and CD). He found the imbalance between IL-1RA and IL-1 to be characteristic of UC and CD, as the ratio in non-IBD inflamed mucosa was similar to that in normal controls (Cominelli, 1994).

Cytokines such as TNF and IL-1 appear to invoke expression of vascular adhesion molecules, which in turn recruit leukocytes from the circulation to the site of intestinal mucosal inflammation in UC and CD. Koizumi et al. (1992) documented increased concentrations of endothelial-leukocyte adherence molecule 1 (ELAM-1) in the inflamed mucosa of patients with these disorders. ELAM-1 was associated with active inflammation and was found in similar concentrations in active UC and CD, leading the investigators to suggest that ELAM-1 is integrally important in sustaining and amplifying inflammation in IBD (Koizumi et al., 1992). Similarly, increased circulating and tissue levels of intercellular adhesion molecule 1 (ICAM-1) have been observed in active IBD (Patel et al., 1995; Nielsen et al., 1996).

Measurements of serum, fecal and mucosal cytokine, cytokine receptor and adhesion molecule profiles have not been useful to date in the clinical management of IBD patients. Reasons are technical as well as biologic. Serum cytokines such as TNF are subject to significant variation in individual subjects. Mucosal cytokine assays are often laborious and therefore not adaptable to screening of large populations. Furthermore, all reported studies in IBD patients share the common finding of extreme heterogeneity in responses. Whether this heterogeneity reflects true biology in patient subsets, assay variability or both is an unresolved question. Future work to define stable serum and fecal measures of inflammatory responses will likely lead to clinically useful markers to classify patient subgroups and gauge responses to therapeutic interventions.

MARKERS OF INTESTINAL PERMEABILITY AND INFLAMMATION

Within families with a positive history of IBD, prevalence rates vary between 5.5 and 22.5 per cent (Ahmad et al., 2001). There has been growing interest in searching for subclinical markers of IBD in families. These markers may reveal clues to genetic and/or environmental factors predisposing to IBD and/or identify an early phase of subclinical disease. Well-studied markers include the serological antibodies and intestinal permeability. Additionally, complement dysfunction, colonic mucin abnormalities and altered immunoglobulin secretion have been found in relatives of patients with IBD (Yang, 1995). Ten to 78 per cent of first-degree relatives of IBD patients may have increased intestinal permeability (Hollander et al., 1986; Katz et al., 1989; Peeters et al., 1997; Soderholm et al., 1999; Irvine and Marshall, 2000). In these studies, intestinal permeability was assessed by gastrointestinal absorption and urinary excretion of poly-ethylene glycol (Ma et al., 1989). Increased intestinal per-meability may in fact be a cause or a consequence of intestinal inflammation. Increased intestinal permeability in relatives of IBD patients may represent a genetically determined defect, or indicate the presence of a com-mon environmental factor leading to inflammation. As discussed, pANCA has been found with increased fre-quency in healthy relatives of UC patients. ASCA has been reported in 9–20 per cent of healthy relatives of CD patients. The lack of ASCA concordance in marital cou-ples may indicate a genetic factor, or perhaps a childhood environmental exposure.

Recent studies in IBD have evaluated the role of fecal calprotectin as a marker of clinical and subclinical inflammation and increased intestinal permeability. Calprotectin comprises 60 per cent of the cytoplasmic protein fraction of circulating neutrophils and it is also found in monocytes, macrophages and intestinal eosinophils (Bjerke et al., 1993; Johne et al., 1997). Calprotectin has antibacterial, antifungal, immunomodu-latory and anti-proliferative effects (Brandtzaeg et al., 1995; Johne et al., 1997). Plasma concentrations of calpro-tectin are elevated in inflammatory diseases, including rheumatoid arthritis, lupus and IBD (Johne et al., 1997). Calprotectin is also detectable in feces. This non-invasive marker has a positive predictive value of 76 per cent for inflammatory gastrointestinal conditions (Tibble et al., 2002). Fecal calprotectin has correlated well with endo-scopic and histologic inflammation in UC and correlates with the gold standard assessment of indium-111 labeled neutrophil excretion in IBD (Roseth et al., 1997, 1999; Tibble 2000a, 2001; Laake et al., 2003). Above 30 mg/ml, it has up to 100 per cent sensitivity for the diagnosis of CD (Tibble et al., 2000b) and above 50 mg/ml, it has 90 per cent sensitivity to predict clinical relapse in CD and UC (Tibble et al., 2000a). Therefore, it may be useful clinically as an early subclinical marker of inflammation. Recently, a study of IBD patients and first-degree relatives from Iceland demonstrated that 49 per cent of healthy relatives of CD patients had fecal calprotectin levels exceeding normal (Thjodleifsson et al., 2003). No association of fecal calprotectin was found with NOD2 mutations or location of inflammatory disease in CD (Thjodleifsson et al., 2003). However, future prospective analyses of IBD patients and their first-degree relatives will be necessary before fecal calprotectin can be advocated as a routine test for sub-clinical inflammatory disease in patients, or as a potential diagnostic and prognostic test in asymptomatic relatives. One potential limitation of fecal calprotectin as a clinical diagnostic is that day-to-day variability in excretion by individual subjects has been documented (Husebye et al., 2001).

C-reactive protein (CRP) was originally named for its capacity to precipitate the C-polysaccharide of *Streptococcus pneumoniae*. It was the first acute phase protein to be described and is a sensitive systemic marker of inflammation. The acute phase response describes the physiological response to most forms of tissue damage, including infection, inflammation and malignancy (Pepys and Hirschfield, 2003). In particular, the synthesis of the number of proteins is rapidly upregulated in hepatocytes under control of cytokines originating at sites of inflamma-tion. Plasma CRP is produced by hepatocytes under the transcriptional control of the cytokine interleukin-6 (IL-6) (Pepys and Hirschfield, 2003). The plasma half-life of CRP is about 19 h and is constant under all conditions of health and disease. When the stimulus for increased production of CRP ceases, the circulating CRP concentration falls rap-idly. There is no significant seasonal variation in baseline CRP and there is no diurnal variation in CRP values (Vigushin et al., 1993). Therefore, CRP concentration is a very useful, albeit non-specific, marker of inflammation that can contribute to screening for inflammatory disease and monitoring of the response to treatment of inflamma-tion. CRP – long dismissed by clinicians – has become an important biomarker for response to anti-TNF based ther-apies, if not all biologic agents in CD. CRP has been demonstrated to drop precipitously following therapy with anti-TNF antibodies and this decrease has correlated with clinical improvement (Targan et al., 1997; Taylor et al., 2001). Interestingly, studies with a humanized anti-TNF monoclonal antibody CDP571 suggested that it may not be as efficacious as the FDA-approved chimeric mono-clonal anti-TNF antibody infliximab, particularly over the long term (Stack et al., 1997; Sandborn et al., 2001b). However, it appeared to work very well in the patient pop-ulation with elevated baseline CRPs (Sandborn et al., 2001b). As placebo responses have been notably higher in studies performed in CD after the initial infliximab trials (Ghosh et al., 2003), the elevated CRP patient population may be the most relevant comparator. The placebo response is much lower in this patient population and they seem to derive benefit from most anti-TNF agents (Ghosh et al., 2003; Ito et al., 2004). Whether differences in efficacy between anti-TNF agents can be demonstrated in patients who do not have elevated baseline CRPs is an interesting question for future study. Given the clear trend toward increasing placebo responses in clinical trials utiliz-ing patients with moderate to severe CD, stratification of studies based on baseline CRP will become standard (Sandborn et al., 2002; Ito et al., 2004).

THERAPEUTIC IMPLICATIONS: ANTI-TNF IN CD

Until recently, the medical management of CD and UC consisted primarily of aminosalicylates and cortico-steroids. Although these agents remain first-line therapy

Table 46.2 Summary of pathogenic mechanisms in CD and UC

Mechanism	Evidence
Genetic	<ul><li>High rates of familial CD and UC</li><li>Concordance for CD and UC in monozygotic twins</li><li>Susceptibility to CD and UC linked with chromosomes 1, 3, 6, 7, 10, 12, 16 and X</li><li>HLA associations: CD – HLA-DR1, DQw5. UC – HLA-DR2</li><li>Increased intestinal permeability in patients and first degree relatives</li></ul>
Serological markers	<ul><li>UC-specific pANCA</li><li>CD-specific ASCA, anti-OmpC, anti-I2</li></ul>
Infectious and environmental triggers	<ul><li>Occurrence of CD and UC associated with foreign travel, enteric infections and perinatal viral infections</li><li>Active CD and UC associated with decreased anaerobic bacteria and *Lactobacillus*</li><li>Serological reactivity against enteric bacterial antigens</li></ul>
Immune system dysregulation	<ul><li>Exaggerated and inappropriate immune responses observed in CD and UC<ul><li>Expression of lymphocyte activation antigens increased in B cells, T cells, CD4+ T cells and CD8+ T cells in UC and CD</li><li>Activated T cells and macrophages secrete pro-inflammatory and immunoregulatory cytokines, e.g. TNF, IL-2, IL-2 receptors</li><li>CD more Th1 predominant</li><li>UC more Th2 predominant?</li><li>Increased expression of vascular adhesion molecules, e.g. ELAM-1 and ICAM-1 in CD and UC</li></ul></li></ul>

for UC, immunomodulators, antibiotics and biologic response modifiers are being used earlier in the treatment of CD (Regueiro, 2000).

Several biologic response modifiers have been evaluated predominantly in patients with CD. These agents include antibodies specific for cytokines known to be key to the pathogenesis of mucosal inflammation in IBD such as anti-TNF agents, anti-inflammatory cytokines such as IL-10 and therapies that inhibit adhesion molecules. Use of such agents that more specifically target major elements of the immune system and inflammatory cascade may offer the greatest promise for a reduction in the morbidity and mortality of IBD.

Infliximab, a chimeric monoclonal antibody directed against TNF is currently the only clinically available biologic therapy for IBD. In controlled clinical studies, infliximab has been used successfully to induce and maintain clinical remission in patients with moderately to severely active CD resistant to conventional treatment, as well as in fistulizing Crohn's disease (Targan et al., 1997; Present et al., 1999; Hanauer et al., 2002; Sands et al., 2004). Recent studies have investigated whether serologic antibody markers or genotype predict response to anti-TNF therapy with infliximab (Vermeire et al., 2000, 2002; Taylor

et al., 2001). In 85 patients who received infliximab for treatment of refractory and fistulizing CD, ASCA and pANCA assays were obtained at baseline and 4 weeks after treatment (Vermeire et al., 2000). ASCA was not predictive for response to the anti-TNF therapy, but the combination of pANCA-positive and ASCA-negative findings was associated with non-response. Taylor et al. (2001) evaluated marker patterns and TNF genotype in 59 patients with CD who did not respond to a single infusion of either placebo or infliximab in a controlled clinical trial (Targan et al., 1997) and were subsequently given another infusion of the biologic agent in an open-label extension. Their observations suggested that a cytoplasmic ANCA is predictive for a CD subgroup with a better response to infliximab; in contrast, pANCA and homozygosity for the lymphotoxin α 1-1-1-1 haplotype appeared to identify subgroups of patients with a poorer response. Furthermore, TNF receptor polymorphisms may correlate with clinical responses to infliximab in CD (Mascheretti et al., 2002). However, no definitive conclusions can be made based on these studies because of the small sample sizes. Larger studies are required better to define the associations between response to anti-TNF therapy and different immunologic markers or lymphotoxin/TNF receptor genotype. Two large studies demonstrated that NOD2 genotype failed to predict responses to infliximab therapy in CD (Taylor et al., 2001; Vermeire et al., 2002).

Fc gamma RIIIa is expressed on macrophages and natural killer cells and is involved in antibody-dependent cell-mediated cytotoxicity. Polymorphisms in the gene for Fc gamma RIIIa have recently been associated with a positive response to rituximab (Cartron et al., 2002), a recombinant IgG1 antibody used in non-Hodgkin's lymphomas. A single nucleotide Fc gamma IIIa polymorphism was determined in 200 CD patients who had received infliximab for refractory CD. Genotypes V/V, V/F and F/F were defined in this population. Decreases in CRP following infliximab were significantly higher in V/V patients. In the subgroup of patients with elevated CRP before treatment, immunosuppressive drugs and FCGR3A genotype were independent factors influencing the clinical response to infliximab (Cartron et al., 2002). Mechanistically, Fc receptor polymorphisms may alter interactions of host Fc receptors with monoclonal antibodies, affecting their biologic activity, or perhaps modulating clearance/half-life of a biologic compound.

KEYS TO FUTURE RESEARCH

The most immediate hope better to understand immune responses in IBD comes from the rapid progress in elucidating the genetics of these disorders. High throughput assays for genetic polymorphisms make the rapid genotyping of large patient populations with IBD a relatively simple task. Many groups have accumulated or are in the process of accumulating cohorts of patients who are well phenotyped clinically. Serological markers which can be qualitatively and quantitatively assayed have provided insights into immune reactivity against the enteric bacterial flora and have begun to define clinically important subgroups of IBD patients. To translate these scientific advances into the clinic, large prospective studies evaluating clinically meaningful endpoints such as natural history and response to medical or surgical therapy are mandated. Immunophenotyping of IBD patients will be greatly facilitated in the future by the development of better assays for T cell reactivity against enteric antigens. The development of these assays will be essential, particularly in the context of clinical studies of new biologic compounds, many of which target T cells. Large-scale genomic and proteomic approaches are being utilized to identify new serum and mucosal markers of disease activity and disease phenotype. As the immunogenetics of the IBDs are further elucidated, clinical definitions established in the 1920s will certainly be revised, as distinct, clinically important subgroups of patients emerge.

REFERENCES

Abreu, M.T., Taylor, K.D., Lin, Y.C. et al. (2002). Mutations in NOD2 are associated with fibrostenosing disease in patients with Crohn's disease. Gastroenterology 123, 679–688.

Ahmad, T.S.J., McGovern, D. et al. (2001). The genetics of inflammatory bowel disease. Aliment Pharmacol Ther 731–748.

Aisenberg, J., Legnani, P.E., Nilubol, N. et al. (2004). Are pANCA, ASCA, or cytokine gene polymorphisms associated with pouchitis? Long-term follow-up in 102 ulcerative colitis patients. Am J Gastroenterol 99, 432–441.

Andres, P.G. and Friedman, L.S. (1999). Epidemiology and the natural course of inflammatory bowel disease. Gastroenterol Clin North Am 28, 255–281, vii.

Andus, T., Targan, S.R., Deem, R. and Toyoda, H. (1993). Measurement of tumor necrosis factor alpha mRNA in small numbers of cells by quantitative polymerase chain reaction. Reg Immunol 5, 11–17.

Angulo, P., Peter, J.B., Gershwin, M.E. et al. (2000). Serum autoantibodies in patients with primary sclerosing cholangitis. J Hepatol 32, 182–187.

Annese, V., Andreoli, A., Andriulli, A. et al. (2001). Familial expression of anti-Saccharomyces cerevisiae Mannan antibodies in Crohn's disease and ulcerative colitis: a GISC study. Am J Gastroenterol 96, 2407–2412.

Arashi, M., Konno, K. and Yachi, A. (1995). Immunoglobulin subclass distribution of anti-LPS antibody-secreting cells of colonic mucosa from patients with inflammatory bowel disease. Adv Exp Med Biol 371B, 1277–1280.

Armuzzi, A., Ahmad, T., Ling, K.L. et al. (2003). Genotype-phenotype analysis of the Crohn's disease susceptibility haplotype on chromosome 5q31. Gut 52, 1133–1139.

Barton, J.G., Paden, M.A., Lane, M. and Postier R.G. (2001). Comparison of postoperative outcomes in ulcerative colitis and familial polyposis patients after ileoanal pouch operations. Am J Surg 182, 616–620.

Bayless, T.M., Tokayer, A.Z., Polito, J.M. 2nd, Quaskey, S.A., Mellits, E.D. and Harris, M.L. (1996). Crohn's disease: concordance

for site and clinical type in affected family members – potential hereditary influences. Gastroenterology 111, 573–579.

Biancone, L., Mandal, A., Yang, H. et al. (1995). Production of immunoglobulin G and G1 antibodies to cytoskeletal protein by lamina propria cells in ulcerative colitis. Gastroenterology 109, 3–12.

Billing, P., Tahir, S., Calfin, B. et al. (1995). Nuclear localization of the antigen detected by ulcerative colitis-associated perinuclear antineutrophil cytoplasmic antibodies. Am J Pathol 147, 979–987.

Bjerke, K., Halstensen, T.S., Jahnsen, F., Pulford, K. and Brandtzaeg, P. (1993). Distribution of macrophages and granulocytes expressing L1 protein (calprotectin) in human Peyer's patches compared with normal ileal lamina propria and mesenteric lymph nodes. Gut 34, 1357–1363.

Braegger, C.P., Nicholls, S., Murch, S.H., Stephens, S. and MacDonald, T.T. (1992). Tumour necrosis factor alpha in stool as a marker of intestinal inflammation. Lancet 339, 89–91.

Brandtzaeg, P., Gabrielsen, T.O., Dale, I., Muller, F., Steinbakk, M. and Fagerhol, M.K. (1995). The leucocyte protein L1 (calprotectin): a putative nonspecific defence factor at epithelial surfaces. Adv Exp Med Biol 371A, 201–206.

Brandwein, S.L., McCabe, R.P., Cong, Y. et al. (1997). Spontaneously colitic C3H/HeJBir mice demonstrate selective antibody reactivity to antigens of the enteric bacterial flora. J Immunol 159, 44–52.

Breese, E.J., Michie, C.A., Nicholls, S.W. et al. (1994). Tumor necrosis factor alpha-producing cells in the intestinal mucosa of children with inflammatory bowel disease. Gastroenterology 106, 1455–1466.

Brett, P.M., Yasuda, N., Yiannakou, J.Y. et al. (1996). Genetic and immunological markers in pouchitis. Eur J Gastroenterol Hepatol 8, 951–955.

Broekroelofs, J., Mulder, A.H., Nelis, G.F., Westerveld, B.D., Tervaert, J.W. and Kallenberg, C.G. (1994). Anti-neutrophil cytoplasmic antibodies (ANCA) in sera from patients with inflammatory bowel disease (IBD). Relation to disease pattern and disease activity. Dig Dis Sci 39, 545–549.

Calkins, B. (1994). Inflammatory bowel disease. In Digestive Diseases in the United States: Epidemiology and Impact, Je, E., ed. Publication No. 94–1447. Washington, DC: Dept of Health & Human Services.

Calkins, B.M., Lilienfeld, A.M., Garland, C.F. and Mendeloff, A.I. (1984). Trends in incidence rates of ulcerative colitis and Crohn's disease. Dig Dis Sci 29, 913–920.

Carter, M.J., Jones, S., Camp, N.J. et al. (2004). Functional correlates of the interleukin-1 receptor antagonist gene polymorphism in the colonic mucosa in ulcerative colitis. Genes Immun 5, 8–15.

Cartron, G., Dacheux, L., Salles, G. (2002). Therapeutic activity of humanized anti-CD20 monoclonal antibody and polymorphism in IgG Fc receptor FcgammaRIIIa gene. Blood 99, 754–758.

Casini-Raggi, V., Kam, L., Chong, Y.J., Fiocchi, C., Pizarro, T.T. and Cominelli, F. (1995). Mucosal imbalance of IL-1 and IL-1 receptor antagonist in inflammatory bowel disease. A novel mechanism of chronic intestinal inflammation. J Immunol 154, 2434–2440.

Cohavy, O., Harth, G., Horwitz, M. et al. (1999). Identification of a novel mycobacterial histone H1 homologue (HupB) as an antigenic target of pANCA monoclonal antibody and serum immunoglobulin A from patients with Crohn's disease. Infect Immun 67, 6510–6517.

Cohavy, O., Bruckner, D., Gordon, L.K. et al. (2000). Colonic bacteria express an ulcerative colitis pANCA-related protein epitope. Infect Immun 68, 1542–1548.

Cominelli, F. (1994). Specific mucosal imbalance of IL-1 and IL-1 receptor antagonist (IL-Ira) in IBD: a potential mechanism of chronic inflammation. Gastroenterology 106.

Cong, Y., Brandwein, S.L., McCabe, R.P. et al. (1998). CD4+ T cells reactive to enteric bacterial antigens in spontaneously colitic C3H/HeJBir mice: increased T helper cell type 1 response and ability to transfer disease. J Exp Med 187, 855–864.

Cong, Y., Weaver, C.T., Lazenby, A. and Elson, C.O. (2002). Bacterial-reactive T regulatory cells inhibit pathogenic immune responses to the enteric flora. J Immunol 169, 6112–6119.

Crohn, B.B., Ginzburg, L. and Oppenheimer, G.D. (1984). Landmark article Oct 15, 1932. Regional ileitis. A pathological and clinical entity. By Burril B. Crohn, Leon Ginzburg and Gordon D. Oppenheimer. J Am Med Assoc 251, 73–79.

Cuthbert, A.P., Fisher, S.A., Mirza, M.M. et al. (2002). The contribution of NOD2 gene mutations to the risk and site of disease in inflammatory bowel disease. Gastroenterology 122, 867–874.

Dalwadi, H., Wei, B., Kronenberg, M., Sutton, C.L. and Braun, J. (2001). The Crohn's disease-associated bacterial protein I2 is a novel enteric t cell superantigen. Immunity 15, 149–158.

Desreumaux, P., Brandt, E., Gambiez, L. et al. (1997). Distinct cytokine patterns in early and chronic ileal lesions of Crohn's disease. Gastroenterology 113, 118–126.

Dubinsky, M.C., Ofman, J.J., Urman, M., Targan, S.R. and Seidman, E.G. (2001). Clinical utility of serodiagnostic testing in suspected pediatric inflammatory bowel disease. Am J Gastroenterol 96, 758–765.

Duchmann, R., Kaiser, I., Hermann, E., Mayet, W., Ewe, K. and Meyer zum Buschenfelde, K.H. (1995). Tolerance exists towards resident intestinal flora but is broken in active inflammatory bowel disease (IBD). Clin Exp Immunol 102, 448–455.

Duchmann, R., Schmitt, E., Knolle, P. et al. (1996). Tolerance towards resident intestinal flora in mice is abrogated in experimental colitis and restored by treatment with interleukin-10 or antibodies to interleukin-12. Eur J Immunol 26, 934–938.

Duchmann, R., Neurath, M.F. and Meyer zum Buschenfelde, K.H. (1997). Responses to self and non-self intestinal microflora in health and inflammatory bowel disease. Res Immunol 148, 589–594.

Dumonceau, J.M., Van Gossum, A., Adler, M. et al. (1996). No Mycobacterium paratuberculosis found in Crohn's disease using polymerase chain reaction. Dig Dis Sci 41, 421–426.

Eggena, M., Cohavy, O., Parseghian, M.H. et al. (2000). Identification of histone H1 as a cognate antigen of the ulcerative colitis-associated marker antibody pANCA. J Autoimmun 14, 83–97.

Elliott, D.E., Urban, J.J., Argo, C.K. and Weinstock, J.V. (2000). Does the failure to acquire helminthic parasites predispose to Crohn's disease? Faseb J 14, 1848–1855.

Elliott, D.E., Li, J., Blum, A. et al. (2003). Exposure to schistosome eggs protects mice from TNBS-induced colitis. Am J Physiol Gastrointest Liver Physiol 284, G385–391.

Facklis, K., Plevy, S.E., Vasiliauskas, E.A. et al. (1999). Crohn's disease-associated genetic marker is seen in medically unresponsive ulcerative colitis patients and may be associated with pouch-specific complications. Dis Colon Rectum 42, 601–605; discussion 605–606.

Falk, R.J., Hogan, S.L., Wilkman, A.S. et al. (1990). Myeloperoxidase specific anti-neutrophil cytoplasmic autoantibodies (MPO-ANCA). Neth J Med 3, 121–125.

Farmer, R. (1986). Association of inflammatory bowel disease in families. Gastrointest Res 11, 17–26.

Fiocchi, C. (1998). Inflammatory bowel disease: etiology and pathogenesis. Gastroenterology 115, 182–205.

Fiocchi, C., Roche, J.K. and Michener, W.M. (1989). High prevalence of antibodies to intestinal epithelial antigens in patients with inflammatory bowel disease and their relatives. Ann Intern Med 110, 786–794.

Fleshner, P.R., Vasiliauskas, E.A., Kam, L.Y. et al. (2001). High level perinuclear antineutrophil cytoplasmic antibody (pANCA) in ulcerative colitis patients before colectomy predicts the development of chronic pouchitis after ileal pouch-anal anastomosis. Gut 49, 671–677.

Fonkalsrud, E.W. (1996). Long-term results after colectomy and ileoanal pull-through procedure in children. Arch Surg 131, 881–885; discussion 885–886.

Fuss, I.J., Neurath, M., Boirivant, M. et al. (1996). Disparate CD4+ lamina propria (LP) lymphokine secretion profiles in inflammatory bowel disease. Crohn's disease LP cells manifest increased secretion of IFN-gamma, whereas ulcerative colitis LP cells manifest increased secretion of IL-5. J Immunol 157, 1261–1270.

Geboes, K. and De Hertogh, G. (2003). Indeterminate colitis. Inflamm Bowel Dis 9, 324–331.

Geng, X., Biancone, L., Dai, H.H. et al. (1998). Tropomyosin isoforms in intestinal mucosa: production of autoantibodies to tropomyosin isoforms in ulcerative colitis. Gastroenterology 114, 912–922.

Ghosh, S., Goldin, E., Gordon, F.H. et al. (2003). Natalizumab for active Crohn's disease. N Engl J Med 348, 24–32.

Gionchetti, P., Campieri, M., Belluzzi, A. et al. (1994). Mucosal concentrations of interleukin-1 beta, interleukin-6, interleukin-8, and tumor necrosis factor-alpha in pelvic ileal pouches. Dig Dis Sci 39, 1525–1531.

Gionchetti, P., Rizzello, F., Venturi, A. et al. (2000). Oral bacteriotherapy as maintenance treatment in patients with chronic pouchitis: a double-blind, placebo-controlled trial. Gastroenterology 119, 305–309.

Gionchetti, P., Rizzello, F., Helwig, U. et al. (2003). Prophylaxis of pouchitis onset with probiotic therapy: a double-blind, placebo-controlled trial. Gastroenterology 124, 1202–1209.

Gitnick, G., Collins, J., Beaman, B. et al. (1989). Preliminary report on isolation of mycobacteria from patients with Crohn's disease. Dig Dis Sci 34, 925–932.

Gross, W.L. and Csernok, E. (1995). Immunodiagnostic and pathophysiologic aspects of antineutrophil cytoplasmic antibodies in vasculitis. Curr Opin Rheumatol 7, 11–19.

Gross, W.L., Csernok, E. and Helmchen, U. (1995). Antineutrophil cytoplasmic autoantibodies, autoantigens, and systemic vasculitis. Apmis 103, 81–97.

Hajeer, A.H. and Hutchinson, I.V. (2001). Influence of TNFalpha gene polymorphisms on TNFalpha production and disease. Hum Immunol 62, 1191–1199.

Hampe, J., Grebe, J., Nikolaus, S. et al. (2002). Association of NOD2 (CARD 15) genotype with clinical course of Crohn's disease: a cohort study. Lancet 359, 1661–1665.

Hanauer, S.B., Feagan, B.G., Lichtenstein, G.R. et al. (2002). Maintenance infliximab for Crohn's disease: the ACCENT I randomised trial. Lancet 359, 1541–1549.

Hardarson, S., Labrecque, D.R., Mitros, F.A., Neil, G.A. and Goeken, J.A. (1993). Antineutrophil cytoplasmic antibody in inflammatory bowel and hepatobiliary diseases. High prevalence in ulcerative colitis, primary sclerosing cholangitis, and autoimmune hepatitis. Am J Clin Pathol 99, 277–281.

Henderson, C.A., Greenlee, L., Williams, R.C. Jr and Strickland, R.G. (1976). Characterization of anti-lymphocyte antibodies in inflammatory bowel disease. Scand J Immunol 5, 837–844.

Higashi, A., Watanabe, Y., Ozasa, K., Hayashi, K., Aoike, A. and Kawai, K. (1988). Prevalence and mortality of ulcerative colitis and Crohn's disease in Japan. Gastroenterol Jpn 23, 521–526.

Hollander, D., Vadheim, C.M., Brettholz, E., Petersen, G.M., Delahunty, T. and Rotter, J.I. (1986). Increased intestinal permeability in patients with Crohn's disease and their relatives. A possible etiologic factor. Ann Intern Med 105, 883–885.

Hugot, J.P. and Thomas, G. (1998). Genome-wide scanning in inflammatory bowel diseases. Dig Dis 16, 364–369.

Hugot, J.P., Chamaillard, M., Zouali, H. et al. (2001). Association of NOD2 leucine-rich repeat variants with susceptibility to Crohn's disease. Nature 411, 599–603.

Hulten, K., Karttunen, T.J., El-Zimaity, H.M. et al. (2000a). Identification of cell wall deficient forms of M. avium subsp. paratuberculosis in paraffin embedded tissues from animals with Johne's disease by in situ hybridization. J Microbiol Methods 42, 185–195.

Hulten, K., Almashhrawi, A., El-Zaatari, F.A. and Graham, D.Y. (2000b). Antibacterial therapy for Crohn's disease: a review emphasizing therapy directed against mycobacteria. Dig Dis Sci 45, 445–456.

Hurst, R.D., Molinari, M., Chung, T.P., Rubin, M. and Michelassi, F. (1996). Prospective study of the incidence, timing and treatment of pouchitis in 104 consecutive patients after restorative proctocolectomy. Arch Surg 131, 497–500; discussion 501–502.

Husebye, E., Ton, H. and Johne, B. (2001). Biological variability of fecal calprotectin in patients referred for colonoscopy without colonic inflammation or neoplasm. Am J Gastroenterol 96, 2683–2687.

Ibbotson, J.P., Lowes, J.R., Chahal, H. et al. (1992). Mucosal cell-mediated immunity to mycobacterial, enterobacterial and other microbial antigens in inflammatory bowel disease. Clin Exp Immunol 87, 224–230.

Inohara, N., Ogura, Y., Fontalba, A. et al. (2003). Host recognition of bacterial muramyl dipeptide mediated through NOD2. Implications for Crohn's disease. J Biol Chem 278, 5509–5512.

Irvine, E.J. and Marshall, J.K. (2000). Increased intestinal permeability precedes the onset of Crohn's disease in a subject with familial risk. Gastroenterology 119, 1740–1744.

Ito, H., Takazoe, M., Fukuda, Y. et al. (2004). A pilot randomized trial of a human anti-interleukin-6 receptor monoclonal antibody in active Crohn's disease. Gastroenterology 126, 989–996.

Jennette, J.C., Hoidal, J.R. and Falk, R.J. (1990). Specificity of anti-neutrophil cytoplasmic autoantibodies for proteinase 3. Blood 75, 2263–2264.

Johne, B., Fagerhol, M.K., Lyberg, T. et al. (1997). Functional and clinical aspects of the myelomonocyte protein calprotectin. Mol Pathol 50, 113–123.

Joossens, S., Reinisch, W., Vermeire, S. et al. (2002). The value of serologic markers in indeterminate colitis: a prospective follow-up study. Gastroenterology 122, 1242–1247.

Katz, K.D., Hollander, D., Vadheim, C.M. et al. (1989). Intestinal permeability in patients with Crohn's disease and their healthy relatives. Gastroenterology 97, 927–931.

Khan, W.I., Blennerhasset, P.A., Varghese, A.K. et al. (2002). Intestinal nematode infection ameliorates experimental colitis in mice. Infect Immun 70, 5931–5937.

Kirsner, J.B. (1988). Historical aspects of inflammatory bowel disease. J Clin Gastroenterol 10, 286–297.

Kobayashi, K., Brown, W.R., Brennan, P.J. and Blaser, M.J. (1988). Serum antibodies to mycobacterial antigens in active Crohn's disease. Gastroenterology 94, 1404–1411.

Koizumi, M., King, N., Lobb, R., Benjamin, C. and Podolsky, D.K. (1992). Expression of vascular adhesion molecules in inflammatory bowel disease. Gastroenterology 103, 840–847.

Korsmeyer, S., Strickland, R.G., Wilson, I.D. and Williams, R.C. Jr (1974). Serum lymphocytotoxic and lymphocytophilic antibody activity in inflammatory bowel disease. Gastroenterology 67, 578–583.

Kossa, K., Coulthart, A., Ives, C.T., Pusey, C.D. and Hodgson, H.J. (1995). Antigen specificity of circulating anti-neutrophil cytoplasmic antibodies in inflammatory bowel disease. Eur J Gastroenterol Hepatol 7, 783–789.

Kugathasan, S., Judd, R.H., Hoffmann, R.G. et al. (2003). Epidemiologic and clinical characteristics of children with newly diagnosed inflammatory bowel disease in Wisconsin: a statewide population-based study. J Pediatr 143, 525–531.

Kullberg, M.C., Rothfuchs, A.G., Jankovic, D. et al. (2001). Helicobacter hepaticus-induced colitis in interleukin-10-deficient mice: cytokine requirements for the induction and maintenance of intestinal inflammation. Infect Immun 69, 4232–4241.

Kusugami, K., Youngman, K.R., West, G.A. and Fiocchi, C. (1989). Intestinal immune reactivity to interleukin 2 differs among Crohn's disease, ulcerative colitis, and controls. Gastroenterology 97, 1–9.

Laake, K.O., Line, P.D., Aabakken, L. et al. (2003). Assessment of mucosal inflammation and circulation in response to probiotics in patients operated with ileal pouch anal anastomosis for ulcerative colitis. Scand J Gastroenterol 38, 409–414.

Lala, S., Ogura, Y., Osborne, C. et al. (2003). Crohn's disease and the NOD2 gene: a role for paneth cells. Gastroenterology 125, 47–57.

Lammers, K.M., Helwig, U., Swennen, E. et al. (2002). Effect of probiotic strains on interleukin 8 production by HT29/19A cells. Am J Gastroenterol 97, 1182–1186.

Landers, C.J., Cohavy, O., Misra, R. et al. (2002). Selected loss of tolerance evidenced by Crohn's disease-associated immune responses to auto- and microbial antigens. Gastroenterology 123, 689–699.

Langholz, E., Munkholm, P., Nielsen, O.H., Kreiner, S. and Binder, V. (1991). Incidence and prevalence of ulcerative colitis in Copenhagen county from 1962 to 1987. Scand J Gastroenterol 26, 1247–1256.

Lesage, S., Zouali, H., Cezard, J.P. et al. (2002). CARD15/NOD2 mutational analysis and genotype-phenotype correlation in 612 patients with inflammatory bowel disease. Am J Hum Genet 70, 845–857.

Loftus, E. (2004). Epidemiology of inflammatory bowel disease. Gastroenterol Clin North Am In Press.

Loftus, E.V. Jr, Silverstein, M.D., Sandborn, W.J., Tremaine, W.J., Harmsen, W.S. and Zinsmeister, A.R. (2000). Ulcerative colitis in Olmsted County, Minnesota, 1940–1993: incidence, prevalence, and survival. Gut 46, 336–343.

Louis, E., Michel, V., Hugot, J.P. et al. (2003). Early development of stricturing or penetrating pattern in Crohn's disease is influenced by disease location, number of flares, and smoking but not by NOD2/CARD15 genotype. Gut 52, 552–557.

Ma, T., Hollander, D., Krugliak, P. and Katz, K. (1989). Gastrointestinal permeability to polyethylene glycol: an evaluation of urinary recovery of an oral load of polyethylene glycol as a parameter of intestinal permeability in man. Eur J Clin Invest 19, 412.

MacDonald, T.T., Hutchings, P., Choy, M.Y., Murch, S. and Cooke, A. (1990). Tumour necrosis factor-alpha and interferon-gamma production measured at the single cell level in normal and inflamed human intestine. Clin Exp Immunol 81, 301–305.

Madsen, K.L., Doyle, J.S., Jewell, L.D., Tavernini, M.M. and Fedorak, R.N. (1999). Lactobacillus species prevents colitis in interleukin 10 gene-deficient mice. Gastroenterology 116, 1107–1114.

Madsen, K., Cornish, A., Soper, P. et al. (2001). Probiotic bacteria enhance murine and human intestinal epithelial barrier function. Gastroenterology 121, 580–591.

McFadden, J.J., Butcher, P.D., Chiodini, R. and Hermon-Taylor, J. (1987). Crohn's disease-isolated mycobacteria are identical to Mycobacterium paratuberculosis, as determined by DNA probes that distinguish between mycobacterial species. J Clin Microbiol 25, 796–801.

McFadden, J., Collins, J., Beaman, B., Arthur, M. and Gitnick, G. (1992). Mycobacteria in Crohn's disease: DNA probes identify the wood pigeon strain of Mycobacterium avium and Mycobacterium paratuberculosis from human tissue. J Clin Microbiol 30, 3070–3073.

Mascheretti, S., Hampe, J., Kuhbacher, T. et al. (2002). Pharmacogenetic investigation of the TNF/TNF-receptor system in patients with chronic active Crohn's disease treated with infliximab. Pharmacogenomics J 2, 127–136.

Mimura, T., Rizzello, F., Helwig, U. et al. (2004). Once daily high dose probiotic therapy (VSL 3) for maintaining remission in recurrent or refractory pouchitis. Gut 53, 108–114.

Monteleone, G., Biancone, L., Marasco, R. et al. (1997). Interleukin 12 is expressed and actively released by Crohn's disease intestinal lamina propria mononuclear cells. Gastroenterology 112, 1169–1178.

Mow, W.S., Vasiliauskas, E.A., Lin, Y.C. et al. (2004). Association of antibody responses to microbial antigens and complications of small bowel Crohn's disease. Gastroenterology 126, 414–424.

Mulder, A.H., Horst, G., Haagsma, E.B., Limburg, P.C., Kleibeuker, J.H. and Kallenberg, C.G. (1993). Prevalence and characterization of neutrophil cytoplasmic antibodies in autoimmune liver diseases. Hepatology 17, 411–417.

Muller-Ladner, U., Gross, V., Andus, T. et al. (1996). Distinct patterns of immunoglobulin classes and IgG subclasses of autoantibodies in patients with inflammatory bowel disease. Eur J Gastroenterol Hepatol 8, 579–584.

Mullin, G.E., Lazenby, A.J., Harris, M.L., Bayless, T.M. and James, S.P. (1992). Increased interleukin-2 messenger RNA in the intestinal mucosal lesions of Crohn's disease but not ulcerative colitis. Gastroenterology 102, 1620–1627.

Murch, S.H., Braegger, C.P., Walker-Smith, J.A. and MacDonald, T.T. (1993). Location of tumour necrosis factor alpha by immunohistochemistry in chronic inflammatory bowel disease. Gut 34, 1705–1709.

Nielsen, O.H., Brynskov, J. and Vainer, B. (1996). Increased mucosal concentrations of soluble intercellular adhesion molecule-1 (sICAM-1), sE-selectin, and interleukin-8 in active ulcerative colitis. Dig Dis Sci 41, 1780–1785.

Ogura, Y., Bonen, D.K., Inohara, N. et al. (2001a). A frameshift mutation in NOD2 associated with susceptibility to Crohn's disease. Nature 411, 603–606.

Ogura, Y., Inohara, N., Benito, A., Chen, F.F., Yamaoka, S. and Nunez, G. (2001b). Nod2, a Nod1/Apaf-1 family member that is restricted to monocytes and activates NF-kappaB. J Biol Chem 276, 4812–4818.

Ogura, Y., Lala, S., Xin, W et al. (2003). Expression of NOD2 in Paneth cells: a possible link to Crohn's ileitis. Gut 52, 1591–1597.

Olsen, I., Wiker, H.G., Johnson, E., Langeggen H. and Reitan, L.J. (2001). Elevated antibody responses in patients with Crohn's disease against a 14-kDa secreted protein purified from Mycobacterium avium subsp. paratuberculosis. Scand J Immunol 53, 198–203.

Onuma, E.K., Amenta, P.S., Ramaswamy, K., Lin, J.J. and Das, K.M. (2000). Autoimmunity in ulcerative colitis (UC): a predominant colonic mucosal B cell response against human tropomyosin isoform 5. Clin Exp Immunol 121, 466–471.

Orholm, M., Munkholm, P., Langholz, E., Nielsen, O.H., Sorensen, I.A. and Binder, V. (1991). Familial occurrence of inflammatory bowel disease. N Engl J Med 324, 84–88.

Orholm, M., Binder, V., Sorensen, T.I., Rasmussen, L.P. and Kyvik, K.O. (2000). Concordance of inflammatory bowel disease among Danish twins. Results of a nationwide study. Scand J Gastroenterol 35, 1075–1081.

Papadakis, K.A. and Targan, S.R. (1999). Serologic testing in inflammatory bowel disease: its value in indeterminate colitis. Curr Gastroenterol Rep 1, 482–485.

Papo, M., Quer, J.C., Gutierrez, C. et al. (1999). Genetic heterogeneity within ulcerative colitis determined by an interleukin-1 receptor antagonist gene polymorphism and antineutrophil cytoplasmic antibodies. Eur J Gastroenterol Hepatol 11, 413–420.

Patel, R.T., Pall, A.A., Adu, D. and Keighley, M.R. (1995). Circulating soluble adhesion molecules in inflammatory bowel disease. Eur J Gastroenterol Hepatol 7, 1037–1041.

Peetermans, W.E., D'Haens, G.R., Ceuppens, J.L., Rutgeerts, P. and Geboes, K. (1995). Mucosal expression by B7-positive cells of the 60-kilodalton heat-shock protein in inflammatory bowel disease. Gastroenterology 108, 75–82.

Peeters, M., Nevens, H., Baert, F. et al. (1996). Familial aggregation in Crohn's disease: increased age-adjusted risk and concordance in clinical characteristics. Gastroenterology 111, 597–603.

Peeters, M., Geypens, B., Claus, D. et al. (1997). Clustering of increased small intestinal permeability in families with Crohn's disease. Gastroenterology 113, 802–807.

Peeters, M., Joossens, S., Vermeire, S., Vlietinck, R., Bossuyt, X. and Rutgeerts, P. (2001). Diagnostic value of anti-Saccharomyces cerevisiae and antineutrophil cytoplasmic autoantibodies in inflammatory bowel disease. Am J Gastroenterol 96, 730–734.

Penna, C., Dozois, R., Tremaine, W. et al. (1996). Pouchitis after ileal pouch-anal anastomosis for ulcerative colitis occurs with increased frequency in patients with associated primary sclerosing cholangitis. Gut 38, 234–239.

Pepys, M.B. and Hirschfield, G.M. (2003). C-reactive protein: a critical update. J Clin Invest 111, 1805–1812.

Plevy, K. TKDTSDSSTS. (1997). Tumor necrosis factor microsatellite (TNF) haplotypes and perinuclear anti-neutrophil cytoplasmic antibody identify Crohn's disease patients with poor clinical responses to anti-TNF monoclonal antibody (cA2). Gastroenterology 112, A1062.

Plevy, S.E., Landers, C.J., Prehn, J. et al. (1997). A role for TNF-alpha and mucosal T helper-1 cytokines in the pathogenesis of Crohn's disease. J Immunol 159, 6276–6282.

Podolsky, D.K. (2002). Inflammatory bowel disease. N Engl J Med 347, 417–429.

Prantera, C., Berto, E., Scribano, M.L. and Falasco, G. (1998). Use of antibiotics in the treatment of active Crohn's disease: experience with metronidazole and ciprofloxacin. Ital J Gastroenterol Hepatol 30, 602–606.

Prantera, C., Kohn, A., Mangiarotti, R., Andreoli, A. and Luzi, C. (1994). Antimycobacterial therapy in Crohn's disease: results of a controlled, double-blind trial with a multiple antibiotic regimen. Am J Gastroenterol 89, 513–518.

Prantera, C., Zannoni, F., Scribano, M.L. (1996). An antibiotic regimen for the treatment of active Crohn's disease: a randomized, controlled clinical trial of metronidazole plus ciprofloxacin. Am J Gastroenterol 91, 328–332.

Present, D.H., Rutgeerts, P., Targan, S. et al. (1999). Infliximab for the treatment of fistulas in patients with Crohn's disease. N Engl J Med 340, 1398–1405.

Quinton, J.F., Sendid, B., Reumaux, D. et al. (1998). Anti-Saccharomyces cerevisiae mannan antibodies combined with antineutrophil cytoplasmic autoantibodies in inflammatory bowel disease: prevalence and diagnostic role. Gut 42, 788–791.

Rath, H.C., Schultz, M., Freitag, R. (2001). Different subsets of enteric bacteria induce and perpetuate experimental colitis in rats and mice. Infect Immun 69, 2277–2285.

Rath, H.C., Herfarth, H.H., Ikeda, J.S. et al. (1996). Normal luminal bacteria, especially Bacteroides species, mediate chronic colitis, gastritis, and arthritis in HLA-B27/human beta2 microglobulin transgenic rats. J Clin Invest 98, 945–953.

Rath, H.C., Wilson, K.H. and Sartor, R.B. (1999). Differential induction of colitis and gastritis in HLA-B27 transgenic rats selectively colonized with Bacteroides vulgatus or Escherichia coli. Infect Immun 67, 2969–2974.

Regueiro, M.D. (2000). Update in medical treatment of Crohn's disease. J Clin Gastroenterol 31, 282–291.

Reinecker, H.C., Steffen, M., Witthoeft, T. et al. (1993). Enhanced secretion of tumour necrosis factor-alpha, IL-6, and IL-1 beta by isolated lamina propria mononuclear cells from patients with ulcerative colitis and Crohn's disease. Clin Exp Immunol 94, 174–181.

Reumaux, D., Sendid, B., Poulain, D., Duthilleul, P., Dewit, O. and Colombel, J.F. (2003). Serological markers in inflammatory bowel diseases. Best Pract Res Clin Gastroenterol 17, 19–35.

Roseth, A.G., Aadland, E., Jahnsen, J. and Raknerud, N. (1997). Assessment of disease activity in ulcerative colitis by faecal calprotectin, a novel granulocyte marker protein. Digestion 58, 176–180.

Roseth, A.G., Schmidt, P.N. and Fagerhol, M.K. (1999). Correlation between faecal excretion of indium-111-labelled granulocytes and calprotectin, a granulocyte marker protein, in patients with inflammatory bowel disease. Scand J Gastroenterol 34, 50–54.

Rowbotham, D.S., Mapstone, N.P., Trejdosiewicz, L.K., Howdle, P.D. and Quirke, P. (1995). Mycobacterium paratuberculosis DNA not detected in Crohn's disease tissue by fluorescent polymerase chain reaction. Gut 37, 660–667.

Roussomoustakaki, M., Satsangi, J., Welsh, K. et al. (1997). Genetic markers may predict disease behavior in patients with ulcerative colitis. Gastroenterology 112, 1845–1853.

Rozen, P., Zonis, J., Yekutiel, P. and Gilat, T. (1979). Crohn's disease in the Jewish population of Tel-Aviv-Yafo. Epidemiologic and clinical aspects. Gastroenterology 76, 25–30.

Ruemmele, F.M., Targan, S.R., Levy, G., Dubinsky, M., Braun, J. and Seidman, E.G. (1998). Diagnostic accuracy of serological assays in pediatric inflammatory bowel disease. Gastroenterology 115, 822–829.

Rutgeerts, P., Goboes, K., Peeters, M. et al. (1991). Effect of faecal stream diversion on recurrence of Crohn's disease in the neoterminal ileum. Lancet 338, 771–774.

Rutgeerts, P. and Vermeire, S. (2000). Serological diagnosis of inflammatory bowel disease. Lancet 356, 2117–2118.

Salemans, J.M., Nagengast, F.M., Lubbers, E.J. and Kuijpers, J.H. (1992). Postoperative and long-term results of ileal pouch-anal anastomosis for ulcerative colitis and familial polyposis coli. Dig Dis Sci 37, 1882–1889.

Sandborn, W.J., Landers, C.J., Tremaine, W.J. and Targan, S.R. (1996). Association of antineutrophil cytoplasmic antibodies with resistance to treatment of left-sided ulcerative colitis: results of a pilot study. Mayo Clin Proc 71, 431–436.

Sandborn, W.J. and Targan, S.R. (2002). Biologic therapy of inflammatory bowel disease. Gastroenterology 122, 1592–1608.

Sandborn, W.J., Landers, C.J., Tremaine, W.J. and Targan, S.R. (1995). Antineutrophil cytoplasmic antibody correlates with chronic pouchitis after ileal pouch-anal anastomosis. Am J Gastroenterol 90, 740–747.

Sandborn, W.J., Loftus, E.V. Jr, Colombel, J.F. et al. (2001a). Evaluation of serologic disease markers in a population-based cohort of patients with ulcerative colitis and Crohn's disease. Inflamm Bowel Dis 7, 192–201.

Sandborn, W.J., Feagan, B.G., Hanauer, S.B. et al. (2001b). An engineered human antibody to TNF (CDP571) for active Crohn's disease: a randomized double-blind placebo-controlled trial. Gastroenterology 120, 1330–1338.

Sands, B.E., Anderson, F.H., Bernstein, C.N. et al. (2004). Infliximab maintenance therapy for fistulizing Crohn's disease. N Engl J Med 350, 876–885.

Sartor, R.B. (1995). Current concepts of the etiology and pathogenesis of ulcerative colitis and Crohn's disease. Gastroenterol Clin North Am 24, 475–507.

Sartor, RBRHCSR. (1996). Microbial factors in chronic intestinal inflammation. Curr Opin Gastroenterol 12, 327.

Satsangi, J., Parkes, M., Louis, E. et al. (1996). Two stage genome-wide search in inflammatory bowel disease provides evidence for susceptibility loci on chromosomes 3, 7 and 12. Nat Genet 14, 199–202.

Saxon, A., Shanahan, F., Landers, C., Ganz, T. and Targan, S. (1990). A distinct subset of antineutrophil cytoplasmic antibodies is associated with inflammatory bowel disease. J Allergy Clin Immunol 86, 202–210.

Schreiber, S., MacDermott, R.P., Raedler, A., Pinnau, R., Bertovich, M.J. and Nash, G.S. (1991). Increased activation of isolated intestinal lamina propria mononuclear cells in inflammatory bowel disease. Gastroenterology 101, 1020–1030.

Schultz, M., Veltkamp, C., Dieleman, L.A. et al. (2002). Lactobacillus plantarum 299V in the treatment and prevention of spontaneous colitis in interleukin-10-deficient mice. Inflamm Bowel Dis 8, 71–80.

Schwarze, C., Terjung, B., Lilienweiss, P. et al. (2003). IgA class antineutrophil cytoplasmic antibodies in primary sclerosing cholangitis and autoimmune hepatitis. Clin Exp Immunol 133, 283–289.

Sellon, R.K., Tonkonogy, S., Schultz, M. et al. (1998). Resident enteric bacteria are necessary for development of spontaneous colitis and immune system activation in interleukin-10-deficient mice. Infect Immun 66, 5224–5231.

Shivananda, S., Lennard-Jones, J., Logan, R. et al. (1996). Incidence of inflammatory bowel disease across Europe: is there a difference between north and south? Results of the European Collaborative Study on Inflammatory Bowel Disease (EC-IBD). Gut 39, 690–697.

Skogh, T. and Peen, E. (1993). Lactoferrin, anti-lactoferrin antibodies and inflammatory disease. Adv Exp Med Biol 336, 533–538.

Smith, K.M., Eaton, A.D., Finlayson, L.M. and Garside, P. (2000). Oral tolerance. Am J Respir Crit Care Med 162, S175–178.

Sobajima, J., Ozaki, S., Uesugi, H. et al. (1998). Prevalence and characterization of perinuclear anti-neutrophil cytoplasmic antibodies (P-ANCA) directed against HMG1 and HMG2 in ulcerative colitis (UC). Clin Exp Immunol 111, 402–407.

Sobajima, J., Ozaki, S., Uesugi, H. et al. (1999). High mobility group (HMG) non-histone chromosomal proteins HMG1 and HMG2 are significant target antigens of perinuclear anti-neutrophil cytoplasmic antibodies in autoimmune hepatitis. Gut 44, 867–873.

Soderholm, J.D., Olaison, G., Lindberg, E. et al. (1999). Different intestinal permeability patterns in relatives and spouses of patients with Crohn's disease: an inherited defect in mucosal defence? Gut 44, 96–100.

Stack, W.A., Mann, S.D., Roy, A.J. et al. (1997). Randomised controlled trial of CDP571 antibody to tumour necrosis factor-alpha in Crohn's disease. Lancet 349, 521–524.

Stainsby, K.J., Lowes, J.R., Allan, R.N. and Ibbotson, J.P. (1993). Antibodies to Mycobacterium paratuberculosis and nine species of environmental mycobacteria in Crohn's disease and control subjects. Gut 34, 371–374.

Stokkers, P.C., Reitsma, P.H., Tytgat, G.N. and van Deventer, S.J. (1999). HLA-DR and -DQ phenotypes in inflammatory bowel disease: a meta-analysis. Gut 45, 395–401.

Sugi, K., Saitoh, O., Matsuse, R. et al. (1999). Antineutrophil cytoplasmic antibodies in Japanese patients with inflammatory bowel disease: prevalence and recognition of putative antigens. Am J Gastroenterol 94, 1304–1312.

Summers, R.W., Elliott, D.E., Qadir, K., Urban, J.F. Jr, Thompson, R. and Weinstock, J.V. (2003). Trichuris suis seems to be safe and possibly effective in the treatment of inflammatory bowel disease. Am J Gastroenterol 98, 2034–2041.

Sutton, C.L., Kim, J., Yamane, A. et al. (2000). Identification of a novel bacterial sequence associated with Crohn's disease. Gastroenterology 119, 23–31.

Taniguchi, M., Geng, X., Glazier, K.D., Dasgupta, A., Lin, J.J. and Das, K.M. (2001). Cellular immune response against tropomyosin isoform 5 in ulcerative colitis. Clin Immunol 101, 289–295.

Targan, S.R. (1999). The utility of ANCA and ASCA in inflammatory bowel disease. Inflamm Bowel Dis 5, 61–63; discussion 66–67.

Targan, S.R., Landers, C.J., Cobb, L., MacDermott, R.P. and Vidrich, A. (1995a). Perinuclear anti-neutrophil cytoplasmic

antibodies are spontaneously produced by mucosal B cells of ulcerative colitis patients. J Immunol 155, 3262–3267.

Targan, S.R., Landers, C., Vidrich, A. and Czaja, A.J. (1995b). High-titer antineutrophil cytoplasmic antibodies in type-1 autoimmune hepatitis. Gastroenterology 108, 1159–1166.

Targan, S.R., Hanauer, S.B., van Deventer, S.J. et al. (1997). A short-term study of chimeric monoclonal antibody cA2 to tumor necrosis factor alpha for Crohn's disease. Crohn's Disease cA2 Study Group. N Engl J Med 337, 1029–1035.

Taylor, K.D., Plevy, S.E., Yang, H. et al. (2001). ANCA pattern and LTA haplotype relationship to clinical responses to anti-TNF antibody treatment in Crohn's disease. Gastroenterology 120, 1347–1355.

Terjung, B., Herzog, V., Worman, H.J. et al. (1998). Atypical antineutrophil cytoplasmic antibodies with perinuclear fluorescence in chronic inflammatory bowel diseases and hepatobiliary disorders colocalize with nuclear lamina proteins. Hepatology 28, 332–340.

Terjung, B., Spengler, U., Sauerbruch, T. and Worman, H.J. (2000). Atypical p-ANCA in IBD and hepatobiliary disorders react with a 50-kilodalton nuclear envelope protein of neutrophils and myeloid cell lines. Gastroenterology 119, 310–322.

Thjodleifsson, B., Sigthorsson, G., Cariglia, N. et al. (2003). Subclinical intestinal inflammation: an inherited abnormality in Crohn's disease relatives? Gastroenterology 124, 1728–1737.

Thomas, G.A., Swift, G.L., Green, J.T. et al. (1998). Controlled trial of antituberculous chemotherapy in Crohn's disease: a five year follow up study. Gut 4, 497–500.

Thompson, N.P., Driscoll, R., Pounder, R.E. and Wakefield, A.J. (1996). Genetics versus environment in inflammatory bowel disease: results of a British twin study. Br Med J 312, 95–96.

Tibble, J.A., Sigthorsson, G., Foster, R., Forgacs, I. and Bjarnason, I. (2002). Use of surrogate markers of inflammation and Rome criteria to distinguish organic from nonorganic intestinal disease. Gastroenterology 123, 450–460.

Tibble, J.A., Sigthorsson, G., Bridger, S., Fagerhol, M.K. and Bjarnason, I. (2000a). Surrogate markers of intestinal inflammation are predictive of relapse in patients with inflammatory bowel disease. Gastroenterology 119, 15–22.

Tibble, J.A. and Bjarnason, I. (2001). Non-invasive investigation of inflammatory bowel disease. World J Gastroenterol 7, 460–465.

Tibble, J., Teahon, K., Thjodleifsson, B. et al. (2000b). A simple method for assessing intestinal inflammation in Crohn's disease. Gut 47, 506–513.

Timmer, A. and Goebell, H. (1999). Incidence of ulcerative colitis, 1980–1995 – a prospective study in an urban population in Germany. Z Gastroenterol 37, 1079–1084.

Tountas, N.A., Casini-Raggi, V., Yang, H. et al. (1999). Functional and ethnic association of allele 2 of the interleukin-1 receptor antagonist gene in ulcerative colitis. Gastroenterology 117, 806–813.

Trallori, G., Palli, D., Saieva, C. et al. (1996). A population-based study of inflammatory bowel disease in Florence over 15 years (1978–92). Scand J Gastroenterol 31, 892–899.

Tysk, C., Lindberg, E., Jarnerot, G. and Floderus-Myrhed, B. (1988). Ulcerative colitis and Crohn's disease in an unselected population of monozygotic and dizygotic twins. A study of heritability and the influence of smoking. Gut 29, 990–996.

Van de Merwe, J.P., Schroder, A.M., Wensinck, F. and Hazenberg, M.P. (1988). The obligate anaerobic faecal flora of patients with Crohn's disease and their first-degree relatives. Scand J Gastroenterol 23, 1125–1131.

Van Kruiningen, H.J. (1999). Lack of support for a common etiology in Johne's disease of animals and Crohn's disease in humans. Inflamm Bowel Dis 5, 183–191.

Vasiliauskas, E.A., Plevy, S.E., Landers, C.J. et al. (1996). Perinuclear antineutrophil cytoplasmic antibodies in patients with Crohn's disease define a clinical subgroup. Gastroenterology 110, 1810–1819.

Vermeire, S.J.S., Peeters, M. et al. (2000). ASCA and pANCA do not predict resonse to anti-TNF-alpha (Remicade) treatment (abstr). Gastroenterology 118.

Vermeire, S., Louis, E., Rutgeerts, P. et al. (2002). NOD2/CARD15 does not influence response to infliximab in Crohn's disease. Gastroenterology 123, 106–111.

Vermeire, S., Satsangi, J., Peeters, M. et al. (2001). Evidence for inflammatory bowel disease of a susceptibility locus on the X chromosome. Gastroenterology 120, 834–840.

Vidrich, A., Lee, J., James, E., Cobb, L. and Targan, S. (1995). Segregation of pANCA antigenic recognition by DNase treatment of neutrophils: ulcerative colitis, type 1 autoimmune hepatitis, and primary sclerosing cholangitis. J Clin Immunol 15, 293–299.

Vigushin, D.M., Pepys, M.B. and Hawkins, P.N. (1993). Metabolic and scintigraphic studies of radioiodinated human C-reactive protein in health and disease. J Clin Invest 91, 1351–1357.

Walmsley, R.S., Ibbotson, J.P., Chahal, H. and Allan, R.N. (1996). Antibodies against Mycobacterium paratuberculosis in Crohn's disease. Q J Med 89, 217–221.

Walmsley, R.S., Zhao, M.H., Hamilton, M.I. et al. (1997). Antineutrophil cytoplasm autoantibodies against bactericidal/permeability-increasing protein in inflammatory bowel disease. Gut 40, 105–109.

Wayne, L.G., Hollander, D., Anderson, B. (1992). Immunoglobulin A (IgA) and IgG serum antibodies to mycobacterial antigens in Crohn's disease patients and their relatives. J Clin Microbiol 30, 2013–2018.

Wei, B., Huang, T., Dalwadi, H., Sutton, C.L., Bruckner, D. and Braun, J. (2002). Pseudomonas fluorescens encodes the Crohn's disease-associated I2 sequence and T-cell superantigen. Infect Immun 70, 657–675.

Yang, J.R.H. (1995). Genetic aspects of idiopathic inflammatory bowel disease. In Inflammatory Bowel Diseases, Shorter K, ed.

Yang, H., Rotter, J.I., Toyoda, H. et al. (1993). Ulcerative colitis: a genetically heterogeneous disorder defined by genetic (HLA class II) and subclinical (antineutrophil cytoplasmic antibodies) markers. J Clin Invest 92, 1080–1084.

Yang, H., Vora, D.K., Targan, S.R., Toyoda, H., Beaudet, A.L. and Rotter, J.I. (1995). Intercellular adhesion molecule 1 gene associations with immunologic subsets of inflammatory bowel disease. Gastroenterology 109, 440–448.

Yapp, T.R., Stenson, R., Thomas, G.A., Lawrie, B.W., Williams, G.T. and Hawthorne, A.B. (2000). Crohn's disease incidence in Cardiff from 1930: an update for 1991–1995. Eur J Gastroenterol Hepatol 12, 907–911.

Autoimmunity – Endocrine

Chapter 47

Michael T. Stang and John H. Yim

Department of Surgery, University of Pittsburgh School of Medicine, Pittsburgh, PA, USA

Men occasionally stumble over truth, but most of them pick themselves up and hurry off as if nothing had happened.

Winston Churchill

INTRODUCTION

Autoimmune diseases are characterized by autoreactive lymphocytes which can cause a spectrum of disease pathology, either through the formation of antibodies that react against host tissues or effector T cells which are specific for endogenous self-peptides (Sinha et al., 1990). Autoimmunity can be either organ specific or systemic. Systemic autoimmunity, including disorders such as systemic lupus erythematosus (SLE), is characterized by a lack of immunologic tolerance and deleterious immune response directed against a panoply of individual self-antigens (Sinha et al., 1990). Endocrine autoimmune disorders, however, are largely organ specific and sometimes cell type specific. They generally involve chronic T cell or antibody targeting of a particular organ or cell type with a subsequent varied clinical expression of hormonal dysfunction. It appears that apoptosis is a central mechanism associated with the development of many autoimmune disorders, either as a failure of elimination of autoreactive lymphocytes or as the means of mediating tissue damage.

Autoimmune endocrine disorders are the most prevalent of the autoimmune disorders. The three most common autoimmune endocrine disorders are autoimmune thyroid disease, type I diabetes mellitus and autoimmune adrenalitis. Together, these diseases account for half of all organ specific autoimmune diseases (Jacobson et al., 1997). The autoimmune thyroid diseases have been studied extensively and will predominate in the discussion of this chapter. Type I diabetes has been covered in a previous chapter.

Animal models have been developed for each of the autoimmune endocrinopathies with some success. These models have greatly advanced our understanding of the effector mechanisms involved in disease expression and have allowed investigation into defining the important serologic markers of each disease. Despite this, there is still a paucity of data that lend themselves to understanding the actual initiation of the aberrant immune response and breach of tolerance of the various autoimmune endocrinopathies. Assays for serologic markers have been developed for each of the respective autoimmune endocrinopathies. However, the sensitivity, specificity and technical reproducibility of these assays vary and, unfortunately, in several instances do not provide clinical benefit in monitoring or managing the disease.

Besides some shared genetic and immunologic predisposition, endocrine autoimmune disorders occur together more frequently than would be expected. These patterns of disease expression have been labeled the autoimmune polyglandular syndromes (APS). Recent investigations into these syndromes have provided some exciting insights into the potential role of central tolerance mechanisms in the development of organ specific

Measuring Immunity, edited by Michael T. Lotze and Angus W. Thomson
ISBN 0-12-455900-X, London

immunity. Hopefully with time, these studies will allow us to understand better why the individual endocrine organs are susceptible to autoimmune attack and help us refine our ability to measure the immune process for these endocrinopathies.

AUTOIMMUNE THYROID DISEASE (AITD)

Thyroid disorders are the most common of the autoimmune endocrinopathies with Graves' disease being the most prevalent of all autoimmune diseases (Jacobson et al., 1997). Our classical understanding of the autoimmune thyroid disorders is that of local infiltration of active lymphocytes into the thyroid gland with subsequent inflammation, production of various autoantibodies and destruction of the gland architecture following immigration of the immune cells. The variants of autoimmune thyroid disease include several conditions with widely disparate clinical and laboratory expression (Weetman, 1994).

The categorization of the thyroid disorders has classically been based on physical findings (presence or absence of goiter, pain, dermatologic sequelae, ophthalmopathy) and the overall physiologic thyroid state (hypothyroid, euthyroid or hyperthyroid). Although with the advent of our understanding that the majority of thyroid disorders are autoimmune in nature, the previous classifications become less satisfying. Investigations have demonstrated a considerable degree of overlap between the various autoimmune thyroid diseases with respect to their autoantibody profiles and histopathologic characteristics. Yet, both hypothyroidism and hyperthyroidism are potential clinical outcomes. As such, it may be more important to understand that most of the immune processes described to date are present in varying degrees and the actual observed clinical state is dependent on the most dominant pathogenic process.

Graves' disease (GD) is typically marked by a thyrotoxic state and gland enlargement (goiter) and is the result of a predominantly stimulating autoimmune process (Weetman, 2000). In contrast, autoimmune thyroiditis represents a spectrum of clinical outcomes that predominantly result in a hypothyroid state (Dayan and Daniels, 1996). The more common chronic autoimmune thyroiditis diseases generally exhibit either goiter as in Hashimoto's thyroiditis (HT) or a normal to small gland with atrophic thyroiditis (AT), which is also known as idiopathic/primary myxedema (Dayan and Daniels, 1996; Weetman et al., 1998). Other thyroiditis diseases may be more acute in nature with an eventual spontaneous remission as with silent (painless) thyroiditis and post-partum thyroiditis (Weetman et al., 1998). Graves' disease is not typically considered a thyroiditis. However, some GD patients will exhibit biochemical qualities and histopathologic features that overlap with the other autoimmune thyroiditis diseases (Dayan and Daniels, 1996; Prummel and Wiersina, 2002).

In addition to the diseases discussed here, which may be strictly labeled as primary autoimmune disorders, other thyroid conditions may manifest secondary immunologic disturbances including those seen with subacute or De Quervain's thyroiditis (post viral inflammation of the thyroid), non-toxic nodular goiter and papillary thyroid carcinoma (Mariotti and Pinna, 2003). In such conditions, focal and occasionally diffuse lymphoid infiltration may be encountered on pathologic review and autoantibodies are present in serologic testing; yet, these conditions are not currently known to be autoimmune in nature (Mariotti and Pinna, 2003).

Histopathology

Autoimmune hyperthyroid disease (GD) is marked by diffuse enlargement of the thyroid gland from parenchymal hypertrophy and hyperplasia with an increase in the size of the organ due to an increase in the number of component cells (Weetman, 2000). Such gland enlargement produces the clinical finding of goiter and the thyroid is often at least double its normal size (Foulis and Riley, 2003). Common abnormalities found in resected glands include the epithelial cells lining the follicle being taller with relatively more cytoplasm and the amount of stored colloid in the follicle being often reduced (Foulis and Riley, 2003). The hyperplasia of the epithelial cells can also manifest as papillary ingrowths (Foulis and Riley, 2003). There may often be a full range of lymphoid cells present including a plasma-cell infiltration (Foulis and Riley, 2003). The lymphocyte infiltration is more commonly observed as nodules of lymphocytes and occasional germinal center formations (Foulis and Riley, 2003). The extent of lymphoid infiltration between glands varies considerably from a paucity of lymphocytes to some glands resembling Hashimoto's disease (Foulis and Riley, 2003).

In Hashimoto's thyroiditis there is an autoimmune destruction of thyroid epithelial cells balanced by a compensatory proliferation (Foulis and Riley, 2003). The combination of massive lymphoid infiltrate and compensatory thyroid hyperplasia results in enlargement of the gland. In HT the thyroid gland shows a diffuse infiltration by mononuclear cells, mainly consisting of lymphocytes (Livolsi, 1994). These may aggregate to form lymphoid follicles with germinal centers (Livolsi, 1994). Plasma cells and macrophages are also present (Foulis and Riley, 2003). The normal architecture of the gland is disrupted and the thyroid follicles are reduced in size containing only sparse amounts of colloid (Foulis and Riley, 2003). Despite the relatively small size of the follicles some thyrocytes often appear enlarged and contain cytoplasm that is granular and pink (oxyphilic changes – secondary to excessive numbers of mitochondria). These metaplastic cells have been referred to as Askenazy or Hürthle cells and a variable degree of fibrosis is present in most cases (Livolsi, 1994). In the chronic fibrous thyroiditis variant, fibrosis predominates and lymphocytic infiltration is less marked (Foulis and Riley, 2003).

Atrophic thyroiditis demonstrates a gland that is markedly reduced in size as a result of atrophy of the follicular epithelium. There is an extensive fibrosis associated with a variable lymphocytic infiltration similar to that seen in Hashimoto's thyroiditis (Dayan and Daniels, 1996). One could conceptually imagine that AT is simply the end stage or further progression of Hashimoto's thyroiditis; however, longitudinal studies have shown little histologic progression of HT for as long as 20 years after initial diagnosis (Hayashi et al., 1985). Thus, atrophic thyroiditis and Hashimoto's are likely unique entities.

In asymptomatic thyroiditis (focal/silent thyroiditis), the thyroid gland is infiltrated with lymphocytes, but germinal centers and Hürthle cells are generally absent (Foulis and Riley, 2003). Approximately 10 per cent of asymptomatic elderly patients, particularly women, will show evidence of focal lymphoid infiltration at autopsy and this has been correlated with the presence of serum thyroid autoantibodies (Dayan and Daniels, 1996). Lymphocytic thyroiditis of childhood and adolescence exhibits less evident Hürthle cells, fibrosis and germinal centers than in the adult form and anti-thyroid antibodies are often absent or present in very low titers (Foulis and Riley, 2003).

Effector mechanisms in autoimmune thyroid disease

Several mechanisms, such as complement-mediated cytotoxicity, antibody-dependent cell-mediated cytotoxicity

Endocrine organ	Autoantigens	Autoantibodies		Pathologic role	Detection method	Disease
Thyroid	Tg		TgAb	Unlikely	ELISA, RIA	AT, HT, GD
	TPO		TPOAb	Unknown; ?ADCC, ?Complement, ?Enzyme Inhibition	ELISA, RIA	AT, HT, GD
	TSHR	TRAbs	TSAb	YES, Hormone receptor stimulation	Functional stimulatory Bioassay (cAMP accumulation)	GD
			TBAb	YES; Hormone receptor blocking	Funtional inhibitory Bioassay (cAMP accumulation)	GD, AT, HT
			TBII	YES; Varies (Combination of TSAbs and TBAbs)	Receptor competition	GD, AT, HT
Adrenal	21-OH	ACA	21-OHAb	Unknown	IIF, IP	AD +/− APS-1,2
	17α-OH		StCA 17α-OHAb	Unknown	IIF, IP	APS-1,2
	P450Scc		P450SccAb			APS-1,2
Ovary	Multiple undefined		Multiple undefined	Unknown	IIF, ELISA	POF
	17α-OH		StCA 17α-OHAb	Unknown	IIF, IP	POF + APS-1
	P450Scc		P450SccAb			
Parathyroid	CaSR?		CaSR antibody	Unknown	None	Autoimmune Hypoparathyroidism

Abbreviations: AT: atrophic thyroiditis, HT: Hashimoto's thyroiditis, GD: Graves' disease, AD: Addison's disease, APS: autoimmune polyglandular syndrome, POF: premature ovarian failure, Tg: thyroglobulin, TPO: thyroperoxidase, TSHR: TSH receptor, TRAbs: TSH receptor antibodies, TSAbs: TSH stimulating antibodies, TBAbs: TSH blocking antibodies, TBII: TSH binding inhibition immunoglobulin, ACA: adrenal cortex antibodies, StCA: steroid cell antibodies, CaSR: calcium sensitive receptor, IIF: indirect immunofluorescence, ELISA: enzyme linked immunosorbent assay, RIA: radioimmunoassay, IP: immunoprecipitation.

(ADCC) and antigen specific T cell cytotoxicity may be involved in the pathogenesis of thyroid damage and gland dysfunction in AITD. Some antibodies can stimulate hormone receptors and induce a hyperfunctional state of the gland. Cytokines produced in the course of the autoimmune reaction may themselves exert cytotoxic or other functional activities on thyroid cells (Mariotti and Pinna, 2003). Additionally, there is mounting evidence that apoptosis mediated via Fas/FasL expression from either thyroid cells or the infiltrating lymphocytes may play an important role in the destructive phenomena of AITD (Stassi and De Maria, 2002).

The autoimmune process is believed to begin with the activation of CD4 (helper) lymphocytes specific for thyroid antigens (Weetman, 1994; Dayan and Daniels, 1996). Thyroid reactive T cells have been readily detected in the peripheral blood of patients with AITD using assay methods based on measuring T cell proliferation and expression of leukocyte migration inhibition factor (Weetman, 1994; Weetman et al., 1998). T lymphocytes and T cell lines isolated from intrathyroidal infiltrates as well have been shown to proliferate when co-cultured with autologous thyroid cells (Mariotti and Pinna, 2003). Indirect evidence for T cell involvement in AITD is also provided by the increased number of intrathyroidal T cells bearing HLA-DR antigen, a marker of T cell activation (Zeki et al., 1987). Within the thyroid infiltrate, CD4+ T cells predominate and many of these are HLA-DR+ (Weetman et al., 1998). How these cells become activated is not known (Dayan and Daniels, 1996). Some hypotheses include molecular mimicry by a bacterial or viral protein product, variations in iodine intake or aberrant autoantigen presentation by dendritic cells or thyrocytes and subsequent failure in normal tolerance mechanisms (Dayan and Daniels, 1996; Prummel and Wiersina, 2002). Nonetheless, once CD4+ T cells are activated, they can then recruit and stimulate other self-reactive immune cell types and provide the resultant antibody or cell-mediated responses.

The thyroid epithelial cells also express several molecules that may modulate thyroid autoimmunity (Hanafusa et al., 1983; Bottazzo et al., 1983). In response to interferon-γ (IFN-γ) produced by infiltrating T cells, the thyroid cells express HLA class II molecules which allows the cells to present antigens (Hanafusa et al., 1983; Bottazzo et al., 1983). Such findings led to the hypothesis that this could initiate or perpetuate the autoimmune response with the thyrocytes acting as antigen presenting cells (Bottazzo et al., 1983). However, IFN-γ is the key regulator of class II expression and the close correlation between the presence of IFN-γ producing T cells and HLA class II+ thyrocytes demonstrates that a lymphocyte infiltrative process is likely a prerequisite for class II expression in thyroid follicular cells (Hamilton et al., 1991). Thus, thyrocytes are unlikely to initiate autoimmune thyroid disease (Weetman et al., 1998). Indeed, naive T cells, which require a co-stimulatory signal, do not respond to thyroid cells presenting antigen (Marelli-Berg et al., 1997). Thyrocytes lack important B-7 co-stimulatory molecules (CD80 and CD86) that stimulate T cells by means of CD28 (Weetman et al., 1998). Therefore, the initiation of AITD is likely to involve antigen-presenting cells that express CD80 and CD86 (Marelli-Berg et al., 1997). With the progression of disease, however, the presentation of antigen by thyroid cells may exacerbate the autoimmune process, as may the expression of other molecules by thyroid cells, such as CD40, CD54, IL-1 and IL-6 (Weetman, 1994).

In contrast to the primary role of T cells in autoantigen presentation and the subsequent orchestration of the immune response, there is little evidence that T cells can actually damage thyrocytes (Weetman, 1994). Cytotoxic T cells recognize autoantigens directly on target cells when these antigens are present in the context of HLA class I molecules and induce cell death through the use of perforin/granzymes and other cell membrane ligands inducing cytotoxicity (Parkin and Cohen, 2001). However, the importance of specifically sensitized cytotoxic T cells as direct mediators of thyroid destruction has only been established in animal models of experimental autoimmune thyroiditis (EAT) (Stafford and Rose, 2000; Mariotti and Pinna, 2003). The demonstration of this mechanism in humans has been elusive owing to the requirement that demonstrating such T cell mediated cytotoxicity requires autologous target cells (Mariotti and Pinna, 2003). One group has shown a specific cytotoxicity toward autologous thyrocytes with at least one CD8+ cell clone derived from a human AITD infiltrate (MacKenzie et al., 1987). The relative prevalence of thyroid specific cytotoxic T cells within the thyroid infiltrate is still unknown (Mariotti and Pinna, 2003). There is indirect evidence which suggests that they could be only a minority (<10 per cent) of the total interglandular lymphoid cells (Mariotti et al., 1989).

Autoantibodies can form immune complexes by binding to their antigen on the thyrocyte and this can activate the complement system leading to the formation of membrane attack complexes (MAC) (Weetman et al., 1998; Prummel and Wiersina, 2002). Increased circulating levels of terminal complement complexes are found in Hashimoto's thyroiditis (Weetman et al., 1998). Furthermore, immune complexes and complement can be visualized around the thyroid follicle by immunohistochemistry in Graves' disease (Werner) and Hashimoto's thyroiditis (Weetman and McGregor, 1984; Weetman et al., 1998). Yet, an argument against complement mediated cell death is supported by the observation that thyrocytes are relatively resistant to the lytic effects of homologous complement attack, due to their expression of complement regulatory proteins (CD46, CD55, CD59 and MAC inhibitory protein) (Tandon et al., 1994). S-protein (vitronectin) is also detectable by immunohistochemistry in HT and probably also regulates MAC formation (Weetman et al., 1998). Nonetheless, complement formation may have several adverse functional effects on thyrocytes including a reduction in their responsiveness to TSH, which could account for gland hypofunction (Tandon et al., 1992). Complement attack on thyrocytes also causes release of reactive oxygen metabolites as well as production of IL-1, IL-6 and prostaglandin E2 all of which could function in the intrathyroidal inflammatory process (Weetman et al., 1992).

Antibody dependent cell-mediated cytotoxicity (ADCC) is a phenomenon of mononuclear cells (MNC) with cytolytic potential (NK cells and other mononuclear cells) binding and lysing target cells coated with IgG antibodies (Parkin and Cohen, 2001). Cell lysis ensues when an antibody has bound to its antigen on the cell surface and the Fc tail on the immunoglobulin is recognized by the Fc-receptor on an NK cell (Parkin and Cohen, 2001). NK cells recognize stressed cells, are inhibited by individual class I MHC molecules and themselves are not antigen specific. NK cells present in a population of peripheral blood lymphocytes can therefore be used in an assay of ADCC (Prummel and Wiersina, 2002). In this assay, lysis of cultured target cells by normal lymphocytes can be measured after incubation with serum containing antibodies (see Chapter 29). The potential importance of ADCC as an effector mechanism in AITD was first described by Calder and colleagues (1973) and later by Bogner et al. (1984). Normal peripheral MNCs were observed to lyse thyroglobulin (Tg) coated erythrocytes or ^{51}Cr-labeled human thyroid cells pre-incubated with sera from Hashimoto's thyroiditis patients (Calder et al., 1973; Bognor et al., 1984). This phenomenon is most likely dependent on the anti-thyroperoxidase fraction of autoantibodies (Rodien et al., 1996). The role of ADCC in AITD is further supported by the observation that a high-proportion of intrathyroidal lymphocytes from AITD display NK-like cytolytic activity (Del Prete et al., 1986).

Thyroid autoantibodies

There are three major thyroid autoantigens that have been extensively studied and described: thyroglobulin, thyroperoxidase and the receptor for thyroid stimulating hormone.

Thyroglobulin

Thyroglobulin (Tg) is a large water soluble glycoprotein with two monomeric 300 kDa subunits each containing four major hormonogenic sites plus a C-terminus region with high homology to acetylcholine esterase (Swillens et al., 1986; Vali et al., 2000). Tg is the most abundant protein in the thyroid and provides the matrix for the synthesis and storage of thyroid hormones thyroxine (T4) and triiodothyronine (T3) (Swillens et al., 1986). As such it is a normal constituent of the serum and its concentration can rise under both physiologic and pathologic conditions.

Anti-thyroglobulin autoantibodies are most often of the IgG2 subclass, but IgG1, IgG4 and IgA antibodies may also be found (Prummel and Wiersina, 2002). Several

methodologies have been executed to identify the specific thyroglobulin epitopes that are recognized by Tg-autoantibodies. Competition studies using monoclonal antibodies and screening of thyroid expression libraries with anti-Tg sera have provided variable results with anti-Tg antibodies showing a significant degree of heterogeneity (Dong et al., 1989; Ludgate et al., 1989; Malthierry et al., 1991; Schultz et al., 1992). Prentice and colleagues (1995) have shown, however, using a competition assay with anti-Tg monoclonal antibodies, some restriction of most patient derived Tg-antibodies to two major conformational epitopes. Overall, the use of these screening methodologies may be impaired because anti-Tg autoantibodies may only recognize three dimensional epitopes (Prentice et al., 1995) and be dependent on the degree of thyroglobulin iodination (Shimojo et al., 1988).

Antibodies to thyroid hormone (anti-T4 and anti-T3) have also been described in patients with autoimmune thyroid disease (Sakata et al., 1985). Such antibodies can interfere with the measurement of serum thyroid hormone levels. They do not appear to interfere with the biologic activity of the hormones themselves (Sakata et al., 1985). These autoantibodies may represent a subset of anti-Tg antibodies that specifically recognize Tg sequences containing iodinated epitopes (Sakata et al., 1985).

The first evidence that Tg may play a role in the pathogenesis of AITD was provided in 1956, when Rose and Witebsky observed autoantibodies to rabbit thyroids and thyroid lesions in rabbits immunized with extracts from normal rabbit thyroids (Witebsky and Rose, 1956; Rose and Witebsky, 1956). Later, Witebsky et al. (1957) and Roitt et al. (1956) independently detected Tg-specific antibodies in sera of patients with Hashimoto's thyroiditis. Immunization with Tg induces experimental autoimmune thyroiditis (EAT) in a number of different animal species (Vali et al., 2000). Indeed, this phenomenon has provided the foundation for the study into the pathogenesis of AITD over the last 40 years in various animal models (Ludgate et al., 1989; Mariotti and Pinna, 2003). Despite this, the role of Tg as an autoantigen with pathologic sequelae has been questioned and is generally regarded as a bystander in human disease (Ludgate, 1998).

Tg antibodies are generally measured using ELISA and RIA methods (Feldt-Rasmussen, 1996). The standardization of these assays and determination of reference ranges has not been consistent among studies owing to varying standards and sources of Tg (Feldt-Rasmussen, 1996). This has resulted in variability of published results of anti-Tg prevalence in autoimmune thyroid disease states and normal population cohorts. Antithyroglobulin antibodies are found in approximately 35–60 per cent of patients with Hashimoto's thyroiditis and 12–30 per cent of patients with Graves' disease (Saravanan and Dayan, 2001). Anti-Tg antibodies can be detected in about 3 per cent of the normal poplulation (Saravanan and Dayan, 2001).

Thyroperoxidase

Thyroperoxidase (TPO) is an essential enzyme in the generation of thyroid hormone with its role in catalyzing the oxidation of iodide and the coupling of iodotyrosil residues of thyroglobulin. It is a membrane bound glycoprotein expressed on the apical membrane of thyrocytes, which line the colloid space within the follicles (McLachlan and Rapoport, 1992).

Autoantibodies directed against TPO are usually of the IgG1 and IgG4 subclasses (Prummel and Wiersina, 2002). The mapping and characterization of the epitopes which are recognized by TPOAbs has provided mixed results and is most likely a function of investigators using either linear peptide segments or conformational components of the TPO protein (Portalano et al., 1992; Chazenbalk et al., 1993; Nishikawa et al., 1994; Tonnacchera et al., 1995; Czarnocka et al., 1997; McIntosh and Weetman, 1997). Using extensive competition assays, several groups have reported marked restriction in TPOAbs from seropositive patients to several conformational epitopes in two regions located on the carboxyl end of the extracellular domain (Portalano et al., 1992; Chazenbalk et al., 1993; Nishikawa et al., 1994; McLachlan and Rapoport, 1995). The epitopes in these two immunodominant regions are recognized by greater than 80 per cent of TPOAbs (Nishikawa et al., 1994). Unfortunately, further investigations have not provided insight into whether different epitopes are preferentially recognized by sera from patients with overt disease and those who are antibody positive without evidence of disease (Portalano et al., 1992; Tonacchera et al., 1995; Jaume et al., 1995).

Anti-TPO antibodies can induce complement-mediated lysis in vitro of cultured thyroid cells (Prummel and Wiersina, 2002). However, Chiovato and colleagues (1993) have shown that complement mediated cytotoxicity could not be completely inhibited after anti-TPO antibodies were removed from sera in patients with AITD. Thus, other autoantibodies may also be involved. The role of these autoantibodies in the cytotoxic process involving thyroid follicular cells in vivo is still controversial (Mariotti and Pinna, 2003). Thyroperoxidase would not be easily available to antibodies in the presence of an intact plasma membrane (Khoury et al., 1984). However, the relevance of this mechanism has been indirectly supported by the observation that TPO is expressed both within the cytoplasm and on the apical surface of the thyroid follicular cells (Khoury et al., 1984). Further, complement-mediated cytotoxicity mediated by anti-TPO antibodies can also be observed in intact thyroid follicles in vitro and in vivo analysis has also demonstrated the presence of anti-TPO antibodies bound to the apical surface of human thyroid follicular cells (Khoury et al., 1984).

Further evidence for the pathogenic role of TPOAbs has been demonstrated by ADCC assays. Rodien and colleagues (1996) have shown that ADCC in autoimmune thyroid disease is most likely dependent on the anti-TPO fraction of autoantibodies. However, not all anti-TPO positive sera are able to induce ADCC in vitro (Rodien et al., 1996). Anti-TPOAbs may also interfere with TPO enzymatic activity that leads to a subsequent impairment of thyroid hormone production independent of complement or antibody mediated cell cytotoxicity. In vitro, the inhibition of thyroperoxidase enzymatic activity by TPOAbs has been observed to varying degrees (Khoury et al., 1984).

Measurement of TPOAb has generally employed ELISA and radioimmunoassay methodologies. Recombinant human TPO generated in eukaryotic cells has provided a pure substrate for detecting TPOAbs with high specificity (Kaufman et al., 1990). However, a clinically functional sensitivity limit has not been established (Feldt-Rasmussen, 1996). Furthermore, approximately 10–15 per cent of the general population shows some degree of TPOAb positivity and this has hampered the development of a clinical reference range (Feldt-Rasmussen, 1996). TPOAbs are frequently present in autoimmune thyroid disease. They are observed in 80–90 per cent of patients with Hashimoto's thyroiditis, approximately 90 per cent of patients with idiopathic myxedema and 45–80 per cent of patients with Graves' disease (Saravanan and Dayan, 2001; Novak and Lernmark, 2002).

Thyroid stimulating hormone receptor

The human TSH receptor (TSHR) is a member of the G-protein-coupled receptor family (Gupta, 2000). It is a large glycoprotein with an extracellular domain and seven transmembrane domains. It shares considerable homology to the luteinizing hormone and follicle stimulating hormone receptors (Gupta, 2000). TSH binding to the TSH receptor stimulates both cAMP and inositol phosphate pathways (Gupta, 2000). These signaling pathways further regulate thyroid hormone secretion, iodide uptake, cell growth and synthesis of thyroid peroxidase, thyroglobulin and prostaglandins (Gupta, 2000).

Autoantibodies directed against the TSH receptor as a whole are a heterogeneous collection of immunoglobulins. The antibodies are capable of interacting with multiple epitopes on the TSH receptor molecule with a variable effect on TSH activities. Taken together the autoantibodies are collectively known as TSHR antibodies (TRAbs). They are capable of either stimulating the native receptor and increasing intracellular cAMP levels, blocking the receptor activity from native TSH, or both (Gupta, 2000).

Adams and Purves first established in 1956 that a factor distinct from TSH was the cause of hyperthyroidism in Graves' disease (Gupta, 2000). They named this the long-acting thyroid stimulator (LATS). Later investigations demonstrated that LATS was actually an immunoglobulin (IgG) (Gupta, 2000). Since then, the stimulating TSHR antibodies have been known as TSAbs. Evidence for functional stimulation of the TSHR by these autoantibodies has been shown through the development of assays which use varying sources of thyroid tissue incubated with sera from patients with TSAbs and subsequent measurement of cAMP accumulation (Rapoport et al., 1998; Gupta, 2000).

Using a different assay method, several groups later independently demonstrated that TRAbs could inhibit the TSH binding on thyroid membranes. This assay was based on a competitive inhibition of radiolabeled TSH to the TSHR (Gupta, 2000). Antibodies measured by this method are known as TSH-binding inhibitory immunoglobulins (TBII). Conceptually, it would follow that both methods would be measuring the same antibodies. If an antibody is binding the TSH receptor and stimulating its function it should also compete with TSH for receptor binding. However, patient sera may be positive for TSAbs but TBII negative and vice versa (Hardisty et al., 1983). This phenomenon is apparently not only due to differences in assay sensitivity but also because these assays are measuring different antibody activities (Prummel and Wiersina, 2002). Indeed, some TRAbs bind to the TSH receptor without a stimulatory response. Instead, these antibodies inhibit the exogenous TSH activation of thyroid adenylate cyclase (Rapoport et al., 1998). Such immunoglobulins are now commonly referred to as TSH blocking antibodies (TBAbs) (Rapoport et al., 1998).

The epitopes recognized by TSAbs tend to segregate toward the N-terminus of the TSH receptor's extracellular domain in at least 95 per cent of patients (Gupta, 2000; Kohn and Harii, 2003). Some of these TSAbs (primarily from GD patients) will also exhibit TBII activity, but the extent of this is unknown (Gupta, 2000). TBII antibodies from Graves' disease patients that do not have stimulating activity (TBAbs) also appear to segregate to the N-terminus in their epitopic recognition (Kohn and Harii, 2003). In contrast, TBII antibodies from patients with atrophic or Hashimoto's thyroiditis tend to recognize epitopes on the C-terminal portion of the extracellular domain (Gupta, 2000; Kohn and Harii, 2003).

There is currently no consistent inter-laboratory standard for TRAb measurement. Different assay methods provide different values and the cutoff for a positive value varies depending on the particular reference population used (Novak and Lernmark, 2002). As previously mentioned, several different methods are used to measure TRAb which include both the stimulatory and inhibitory functional bioassays on human thyroid membranes as well as receptor competition binding assays (Volpe, 1994). COS cells with stable expression of a recombinant TSH receptor appear to allow a more consistent and sensitive measurement (Persani et al., 1993).

Autoimmune hyperthyroidism

The clinical manifestations of Graves' disease involve those symptoms that are common to all forms of hyperthyroidism and those that are specific to the autoimmune process. Hyperthyroidism more commonly results in nervousness, fatigue, rapid heart rate or palpitations, heat intolerance and weight loss. In the older patient, atrial fibrillation may occur. Autoimmune hyperthyroidism is more specifically marked by diffuse goiter, ophthalmopathy and occasionally a localized dermatopathy (Weetman, 2000).

Stimulating TSHR antibodies are the key mediators of autoimmune hyperthyroid disease expression. However, patients with Graves' disease often have a number of thyroid autoantibodies including TBAbs, TPOAbs and TgAbs (Weetman, 2000). The serum concentrations of these antibodies vary among patients and the antibodies themselves may modify the stimulatory effects of thyroid stimulating antibodies (Weetman, 2000). Indeed, the simultaneous production of antibodies that block the TSH receptor in some GD patients reduces the stimulatory action of TSAbs (Gupta, 2000). For these reasons, there is no direct correlation between serum concentrations of TSAbs and serum thyroid hormone concentrations (Weetman, 2000).

Among all patients with hyperthyroidism, 60–80 per cent have Graves' disease (Weetman, 2000). The peak age of occurrence of the disease is during the third and fourth decades of life and it is unusual in children (Brix et al., 1998). The disease occurs 7 to 10 times more frequently in women than in men (Brix et al., 1998). No single gene is known to cause the disease or to be necessary for its development. There are, however, well established associations with certain HLA haplotypes and polymorphisms of the cytotoxic T-lymphocyte antigen 4 (CTLA-4) (Brix et al., 1998).

Despite the advances in understanding the pathogenesis of autoimmune hyperthyroidism, little has changed in diagnosing the disease. The diagnosis of hyperthyroidism is based on clinical and biochemical markers of hyperthyroidism. The appropriate screening test is a TSH level. Almost all hyperthyroidism is accompanied by a suppressed serum TSH (less than 0.1 mIU/l); however, confirmation of a diagnosis of hyperthyroidism should also be made by measurement of serum free thyroxine (T4) (Singer et al., 1995). In the early stage of Graves' disease, patients may have only increased triiodothyronine (T3) (Weetman, 2000). Thus, patients with normal serum free T4 and low TSH should have a free T3 level measured (Singer et al., 1995). Specifying the hyperthyroidism as autoimmune in nature is usually confirmed by any clinical findings of ophthalmopathy (present in about half of Graves' disease patients) and diffuse uptake on radionuclide scan (Weetman, 2000). Over 90 per cent of hyperthyroid patients with Graves' disease are posi-tive for thyroid stimulating antibodies (TSAb) (Zakarija and McKenzie, 1987). Yet, there is limited general clinical application for TSH receptor antibodies (TRAb) with the equally adequate and less expensive laboratory tests available for diagnosing hyperthyroidism (McKenzie and Zakarija, 1989; Bayer, 1991).

Several special instances do exist where TRAbs serve as a useful surrogate marker of clinical disease. TRAb assays are useful in predicting fetal and transient neonatal thyroid dysfunction. As such, the assay is indicated for pregnant women with active Graves' disease or with a history of Graves' disease (McKenzie and Zakarija, 1989). Maternal TSAb values normally decline during the third trimester and an elevated TSAb level at 28–30 weeks of gestation is associated with an increased frequency of Graves' hyperthyroidism in the neonate (McKenzie and Zakarija, 1989; Gupta, 2000). Likewise, thyroid blocking antibody levels can be used to confirm transient neonatal hypothyroidism due to transplacental transfer of maternal TBAbs (McKenzie and Zakarija, 1989; Gupta, 2000).

TSAb activity is also useful in diagnosing Graves' ophthalmopathy. Such ophthalmopathy typically presents with a combination of symptoms including proptosis, periorbital inflammation, congestive oculopathy and optic neuropathy (Weetman, 2000). The etiology has not been completely elucidated; however, it may involve autoantibodies to the thyroid stimulating hormone receptor which is expressed by the pre-adipocyte subpopulation of orbital fibroblasts (Weetman, 2000). Exophthalmos in the presence of hyperthyroidism effectively guarantees that the ophthalmopathy is secondary to autoimmune thyroid disease. However, a Graves' variant with exophthalmos can occur in a euthyroid state and an appropriate diagnosis can be challenging in this situation. Thus, TSAb assays may be valuable in determining the etiology of exophthalmos and proptosis of unknown etiology (Kashiwai et al., 1995).

Current treatments for Graves' hyperthyroidism consist of antithyroid medications, radioactive iodine and surgery (Dayan and Daniels, 1996; Weetman et al., 1998). Antithyroid drugs are effective, but relapses often occur upon discontinuation of therapy (Weetman et al., 1998). In the USA, the favored therapy for adults is radioactive iodine administration. This method is very effective; however, the therapeutic success is often at the expense of iatrogenic hypothyroidism and obligate life-long treatment with thyroid hormone replacement. Murakami and colleagues (1996) have correlated elevated TSAb levels with resistance to radioactive iodine (RAI) therapy for Graves' thyrotoxicosis and this may be a function of TSAbs acting in a trophic manner on the thyrocytes and counteracting the RAI-induced cell destruction. Further, elevated TSAb activity in acutely hypothyroid patients following RAI therapy can predict recovery whereas low TSAb activity can suggest permanent hypothyroidism (Aiziawa et al., 1997). Therefore, TSAb titers may be clinically useful in predicting the dosage of RAI therapy necessary to achieve euthyroidism in addition to predicting outcome following RAI therapy.

Chronic autoimmune thyroiditis

Chronic autoimmune thyroiditis usually manifests as either a goitrous form with or without overt hypothyroidism (Hashimoto's thyroiditis) or as atrophic thyroiditis when symptomatic hypothyroidism is apparent without evidence of thyroid enlargement (Weetman et al., 1998).

However, with the widespread use of TSH assays, biochemical hypothyroidism is being detected earlier and treated prior to the development of obvious symptoms (Weetman et al., 1998). The symptoms of hypothyroidism may be vague such as weakness, fatigue, cold intolerance, constipation, joint pain, mental impairment and depression.

Thyroiditis occurring in the post-partum period (post-partum thyroid dysfunction – PPTD) is a transient, silent and usually painless condition. It is often associated with a hyperthyroid phase followed by a hypothyroid phase and it usually resolves spontaneously afterwards. Despite the initial recovery, about one-fourth of women will develop overt hypothyroidism within 4 or more years.

The principal pathogenic mechanisms of the individual autoimmune hypothyroid disorders are still not clear and are likely a combination of both humoral and cell-mediated immune responses as previously discussed. Certainly, TPOAbs and TgAbs are readily detectable in most cases of autoimmune thyroiditis but their role and importance in actual disease expression is unknown. TSHR blocking antibodies (TBAbs) have been detected in approximately 20 per cent of patients with atrophic thyroiditis and are considered pathogenic for this subset of patients (Dayan and Daniels, 1996; Gupta, 2000). Yet, TBAbs still do not explain the disease process for the remaining 80 per cent.

Among all patients with non-iatrogenic hypothyroidism, over 90 per cent have some form of autoimmune thyroiditis (Weetman et al., 1998). Hypothyroidism develops gradually and clinically apparent disease represents the culmination of ongoing thyroid damage over many months or years. The majority of cases are diagnosed during the fourth through sixth decades of life (Vanderpump et al., 1995). Women are five to seven times more likely to be affected than men (Vanderpump et al., 1995). Thyroid autoimmunity is familial with as many as 50 per cent of first degree relatives of patients with chronic autoimmune thyroiditis having thyroid antibodies (Dayan and Daniels, 1996). However, as with Graves' disease, no single gene has been identified to be necessary for its development. Weak associations with individual HLA haplotypes and CTLA-4 gene polymorphisms (see Chapters 1 and 2) have been described (Dayan and Daniels, 1996; Kotsa et al., 1997).

Establishing the diagnosis of hypothyroidism should include measurement of serum TSH and free T4 levels (Singer et al., 1995). Further, the cause of the hypothyroidism as autoimmune in nature can be confirmed by the presence of thyroid autoantibodies. Subanalysis of sera positivity for TgAbs shows that a large percentage (approximately 90 per cent) of anti-Tg positive patients are also positive for other thyroid autoantibodies (namely TPO) (Nordyke et al., 1993). However, as much as 65 per cent of anti-TPO positive sera is negative for anti-Tg (Nordyke et al., 1993). Therefore, more recent studies have concluded that measurement of TPO-antibody is generally sufficient when investigating hypothyroidism in a patient (Nordyke et al., 1993; Dayan and Daniels, 1996). It is generally thought that Tg-antibody testing should be reserved for patients with negative TPO-antibody findings but who show clinical signs of thyroid autoimmunity (Feldt-Rasmussen, 1996) or in screening for interference in thyroglobulin assays by anti-Tg antibodies (Saravanan and Dayan, 2001).

All patients with overt hypothyroidism should be treated with thyroid hormone replacement (thyroxine) (Singer et al., 1995; Dayan and Daniels, 1996). The dose may be adjusted to normalize the serum TSH concentration (Singer et al., 1995; Dayan and Daniels, 1996). In elderly patients, treatment should begin with a low dose (12.5–25 μg daily) with escalation of dosing done at 4–6 week intervals (Singer et al., 1995; Dayan and Daniels, 1996). Thyroid hormone replacement should be lifelong. Remissions have been reported in 5–10 per cent of patients; however, the duration of such remissions is unknown and thus withdrawl of thyroxine is not recommended (Weetman et al., 1998). Subclinical hypothyroidism is marked by an elevated TSH value despite normal T4 levels and the role of thyroxine therapy in these patients is more controversial (Mandel et al., 1993).

Euthyroid patients with goitrous autoimmune thyroiditis may also be given thyroxine therapy to decrease the size of the goiter (Dayan and Daniels, 1996). The size of the goiter typically decreases in approximately 50–90 per cent of patients following 6 months of treatment (Hegedus et al., 1991). Thyroidectomy is only indicated if there is a suspicion of tumor or if a patient has persistent painful thyroiditis that has failed medical management.

AUTOIMMUNE ADRENAL DISEASE

Autoimmune adrenalitis

The clinical disorder caused by autoimmune adrenocortical destruction was first described by Dr Addison more than 150 years ago (Peterson et al., 1998; Furmaniak and Smith, 2002). The clinical signs and symptoms of the condition are due to the failure of the adrenal cortex to produce the steroid hormones cortisol and aldosterone. The lack of cortisol results in weight loss, weakness and vomiting and elevated serum levels of ACTH. By the time the diagnosis of autoimmune adrenalitis is made the adrenal cortex is usually completely destroyed (Peterson et al., 1998). Most of the original cases of adrenalitis described were actually a consequence of tuberculosis affecting the adrenal glands, which is still the predominant etiology in developing countries (Peterson et al., 1998). However, the prevalence of tuberculosis in developed countries is much less and an autoimmune form predominates (Laureti et al., 1999). Overall, the incidence of Addison's disease is 40–117 cases per million in developed countries, of which, autoimmune adrenalitis accounts for approximately 90 per cent

(Peterson et al., 1998; Laureti et al., 1999). Other non-immunologic causes of adrenal insufficiency include HIV, cytomegalovirus, amyloidosis, tumors, hemorrhage or adrenal leukodystrophy (Ten et al., 2001).

A main feature of autoimmune endocrine diseases is their tendency to associate with each other and with other organ-specific autoimmune disorders. Addison's disease can present as an isolated disorder or as a component of APS type 1, type 2 or type 4 (see later). Autoimmune Addison's disease is a major part of type-1 and type-2 APS (Ten et al., 2001). The age of onset usually varies for the various disorders with APS-1 developing early in childhood and isolated autoimmune adrenalitis and APS-2 developing in the third decade of life (Ten et al., 2001).

In the early phase of the disease, small areas of hyperplastic and hypertrophic adrenal cortical cells can be found (Muir et al., 1993). There is considerable infiltration with mononuclear cells, lymphocytes, plasma cells and macrophages in the adrenal cortex and destruction of the cortical cells (Muir et al., 1993). The normal zonal architecture of the adrenal cortex is destroyed and the cortex cells show necrosis and pleomorphism (Muir et al., 1993). The adrenal medulla, however, remains intact. In progressed stages, the active destructive process is replaced with fibrosis. Indeed, at autopsy the adrenals of patients with progressed disease often weigh only 1 g each instead of a more normal 4 g (Muir et al., 1993; Furmaniak and Smith, 2002).

Both T and B cells are observed in the lymphocytic infiltrate and deposits of IgG are present in the adrenal cortex (Muir et al., 1993). T cell responses toward adrenal tissue have been examined by the leukocyte migration inhibition assay *in vitro*. The finding of leukocyte migration inhibition with positive reactivity to homogenized adrenal extracts has been found in 40–80 per cent of patient with autoimmune adrenalitis (Peterson et al., 1998). However, leukocyte migration assays did not show a correlation with the presence of adrenocortical antibodies or to the duration of the disease. A delayed type skin reaction assay has also demonstrated an adrenal antigen specific reaction *in vivo* by injection of adrenal extracts in patients with autoimmune adrenalitits (Nerup and Bendixen, 1969). The extent of cell-mediated cytotoxicity in adrenal autoimmune expression has not been described.

As previously discussed with AITD, aberrant HLA class II expression and antigen presentation has been proposed as an initiating mechanism in pathogenesis of autoimmune endocrine diseases (Bottazzo et al., 1983). Expression of HLA class II can be found in 10–20 per cent of cortical cells in normal adrenal glands. In contrast, 50–100 per cent of residual cortical cells in autoimmune adrenalitis are HLA class II positive (Peterson et al., 1998; Furmaniak and Smith, 2002). However, this phenomenon is also observed in infectious forms of Addison's disease indicating that this is likely a secondary event in response to cytokine release (IFN-γ) from inflammatory cells (Peterson et al., 1998; Furmaniak and Smith, 2002).

Autoantibodies against the adrenal cortex were first described in 1957 (Anderson et al., 1957). Initially using indirect immunofluorescence assays, adrenal autoantibodies were found to react with all layers of the adrenal cortex and as a collection are called adrenal cortex autoantibodies (ACA). However, sera from some patients with Addison's disease also react with cells from other steroid-producing organs (ovary, testis and placenta). This specific subset of antibodies has been termed steroid cell antibodies (StCA). Subsequent work done to isolate the specific antigens in autoimmune adrenalitis found that sera from patients with Addison's reacted with various microsomal subfractions of adrenal extracts (Furmaniak et al., 1988). The major antigens were later identified as the steroidogenic cytochrome P450 enzymes: 17a-hydroxylase (17a-OH), 21-hydroxylase (21-OH) and the side-chain cleavage enzyme (P450scc) (Krohn et al., 1992; Bednarek et al., 1992; Winqvist et al., 1992, 1993). All three autoantibodies are likely responsible for the observations of ACA assays; however, the steroid cell antibodies are probably only represented by P450scc and 17a-OH. The originally reported prevalence of these antibodies in patients with Addison's disease varied considerably and this is most likely attributable to different antigen sources and assay methodologies (Novak and Lernmark, 2002). More recent studies employing recombinant antigens found 21-OH to be the most prevalent (Colls et al., 1995; Falorni et al., 1995; Chen et al., 1996; Peterson et al., 1997). Antibodies to 17a-OH and P450scc are less prevalent and are predominantly found in patients with APS types 1 and 2 and only occasionally in patients with solitary Addison's disease (Peterson et al., 1997).

The pathogenic role of adrenal autoantibodies is still not clear. Initial *in vitro* studies suggested that steroidogenic antibodies might participate in the pathogensis of autoimmune Addison's disease because antibody preparations from adrenalitis patient sera were able to inhibit 21-OH activity (Furmaniak et al., 1994). However, later *in vivo* studies found no impairment of 21-OH enzymatic activity in autoantibody positive sera from patients with varying degrees of adrenal failure (Boscaro et al., 1996). Other mechanisms such as complement fixation and ADCC may be of more clinical significance.

The characteristic clinical symptoms of Addison's disease are fatigue, weakness, listlessness, orthostatic dizziness, weight loss, anorexia and salt craving (Oelkers, 1996). Other presenting complaints may include gastrointestinal symptoms such as nausea, vomiting, abdominal cramps and diarrhea (Oelkers, 1996). Varying degrees of changes in skin pigmentation may occur. Laboratory tests often show hyponatremia with hyperkalemia, hypoglycemia, eosinophilia and hypercalcemia (Oelkers, 1996).

As mentioned before, autoimmune adrenalitis affects all steroid-producing cells of the adrenal cortex and, as such, will cause a deficiency in both cortisol and aldosterone. Thus, clinical diagnosis of adrenal insufficiency is usually based on measurement of basal plasma levels of cortisol, aldosterone, ACTH and plasma renin activity (Oelkers, 1996). Measurements of plasma cortisol concentration before and 60 minutes following injection of 250 μg of cosyntropin give nearly 100 per cent sensitivity for detection of adrenal hypofunction (Oelkers, 1996). Detection of adrenal hypofunction in patients with overt disease as well as those with subclinical findings is extremely important in order to prevent the development of an Addisonian crisis. Stress, strenuous physical activity, viral infection, extensive dental work or serious illness can lead to acute and often fatal decompensation of adrenal reserve (Oelkers, 1996).

The standard test for detecting adrenal cortex autoantibodies (ACA) is the indirect immunofluorescence technique used on sections of bovine or human adrenal cortex (Falorni et al., 1995). The sensitivity of this test in patients with autoimmune adrenalitis is about 70 per cent with a high degree of specificity (Falorni et al., 1995); however, this assay has never been standardized (Novak and Lernmark, 2002). The use of measurement of adrenal autoantibodies as a marker of the prediction of development of Addison's disease is probably most useful in children (Novak and Lernmark, 2002).

The main goal in treating autoimmune adrenalitis is to replace the hormone deficiency. Patients with symptomatic adrenal insufficiency should be treated with hydrocortisone or cortisone to replace cortisol deficiency and fludrocortisone for aldosterone. The goal should be to use the smallest dose which relieves the patient's symptoms and drug management can be guided by measurements of urinary cortisol, blood pressure, serum potassium and plasma renin activity (Oelkers, 1996).

AUTOIMMUNE REPRODUCTIVE DISEASE

Lymphocytic oophoritis

Premature ovarian failure (POF) is a condition characterized by amenorrhea, infertility, sex steroid deficiency and elevated serum levels of gonadotropins as are seen in the naturally occurring condition of menopause (Anasti, 1998; Kalantaridou and Nelson, 2002). However, the mean age of menopause in the USA is 50 years and should cessation of ovulation occur prior to the age of 40 the condition is labeled as premature (Hoek et al., 1997). It affects approximately 0.1 per cent of women by age 30 and 1 per cent of women by age 40 (Coulam et al., 1986). It is a heterogeneous disorder with a spectrum of etiologies. Overall, it is marked by either a depletion or dysfunction of ovarian follicles. Such depletion or dysfunction can be the result of gonadal dysgenesis, metabolic derangements, steroid enzyme deficiencies, mutations in gonadotropin receptors, various infectious agents or iatrogenic causes such as chemotherapeutics and radiation (Anasti, 1998; Hoek et al., 1997).

Another less well-defined group of POF is idiopathic in nature and growing evidence suggests that such ovarian failure may be autoimmune mediated and this is marked by evidence of lymphocytic oophoritis (Hoek et al., 1997; Kalantaridou et al., 2002). Isolated cases of lymphocytic oophoritis have been described (Wolfe and Stirling, 1988). However, autoimmune POF is commonly associated with other autoimmune endocrinopathies such as hypothyroidism, Addison's disease and diabetes mellitus (Hoek et al., 1997; Kalantaridou et al., 2002). In females with APS-1, POF will develop in as many as 60 per cent of afflicted patients (Ahonen et al., 1990).

The reported histologic analysis of autoimmune POF is somewhat mixed with small numbers of case reports and findings that vary depending on the presence of other autoimmune diseases (primarily Addison's disease) (Hoek et al., 1997). In general, the pattern of autoimmune infiltration revolves around the steroid producing cells of the ovary. Microscopically, it is characterized by mononuclear infiltration of the theca interna and theca externa of developing follicles. The degree and density of infiltration increases with more mature follicles (Hoek et al., 1997; Kalantaridou et al., 2002). Perineural and perivascular accumulation of lymphocytes may also be present in the ovarian hilum (Hoek et al., 1997; Kalantaridou et al., 2002). Primordial follicles and the ovary cortex are usually spared. In established disease, the infiltrating mononuclear cells are mainly T cells with some B cells, macrophages, natural killer cells and plasma cells (Hoek et al., 1997). In a limited study, Sedmark and colleagues (1987) noted a proportionately higher number of the T cells to be CD4+ than CD8+.

In 1966, Vallotton and Forbes were able to show by indirect immunofluorescence against a rabbit ovarian antigen source the presence of ovarian antibodies from sera in a small number of female patients with POF when compared to controls. Later, Irvine and colleagues (1975) observed anti-steroid cell antibodies were present in women with suspected autoimmune POF and Addison's disease. As discussed previously, these steroid cell antibodies are believed to represent antibodies against 17-alpha hydroxylase, p450scc enzymes and an ill-defined 51 kDa protein. Sera of patients with APS-1 and steroid cell antibodies have been shown to be cytotoxic for culture granulosa cells in the presence of complement (McNatty et al., 1975). However, the role of the steroid cell antibodies in the pathogenesis of autoimmune POF is largely unknown. Further, the presence of these antibodies appears to be restricted to a population of patients with a diagnosis of both POF and Addison's disease or APS-1. Subsequent studies have shown that patients with isolated autoimmune POF do not have steroid cell antibodies (Chen et al., 1996).

Other possible candidates for an ovarian autoantigen have been described. Several investigators have found evidence of IgGs with either binding or blocking potential of the FSH and LH receptors in a small percentage of patients with autoimmune POF (Chiauzzi et al., 1982;

Tang and Faiman, 1983; Moncayo et al., 1989; Van Weissenbruch et al., 1991). These studies however, utilized non-human gonadotropin receptors and the results of these previous studies have largely been refuted by newer assays employing recombinant human receptors (Anasti et al., 1995; Anasti, 1998; Kalantaridou et al., 2002).

The zona pellucida has also been a target of investigation as a putative ovarian autoantigen. The zona pellucida (ZP) is the acellular matrix that surrounds developing and ovulated oocytes and is also detectable in atretic follicles (Hoek et al., 1997). Nelson and colleagues were able to show 50 per cent of patients' sera with autoimmune POF were positive for antibodies against primate ZP (Kalantaridou et al., 2002). However, 30 per cent of controls were also positive. As such, ZP antibodies in autoimmune POF cannot be correlated with disease expression (Kalantaridou et al., 2002).

As shown with other autoimmune endocrinopathies, women with autoimmune premature ovarian failure have increased activation of peripheral T lymphocytes as marked by HLA-DR+ and IL-2 receptor positivity (Nelson et al., 1991; Hoek et al., 1997). Further, this T cell activation may be specific for ovarian antigens. Perkonen and colleagues (1986) have demonstrated an ovarian antigen specific T cell response utilizing a leukocyte migration inhibition factor assay. These data taken together with some suggestion of putative ovarian autoantibodies and the predilection of some POF patients to have associated autoimmune diseases implies that this phenomenon is autoimmune in nature.

Premature ovarian failure is diagnosed by clinical findings of at least 4 months of amenorrhea with two subsequent FSH values greater than 40 mIU/ml obtained at least one month apart in a woman less than 40 years of age (Hoek et al., 1997; Anasti, 1998; Kalantaridou et al., 2002). Ovarian biopsy is the only way to diagnose autoimmune POF with certainty. However, such invasive diagnostic procedures have not been shown to provide clinical benefit and are not warranted in the evaluation of POF (Kalantaridou et al., 2002). Other imaging modalities such as ovarian ultrasound do not change the clinical management of this disease process and are not generally pursued (Kalantaridou et al., 2002).

The principal method for detection of ovarian antibodies has been indirect immunofluorescence (Novak and Lernmark, 2002). As with other assays which use tissue immunofluorescence, there is great variability in the source of ovarian tissue. This has prevented any standardization in the detection and interpretation of this assay (Novak and Lernmark, 2002). Greater sensitivity has been demonstrated in more recent investigations using ELISA based methods for antibody detection (Luborsky et al., 1990; Wheatcroft et al., 1994, 1997). However, because these assays still depend on tissue samples as antigen sources, reproducibility has been variable (Wheatcroft et al., 1997). Other confounding factors for the clinical usefulness of current assays are that ovarian autoantibodies have also been found in iatrogenic forms of POF and in women with infertility secondary to Turner's syndrome (Wheatcroft et al., 1994). Thus, the use of ovarian auto-antibodies as an immunologic surrogate in the diagnosis of autoimmune POF is currently not justified. The diagnosis is a presumptive one based on the aforementioned findings of gonadotropin excess and absence of other causes of POF especially in those patients with associated autoimmune diseases. Indeed, the most important tests in the clinical management of POF is to monitor for other related autoimmune disorders (hypothyroidism, adrenal insufficiency and diabetes) (Kalantaridou et al., 2002).

Treatment of young women with premature ovarian failure should include hormone replacement therapy to relieve the symptoms of estrogen deficiency (vasomotor symptoms and vaginal atrophy) and loss of bone mineral density. About two-thirds of patients with POF have a bone mineral density one standard deviation or more below the mean of similar aged women and this deficiency is associated with a significantly increased risk for hip fracture (Anasti, 1998; Kalantaridou et al., 2002). Women with POF usually require administration of 0.625 mg of conjugated estrogen to maintain bone density; however, younger women may require a higher dose of 1.25 mg to control vasomotor symptoms (Anasti, 1998). Addition of cyclic progesterone dosing is also required to prevent unrestrained endometrial proliferation and potential cancer development (Anasti, 1998). Androgen replacement should also be considered for women experiencing persistent fatigue and low libido (Kalantaridou et al., 2002).

Other management considerations are addressed when patients with POF desire pregnancy. The disease may have a fluctuating course with high gonadotropin levels that periodically return to normal (Kalantaridou et al., 2002). Indeed, women with POF do continue to have intermittent ovarian function and retain at least some chance for spontaneous pregnancy. Some case reports have suggested that glucocorticoid treatment and other immunosuppressive modalities may restore ovarian function in women with POF (Kalantaridou et al., 2002). However, considering 20 per cent of patients with POF ovulate intermittently, immunosuppression or treatment with glucocorticoids has no proven benefit. Other pharmacologic methods of ovulation induction in POF patients have also failed to demonstrate increased ovulation rates when compared to that in untreated patients (Kalantaridou et al., 2002). Thus, for women with a prolonged absence of spontaneous pregnancy, oocyte donation is an option.

AUTOIMMUNE PARATHYROID DISEASE

Idiopathic hypoparathyroidism

Hypoparathyroidism is characterized by a deficiency of parathyroid hormone (PTH) production. Such deficiency can be caused by mutations in the PTH gene, activating mutations in the calcium-sensing receptor gene or developmental defects of the parathyroid glands as are observed in DiGeorge syndrome (Marx, 2000). The most common cause of acute and chronic hypoparathyroidism is iatrogenic damage to the parathyroid glands during surgery (Marx, 2000). An autoimmune process may also incite parathyroid hormone deficiency and this has been classically labeled as idiopathic hypoparathyroidism. Autoimmune hypoparathyroidism may occur in isolation; however, a preponderance of autoimmune parathyroid disease is seen as a component of the autoimmune polyglandular syndromes (APS) and more specifically APS-1 (Marx, 2000). What is not clear is whether these autoimmune entities are the result of similar or disparate pathogenic processes.

The histology seen in autoimmune parathyroid disorders has shown to varying degrees fatty replacement of the gland architecture, atrophy and lymphocyctic infiltration (Kifor et al., 2004). In animal models of this disease, specific disaggregation of the structure of the parathyroid gland and the consequent atrophy has been described in isoimmunized rats with parathyroid tissue (Lupulescu et al., 1965). Hypoparathyroidism has also been described in a similar dog model with histologic findings of disorganization of the columnar structure, extensive zones of fibrosis and lymphocytic and plasma cell infiltrations (Maclaren et al., 2002).

Blizzard and colleagues first described autoantibodies in humans directed against the parathyroid gland in association with hypoparathyroidism in 1966. In this study, 38 per cent of patients with idiopathic hypoparathyroidism demonstrated parathyroid antibodies by indirect immunofluorescence compared to 6 per cent of control patients (Blizzard et al., 1966). The study included positive sera cohorts with isolated hypoparathyroidism and hypoparathyroidism in association with APS. The antibodies were believed to be specific because competitive inhibition occurred with parathyroid gland extracts but not with extracts of gastric, adrenal, thyroid, liver or kidney tissue (Blizzard et al., 1966). Subsequent studies found that anti-mitochondrial antibodies may explain the reactivity seen against parathyroid cells (Swana et al., 1977; Betterle et al., 1985). Moreover, these antibodies appear to be actually directed against mitochondria-rich oxyphil cells of the parathyroid gland rather than to the PTH-secreting parathyroid cells themselves (Swana et al., 1977; Betterle et al., 1985).

Other autoantigens in autoimmune hypoparathyroidism have been described. Fattorossi and colleagues (1988) have described the presence of a 200 kD and 130 kD autoantigen in parathyroid endothelial cells. Later, other groups identified the calcium sensitive receptor (CaSR) as an autoantigen and demonstrated antibodies against the receptor in 56 per cent of patients with hypoparathyroidism (Li et al., 1996). However, they were unable to demonstrate a cytopathologic effect by these CaSR autoantibodies on live HEK-293 cells transfected with the CaSR cDNA (Li et al., 1996). Subsequent investigation has confirmed similar percentages of patients with seropositivity against CaSR in cases of isolated idiopathic hypoparathyroidism and that this is significantly associated with two specific HLA-DR haplotypes (Goswami et al., 2004). These data at least imply an autoimmune component to the disease and that the CaSR antibodies may be involved.

The role of parathyroid autoantibodies in the pathogenesis of the disease has not been determined. It is not known, for instance, whether the CaSR autoantibodies observed in some patients bring about the primary destruction of the parathyroid gland or whether these autoantibodies mark the end stage of a disease process which originally begins with damage to the parathyroid cells mediated through Th1 lymphocytes with activation of local Th2 cells and consequent development of autoantibodies. Indeed, Gylling et al. (2003) analyzed a series of patients with APS associated hypoparathyroidism and found a relatively small percentage of these patients had antibodies to CaSR and even fewer had detectable antibodies at the onset of disease. Serum from patients with type 1 APS associated hypoparathyroidism has demonstrated antibody-dependent cytotoxicity in cultured bovine parathyroid cells (Brandi et al., 1986). Using an in vitro cell system of dispersed human parathyroid tissue, others have found that binding of autoantibodies results in inhibition of parathyroid hormone secretion in a subset of patients with idiopathic hypoparathyroidism (Posillico et al., 1986). This suggests that at least in some individuals the autoantibodies may themselves contribute to the hypoparathyroidism (Possillico et al., 1986). Patients with adult onset hypoparathyroidism have generalized T cell activation, which could be a manifestation of cell-mediated immunity against parathyroid chief cells with consequent parathyroiditis (Worstman et al., 1992). Therefore, both humoral and cell-mediated immunity could contribute to loss of parathyroid cells in hypoparathyroidism.

Hypoparathyroidism is diagnosed on the basis of measurements of serum calcium and parathyroid hormone (Marx, 2000). Overall the use of parathyroid autoantibodies to characterize the disease has been limited and there is currently no accepted clinically relevant assay for this disease process. Further characterization of the autoantibodies present in hypoparathyroidism may eventually allow for the use of antibody markers to diagnose autoimmune parathyroid disease and monitor its progression.

Irrespective of whether hypoparathyroidism is the result of an autoimmune process or other more common causes, the treatment is the same. The major objective in treatment is to elevate the plasma calcium concentration above 9 mg/dl through vitamin D or its associated analogs and calcium supplementation (Marx, 2000). Renal production of 1,25-dihydroxyvitamin D is deficient in all hypoparathyroid states and supplementation with an active vitamin D analog should be done (Marx, 2000). However, with diminished levels of PTH there is less control in renal excretion of calcium and excessive therapy with vitamin D analogs can lead to hypercalciuria, nephrolithiasis and renal damage. Some patients have been treated successfully with synthetic human parathyroid hormone; however, clinical trials are ongoing and such therapies are not currently commercially available.

AUTOIMMUNE POLYENDOCRINE SYNDROMES

APS type 1 (also know as APECED for autoimmune polyendocrinopathy-candidiasis-ectodermal dystrophy) is defined by the presence of three principal components including chronic or recurrent mucocutaneous candidiasis, idiopathic hypoparathyroidism and autoimmune adrenalitis (Peterson et al., 1998; Ten et al., 2001; Furmaniak and Smith, 2002). In order to classify a patient as having APS type-1, at least two of these three components must be present (Peterson et al., 1998; Furmaniak and Smith, 2002). Other characteristics are possible and include hypogonadism, ectodermal dystrophy, chronic active hepatitis, chronic atrophic gastritis with or without pernicious anemia, type-1 diabetes, autoimmune thyroiditis, gastrointestinal malabsorption, alopecia universalis and anterior hypophysitis. Chronic mucocutaneous candidiasis caused by infection with *Candida albicans* is usually the initial feature (Ten et al., 2001). Hypoparathyroidism usually occurs next, but hypocalcemia can be masked by untreated Addison's disease and only become clinically evident after steroid replacement (Ten et al., 2001).

APS-1 affects males and females equally and often first manifests during infancy or early childhood. APS-1 is a rare recessive disease and tends to segregate to specific populations of Finnish and Iranian Jew descent (Perheentupa, 1996). Mutations in AIRE (autoimmune regulatory gene) have been described as the likely cause of this disorder; this is an ill-defined transcription factor with primary expression observed in thymic medullary epithelial cells and monocyte-dendritic cells in the thymus and may play a central role in the maintenance of immune tolerance (Pitkanen and Peterson, 2003).

APS type 2 is characterized by at least two of the three major autoimmune endocrine diseases (adrenal, thyroid and type 1 diabetes). Addison's disease together with autoimmune thyroid disease has also been known as Schmidt's syndrome or with type-1 diabetes as Carpenter's syndrome. It may also be associated with other non-endocrine organ specific autoimmune diseases such as vitiligo, pernicious anemia and alopecia (Betterle et al., 1996). APS-2 has a strong female bias in disease expression and can occur at any age, but the peak onset is at 30 years of age (Betterle et al., 1996). This syndrome shows marked restriction to several HLA haplotypes; however, no specific gene abnormality has been described.

APS-3 is autoimmune thyroid disease in association with atrophic gastritis, pernicious anemia, vitiligo and occasionally type-1 diabetes. APS-3 has a strong female bias in disease expression and can occur at any age, but the peak onset is 30 years of age.

APS-4 is a rare syndrome characterized by the association of autoimmune combinations not falling into the above categories (Betterle et al., 2002).

REFERENCES

Ahonen, P., Myllarniemi, S., Sipila, I. et al. (1990). Clinical variation of autoimmune polyendocrinopathy-candidiasis-ectodermal dystrophy (APECED) in a series of 68 patients. N Engl J Med 322, 1829–1836.

Aiziawa, Y., Yoshida, K., Kaise, N. et al. (1997). The development of transient hypothyroidism after iodine-131 treatment in hyperthyroid patients with Graves' disease: prevelance, mechanism, and prognosis. Clin Endocrinol 78, 98–102.

Anasti, J.N. (1998) Premature ovarian failure. In Endocrine Autoimmunity and Associated Conditions, Weetman, A.P., ed. Dordrecht, Netherlands: Kluwer Academic Publishers, pp. 183–221.

Anasti, J.N., Flack, M.R., Froelich, J. et al. (1995). The use of human recombinant gonadotropin receptors to search for immunoglobulin G-mediated premature ovarian failure. J Clin Endocrinol Metab 80, 824–828.

Anderson, J.R., Goudie, R.B., Gray, K.G. et al. (1957) Autoantibodies in Addison's disease. Lancet 1, 1123–1124.

Bayer, M.F. (1991). Effective laboratory evaluation of thyroid status. Med Clin N Am 75, 1–26.

Bednarek, J., Furmaniak, J., Wedlock, N. et al. (1992). Steroid 21-hydroxylase is a major autoantigen involved in adult onset autoimmune Addison's disease. FEBS Lett 309, 51–55.

Betterle, C., Caretto, A., Zeviani, M., Pedini, B. and Salviati, C. (1985). Demonstration and characterization of anti-human mitochondria autoantibodies in idiopathic hypoparathyroidism and in other conditions. Clin Exp Immunol 62, 353–360.

Betterle, C., Volpato, M., Greggio, A.N. et al. (1996). Type 2 polyglandular autoimmune disease (Schmidt's syndrome). J Pediatr Endocrinol Metab 9, 113–123.

Betterle C., Dal Pra, C., Mantero, F. and Zanchetta, R. (2002). Autoimmune adrenal insufficiency and autoimmune polyendocrine syndromes: autoantibodies, autoantigens, and their applicability in diagnosis and disease prediction. Endocrinol Rev 23, 327–364.

Blizzard, R.M., Chee, D. and Davis, W. (1966). The incidence of parathyroid and other antibodies in the sera of patients with idiopathic hypoparathyroidism. Clin Exp Immunol 1, 119–128.

Bogner, U., Schleusener, H. and Wall, J.R. (1984). Antibody-dependent cell mediated cytotoxicity against human thyroid cells in Hashimoto's thyroiditis but not Graves' disease. J Clin Endocrinol Metab 59, 734–738.

Boscaro, M., Betterle, C., Volpato, M. et al. (1996). Hormonal responses during various phases of autoimmune adrenal failure: no evidence for 21-hydroxylase enzyme activity inhibiton in vivo. J Clin Endocrinol Metab 81, 2801–2804.

Bottazzo, G.F., Pujol-Borrell, R., Hanafusa, T. and Feldman, M. (1983). Role of aberrant HLA-DR expression and antigen presentation in induction of endocrine autoimmunity. Lancet 2, 1115–1119.

Brandi, M.L., Aurbach, G.D., Fattorossi, A., Quarto, R., Marx, S.J. and Fitzpatrick, L.A. (1986). Antibodies cytotoxic to bovine parathyroid cells in autoimmune hypoparathyroidism. Proc Natl Acad Sci USA 83, 8366–8369.

Brix, T.H., Kyvik, K.O. and Hegedus, L. (1998). What is the evidence of genetic factors in the eitiology of Graves' disease? A brief review. Thyroid 8, 627–634.

Calder, E.A., Penhale, W.J., McLeman, D., Barnes, E.W. and Irvine, W.J. (1973). Lymphocyte-dependent antibody-mediated cytotoxicity in Hashimoto thyroiditis. Clin Exp Immunol 14, 153–158.

Chazenbalk, G.D., Portalano, S., Russo, D. et al. (1993). Molecular cloning and expression of an autoantibody gene repertoire for a major autoantigen reveals an antigenic immunodominant region and restricted immunoglobulin gene usage in the target organ. J Clin Invest 92, 62–74.

Chen, S., Sawicka, J., Betterle, C. et al. (1996). Autoantibodies to steroidogenic enzymes in autoimmune polyglandular syndrome, Addison's disease, and premature ovarian failure. J Clin Endocrinol Metab 81, 1871–1876.

Chiovato, L., Bassi, P., Mammoli, C. et al. (1993). Antibodies producing complement-mediated thyroid cytotoxicity in patients with atrophic and goitrous autoimmune thyroiditis. J Clin Endocrinol Metab 77, 1700–1705.

Chiauzzi, V., Cigorraga, S., Escobar, M.E., Rivarola, M.A. and Charreau, E.H. (1982). Inhibition of follicle-stimulating hormone receptor binding by circulating immunoglobulins. J Clin Endocrinol Metab 54, 1221–1228.

Colls, J., Betterle, C., Volpato, M. et al. (1995). Immunoprecipitation assay for autoantibodies to steroid 21-hydroxylase in autoimmune adrenal diseases. Clin Chem 41, 375–380.

Coulam, C.B., Adamson, S.C. and Annergers, J.F. (1986). Incidence of premature ovarian failure. Obstet Gynecol 67, 604–606.

Czarnocka, B., Janota-Bzowski, M., McIntosh, R.S. et al. (1997). Immunoglobulin G kappa anti-thyroid peroxidase antibodies in Hashimoto's thyroiditis: epitope mapping analysis. J Clin Endocrinol Metab 82, 2639–2644.

Dayan, C.M. and Daniels, G.H. (1996). Medical progress: chronic autoimmune thyroiditis. N Engl J Med 335, 99–107.

Del Prete, G.F., Vercelli, D. and Tiri, A. (1986). In vivo activated cytotoxic T cells in the thyroid infiltrate of patients with Hashimoto's thyroiditis. Clin Exp Immunol 65, 140–147.

Dong, Q., Ludgate, M. and Vassart, G. (1989). Towards an antigenic map of thyroglobulin: identification of ten epitope bearing sequences within the primary structure of thyroglobulin. J Endocrinol 122, 169–176.

Falorni, A., Nikosjkov, A., Laureti, S. et al., (1995). High diagnostic accuracy for idiopathic Addison's disease with a sensitive radiobinding assay for autoantibodies against recombinant human 21-hydroxylase. J Clin Endocrinol Metab 80, 2752–2755.

Fattorosi, A., Aurbach, G.D., Sakaguchi, K. et al. (1988). Anti-endothelial cell antibodies: detection and characterization in sera from patients with autoimmune hypoparathyroidism. Proc Natl Acad Sci USA 85, 4015–4019.

Feldt-Rasmussen, U. (1996). Analytical and clinical performance goals for testing autoantibodies to thyroperoxidase, thyroglobulin, and thyrotropin receptor. Clin Chem 42, 160–163.

Foulis, A.K. and Riley, A. (2003). Pathology/histology of organ specific autoimmune diseases. In Diseases of the Thyroid, 2nd edn, Braverman, L.E., ed. Totowa, New Jersey: Humana Press, pp. 499–528.

Furmaniak, J. and Smith, B.R. (2002). Addison's disease. In Immunologically mediated endocrine diseases, Gill, R.G., Harmon, J.T. and Maclaren, N.K., eds. Philadelphia: Lippincott Williams and Wilkins, pp. 431–451.

Furmaniak, J., Talbot, D., Reinwein, D. et al. (1988). Immunoprecipitation of human adrenal microsomal antigen. FEBS Lett 231, 25–28.

Furmaniak, J., Kominami, S., Asawa, T. et al. (1994). Autoimmune Addison's disease – evidence for a role of steroid 21-hydroxy-lase autoanibodies in adrenal insufficiency. J Clin Endocrinol Metab 79, 1517–1521.

Goswami, R., Brown, E.M., Kochupillai, N. et al. (2004). Prevelance of calcium sensing receptor autoantibodies in patients with sporadic idiopathic hypoparathyroidsim. Eur J Endocrinol 150, 9–18.

Gupta, M.K. (2000). Thyrotropin-receptor antibodies in thyroid diseases: advances in detection techniques and clinical applications. Clinica Chemica Acta. 293, 1–29.

Gylling, M., Kaariainen, E., Vaisanen, R. et al. (2003). The hypoparathyroidism of autoimmune polyendocrinopathy-candidiasis-ectodermal-dystrophy, protective effect of male sex. J Clin Endocrinol Metab 88, 4602–4608.

Hamilton, F., Black, M., Farquharson, M.A., Stewart, C. and Foulis, A.K. (1991). Spatial correlation between thyroid epithelial cells expressing class II MHC molecules and interferon-gamma-containing lymphocytes in human thyroid autoimmune disease. Clin Exp Immunol 83, 64–68.

Hanafusa, T., Pujol-Borrell, R., Chiovato, L., Russell, R.C., Doniach, D. and Bottazzo, G.F. (1983). Aberrant expression of HLA-DR antigen on thyrocytes in Graves' disease: relevance for autoimmunity. Lancet 2, 1111–1115.

Hardisty, C.A., Kendall-Taylor, P., Atkinson, S. et al. (1983). The assay of Graves' immunoglobulins: A comparison of different methods. Clin Endocrinol 18, 637–644.

Hayashi, Y., Tamai, H., Fukata, S. et al. (1985) A long-term clinical, immunologic, and histological follow-up study of patients with goitrous chronic lympocytic thyroiditis. J Clin Endocrinol Metab 61, 1172–1178.

Hegedus, L., Hansen, J.M., Feldt-Rasmussen, U., Hansen, B.M. and Hoier-Madsen, M. (1991). Influence of thyroxine treatment on thyroid size and anti-thyroid peroxidase antibodies in Hashimoto's thyroiditis. Clin Endocrinol 35, 235–238.

Hoek, A., Schoemaker, J. and Drexhage, H.A. (1997). Premature ovarian failure and ovarian autoimmunity. Endocrine Rev 18, 107–134.

Irvine W.J. and Barnes, E.W. (1975). Addison's disease, ovarian failure and hypoparathyroidism. Clin Endocrinol Metab 4, 379–434.

Jacobson, D.L., Gange, S.J., Rose, N.R. and Graham, N.M.H. (1997). Epidemiology and estimated population burden of selected autoimmune diseases in the United States. Clin Immunol Immunopathol 84, 223–243.

Jaume, J.C., Parkes, A.B., Lazarus, J.H. et al. (1995). Thyroid perxoidase autoantibody fingerprints in hypothyroid and euthyroid individuals. I. Cross-sectional study in elderly women. J Clin Endocrinol Metab 80, 994–999.

Kalantaridou, S.N. and Nelson, L.M. (2002) Ovarian autoimmunity. In Immunologically Mediated Endocrine Diseases,

Gill, R.G., Harmon, J.T. and Maclaren, N.K., eds. Philadelphia: Lippincott Williams and Wilkins, pp. 475–487.

Kashiwai, T., Tada, H. and Asahi, K. (1995). Significance of thyroid stimulating antibody and long-term follow-up in patients with euthyroid Graves' disease. Endocrinol J 42, 405–412.

Kaufman, K.D., Filetti, S., Seto, P. et al. (1990). Recombinant human thyroid peroxidase generated in eukaryotic cells: a source of specific antigen for the immunological assay of antimicrosomal antibodies in the sera of patients with autoimmune thyroid disease. J Clin Endocrinol Metab 70, 724–728.

Khoury, E.L., Bottazzo, G.F. and Roitt, I.M. (1984). The thyroid 'microsomal' antibody revisted. Its paradoxical binding in vivo to the apical surface of the follicular epithelium. J Exp Med 159, 577–591.

Kifor, O., Mcelduff, A., Leboff, M.S. et al. (2004). Activating antibodies to the calcium-sensing receptor in two patients with autoimmune hypoparathyroidism. J Clin Endocrinol Metab 89, 548–556.

Kohn, L. and Harii, N. (2003). Thryotropin receptor autoantibodies (TSHRAbs): epitopes, origins and clinical significance. Autoimmunity 36, 331–337.

Kotsa, K., Watson, P.F. and Weetman, A.P. (1997). A CTLA-4 gene polymorphism is associated with both Graves' disease and Hashimoto's thyroiditis. Clin Endocrinol 46, 551–554.

Krohn, K., Uibo, R., Aavik, E. et al. (1992). Identification by molecular cloning of an autoantigen associated with Addison's disease as steroid 17 alpha-hydroxylase. Lancet 339, 770–773.

Laureti, S. et al. (1998). Levels of adrenocartical autoantibodies correlate with the degree of adrenal dysfunction in subjects with proclinical Addison's disease. Journal of Clinical Endocrinology and Metabolism 83, 3507–11.

Li, Y., Song, Y-H., Rais, N. et al. (1996). Autoantibodies to the extracellular domain of the calcium sensing receptor in patient with acquired hypoparathyroidism. J Clin Invest 97, 910–914.

Livolsi, V.A. (1994). The pathology of autoimmune thyroid disease: a review. Thyroid 4, 333–339.

Luborsky, J.L., Visintin, I., Boyers, S. et al. (1990). Ovarian antibodies detected by immobilized antigen immunoassay in patients with premature ovarian failure. J Clin Endocrinol Metab 70, 69–75.

Ludgate, M. (1998). Thyroid autoantigens. In Endocrine Autoimmunity and Associated Conditions, Weetman, A.P., ed. Dordrecht, Netherlands: Kluwer Academic Publishers, pp. 25–38.

Ludgate, M., Dong, Q., Dreyfus, P. et al. (1989). Definition at the molecular level of a thyroglobulin-acetylcholinesterase shared epitope: study of its pathophysiological significance in patients with Graves' ophthalmopathy. Autoimmunity 3, 167–176.

Lupulescu, A., Pop, A. and Merculiev, E. (1965). Experimental iso-immune hypoparathyroidism in rats. Nature 206, 415–416.

Maclaren, N.J., Li, Y. and Song, Y-H. (2002). Hypoparathyroidism. In Immunologically Mediated Endocrine Diseases, Gill, R.G., Harmon, J.T. and Maclaren, N.K., eds. Philadelphia: Lippincott Williams and Wilkins, pp. 427–430.

MacKenzie, W.A., Schwartz, A.E., Friedman, E.W. and Davies, T.F. (1987). Intrathyroidal T cell clones form patients with autoimmune thyroid disease. J Clin Endocrinol Metab 64, 818–824.

Malthierry, Y., Henry, M. and Zanelli, E. (1991). Epitope mapping of human thyroglobulin reveals a central immunodominant region. FEBS Lett 279, 190–192.

Mandel, S.J., Brent, G.A. and Larsen, P.R. (1993). Levothyroxine therapy in patients with thyroid disease. Ann Intern Med 119, 492–502.

Marelli-Berg, F.M., Weetman, A.P., Frasca, L. et al. (1997). Antigen presentation by epithelial cells induces anergic immunoregulatory CD45R0+ T cells and deletion of CD45RA+ T cells. J Immunol 159, 5853–5861.

Mariotti, S., Chovato, L., Vitti, P. et al. (1989). Recent advances in the understanding of humoral and cellular mechanisms implicated in thyroid autoimmune disorders. Clin Immunol Immunopathol 50, S73-S84.

Mariotti, S. and Pinna, G. (2003). Autoimmune thyroid diseases. In Diseases of the Thyroid, 2nd edn, Braverman, L.E., ed. Totowa, New Jersey: Humana Press, pp. 107–160.

Marx S.J. (2000). Hyperparathyroid and hypoparathyroid disorders. N Engl J Med 343, 1863–1875.

McKenzie, J.M. and Zakarija, M. (1989). Clinical review III: The clinical use of thyrotropin receptor antibody measurements. J Clin Endocrinol Metab 69, 1093–1096.

McIntosh, R.S. and Weetman, A.P. (1997). Molecular analysis of the antibody response to thyroglobulin and thyroid peroxidase. Thyroid 7, 471–487.

McLachlan, S.M. and Rapaport, B. (1992). The molecular biology of thyroid peroxidase: Cloning, expression and role as autoantigen in autoimmune thyroid disease. Endocrinol Rev 13, 192–206.

McLachlan, S.M. and Rapaport, B. (1995). Genetic and epitopic analysis of thyroid peroxidase (TPO) autoantibodies: Markers of the human thyroid autoimmune response. Clin Exp Immunol 101, 200–206.

McNatty, K.P., Short, R.V., Barnes, E.W. and Irvine, W.J. (1975). The cytotoxic effect of serum from patients with Addson's disease and autoimmune ovarian failure on human granulosa cells in culture. Clin Exp Immunol 22, 378–384.

Moncayo, H., Moncayo, R., Benz, R., Wolf, A. and Lauritzen, C. (1989). Ovarian failure and autoimmunity. J Clin Invest 84, 1857–1865.

Muir, A., Schatz, D.A. and Maclaren, N.K. (1993). Autoimmune Addison's disease. Springer Semin Immunopathol 14, 275–284.

Murakami, Y., Takamatsu, J. and Sakane, S. (1996). Changes in thyroid volume in response to radioactive iodine for Graves' hyperthyroidism correlated with activity of thyroid-stimulating antibody and treatment outcome. J Clin Endocrinol Metab 81, 3257–3260.

Nelson, L.M., Kimzey, L.M., Merriam, G.R. et al. (1991). Increased peripheral T lymphocyte activation in patients with karyotypically normal spontaneous premature ovarian failure. Fertil Steril 55, 1082–1087.

Nerup, J. and Bendixen, G. (1969). Anti-adrenal cellular hypersensitivity in Addison's disease. 2. Correlation with clinical and serological findings. Clin Exp Immunol 5, 341–354,

Nishikawa, T., Constante, G., Prummel, M.F. et al. (1994). Recombinant thyroid peroxidase autoantibodies can be used for epitopic 'fingerprinting' of thyroid peroxidase autoantibodies in the sera of individual patients. J Clin Endocrinol Metab 78, 944–949.

Nordyke, R.A., Gilbert, Jr., F.I., Miyamoto, L.A. et al. (1993). The superiority of anti-microsomal over antithyroglobulin antibodies for detecting Hashimoto's thyroiditis. Arch Intern Med 153, 862–865.

Novak, E.J. and Lernmark, A. (2002). Immunological markers and disease prediction. In Immunologically Mediated Endocrine Diseases, Gill, R.G., Harmon, J.T. and Maclaren, N.K., eds. Philadelphia: Lippincott Williams and Wilkins, pp. 529–548.

Oelkers, W. (1996). Adrenal insufficiency. N Engl J Med 335, 1206–1212.

Parkin, J. and Cohen, B. (2001). An overview of the immune system. Lancet 357, 1777–1789.

Pekonen, F., Siegberg, R., Makinen, T., Miettinen, A. and Yli-Kokala, O. (1986). Immunological disturbances in patients with premature ovarian failure. Clin Endocrinol 25, 1–6.

Perheentupa, J. (1996). Autoimmune polyendocrinopathy-candidiasis-ectodermal dystrophy (APECED). Hormone Metab Res 28, 353–356.

Persani, L., Tonacchera, M. and Beck-Peccoz, P. (1993). Measurement of camp accumulation in Chinese hamster ovary cells transfected with the recombinant human TSH receptor (CHO-R): a new bioassay for human thyrotropin. J Endocrinol Invest 16, 511–519.

Peterson, P., Uibo, R., Peranen, J. et al. (1997). Immuno-precipitation of steroidogenic enzyme autoantigens with autoimmune polyglandular syndrome type 1 (APS 1) sera; further evidence for independent humoral immunity to P450c17 and P450c21. Clin Exp Immunol 107, 335–340.

Peterson, P., Uibo, R. and Krohn, K.J.E. (1998). Addison's disease and related polyendocrinopathies. In Endocrine Autoimmunity and Associated Conditions, Weetman, A.P., ed. Dordrecht, Netherlands: Kluwer Academic Publishers, pp. 163–182.

Pitkanen J. and Peterson P. (2003). Autoimmune regulator: from loss of function to autoimmunity. Genes Immun 4, 12–21.

Portalano, S., Chazenbalk, G.D., Seto, P. et al. (1992). Recognition by recombinant autoimmune thyroid disease-derived Fab fragments of a dominant conformational epitope on human thyroid peroxidase. J Clin Invest 90, 720–726.

Posillico, J.T., Wortsman, J. and Srikanta, S. (1986). Parathyroid cell surface autoantibodies that inhibit parathyroid hormone secretion from dispersed human parathyroid cells. J Bone Mineral Res 1, 475–483.

Prentice, L., Kiso, Y., Fukuma, N. et al. (1995). Monoclonal thyroglobulin autoantibodies: variable region analysis and epitope recognition. J Clin Endocrinol Metab 80, 977–986.

Prummel, M.F. and Wiersina, W.M. (2002). Autoimmnue thyroid diseases. In Immunologically Mediated Endocrine Diseases, Gill, R.G., Harmon, J.T. and Maclaren, N.K., eds. Philadelphia: Lippincott Williams and Wilkins, pp. 373–396.

Rapoport, B., Chazenbalk, G.D., Jaume, J.C. and McLachlan, S.M. (1998). The thyrotropin (TSH) receptor: Interaction with TSH and autoantibodies. Endocrine Rev 19, 673–716.

Rodien, P., Madec, A., Ruf, J. et al. (1996). Antibody-dependent cell-mediated cytotoxicity in autoimmune thyroid disease: Relationship to anti-thyroperoxidase antibodies. J Clin Endocrinol Metab 81, 2595–2600.

Roitt, I.M., Doniach, D., Campbell, P.N. and Hudson, R.V. (1956). Autoantibodies in Hashimoto's disease. Lancet 2, 820–821.

Rose, N.R. and Witebsky, E. (1956). Studies on organ specificity. V. Changes in the thyroid glands of rabbit following active immunization with rabbit thyroid extracts. J Immunol 76, 417–427.

Sakata, S., Nakamura, S. and Mirua, K. (1985). Autoantibodies against thyroid hormones or iodothyronine. Implications in diagnosis, thyroid function, treatment, and pathogenesis. Ann Intern Med 103, 579–589.

Saravanan, P. and Dayan, C.M. (2001). Thyroid autoantibodies. Endocrinol Metab Clin N Am 30, 315–337.

Schultz, E., Benker, G., Bethauser, H., Stempka, L. and Hufner, M. (1992). An auto-immunodominant thyroglobulin epitope characterized by a monoclonal antibody. J Endocrinol Invest 15, 25–30.

Sedmark, D.D., Hart, W.R. and Tubbs, R.R. (1987). Autoimmune oophoritis: a histopathologic study of involved ovaries with immunlogic characterization of the mononuclear cell infiltrate. Int J Gynecol Pathol 6, 73–81.

Shimojo, N., Saito, K., Kohno, Y., Sasaki, N., Tarutani, O. and Nakajima, H. (1988). Antigenic determinants on thyroglobulin: comparison of the reactivities of different thyroglobulin preparations with serum antibodies and T cells of patients with chronic thyroiditis. J Clin Endocrinol Metab 66, 689–695.

Singer, P.A. et al. (1995). Treatment guidelines for patients with hyperthyroidism and hypothyroidism. Standards of Care Committee, American Thyroid Association. JAMA 273, 808–812.

Sinha, A.A., Lopez, M.T. and McDevitt, H.O. (1990). Autoimmune diseases: the failure of self tolerance. Science 248, 1380–1388.

Stafford, E.A. and Rose, N.R. (2000). Newer insights into the pathogenesis of experimental autoimmune thyroiditis. Int Rev Immunol 19, 501–533.

Stassi, G. and De Maria, R. (2002). Autoimmune thyroid disease: new models of cell death in autoimmunity. Nat Rev Immunol 2, 195–204.

Swana, G.T., Swana, M.R., Bottazzo, G.F. and Doniach, D. (1977). A human-specific mitochondrial antibody – its importance in the identification of organ-specific reactions. Clin Exp Immunol 28, 517–525.

Swillens, S., Ludgate, M., Merken, L., Dumont, J.E. and Vassart, G. (1986). Analysis of sequence and structure homologies between thyroglobulin and acetylcholinesterase: possible functional and clinical significance. Biochem Biophys Res Commun 137, 142–148.

Tandon, N., Yan, S.L., Morgan, B.P. and Weetman, A.P. (1994). Expression and function of multiple regulators of complement activation in autoimmune thyroid disease. Immunology 81, 643–647.

Tandon, N., Morgan, B.P. and Weetman, A.P. (1992). Expression and function of membrane attack inhibitory proteins on thyroid follicular cells. Immunology 75, 643–647.

Tang, V.W. and Faiman, C. (1983). Premature ovarian failure: a search for circulating factors against gonadotropin receptors. Am J Obstet Gynecol 146, 816–821.

Ten, S., New, M. and Maclaren, N. (2001). Clinical review 130: Addison's disease 2001. J Clin Endocrinol Metab 86, 2909–2922.

Tonacchera, M., Cetani, F., Costagliola, S. et al. (1995). Mapping thyroid peroxidase epitopes using recombinant protein fragments. Eur J Endocrinol 132, 53–61.

Vali, M., Rose, N. and Caturegli, P. (2000). Thyroglobulin as autoantigen: Structure-function relationships. Rev Endocrine Metab Disord 1, 69–77.

Vallotton, M.B. and Forbes, A.P. (1966). Antibodies to cytoplasm of ova. Lancet 2, 264–265.

Vanderpump, M.P.J., Tunbridge, W.M.G., French, J.M. et al. (1995). The incidence of thyroid disorders in the community: a twenty-year follow-up of the Whickham Survey. Clin Endocrinol 43, 55–68.

Van Weissenbruch, M.M., Hoek, A., van Vlietbleeker, I., Schoemaker, J. and Drexhage, H. (1991). Evidence for existence of immunoglobulins that block ovarian granulose cell growth in vitro. A putative role in resistant ovary syndrome. J Clin Endocrinol Metab 73, 360–367.

Volpe, R. (1994). Autoimmune endocrinopathies: aspects of pathogenesis and the role of immune assays in investigation and management. Clin Chem 40, 2132–2145.

Weetman, A.P. (1994). Autoimmune thyroid disease: further developments in our understanding. Endocrinol Rev 15, 788–830.

Weetman, A.P. (2000). Graves' disease. N Engl J Med 343, 1236–1248.

Weetman, A.P. and McGregor, A.M. (1984). Autoimmune thyroid disease: developments in our understanding. Endocrinol Rev 5, 309–355.

Weetman, A.P., Tandon, N. and Morgan, B.P. (1992). Antithyroid drugs and release of inflammatory mediators by complement-attacked thyroid cells. Lancet 340, 633–636.

Weetman, A.P., McIntosh, R.S. and Watson, P.F. (1998). Autoimmune hypothyroidism. In Endocrine Autoimmunity and Associated Conditions, Weetman, A.P., ed. Dordrecht, Netherlands: Kluwer Academic Publishers, pp. 39–61.

Wheatcroft, N.J., Toogood, A.A., Li, T.C. et al. (1994). Detection of antibodies to ovarian antigens in women with premature ovarian failure. Clin Exp Immunol 96, 122–128.

Wheatcroft, N.J., Salt, C., Milfor-Ward, A. et al. (1997). Identification of ovarian antibodies by immunofluorescence, enzyme-linked immunosorbent assay or immunoblotting in premature ovarian failure. Hum Reprod 12, 2617–2622.

Winqvist, O., Karlsson, F.A. and Kampe, O. (1992). 21-Hydroxylase, a major autoantigen in idiopathic Addison's disease. Lancet 339, 1559–1562.

Winqvist, O., Gustafsson, J., Rorsman, F. et al. (1993). Two different cytochrome P450 enzymes are the adrenal antigens in autoimmune polyendocrine syndrome type1 and Addison's disease. J Clin Invest 92, 2377–2385.

Witebsky, E. and Rose, N.R. (1956). Studies on organ specificity. IV, Production of rabbit thyroid antibodies in the rabbit. J Immunol 76, 408–416.

Witebsky, E., Rose, N.R., Terplan, K., Paine, J.R. and Egan, R.W. (1957). Chronic thyroiditis and autoimmunization. J Am Med Assoc 164, 1439–1447.

Wolfe, C.D.A. and Stirling, R.W. (1988). Premature menopause associated with autoimmune oophoritis. Case report. Br J Obstet Gynaecol 95, 630–632.

Wortsman, J., McConnachie, P., Baker, J.R.J. and Mallette, L.E. (1992). T-lymphocyte activation in adult-onset idiopathic hypoparathyroidism. Am J Med 92, 352–356.

Zakarija, M. and McKenzie, J.M. (1987). The spectrum and significance of autoantibodies reacting with the thyrotropin receptor. Endocrinol Metab Clin N Am 16, 343–363.

Zeki, K., Fujihira, T., Shirakawa, F., Wantanbe, K. and Eto, S. (1987). Existence and immunological significance of circulating Ia+ T cells in autoimmune thyroid diseases. Acta Endocrinol 115, 282–288.

Autoimmunity – Vasculitis

Chapter 48

Jan Willem Cohen Tervaert and Jan Damoiseaux
*Department of Clinical and Experimental Immunology,
University Hospital Maastricht, Maastricht, The Netherlands*

Where there is peace the war man attacks himself.

Friedrich Nietzsche

INTRODUCTION

Vasculitis was recognized in the eighteenth and nineteenth centuries. An important publication was that by Rokitansky in 1852, who reported three cases of polyarteritis (Rokitansky, 1852). However, the best-described first case was a 27-year-old male who died of severe systemic vasculitis and in whom vessels throughout the body were transformed into thickened cords with the formation of nodes. This case, described by Kussmaul and Maier, highlighted very well the severe consequences of polyarteritis (Kussmaul and Maier, 1866). Since then, many different forms of vasculitis have been described, and it has become apparent that there are large regional differences in the types of vasculitis that occur. Furthermore, many different clinical syndromes have been described and many attempts made to classify patients into categories. In 1993, an international consensus group proposed a classification scheme and definitions for the various vasculitic syndromes (Jennette et al., 1994) (Table 48.1). These definitions were not intended to be used as diagnostic criteria. Nowadays, however, many physicians base their diagnoses on these Chapel Hill Consensus Conference definitions. Apart from the so-called primary vasculitides, many vasculitides arise secondary to other conditions. Underlying conditions are infections (such as hepatitis B, hepatitis C, human immunodeficiency virus), connective tissue diseases (such as rheumatoid arthritis, systemic lupus erythematosus, Sjogren syndrome), malignancies or hypersensitivity reactions.

The estimated prevalence of primary vasculitides varies from 2 to 5 per 10 000 people. The estimated prevalence of secondary forms of vasculitis is not known. The annual incidence of secondary forms of vasculitis is, however, 25 per cent of the annual incidence of primary vasculitis (Gonzalez-Gay and Garcia-Porrua, 2001).

Table 48.1 Primary vasculitides

Type of vessels (primarily) involved	Diseases
Large vessels	Giant cell arteritis Takayasu's arteritis
Medium-sized vessels	Polyarteritis nodosa Kawasaki disease
Small vessels 　ANCA-associated	Wegener's granulomatosis Churg-Strauss syndrome Microscopic polyangiitis
Not ANCA-associated	Henoch-Schönlein purpura Essential cryoglobulinemic 　vasculitis Cutaneous leukocytoclastic 　angiitis

ANCA, anti-neutrophil cytoplasmic antibodies.

*Measuring Immunity, edited by Michael T. Lotze and Angus W. Thomson
ISBN 0-12-455900-X, London*

The most important primary vasculitides are:

Giant cell arteritis or temporal arteritis. A common form of vasculitis, particularly in the Caucasian population, in which vessel walls are invaded by macrophages, lymphocytes, plasma cells and giant cells. Clinically, the disease frequently presents with headache, tenderness of the scalp, especially around the temporal arteries and claudication of the jaws and/or tongue. In addition, symptoms related to ischemia, such as loss of vision, may be present. Moreover, about half of the patients have pain and stiffness of the proximal extremities (polymyalgia rheumatica). The disease generally occurs at an older age, i.e. over 50 years, with an annual incidence of 100–250/million persons over 50 years of age.

Takayasu arteritis. This form of vasculitis affects the aorta, its brachiocephalic branches, visceral arteries, arteries of the lower extremities and pulmonary arteries. Lesions are characterized by lymphoplasmacytic infiltrates with eosinophils, histiocytes and Langhans' giant cells. Clinically, most patients have non-specific systemic symptoms such as fatigue, weight loss and fever. Later symptoms are related to the obstruction of the involved vessels and include claudication of upper and lower extremities, cervical symptoms, ischemic bowel disease, renovascular hypertension and many others. The disease occurs at a younger age, particularly in women between 15 and 45 years of age. It is more frequent in Asians, Africans and Latin Americans, and is rare in Caucasians (annual incidence varies between countries from 0.2 to 20/million).

Polyarteritis nodosa. This form of vasculitis is confined to medium-sized arteries without involvement of smaller vessels. Histopathologically, the disease is characterized by fibrinoid necrosis of the vessel wall frequently accompanied by microaneurysm formation. Clinically, systemic symptoms include fever, fatigue, weight loss, arthralgias and myalgias. Furthermore, renovascular hypertension, ischemic bowel disease, neuropathy and nodular skin lesions are often present. The disease is nowadays rare with an estimated annual incidence rate of 2–9/million. Higher incidences, however, are being reported in areas where hepatitis B is still endemic, such as Alaska.

Kawasaki syndrome. This form of vasculitis particularly affects children. Histopathologically, panarteritis with thrombosis of coronary arteries can often be found. Also in this form of vasculitis, aneurysm formation frequently occurs. Clinically, the disease presents with fever, exanthema, reddening of the lips, oral cavity, palms and soles, bilateral congestion of ocular conjunctivae and cervical lymphadenopathy. The annual incidence in Western countries is 30–150 cases/million children less than 5 years of age, whereas in Japan the annual incidence is 1000–2000/million children younger than 5 years of age.

ANCA associated vasculitis. Within the spectrum of small-vessel vasculitides, Wegener's granulomatosis (WG), microscopic polyangiitis (MPA) and the Churg-Strauss syndrome (CSS) are strongly associated with the presence of anti-neutrophil cytoplasmic antibodies (ANCA). WG is characterized by the triad of chronic destructive inflammation of the respiratory tract, systemic vasculitis and glomerulonephritis. Histopathologically, focal granulomatous lesions and necrotizing vasculitis with fibrinoid necrosis may be found. The disease generally follows a biphasic course. Initially, symptoms of the upper respiratory tract occur such as rhinitis, bloody nasal discharge, sinusitis and otitis. Systemic symptoms such as malaise, arthralgias and myalgias are also frequently present initially. Later on, systemic vasculitis with rapidly progressive glomerulonephritis develops in many patients. Other organs such as the lungs, the eyes, the skin and the peripheral nervous system are frequently involved as well.

In contrast to WG, MPA is a form of systemic vasculitis and glomerulonephritis without granulomatous inflammation and/or destructive lesions in the respiratory tract. Most frequently affected organs are the lungs, the kidneys, the eyes, the skin and the peripheral nervous system.

The CSS is a form of systemic vasculitis in which patients also have asthma, nasal polyps and hypereosinophilia. Histopathologically, many eosinophils are found in the biopsies which may also contain granulomas and signs of vasculitis. Clinical manifestations of vasculitis include mononeuritis multiplex, ischemic bowel disease and purpura or nodules of the skin. Cardiomyopathy also occurs frequently in this form of vasculitis.

The annual incidence of the three ANCA-associated vasculitides is 10–30/million. Roughly, about 60 per cent of the cases with ANCA associated vasculitis have WG, 30 per cent MPA and 10 per cent the CSS.

Other forms of small vessel vasculitis. These forms include Henoch Schönlein purpura, essential cryoglobulinemic vasculitis and cutaneous leukocytoclastic angiitis. Henoch Schönlein purpura is a form of vasculitis that predominantly occurs in children. It is clinically characterized by attacks of purpura, arthralgias/arthritis, gastrointestinal symptoms and glomerulonephritis. Histopathologically, the vasculitic lesions are characterized by deposits of IgA in the vessel wall. The annual incidence in children ranges between 135 and 180/million and in adults between 3 and 15/million.

Essential mixed cryoglobulinemia is a form of vasculitis that is in most cases secondary to hepatitis C virus infection. Idiopathic cases, however, also occur in which cryoglobulins consist of polyclonal IgG and monoclonal (type II) or polyclonal (type III) IgM with rheumatoid factor activity. IgG and IgM deposits are detectable in the lesions. Clinically, purpura, arthralgias and neuropathy are most prominent. Glomerulonephritis also occurs frequently. The annual incidence is 1–5/million.

Cutaneous leukocytoclastic angiitis is a form of primary vasculitis that is confined to the skin. This form is rare since most patients with skin vasculitis appear to have either one of the other forms of primary vasculitis or one of the secondary forms of vasculitis.

AUTOIMMUNITY AND VASCULITIS

There is circumstantial evidence of the autoimmune nature of systemic vasculitides: immunosuppressive treatment is, generally, effective and, more importantly, autoimmune phenomena occur and are involved in disease pathophysiology (Kallenberg and Cohen Tervaert, 2002). T cells infiltrating the vessel walls have been observed in different forms of vasculitis. These T cells are especially well studied in giant cell arteritis. In this form of vasculitis they are clonally expanded. Sequencing showed a diversity of TCR Vβ chain sequences. The antigen that is recognized is not well characterized, but may be a modified antigen in the temporal artery. Both anti-endothelial cell antibodies (AECA) and ANCA have been described in patients with different forms of systemic vasculitis. AECA are a group of autoantibodies directed against a variety of ill-defined endothelial antigens. In most cases AECA react not only with endothelial cells but also with other cells such as peripheral blood mononuclear cells and/or fibroblasts. The antigens from the endothelial cells may be constitutively expressed or cryptic (Belizna and Cohen Tervaert, 1997). Furthermore, antigenic determinants for AECA may be molecules that adhere to endothelial cells. Examples of these latter are DNA, β_2-glycoprotein I (β_2 GPI), proteinase 3 (PR-3) and/or myeloperoxidase (MPO). AECA binding to endothelial cells may result in activation of endothelial cells. Also, AECAs may induce apoptosis of endothelial cells. Alternative mechanisms by which AECA could trigger endothelial cell damage are by complement dependent cytotoxicity (CDC) and/or antibody dependent cell cytotoxicity (ADCC). AECAs may be present in all forms of vasculitis. Frequencies range between 33 and 100 per cent. Results vary between the different forms of vasculitides that are being studied and the techniques used to detect AECA (Belizna and Cohen Tervaert, 1997). AECA are, however, not specific for vasculitis and can also be found in many other inflammatory disorders such as systemic lupus erythematosus.

ANCA, particularly those reacting with PR-3 and MPO, are sensitive and specific for WG, MPA and the CSS.

Furthermore, it has been demonstrated in an experimental model that these antibodies induce vasculitis and glomerulonephritis. Therefore, these antibodies will be discussed in greater detail.

ANTINEUTROPHIL CYTOPLASMIC ANTIBODIES (ANCA)

In patients with vasculitis and/or glomerulonephritis, ANCA were first described in 1982 (Davies et al., 1982). The link between ANCA and active WG became apparent in 1985 (van der Woude et al., 1985). The antibodies that are found in patients with WG produce a cytoplasmic fluorescence pattern with accentuation of the area within the nuclear lobes when tested by indirect immunofluorescence (IIF) on ethanol fixed neutrophils (Figure 48.1). These antibodies were later designated as c-ANCA. Goldschmeding et al. (1989) demonstrated that the target antigen of c-ANCA was a 29 kDa serine protease contained within the azurophilic or α-granules of neutrophils that was different from elastase and cathepsin G, the other serine proteases in these granules. It was later confirmed that this 29 kDa serine protease was identical to PR-3. PR-3 is present both in monocytes and granulocytes and appears early in mono-myeloid differentiation. The presence of PR-3 in other cells such as endothelial cells is still controversial (Cohen Tervaert, 2000). On endothelial cells a specific receptor for PR-3 is present and as such PR-3 may be bound to endothelial cells and targeted by autoantibodies to PR-3 (Taekema-Roelvink et al., 2000). PR-3 is a slightly cationic serine protease with proteolytic activity, which is inhibited by α-1-antitrypsin. PR-3 is expressed on the surface of resting neutrophils in most individuals in a low percentage and is present on apoptotic neutrophils. Furthermore, after neutrophil activation with pro-inflammatory cytokines such as TNF-α, IL-1 or IL-8, membrane expression of PR-3 is increased. Binding of PR-3 to neutrophils may be due to charge interaction, via the serine protease inhibitor enzyme complex (SEC) receptor on neutrophils or via β_2-integrins (Muller Kobold et al., 1999).

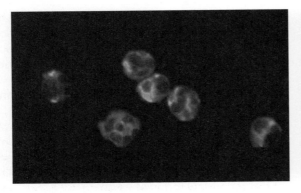 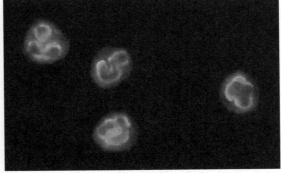

Figure 48.1 Distinct ANCA patterns by indirect immunofluorescence revealing c-ANCA (left) and p-ANCA (right).

Following the description of c-ANCA as a marker for WG, several groups observed that sera from a number of patients suspected of suffering from vasculitis produced a perinuclear fluorescence pattern on ethanol-fixed neutrophils (see Figure 48.1). In these patients, myeloperoxidase (MPO) appeared to be the most important antigen. MPO (EC 1.11.1.7) is a highly cationic protein present in neutrophils and monocytes with a molecular weight of 146 kDa. MPO plays a critical role in the generation of reactive oxygen species by catalyzing the formation of bleach (hypochlorous acid; HOCl) out of chloride ions and hydrogen peroxide (H_2O_2). In serum, ceruloplasmin is the natural inhibitor. Resting neutrophils do not have surface expression of MPO, but after priming of neutrophils with low concentrations of pro-inflammatory cytokines surface expression of MPO can be detected.

ANCA testing

Detection of ANCA is classically done by IIF on ethanol fixed neutrophils. Two patterns can be recognized: either a cytoplasmic (c-ANCA) pattern or a perinuclear (p-ANCA) pattern. In patients with vasculitis and/or glomerulonephritis the c-ANCA pattern is related to autoantibodies against PR-3, whereas the p-ANCA pattern is related to MPO. The p-ANCA pattern of MPO is an artifact of ethanol fixation. When neutrophils are fixed with a cross-linking fixative, such as paraformaldehyde, MPO-ANCA positive sera produce a cytoplasmic staining pattern. Since MPO is a highly cationic protein (PI 11.0), it moves during ethanol fixation to the negatively charged nuclear membrane, causing the perinuclear pattern. The c-ANCA pattern is not always identical with autoantibodies to PR-3 and the p-ANCA pattern not with antibodies to MPO. Other autoantibodies that may cause a perinuclear or cytoplasmic staining pattern are antibodies to lactoferrin, elastase and many others. These latter autoantibodies, however, are not specifically found in patients with vasculitis and/or glomerulonephritis, but in patients with other inflammatory disorders. Thus, the detection of ANCA as a sensitive and/or specific test for vasculitis and/or glomerulonephritis requires antigen specific assays. These assays use either purified or recombinant PR-3 and/or MPO in a directly coated system ('direct ELISA'), or PR-3 or MPO specific monoclonal antibodies to capture the antigen from an extract of neutrophil granules, and/or purified PR-3 or MPO ('capture ELISA'). Capture ELISA has the advantage of having the antigen presented in its native configuration, which is important because the autoantibodies react primarily with conformational epitopes. As shown in several collaborative European studies, standardization of the assays is of the utmost importance (Hagen et al., 1996). Recently, it was found for PR-3 ANCA, that within different laboratories, the capture ELISA produced the best comparable results (Csernok et al., 2004).

ANCA as diagnostic markers

Several groups have investigated the sensitivity and specificity of ANCA for small vessel vasculitides. A meta-analysis revealed that a testing system combining the IIF technique with antigen specific ELISAs yields a pooled sensitivity of 88.5 per cent and a pooled specificity of 98.6 per cent of p-ANCA/MPO-ANCA and c-ANCA/PR-3 ANCA for small vessel vasculitides (Choi et al., 2001). However, the sensitivity and specificity of PR-3 ANCA and/or MPO-ANCA may vary with the disease condition studied. For WG, the presence of the classical c-ANCA pattern at any time during the disease has a pooled sensitivity of 66 per cent, which increases to 91 per cent during active disease with a specificity of 99 per cent (Rao et al., 1995). Whereas ANCA as detected by IIF is found frequently in other inflammatory diseases, PR-3 ANCA and MPO-ANCA are only rarely detected in other conditions than small vessel vasculitides (Merkel et al., 1997). MPO-ANCA is, however, also found in patients with drug-induced vasculitis and in 30–50 per cent of patients with anti-GBM disease. Furthermore, false positive MPO-ANCA may be found occasionally in patients with systemic lupus erythematosus or rheumatoid arthritis and in other inflammatory disorders such as autoimmune liver disease and inflammatory bowel disease (Boomsma et al., 2001). These latter false positive results, however, can be avoided by using a capture ELISA to detect MPO-ANCA. Therefore, it is our current policy to confirm all positive MPO-ANCA results, obtained in a direct ELISA, by performing a capture ELISA. For PR-3 ANCA, the capture ELISA system does not seem to differ much from a direct ELISA system with respect to specificity but the capture ELISA seems to be more sensitive (Csernok et al., 2004). Even though the presence of PR3-ANCA/MPO-ANCA is highly specific for WG, MPA and/or CSS, a positive ANCA result should always be interpreted with consideration of the clinical setting since the presence of specific clinical features plays a major role in determining the diagnostic probability of vasculitis (Choi et al., 2001).

Prognostic value of ANCA during follow up

ANCA-associated vasculitis has a 1-year survival of at least 80–90 per cent. Treatment consists generally of a combination of prednisolone and cyclophosphamide. During the last decade, attempts have been made to replace cyclophosphamide with other immunosuppressive drugs (Cohen Tervaert et al., 2001; Jayne et al., 2003; Langford, 2003). Since all drugs that are used produce toxic side effects, medications are generally tapered and eventually eliminated in most cases. However, during follow up, up to 80 per cent of the patients in remission experience relapses. Patients with WG relapse more frequently than patients with MPA. In addition, patients with PR-3 ANCA have more frequent relapses than patients with MPO-ANCA. This is also true when patients are subdivided into groups according to their diagnosis. So, patients with either WG or MPA who are PR-3 ANCA positive have a higher relapse rate than patients with MPO-ANCA associated with the respective disease type. Thus, ANCA testing is not only a highly sensitive and specific test for making a diagnosis of WG, MPA or CSS, but ANCA specificity (either PR-3 ANCA or MPO-ANCA) has also a prognostic value with respect to the development of relapses during follow up.

Next to the difference in relapse rates between PR-3 and MPO-ANCA positive patients, differences in both patient and renal survival have been described for the ANCA subtypes. Patients with PR-3 ANCA may be at higher risk of death as was found by the Chapel Hill group (Hogan et al., 1996), but not by others (Geffriaud-Ricouard et al., 1993, Franssen et al., 1995) and patients with MPO-ANCA may be at higher risk for renal failure as was recently reported by Vizjak (Vizjak et al., 2003), but not by others (Falk et al., 1990a; Geffriaud-Ricouard et al., 1993; Franssen et al., 1995). Differences between the various studies could be explained by local differences in therapy and follow up of these patients. Furthermore, relapses in PR-3 positive patients are much more fulminant than relapses in MPO-ANCA positive patients. Indeed, the causes of progression of renal failure differ between PR-3 and MPO-ANCA positive patients. In patients with PR-3 ANCA, renal function is stable during remission, but declines with every relapse (Slot et al., 2003). In patients with MPO-ANCA, a slowly progressive course is often observed with patients developing dialysis dependency during follow up without signs of clinically active disease. In these patients, proteinuria is the most important risk factor for renal failure during follow up (Franssen et al., 1998). In addition to ANCA specificity, ANCA levels at diagnosis and during follow up have been shown to be predictive for patients' renal and disease-free survival. A high PR-3 ANCA level in capture ELISA at diagnosis is a risk factor for poor patient and renal survival (Westman et al., 2003) and a constantly elevated MPO-ANCA level is a risk factor for poor renal survival (Franssen et al., 1998). During induction therapy with cyclophosphamide and prednisolone, ANCA levels fall and become negative in many patients within the first few months. Persistent or recurring c-ANCA during the first year is significantly related to subsequent relapse (Stegeman et al., 1994). This is even more pronounced when induction therapy is switched from cyclophosphamide to azathioprine. We recently found that a positive c-ANCA titer at the moment of switch is strongly associated with risk for relapse during follow up, with a disease-free survival of 17 per cent at 5 years in patients who were positive for c-ANCA when switched to azathioprine (Slot et al., 2004) compared to a disease-free survival of 41 per cent at 5 years when patients were ANCA negative at the moment of switch. More than 80 per cent of the patients who were ANCA positive at diagnosis and who experience a relapse, are testing positive for ANCA at the time of relapse. So, patients persistently negative for ANCA have a very low risk of development of a relapse, although relapses localized to the respiratory tract can occur in these patients.

Prediction of disease activity by serial measurement of ANCA levels

The usefulness of serially measuring ANCA titers in predicting disease activity and in guiding therapy is at present still controversial. Rising titers of PR-3 ANCA occurring during clinical remission often predict relapses in patients with WG (Boomsma et al., 2000; Cohen Tervaert, 2003). This is also probably true for MPO-ANCA in patients with ANCA-associated vasculitis (Cohen Tervaert, 2003), but large prospective studies with respect to MPO-ANCA are lacking.

Many studies have been published in which the relation between rises in ANCA levels as measured by IIF or by ELISA and disease activity of ANCA associated vasculitis was studied (Tables 48.2 and 48.3). Some studies clearly show an association between rise in ANCA titer and renewed disease activity, but in other studies this is not so clear. When comparing the IIF techniques, the direct ELISA technique and the capture ELISA technique for the prediction of relapses, it is found that the capture ELISA technique is somewhat more accurate in predicting relapses than the other techniques (Boomsma et al., 2003a) (Table 48.4). The best way to monitor PR-3 ANCA, however, is probably when a combination of two methods is used. In the study by Boomsma et al., the best combination was direct ELISA together with capture ELISA (Boomsma et al., 2003a). Nonetheless, two studies show

Table 48.2 Relation between rises in ANCA as determined by IIF and relapse of ANCA-related small-vessel vasculitis as reported by different studies

Number of patients	ANCA pattern on IIF	ANCA rise prior or at moment of relapse (%)	ANCA rise followed by relapse (%)	Reference
35	c-ANCA	100	77	Cohen Tervaert et al., 1989
10	c-ANCA	100	75	Egner and Chapel, 1990
58	c-ANCA	90	82	Cohen Tervaert et al., 1990
10	NR	82	65	Chan et al., 1993
68	c-ANCA	24	56	Kerr et al., 1993
37	c-/p-ANCA	43	23	Davenport et al., 1995
19	c-ANCA	NR	57	Kyndt et al., 1999
85	c-ANCA	52	57	Boomsma et al., 2000
18	c-/p-ANCA	37	NR	Nowack et al., 2001

NR = Not reported.

Table 48.3 Relation between rises in ANCA as measured by ELISA and relapse of ANCA-related small-vessel vasculitis as reported by different studies

Number of patients	ANCA antigenic specificity	ANCA rise prior or at moment of relapse (%)	ANCA rise followed by relapse (%)	Reference
56	Extract	41	62	De'Oliviera et al., 1995
60	NR	74	79	Jayne et al., 1995
17	PR3	33	59	Kyndt et al., 1999
19	MPO	73	79	Kyndt et al., 1999
25	MPO	100	80	Ara et al., 1999
85	PR3	81	71	Boomsma et al., 2000
15	MPO	75	100	Boomsma et al., 2000
14	PR3 (capture)	43	NR	Nowack et al., 2001
18	MPO/PR3 (direct)	32	NR	Nowack et al., 2001
10	PR3 (direct)	79	92	Gisslen et al., 2002
10	PR3 (capture)	100	83	Gisslen et al., 2002
48	MPO/PR3 (direct/ capture)	61	100	Han et al., 2003
100	PR3 (direct)	74	60	Boomsma et al., 2003b

NR = Not reported

Table 48.4 Rises in ANCA in relation to the occurrence of relapses in 16 patients with Wegener's granulomatosis with a relapse and 16 patients with Wegener's granulomatosis without a relapse (Boomsma et al., 2003a)

Detection system	Rises in ANCA	Relapse/rise in ANCA (%)	No relapse/no rise in ANCA (%)
Image analysis	16	11/16 (69)	11/16 (69)
IIF	18	11/18 (56)	9/14 (64)
Direct ELISA	17	12/17 (71)	11/15 (73)
Capture ELISA	16	12/16 (75)	12/16 (75)
Direct plus capture ELISA	20	15/20 (75)	11/12 (92)

ANCA = antineutrophil cytoplasmic antibodies; ELISA = enzyme-linked immunosorbent assay; IIF = indirect immunofluorescence.

that when a rise in ANCA titer of fourfold or greater is found in a patient, pre-emptive treatment reduces the risk of relapses and may lead to a reduced exposure to immunosuppressive drugs (Cohen Tervaert et al., 1990; Han et al., 2003). Furthermore, we recently performed a large prospective study in which 100 PR-3 ANCA positive patients were followed during a period of 3 years. Once an ANCA rise of 75 per cent or more, as measured by ELISA, occurred, patients were randomized to receive pre-emptive therapy (9 months' course of azathioprine

and a 4½ month course of prednisolone) or no treatment. Also in this study, pre-emptive therapy clearly reduced the risk to relapse. However, during follow up, when azathioprine was tapered and/or stopped, ANCA titers rose again and relapses occurred. Therefore, in this study relapses were only postponed by pre-emptive therapy (Boomsma et al., 2003b). Altogether the predictive value of measuring ANCA levels in individual patients is not yet completely clear. As it stands now, treatment based on ANCA levels alone is not yet recommended, but significant increases should prompt the clinician to monitor more closely the condition of the patient.

Pathogenic potential of ANCA

ANCA are capable of activating the cells that are the source of the ANCA antigens (i.e. neutrophils and monocytes). In addition, ANCA may stimulate endothelial cells. For these latter cells, it is not yet clear whether they themselves could be the source of the ANCA antigens or that ANCA antigens bind via a specific receptor to these cells (see above). The best studied *in vitro* effects of ANCA are the induction of the respiratory burst and the extracellular release of lysosomal enzymes by neutrophils. Falk et al. demonstrated that neutrophils have to be primed before they can be activated by ANCA (Falk et al., 1990b). Priming is a process of pre-activation that can be accomplished *in vitro* with low doses of pro-inflammatory cytokines, such as TNF-α, IL-1 or IL-8. This priming results in increased surface expression of the target antigens of ANCA. In this way, the antigens are available for interaction with the antibodies. Moreover, co-incubation of ANCA activated neutrophils with endothelial cells results in endothelial cell lysis, suggesting that these effector pathways are responsible for the vessel injury observed in patients (Savage et al., 1992; Ewert et al., 1992). Activation of neutrophils generally occurs via the simultaneous engagement of the ANCA antigens and Fc receptors by ANCA. Furthermore, the activation is β_2-integrin dependent. Investigations into the signal transduction pathways have demonstrated the involvement of P38 mitogen activated protein kinases (MAPK), extracellular signal-regulated kinases (ERK), as well as phosphatidyl inositol 3 (PI$_3$) kinase signaling systems (Kettritz et al., 2001, 2002; Ben-Smith et al., 2001).

In vivo most work has been done with respect to MPO-ANCA vasculitis. MPO-ANCA can be found in various vasculitis models where polyclonal B cell activation is present such as in mercury chloride-treated rats and autoimmune prone mouse strains such as MRL-lpr and SCG-Kj mice. In addition, active immunization of rats with human MPO induces antibodies to human MPO that cross-react with rat MPO. In most rat strains, however, this does not result in vasculitis and/or glomerulonephritis. Subsequent renal perfusion or systemic administration of human neutrophil lysosomal extracts, however, induces crescentic glomerulonephritis or pulmonary and intestinal vasculitis, respectively (Brouwer et al., 1993; Heeringa et al., 1997). Furthermore, Smyth et al. recently found that Wistar Kyoto (WKY) rats, 8 weeks after immunization with human MPO, develop alveolar lung hemorrhage and a mild glomerulonephritis without crescent formation (Smyth et al., 2002). Moreover, recently Xiao et al. (2002) provided firm evidence that MPO-ANCA alone induce pauci-immune glomerulonephritis and vasculitis in mice. In these studies, MPO deficient mice were immunized with mouse MPO and circulating anti-murine MPO antibodies developed. Adoptive transfer, either of splenocytes or purified IgG derived from the MPO-immunized MPO-deficient mice, resulted in the development of crescentic glomerulonephritis and systemic vasculitis mimicking the human disease (Xiao et al., 2002). These studies provided direct evidence that MPO-ANCA are indeed pathogenic. Recently, similar experiments were performed by immunizing PR-3/elastase deficient mice with recombinant murine PR-3. Antibodies developed in these mice that recognized both recombinant and native murine PR-3. By transferring mouse PR-3 ANCA antiserum to wild type mice, it was demonstrated that PR-3 ANCA were able to exacerbate a local TNF-α induced subcutaneous panniculitis (Pfister et al., 2003), although mouse PR-3 ANCA did not induce nephritis and/or vasculitis. Thus, PR-3 ANCA also contribute to tissue damage by enhancing inflammatory responses. Further studies, however, are needed to confirm the pathogenic potential of PR-3 ANCA.

CONCLUSION

Primary vasculitides are probably autoimmune diseases. Proof of the autoimmune nature, however, for most forms is lacking. The best-studied vasculitides are ANCA-associated vasculitides in which predominantly small vessels are affected. It has been shown that both PR-3 ANCA and MPO-ANCA as tested by ELISA, but not ANCA detected only by IIF, are important diagnostic markers for these forms of vasculitis. Changes in levels of PR-3 ANCA and possibly also MPO-ANCA, are related to changes in disease activity although this correlation is far from absolute. In *in vitro* studies, it has been clearly demonstrated that these antibodies interact with myeloid cells resulting in the activation of these cells enhancing their destructive activity towards endothelial cells. *In vivo* experimental models have demonstrated that MPO-ANCA induces glomerulonephritis and vasculitis. The pathogenic potential of PR-3 ANCA as tested in animal models is not yet completely clear, but also there is the suggestion that the PR-3 ANCA enhance inflammatory responses.

REFERENCES

Ara, J., Mirapeix, E., Rodriguez, R., Saurina, A. and Darnell, A. (1999). Relationship between ANCA and disease activity in small vessel vasculitis patients with anti-MPO ANCA. Nephrol Dial Transplant 14, 1667–1672.

Belizna, C. and Cohen Tervaert, J.W. (1997). Specificity, pathogenecity, and clinical value of antiendothelial cell antibodies. Semin Arthritis Rheum 27, 98–109.

Ben-Smith, A., Dove, S.K., Martin, A., Wakelam, M.J. and Savage, C.O. (2001). Antineutrophil cytoplasm autoantibodies from patients with systemic vasculitis activate neutrophils through distinct signaling cascades: comparison with conventional Fcgamma receptor ligation. Blood 98, 1448–1455.

Boomsma, M.M., Damoiseaux, J.G., Stegeman, C.A. et al. (2003a). Image analysis: a novel approach for the quantification of antineutrophil cytoplasmic antibody level in patients with Wegener's granulomatosis. J Immunol Methods 274, 27–35.

Boomsma, M.M., Stegeman, C.A., Hermans, J. et al. (2003b). Prevention of relapses in PR3 anti-neutrophil antibody (ANCA) associated vasculitis by treatment with azathioprine and corticosteroids: a multi-centre, randomized study (abstract). Kidney and Blood Press Res 26, 276.

Boomsma, M.M., Stegeman, C.A., Oost-Kort, W.W. et al. (2001). Native and recombinant proteins to analyze auto-antibodies to myeloperoxidase in pauci-immune crescentic glomerulonephritis. J Immunol Methods 254, 47–58.

Boomsma, M.M., Stegeman, C.A., van der Leij, M.J. et al. (2000). Prediction of relapses in Wegener's granulomatosis by measurement of antineutrophil cytoplasmic antibody levels: a prospective study. Arthritis Rheum 43, 2025–2033.

Brouwer, E., Huitema, M.G., Klok, P.A. et al. (1993). Antimyeloperoxidase-associated proliferative glomerulonephritis: an animal model. J Exp Med 177, 905–914.

Chan, T.M., Frampton, G., Jayne, D.R., Perry, G.J., Lockwood, C.M. and Cameron, J.S. (1993). Clinical significance of anti-endothelial cell antibodies in systemic vasculitis: a longitudinal study comparing anti-endothelial cell antibodies and anti-neutrophil cytoplasm antibodies. Am J Kidney Dis 22, 387–392.

Choi, H.K., Liu, S., Merkel, P.A., Colditz, G.A. and Niles, J.L. (2001). Diagnostic performance of antineutrophil cytoplasmic antibody tests for idiopathic vasculitides: metaanalysis with a focus on antimyeloperoxidase antibodies. J Rheumatol 28, 1584–1590.

Cohen Tervaert, J.W. (2000). Proteinase 3: A cofactor for the binding of antineutrophil cytoplasm antibodies (ANCA) to endothelial cells? Kidney Int 57, 2171–2172.

Cohen Tervaert, J.W. (2003). ANCA testing in monitoring the activity of the disease. Kidney Blood Press Res 26, 226–230.

Cohen Tervaert, J.W., Huitema, M.G., Hene, R.J. et al. (1990). Prevention of relapses in Wegener's granulomatosis by treatment based on antineutrophil cytoplasmic antibody titre. Lancet 336, 709–711.

Cohen Tervaert, J.W., Stegeman, C.A. and Kallenberg, C.G. (2001). Novel therapies for anti-neutrophil cytoplasmic antibody-associated vasculitis. Curr Opin Nephrol Hypertens 10, 211–217.

Cohen Tervaert, J.W., van der Woude, F.J., Fauci, A.S. et al. (1989). Association between active Wegener's granulomatosis and anticytoplasmic antibodies. Arch Intern Med 149, 2461–2465.

Csernok, E., Holle, J., Hellmich, B. et al. (2004). Evaluation of capture ELISA for detection of antineutrophil cytoplasmic antibodies directed against proteinase 3 in Wegener's granulomatosis: first results from a multicentre study. Rheumatology (Oxford) 43, 174–180.

Davenport, A., Lock, R.J. and Wallington, T. (1995). Clinical significance of the serial measurement of autoantibodies to neutrophil cytoplasm using a standard indirect immunofluorescence test. Am J Nephrol 15, 201–207.

Davies, D.J., Moran, J.E., Niall, J.F. and Ryan, G.B. (1982). Segmental necrotising glomerulonephritis with antineutrophil antibody: possible arbovirus aetiology? Br Med J (Clin Res Ed) 285, 606.

De'Oliviera, J., Gaskin, G., Dash, A., Rees, A.J. and Pusey, C.D. (1995). Relationship between disease activity and anti-neutrophil cytoplasmic antibody concentration in long-term management of systemic vasculitis. Am J Kidney Dis 25, 380–389.

Egner, W. and Chapel, H.M. (1990). Titration of antibodies against neutrophil cytoplasmic antigens is useful in monitoring disease activity in systemic vasculitides. Clin Exp Immunol 82, 244–249.

Ewert, B.H., Jennette, J.C. and Falk, R.J. (1992). Anti-myeloperoxidase antibodies stimulate neutrophils to damage human endothelial cells. Kidney Int 41, 375–383.

Falk, R.J., Hogan, S., Carey, T.S. and Jennette, J.C. (1990a). Clinical course of anti-neutrophil cytoplasmic autoantibody-associated glomerulonephritis and systemic vasculitis. The Glomerular Disease Collaborative Network (see comments). Ann Intern Med 113, 656–663.

Falk, R.J., Terrell, R.S., Charles, L.A. and Jennette, J.C. (1990b). Anti-neutrophil cytoplasmic autoantibodies induce neutrophils to degranulate and produce oxygen radicals in vitro. Proc Natl Acad Sci USA 87, 4115–4119.

Franssen, C.F.M., Gans, R.O., Arends, B. et al. (1995). Differences between anti-myeloperoxidase- and anti-proteinase 3-associated renal disease. Kidney Int 47, 193–199.

Franssen, C.F.M., Stegeman, C.A., Oost-Kort, W.W. et al. (1998). Determinants of renal outcome in anti-myeloperoxidase-associated necrotizing crescentic glomerulonephritis. J Am Soc Nephrol 9, 1915–1923.

Geffriaud-Ricouard, C., Noel, L.H., Chauveau, D., Houhou, S., Grunfeld, J. P. and Lesavre, P. (1993). Clinical spectrum associated with ANCA of defined antigen specificities in 98 selected patients. Clin Nephrol 39, 125–136.

Gisslen, K., Wieslander, J., Westberg, G. and Herlitz, H. (2002). Relationship between anti-neutrophil cytoplasmic antibody determined with conventional binding and the capture assay, and long-term clinical course in vasculitis. J Intern Med 251, 129–135.

Goldschmeding, R., van der Schoot, C.E., ten Bokkel Huinink, D. et al. (1989). Wegener's granulomatosis autoantibodies identify a novel diisopropylfluorophosphate-binding protein in the lysosomes of normal human neutrophils. J Clin Invest 84, 1577–1587.

Gonzalez-Gay, M.A. and Garcia-Porrua, C. (2001). Epidemiology of the vasculitides. Rheum Dis Clin North Am 27, 729–749.

Hagen, E.C., Andrassy, K., Csernok, E. et al. (1996). Development and standardization of solid phase assays for the detection of anti-neutrophil cytoplasmic antibodies (ANCA). A report on the second phase of an international cooperative study on the standardization of ANCA assays. J Immunol Methods 196, 1–15.

Han, W.K., Choi, H.K., Roth, R.M., McCluskey, R.T. and Niles, J.L. (2003). Serial ANCA titers: useful tool for prevention of relapses in ANCA-associated vasculitis. Kidney Int 63, 1079–1085.

Heeringa, P., Foucher, P., Klok, P.A. et al. (1997). Systemic injection of products of activated neutrophils and H_2O_2 in myeloperoxidase-immunized rats leads to necrotizing vasculitis in the lungs and gut. Am J Pathol 151, 131–140.

Hogan, S.L., Nachman, P.H., Wilkman, A.S., Jennette, J.C. and Falk, R.J. (1996). Prognostic markers in patients with antineutrophil cytoplasmic autoantibody-associated microscopic polyangiitis and glomerulonephritis. J Am Soc Nephrol 7, 23–32.

Jayne, D., Rasmussen, N., Andrassy, K. et al. (2003). A randomized trial of maintenance therapy for vasculitis associated with antineutrophil cytoplasmic autoantibodies. N Engl J Med 349, 36–44.

Jayne, D.R., Gaskin, G., Pusey, C.D. and Lockwood, C.M. (1995) ANCA and predicting relapse in systemic vasculitis. Q J Med 88, 127–133.

Jennette, J.C., Falk, R.J., Andrassy, K. et al. (1994). Nomenclature of systemic vasculitides. Proposal of an international consensus conference. Arthritis Rheum 37, 187–192.

Kallenberg, C.G. and Cohen Tervaert, J.W. (2002). In The Molecular Pathology of Autoimmune Diseases, 2nd edn, Theofilopoulos, A.N. and Bona, C.A., eds. New York: Taylor & Francis, pp. 483–503.

Kerr, G.S., Fleisher, T.A., Hallahan, C.W., Leavitt, R.Y., Fauci, A.S. and Hoffman, G.S. (1993). Limited prognostic value of changes in antineutrophil cytoplasmic antibody titer in patients with Wegener's granulomatosis. Arthritis Rheum 36, 365–371.

Kettritz, R., Choi, M., Butt, W. et al. (2002). Phosphatidylinositol 3-kinase controls antineutrophil cytoplasmic antibodies-induced respiratory burst in human neutrophils. J Am Soc Nephrol 13, 1740–1749.

Kettritz, R., Schreiber, A., Luft, F.C. and Haller, H. (2001). Role of mitogen-activated protein kinases in activation of human neutrophils by antineutrophil cytoplasmic antibodies J Am Soc Nephrol 12, 37–46.

Kussmaul, A. and Maier, R. (1866). Ueber eine bisher nicht beschreibene eigenthuemliche Arterienerkrankung (Periateriitis nodosa), die mit Morbus Brightii und rapid fortschreitender allgemeiner Muskellaehmung einhergeht. Dtsch Arch Klin Med 1, 484–517.

Kyndt, X., Reumaux, D., Bridoux, F. et al. (1999). Serial measurements of antineutrophil cytoplasmic autoantibodies in patients with systemic vasculitis. Am J Med 106, 527–533.

Langford, C.A. (2003). Treatment of ANCA-associated vasculitis. N Engl J Med 349, 3–4.

Merkel, P.A., Polisson, R.P., Chang, Y., Skates, S.J. and Niles, J.L. (1997). Prevalence of antineutrophil cytoplasmic antibodies in a large inception cohort of patients with connective tissue disease. Ann Intern Med 126, 866–873.

Muller Kobold, A.C., van der Geld, Y.M., Limburg, P.C., Cohen Tervaert, J.W. and Kallenberg, C.G. (1999). Pathophysiology of ANCA-associated glomerulonephritis. Nephrol Dial Transplant 14, 1366–1375.

Nowack, R., Grab, I., Flores-Suarez, L.F., Schnulle, P., Yard, B. and van der Woude, F.J. (2001). ANCA titres, even of IgG subclasses, and soluble CD14 fail to predict relapses in patients with ANCA-associated vasculitis. Nephrol Dial Transplant 16, 1631–1637.

Pfister, H., Ollert, M.W., Frohlich, L., Quantanilla-Martinez, L., Colby, T.V., Specks, U. and Jenne, D.E. (2004). Anti-neutrophil cytoplasmic autoantibodies (ANCA) against the murine homolog of proteinase 3 are pathogenic in vivo. Blood 104, 1411–1418.

Rao, J.K., Weinberger, M., Oddone, E.Z., Allen, N.B., Landsman, P. and Feussner, J.R. (1995). The role of antineutrophil cytoplasmic antibody (c-ANCA) testing in the diagnosis of Wegener granulomatosis. A literature review and meta-analysis. Ann Intern Med *123*, 925–932.

Rokitansky, K. (1852). Ueber einige der wichtigsten Krankheiten der Arterien. Denksh. dK Akad d Wissensch *4*, 49.

Savage, C.O., Pottinger, B.E., Gaskin, G., Pusey, C.D. and Pearson, J.D. (1992). Autoantibodies developing to myeloperoxidase and proteinase 3 in systemic vasculitis stimulate neutrophil cytotoxicity toward cultured endothelial cells. Am J Pathol *141*, 335–342.

Slot, M.C., Cohen Tervaert, J.W., Boomsma, M.M. and Stegeman, C.A. (2004). A positive cANCA titer at switch to azathioprine therapy is associated with a disquieting relapse rate in PR3-ANCA-related vasculitis. Arthritis Rheum *15*, 269–273.

Slot, M.C., Cohen Tervaert, J.W., Franssen, C.F. and Stegeman, C.A. (2003). Renal survival and prognostic factors in patients with PR3-ANCA associated vasculitis with renal involvement. Kidney Int *63*, 670–677.

Smyth, C.L., Smith, J., Cook, H.T., Haskard, D.O. and Pusey, C.D. (2002). Immunisation with MPO directly induces small vessel vasculitis with pauci-immune focal segmental glomerulonephritis and alveolar haemorrhage in rats. J Am Soc Nephrol *13s*, 170A.

Stegeman, C.A., Cohen Tervaert, J.W., Sluiter, W.J., Manson, W.L., de Jong, P.E. and Kallenberg, C.G.M. (1994). Association of chronic nasal carriage of Staphylococcus aureus and higher relapse rates in Wegener granulomatosis. Ann Intern Med *120*, 12–17.

Taekema-Roelvink, M.E., Kooten Van, C., Heemskerk, E. and Schroeijers, W.M.R. (2000). Proteinase 3 interacts with a 111-kD membrane molecule of human umbilical vein endothelial cells. J Am Soc Nephrol *11*, 640–648.

van der Woude, F.J., Rasmussen, N., Lobatto, S. et al. (1985). Autoantibodies against neutrophils and monocytes: tool for diagnosis and marker of disease activity in Wegener's granulomatosis. Lancet *1*, 425–429.

Vizjak, A., Rott, T., Koselj-Kajtna, M., Rozman, B., Kaplan-Pavlovcic, S. and Ferluga, D. (2003). Histologic and immunohistologic study and clinical presentation of ANCA-associated glomerulonephritis with correlation to ANCA antigen specificity. Am J Kidney Dis *41*, 539–549.

Westman, K.W., Selga, D., Isberg, P.E., Bladstrom, A. and Olsson, H. (2003). High proteinase 3-anti-neutrophil cytoplasmic antibody (ANCA) level measured by the capture enzyme-linked immunosorbent assay method is associated with decreased patient survival in ANCA-associated vasculitis with renal involvement. J Am Soc Nephrol *14*, 2926–2933.

Xiao, H., Heeringa, P., Hu, P. et al. (2002). Antineutrophil cytoplasmic autoantibodies specific for myeloperoxidase cause glomerulonephritis and vasculitis in mice. J Clin Invest *110*, 955–963.

Transplantation

Darshana Dadhania, Choli Hartono and Manikkam Suthanthiran

Department of Transplantation Medicine, The New York Presbyterian Hospital – Weill Cornell Medical Center, New York, NY, USA

You have to know how to accept rejection and reject acceptance.

Ray Bradbury, US science fiction author (1920–)

INTRODUCTION

Measurements of organ graft recipient's immune activity can lead to personalized medicine. Herein, we provide an overview of the innate and adaptive immune process as it relates to solid organ transplantation and discuss immune and molecular parameters informative of a patient's status.

The innate and adaptive immunity

Innate as well as adaptive immunity contributes to the anti-allograft repertoire (Fox and Harrison, 2000; Dallman, 2001; Luster, 2002; He et al., 2002). The innate immune system, comprised of monocyte/macrophages, neutrophils and other granulocytes, is triggered via pattern-recognition receptors (PRRs) expressed on their cell surface. Toll-like receptors (TLRs), displayed on antigen presenting cells (APCs) such as dendritic cells, play an important role in eliciting innate immunity. The elicited response includes phagocytosis, release of cytotoxic granules, direct cell-mediated cytotoxicity and complement activation.

Engagement of TLRs activates the NF-κB pathway and expression of chemoattractants: IL-8, a recruiter of neutrophils, MIP-1α and MIP-1β, recruiters of NK cells and immature dendritic cells and IP-10, a chemoattractant of activated T cells. TLR stimulation leads to dendritic cell maturation and homing to lymph nodes where they encounter and stimulate antigen specific T and B cells. T cells contribute to the activation of effector cells of innate immunity.

The antigen specific immune response is initiated when the host immune cells encounter alloantigens within the allograft and/or the host lymphoid organs. Antigen experienced cells are recruited to the site of inflammation by the chemoattractants. IFN-γ inducible chemokines, IP-10, Mig and I-TAC are all important for the trafficking of the Th1 response whereas chemokines such as exotaxin -1, -2, -3, CCL1 and CCL17 are responsible for Th2 cells. Chemotactic factors provide the invitational signal and the increased expression of adhesion molecules assists in the migration as well. Blockade of CCR5, CXCR3 prevents cellular traffic into the allograft and prolongs allograft survival (Hancock et al., 2000; Gao et al., 2001; Colvin and Thomson, 2002); blockade of ICAM-1 minimizes neutrophilic infiltration into the kidney and protects the kidney against ischemic injury in a rat model (Kelly et al., 1994). Larsen and colleagues have demonstrated that passenger dendritic cells upregulate expression of MHC class II molecules and migrate to recipient lymphoid organs (Larsen et al., 1990a,b). Presentation of alloantigens by passenger dendritic cells provides a powerful stimulus for the development of adaptive immunity.

Measuring Immunity, edited by Michael T. Lotze and Angus W. Thomson
ISBN 0-12-455900-X, London

Allograft recognition

The major determinants of an allograft specific immune response are the major and minor histocompatibility antigens. In humans, the genes for the major histocompatibility complex (MHC) are located on the short arm of chromosome 6 and encode for cell surface proteins, human leukocyte antigens (HLA). HLA class I molecules consisting of HLA-A, HLA-B and HLA-C are found on all nucleated cells while HLA class II molecules consisting of HLA-DR, HLA-DP and HLA-DQ are found mostly on antigen presenting cells (APCs). Naive T cells recognize foreign antigens in the context of MHC molecules present on APCs. CD8+ T cells recognize foreign peptides in the context of MHC class I molecules whereas CD4+ T cells recognize foreign peptides in the context of MHC class II molecules.

The frequency of alloreactive T cells increases with increasing HLA disparity between the donor and the recipient. The number of alloreactive precursor T cells is significantly larger compared to the number of T cells reacting against other natural antigens (Krensky, 2001). T cell recognition of the HLA antigens can occur via direct and/or indirect presentation of alloantigens. Initially, direct recognition of both donor derived MHC molecules alone and donor derived MHC molecules + peptide (recipient or donor) predominates. The magnitude of this direct T cell response is attributed to the high density of cell surface alloantigens, affinity of the T cell receptor for the MHC molecules as well as the large number of potential combinations of donor MHC molecules and (allo- or self-) peptides. Indirect recognition occurs via processing and presentation of donor alloantigens in the context of self class-II MHC molecules expressed on the recipient's antigen presenting cells (Slavcev, 2001).

The stimulation of the adaptive immune response by foreign antigens leads to T cell activation via TCR (T cell receptor). TCR consists of clonotypic α/β chains or γ/δ chains that are associated with the lineage specific CD3 complex. CD3 proteins participate in T cell signal transduction via tyrosine kinases and phosphatases, activation of transcriptional factors such as STAT, NFAT and NF-κB and production of cytokines, growth factors and receptors. However, to activate fully the T cell, additional co-stimulatory signals are obligatory. T cell co-stimulatory molecule CD28, via its interactions with B7-1/B7-2 molecules on APCs, increases the expression of IL-2 and IFN-γ and GM-CSF. Other interactions such as CD2 with CD59, CD154 with CD40 and LFA1 with ICAM-1 contribute to the informative interactions between the T cell and APCs (Watts and DeBenedette, 1999). Interruption of the co-stimulatory signal in the presence of TCR engagement by an alloantigen aborts T cell activation and promotes antigen specific anergy. This property is being explored to promote allograft survival in experimental models of transplantation (Suthanthiran, 1996; Alegre et al., 2001; Yamada and Sayegh, 2002).

The anti-allograft repertoire

CD4+ T helper cells differentiate into either Th1 or Th2 type cells depending on the cytokine environment. Presence of IL-12 and IFN-γ promotes Th1 type generation and production of IL-2 and IFN γ, whereas IL-4 promotes Th2 type differentiation and production of IL-4, IL-5, IL-6, IL-10 and IL-13. Th1 response is associated with macrophage activation and delayed type hypersensitivity while Th2 response is associated with B cell activation. CD8+ cytotoxic T cells are activated in the presence of cytokines such as IL-2 and IFN-γ. Cytokines such as IFN γ and TNF-α increase the expression of adhesion molecules ICAM-1, VCAM-1 and E-selectin (Krensky, 2001).

T cells make up the majority of the graft infiltrating cells. Cytotoxic T cells induce cell death via release of cytotoxic proteins like perforin and granzyme B, TNF-β and TNF-α. Cytotoxic T cells as well as Th1 cells can induce target cell death via interaction of Fas ligand (present on activated T cells) with Fas (present on target cells). B cells, NK cells and macrophages are also important in the effector phase. The unstimulated B cells present foreign antigens in the context of shelf MHC class II molecule to T cells. After binding the foreign antigen via TCR, CD4+ T cells help activate the B cells by providing an accessory signal via CD40/CD40 ligand interaction and release of IL 2 and IL 4. The activated B cells mature into either antibody secreting plasma cells or memory cells. Secreted antibodies bind donor antigens and cause allograft damage via complement activation or activation and degranulation of effector cells. The antibodies can also function as receptors for phagocytosis by host macrophages or cell mediated antibody dependent cellular cytotoxicity by Fc receptor bearing cells. Allograft destruction by specific alloantibodies can occur over hours or much more slowly depending on the antibody titer, the antibody specificity, the ability to fix complement and how soon they appear following transplantation. NK cells cause damage when they recognize that the expression of self-MHC class I molecules is absent, reduced or altered in some way.

MEASUREMENT OF IMMUNITY IN ORGAN TRANSPLANTATION

Immune parameters that predict allograft outcome as well as those that identify individuals requiring modulation of their immune system are beginning to be resolved. The following are worthy of assessment in the transplantation setting:

1 genomic factors that may influence immune responsiveness of the organ graft recipient
2 host humoral immunity
3 host cellular immunity
4 molecular correlates of the host immune response.

Genomic factors that may influence immune responsiveness of the graft recipient

Single nucleotide polymorphisms (SNPs), dinucleotide repeats and microsatellites in genes encoding cytokines, cytokine receptors, chemokines and their receptors and adhesion molecules have been identified. Several of the polymorphisms are located in the promoter region of the gene, affect transcription and/or translation and, not infrequently, determine the level of expression of the protein product and adverse graft outcome (Table 49.1).

A number of methodologies, mostly polymerase chain reaction (PCR) based, are used to detect the genetic variations. Allele discrimination can be accomplished with sequence specific oligonucleotide probes (SSOP), reverse dot blot, reverse line blot, oligonucleotide ligation assay and with amplification refractory mutation system PCR (Turner et al., 1997; Awad et al., 1998; Sankaran et al., 1999; Kobayashi et al., 1999).

Cytokine gene polymorphisms and allograft rejection

TNF-α genotype is reported to be a correlate of cardiac allograft rejection (Turner et al., 1997). In their studies, the incidence and severity of rejection and death from severe allograft rejection were associated with the high producer genotype, especially when HLA-DR compatibility and IL-10 genotype were taken into consideration. In a series of 115 cardiac allograft recipients, it was found that five of 19 patients who experienced severe rejection were typed as high TNF-α and low IL-10 producers. Pediatric heart recipients with acute rejection were also more likely to be high TNF-α and low IL-10 producers (Awad et al., 2001).

TNF-α high producer genotype has been associated with steroid-resistant acute renal allograft rejection and multiple rejection episodes in the HLA-DR mismatched recipients were more frequent in those genotyped as TNF-α high producers (Sankaran et al., 1999). In contrast to cardiac allograft recipients, IL-10 high producer genotype was a correlate of acute renal allograft rejection.

Two polymorphic dinucleotide repeats (IL-10.G and IL-10.R microsatellites) in the IL-10 promoter region have been studied in 120 pairs of donor-recipients matched for one HLA-haplotype and one DRB1-mismatched combination (Kobayashi et al., 1999). The allograft recipients were classified as rejection-free ($n = 53$), as a steroid-sensitive rejection group ($n = 32$) or as a steroid-resistant group ($n = 35$). The frequency of IL-10.G12 allele was significantly higher in recipients with steroid-resistant rejection compared to the no rejection group or the steroid-sensitive rejection group. IL-10 genotyping of organ donors was not informative in this investigation.

TGF-β_1 gene polymorphisms

Awad et al. (1998) reported that the frequency of Arg[25] allele (the high producer type) is higher in those who developed allograft fibrosis following lung transplantation compared to patients without allograft fibrosis. Interestingly, the frequency of Arg[25] allele was also found to be higher in lung transplant candidates with pretransplant fibrotic lung disease compared to those with nonfibrotic lung disease.

Additional polymorphisms

Polymorphisms in the TAP1, TAP2, LMP2, HLA-DMA and HLA-DMP were not found to be a correlate of renal allograft outcome in the study of Chervier et al. (1998). A significant increase in the frequency of HLA-DMA* 0102 allele, however, was found in the rejection group compared to the non-rejection group.

A polymorphism located in exon 4 of the ICAM-1 gene was found to be more frequent in patients with chronic allograft failure compared to recipients with long-term (>10 years) graft function and an additional polymorphism located in exon 6 was associated with a rapid progression to allograft failure (McLaren et al., 1999). Murphy and colleagues (Slavcheva et al., 2001) have

Table 49.1 Cytokine SNPs and allograft outcome

Gene	Location	Genotype	Phenotype	Allograft	Impact on allograft
TNF-α[a]	−308 bp	G/A, A/A	Increased production	Cardiac	Increased acute rejection
IL-10[a]	−1082 bp	ACC/ACC, ACC/ATA, ATA/ATA	Lower production	Cardiac	Increased acute rejection
TGF-β_1[b]	915 bp	G/G	Increased production	Lung	Increased fibrosis
ICAM-1[c]	241 bp	GGG/AGG	? Increased cellular recruitment	Kidney	Increased chronic allograft failure
CTLA-4[d]	642 bp	(AT)n repeat – allele 3 and 4	? Decreased expression	Kidney and liver	Increased acute rejection
MCP-1[e]	−2518 bp	G/G	Increased production	Kidney	Decreased allograft survival
CCR5[f]	794–825	32 bp deletion – homozygous	Defective function	Kidney	Improved allograft survival

[a] Awad et al., 2001; [b] Awad et al., 1998; [c] McLaren et al., 1999; [d] Slavcheva et al., 2001; [e] Kruger et al., 2002; [f] Fischereder et al., 2001.

explored the association between CTLA-4 polymorphisms and allograft rejection and found that the alleles 3 and 4 in kidney and liver graft recipients is associated with a higher risk of rejection. Interestingly, the allele 1 was associated with a lesser risk of acute rejection and was less frequent in the African Americans compared to Caucasians.

Akalin and Neylan (2003) evaluated the influence of different duffy antigen phenotypes on renal allograft survival. The majority of African Americans (65–68 per cent) have the Fy(a-b-) phenotype while it is present in only 1 per cent of whites. Among patients who experienced delayed graft function, the Fy(a-b-) phenotype was associated with a significantly lower renal allograft survival ($P = 0.003$). Duffy antigens are receptors on red blood cells which have recently been demonstrated to bind chemokines from both the CXC and CC family. The duffy antigens are believed to act as chemokine sinks since the binding of the chemokine to the duffy antigen does not lead to signal transduction in red blood cells.

Hutchings et al. (2001) described increased expression of B7 co-stimulatory molecules CD80 and CD86 in African Americans compared to Caucasians. Hutchings et al. have linked the increased expression of CD80 and CD86 on resting APCs to IL-6 and IL-10 polymorphisms. Individuals who demonstrated IL-6 polymorphism associated with increased IL-6 production and individuals who demonstrated IL-10 polymorphism associated with decreased IL-10 production had significantly increased CD80 and CD86 expression (Hutchings et al., 2002).

Polymorphisms in chemokine and chemokine receptors have been linked to altered renal allograft survival. Kruger et al. (2002) evaluated the polymorphic variation in MCP-1 in 232 renal allograft recipients and reported that those homozygous for the mutation had significantly shorter graft survival times ($P = 0.0052$). CCR5 deletion mutation that leads to a non-functional receptor has been associated with improved allograft survival in transplant recipients (Fischereder et al., 2001). Polymorphisms in genes encoding ACE, and factor 5 Lieden have all been reported to alter allograft survival and/or function (Filler and Hocher, 2002).

Humoral immunity

The complement-dependent cytotoxicity assay (CDC) detects antibodies that utilize and activate complement and mediate complement-dependent cytotoxicity. The CDC assay can be used to detect antigenic specificities at which the antibodies are directed by using appropriate target cells and with sera that are specifically absorbed with platelets or B lymphoblastoid cell lines.

A positive CDC cross-match using current serum is a contraindication to renal transplantation since preformed class I HLA antibodies are associated with hyperacute rejection and early graft loss (Kissmeyer-Nielsen et al., 1966). In renal allograft recipients, even a historical positive CDC cross-match with sera obtained more than 6 months prior to transplantation has been reported to be associated with a higher incidence of acute rejection episodes, increased rate of delayed graft function and poorer 10-year graft survival (Noreen et al., 2003). Poor allograft survival in the presence of a positive T cell CDC cross-match has been demonstrated with other solid organ transplants as well (Ratkovec et al., 1992).

Panel reactive antibodies

Screening of recipients' serum for the presence of antibodies against a panel of lymphocytes representing almost all known HLA antigens (PRA) is used to monitor patients awaiting transplantation. The PRA test can also be performed using beads coated with HLA antigens. Patients with a high PRA value wait longer to receive a kidney allograft as compared to those with low PRA values, due to the increased likelihood of a positive cross-match. A high PRA value is associated with a high incidence of acute rejection and poor graft outcome. UNOS registry analysis of patients with similar etiologies for ESRD has shown that those with >50 per cent PRA demonstrate approximately 5–10 per cent lower 3-year graft survival (Hardy et al., 2001). Barama et al. (2000) demonstrated that kidney allograft recipients with >50 per cent PRA were more likely to suffer acute rejection related allograft loss within the first 6 months as compared to those with lower PRA values. Cardiac allograft recipients with >10% PRA experienced a 77% graft rejection rate compared to 56% in those with PRA <10%; 92% of graft rejections in recipients with PRA > 10% occurred within the first 30 days post-cardiac transplantation (Kerman et al., 1998).

Donor specific antibodies have been associated with both acute and chronic rejection of solid organ grafts. For example, the presence of donor specific antibodies in cardiac allograft recipients is a correlate of acute rejection and associated with increased requirement for antibody therapy (Ratkovec et al., 1992; Smith et al., 1992). The development of anti-HLA antibodies post-transplant correlated also with lower 5-year survival rates of cardiac allografts and renal allografts (Barr et al., 1993). Selected investigations demonstrating the adverse impact of donor-specific anti-HLA antibodies on allograft function and status have been summarized (Table 49.2). The detection of these antibodies is also helpful in organs that are less likely to stimulate the recipient's immune system such as the liver and cornea (Hahn et al., 1995; Kasahara et al., 1999). Often, donor-specific anti-HLA antibodies precede the development of acute rejection and are a poor prognostic sign (Worthington et al., 2003).

Central to the development of chronic damage is the proliferation of smooth muscle cells, endothelial cells and fibroblasts and release of growth factors that contribute to fibrosis and vascular sclerosis. Recent evidence suggests that anti-HLA antibodies may induce the expression of growth factor receptors and contribute to increased proliferation of fibroblasts and smooth muscle cells. In

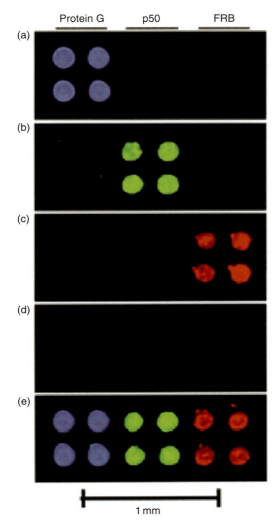

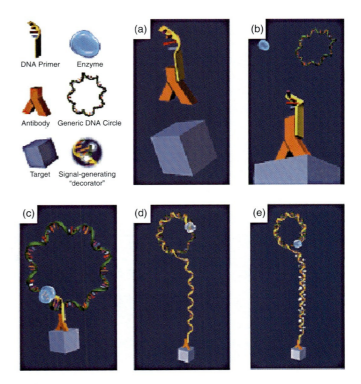

Figure 59.4 Schematic representation of immunoassays with RCA signal amplification. (a) In the adaptation of RCA used for protein signal amplification, the 5 end of an oligonucleotide primer is attached to an antibody. (b) The antibody-DNA conjugate binds to its specific target molecule; in the multiplexed microarray immunoassay, the targets are biotinylated secondary antibodies and the conjugate is an anti-biotin antibody. (c) A circular DNA molecule hybridizes to its complementary primer on the conjugate, and in the presence of DNA polymerase and nucleotides, rolling-circle replication occurs. (d) A long single DNA molecule that represents a concatamer of complements of the circle DNA sequence is generated that remains attached to the antibody. (e) This RCA product is detected by hybridization of multiple fluorescent, complementary oligonucleotide probes. RCA product fluorescence is measured with a conventional microarry scanning device. The amount of florescence at each spot is directly proportional to the amount of specific protein in the original sample.

Figure 59.1 Detecting protein-protein interactions on glass slides. (a) Slide probed with BODIPY-FL-IgG (0.5 μg/ml). (b) Slide probed with Cy3-IkBα (0.1 μg/ml). (c) Slide probed with Cy5-FKBP12(0.5 μg/ml) and no rapamycin. (d) Slide probed with Cys-FKBP12 (0.5 μg/ml) and no rapamycin. (e) Slide probed with BODIPY-FL-IgG(0.5 μg/ml)). Cy3-IkBα (0.1 μg/ml). Cy5-FKBP12 (0.5 μg/ml), and 100 nM rapamycin. In all panels, BODIPY-FL, Cy3, and Cy5 fluorescence were false-colored blue, green, and red, respectively.

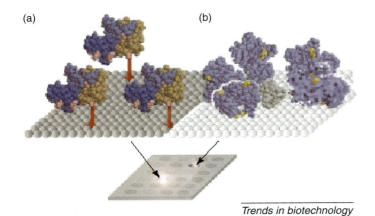

Trends in biotechnology

Figure 59.3 An illustration of the presentation of immobilized proteins in an array. (a) An idealized illustration of the presentation of immobilized proteins in an array. The proteins are all iniformly oriented, properly folded and optimally spaced to allow protein-protein interactions. (b) Current technologies present proteins in a range of orientations, with varying degrees of denaturation and with the presence of non-specifically absorbed proteins.

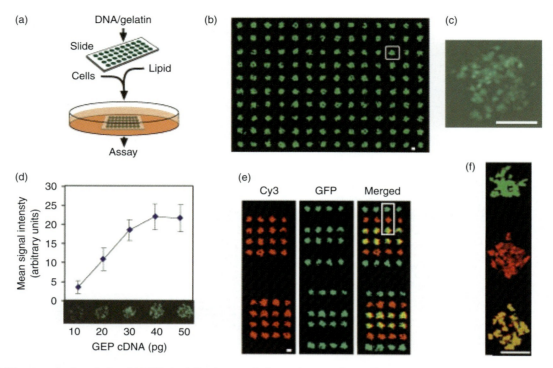

Figure 59.5 Well-less transfection of plasmid DNAs in defined areas of a lawn of mammalian cells. (a) Protocol for making microarrays of transfected cells. (b) Laser scan image of a GFP-expressing microarray made from a slide printed in a 14 10 pattern with a GFP expression construct. (c) Higher magnification image obtained with fluorescence microscopy of the cell cluster boxed in b. Scale bar, 100 μm. (d) Expression levels of cell clusters in a microarray are proportional, over a fourfold range, to the amount of plasmid DNA printed on the slide. Indicated amounts of the GFP construct assume a 1-nl printing volume. The graph shows the mean s.d. of the fluorescence intensities of the cell clusters ($n = 6$). The fluorescent image is from a representative expirement. (e) CO-transfection is possible with transfected cell microarrays. Arrays with elements containing expression constructs for HA-GST, GFP of both were transfected and processed for immunofluorescence and imaged with a laser scanner. Cy3, cell clusters expressing HA-GST; GFP, cell clusters expressing GFP; merged, superimposition of Cy3 and GFP signals. Yellow colour indicates co-expression. Scale bar, 100 μm. (f) Enlarged view of boxed area of scan image from (e).

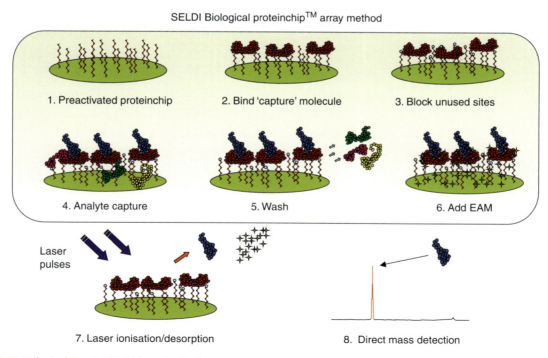

Figure 59.6 SELDI Biological ProteinChip™ Array Method.

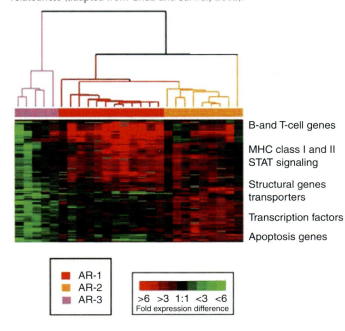

Figure 60.1 The generation of a microarray experiment begins with the labeling and reverse transcription of sample and reference mRNA. After competitive hybridization to a pre-formed cDNA or oligonucleotide microarray, data are scanned and subsequently analyzed according to a variety of protocols. Among the most popular is 'clustering' of data, or organizing genes and experimental samples according to their expression patterns and relatedness (adapted from Chua and Sarwal, 2002).

Reference mRNA

Sample mRNA

Reverse transcription fluorescent labeling

Hybridize to microarray

Prepare microarray

Analysis

Experimental samples

Genes

Identification of differentially-expressed genes; functionally-related genes; disease classificaton

B-and T-cell genes

MHC class I and II STAT signaling

Structural genes transporters

Transcription factors

Apoptosis genes

- AR-1
- AR-2
- AR-3

>6 >3 1:1 <3 <6
Fold expression difference

Figure 60.3 Classification of renal allograft acute rejection samples into three categories based on microarray clustering. Each rejection subtype demonstrates differential expression of genes involved in biological processes such as apoptosis and cell signaling. With this information, novel therapies can be developed and tailored according to patient subtype (adapted from Sarwal et al., 2003a).

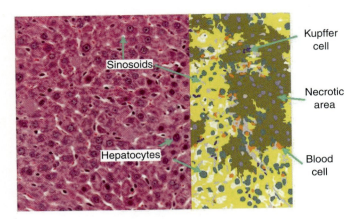

Figure 61.2 Image segmentation in liver. The right hand side displays an overlay that shows how the image can be broken down and classified into different tissue objects. These components are a prerequisite for a high-content morphometric quantification.

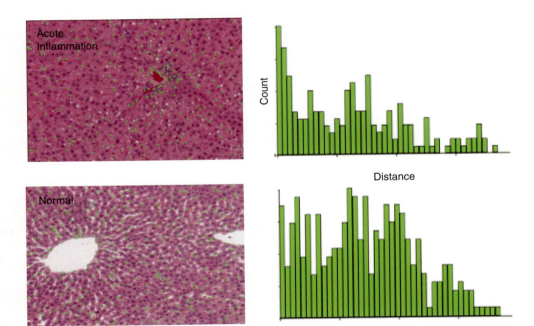

Figure 61.3 Distance distribution of monocytes in normal and acute inflamed liver. Assessments like these are consistent with pathological diagnosis.

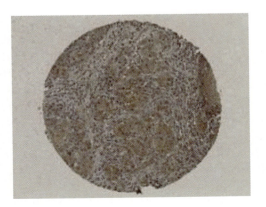
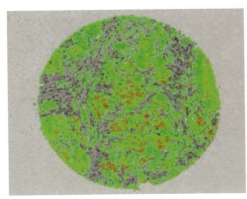

Figure 61.5 Displayed is an immunoperoxidase stained tissue core and the computer processed false color image that gives the concentration of the stain. Colors are graded from green to red, with red representing the highest intensity staining. The automated stain analysis allows efficient high-throughput evaluation of expressions in TMAs.

Table 49.2 Impact of positive donor-specific antibodies in the post-transplant period (selected studies)

Assay	Antibodies detected (n = number of recipients)		Allograft	Clinical impact
CDC[a]	HLA class I and II	Present (n = 18) Absent (n = 27)	Heart	56% of recipients with HLA antibodies experienced steroid-resistant acute rejection compared to 15% of those without HLA antibodies
CDC and ELISA[b]	HLA class I and II	Present (n = 59) Absent (n = 176)	Kidney	97% graft failure rate in recipients with HLA antibodies over a mean of 6 years versus 31% in patients without HLA antibodies who were followed for a mean of 9 years
Flow cytometry[c]	HLA class II	Present (n = 30) Absent (n = 32)	Kidney	86% of recipients with HLA antibodies had developed chronic rejection rate

[a] Smith et al., 1992; [b] Worthington et al., 2003; [c] Abe et al., 1997.

renal transplantation, the presence of anti-donor HLA antibodies was found in 51–86 per cent of recipients diagnosed with chronic rejection as compared to 2–15 per cent of those with stable function (Abe et al., 1997). The 5-year renal and cardiac allograft survival is 17 per cent and 13 per cent lower respectively in recipients who developed anti-HLA alloantibodies in the first post-transplant year as compared to those without alloantibodies (Barr et al., 1993). Suciu-Foca and colleagues (1991a,b) have also demonstrated that allograft recipients with anti-idiotypic antibodies maintain stable graft function despite the presence of anti-donor antibodies. The authors postulate that the development of anti-idiotypic antibodies may play a protective role.

The diagnosis of humoral component in the acute or chronic rejection process has been aided by the detection of complement fragment C4d in the allograft biopsies. A positive C4d staining during an acute rejection episode is associated with increased rate of graft loss in both renal and cardiac allograft recipients. In renal allograft recipients with chronic rejection, those with positive C4d staining had an inferior 1-year graft survival compared to those with negative C4d staining (Behr et al., 1999; Collins et al., 1999; Mauiyyedi et al., 2001).

In liver transplantation, the presence of donor specific cytotoxic antibodies does not appear to have a significant impact on short-term survival or acute rejection rates; this may be a result of immune absorption of antibodies by the liver graft or the presence of soluble donor HLA antigens. It is noteworthy that peripheral T cell stimulation by soluble donor antigens in the absence of co-stimulatory signal may induce T cell anergy (Donaldson and Williams, 1997). The precise impact of preformed antibodies or HLA matching on liver allografts is not known (Bishara et al., 2002; Neumann et al., 2003).

Flow cytometry and ELISA

Flow cytometry and ELISA facilitate the detection of low levels of both complement-fixing and non-complement-fixing antibodies. In the UNOS data, a positive cross-match test by flow cytometry, despite a negative standard cross-match test, was associated with a 5 per cent survival disadvantage for subsequent but not for primary renal grafts (Ogura, 1992). UCLA data suggest a positive cross-match by flow cytometry may also be an adverse risk factor for primary renal grafts (Ogura, 1992).

Flow cytometry has been used to detect antibodies in recipients of liver or cardiac allografts. The flow cytometry cross-match is a more sensitive indicator of rejection, compared to standard cross-match, in liver allograft recipients. The flow cytometry technique is also useful in monitoring patients following transplantation.

Class I antibodies, undetected by the CDC assay but detected using flow cytometry, have been associated with increased incidence of early acute rejection and subclinical rejection episodes, increased chronic rejection and lower renal allograft function and survival (Ogura, 1992; Abou El Fettouh et al., 2001). Detection of class I and class II antibodies, with the use of ELISA, have also been correlated with acute rejection as well as immunological graft loss in kidney transplantation (Emonds et al., 2000).

The significance of anti-HLA class II antibodies alone is not clear; some studies have demonstrated a trend towards increased chronic rejection and lower graft survival (Scornik et al., 2001; Susal and Opelz, 2002). In heart transplantation, Itescu et al. (1998) demonstrated that the presence of HLA class II antibodies pre-transplant results in a twofold increased risk of developing high-grade cellular rejection.

Cellular immunity

The lymphocyte-mediated cytotoxicity (LMC) assay is designed to detect the presence of cytotoxic effector cells. By using appropriate target cell populations, the nature of cellular immunity can be assessed and by using precisely identified lymphoid cells as effector cells in the lymphocyte-mediated cytotoxicity assay, the pedigree of the effector cells mediating cytotoxicity can be discerned. The rationale for the use of this assay in the renal allograft recipient is based on considerable clinical and experimental evidence for the participation of cytotoxic T cells in the destruction of allografts.

Several transplant groups have reported that a positive LMC assay is a correlate of acute rejection (Suthanthiran et al., 1997). Also, a persistently positive assay, especially in the first month post-transplantation, is associated with graft failure within 3 months post-transplantation. Assays tend to be positive in rejection episodes characterized by a greater degree of cellular infiltration and a correlation between lymphocyte-mediated cytotoxic activity and the intensity of cell infiltration can also be demonstrated. Recent molecular studies demonstrating heightened expression of genes that code for cytotoxic T cell effector molecules are discussed in the latter sections of this chapter.

Molecular characterization of solid organ graft recipients

A highly sensitive molecular technique, reverse transcription assisted polymerase chain reaction (RT-PCR), permits identification and quantification of mRNA of low abundance. In this procedure, total RNA is isolated from the tissues or the cells and reverse transcribed into first strand cDNA. The cDNA is then amplified by PCR using sequence-specific oligonucleotide primer pairs, Taq DNA polymerase and dNTPs (dATP, dTTP, dCTP and dGTP).

RT-PCR has been used for mRNA phenotyping of allograft biopsies obtained from organ graft recipients (Suthanthiran and Strom, 1996, Suthanthiran et al., 1997). The existing data suggest that mRNA encoding cytotoxic attack molecules and mRNA encoding immunoregulatory cytokines are usually detectable at the time of allograft rejection. In studies performed with renal allograft biopsy specimens, intragraft expression of granzyme B mRNA has been found to be a significant correlate of acute rejection. Additional molecules involved in the cytolytic pathway, perforin (a pore-forming protein), TIA-1 (a potential activator of endogenous nuclease) and the ligand for Fas (APO-1, CD95) antigen, are all present in the renal allograft during acute rejection. Among the immunoregulatory cytokines, intragraft expression of mRNA encoding IL-2, IFN-γ, IL-6 or IL-10 has been correlated with acute rejection in some but not all studies. Intragraft expression of mRNA encoding IL-1β, IL-2 receptor β, IL-4, IL-7, IL-8 or TNF-α has not been informative regarding the immunological status of renal allografts.

mRNAs encoding cytotoxic attack molecules have been found to be correlates of liver, cardiac or lung rejection. The cytotoxic T cell specific granzyme A and perforin have been detected by RT-PCR and by in situ hybridization during cardiac allograft rejection. The intragraft expression of granzyme A has been correlated also with a decrease in diastolic function. As reported with renal allograft biopsy specimens, intragraft expression of IL-6 mRNA is a correlate of acute cardiac rejection and the TCR α/β repertoire is broader in acute rejection biopsies compared to cardiac biopsies without rejection.

Intragraft expression of granzyme B mRNA has also been observed with liver allograft rejection and with rejection of lung allografts. In addition to granzyme B expression, a significant correlation between intrahepatic IL-5 mRNA expression and acute liver allograft rejection has been reported. Intragraft expression of IL-2 mRNA, as reported with renal allograft specimens, correlated also with acute rejection. However, IL-2 mRNA is infrequently detected and when expressed, transient in nature. The expression of IL-1β, IL-6 or TNF-α mRNA does not appear to reflect immunological rejection of hepatic allografts. Cells obtained by bronchoalveolar lavage have been analyzed by RT-PCR and a decrease in the level of expression of IL-6 mRNA and IFN-α mRNA following cyclosporine inhalation therapy for rejection has been reported.

An important refinement of the RT-PCR methodology is the development of quantitative PCR. The quantitative PCR avoids many of the pitfalls of the standard PCR (e.g. tube-to-tube variation) and provides precise information regarding mRNA abundance. Indeed, data that the level of expression of granzyme B is a correlate of the intensity of acute rejection have already been generated in studies of renal allograft recipients.

Non-invasive and molecular biomarkers

Given the invasive nature of allograft biopsies, recent studies have focused on the development of non-invasive protocols for the measurement of the immune status of the organ recipients.

Peripheral blood molecular biomarkers

Peripheral blood cell expression of mRNA encoding cytotoxic attack molecules granzyme B, perforin and fas ligand as well as transcripts for INF-γ, IL-2 and IL-6 have all been associated with acute allograft rejection (Gorczynski et al., 1996; Vasconcellos et al., 1998; Dugre et al., 2000). Simon et al. (2003) have compared serial expression of cytotoxic genes, perforin and granzyme B in blood samples from patients with and without early acute rejection episodes (Table 49.3). Based on the change in the level of expression of cytotoxic attack molecules on postoperative days 8–10, recipients likely to reject were identified with a sensitivity of 72 per cent and 82 per cent and specificity of 87 per cent and 90 per cent for granzyme B and perforin, respectively. The levels of expression of mRNAs decreased in response to anti-rejection therapy. The effect of systemic infection however has not been evaluated in many of these studies.

Urinary molecular biomarkers

Analysis of gene expression in urinary cells has been helpful in the diagnosis of acute renal allograft rejection

Table 49.3 Molecular correlates of acute renal allograft rejection measured with real time PCR assays

	Sensitivity (%)	Specificity (%)
Blood		
Granzyme B[a]	72	82
Perforin[a]	87	90
Urine		
Granzyme B[b]	88	79
Perforin[b]	88	79
PI-9[b]	76	79
CD103[c]	59.4	75.5

[a] Simon et al., 2003; [b]Muthukumar et al., 2003; [c]Ding et al., 2003

(see Table 49.3). In our study, elevated levels of mRNA for cytotoxic attack molecules, perforin and granzyme B, were a correlate of acute renal allograft rejection (Li et al., 2001). Furthermore, mRNA levels in urinary cells predicted subsequent development of acute allograft rejection. The heightened expression of a natural antagonist of granzyme B, proteinase inhibitor-9 (PI-9), distinguished acute rejection and the magnitude of the increase correlated with renal function 6 months post the rejection episode (Muthukumar et al., 2003). CD103 plays a critical role in the homing of CD8+ CTLs to the intratubular space via its interaction with E-cadherin and intratubular infiltration (tubulitis) can be readily detected by the measurements of CD103 mRNA in urinary cells (Ding et al., 2003). Bacterial urinary tract infections are not a confounding factor (Dadhania et al., 2003). Whether urinary cell mRNA profiling informs immunosuppression weaning remains to be determined.

SUMMARY

We have reviewed immune factors considered to play a deterministic role in allograft outcome. Assessment of host immune repertory at the cellular, humoral and molecular levels may open the door for pre-emptive therapy.

REFERENCES

Abe, M., Kawai, T., Futatsuyama, K. et al. (1997). Postoperative production of anti-donor antibody and chronic rejection in renal transplantation. Transplantation 63, 1616–1619.

Abou El Fettouh, H., Cook, D.J., Flechner, S. et al. (2001). Early and late impact of a positive flow cytometry crossmatch on graft outcome in primary renal transplant. Transplant Proc 33, 2968–2970.

Akalin, E. and Neylan, J. F. (2003). The influence of Duffy blood group on renal allograft outcome in African Americans. Transplantation 75, 1496–1500.

Alegre, M., Fallarino, F., Zhou, P. et al. (2001). Transplantation and the CD28/CTLA4/B7 pathway. Transplant Proc 33, 209–211.

Awad, M.R., El-Gamel, A., Hasleton, P., Turner, D.M., Sinnott, P.J. and Hutchinson, I.V. (1998). Genotypic variation in the transforming growth factor-beta1 gene: association with transforming growth factor-beta1 production, fibrotic lung disease, and graft fibrosis after lung transplantation. Transplantation 66, 1014–1020.

Awad, M.R., Webber, S., Boyle, G. et al. (2001). The effect of cytokine gene polymorphisms on pediatric heart allograft outcome. J Heart Lung Transplant 20, 625–630.

Barama, A., Oza, U., Panek, R. et al. (2000). Effect of recipient sensitization (peak PRA) on graft outcome in haploidentical living related kidney transplants. Clin Transplant 14, 212–217.

Barr, M.L., Cohen, D.J., Benvenisty, A.I. et al. (1993). Effect of anti-HLA antibodies on the long-term survival of heart and kidney allografts. Transplant Proc 25, 262–264.

Behr, T.M., Feucht, H.E., Richter, K. et al. (1999). Detection of humoral rejection in human cardiac allografts by assessing the capillary deposition of complement fragment C4d in endomyocardial biopsies. J Heart Lung Transplant 18, 904–912.

Bishara, A., Brautbar, C., Eid, A., Scherman, L., Ilan, Y. and Safadi, R. (2002). Is presensitization relevant to liver transplantation outcome? Hum Immunol 63, 742–750.

Chevrier, D., Giral, M., Muller, J.Y., Bignon, J.D. and Soulillou, J.P. (1998). Impact of the MHC-encoded HLA-DMA, DMB, and LMP2 gene polymorphisms on kidney graft outcome. Hum Immunol 59, 650–655.

Collins, A.B., Schneeberger, E.E., Pascual, M.A. et al. (1999). Complement activation in acute humoral renal allograft rejection: diagnostic significance of C4d deposits in peritubular capillaries. J A S N 10, 2208–2214.

Colvin, B.L. and Thomson, A.W. (2002). Chemokines, their receptors, and transplant outcome. Transplantation 74, 149–155.

Dadhania, D., Muthukumar, T., Ding, R et al. (2003). Molecular signatures of urinary cells distinguish acute rejection of renal allografts from urinary tract infection. Transplantation 75, 1752–1754.

Dallman, M. (2001). Immunobiology of graft rejection. In Pathology and Immunology of Transplantation and Rejection, Thiru, S. and Waldmann, H., eds. London: Blackwell Science Ltd, pp. 1–28.

Ding, R., Li, B., Muthukumar, T et al. (2003). CD103 mRNA levels in urinary cells predict acute rejection of renal allografts. Transplantation 75, 1307–1312.

Donaldson, P.T. and Williams, R. (1997). Cross-matching in liver transplantation. Transplantation 63, 789–794.

Dugre, F.J., Gaudreau, S., Belles-Isles, M., Houde, I. and Roy, R. (2000). Cytokine and cytotoxic molecule gene expression determined in peripheral blood mononuclear cells in the diagnosis of acute renal rejection. Transplantation 70, 1074–1080.

Emonds, M.P., Herman, J., Dendievel, J., Waer, M. and Van Damme-Lombaerts, R. (2000). Evaluation of anti-human leukocyte antigen allo-immunization in pediatric cadaveric kidney transplantation. Pediatr Transplantation, 4, 6–11.

Filler, G. and Hocher, B. (2002). The emerging role of gene polymorphisms determining outcome after solid-organ transplantation (comment). Pediatr Transplantation 6, 12–14.

Fischereder, M., Luckow, B., Hocher, B. et al. (2001). CC chemokine receptor 5 and renal-transplant survival. Lancet 357, 1758–1761.

Fox, A. and Harrison, L.C. (2000). Innate immunity and graft rejection. Immunol Rev 173, 141–147.

Gao, W., Faia, K.L., Csizmadia, V. et al. (2001). Beneficial effects of targeting CCR5 in allograft recipients. Transplantation 72, 1199–1205.

Gorczynski, R.M., Adams, R.B., Levy, G.A. and Chung, S.W. (1996). Correlation of peripheral blood lymphocyte and intragraft cytokine mRNA expression with rejection in orthotopic liver transplantation. Surgery 120, 496–502.

Hahn, A.B., Foulks, G.N., Enger, C. et al. (1995). The association of lymphocytotoxic antibodies with corneal allograft rejection in high risk patients. The Collaborative Corneal Transplantation Studies Research Group. Transplantation 59, 21–27.

Hancock, W.W., Lu, B., Gao, W. et al. (2000). Requirement of the chemokine receptor CXCR3 for acute allograft rejection. J Exp Med 192, 1515–1520.

Hardy, S., Lee, S.H. and Terasaki, P.I. (2001). Sensitization 2001. In Clinical Transplants, Cecka, J.M. and Terasaki, P.I., eds. Los Angeles, pp. 271–278.

He, H., Stone, J.R. and Perkins, D.L. (2002). Analysis of robust innate immune response after transplantation in the absence of adaptive immunity. Transplantation 73, 853–861.

Hutchings, A., Guay-Woodford, L., Thomas, J.M. et al. (2002). Association of cytokine single nucleotide polymorphisms with B7 costimulatory molecules in kidney allograft recipients (see comment). Pediatr Transplantation 6, 69–77.

Hutchings, A., Purcell, W.M. and Benfield, M.R. (2001). Increased costimulatory responses in African-American kidney allograft recipients. Transplantation 71, 692–695.

Itescu, S., Tung, T.C., Burke, E.M. et al. (1998). Preformed IgG antibodies against major histocompatibility complex class II antigens are major risk factors for high-grade cellular rejection in recipients of heart transplantation. Circulation 98, 786–793.

Kasahara, M., Kiuchi, T., Takakura, K. et al. (1999). Postoperative flow cytometry crossmatch in living donor liver transplantation: clinical significance of humoral immunity in acute rejection. Transplantation 67, 568–575.

Kelly, K.J., Williams, W.W. Jr, Colvin, R.B. and Bonventre, J.V. (1994). Antibody to intercellular adhesion molecule 1 protects the kidney against ischemic injury. Proc Natl Acad Sci USA 91, 812–816.

Kerman, R.H., Susskind, B., Kerman, D. et al. (1998). Comparison of PRA-STAT, sHLA-EIA, and anti-human globulin-panel reactive antibody to identify alloreactivity in pretransplantation sera of heart transplant recipients: correlation to rejection and posttransplantation coronary artery disease. J Heart Lung Transplant 17, 789–794.

Kissmeyer-Nielsen, F., Olsen, S., Petersen, V.P. and Fjeldborg, O. (1966). Hyperacute rejection of kidney allografts, associated with pre-existing humoral antibodies against donor cells. Lancet 2, 662–665.

Kobayashi, T., Yokoyama, I., Hayashi, S. et al. (1999). Genetic polymorphism in the IL-10 promoter region in renal transplantation. Transplant Proc 31, 755–756.

Krensky, A. (2001). Immunobiology and transplantation research. In Primer on Transplantation, 2nd edn, Norman, D.J. and Turka, L., eds. Mt. Laurel: American Society of Transplantation, pp. 1–60.

Kruger, B., Schroppel, B., Ashkan, R. et al. (2002). A monocyte chemoattractant protein-1 (MCP-1) polymorphism and outcome after renal transplantation. J A S N 13, 2585–2589.

Larsen, C.P., Morris, P.J. and Austyn, J.M. (1990a). Migration of dendritic leukocytes from cardiac allografts into host spleens.

A novel pathway for initiation of rejection. J Exp Med 171, 307–314.

Larsen, C.P., Steinman, R.M., Witmer-Pack, M., Hankins, D.F., Morris, P.J. and Austyn, J.M. (1990b). Migration and maturation of Langerhans cells in skin transplants and explants. J Exp Med 172, 1483–1493.

Li, B., Hartono, C., Ding, R. et al. (2001) Noninvasive diagnosis of renal-allograft rejection by measurement of messenger RNA for perforin and granzyme B in urine (see comment). N Engl J Med 344, 947–954.

Luster, A.D. (2002). The role of chemokines in linking innate and adaptive immunity. Curr Opin Immunol 14, 129–135.

Mauiyyedi, S., Pelle, P.D., Saidman, S. et al. (2001). Chronic humoral rejection: identification of antibody-mediated chronic renal allograft rejection by C4d deposits in peritubular capillaries. J A S N 12, 2574–2582.

McLaren, A.J., Marshall, S.E., Haldar, N.A. et al. (1999). Adhesion molecule polymorphisms in chronic renal allograft failure. Kidney Int 55, 1977–1982.

Muthukumar, T., Ding, R., Dadhania, D. et al. (2003). Serine proteinase inhibitor-9, an endogenous blocker of granzyme B/perforin lytic pathway, is hyperexpressed during acute rejection of renal allografts. Transplantation 75, 1565–1570.

Neumann, U.P., Guckelberger, O., Langrehr, J.M. et al. (2003). Impact of human leukocyte antigen matching in liver transplantation. Transplantation 75, 132–137.

Noreen, H.J., McKinley, D.M., Gillingham, K.J., Matas, A.J. and Segall, M. (2003). Positive remote crossmatch: impact on short-term and long-term outcome in cadaver renal transplantation. Transplantation 75, 501–505.

Ogura, K. (1992). Sensitization. In Clinical Transplantation, Checka, J.M. and Terasaki, P., eds. Los Angeles, pp. 357–369.

Ratkovec, R.M., Hammond, E.H., O'Connell, J.B. et al. (1992). Outcome of cardiac transplant recipients with a positive donor-specific crossmatch – preliminary results with plasmapheresis. Transplantation 54, 651–655.

Sankaran, D., Asderakis, A., Ashraf, S. et al. (1999). Cytokine gene polymorphisms predict acute graft rejection following renal transplantation. Kidney Int 56, 281–288.

Scornik, J.C., Clapp, W., Patton, P.R. et al. (2001). Outcome of kidney transplants in patients known to be flow cytometry crossmatch positive. Transplantation 71, 1098–1102.

Simon, T., Opelz, G., Wiesel, M., Ott, R.C. and Susal, C. (2003). Serial peripheral blood perforin and granzyme B gene expression measurements for prediction of acute rejection in kidney graft recipients. Am J Transplant 3, 1121–1127.

Slavcev, A. (2001). Mechanisms of allorecognition and organ transplant rejection. Ann Transplant 6, 5–8.

Slavcheva, E.A.E., Jiao, Q., Tran, H. et al. (2001). The effect of CTLA4 gene polymorphisms in transplant patients. Transplantation 72, 935–940.

Smith, J.D., Danskine, A.J., Rose, M.L. and Yacoub, M.H. (1992). Specificity of lymphocytotoxic antibodies formed after cardiac transplantation and correlation with rejection episodes. Transplantation 53, 1358–1362.

Suciu-Foca, N., Ho, E., King, D.W. et al. (1991a). Soluble HLA and anti-idiotypic antibodies in transplantation: modulation of anti-HLA antibodies by soluble HLA antigens from the graft and anti-idiotypic antibodies in renal and cardiac allograft recipients. Transplant Proc 23, 295–296.

Suciu-Foca, N., Reed, E., D'Agati, V.D. et al. (1991b). Soluble HLA antigens, anti-HLA antibodies, and antiidiotypic antibodies in the circulation of renal transplant recipients. Transplantation 51, 593–601.

Susal, C. and Opelz, G. (2002). Kidney graft failure and presensitization against HLA class I and class II antigens. Transplantation 73, 1269–1273.

Suthanthiran, M. (1996). Transplantation tolerance: fooling mother nature. Proc Natl Acad Sci USA 93, 12072–12075.

Suthanthiran, M. and Strom, T.B. (1996). Human renal graft rejection: immune mechanisms, molecular correlates and management strategies. Nephrology 2, 1–12.

Suthanthiran, M., Garovoy, M.R. and Strom, T.B. (1997). Immunological characterization of solid organ graft recipients. In Manual of Clinical Laboratory Immunology, 5th edn, Rose, N.R. et al., eds. Washington, DC: ASM Press, pp. 1117–1122.

Turner, D., Grant, S.C., Yonan, N. et al. (1997). Cytokine gene polymorphism and heart transplant rejection. Transplantation 64, 776–779.

Vasconcellos, L.M., Schachter, A.D., Zheng, X.X. et al. (1998). Cytotoxic lymphocyte gene expression in peripheral blood leukocytes correlates with rejecting renal allografts. Transplantation 66, 562–566.

Watts, T.H. and DeBenedette, M.A. (1999). T cell co-stimulatory molecules other than CD28. Curr Opin Immunol 11, 286–293.

Worthington, J.E., Martin, S., Al-Husseini, D.M., Dyer, P.A. and Johnson, R.W. (2003). Posttransplantation production of donor HLA-specific antibodies as a predictor of renal transplant outcome. Transplantation 75, 1034–1040.

Yamada and Sayegh, M.H. (2002). The CD154-CD40 costimulatory pathway in transplantation. Transplantation 73, S36–39.

Viral Responses – HIV-1

Chapter

50

Bonnie A. Colleton, Paolo Piazza and Charles R. Rinaldo Jr
Department of Pathology, University of Pittsburgh, PA, USA

Science baits laws with stars to catch telescopes.

E.E. Cummings, New Poems 16

INTRODUCTION

From an evolutionary standpoint, viral infections can be viewed as a competition between the pathogen and the host: in order for the latter to survive, the spread of the virus must be cleared or at the very least kept under strict control. For this to occur, an array of immune responses, both innate and adaptive, has to be implemented and, in particular, cell-mediated immunity has to develop faster than the spread of the pathogen within the host.

In human immunodeficiency virus type 1 (HIV-1) infection, in spite of the appearance of virus-specific CD8+ T cells that coincides with a rapid decline of plasma viremia, the virus continues to proliferate and eludes eradication by the immune system. Over the months following sero-conversion, a chronic, slowly progressive infection takes hold as a viral setpoint is established. With the exception of individuals who have a delay in disease progression due, for instance, to mutations in one of the viral receptors (CCR5 delta 32) (Dean et al., 1996; Liu et al., 1997), most individuals who are infected with HIV-1 will, if left untreated, eventually succumb to AIDS within an average of 10 years after a period of apparent quiescence. The variable rate of disease progression among infected subjects is influenced by virologic and host factors. The host's limited ability to control HIV-1 replication is attributed

to the unique propensity of the virus to infect the very cells that are responsible for fighting it, i.e. CD4+ T lymphocytes. This pathogenicity profile causes profound perturbations of the immune system – most notably, the hallmark of HIV-1 progressive infection is the depletion of CD4+ T cells. Yet, the nature and mechanisms by which this depletion occurs remain highly controversial.

As will be detailed below, the decision when to initiate combination anti-retroviral drug therapy (ART) is currently based on two well established parameters, or endpoints of HIV-1 infection, namely viral load and CD4+ T cell count measurements. However, to tailor better such toxic and costly treatment to individual needs, newer, improved surrogates of disease progression are needed. This review focuses on the assessment of immunity measured by the enumeration of HIV-1 specific CD8+ and CD4+ T cells.

CD4+ T CELL COUNTS AND HIV-1 RNA LOAD: STILL *SINE QUA NON* FOR PREDICTING HIV-1 DISEASE PROGRESSION

The sequence of events that takes place in the acute phase of HIV-1 infection has only recently been studied in detail in humans and non-human primates, particularly the SIV rhesus macaque model. The characteristics of the disease are essentially the same in both the human and the animal model, even though immunosuppression is considerably more rapid in monkeys. In humans, an acute

Measuring Immunity, edited by Michael T. Lotze and Angus W. Thomson
ISBN 0-12-455900-X, London

or primary HIV-1 infection is either asymptomatic or manifests itself as mononucleosis-like illness that lasts for several weeks (Fauci, 1988; Tindall et al., 1989) and is associated with high viremia and a significant drop in peripheral blood CD4$^+$ T cell counts (Lyles et al., 2000), resulting in the inversion of the normal CD4$^+$/CD8$^+$ ratio. In addition to the reduction of CD4$^+$ T cell numbers, the ratio inversion is due to an increase of CD8$^+$ T cell numbers, particularly those displaying an activated phenotype which is suggestive of a mounting cell mediated response to infection. However, the most convincing evidence for the fundamental role that CD8$^+$ T cells play in viral control comes from the SIV model in rhesus macaques, where in vivo ablation of CD8$^+$ T cells results in much higher levels of viral replication and faster development of full blown, irreversible immunosuppression (Matano et al., 1998; Jin et al., 1999; Schmitz et al., 1999). The transition between the acute and chronic phases is marked by a sharp fall in viral load which is associated with the rise in antigen-specific CTL (Koup et al., 1994; Borrow et al., 1994).

Acute infection shows an elevated increase in viral load and a rapid CD4$^+$ T cell depletion which results in a set point when a balance between the immune response and viral replication is reached. The chronic phase of the infection is characterized by very different viral and T cell dynamics. Plasma viral loads are lower but then rise slowly; peripheral blood CD4$^+$ T cell counts often recover partially from their lowest point during acute infection but then fall slowly over a period of years before the onset of AIDS. Infected individuals can develop AIDS after an average of 10 years of asymptomatic chronic infection without therapeutic intervention. However, the chronic phase is not immunologically silent, rather, it is marked by a high level of activation of both CD4$^+$ and CD8$^+$ T cells.

Mellors and associates (Mellors et al., 1995, 1996, 1997) were the first to define in depth a set of surrogate markers that have become crucial in predicting disease progression and helping establish therapeutic regimens. This body of work shows that plasma viral load is the single best predictor of progression to AIDS and death, followed by absolute counts of circulating CD4$^+$ lymphocytes. However, while plasma viral load is a strong independent predictor of the rate of decrease in CD4$^+$ lymphocyte counts and progression to AIDS and death, the prognosis of HIV-infected persons is more accurately defined when measurements of plasma HIV-1 RNA and circulating CD4$^+$ lymphocytes are combined (Geskus et al., 2003).

Other investigations have suggested that chronic activation, particularly manifested as expression of CD38 or CD28 and HLA DR on T cells, may be a better predictor of disease progression than plasma viral load (Simmonds et al., 1991; Giorgi et al., 1999; Roussanov et al., 2000; Leng et al., 2001; Choi et al., 2002). However, the interpretation of T cell dynamics in chronic HIV-1 infection is difficult due to contradictory studies and complicated methodologies. In some cases, 'high turnover' levels affect both CD4$^+$ and CD8$^+$ T cells (Mohri et al., 1998; Sachsenberg et al., 1998; Hellerstein et al., 1999; McCune et al., 2000), while other studies have not found this effect (Kovacs et al., 2001). Persistent hyperactivation has also been linked to loss of naive CD4$^+$ T cells (Hazenberg et al., 2003). In contrast, the SIV model has shown increased turnover rates in vivo in all T cell populations, with memory T cells being affected far more than naive (Rosenzweig et al., 1998; Mohri et al., 2001). Studies using Ki67 expression as a marker of cell proliferation have indicated that CD4$^+$ and CD8$^+$ T cell turnover increases in both naive and memory subsets during HIV-1 infection (Sachsenberg et al., 1998; Fleury et al., 2000; Hazenberg et al., 2000).

Treatment of HIV-1 infection has been revolutionized since the mid-1990s by the advent of potent combination antiretroviral therapy, termed ART (Volberding, 2003). Presently, AIDS is a manageable disease, albeit incurable. These treatments, however, should not be used indiscriminately as they have significant drawbacks including toxicity, development of antiviral drug resistance, adherence to complicated regimens and high expense. Thus, there is need to define laboratory parameters that signal when to introduce antiviral drug therapy in an HIV-1 infected person. To date, the most valuable laboratory parameters for deciding when to initiate or alter antiretroviral drug treatments are blood CD4$^+$ T cell numbers and viral RNA loads. Cohort studies of treatment efficacy have shown that low CD4$^+$ T cell numbers and not viral load at the initiation of treatment is the most powerful predictor of poor outcome (Bennett et al., 2002; Egger et al., 2002). Once on therapy, however, drug regimens may have to be altered depending on decreases in levels of HIV-1 RNA and increases in numbers of CD4$^+$ T cells over the first months (Hughes et al., 1997; Group, 2000; Demeter et al., 2001). If viral load on ART fails to go below a pre-therapy setpoint, CD4$^+$ T cell counts can eventually decrease (Deeks et al., 2002). A recent analytical review of the literature concluded that there is some clinical benefit in instituting immediate antiretroviral therapy in persons with CD4$^+$ T cell counts of 350×10^6 per liter (Phillips et al., 2003).

Immune responses mediated by CD4$^+$ T lymphocytes are a critical component in most viral infections but their importance in HIV-1 infected subjects has been controversial (Picker and Maino, 2000). In the course of chronic HIV-1 infection, an elevated impairment of CD4$^+$ T cell lymphoproliferative responses is common, with a strong negative association between the magnitude of the response and HIV viral load. The earliest T cell reactivity is specific for Env, with Gag specificity emerging thereafter (Malhotra et al., 2003). This early anti-Gag CD4$^+$ T cell response correlates with a lower viral set point (Patke et al., 2002). In long-term non-progressors, these T cell responses are preserved at high levels, as assessed by lymphoproliferation and production of IFN-γ and other cytokines (Rosenberg et al., 1997; Wilson et al., 2000).

Also, a restoration of CD4[+] T cell responses can be observed in patients on ART following acute infection (Rosenberg et al., 1997) but declines with prolonged ART (Pitcher et al., 1999). Intact anti-HIV-1 CD4[+] T cell responses are also necessary for maintenance of anti-HIV-1 CD8[+] T cell responses. In HIV-1 chronically infected persons, a positive correlation has been observed between gag p24 specific lymphoproliferation and anti-p24 CTLs, and a negative correlation with viral load (Kalams et al., 1999a). Moreover, the HIV-1 specificity of the repertoire of CD4[+] T cells during ART is quite diverse (Boritz et al., 2003). The capacity of CD4[+] T cells to produce IL-2 in response to HIV-1 antigen appears critical to maintenance of T cell lymphoproliferation and control of viral load in all phases of HIV-1 infection (Boaz et al., 2002; Iyasere et al., 2003; Hardy et al., 2003). These studies support the requirement of anti-HIV-1 CD4[+] T cell immune reactivity for control of HIV-1 infection.

Some investigations have not found a significant role of anti-HIV-1 CD4[+] T cells in control of HIV-1 infection (Betts et al., 2001a). Discrepancies among studies of anti-HIV-1 CD4[+] T cell function appear to be in part due to differences in assays. Indeed, when CD4[+] T cell IFN-γ production and lymphoproliferation were compared, differences in the estimate of antigen specific CD4[+] frequencies were shown. Furthermore, differences in CD4[+] T cell function among subjects on ART and those with high viral loads are evident only when lymphoproliferation and not IFNγ release is measured (Palmer et al., 2002). In another study (Wilson et al., 2000), IFN-γ production was detectable while proliferation was not in subjects with progressive infection.

MEASUREMENTS OF HIV SPECIFIC CD8[+] T CELL RESPONSES AND THEIR VALUE AS SURROGATE MARKERS

The development of highly sophisticated assays to determine the number and function of antigen specific CD8[+] T cells has helped to characterize the immune response more accurately in infected individuals. Hereafter, we will briefly describe these novel techniques and how they are changing our understanding of HIV infection.

Cytotoxic T lymphocytes

The most traditional way to measure the killing capacity of CD8[+] effector T cells, i.e. cytolytic T lymphocytes (CTLs), is the chromium release assay (CRA). This assay consists of incubating CTLs with radiolabeled autologous targets that express HIV-1 antigens by which the killing capacity is quantified through the measuring of the radioactivity released upon specific lysis of these targets. With the exception of a very few instances, effector T cells are, for the most part, too few or weak to be revealed when lymphocytes are measured directly from the peripheral

blood. Therefore a period of *in vitro* activation is required through which the CTLs are expanded in the presence of growth factors such as IL-2 and/or IL-15, as well as HIV antigens. However, interpretation of the immune response may be distorted due to *in vitro* activation. Culture conditions could change the immune response profile by either positively selecting activated rather than resting cells or by inducing cell death due to over stimulation. The relatively poor sensitivity of this assay is revealed by the necessity of greater than 1 per cent of circulating, antigen specific T cell frequencies that are needed to detect lytic function (Gotch et al., 1990; Moss et al., 1995).

The obvious result of these cell culture techniques is the great variability observed among studies and the relatively poor predictive power of these assays, which at best can be considered semi-quantitative. A refinement of bulk CTL assays, known as limiting dilution analysis or LDA, consists of culturing responder cells in decreasing numbers (from a few thousand to a few hundred) in several replicate wells for 2 weeks, which allows for an estimate of the frequency of precursor lymphocytes (pCTL). However, the same *in vitro* limitations exist for the bulk CTL assays: 10–15 cycles of cell division are required before sufficient proliferation occurs and one can ascertain measurement. Indeed, when LDA is compared to a more sophisticated and accurate enumeration of CTLs, such as tetramer staining or single cell enzyme immunoassay (ELISPOT), a 10- to 100-fold lower frequency is observed (Murali-Krishna et al., 1998; Kuroda et al., 1998). It should be noted that these discrepancies tend to disappear when improved culture techniques are employed (Goulder et al., 2000). Finally, the LDA method is extremely tedious, technically demanding and has resulted in great variability among different laboratories.

CTL reactivity, measured by these various methods, increases during acute infection in association with decline of HIV-1 load to a 'setpoint' (Borrow et al., 1994; Koup et al., 1994), suggesting that CTLs are involved in controlling HIV-1 replication. Notably, extremely rapid disease progression is associated with failure to mount an anti-HIV-1 CTL response (Demarest et al., 2001). Others have shown that in early HIV-1 infection, only the levels of Env specific memory CTLs and not Gag or Pol specific CTLs, are inversely correlated with RNA viral load (Musey et al., 1997). It has also been shown that the CTL response, which is highly focused toward a few epitopes during primary HIV infection, later broadens during the chronic phase (Dalod et al., 1999). However, only suggestive correlations have been found between levels of direct, circulating anti-HIV-1 CTL activity or CTL precursors and HIV RNA load (Grant et al., 1992; Klein et al., 1995; Cao et al., 1995; Rinaldo et al., 1995a, b; Harrer et al., 1996; Greenough et al., 1997). Inveritably, the level and diversity of CTL responses during progressive HIV-1 infection appear to be driven by the viral antigen burden (Rinaldo et al., 1998; Connick et al., 2001). Thus, increases in CTL precursor frequency, as well as IFN-γ producing

CD8+ T cells are linked to increases in viral load during the first years of infection, when the host's immune response is attempting to control the persistent, high-level turnover of viral antigen. In chronic progressive infection without treatment intervention, these CTL levels eventually decline as the viral load peaks and leads to AIDS (Klein et al., 1995). However, levels of CTLp decrease in relation to lowering of the viral burden during long-term ART (Kalams et al., 1999b). Therefore, during progressive HIV-1 infection, there is likely an antigenic threshold for maintaining a high level of CTL, whereas during successful antiviral treatment, the limited amount of antigen eventually leads to lower CTL levels (Jin et al., 2000).

Tetramer staining

Perhaps the most powerful new tool available to immunologists is the tetramer staining technique. Briefly, tetrameric molecular complexes of MHC class I that have previously been loaded with optimal peptide epitopes will directly bind to the T cell receptors (TCRs) present on the surface of antigen-specific CD8+ T cells (Altman et al., 1996). It is important to note that the binding event is independent of the functional capacity of tetramer positive T cells and does not require in vitro activation. Therefore, it is a representative snapshot of the magnitude of antigen-specific CD8+ T cells circulating in the periphery of an infected individual. The addition of an activation step has allowed for identification of defects in functional activity of antigen-specific cells. This is revealed by lower expression of the cytolytic function-associated molecule, perforin, in CD8+ T cells specific for HIV-1 as compared to cytomegalovirus (Appay et al., 2000). Although not a functional assay per se, tetramer staining correlates with other known techniques that evaluate ex vivo functional activity of lymphocytes. Importantly, this technique allows one to analyze, within a population of tetramer positive CD8+ T cells, the co-expression of cell surface markers. Notably, this is useful in the identification of the various phenotypic maturation states of lymphocytes (Mueller et al., 2001) and of intracellular cytokines or other effector molecules (Appay et al., 2000).

A significant association was found between slower disease progression and high frequencies of p17 gag tetramer binding CD8+ T cells (Ogg et al., 1999b). Individuals progressing to AIDS had lower frequencies of these cells. Up to 5 per cent tetramer positive CD8+ T cells can be detected in chronic infection, but a large proportion of these have been shown to be functionally impaired (Altman et al., 1996; Ogg and McMichael, 1999; Appay et al., 2000). There is one drawback to this powerful technique, however, in that each tetramer is unique for a particular TCR and therefore only allows detection of one HLA class I epitope, ultimately limiting the assay to known epitopes. Consequently, tetramers can measure the intensity but not the breadth of a T cell response.

Early data supported an association between a loss in the percentage of HIV-1 tetramer positive CD8+ T cells and increase in HIV-1 burden in the blood in HIV-1 disease progression (Ogg et al., 1998, 1999a). Subsequent work, however, indicated that the number of HIV-1 specific CD8+ T cells determined by tetramer staining persisted at high levels in progressors, while their anti-viral function declined (Kostense et al., 2001, 2002). Moreover, similar high levels of HIV-1 tetramer positive CD8+ T cells have been detected in long-term slow progressors as in non-progressors (Papagno et al., 2002). Chronically infected individuals on ART may demonstrate a decline in the level of T cells binding HIV-1 specific tetramers (Ogg et al., 1998), although this is less pronounced in some patients (Kalams et al., 1999b).

The loss of control of HIV-1 infection has further been linked to impaired maturation of CD8+ T cells, as shown by predominance of perforin negative, CD8+CD27+ T cells during HIV-1 infection (Appay et al., 2000). This has led to a more refined definition of memory and effector CD8+ T cells that may be a more competent measure of impaired T cell function during HIV-1 infection, with the loss of CD8+CD27- effector cells correlating with disease progression (van Baarle et al., 2002; Appay et al., 2002). Nevertheless, as revolutionary as the tetramer assay has been for defining T cell immunity, the level of tetramer positive CD8+ T cells has not yet proven to be a consistently strong correlate of immunity for HIV-1 infection.

ELISPOT and intracellular cytokine staining (ICS)

T lymphocytes respond to foreign antigen by proliferation and synthesis of cytokines – characteristically, CD8+ T cells synthesize IL-2 and IFN-γ. The production of IFN-γ is exploited as representative of function of cytotoxic CD8+ T cells. The enzyme-linked immunospot (ELISPOT) assay was developed as an adaptation of an ELISA and is delineated through the capture of cytokine secretion. The ELISPOT is capable of detecting very low frequencies of uncultured peptide-specific CD8+ T cells freshly isolated from peripheral blood (Mwau et al., 2002). Secretion of cytokine, in this case IFN-γ, is captured by antibody coated to the plate and then revealed through the use of a secondary antibody coupled to a chromogenic substrate. The locally secreted cytokine molecules form spots, with each one corresponding to an IFN-γ secreting cell. The number of spots detected allows one to determine the frequency of IFN-γ secreting cells specific for a given antigen in the analyzed sample.

This assay has been expanded from earlier use of viral vectors expressing single HIV-1 proteins to include the use of large libraries of HIV-1 peptides representing either known CTL epitopes for particular HLA class I haplotypes or 15 amino acid peptides overlapping by 11 amino acids for different HIV-1 proteins. This allows for simultaneous delineation of the quantity and breadth of the CD8+ T cell response to various HIV-1 proteins. These may be used in a matrix format consisting of multiple pools of up to 15 peptides each for screening purposes and used to fine-map the epitopes (Betts et al., 2001b; Mwau et al., 2002; Draenert et al., 2003).

Cytokine production by T cells can also be analyzed by ICS. When T cells are treated with inhibitors of secretion, such as brefeldin A (BFA) or monensin, they retain cytokine in the cytoplasm after antigen activation (Nylander and Kalies, 1999). Intracellular cytokine measurement usually requires larger cell numbers than does the ELISPOT assay. However, it remains the only reliable assay that determines simultaneously the type of cytokine produced by different cell phenotypes. In most situations, functional assays detect fewer cells than tetramer stains, although contradictory data have been reported. Nevertheless, the actual threshold of detection in human ELISPOT assays is generally very low – ~20 to 50 spots per million PBMC (0.002–0.005 per cent). Given that, on average, one in 3–10 tetramer positive T cells are positive in ELISPOT asays, this is often approximately the same end point as for detection by tetramers (0.01 per cent of PBMCs). In other words, in terms of ability to detect very low cell numbers, the assays are fairly similar.

Early work showed that stimulation with vaccinia virus vectors expressing HIV-1 proteins could quantitate HIV-1 specific CD8+ T cells by ELISPOT (Larsson et al., 1999; Huang et al., 2000), in weak association with disease progression. Recently, investigators have used pools of overlapping 15 mer or 20 mer HIV-1 peptides representing the whole length of HIV-1 proteins as stimulators in IFN-γ ELISPOT and ICS assays. This approach presumes that these peptides will not differentially compete for processing in antigen-presenting cells (APCs). In fact, most of these assays do not control for the number and function of APCs, ignoring the fundamental role of antigen presentation in T cell activation. In this regard, we have recently found that optimal presentation of exogenous peptides representing minimal 9 mer HLA class I epitopes requires uptake and vesicular trafficking in dendritic cells (Huang et al., 2004). This processing was comparable in dendritic cells from HIV-1 infected and uninfected persons. Moreover, autologous mature dendritic cells were the most potent APCs for stimulating HIV-1 specific CD8+ T cells.

Given these caveats, an inverse association has been reported for Gag-specific IFN-γ producing, CD8+ T cells and viral load in HIV-1 disease progression (Edwards et al., 2002). This procedure has also been advanced to assess the fine specificity of anti-HIV-1 T cell responses, using matrices of overlapping peptides for the whole HIV-1 genome (Addo et al., 2003). Interestingly, neither the breadth nor the magnitude of the CD8+ T cell response was associated with plasma virus load. This lack of association could be due in part to use of peptides representing sequences of proteins derived from laboratory strains of HIV-1. Given the huge genetic diversity of HIV-1, use of peptides based on autologous viral sequences may

improve the sensitivity and specificity of T cell assays, as suggested in a recent study of primary HIV-1 infection (Altfeld et al., 2003). Finally, initiating ART during early, primary HIV-1 infection can preserve anti-HIV-1 CTL responses in association with lowering of viral burden (Alter et al., 2003), although these CTL may have a limited breadth of antigenic reactivity (Altfeld et al., 2001).

T cell receptor (TCR) V analysis

The ability of the adaptive immune system to respond to a pathogen rests in the broad diversity of the TCR repertoire. When naive T cells are activated by the interaction between a TCR and its recognition of presented antigen that is bound to the MHC molecule, the T cell is instructed to proliferate and expand oligoclonally into differentiated memory cells.

However, HIV-1 infection affects T cell development; the virus impairs thymic output, thereby decreasing the number of both the CD4+ and CD8+ T cell populations (McCune, 2001). Persistent virus replication incites a chronic state of T cell activation that may ultimately result in clonal exhaustion due to continuous antigenemia (Lieberman et al., 2001). It is the combination of these events that enables HIV-1 to skew CD8+ T cell maturation and leads to an accumulation of CD8+ T cells that are activated and cannot effectively control the viral burden (Champagne et al., 2001). This may be manifested early in HIV-1 infection by oligoclonal V expansions of CD8+ T cells mediating HIV-1-specific cytotoxicity (Pantaleo et al., 1994, 1997). However, effective control of the high level of plasma viremia that occurs in primary infection is seen in individuals with oligoclonal (restricted TCR repertoire), as well as in those with polyclonal T cell responses. Moreover, perturbations in the CD8+ TCR repertoire are independent of clinical status or plasma viral load. Nonetheless, an association has been shown between the number of CD8+ V dominant clones and the percentage of CD4+ T cell HIV-1-infected children (Than et al., 1999). Recently, a concordance has been found between skewing of the TCR V repertoire within the CD45RA subset of CD8+ T cells and high viral load, low CD4+ T cell numbers in HIV-1 infected children (Kou et al., 2003). Potentially with more refined CDR3 length approaches, this method could be used as a predictor of HIV-1 disease progression.

CONCLUSIONS

To date we do not have a set of surrogate markers of immunological function that reliably predicts HIV-1 disease outcome or correlate with protection after vaccination. However, the assays have provided us with fundamental insights into the mechanisms responsible for the failure of the immune system to control HIV-1 infection, such as chronic immune activation and the exhaustion of effector memory cell pool. This has paved the way for potential interventions through immune reconstitution. Further refinement of these techniques should lead to suitable surrogates for predicting the efficacy of therapeutic regimens and tailoring treatment to individual patient needs.

REFERENCES

Addo, M. M., Yu, X. G., Rathod, A. et al. (2003). Comprehensive epitope analysis of human immunodeficiency virus type 1 (HIV-1)-specific T-cell responses directed against the entire expressed HIV-1 genome demonstrate broadly directed responses, but no correlation to viral load. J Virol 77, 2081–2092.

Alter, G., Hatzakis, G., Tsoukas, C. M. et al. (2003). Longitudinal assessment of changes in HIV-specific effector activity in HIV-infected patients starting highly active antiretroviral therapy in primary infection. J Immunol 171, 477–488.

Altfeld, M., Addo, M. M., Shankarappa, R. et al. (2003). Enhanced detection of human immunodeficiency virus type 1-specific T-cell responses to highly variable regions by using peptides based on autologous virus sequences. J Virol 77, 7330–7340.

Altfeld, M., Rosenberg, E. S., Shankarappa, R. et al. (2001). Cellular immune responses and viral diversity in individuals treated during acute and early HIV-1 infection. J Exp Med 193, 169–180.

Altman, J. D., Moss, P. A., Goulder, P. J. et al. (1996). Phenotypic analysis of antigen-specific T lymphocytes. Science 274, 94–96.

Appay, V., Dunbar, P. R., Callan, M. et al. (2002). Memory CD8+ T cells vary in differentiation phenotype in different persistent virus infections. Nat Med 8, 379–385.

Appay, V., Nixon, D. F., Donahoe, S. M. et al. (2000). HIV-specific CD8(+) T cells produce antiviral cytokines but are impaired in cytolytic function. J Exp Med 192, 63–75.

Bennett, K. K., DeGruttola, V. G., Marschner, I. C., Havlir, D. V. and Richman, D. D. (2002). Baseline predictors of CD4 T-lymphocyte recovery with combination antiretroviral therapy. J Acquir Immune Defic Syndr 31, 20–26.

Betts, M. R., Ambrozak, D. R., Douek, D. C. et al. (2001a). Analysis of total human immunodeficiency virus (HIV)-specific CD4(+) and CD8(+) T-cell responses: relationship to viral load in untreated HIV infection. J Virol 75, 11983–11991.

Betts, M. R., Casazza, J. P. and Koup, R. A. (2001b). Monitoring HIV-specific CD8+ T cell responses by intracellular cytokine production. Immunol Lett 79, 117–125.

Boaz, M. J., Waters, A., Murad, S., Easterbrook, P. J. and Vyakarnam, A. (2002). Presence of HIV-1 Gag-specific IFN-gamma+IL-2+ and CD28+IL-2+ CD4 T cell responses is associated with nonprogression in HIV-1 infection. J Immunol 169, 6376–6385.

Boritz, E., Palmer, B. E., Livingston, B., Sette, A. and Wilson, C. C. (2003). Diverse repertoire of HIV-1 p24-specific, IFN-gamma-producing CD4+ T cell clones following immune reconstitution on highly active antiretroviral therapy. J Immunol 170, 1106–1116.

Borrow, P., Lewicki, H., Hahn, B. H., Shaw, G. M. and Oldstone, M. B. (1994). Virus-specific CD8+ cytotoxic T-lymphocyte activity associated with control of viremia in primary human immunodeficiency virus type 1 infection. J Virol 68, 6103–6110.

Cao, Y., Qin, L., Zhang, L., Safrit, J. and Ho, D. D. (1995). Virologic and immunologic characterization of long-term survivors of human immunodeficiency virus type 1 infection. N Engl J Med 332, 201–208.

Champagne, P., Ogg, G. S., King, A. S. et al. (2001). Skewed maturation of memory HIV-specific CD8 T lymphocytes. Nature 410, 106–111.

Choi, B. S., Park, Y. K. and Lee, J. S. (2002). The CD28/HLA-DR expressions on CD4+T but not CD8+T cells are significant predictors for progression to AIDS. Clin Exp Immunol 127, 137–144.

Connick, E., Schlichtemeier, R. L., Purner, M. B. et al. (2001). Relationship between human immunodeficiency virus type 1 (HIV-1)-specific memory cytotoxic T lymphocytes and virus load after recent HIV-1 seroconversion. J Infect Dis 184, 1465–1469.

Dalod, M., Dupuis, M., Deschemin, J. C. et al. (1999). Weak anti-HIV CD8(+) T-cell effector activity in HIV primary infection. J Clin Invest 104, 1431–1439.

Dean, M., Carrington, M., Winkler, C. et al. (1996). Genetic restriction of HIV-1 infection and progression to AIDS by a deletion allele of the CKR5 structural gene. Hemophilia Growth and Development Study, Multicenter AIDS Cohort Study, Multicenter Hemophilia Cohort Study, San Francisco City Cohort, ALIVE Study. Science 273, 1856–1862.

Deeks, S. G., Barbour, J. D., Grant, R. M. and Martin, J. N. (2002). Duration and predictors of CD4 T-cell gains in patients who continue combination therapy despite detectable plasma viremia. Aids 16, 201–207.

Demarest, J. F., Jack, N., Cleghorn, F. R. et al. (2001). Immunologic and virologic analyses of an acutely HIV type 1-infected patient with extremely rapid disease progression. AIDS Res Hum Retroviruses 17, 1333–1344.

Demeter, L. M., Hughes, M. D., Coombs, R. W. et al. (2001). Predictors of virologic and clinical outcomes in HIV-1-infected patients receiving concurrent treatment with indinavir, zidovudine, and lamivudine. AIDS Clinical Trials Group Protocol 320. Ann Intern Med 135, 954–964.

Draenert, R., Altfeld, M., Brander, C. et al. (2003). Comparison of overlapping peptide sets for detection of antiviral CD8 and CD4 T cell responses. J Immunol Methods 275, 19–29.

Edwards, B. H., Bansal, A., Sabbaj, S., Bakari, J., Mulligan, M. J. and Goepfert, P. A. (2002). Magnitude of functional CD8+ T-cell responses to the gag protein of human immunodeficiency virus type 1 correlates inversely with viral load in plasma. J Virol 76, 2298–2305.

Egger, M., May, M., Chene, G. et al. (2002). Prognosis of HIV-1-infected patients starting highly active antiretroviral therapy: a collaborative analysis of prospective studies. Lancet 360, 119–129.

Fauci, A. S. (1988). The human immunodeficiency virus: infectivity and mechanisms of pathogenesis. Science 239, 617–622.

Fleury, S., Rizzardi, G. P., Chapuis, A. et al. (2000). Long-term kinetics of T cell production in HIV-infected subjects treated with highly active antiretroviral therapy. Proc Natl Acad Sci USA 97, 5393–5398.

Geskus, R. B., Miedema, F. A., Goudsmit, J., Reiss, P., Schuitemaker, H. and Coutinho, R. A. (2003). Prediction of residual time to AIDS and death based on markers and cofactors. J Acquir Immune Defic Syndr 32, 514–521.

Giorgi, J. V., Hultin, L. E., McKeating, J. A. et al. (1999). Shorter survival in advanced human immunodeficiency virus type 1 infection is more closely associated with T lymphocyte activation than with plasma virus burden or virus chemokine coreceptor usage. J Infect Dis 179, 859–870.

Gotch, F. M., Nixon, D. F., Alp, N., McMichael, A. J. and Borysiewicz, L. K. (1990). High frequency of memory and effector gag specific cytotoxic T lymphocytes in HIV seropositive individuals. Int Immunol 2, 707–712.

Goulder, P. J., Tang, Y., Brander, C. et al. (2000). Functionally inert HIV-specific cytotoxic T lymphocytes do not play a major role in chronically infected adults and children. J Exp Med 192, 1819–1832.

Grant, M. D., Smaill, F. M., Singal, D. P. and Rosenthal, K. L. (1992). The influence of lymphocyte counts and disease progression on circulating and inducible anti-HIV-1 cytotoxic T-cell activity in HIV-1-infected subjects. AIDS 6, 1085–1094.

Greenough, T. C., Brettler, D. B., Somasundaran, M., Panicali, D. L. and Sullivan, J. L. (1997). Human immunodeficiency virus type 1-specific cytotoxic T lymphocytes (CTL), virus load, and CD4 T cell loss: evidence supporting a protective role for CTL in vivo. J Infect Dis 176, 118–125.

Group, H. S. M. C. (2000). Human immunodeficiency virus type 1 RNA level and CD4 count as prognostic markers and surrogate end points: a meta-analysis. HIV Surrogate Marker Collaborative Group. AIDS Res Hum Retroviruses 16, 1123–1133.

Hardy, G. A., Imami, N., Sullivan, A. K. et al. (2003). Reconstitution of CD4+ T cell responses in HIV-1 infected individuals initiating highly active antiretroviral therapy (HAART) is associated with renewed interleukin-2 production and responsiveness. Clin Exp Immunol 134, 98–106.

Harrer, T., Harrer, E., Kalams, S. A. et al. (1996). Cytotoxic T lymphocytes in asymptomatic long-term nonprogressing HIV-1 infection. Breadth and specificity of the response and relation to in vivo viral quasispecies in a person with prolonged infection and low viral load. J Immunol 156, 2616–2623.

Hazenberg, M. D., Otto, S. A., van Benthem, B. H. et al. (2003). Persistent immune activation in HIV-1 infection is associated with progression to AIDS. AIDS 17, 1881–1888.

Hazenberg, M. D., Stuart, J. W., Otto, S. A. et al. (2000). T-cell division in human immunodeficiency virus (HIV)-1 infection is mainly due to immune activation: a longitudinal analysis in patients before and during highly active antiretroviral therapy (HAART). Blood 95, 249–255.

Hellerstein, M., Hanley, M. B., Cesar, D. et al. (1999). Directly measured kinetics of circulating T lymphocytes in normal and HIV-1-infected humans. Nat Med 5, 83–89.

Huang, X.-L., Fan, Z., Colleton, B.A. et al. (2004). Processing and presentation of exogenous HLA class I peptides by dendritic cells from HIV-1 infected and uninfected persons. J. Virol, in press.

Huang, X. L., Fan, Z., Kalinyak, C., Mellors, J. W. and Rinaldo, C. R. Jr (2000). CD8(+) T-cell gamma interferon production specific for human immunodeficiency virus type 1 (HIV-1) in HIV-1-infected subjects. Clin Diagn Lab Immunol 7, 279–287.

Hughes, M. D., Johnson, V. A., Hirsch, M. S. et al. (1997). Monitoring plasma HIV-1 RNA levels in addition to CD4+ lymphocyte count improves assessment of antiretroviral therapeutic response. ACTG 241 Protocol Virology Substudy Team. Ann Intern Med 126, 929–938.

Iyasere, C., Tilton, J. C., Johnson, A. J. et al. (2003). Diminished proliferation of human immunodeficiency virus-specific CD4+ T cells is associated with diminished interleukin-2 (IL-2) production and is recovered by exogenous IL-2. J Virol 77, 10900–10909.

Jin, X., Bauer, D. E., Tuttleton, S. E. et al. (1999). Dramatic rise in plasma viremia after CD8(+) T cell depletion in simian immunodeficiency virus-infected macaques. J Exp Med 189, 991–998.

Jin, X., Ogg, G., Bonhoeffer, S. et al. (2000). An antigenic threshold for maintaining human immunodeficiency virus type 1-specific cytotoxic T lymphocytes. Mol Med 6, 803–809.

Kalams, S. A., Buchbinder, S. P., Rosenberg, E. S. et al. (1999a). Association between virus-specific cytotoxic T-lymphocyte and helper responses in human immunodeficiency virus type 1 infection. J Virol 73, 6715–6720.

Kalams, S. A., Goulder, P. J., Shea, A. K. et al. (1999b). Levels of human immunodeficiency virus type 1-specific cytotoxic T-lymphocyte effector and memory responses decline after suppression of viremia with highly active antiretroviral therapy. J Virol 73, 6721–6728.

Klein, M. R., van Baalen, C. A., Holwerda, A. M. et al. (1995). Kinetics of Gag-specific cytotoxic T lymphocyte responses during the clinical course of HIV-1 infection: a longitudinal analysis of rapid progressors and long-term asymptomatics. J Exp Med 181, 1365–1372.

Kostense, S., Ogg, G. S., Manting, E. H. et al. (2001). High viral burden in the presence of major HIV-specific CD8(+) T cell expansions: evidence for impaired CTL effector function. Eur J Immunol 31, 677–686.

Kostense, S., Vandenberghe, K., Joling, J. et al. (2002). Persistent numbers of tetramer+ CD8(+) T cells, but loss of interferon-gamma+ HIV-specific T cells during progression to AIDS. Blood 99, 2505–2511.

Kou, Z. C., Puhr, J. S., Wu, S. S., Goodenow, M. M. and Sleasman, J. W. (2003). Combination antiretroviral therapy results in a rapid increase in T cell receptor variable region beta repertoire diversity within CD45RA CD8 T cells in human immunodeficiency virus-infected children. J Infect Dis 187, 385–397.

Koup, R. A., Safrit, J. T., Cao, Y. et al. (1994). Temporal association of cellular immune responses with the initial control of viremia in primary human immunodeficiency virus type 1 syndrome. J Virol 68, 4650–4655.

Kovacs, J. A., Lempicki, R. A., Sidorov, I. A. et al. (2001). Identification of dynamically distinct subpopulations of T lymphocytes that are differentially affected by HIV. J Exp Med 194, 1731–1741.

Kuroda, M. J., Schmitz, J. E., Barouch, D. H. et al. (1998). Analysis of Gag-specific cytotoxic T lymphocytes in simian immunodeficiency virus-infected rhesus monkeys by cell staining with a tetrameric major histocompatibility complex class I-peptide complex. J Exp Med 187, 1373–1381.

Larsson, M., Jin, X., Ramratnam, B. et al. (1999). A recombinant vaccinia virus based ELISPOT assay detects high frequencies of Pol-specific CD8 T cells in HIV-1-positive individuals. AIDS 13, 767–777.

Leng, Q., Borkow, G., Weisman, Z., Stein, M., Kalinkovich, A. and Bentwich, Z. (2001). Immune activation correlates better than HIV plasma viral load with CD4 T-cell decline during HIV infection. J Acquir Immune Defic Syndr 27, 389–397.

Lieberman, J., Shankar, P., Manjunath, N. and Andersson, J. (2001). Dressed to kill? A review of why antiviral CD8 T lymphocytes fail to prevent progressive immunodeficiency in HIV-1 infection. Blood 98, 1667–1677.

Liu, S. L., Schacker, T., Musey, L. et al. (1997). Divergent patterns of progression to AIDS after infection from the same source: human immunodeficiency virus type 1 evolution and antiviral responses. J Virol 71, 4284–4295.

Lyles, R. H., Munoz, A., Yamashita, T. E. et al. (2000). Natural history of human immunodeficiency virus type 1 viremia after seroconversion and proximal to AIDS in a large cohort of homosexual men. Multicenter AIDS Cohort Study. J Infect Dis 181, 872–880.

Malhotra, U., Holte, S., Zhu, T. et al. (2003). Early induction and maintenance of Env-specific T-helper cells following human immunodeficiency virus type 1 infection. J Virol 77, 2663–2674.

Matano, T., Shibata, R., Siemon, C., Connors, M., Lane, H. C. and Martin, M. A. (1998). Administration of an anti-CD8 monoclonal antibody interferes with the clearance of chimeric simian/human immunodeficiency virus during primary infections of rhesus macaques. J Virol 72, 164–169.

McCune, J. M. (2001). The dynamics of CD4+ T-cell depletion in HIV disease. Nature 410, 974–979.

McCune, J. M., Hanley, M. B., Cesar, D. et al. (2000). Factors influencing T-cell turnover in HIV-1-seropositive patients. J Clin Invest 105, R1–8.

Mellors, J. W., Kingsley, L. A., Rinaldo, C. R. Jr et al. (1995). Quantitation of HIV-1 RNA in plasma predicts outcome after seroconversion. Ann Intern Med 122, 573–579.

Mellors, J. W., Munoz, A., Giorgi, J. V. et al. (1997). Plasma viral load and CD4+ lymphocytes as prognostic markers of HIV-1 infection. Ann Intern Med 126, 946–954.

Mellors, J. W., Rinaldo, C. R. Jr, Gupta, P., White, R. M., Todd, J. A. and Kingsley, L. A. (1996). Prognosis in HIV-1 infection predicted by the quantity of virus in plasma. Science 272, 1167–1170.

Mohri, H., Bonhoeffer, S., Monard, S., Perelson, A. S. and Ho, D. D. (1998). Rapid turnover of T lymphocytes in SIV-infected rhesus macaques. Science 279, 1223–1227.

Mohri, H., Perelson, A. S., Tung, K. et al. (2001). Increased turnover of T lymphocytes in HIV-1 infection and its reduction by antiretroviral therapy. J Exp Med 194, 1277–1287.

Moss, P. A., Rowland-Jones, S. L., Frodsham, P. M. et al. (1995). Persistent high frequency of human immunodeficiency virus-specific cytotoxic T cells in peripheral blood of infected donors. Proc Natl Acad Sci USA 92, 5773–5777.

Mueller, Y. M., De Rosa, S. C., Hutton, J. A. et al. (2001). Increased CD95/Fas-induced apoptosis of HIV-specific CD8(+) T cells. Immunity 15, 871–882.

Murali-Krishna, K., Altman, J. D., Suresh, M. et al. (1998). Counting antigen-specific CD8 T cells: a reevaluation of bystander activation during viral infection. Immunity 8, 177–187.

Musey, L., Hughes, J., Schacker, T., Shea, T., Corey, L. and McElrath, M. J. (1997). Cytotoxic-T-cell responses, viral load, and disease progression in early human immunodeficiency virus type 1 infection. N Engl J Med 337, 1267–1274.

Mwau, M., McMichael, A. J. and Hanke, T. (2002). Design and validation of an enzyme-linked immunospot assay for use in clinical trials of candidate HIV vaccines. AIDS Res Hum Retroviruses 18, 611–618.

Nylander, S. and Kalies, I. (1999). Brefeldin A, but not monensin, completely blocks CD69 expression on mouse lymphocytes: efficacy of inhibitors of protein secretion in protocols for intracellular cytokine staining by flow cytometry. J Immunol Methods 224, 69–76.

Ogg, G. S., Jin, X., Bonhoeffer, S. et al. (1998). Quantitation of HIV-1-specific cytotoxic T lymphocytes and plasma load of viral RNA. Science 279, 2103–2106.

Ogg, G. S., Jin, X., Bonhoeffer, S. et al. (1999a). Decay kinetics of human immunodeficiency virus-specific effector cytotoxic T lymphocytes after combination antiretroviral therapy. J Virol 73, 797–800.

Ogg, G. S., Kostense, S., Klein, M. R. et al. (1999b). Longitudinal phenotypic analysis of human immunodeficiency virus type 1-specific cytotoxic T lymphocytes: correlation with disease progression. J Virol 73, 9153–9160.

Ogg, G. S. and McMichael, A. J. (1999). Quantitation of antigen-specific CD8+ T-cell responses. Immunol Lett 66, 77–80.

Palmer, B. E., Boritz, E., Blyveis, N. and Wilson, C. C. (2002). Discordance between frequency of human immunodeficiency virus type 1 (HIV-1)-specific gamma interferon-producing CD4(+) T cells and HIV-1-specific lymphoproliferation in HIV-1-infected subjects with active viral replication. J Virol 76, 5925–5936.

Pantaleo, G., Demarest, J. F., Soudeyns, H. et al. (1994). Major expansion of CD8+ T cells with a predominant V beta usage during the primary immune response to HIV. Nature 370, 463–467.

Pantaleo, G., Soudeyns, H., Demarest, J. F. et al. (1997). Evidence for rapid disappearance of initially expanded HIV-specific CD8+ T cell clones during primary HIV infection. Proc Natl Acad Sci USA 94, 9848–9853.

Papagno, L., Appay, V., Sutton, J. et al. (2002). Comparison between HIV- and CMV-specific T cell responses in long-term HIV infected donors. Clin Exp Immunol 130, 509–517.

Patke, D. S., Langan, S. J., Carruth, L. M. et al. (2002). Association of Gag-specific T lymphocyte responses during the early phase of human immunodeficiency virus type 1 infection and lower virus load set point. J Infect Dis 186, 1177–1180.

Phillips, A. N., Lepri, A. C., Lampe, F., Johnson, M. and Sabin, C. A. (2003). When should antiretroviral therapy be started for HIV infection? Interpreting the evidence from observational studies. AIDS 17, 1863–1869.

Picker, L. J. and Maino, V. C. (2000). The CD4(+) T cell response to HIV-1. Curr Opin Immunol 12, 381–386.

Pitcher, C. J., Quittner, C., Peterson, D. M. et al. (1999). HIV-1-specific CD4+ T cells are detectable in most individuals with active HIV-1 infection, but decline with prolonged viral suppression. Nat Med 5, 518–525.

Rinaldo, C., Huang, X. L., Fan, Z. F. et al. (1995a). High levels of anti-human immunodeficiency virus type 1 (HIV-1) memory cytotoxic T-lymphocyte activity and low viral load are associated with lack of disease in HIV-1-infected long-term nonprogressors. J Virol 69, 5838–5842.

Rinaldo, C. R. Jr, Beltz, L. A., Huang, X. L., Gupta, P., Fan, Z. and Torpey, D. J. 3rd (1995b). Anti-HIV type 1 cytotoxic T lymphocyte effector activity and disease progression in the first 8 years of HIV type 1 infection of homosexual men. AIDS Res Hum Retroviruses 11, 481–489.

Rinaldo, C. R. Jr, Gupta, P., Huang, X. L. et al. (1998). Anti-HIV type 1 memory cytotoxic T lymphocyte responses associated with changes in CD4+ T cell numbers in progression of HIV type 1 infection. AIDS Res Hum Retroviruses 14, 1423–1433.

Rosenberg, E. S., Billingsley, J. M., Caliendo, A. M. et al. (1997). Vigorous HIV-1-specific CD4+ T cell responses associated with control of viremia. Science 278, 1447–1450.

Rosenzweig, M., DeMaria, M. A., Harper, D. M., Friedrich, S., Jain, R. K. and Johnson, R. P. (1998). Increased rates of CD4(+) and CD8(+) T lymphocyte turnover in simian immunodeficiency virus-infected macaques. Proc Natl Acad Sci USA 95, 6388–6393.

Roussanov, B. V., Taylor, J. M. and Giorgi, J. V. (2000). Calculation and use of an HIV-1 disease progression score. AIDS 14, 2715–2722.

Sachsenberg, N., Perelson, A. S., Yerly, S. et al. (1998). Turnover of CD4+ and CD8+ T lymphocytes in HIV-1 infection as measured by Ki-67 antigen. J Exp Med 187, 1295–1303.

Schmitz, J. E., Kuroda, M. J., Santra, S. et al. (1999). Control of viremia in simian immunodeficiency virus infection by CD8+ lymphocytes. Science 283, 857–860.

Simmonds, P., Beatson, D., Cuthbert, R. J. et al. (1991). Determinants of HIV disease progression: six-year longitudinal study in the Edinburgh haemophilia/HIV cohort. Lancet 338, 1159–1163.

Than, S., Kharbanda, M., Chitnis, V., Bakshi, S., Gregersen, P. K. and Pahwa, S. (1999). Clonal dominance patterns of CD8 T cells in relation to disease progression in HIV-infected children. J Immunol 162, 3680–3686.

Tindall, B., Hing, M., Edwards, P., Barnes, T., Mackie, A. and Cooper, D. A. (1989). Severe clinical manifestations of primary HIV infection. AIDS 3, 747–749.

van Baarle, D., Kostense, S., Hovenkamp, E. et al. (2002). Lack of Epstein-Barr virus- and HIV-specific CD27−CD8+ T cells is associated with progression to viral disease in HIV-infection. AIDS 16, 2001–2011.

Volberding, P. A. (2003). HIV therapy in 2003: consensus and controversy. AIDS 17, S4–11.

Wilson, J. D., Imami, N., Watkins, A. et al. (2000). Loss of CD4+ T cell proliferative ability but not loss of human immunodeficiency virus type 1 specificity equates with progression to disease. J Infect Dis 182, 792–798.

Viral Responses – Epstein-Barr Virus

Chapter 51

David Rowe

Department of Infectious Diseases and Microbiology, Graduate School of Public Health, Pittsburgh, PA, USA

A flea and a fly in a flue,
Were imprisoned, so what could they do?
Said the fly, 'Let us flee!'
'Let us fly!' said the flea,
And they flew through a flaw in the flue.

A little fire is quickly trodden out;
Which, being suffered, rivers cannot quench

William Shakespeare, King Henry VI

INTRODUCTION

The human herpesviruses, as a group, all employ a similar acute/persistent strategy. Naive susceptible hosts are infected by transmission of virus through close contact with a shedding and possibly asymptomatic human carrier. Acute infection is characterized by a burst of virus replication accompanied by symptoms of disease that are usually mild but could be severe and that only end when specific cell-mediated immune responses isolate and eliminate virus-producing cells. Regardless of how vigorous it is, the immune response is always insufficient to eliminate all the virus infected cells and the new host becomes one more life-long persistent carrier. Persistent infection is characterized by a latent infection with episodic reactivation and a strong antiviral immune surveillance. Members of the α-, β- and γ-subfamilies of the Herpesviridae can be distinguished by the types of tissues within which the acute lytic replication occurs and the types of tissues within which viral genomes persist in the latent state (Rowe, 1999). These pathogenic tropisms are considered to be the consequence of an evolutionary process that adapts the acute/persistent strategy to the demands of different tissue environments.

Human herpesvirus 4 is one of the most widely distributed human herpesviruses (Rickinson and Kieff, 1996). More commonly known as Epstein-Barr virus (EBV), it is a lymphotropic gamma herpesvirus that replicates in B lymphocytes and is the causative agent of infectious mononucleosis. The virus is excreted in saliva and spread by close contact beginning at an early age. Primary infection is usually asymptomatic, but can manifest as a mononucleosis in young adults involving fever, sore throat and swollen lymph glands. Enlarged spleen or liver may be complications limiting a return to a fully active lifestyle during convalescence. There are no known complications (miscarriages or birth defects) affecting pregnancy. Over 95 per cent of adults in the USA are seropositive for EBV infection and thus have a persistent latent virus infection accompanied by periodic asymptomatic reactivation. The prevalence of infection is similar globally. This fact taken together with the generally mild course of disease and remarkable conservation of the viral genome (only two closely related strains are known) makes EBV the model for a successful parasite using the acute/persistent strategy. Understanding the mechanisms of establishing a persistent infection in the face of a targeted immune response has been a decades-long focus of research into the molecular biology of EBV infection.

Measuring Immunity, edited by Michael T. Lotze and Angus W. Thomson
ISBN 0-12-455900-X, London

One of the early realizations of this investigation was that vigilant immune surveillance against the virus is actually essential to health and well-being. An EBV infection in an immunocompromised host is a dangerous prospect accompanied by the constant risk of developing a fatal virus-driven lymphoproliferative disease. Indeed, an underlying immunodeficiency is the root cause of most of the tumors and lymphoproliferative diseases in which EBV seems to play a role. Immunosuppression accompanying solid organ transplantation creates an elevated risk of EBV disease with complications associated with B lymphocyte proliferation. Estimates of EBV-related post-transplant lymphoproliferative disease (PTLD) frequency range from 0.5 to 23 per cent depending on the organ grafted, the immunosuppressive regimen and the characteristics of the recipient (Kocoshis, 1994; Leblond et al., 1995; Lumbreras et al., 1995; Walker et al., 1995; Nalesnik, 1998). Over the course of the last decade, measuring the status of the EBV/host interaction has become an essential part of transplant patient management. Improving the means of assessing this interaction is a major goal of transplant-related clinical research. The available assays and those in development are aimed at measuring one or other of the factors in the virus/host balance. They examine either the activity of the virus or the response of the host.

MEASUREMENT OF EPSTEIN-BARR VIRUS ACTIVITY

Quantitating viral load in the peripheral blood of transplant recipients

A number of studies have shown that measurements of viral load in the peripheral blood by PCR can provide valuable supporting evidence in the diagnosis of PTLD (Wagner et al., 1992; Rowe et al., 1997; Green et al., 1998; Lucas et al., 1998; McDiarmid et al., 1998; Nalesnik, 1998; Kimura et al., 1999; Middledorp, 1999; Mutimer et al., 2000; Niesters et al., 2000; Vajro et al., 2000). The consensus of these studies is that EBV viral loads in the peripheral blood are elevated at the time of a diagnosis of PTLD. When measured by quantitative PCR assays, there is consistently a three to four orders of magnitude difference between the normal latent viral load of a healthy carrier and the load detected in a PTLD patient. Monitoring viral load in the peripheral blood by quantitative PCR provides early detection of infection and allows a means of gauging the effectiveness of therapeutic strategies aimed at treating EBV infections and lymphoproliferative diseases. Consequently, a number of reports describe a plethora of techniques to arrive at a measure of the load in the peripheral blood. Fractionation studies have shown that the load is primarily cell-associated and carried by B lymphocytes (Babcock et al., 1999; Rose et al., 2001). Quantitative assays which sample this compartment (those based on whole blood or PBMCs)

provide the most reproducible and readily interpretable results (Wadowsky et al., 2003). The type of assay (LightCycler, Taqman or qcPCR) and DNA target sequence, the standards employed and the denominator used (commonly/μDNA,/ml blood, /10^5 or /10^6 PBMCs) for reporting make inter-laboratory interpretation virtually impossible (Rowe et al., 2001). Thus, the values and thresholds described below apply only to the qcPCR assay performed on PBMCs. However, the general trends, with the rises and falls in load associated with various stages of disease, are also observed in serial monitoring with other assays.

A viral load immediately after transplant is very rare (sensitivity: 1 genome/10^5 PBMCs), however, most pediatric transplant recipients (approximately 70 per cent) become viral load positive within the first year post-transplant. Using the qcPCR assay we have established a threshold value of >200 genome copies/10^5 PBMCs as the threshold value for symptomatic EBV disease and/or PTLD (Green et al., 1999). Initial detection of the rising viral load still below the threshold value may be obtained with a telescoping series of load measurements (every 2 weeks for the first 3 months post-transplant, monthly for the next 3 months post-transplant and every 2 months thereafter to the end of the first year post-transplant). Our experience with intestinal transplant recipients prior to PCR monitoring was a 40 per cent incidence of PTLD. After the introduction of viral load monitoring, we followed 30 pediatric intestinal transplant recipients with survival greater than 3 months under a pre-emptive therapy protocol. Viral loads of 40 copies/10^5 PBLs in pre-transplant seronegatives and 200 copies/10^5 PBLs in pre-transplant seropositives were treated with i.v. ganciclovir (10 mg/kg in two divided doses) and i.v. CMV-IG (CytoGam, Medimmune, Inc. Gaithersburgh, MD) in three separate 100 mg/kg doses during the first 7 days after initiation of therapy. When possible, the level of immunosuppression was also reduced at or near the time of therapy. Eighteen patients experienced elevated viral loads which were treated. In 13 patients the viral load fell and none developed PTLD. PTLD developed in five patients. Two of the five patients developing PTLD violated the protocol and did not receive timely pre-emptive therapy after the rising viral loads were identified. The three other patients received appropriate pre-emptive therapy which failed to prevent the development of disease. When the two protocol violators are removed, the incidence of PTLD in the pediatric intestinal transplant population at our center had dropped to 11 per cent (21). In another study, we examined liver transplant recipients presenting with a diagnosis of PTLD and a high viral load (between 1000 and 20 000 copies/10^5 PBMCs). The viral load dropped below 200 copies/10^5 cells in all patients a mean 19 days following withdrawal or reduction in immune suppression. The decline in viral load correlated with regression in PTLD and with the onset of rejection (Green et al., 1998).

Regardless of whether patients have been pre-emptively treated or not, or whether there is a history of PTLD, about two-thirds of the pediatric transplant recipients we have monitored serially eventually developed a persistently elevated viral load. An elevated load is one that is at least detectable in the qcPCR assay which becomes sensitive at two to three orders of magnitude above the value expected for a normal healthy carrier. Most of these loads (80 per cent) are below the threshold value of 200 copies/10^5 PBMCs, but some are above the threshold. Fluorescence *in situ* hybridization (FISH) studies with peripheral blood B cells from load carriers below the threshold value revealed that the circulating virus-infected B cells harbored one or two genome copies/cell, in line with the estimated per cell copy numbers for latently infected cells in healthy carriers (Miyashita et al., 1995, 1997; Rose et al., 2002). The load in these carriers seems to be due to a higher number of essentially normal latently infected B cells. Load carriers above the threshold also had low copy cells but, in addition, carried a distinct population of B cells with high numbers of viral genome copies. Higher viral loads were associated with more high copy cells in the circulation. Not surprisingly, high copy cells also predominated in FISH analyses of peripheral blood from PTLD patients with very high viral loads (Rose et al., 2002).

These studies clearly indicate that the EBV load measurements made on peripheral blood specimens do not simply measure a continuum of identically infected B cells. There are at least two types readily identifiable. This helps to explain why antiviral therapies can reduce the very high loads of PTLD, but cannot eliminate the residual persistent viral loads that most assays are able to detect in convalescing PTLD patients.

Profiling viral gene expression in the peripheral blood of transplant recipients

One lesson from viral load monitoring is that there are circumstances when the number of circulating viral genomes is not sufficiently informative to allow a diagnostic or prognostic interpretation. Some additional information that would allow us to know the state of the virus infection (e.g. is it a latent infection, a lymphoproliferative state or an acute virus-productive infection?) would provide a better assessment of the condition of the patient. Since different genes are expressed in latent versus proliferative or virus-productive states, a measure of the patterns of viral gene expression could reveal what is happening. While there are over 85 open reading frames (ORFs) in the EBV genome, expression of only around 10 genes is detected in proliferating B cells *in vitro* and different subsets of these are characteristically expressed in latency, EBV-associated tumors and lymphoproliferative diseases (Tierney et al., 1994; Rowe, 1998; Küppers, 2003). Thus, detecting expression of a panel of these genes by RT-PCR might provide an adjunct to viral load

measurements that would clearly reveal the status of the virus/host balance. EBNA1, EBNA2, LMP1 and LMP2a are the most likely candidate genes as their expression was often detected in PBL specimens collected close to the diagnosis of PT-LPD (Qu et al., 2000). Among these, EBNA2 and LMP2a were the most consistently detectable gene products. In addition, two distinct expression patterns related to the level of persistent viral load were identified. Patients carrying persistent viral loads up to 200 copies/10^5 lymphocytes expressed LMP2a only, a state of viral infection transcriptionally indistinguishable from the latency that has been described in healthy individuals (Babcock et al., 1999; Qu et al., 2000). Patients carrying persistent viral loads above 200 copies/10^5 lymphocytes expressed LMP2a and LMP1, a unique pattern of transcription. Since EBNA2 expression was always associated with PTLD and was not detected in the persistent load carrier state, an assay based on detection of EBNA2 gene expression is under investigation as a useful RNA marker for distinguishing an elevated load carrier state from an active disease process.

MEASUREMENT OF ANTI-EPSTEIN-BARR VIRUS IMMUNE RESPONSES

Humoral immune responses

Before a causative agent was known, a diagnosis of infectious mononucleosis was made when the typical symptoms appeared (fever, sore throat and swollen lymph glands) and a routine CBC showed an elevated white blood cell count and the presence of atypical (activated) lymphocytes. A positive reaction in a 'mono-spot' test for non-specific sheep-red-blood-cell agglutinating antibodies confirmed the diagnosis (Thiele and Okano, 1993; Obel et al., 1996). Once EBV was discovered in the late 1960s, the association between the stages of disease and the EBNA (Epstein-Barr nuclear antigen), EA (early antigen) and VCA (viral capsid antigen) specific antibody responses was determined. These three 'antigen' designations do not represent individual epitopes or proteins but classes of proteins derived from the more than 85 open reading frames present in the viral genome (Rickinson and Kieff, 1996). Linking the major epitopes within each class to the products of specific viral ORFs has led to the production of a number of ELISA assays employing purified recombinant proteins (Thiele and Okano, 1993; Nebel-Schickel et al., 1994; van Grunsven et al., 1994; Shedd et al., 1995; Votava et al., 1996; Obel et al., 1996; Mitchell et al., 1998; Buisson et al., 1999; Bruu et al., 2000; Schaade et al., 2001; Rea et al., 2002; Gartner et al., 2003). Not surprisingly, these tests have greater sensitivity (100 per cent) and specificity (97 per cent) than the mono-spot assay, particularly in young children where mono-spot tests are sometimes negative (Votava et al., 1996; Schaade et al., 2001).

In general, IgM antibodies against EA and VCA are detected 1–2 weeks after infection while IgG antibody titers against these antigens peak in the acute phase of mononucleosis. EBNA responses emerge later during convalescence when anti-EA disappears and anti-VCA becomes very low or non-detectable. When researchers talk about human subjects and their seroconversion to an EBV positive status, they are usually referring to the persistent low titer IgG anti-EBNA1 response that nearly all individuals develop after infection (Nebel-Schickel et al., 1994). In addition to this, there often persists a low level anti-VCA response dominated by an epitope on the BFRF3 ORF (van Grunsven et al., 1994; Shedd et al., 1995). Because the anti-EA response is transient, a lack of EA antibodies is usually considered indicative of a latent infection, while the presence of anti-EA indicates a recent or ongoing active replicative process. Current serological methods based on detection of IgM antibodies to VCA and EBNA do not clearly differentiate between a primary infection and a reactivation of latent virus (Robertson et al., 2003). IgG avidity state (a measure of affinity maturation) may have the potential to distinguish a recent from past or reactivated infection. In one study, avidity measurement improved the sensitivity of serologic diagnosis of primary EBV infection from 93 to 100 per cent. The specificity of IgM anti-VCA testing alone was poor (49 per cent false-positive results), but improved to 97 per cent by the demonstration of high-avidity IgG anti-VCA. The combination of negative IgG anti-EBNA and low-avidity IgG anti-VCA had a sensitivity and specificity of 100 per cent (Robertson et al., 2003).

The persistent anti-EBV antibody responses seen in adults are generally considered to be of little or no consequence in protecting against infection or reactivation. For this reason there has been essentially no effort made to develop vaccines that recreate these humoral responses in naive hosts. However, a recent study of EBV infection in infancy showed that maternal anti-EBV antibodies were readily detected in cord blood and infant serum (Chan et al., 2001). The most remarkable observation from the infant study was the abrupt onset of primary infection after a delay of 8 months, implying a protective role for the maternal anti-EBV antibodies. Regardless of whether humoral responses are immunologically useful or not, the antibodies raised against EBV after infection have been exploited in a steady stream of publications over the last three decades to attempt to make correlations between EBV and various diseases, syndromes and cancers. The ultimate objective of a serological study would be an assay that in clinical settings was able to either exclude or confirm the diagnosis of a particular EBV associated disease. Perhaps the most intense search has been for a means of serologically screening large populations of Chinese for nasopharyngeal carcinoma (NPC). In this quest, assays for IgA antibodies to either EBNA or VCA appear to have the most utility, but none of the plethora of assays for Igs with varying heavy chain isotype and antigenic specificity has individually met this objective (Sigel et al., 1994; Liu et al., 1997; Chan et al., 1998, 2003; Ho et al., 1998; Liu and Yeh, 1998; Kantakamalakul et al., 2000; Tiwawech et al., 2003; Leung et al., 2004). A recent study combining an anti-EBNA1 IgA assay and an anti-Zta (one of the EA antigens) IgG assay produced a confirmed negative result with a negative predictive value of 99.1 per cent, providing a clear indicator that excludes a diagnosis of NPC. A confirmed positive result was associated with a positive predictive value of 86.8 per cent providing a clear indicator to proceed with a more expensive diagnostic work-up of NPC (Chan et al., 2003). The addition of a viral DNA load PCR assay to an IgA anti-VCA serological assay improves the accuracy of detection of NPC by identifying serological false positives (Leung et al., 2004).

In other diseases under investigation, the associations between the disease and anti-EBV humoral responses are less clear. EBV is associated with a variety of lymphoid malignancies including Burkitt's lymphoma, B non-Hodgkin's lymphomas, T/NK cell lymphomas and more than half of Hodgkin's lymphomas (Levine et al., 1994; Mitarnun et al., 2002; Wakiguchi, 2002). For Hodgkin's lymphoma, individuals with a history of mononucleosis and elevated EBNA and VCA antibodies are at greater risk of disease but there is not a strong correlation between EBV serology and presence of EBV in the Reed-Sternberg (RS) cells of Hodgkin's patients (Levine et al., 1994; Alexander et al., 1995; Enblad et al., 1997; Meij et al., 2002). Antibodies to LMP1 (a viral protein that is often highly expressed in RS cells) were detected in 30 per cent of the EBV-seropositive Hodgkin's disease patients. LMP1 epitopes are not typically part of the humoral response to EBV infection and the anti-LMP1 response detected was not part of a distinct anti-EBV antibody profile. While significantly more patients with EBV-positive tumors had anti-LMP1 responses, antibodies to LMP1 did not correlate with expression of LMP1 in the RS cells. The strongest antibody responses to LMP1 were among patients with EBV-negative RS cells, suggesting that the response might directly or indirectly be associated with immune surveillance (Meij et al., 2002). Many of the malignancies with an EBV association show elevations of anti-EA responses reminiscent of viral reactivation and may be the consequence of reduced immune surveillance. Serological studies have shown an association between EBV humoral responses and T cell lymphoma, hairy cell leukemia and gastric carcinoma (Jumbou et al., 1997; Nordstrom et al., 1999; Shinkura et al., 2000; Szkaradkiewicz et al., 2002; Chan et al., 2003). Diseases with clearly recognized underlying immunologic dysregulation such as rheumatoid arthritis, autoimmune thyroiditis, multiple sclerosis, chronic fatigue syndrome and AIDS also show elevation of anti-EBV antibodies with profiles suggestive of virus reactivation (Vrbikova et al., 1996; Myhr et al., 1998; Blaschke et al., 2000; O'Sullivan et al., 2002; Stevens et al., 2002; Hollsberg et al., 2003).

Even healthy individuals can develop similar serological signs of EBV reactivation when placed under psychological or physical stress (Glaser et al., 1999; Stowe et al., 2000). These findings serve to emphasize the point that constant immunosurveillance against EBV is essential to the health and well-being of an individual and that altered serological responses to EBV are not sufficient evidence of a causative link between the virus and a particular disease.

Therapeutic immunosuppression to prevent graft rejection following organ transplantation places the patient at risk for PTLD and other complications associated with EBV reactivation (Harwood et al., 1999; Webber, 1999; Schwab et al., 2000; Loren et al., 2003; Verschuuren et al., 2003). Serologically, no clear pattern of anti-EBV responses has been suggested to presage the development of PTLD. Early studies indicated that anti-EBNA titers often decreased and anti-VCA titers rose slightly following transplant (Preiksaitis et al., 1992; McKnight et al., 1994; Riddler et al., 1994; Rogers et al., 1997). Recent work shows that because of the immunosuppression, there is a rather limited humoral response to primary EBV infection in transplant recipients (Verschuuren et al., 2003). It is dominated by anti-VCA antibodies with little or no anti-EA and no anti-EBNA. There is also no striking change in antibody profile or titers preceding a clinical diagnosis of PTLD. These results suggest that direct measures of viral load are more sensitive at detecting the onset of PTLD than serological assays. One recent study showed that when transplant patients developed anti-EA antibodies concomitant with a rising EBV DNA load they did not go on to develop PTLD, making the anti-EA response a potentially useful tool for discriminating the high EBV loads associated with persistent infections under control from the high EBV loads preceding development of lymphoproliferative states (Carpentier et al., 2003).

Cell-mediated immune responses

In the immunocompetent host, cell-mediated, rather than humoral, responses are presumed to be responsible for controlling EBV infection. Acute infection with EBV elicits a pronounced cellular immune response which results in the production of large numbers of specific CD8+ cytotoxic T cells (CTL) (Catalina et al., 2002; Callan, 2003; Precopio et al., 2003). EBV-specific CTL responses have been characterized in immunocompetent individuals for both the primary response during infectious mononucleosis and for the long-term immunosurveillance in persistent carrier state (Catalina et al., 2002; Hislop et al., 2002; Rickinson, 2002; Callan, 2003). The primary response is dominated by epitope specificities drawn from proteins expressed during virus production (particularly from the genes BZLF1 and BMLF1). The frequency of T cells in the circulation with these epitope specificities can exceed 40 per cent of the total CD8$^+$ T cell population (Callan et al., 1998). These viral gene products also contribute to

the humoral anti-EA antibody response, and like the antibody response, the frequency of BZLF1 and BMLF1 specific T cells is significantly reduced upon resolution of acute infection (Catalina et al., 2002; Macallan et al., 2003). CD8$^+$ T cells with epitope specificities to the EBNA proteins are less abundant in acute phase mononucleosis but increase during convalescence and predominate in healthy carriers (Hislop et al., 2002).

Healthy carriers of a latent infection maintain circulating CTL precursors (CTLp) at frequencies in the range of 1/100 to 1/500 circulating T cells when measured by functional assays (Yang et al., 2000). The frequency of T cells specific for EBV epitopes is much higher (1/400 to 1/42 000) when analyses are based on peptide loaded HLA tetramer staining, but it is likely that not all the positive cells are functional (Bourgeault et al., 1991; Redchenko and Rickinson, 1999; Munz et al., 2000; Catalina et al., 2002; Ouyang et al., 2003). This large pool of CTLp is apparently needed for surveillance against virus reactivation. Although the frequency of CTLp is high, the range of specificity for EBV target antigens is rather narrow. Peptide epitopes are drawn primarily from the three EBNA3 proteins (EBNA3A, EBNA3B and EBNA3C) (Murray et al., 1992; Tamaki et al., 1995; Rickinson et al., 1998; Tan et al., 1999; Leen et al., 2001) and CTLs from any given latent virus carrier predominantly target just one or two EBNA3 epitopes. Subdominant epitopes are mainly derived from the protein products of the LMP2 gene. CTL epitope dominance in immune responses is HLA allele-specific, with each HLA allele presenting a particular set of epitopes. HLA-B alleles appear to be more efficient in presenting antigens to CD8$^+$ T cells than the HLA-A alleles (Albert et al., 1998; Blake et al., 2000). By their expression of co-stimulatory markers (CD27 and CD28), anti-EBV memory T cells appear to retain the phenotype of T cells in an early stage of differentiation (Appay et al., 2002). After comparison with other viruses that also have acute/persistent infection strategies, it appears likely that, in each case, distinct and characteristic CD8+ T cell phenotypes arise depending on the pathogen. Ascribing strict effector and memory functions to T cell subsets with different differentiation phenotypes is probably inappropriate (Appay et al., 2002).

Interestingly, EBNA1, which dominates in the humoral response of healthy carriers, evades proteolytic antigen processing and largely escapes CD8$^+$ CTL-mediated immune surveillance. Recent reports demonstrate the existence of EBV-specific CD4$^+$ T cells mediating IFNγ and cytolytic responses against EBNA1 expressing cells (Munz et al., 2000; Leen et al., 2001; Paludan et al., 2002; Nikiforow et al., 2003). CD4$^+$ T cells recognizing a major HLA DR presented peptide from the EA antigen BHRF1 also efficiently killed EBV infected B cells (Landais et al., 2004). Primary infection with EBV stimulates a significant, early CD4$^+$ T cell response with the frequency of responding CD4$^+$ T cells ranging from 0.04 to 5.2 per cent.

Because healthy latent carriers have very low or undetectable EBV specific CD4+ T cells, it has been suggested that many of the primary CD4+ effector cells die or lose functional capacity. A smaller population of CD4+ T cells is apparently sufficient to provide surveillance during the persistent phase of infection (Amyes et al., 2003). The levels of cytokines produced by CD4+ T cells in response to viral antigens, with predominance of Th1 (IFNγ) versus Th2 (IL4) profiles, are good predictors of the outcome of virus infection (Yang et al., 2000; Catalina et al., 2002; Attarbaschi et al., 2003). This type of response to EBV antigens highlights the potential importance of CD4+ T cells in the control of EBV latency and suggests that eliciting or augmenting CD4+ all responses could have major therapeutic significance (Gao et al., 2002).

There are EBV-specific CD8+ T cells in transplant recipients when EBV infection occurs in the context of impaired immunity. CD8+ T cells specific for both BZLF1 and EBNA3A epitopes were detected by tetramer staining of blood from a small cohort of seronegative pediatric liver and kidney organ transplant patients a few weeks after receiving an organ from a seropositive donor (Falco et al., 2002). The cells had an activated/memory phenotype, but their frequency was an order of magnitude lower than expected for an immunocompetent response. This demonstrates that CTL responses can be generated in solid organ transplant recipients and suggests that immunosuppression is reducing the magnitude of the response while not eliminating it entirely. Consistent with this is the observation that the frequency of PTLD is directly correlated with the intensity and duration of the immunoablative therapy prior to bone marrow transplantation (BMT) (Meijer et al., 2002; Carpentier et al., 2003). The probability of developing PTLD in BMT recipients is directly correlated to the time required post-transplant for the recipient to develop CTLp frequencies comparable to those of normal seropositive adults. PTLD is extremely rare when BMT patients receive non-T cell depleted marrow (Patton et al., 1990; Papadopoulos et al., 1994; Lucas et al., 1996; Heslop et al., 1999; Meijer et al., 2002). Not surprisingly, low dose immunosuppression also reduces the incidence of PTLD in pediatric solid organ transplant recipients (Ganschow et al., 2004). In transplant patients, EBV specific CD8+ T cell frequencies inversely correlate with positivity in an assay for spontaneous outgrowth of EBV infected B cells. Reduction in immunosuppression increases the CD8+ all frequency while reducing the spontaneous outgrowth frequency. Measuring the EBV specific T cell response in immunocompromised patients with a primary EBV infection has been suggested as a predictive marker for the risk for post-transplant lymphoproliferative disease (Smets et al., 2002).

It is clearly understandable that the most effective approach to the treatment of EBV-associated lymphoproliferative disease in transplant recipients is reduction and/or withdrawal of immunosuppression (Meijer et al., 2003). However, this therapeutic approach is limited by a number of factors, the most serious of which is development of acute or chronic allograft rejection. Antiviral therapy with acyclovir and gancyclovir has been shown to be effective when administered prophylactically for polyclonal lymphoproliferations or/and in conjunction with reduction in immunosuppression (Armitage et al., 1991; Aris et al., 1996). Surgical resection or emergency radiotherapy has also been employed to treat rapidly growing circumscribed tumors, with variable outcome. However, PTLD is a systemic disease that cannot be dealt with by local therapy alone. For PTLD that is refractory to the interventions described above, chemotherapy is employed. There is significant morbidity and further suppression of the function of cytotoxic T cells (Chen et al., 1993; Cockfield et al., 1993). As a consequence, the use of immunotherapeutic approaches together with reduction in immunosuppression and/or antiviral therapy to treat refractory PTLD has gained considerable recent support. Adoptive immunotherapy with *ex vivo* generated donor EBV-specific T lymphocytes for PTLD following bone marrow transplantation (BMTx) has been shown efficiently to control B cell lymphoproliferations by restoring antitumor/antiviral immune surveillance (Slobod et al., 2001; Wagner et al., 2002; Sherritt et al., 2003). Adoptive immunotherapy with bulk unselected T cells was first described by Papadopoulos et al. (1994) and was designed to restore anti-EBV CTL responses in transplant patients. Since then, several groups have used the same approach to treat PTLD in BMTx (Slobod et al., 2001; Wagner et al., 2002; Sherritt et al., 2003). The procedure involves generating autologous B lymphoblastoid cell lines (LCLs) that express and present latency associated viral proteins which are used to expand a population of donor provided EBV-specific CTLs *in vitro*. After infusion, these polyclonal EBV-specific CTLs provide the anti-EBV immune surveillance that targets proliferating virus infected B cells. Infused T cells persist for up to 18 months after administration and offer long-term protection against subsequent EBV challenges (Wagner et al., 2002; Gottschalk et al., 2002; Meijer et al., 2003; Sherritt et al., 2003). Adoptive immunotherapy for PTLD following solid organ transplant involves generating LCLs and CTLs from the immunosuppressed recipient and requires that the patient have a pre-existing circulating pool of anti-EBV memory T cells (Savoldo et al., 2001; Comoli et al., 2002; Gottschalk et al., 2002; Porcu et al., 2002; Sherritt et al., 2003). For patients who are EBV-seronegative at the time of the transplant (the group at highest risk), this approach is not suitable, since there is no expandable memory T cell pool. Two approaches are under consideration to solve this problem. The first involves the transfer of heterologous but HLA-matched EBV specific CD8+ T cells (Haque et al., 2001). Investigators envision one day having a bank of anti-EBV T cells with different histotypes that could be tapped for immunotherapy for almost anyone. The second strategy uses novel strategies for *ex vivo* generation of autologous EBV-specific CTLs from naive T cell pools using EBV peptide loaded dendritic cells (DCs). Both strategies hold the promise that T cell therapy may soon be extended to the highest risk patients (Savoldo et al., 2001, 2002; Popescu et al., 2003).

Vaccines

Our knowledge of the natural humoral and cell-mediated responses that control EBV infection has been employed in developing various vaccine strategies. In the humoral immunity approach, it has been shown that antibodies to a recombinant viral envelope glycoprotein gp350 are neutralizing (Jackman et al., 1999) and a gp350 subunit vaccine did confer protection in a model of EBV-induced B cell lymphoma in cotton-top tamarins (Morgan, 1992; Finerty et al., 1994; Cox et al., 1998). A DNA-based gp350 vaccine raised humoral and cell-mediated responses in mice (Jung et al., 2001). In the most advanced study to date, a live recombinant vaccinia vaccine expressing gp350 has been constructed and tested in humans. All vaccinated infants developed neutralizing antibodies to gp350, and over a 16-month follow-up period all 10 unvaccinated control infants became infected while only three of nine vaccinated infants became infected (Gu et al., 1995). This is the first demonstration of protection against and/or delay of EBV infection by a vaccine in humans.

Because of the pivotal role of $CD8^+$ T cell responses in controlling the proliferation of EBV infected cells, T cell vaccines have been pursued with the aim of curbing or controlling the excesses of infectious mononucleosis, PTLD, Burkitt's lymphoma (BL), NPC and HD (Moss et al., 1998; Bharadwaj and Moss, 2002; Lin et al., 2002). Direct peptide immunization approaches have been tried first with limited but encouraging efficacy (Moss et al., 1998; Lin et al., 2002). A first attempt at therapeutic vaccination of nasopharyngeal carcinoma patients with peptides representing T cell epitopes loaded onto dendritic cells (DCs) produced mixed results (Lin et al., 2002). Adenoviral-mediated gene transfer of the LMP2A protein into DCs efficiently directed $CD8^+$ effector cell production in vitro and could be a better approach to vaccine-mediated augmentation of immune responses to tumors expressing EBV antigens (Gahn et al., 2001). Much effort has recently gone into tailoring virus vectors to deliver immunodominant class I and class II epitopes (Thomson et al., 1998; Taylor et al., 2004). There is a recombinant vaccinia candidate vaccine that encodes a polyepitope protein comprising six HLA A2-restricted epitopes derived from LMP1 that is designed specifically for therapeutic augmentation of CTL responses in patients with HD and NPC (Duraiswamy et al., 2003). There is also a recently described vaccinia vaccine recombinant that expresses the CD4 epitope-rich C-terminal domain of EBNA1 fused to full-length LMP2. This vaccine candidate reactivated $CD4^+$ and $CD8^+$ T cells in vitro, an ideal effect if one is hoping for a strong and sustained T cell response akin to natural immunosurveillance (Taylor et al., 2004).

More T cell-based immunotherapies and vaccine trials in humans lie just ahead as our efforts to understand EBV biology and immunology begin to pay dividends.

REFERENCES

Albert, M.L., Sauter, B. and Bhardwaj, N. (1998). Dendritic cells acquire antigen from apoptotic cells and induce class I-restricted CTLs. Nature 392, 86.

Alexander, F.E., Daniel, C.P., Armstrong, A.A. et al. (1995). Case clustering, Epstein-Barr virus Reed-Sternberg cell status and herpes virus serology in Hodgkin's disease: results of a case-control study. Eur J Cancer 31A, 1479–1486.

Amyes, E., Hatton, C., Montamat-Sicotte, D. et al. (2003). Characterization of the $CD4^+$ T cell response to Epstein-Barr virus during primary and persistent infection. J Exp Med 198, 903–911.

Appay, V., Dunbar, P.R., Callan, M. et al. (2002). Memory $CD8^+$ T cells vary in differentiation phenotype in different persistent virus infections. Nat Med 8, 379–385.

Aris, R.M., Maia, D.M., Neuringer, I.P. et al. (1996). Post-transplantation lymphoproliferative disorder in the Epstein-Barr virus-native lung transplant recipient. Am J Respir Crit Care Med 154, 1712.

Armitage, J.M., Kormos, R.L., Stuart, R.S. et al. (1991). Posttransplant lymphoproliferative disease in thoracic organ transplant patients: ten years of cyclosporine-based immunosuppression. J Heart Lung Transplant 10, 877.

Attarbaschi, T., Willheim, M., Ramharter, M. et al. (2003). T cell cytokine profile during primary Epstein-Barr virus infection (infectious mononucleosis). Eur Cytokine Netw 14, 34–39.

Babcock, G.J., Decker, L.L., Freeman, R.B. and Thorley-Lawson, D.A. (1999). EBV-infected resting memory B cells, not proliferating B lymphoblasts, accumulate in the peripheral blood of immunosuppressed patients. J Exp Med 190, 567–576.

Bharadwaj, M. and Moss, D.J. (2002). Epstein-Barr virus vaccine: a cytotoxic T-cell-based approach. Expert Rev Vaccines 1, 467–476.

Blake, N., Haigh, T., Shaka'a, G., Croom-Carter, D. and Rickinson, A. (2000). The importance of exogenous antigen in priming the human $CD8^+$ T cell response: lessons from the EBV nuclear antigen EBNA1. J Immunol 165, 7078–7087.

Blaschke, S., Schwarz, G., Moneke, D., Binder, L., Muller, G. and Reuss-Borst, M. (2000). Epstein-Barr virus infection in peripheral blood mononuclear cells, synovial fluid cells, and synovial membranes of patients with rheumatoid arthritis. J Rheumatol 27, 866–873.

Bourgeault, I., Gomez, A. and Gomarrd, E. (1991). Limiting dilution analysis of the HLA restriction of anti-EBV specific CTLs. Clin Exp Immunopath 84, 501–509.

Bruu, A.L., Hjetland, R., Holter, E. et al. (2000). Evaluation of 12 commercial tests for detection of Epstein-Barr virus-specific and heterophile antibodies. Clin Diagn Lab Immunol 7, 451–456.

Buisson, M., Fleurent, B., Mak, M. et al. (1999). Novel immunoblot assay using four recombinant antigens for diagnosis of Epstein-Barr virus primary infection and reactivation. J Clin Microbiol 37, 2709–2714.

Callan, M.F. (2003). The evolution of antigen-specific $CD8^+$ T cell responses after natural primary infection of humans with Epstein-Barr virus. Viral Immunol 16, 3–16.

Callan, M.F., Tan, L., Annels, N. et al. (1998). Direct visualization of antigen-specific CD8+ T cells during the primary immune response to Epstein-Barr virus In vivo. J Exp Med 187, 1395–1402.

Carpentier, L., Tapiero, B., Alvarez, F., Viau, C. and Alfieri, C. (2003). Epstein-Barr Virus (EBV) early-antigen serologic testing in conjunction with peripheral blood EBV DNA load as a marker for risk of posttransplantation lymphoproliferative disease. J Infect Dis 188, 1853–1864.

Catalina, M.D., Sullivan, J.L., Brody, R.M. and Luzuriaga, K. (2002). Phenotypic and functional heterogeneity of EBV epitope-specific CD8+ T cells. J Immunol 168, 4184–4191.

Chan, K.H., Gu, Y.L., Ng, F. et al. (2003). EBV specific antibody-based and DNA-based assays in serologic diagnosis of nasopharyngeal carcinoma. Int J Cancer 105, 706–709.

Chan, K.H., Tam, J.S., Peiris, J.S., Seto, W.H. and Ng, M.H. (2001). Epstein-Barr virus (EBV) infection in infancy. J Clin Virol 21, 57–62.

Chan, S.H., Soo, M.Y., Gan, Y.Y. et al. (1998). Epstein Barr virus (EBV) antibodies in the diagnosis of NPC – comparison between IFA and two commercial ELISA kits. Singapore Med J 39, 263–265.

Chen, J.M.B., Barr, M.L., Chadburn, A. et al. (1993). Management of lymphoproliferative disorders after cardiac transplantation. Ann Thorac Surg 56, 527–536.

Cockfield, S.M., Preiksaitis, J.K., Jewell, L.D. and Parfrey, N.A. (1993). Post-transplant lymphoproliferative disorder in renal allograft recipients. Transplantation 56, 88–94.

Comoli, P., Labirio, M., Basso, S. et al. (2002). Infusion of autologous Epstein-Barr virus (EBV)-specific cytotoxic T cells for prevention of EBV-related lymphoproliferative disorder in solid organ transplant recipients with evidence of active virus replication. Blood 99, 2592–2598.

Cox, C., Naylor, B.A., Mackett, M., Arrand, J.R., Griffin, B.E. and Wedderburn, N. (1998). Immunization of common marmosets with Epstein-Barr virus (EBV) envelope glycoprotein gp340: effect on viral shedding following EBV challenge. Med Virol 55, 255–261.

Duraiswamy, J., Sherritt, M., Thomson, S. et al. (2003). LMP1 polyepitope vaccine for EBV-associated Hodgkin disease and nasopharyngeal carcinoma. Blood 101, 3150–3156.

Enblad, G., Sandvej, K., Lennette, E. et al. (1997). Lack of correlation between EBV serology and presence of EBV in the Hodgkin and Reed-Sternberg cells of patients with Hodgkin's disease. Int J Cancer 72, 394–397.

Falco, D.A., Nepomuceno, R.R., Krams, S.M. et al. (2002). Identification of Epstein-Barr virus-specific CD8+ lymphocytes in the circulation of pediatric transplant recipients. Transplantation 74, 501–510.

Finerty, S., Mackett, M., Arrand, J.R., Watkins, P.E., Tarlton, J. and Morgan, A.J. (1994). Immunization of cottontop tamarins and rabbits with a candidate vaccine against the Epstein-Barr virus based on the major viral envelope glycoprotein gp340 and alum. Vaccine 12, 1180–1184.

Gahn, B., Siller-Lopez, F., Pirooz, A.D. et al. (2001). Adenoviral gene transfer into dendritic cells efficiently amplifies the immune response to LMP2A antigen: a potential treatment strategy for Epstein-Barr virus–positive Hodgkin's lymphoma. Int J Cancer 93, 706–713.

Ganschow, R., Schulz, T., Meyer, T., Broering, D.C. and Burdelski, M. (2004). Low-dose immunosuppression reduces the incidence of post-transplant lymphoproliferative disease in pediatric liver graft recipients. J Pediatr Gastroenterol Nutr 38, 198–203.

Gao, F.G., Khammanivong, V., Liu, W.J., Leggatt, G.R., Frazer, I.H. and Fernando, G.J. (2002). Antigen-specific CD4+ T-cell help is required to activate a memory CD8+ T cell to a fully functional tumor killer cell. Cancer Res 62, 6438–6441.

Gartner, B.C., Hess, R.D., Bandt, D. et al. (2003). Evaluation of four commercially available Epstein-Barr virus enzyme immunoassays with an immunofluorescence assay as the reference method. Clin Diagn Lab Immunol 10, 78–82.

Glaser, R., Friedman, S.B., Smyth, J. et al. (1999). The differential impact of training stress and final examination stress on herpesvirus latency at the United States Military Academy at West Point. Brain Behav Immun 13, 240–251.

Gottschalk, S., Heslop, H.E. and Rooney, C.M. (2002). Treatment of Epstein-Barr virus-associated malignances with specific T cells. Adv Cancer Res 84, 175–201.

Green, M., Cacciarelli, T.V., Mazariegos, G. et al. (1998). Serial measurement of EBV viral load in peripheral blood in pediatric liver transplant recipients during treatment for post transplant lymphoproliferative disease. Transplantation 66, 1641–1644.

Green, M., Michaels, M.G., Webber, S.A., Rowe, D. and Reyes, J. (1999). The management of Epstein-Barr virus associated post-transplant lymphoproliferative disorders in pediatric solid-organ transplant recipients. Pediatr Transplantation 3, 271–281.

of viral load in the diagnosis, management and possible prevention of Epstein-Barr virus-associated post-transplant lymphoproliferative disease following solid organ transplantation. Curr Opin Organ Transplant 4, 292–296.

Gu, S.Y., Huang, T.M., Ruan, L. et al. (1995). First EBV vaccine trial in humans using recombinant vaccinia virus expressing the major membrane antigen. Dev Biol Stand 84, 171–177.

Haque, T., Taylor, C., Wilkie, G.M. et al. (2001). Complete regression of posttransplant lymphoproliferative disease using partially HLA-matched Epstein Barr virus-specific cytotoxic T cells. Transplantation 72, 1399–1402.

Harwood, J.S., Gould, F.K., McMaster, A. et al. (1999). Significance of Epstein-Barr virus status and post-transplant lymphoproliferative disease in pediatric thoracic transplantation. Pediatr Transplant 3, 100–103.

Heslop, H.E., Perez, M., Benaim, E., Rochester, R., Brenner, M.K. and Rooney, C.M. (1999). Transfer of EBV-specific CTL to prevent EBV lymphoma post marrow transplant. J Clin Apheresis 14, 154–164.

Hislop, A.D., Annels, N.E., Gudgeon, N.H., Leese, A.M. and Rickinson, A.B. (2002). Epitope-specific evolution of human CD8(+) T cell responses from primary to persistent phases of Epstein-Barr virus infection. J Exp Med 195, 893–905.

Ho, S., Teo, P., Kwan, W.H., Choi, P., Tjong, J. and Johnson, P.J. (1998). Staging and IgA VCA titre in patients with nasopharyngeal carcinoma: changes over a 12-year period. Oral Oncol 34, 491–495.

Hollsberg, P., Hansen, H.J. and Haahr, S. (2003). Altered CD8+ T cell responses to selected Epstein-Barr virus immunodominant epitopes in patients with multiple sclerosis. Clin Exp Immunol 132, 137–143.

Jackman, W.T., Mann, K.A., Hoffmann, H.J. and Spaete, R.R. (1999). Expression of Epstein-Barr virus gp350 as a single chain glycoprotein for an EBV subunit vaccine. Vaccine 17, 660–668.

Jung, S., Chung, Y.K., Chang, S.H. et al. (2001). DNA-mediated immunization of glycoprotein 350 of Epstein-Barr virus induces the effective humoral and cellular immune responses against the antigen. Mol Cells 12, 41–49.

Jumbou, O., Mollat, C., N'Guyen, J.M., Billaudel, S., Litoux, P. and Dreno, B. (1997). Increased anti-Epstein-Barr virus antibodies in epidermotropic cutaneous T-cell lymphoma: a study of 64 patients. Br J Dermatol 136, 212–216.

Kantakamalakul, W., Chongkolwatana, C., Naksawat, P. et al. (2000). Specific IgA antibody to Epstein-Barr viral capsid antigen: a better marker for screening nasopharyngeal carcinoma than EBV-DNA detection by polymerase chain reaction. Asian Pac J Allergy Immunol 18, 221–226.

Kimura, H., Morita, M. and Yabuta, Y. (1999). Quantitative analysis of Epstein-Barr virus load by using a real-time PCR assay. J Clin Microbiol 37, 132–136.

Kocoshis, S.A. (1994). Small bowel transplantation in infants and children. Pediatr Gastroenterol 23, 727–733.

Küppers, R. (2003). B cells under influence: transformation of B cells by Epstein Barr virus. Nat Rev (Immunol) 3, 801–812.

Landais, E., Saulquin, X., Scotet, E. et al. (2004). Direct killing of Epstein-Barr virus (EBV)-infected B cells by CD4 T cells directed against the EBV lytic protein BHRF1. Blood 103, 1408–1416.

Leblond, V., Sutton, L., Dorent, R. et al. (1995). Lymphoproliferative disorders after organ transplantation: a report of 24 cases observed in a single center. J Clin Oncol 13, 961–969.

Leen, A., Meij, P., Redchenko, I. et al. (2001). Differential immunogenecity of Epstein-Barr virus latent-cycle proteins for human CD4+ T-helper 1 responses. J Virol 75, 8649–8659.

Leung, S.F., Tam, J.S., Chan, A.T., et al. (2004). Improved accuracy of detection of nasopharyngeal carcinoma by combined application of circulating Epstein-Barr virus DNA and anti-Epstein-Barr viral capsid antigen IgA antibody. Clin Chem 50, 339–345.

Levine, P.H., Pallesen, G., Ebbesen, P., Harris, N., Evans, A.S. and Mueller, N. (1994). Evaluation of Epstein-Barr virus antibody patterns and detection of viral markers in the biopsies of patients with Hodgkin's disease. Int J Cancer 59, 48–50.

Lin, C.L., Lo, W.F., Lee, T.H. et al. (2002). Immunization with Epstein-Barr Virus (EBV) peptide-pulsed dendritic cells induces functional CD8+ T-cell immunity and may lead to tumor regression in patients with EBV-positive nasopharyngeal carcinoma. Cancer Res 62, 6952–6958.

Liu, M.T. and Yeh, C.Y. (1998). Prognostic value of anti-Epstein-Barr virus antibodies in nasopharyngeal carcinoma (NPC). Radiat Med 16, 113–117.

Liu, M.Y., Chang, Y.L., Ma, J. et al. (1997). Evaluation of multiple antibodies to Epstein-Barr virus as markers for detecting patients with nasopharyngeal carcinoma. J Med Virol 52, 262–269.

Loren, A.W., Porter, D.L., Stadtmauer, E.A. and Tsai, D.E. (2003). Post-transplant lymphoproliferative disorder: a review. Bone Marrow Transplant 31, 145–155.

Lucas, K., Small, T., Heller, G., Dupont, B. and O'Reilly, R. (1996). The development of cellular immunity to EBV following allogeneic bone marrow transplantation. Blood 91, 3654–3661.

Lucas, K.G., Burton, R.L. and Zimmerman, S.E. (1998). Semi-quantitative Epstein-Barr virus (EBV) polymerase chain reaction for the determination of patients at risk for EBV-induced lymphoproliferative disease after stem cell transplantation. Blood 91, 3654–3661.

Lumbreras, C., Fernandez, I., Velosa, J., Munn, S., Sterioff, S. and Paya, C.V. (1995). Infectious complications following pancreatic transplantation: incidence, microbiological and clinical characteristics, and outcome. Clin Infect Dis 20, 514–521.

Macallan, D.C., Wallace, D.L., Irvine, A.J. et al. (2003). Rapid turnover of T cells in acute infectious mononucleosis. Eur J Immunol 33, 2655–2665.

Manian, F.A. (1994). Simultaneous measurement of antibodies to Epstein-Barr virus, human herpesvirus 6, herpes simplex virus types 1 and 2, and 14 enteroviruses in chronic fatigue syndrome: is there evidence of activation of a non-specific polyclonal immune response? Clin Infect Dis 19, 448–453.

McDiarmid, S.V., Jordan, S. and Lee, G.S. (1999). Prevention and preemptive therapy of posttransplant lymphoproliferative disease in pediatric liver recipients. Transplantation 66, 1604–1611.

McKnight, J.L., Cen, H., Riddler, S.A. et al. (1994). EBV gene expression, EBNA antibody responses and EBV+ peripheral blood lymphocytes in post-transplant lymphoproliferative disease. Leuk Lymphoma 15, 9–16.

Meij, P., Vervoort, M.B., Bloemena, E. et al. (2002). Antibody responses to Epstein-Barr virus-encoded latent membrane protein-1 (LMP1) and expression of LMP1 in juvenile Hodgkin's disease. J Med Virol 68, 370–377.

Meijer, E., Dekker, A.W., Weersink, A.J., Rozenberg-Arska, M. and Verdonck, L.F. (2002). Prevention and treatment of Epstein-Barr virus-associated lymphoproliferative disorders in recipients of bone marrow and solid organ transplants. Br J Haematol 119, 596–607.

Middledorp, J. M. (1999). Monitoring of Epstein-Barr virus DNA load in the peripheral blood by quantitative competitive PCR. J Clin Microbiol 37, 2852–2857.

Mitarnun, W., Praduktkanchana, J., Takao, S., Saechan, V., Suwiwat, S. and Ishida, T. (2002). Epstein-barr virus-associated non-Hodgkin's lymphoma of B-cell origin, Hodgkin's disease, acute leukemia, and systemic lupus erythematosus: a serologic and molecular analysis. J Med Assoc Thai 85, 552–559.

Mitchell, J.L., Doyle, C.M., Land, M.V. and Devine, P.L. (1998). Comparison of commercial ELISA for detection of antibodies to the viral capsid antigen (VCA) of Epstein-Barr virus (EBV). Dis Markers 13, 245–249.

Miyashita, E., Yang, B., Lam, K., Crawford, D. and Thorley-Lawson, D. (1995). A novel form of Epstein-Barr virus latency in normal B cells in vivo. Cell 80, 593–601.

Miyashita, E., Yang, B., Babcock, G. and Thorley-Lawson, D. (1997). Identification of the site of Epstein-Barr persistence in vivo as a resting B cell. J Virol 71, 4882–4891.

Morgan, A.J. (1992). Epstein-Barr virus vaccines. Vaccine 10, 563–571.

Moss, D.J., Burrows, S.R., Suhrbier, A. and Khanna, R. (1994). Potential antigenic targets on Epstein-Barr virus-associated tumours and the host response. Ciba Found Symp 187, 4–20.

Moss, D.J., Suhrbier, A. and Elliott, S.L. (1998). Candidate vaccines for Epstein-Barr virus. Brit Med J 317, 423–424.

Munz, C., Bickham, K., Subklewe, M. et al. (2000). Human CD4+ T lymphocytes consistently respond to the latent Epstein Barr Virus nuclear antigen EBNA1. J Exp Med 191, 1610–1649.

Murray, R., Kurila, M. and Brooks, J. (1992). Identification of target antigens for the human CTL response to EBV: implications for the immune contol of EBV-positive malignancies. J Exp Med 176, 157–167.

Mutimer, D., Kaur, N., Tang, H. et al. (2000). Quantitation of Epstein-Barr virus DNA in the blood of adult liver transplant recipients. Transplantation 69, 954–959.

Myhr, K.M., Riise, T., Barrett-Connor, E. et al. (1998). Altered antibody pattern to Epstein-Barr virus but not to other herpesviruses in multiple sclerosis: a population based case-control study from western Norway. J Neurol Neurosurg Psychiatr 64, 539–542.

Nalesnik, M. (1998). Clinical and pathological features of post-transplant lymphoproliferative disorders. Springer Semin. Immunopathol 20, 325–346.

Nebel-Schickel, H., Hinderer, W., Saavedra, C. et al. (1994). Anti-EBNA-1 (carboxy-half) IgG antibodies as a seroepidemiological marker for Epstein-Barr virus infection. Beitr Infusionsther Transfusionsmed 32, 134–137.

Niesters, H.G., Van Esser, J., Fries, E., Wolhers, K.C., Corneilissen. J. and Osterhaus, A.D. (2000). Development of a real-time quantitaive assay for detection of Epstein-Barr virus. J Clin Microbiol 38, 712–715.

Nikiforow, S., Bottomly, K., Miller, G. and Munz, C. (2003). Cytolytic CD4(+)-T-cell clones reactive to EBNA1 inhibit Epstein-Barr virus-induced B-cell proliferation. J Virol 77, 12088–12104.

Nordstrom, M., Hardell, L., Linde, A., Schloss, L. and Nasman, A. (1999). Elevated antibody levels to Epstein-Barr virus antigens in patients with hairy cell leukemia compared to controls in relation to exposure to pesticides, organic solvents, animals, and exhausts. Oncol Res 11, 539–544.

Obel, N., Hoier-Madsen, M. and Kangro, H. (1996). Serological and clinical findings in patients with serological evidence of reactivated Epstein-Barr virus infection. APMIS 104, 424–428.

O'Sullivan, C.E., Peng, R., Cole. K.S. et al. (2002). Epstein-Barr virus and human immunodeficiency virus serological responses and viral burdens in HIV-infected patients treated with HAART. J Med Virol 67, 320–326.

Ouyang, Q., Wagner, W.M., Walter, S. et al. (2003). An age-related increase in the number of CD8+ T cells carrying receptors for an immunodominant Epstein-Barr virus (EBV) epitope is counteracted by a decreased frequency of their antigen-specific responsiveness. Mech Ageing Dev 124, 477–485.

Paludan, C., Bickham, K., Nikiforow, S. et al. (2002). Epstein-Barr nuclear antigen 1-specific CD4+ Th1 cells kill Burkitt's lymphoma cells. J Immunol 169, 1593–1603.

Papadopoulos, E.B., Ladanyi, M. and Emanuel, D. (1994). Infusions of donor leukocytes as treatment of EBV associated lymphoproliferative disorders complicating allogeneic bone marrow transplantation. N Engl J Med 330, 1185–1189.

Patton, D., Wilkowski, C. and Hanson, C. (1990). EBV, immunodeficiency and B cell proliferation. Transplantation 49, 1080–1085.

Popescu, I., Macedo, C., Zeevi, A. et al. (2003). Ex vivo priming of naive T cells into EBV-specific Th1/Tc1 effector cells by mature autologous DC loaded with apoptotic/necrotic LCL. Am J Transplant 3,1369–1377.

Porcu, P., Eisenbeis, C.F., Pelletier, R.P. et al. (2002). Successful treatment of posttransplantation lymphoproliferative disorder (PTLD) following renal allografting is associated with sustained CD8(+) T-cell restoration. Blood 100, 2341–2348.

Precopio, M.L., Sullivan, J.L., Willard, C., Somasundaran. M. and Luzuriaga, K. (2003). Differential kinetics and specificity of EBV-specific CD4+ and CD8+ T cells during primary infection. J Immunol 170, 2590–2598.

Preiksaitis, J.K., Diaz-Mitoma, F., Mirzayans, F., Roberts, S. and Tyrrell, D.L. (1992). Quantitative oropharyngeal Epstein-Barr virus shedding in renal and cardiac transplant recipients: relationship to immunosuppressive therapy, serologic responses, and the risk of posttransplant lymphoproliferative disorder. J Infect Dis 166, 986–994.

Qu, L., Green, M., Webber, S., Reyes, J., Ellis, D. and Rowe, D. (2000). EBV gene expression in the peripheral blood of transplant recipients with persistent circulating viral loads. J Infect Dis 182, 1013–1021.

Qu, L. and Rowe, D.T. (1992). Epstein-Barr virus latent gene expression in uncultured peripheral blood lymphocytes. J Virol 66, 3715–3724.

Rea, T.D., Ashley, R.L., Russo, J.E. and Buchwald, D.S. (2002). A systematic study of Epstein-Barr virus serologic assays following acute infection. Am J Clin Pathol 117, 156–161.

Redchenko, I.V. and Rickinson, A.B. (1999). Accessing Epstein-Barr virus-specific T-cell memory with peptide-loaded dendritic cells. J Virol 73, 334–342.

Rickinson, A. (2002). Epstein-Barr virus. Virus Res 82, 109–113.

Rickinson, A. and Kieff, E. (1996). Epstein-Barr virus. In Fields virology, 3rd edn. Fields, B. N., Knipe, D. M., Howley, P. M. et al., eds. Raven Press, New York, pp. 2397–2436.

Rickinson, A., Lee, S. and Steven, N. (1998). CTL responses to EBV Curr. Opin Immunol 8, 492–501.

Riddler, S.A., Breinig, M.D. and McKnight, J.L.C. (1994). Increased levels of circulating Epstein-Barr virus (EBV)-infected lymphocytes and decreased EBV nuclear antigen antibody responses are associated with the development of posttransplant lymphoproliferative disease in solid-organ transplant recipients. Blood 84, 1972–1984.

Robertson, P., Beynon, S., Whybin, R. et al. (2003). Measurement of EBV-IgG anti-VCA avidity aids the early and reliable diagnosis of primary EBV infection. J Med Virol 70, 617–623.

Rogers, B.B., Conlin, C., Timmons, C.F., Dawson. D.B., Krisher, K. and Andrews W.S. (1997). Epstein-Barr virus PCR correlated with viral histology and serology in pediatric liver transplant patients. Pediatr Pathol Lab Med 17, 391–400.

Rose, C., Green, M., Webber, S., Ellis, D., Reyes, J. and Rowe, D. (2001). Pediatric solid organ transplant recipients carry chronic loads of EBV exclusively in IgD-negative B cell compartments. J Clin Microbiol 39, 1407–1415.

Rose, C., Green, M., Webber, S.A. et al. (2002). Detection of EBV genomes in peripheral blood B cells from solid organ recipients by fluorescence in situ hybridization. J Clin Microbiol 40, 2533–2544.

Rowe, D.T. (1999). Epstein-Barr virus immortalization and latency. Frontiers Biosci 4, 346–371.

Rowe, D.T., Qu, L., Reyes, J. and Green, M. (1997). Use of quantitative competitive PCR to measure Epstein-Barr virus genome load in the peripheral blood of pediatric transplant patients with lymphoproliferative disorders. J Clin Microbiol 35, 1612–1615.

Rowe, D.T., Webber, S., Schauer, E.M., Reyes, J. and Green, M. (2001). Epstein-Barr virus load monitoring: its role in the prevention and management of post-transplant lymphoproliferative disease. Transpl Infect Dis 3, 79–87.

Savoldo, B., Cubbage, M.L., Durett, A.G. et al. (2002). Generation of EBV-specific CD4+ cytotoxic T cells from virus naive individuals. J Immunol 168, 909–918.

Savoldo, B., Goss, J., Liu, Z. et al. (2001). Generation of autologous Epstein-Barr virus-specific cytotoxic T cells for adoptive immunotherapy in solid organ transplant recipients. Transplantation 72, 1078–1086.

Schaade, L., Kleines, M. and Häusler, M. (2001). Application of virus-specific immunoglobulin M (IgM), IgG, and IgA antibody detection with a polyantigenic enzyme-linked immunosorbent assay for diagnosis of Epstein-Barr virus infections in childhood. J Clin Microbiol 39, 3902–3905.

Schwab, M., Boswald, M., Korn, K. and Ruder, H. (2000). Epstein-Barr virus in pediatric patients after renal transplantation. Clin Nephrol 53, 132–139.

Shedd, D., Angeloni, A., Niederman, J. and Miller, G. (1995). Detection of human serum antibodies to the BFRF3 Epstein-Barr virus capsid component by means of a DNA-binding assay. J Infect Dis 172, 1367–1370.

Sherritt, M.A., Bharadwaj, M., Burrows, J.M. et al. (2003). Reconstitution of the latent T-lymphocyte response to Epstein-Barr virus is coincident with long-term recovery from posttransplant lymphoma after adoptive immunotherapy. Transplantation 75, 1556–1560.

Shinkura, R., Yamamoto, N., Koriyama, C., Shinmura, Y., Eizuru, Y. and Tokunaga, M. (2000). Epstein-Barr virus-specific antibodies in Epstein-Barr virus-positive and -negative gastric carcinoma cases in Japan. J Med Virol 60, 411–416.

Sigel, G., Schillinger, M., Henninger, K. and Bauer, G. (1994). IgA directed against early antigen of Epstein-Barr virus is no specific marker for the diagnosis of nasopharyngeal carcinoma. J Med Virol 43, 222–227.

Slobod, K.S., Benaim, E., Woodruff, L. et al. (2001). T cell immunotherapeutic populations control viral infections in bone marrow transplant recipients. Immunol Res 24, 289–301.

Smets, F., Latinne, D., Bazin, H. et al. (2002). Ratio between Epstein-Barr viral load and anti-Epstein-Barr virus specific T-cell response as a predictive marker of posttransplant lymphoproliferative disease. Transplantation 73, 1603–1610.

Stevens, S.J., Blank, B.S., Smits, P.H., Meenhorst, P.L. and Middeldorp, J.M. (2002). High Epstein-Barr virus (EBV) DNA loads in HIV-infected patients: correlation with antiretroviral therapy and quantitative EBV serology. AIDS 16, 993–1001.

Stowe, R.P., Pierson, D.L., Feeback, D.L. and Barrett, A.D. (2000). Stress-induced reactivation of Epstein-Barr virus in astronauts. Neuroimmunomodulation 8, 51–58.

Szkaradkiewicz, A., Kruk-Zagajewska, A., Wal, M., Jopek, A., Wierzbicka, M. and Kuch, A. (2002). Epstein-Barr virus and human papillomavirus infections and oropharyngeal squamous cell carcinomas. Clin Exp Med 2, 137–141.

Tamaki, H., Beaulieu, B., Somasunrdaran, M. and Sullivan, J. (1995). Major histocompatibility complex Class I restricted CTL responses to EBV in children. J Inf Dis 172, 7397–48.

Taylor, G.S., Haigh, T.A., Gudgeon, N.H. et al. (2004). Dual stimulation of Epstein-Barr virus (EBV)-specific CD4+- and CD8+ T-cell responses by a chimeric antigen construct: potential therapeutic vaccine for EBV-positive nasopharyngeal carcinoma. J Virol 78, 768–778.

Tan, L.C., Gudgeon, N., Annels, N.E. et al. (1999). A re-evaluation of the frequency of CD8+ T cells specific for EBV in healthy virus carriers. J Immunol 162, 1827–1835.

Thiele, G. M. and Okano, M. (1993). Diagnosis of Epstein-Barr virus infections in the clinical laboratory. Clin Microbiol News 15, 41–46.

Thomson, S.A., Burrows, S.R., Misko, I.S., Moss, D.J., Coupar, B.E. and Khanna, R. (1998). Targeting a polyepitope protein incorporating multiple class II-restricted viral epitopes to the secretory/endocytic pathway facilitates immune recognition by CD4+ cytotoxic T lymphocytes: a novel approach to vaccine design. J Virol 72, 2246–2252.

Tierney, R. J., Steven, N., Young, L.S. and Rickinson, A.B. (1994). EBV latency in blood mononuclear cells: analysis of viral gene transcription during primary infection and in the carrier state. J Virol 68, 7374–7383.

Tiwawech, D., Srivatanakul, P., Karaluk, A. and Ishida, T. (2003). Significance of plasma IgA and IgG antibodies to Epstein-Barr virus early and viral capsid antigens in Thai nasopharyngeal carcinoma. Asian Pac J Cancer Prev 4, 113–118.

Vajro, P., Lucariello, S. and Migliaro, F. (2000). Predictive value of Epstein-Barr virus genome copy number and BZLF1 expression in blood lymphocytes of transplant receipients at risk for lymphoproliferative disease. J Infect Dis 181, 2050–2054.

van Grunsven, W.M., Spaan, W.J. and Middeldorp, J.M. (1994). Localization and diagnostic application of immunodominant domains of the BFRF3-encoded Epstein-Barr virus capsid protein. J Infect Dis 170, 13–19.

Verschuuren, E., van der Bij, W., de Boer, W., Timens, W., Middeldorp, J. and The, T.H. (2003). Quantitative Epstein-Barr virus (EBV) serology in lung transplant recipients with primary EBV infection and/or post-transplant lymphoproliferative disease. J Med Virol 69, 258–266.

Votava, M., Bartosova, D., Krchnakova, A., Crhova, K. and Kubinova, L. (1996). Diagnostic importance of heterophile antibodies and immunoglobulins IgA, IgE, IgM and low-avidity IgG against Epstein-Barr virus capsid antigen in children. Acta Virol 40, 99–101.

Vrbikova, J., Janatkova, I., Zamrazil, V., Tomiska, F. and Fucikova, T. (1996). Epstein-Barr virus serology in patients with autoimmune thyroiditis. Exp Clin Endocrinol Diabetes 104, 89–92.

Wadowsky, R.M., Laus, S., Green, M., Webber, S.A. and Rowe, D. T. (2003). Measurement of Epstein-Barr virus DNA loads in whole blood and plasma by TaqMan PCR and in peripheral blood lymphocytes by competitive PCR. J Clin Microbiol 41, 5245–5249.

Wagner, H.J., Bein, G., Bitsch, A. and Kirchner, H. (1992). Detection and quantitation of latently infected B lymphocytes in EBV seropositive healthy individuals by polymerase chain reaction. J Clin Microbiol 30, 2826–2831.

Wagner, H.J., Rooney, C.M. and Heslop, H.E. (2002). Diagnosis and treatment of posttransplantation lymphoproliferative disease after hematopoietic stem cell transplantation. Biol Blood Marrow Transplant 8, 1–8.

Wakiguchi, H. (2002). Overview of Epstein-Barr virus-associated diseases in Japan. Crit Rev Oncol Hematol 44, 193–202.

Walker, R.C., Marshall, W.F., Strickler, J.G. et al. (1995). Pretransplantation assessment of the risk of lymphoproliferative disorder. Clin Infect Dis 20, 1346–1353.

Webber, S. (1999). Posttransplant lymphoproliferative disorders: A preventable complication of solid organ transplantation? Pediatr Transplantation 3, 95–99.

Yang, J., Lemas. V.M., Flinn, I.W., Krone, C. and Ambinder, R.F. (2000). Application of the ELISPOT assay to the characterization of CD8(+) responses to Epstein-Barr virus antigens. Blood 95, 241–248.

Viral Responses – Hepatitis

Chapter 52

Tatsuya Kanto

Department of Molecular Therapeutics, Department of Dendritic Cell Biology and Clinical Application, Osaka University Graduate School of Medicine, Osaka, Japan

Jaundice is the disease that your friends diagnose.
There are regions, in partibus infidelium, to which you will go as missionaries, carrying the gospel of loyalty to truth in the science and in the art of medicine, and your lives of devotion may prove to many a stimulating example.

Sir William Osler, The Army Surgeon, 1894

INTRODUCTION

Hepatitis B virus (HBV) and hepatitis C virus (HCV) are two major causes of chronic liver disease worldwide. Both viruses are hepatotrophic, but not directly cytopathic and elicit progressive liver injuries resulting in end-stage liver disease unless effectively eradicated (Liang et al., 2000; Lok and McMahon, 2001). Epidemiological studies revealed that the relative percentages of acutely infected patients developing chronic hepatitis are different when comparing HBV and HCV infection. Less than 10 per cent of HBV-infected patients develop chronic hepatitis, while more than 80 per cent of those infected with HCV do so (Liang et al., 2000; Lok and McMahon, 2001). Such a difference may in part rely on the differences in the immunogenicity of viral proteins and the kinetics of viral replication during the early stages of infection (Bertoletti and Ferrari, 2003). One of the major determinants in the clinical course of viral hepatitis is the host immune response. It has been proposed that the ability of infected hosts to mount vigorous and sustained cellular immune reactions to HBV and HCV is required for control in primary infection (Bertoletti and Ferrari, 2003). Once HBV or HCV survives the initial interaction with the host immune system, it uses several means to nullify the selective immunological pressure during the later phases of infection. First, these viruses alter their antigenic epitopes recognized by T cells and neutralizing antibodies to escape immune surveillance (Liang et al., 2000; Lok and McMahon, 2001). HBV and HCV also subvert immune functions, including those of NK cells, dendritic cells (DC) and T cells. Antiviral agents, IFN-α, ribavirin and lamivudine, widely used for the treatment of chronic HBV or HCV infection either reduce the viral load or enhance immunity in order to prevent the subsequent development of liver cirrhosis or hepatocellular carcinoma (HCC) (Liang et al., 2000; Lok and McMahon, 2001). In addition to providing direct inhibition of viral replication, these agents modulate antiviral immune responses, which greatly contribute to the successful therapeutic response.

Sensitive assays to measure antigen-specific CD4 and CD8 T cell responses have been developed and serve as a means to monitor the relationship of T-cell responses in the setting of acute or chronic viral hepatitis in patients under treatment. These techniques, including enzyme-linked immunospot (ELISPOT) and MHC-peptide tetramer assays, are able to measure T cell responses without culturing cells *in vitro*, thus providing direct assessment of the immune response presumably occurring within the liver. In this chapter, the current concepts of immunopathogenesis of viral hepatitis are discussed and to which validated

Measuring Immunity, edited by Michael T. Lotze and Angus W. Thomson
ISBN 0-12-455900-X, London

bioassays for hepatitis virus-specific cell-mediated immunity have significantly contributed. In addition we include information about the critical role of dendritic cells in the host and how they serve as immune sentinels, capable of modifying immunity.

KEY ELEMENTS IN IMMUNE RESPONSES TO VIRAL HEPATITIS

After HBV or HCV infects the liver, viral replication continues and viral particles are continuously released into the circulation. The first lines of defense are provided by cells of the innate immune response. It has been suggested that activation of NK and NKT cells occurs in the liver as well, where expression of IFN-α and IFN-inducible genes are extremely high during the early phase of hepatitis virus infection (Su et al., 2002). Activated NK and NKT cells secrete IFN-γ, which inhibits replication of HBV and HCV through a non-cytolytic mechanism (Guidotti and Chisari, 2001). During HBV infection, those cells involved in innate immunity contribute significantly to the suppression of viral replication (Kakimi et al., 2000; Webster et al., 2000). Their roles however, during the acute or chronic phase of HCV infection remain elusive.

Blood DC or resident macrophages in the liver are capable of taking up viral antigens, processing and presenting them to other immune cells (Banchereau et al., 2000). Since DC express distinct sets of toll-like receptors (TLRs) (Kadowaki et al., 2001), it is likely that some viral components stimulate DC through cytosolic ligation of TLRs, presumably TLR7-9 (Heil et al., 2003). DC develop a mature phenotype and migrate to lymphoid tissues, where they stimulate NK cells, NKT cells, T cells and B cells. Following encounter of DC with other cells, DC secrete various cytokines (IL-12, TNF-α, IFN-α and IL-10) instructing or regulating the functions of the adjacent cells (Banchereau et al., 2000). Besides these cytokines, DC express various co-stimulatory molecules and ligands to enhance or limit the functions of immune and infected cells. The existence of functionally and ontogenetically distinct DC subsets has been reported, i.e. myeloid DC (MDC) and plasmacytoid DC (PDC) (Shortman and Liu, 2002). MDC predominantly produce IL-12 or TNF-α following pro-inflammatory stimuli, while PDC release considerable amounts of IFN-α upon virus infection (Liu et al., 2000) depending on the immune stimulus; both cytokines in actuality can be made by both cells. Helper T cells have an immunoregulatory function mediated by the secretion of cytokines that support either cytotoxic T lymphocyte (CTL) generation (Th1 with secretion of IL-2, IFN-γ and TNF-α) or B cell function and antibody production (Th2 with secretion of IL-4, IL-5, IL-10 and IL-13). DC ontogeny and DC-derived cytokines are crucially associated with polarization of helper T cell subsets. In this regard, MDC potently polarize helper T cells to attain a Th1 phenotype, while PDC are able to induce Th2 responses, although

their roles in T cell instruction of DC subsets are flexible *in vivo* (Shortman and Liu, 2002).

It is generally accepted that adaptive immunity performs a critical role during the clinical courses of hepatitis. The involvement of antigen-specific CD4 T cells in HBV and HCV eradication has been well described both during acute or chronic infection (Penna et al., 1996; Day et al., 2002). However, there is little evidence that CD4 T cells mediate direct liver cell injury either in HBV or HCV infection. Thus, it is likely that CD4 T cells play a critical role in facilitating other antiviral immune mechanisms, such as enhancing CD8 effector function. In general, the antigen-specific CD8 T cell is the critical element in the eradication of virus-infected cells. Recent technical advances in measuring CD8 T cell responses disclosed the distinct properties of CD8 T cells when comparing HBV and HCV infection (Rehermann et al., 1996a). It has been clearly demonstrated that HBV-specific CTL are able to eliminate HBV either by inducing apoptosis in infected hepatocytes (cytolytic mechanism) or by releasing IFN-γ (non-cytolytic mechanism) (Guidotti and Chisari, 2001). However, there are conflicting reports regarding the involvement of HCV-specific CD8 T cells in the control of HCV replication during the chronic state (Rehermann et al., 1996a; Hiroishi et al., 1997; Wong et al., 1998). Analyses of mononuclear cells infiltrated in chronically HCV-infected liver reveals that CD8 T cells are directly related to liver inflammation but not virus elimination (Leroy et al., 2003). Cellular components of immune response in hepatitis virus infection are shown in Figure 52.1.

MEASURING IMMUNE RESPONSE IN VIRAL HEPATITIS

Understanding the interaction between host and virus relies crucially on quantitative measurements of immune responses. The applications, advantages and drawbacks of currently used T cell immunological assays are summarized in Table 52.1. Similarly, Table 52.2 provides means to assess MDC and PDC function.

Measuring T cell response

Proliferation assay (CD4)

Memory T cells are able to proliferate following recognition of the relevant antigen. This phenomenon has been widely used as an indicator of the presence of antigen-specific CD4 T cells in various clinical samples. In brief, CD4 T cells or PBMC are mixed with antigens and cultured for 3–5 days. After culture, DNA synthesis is measured to quantify the amount of [^{3}H]-thymidine incorporated into cells. A stimulation index (SI) can be calculated by dividing the numbers of counts per minute (cpm) for the specimen by those in cells incubated without antigen as control.

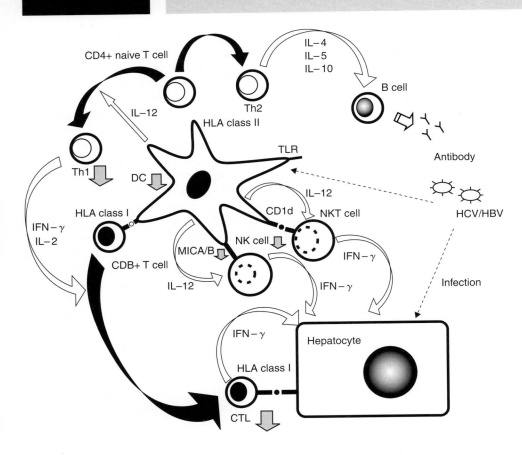

Figure 52.1 Key elements and reported defects in immune responses to viral hepatitis. There are several important cellular functions which promote immunity to viral pathogens which appear in some individuals to be altered in viral hepatitis. Measures of immunity reflect the cells and factors in the blood reflecting the intrahepatic environment. CTL, cytotoxic T lymphocyte; DC, dendritic cell; MIC A/B, MHC class I-related chain A/B; HBV, hepatitis B virus; HCV, hepatitis C virus; NK, natural killer cell; NKT, natural killer T cell; Th, helper T cell; TLR, Toll-like receptors; white arrows, secretion of cytokines; black arrows, differentiation; gray arrows, decrease in function in chronic viral hepatitis.

For the analysis of HBV or HCV-specific responses, recombinant viral proteins are usually used as the antigen source (Penna et al., 1996; Chang et al., 2001). Although certain proteins have been considered to be immunogenic as targets for virus elimination (Diepolder et al., 1995; Wertheimer et al., 2003), such studies utilizing limited numbers of antigens is not sufficient to estimate the CD4 T cell response as a whole. The major advantage of this assay is the ability to use directly peripheral blood samples, gaining insights into T cell activity within the blood. The possibility exists, however, that the SI correlates imperfectly with the number of antigen-specific T cells present *in vivo*.

Cell division assay (CD4, CD8)

This technique allows the visualization of eight to 10 discrete cycles of cell division by flow cytometry (Lyons, 2000). A membrane-bound vital dye, CFSE (carboxyfluorescein diacetate, succinimidyl ester) is successfully diluted with daughter cells after replication, which is useful to assess T cell proliferation in response to specific antigens. Poor proliferative capacity of HCV-specific CD8 T cells in chronic hepatitis C patients can be demonstrated by dual staining with MHC class I tetramer and CFSE (Wedemeyer et al., 2002). Alternatively, this assay is also used to track cell division after stimulation *in vivo* following adoptive transfer.

Intracellular cytokine staining (CD4, CD8)

By using multicolor staining techniques, monitoring the quality of T cell responses (Th1 or Th2) becomes possible by characterizing their cytokine secretion patterns (Day et al., 2002). Staining antigen-specific CD8 T cells for expression of the death-inducing molecules, perforin or granzyme, provides a functionally relevant assay for CTL (Urbani et al., 2002). Practically, after a short period of *in vitro* T cell activation, either with antigen or mitogen, cells are stained with phenotypic markers and then permeabilized for intracellular cytokine detection. A combination of MHC class-I tetramer and intracellular cytokine staining technique has significantly contributed thus far to the understanding of the roles of HBV- or HCV-specific CTL in the pathogenesis of hepatitis (Lechner et al., 2000; Urbani et al., 2002). One of the major drawbacks of this assay is that the detected cells are no longer viable, thus they cannot be sorted and cultured for cloning.

Cytotoxicity assay (CD8)

Traditionally, in the assessment of killing activity mediated by CD8 T cells, PBMC are cultured for several weeks with repetitive antigen stimulation in the presence of IL-2 (Hiroishi et al., 1997). Although this assay is a function-based method, it allows assessment of a single epitope associated with a specific HLA molecule. More importantly, there is

Table 52.1 Immunological assays used to monitor antigen-specific T cell responses in viral hepatitis

T-cell Assay	Cell type	In vitro culture	Frequency	Function	Advantages	Disadvantages	References
Proliferation	CD4	Yes	No	Yes	• Simple	• Low sensitivity • Stimulation index correlates imperfectly with antigen-specific T cell numbers in vivo	Penna et al. 1996 Chang et al. 2001 Wertheimer et al. 2003
Cell division / CFSE*	CD4 CD8	Yes (in vitro) /No (in vivo)	No	Yes	• Applicable for tracking cell division in vivo	• Not quantitative	Wedemeyer et al. 2002
Cytotoxicity / CTL response index	CD8	Yes	No	Yes	• Simple	• Low sensitivity • Results are semi-quantitative.	Hiroishi et al. 1997 Wong et al. 1998 Rehermann et al. 1996a, b
LDA# / CTL precursor frequency	CD8	Yes	Yes	No	• Measures precursor frequency	• Low sensitivity • Cumbersome • Operator-dependent	Rehermann et al. 1996b, c Scognamiglio et al. 1999
Intracellular cytokine staining	CD4 CD8	No	Yes	Yes	• Simple • Measures frequency and function	• Analyzed cells are not viable	Day et al. 2002 Urbani et al. 2002
ELISPOT&	CD4 CD8	No	Yes	Yes	• Increased sensitivity • Applied in a high throughput mode • Measures frequency and function • Either peptide or protein can be used for antigens	• Unable to analyze the phenotypes of spot-forming cells • The results do not always correlate with killing activity	Lechner et al. 2000 Lauer et al. 2002 Nascimbeni et al. 2003 Wertheimer et al. 2003
Peptide- MHC tetramer	CD4 CD8	No No	Yes Yes	Yes (When combined with other functional assays)	• Increased sensitivity • Measures frequency and function • Tetramer-positive cells can be analyzed for phenotypes and functions • Tetramer-positive cells can be sorted for cloning	• Requires specialized agents for the relevant epitopes • Tetramer-positive cells are not always functional • Cross-reactive with other TCR/peptide/MHC combinations	Lechner et al. 2001 Reignat et al. 2002 Day et al. 2003

*CFSE, carboxyfluorescein diacetate succinimidyl ester; # LDA, limiting dilution analysis; & ELISPOT, enzyme-linked immunospot assay

Table 52.2 Immunological assays used to monitor dendritic cell frequency and function in viral hepatitis

Assays	DC type[+]	Requirement of in vitro DC culture	Frequency	Function	Readouts	References
Frequency	MDC PDC	No	Yes	No	• MDC: Lineage marker*[−], HLA-DR[+], CD11c[+], CD123[+] • PDC: Lineage marker[−], HLA-DR[+], CD11c[−], CD123[++]	Kanto et al. 2003 Beckebaum et al. 2002
Phenotype	Mo-DC MDC PDC	Yes	No	No	• Subset-specific markers: BDCA1,2,3,4 • Maturation markers: CD1a, CD40, CD83, CD86, HLA-DR, DC-LAMP, CCR7	Dzionek et al. 2000 Rollier et al. 2003
Phagocytic activity	Mo-DC	Yes	No	Yes	• Uptake of fluorescein-labeled dextran or microparticles	Kanto et al. 1999
Cytokine production	Mo-DC MDC PDC	Yes	No	Yes	• ELISA • Intracellular cytokine staining	Beckebaum et al. 2002
Stimulatory capacity of T cells	Mo-DC MDC PDC	Yes	No	Yes	• Allogeneic MLR[$] • T cell polarization (Th1/Th2) • Antigen-specific CD4 T cell response	Romani et al. 1994 Kanto et al. 1999, 2003 Bain et al. 2001 Lohr et al. 2002
Stimulatory capacity of NK cells	Mo-DC MDC PDC	Yes	No	Yes	• MICA/B expression • Killing activity and IFN-γ production of NK cells co-cultured with DC	Jinushi et al. 2003

[+] Mo-DC, monocyte-derived DC; MDC, myeloid DC; PDC, plasmacytoid DC; * Lineage marker, CD3, CD14, CD16, CD19, CD20, CD56; [$] MLR, mixed lymphocyte reaction no evidence that the results with selected epitopes are representative of the response as a whole. As a substitute for PBMC, liver-infiltrated mononuclear cells were polyclonally expanded to detect liver-infiltrated HCV-specific CTL activity (Wong et al., 1998). To examine the breadth of antigen-specific CTL responses, a CTL response index (CRI) was introduced, which is determined by the sum of killing activity against multiple epitopes (Rehermann et al., 1996a,b). However, the drawbacks of these cytotoxicity assays are that they are relatively insensitive and are not able to assess the frequency of killer cells.

CTL precursor frequency (CD8)

The frequency of antigen-specific CTL precursors (CTLpf) can be calculated based on limiting dilution analysis (LDA) (Rehermann et al., 1996b,c). LDA is a cumbersome method that involves the serial dilution of T cells in a large number of wells. The cells are stimulated repetitively with peptides and IL-2 and are then placed in a microcytotoxicity assay. Poisson distribution analysis is applied to determine the proportion of wells at a particular T cell dilution that have more than one precursor at the start of stimulation. This assay is operator-dependent and may not directly relate to the quality of the T cell response because of the potential for precursor modulation following *in vitro* culture with IL-2. Furthermore, it requires that cells proliferate prior to lysing target cells, thus suggesting that this assay considerably underestimates the number of existing CTL. Direct comparison between CTLpf and ELISPOT assay for the determination of HCV-specific CTL numbers demonstrated that the CTLpf was ten times less sensitive than the ELISPOT (Scognamiglio et al., 1999).

Detection of secreted cytokines by ELISA and ELISPOT (CD4, CD8)

Cytokines released from T cells in response to antigens are measured either by bulk production (ELISA) or following enumeration of individual cytokine-producing cells (ELISPOT). The ELISPOT assay is a method for identifying cells through the detection of cytokine release. IFN-γ is used for the detection of Th1 or CD8 T cells and IL-4, IL-5 or IL-10 are used for Th2, respectively. The cells are offered antigen in antibody-coated wells; secreted cytokines are trapped and visualized by means of a sandwich technique. This method is particularly sensitive, since as few as 15 antigen-specific cells per million PBMC can be detected (Lechner et al., 2001). ELISPOT techniques have been frequently used for the analyses of HBV- and HCV-specific CD4 as well as CD8 T cell responses both in humans and chimpanzees (Lechner et al., 2000; Nascimbeni et al., 2003). This method can be applied either with protein or peptide antigens and the results are quantitative and qualitative. Since ELISPOT assays can be applied in a high throughput mode when a specialized

spot reader is available, it can be used for the screening of unknown epitopes (Lauer et al., 2002; Wertheimer et al., 2003). The ELISPOT analysis however relies on IFN-γ release, which does not always correlate directly with killing activity.

Tetramers (CD8, CD4)

Recently, visualization of antigen-specific T cells under flow cytometry became possible using soluble, fluorescent labeled and multimeric MHC-peptide complexes. HLA class-I tetramers are a powerful tool for the direct enumeration of peptide-specific CD8 T cells without culture *in vitro* (Lechner et al., 2001). It allows the investigator the opportunity to characterize further antigen-specific T cells by staining with activation markers (CD38, CD69 and class-II), memory markers (CD45RO, CD62L and CCR7) (Nascimbeni et al., 2003) or effector molecules (perforin) (Urbani et al., 2002). It is also applicable for CTL cloning with selection of tetramer-positive cells. The major problems of this assay are as follows:

1. tetramers are of limited utility for only known antigens
2. it is difficult to select epitopes
3. tetramer-positive cells are not always functional
4. the tetramer reagents may cross-react with other T cell receptors responsive to other MHC/peptide combinations.

Discrepancy of the CD8 T cell frequency when comparing ELISPOT and tetramer staining has been reported (Rubio-Godoy et al., 2001). One of the reasons for such different outcomes is the alteration of CD8 T cell binding ability to tetramers. In situations of high-dose viral antigens including chronic HBV infection, CD8 T cells with altered HLA/peptide tetramer binding have been observed (Reignat et al., 2002). Despite these drawbacks, ELISPOT and tetramer assays have been widely used for monitoring of antigen-specific T cell responses in cancer patients who undergo immune adjuvant therapy. When MHC class-II peptide tetramers came into use in clinical settings (Day et al., 2003), much additional information became available on the role of antigen-specific CD4 T cells in hepatitis and various other diseases.

Measuring APC/DC function

Dendritic cells (DC) are arguably the most potent professional APC *in vivo* that play pivotal roles in the orchestration of immune reactions (Banchereau et al., 2000). To assess DC function in humans, monocytes have been widely used as a DC source. They develop into DC in the presence of GM-CSF and IL-4 (Romani et al., 1994). Although monocyte-derived DC (Mo-DC) is a well-acknowledged source of cells for the analysis of DC biology, criticism has been raised with respect to the validity of this model as a surrogate for *in vivo* DC function.

Blood DC subsets are identified from the expression pattern of lineage (Lin-) markers (CD3, CD14, CD16, CD19, CD56), HLA-DR, CD11c and CD123. MDC are Lin-negative, HLA-DR$^+$, CD11c$^+$, CD123$^+$ and PDC are Lin-negative, HLA-DR$^+$, CD11c$^-$, CD123^{++}, respectively (Liu et al., 2000). The frequency of DC subsets is measured in infectious disease or cancer patients where decreases in some DCs are associated with generalized immunosuppression (Soumelis et al., 2001). Separation of DC from PBMC is possible using a cell sorter or with subset-specific antibodies conjugated with magnetic beads (Dzionek et al., 2000). DC change their function according to the maturation status, which is determined by their altered phenotypes and phagocytic activity (Banchereau et al., 2000). Co-culture of DC with allogeneic CD4 T cells (mixed lymphocyte reaction, MLR) has been traditionally used for the assessment of DC ability to stimulate T cells (Romani et al., 1994). Several groups have reported that DC from HCV-infected patients were impaired in MLR (Kanto et al., 1999; Bain et al., 2001). Although these assays are easy and reliable ways to analyze DC function, the results need to be interpreted carefully. DC capacity to stimulate allogeneic cells is not necessarily parallel with capacity to stimulate antigen-reactive autologous T cells (Kanto et al., 1999).

IMMUNOPATHOGENESIS OF VIRAL HEPATITIS

Natural course of acute HBV or HCV infection

Acute HBV infection

During the early phase of primary HBV infection, HBV-DNA is not detectable in serum or the liver for 4–7 weeks following exposure (Fong et al., 1994). HBV infection of the liver directly induces type I IFN, which subsequently activates NK cells. Thus, even in the incubation phase, activated NK cells are thought to play a crucial role in the control of HBV replication by producing IFN-γ. This is supported by the observation that circulating NK cells increase before the peak of HBV replication, which subsides following HBV reduction (Webster et al., 2000). Activated NKT cells are involved in the inhibition of HBV replication, as evidenced by the HBV transgenic mouse model (Kakimi et al., 2000). Subsequently a rapid increase in HBV replication occurs at 10–12 weeks of infection, which is accompanied by induction of adaptive immunity. HBV-specific CD4 and CD8 T cells are detectable in the blood even before the onset of overt hepatitis (Webster et al., 2000). Generally, a strong and Th1-biased CD4 T cell response and a multi-specific CD8 response are associated with HBV clearance (Penna et al., 1996; Maini et al., 1999). HBV-specific CD8 T cells continue to increase after a marked reduction in HBV-DNA and reach their highest number at the time of maximal ALT levels (0.1–1.3 per cent of peripheral CD8 T cells), then decline during the recovery phase, in parallel with a resolution of hepatitis

(Maini et al., 1999; Webster et al., 2000). From a CD4 or CD8 T cell depletion study in chimpanzees, HBV-specific CD8 T cells, but not CD4, are the main effectors responsible for viral clearance (Thimme et al., 2003). In comparison with HCV-specific CD8 T cells using tetramers, HBV-specific CD8 T cells are highly activated and capable of proliferating and secreting much IFN-γ (Urbani et al., 2002).

Acute HCV infection

In clear contrast with HBV, HCV-RNA levels rapidly increase during the first few days of HCV infection and continue to be high during the incubation period (Thimme et al., 2001) which lasts for up to 10–12 weeks following infection. Although HCV triggers expression of type I IFN and IFN-induced genes in the liver during this phase (Su et al., 2002), the HCV viral load does not decrease. This suggests that HCV impedes the execution of antiviral molecular mechanisms, including interferon regulatory factor (IRF)-3 (Foy et al., 2003), as well as NF-κB and RNA-dependent protein kinases (PKR) (Taylor et al., 1999). In parallel with the onset of acute hepatitis, activated HCV-specific T cells enter the liver (Thimme et al., 2002). HCV-specific CD4 and CD8 T cell responses and IFN-γ co-expression coincide with decreases in HCV quantity (Thimme et al., 2002). Vigorous, multi-epitope-specific, Th1 type and sustained CD4 T cell responses are detected in resolved cases (Thimme et al., 2001; Day et al., 2002). By contrast, in cases that progress to chronic hepatitis, CD4 T cell responses are weak, narrowly selected and short-lived (Day et al., 2002). The frequency of HCV-specific CD8 T cells is high during the acute phase of infection (2–8 per cent of peripheral CD8 T cells), however, it decreases after HCV persistence develops (0.01–1.2 per cent) (He et al., 1999; Lechner et al., 2000). Despite the high numbers of CTL, some of these cells are "stunned" in the acute phase, as demonstrated by an inability to produce IFN-γ and to proliferate in response to HCV antigens (Lechner et al., 2000; Gruener et al., 2001).

Immune response in resolved cases of acute HBV or HCV infection

HBV- or HCV-specific antibodies are detectable in the serum following appearance of the cellular immune response. Significant HBV-specific CD4 and CD8 T cell responses are detectable in self-limited acute hepatitis B patients more than 10 years after the primary infection, suggesting that long-term T cell memory persists in these cases (Penna et al., 1996; Rehermann et al., 1996c). In HCV infection, limited *in vivo* studies on chimpanzees report that HCV-specific antibodies with *in vitro* neutralizing ability exert a protective role against HCV infection (Farci et al., 1994). In a comparative analysis in chimpanzees that resolved after acute HCV infection and chimpanzees that did not, strong and multi-specific CTL are better correlated with protection against HCV than antibodies

(Cooper et al., 1999). Longitudinal analysis of resolved HCV infection reveals that HCV-specific antibody titers decrease within 10 to 20 years. HCV-specific CD4 and CD8 responses persist even after several decades (Takaki et al., 2000; Wertheimer et al., 2003). Long-lasting memory of CD4 or CD8 T cells against hepatitis virus in the absence of antibody is confirmed in observations on health-care workers (Koziel et al., 1997), spouses and healthy family members of chronic hepatitis C patients (Scognamiglio et al., 1999).

A question has been raised whether or not sterilizing or protective immunity against HCV exists in resolved cases. Reinfection of HCV in once-recovered chimpanzees suggests that sterilizing immunity to HCV does not exist (Nascimbeni et al., 2003). In terms of protective immunity, rechallenge of HCV inocula to recovered chimpanzees demonstrates that memory CD4 and CD8 T cells play a primary role in the prevention of persistent HCV infection (Nascimbeni et al., 2003; Shoukry et al., 2003).

Mechanisms of virus escape from immunity in the chronically infected state

Chronic HBV infection

HBV and HCV possess diverse strategies to escape from immune surveillance. Extensive work has been done on CD4 and CD8 T cell dysfunction. Patients with chronic HBV infection are generally hyporesponsive to HBV proteins and the level of T cell reactivity at this stage is significantly weaker than in acute self-limited hepatitis B (Rehermann et al., 1996c). Even with tetramers, HBV-specific CD8 T cells are barely detected in the circulation of HBe antigen-positive patients (Maini et al., 2000). The importance of HBV-specific CD8 T cells in the control of virus replication and the suppression of liver inflammation has been well established (Maini et al., 2000). In HBe antigen-negative chronic hepatitis B patients without liver inflammation, tetramer positive CD8 T cells were highly active and more frequently observed both in the liver and PBMC than in HBe antigen-positive patients with active hepatitis (Maini et al., 2000). It has been speculated that one of the mechanisms of T cell hyporeactivity in chronic HBV infection is the exhaustion of antigen-specific T cells due to the presence of large quantity of virus or viral proteins, such as HBe antigen (Reignat et al., 2002). In support of this, reduction of HBV-DNA in patients treated with lamivudine coincided with a significant increase in HBV-specific CD4 and CD8 T cell responses (Boni et al., 2001).

Chronic HCV infection

The relevance of CD4 and CD8 T cells in chronic HCV infection is different from that observed with HBV. Many reports have been published on the importance of CD4 T cell response in the clearance and control of HCV. In chronic hepatitis C patients, HCV-specific CD4 T cells

were functionally impaired and their activity was not sustained (Ulsenheimer et al., 2003), which was in clear contrast with resolved cases. Inoculation studies of infectious HCV to recovered chimpanzees demonstrated that CD4 T cell help was indispensable for the development of an effective CD8 T cell response to protect from HCV persistence (Grakoui et al., 2003). Since the liver is the major site where the hepatitis virus replicates, analyses of liver-infiltrated lymphocytes gives quite distinct perspectives from that obtained with PBMC (Grabowska et al., 2001). Compartmentalization of specific Th1 type CD4 T cells occurs in the chronic HCV-infected liver and can be distinguished from cells found in the periphery (Schirren et al., 2000; Penna et al., 2002). The immunological environment in the liver is potentially tolerogenic to infiltrating T cells (Crispe, 2003). Liver sinusoidal endothelial cells (LSEC), Kupffer cells, stellate cells and liver DC may mediate this tolerogenic effect (Lau and Thomson, 2003) (Figure 52.2).

With regard to HCV-specific CD8 T cells observed during the chronic stages of disease, conflicting results have been reported for their roles in HCV replication and liver inflammation. Several investigators have shown that the HCV-specific CTL response is inversely correlated with viral load, suggesting its inhibitory capacity on HCV replication (Hiroishi et al., 1997; Nelson et al., 1997). However, others did not find a significant relationship between these parameters (Rehermann et al., 1996a; Wong et al., 1998). HCV-specific CD8 T cells in chronic hepatitis C patients possess lesser capacity to proliferate and produce less IFN-γ in response to HCV antigens (Wedemeyer et al., 2002). Since CD8 T cells are reported to be involved in HCV-induced liver inflammation (Leroy et al., 2003), inefficient CD8 T cells may evoke only milder hepatocyte injury, at a level which is not sufficient for HCV eradication (Prezzi et al., 2001).

The immunosuppressive potential of HCV-derived core and envelope proteins has been implicated as a mechanism for T cell functional subversion. HCV core proteins are elevated in the serum of chronic hepatitis C patients. The association of core proteins with the globular domain of C1q receptor (gC1qR) on T cells downregulates T cell proliferation and IL-2 production (Kittlesen et al., 2000). The HCV E2 protein also displays high affinity binding to the tetraspanin cell surface molecule CD81, which is considered a likely HCV entry co-receptor (Zhang et al., 2004). Recently, it has been demonstrated that E2-mediated cross-linking of CD81 on NK cells directly inhibits NK cell activation (Crotta et al., 2002). Serial analyses of HCV-specific CD4 and CD8 T cell responses during the course of IFN-α and ribavirin therapy reveal significant increases in the CD4 response in parallel with HCV reduction (Barnes et al., 2002). These observations suggest that antigen-specific CD4 T cells are exhausted in the presence of a high viral load but recover when the viral burden decreases, as has been observed in patients with chronic HBV infection following treatment with lamivudine (Boni et al., 2001).

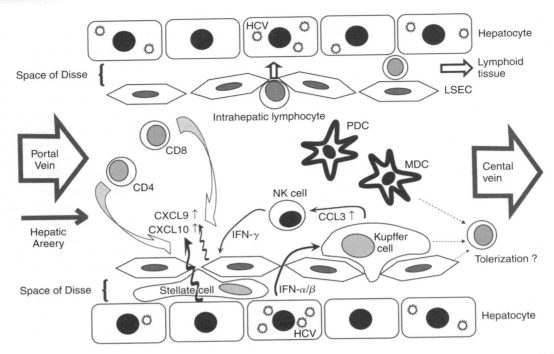

Figure 52.2 Sinusoidal microenvironment in the hepatitis C virus (HCV)-infected liver. Hepatocytes produce IFN-α/β in response to HCV infection, which induces resident macrophages (Kupffer cells) to produce CCL3 (monocyte inflammatory protein-1α, MIP1-α). CCL3 stimulates NK cells to release IFN-γ, which subsequently induces liver sinusoidal endothelial cells (LSECs) and hepatocytes to produce CXCL9 (monokine induced by IFN-γ, Mig) and CXCL10 (IFN-inducible protein-10, IP-10). Activated CD4 and CD8 T cells are attracted by CXCL9 and CXCL10, which gain access to LSECs, stellate cells and hepatocytes (Crispe, 2003). LSECs, Kupffer cells and liver dendritic cells (DCs) induce tolerance rather than full activation of incoming T cells (Lau and Thomson, 2003).

DC dysfunction in chronic HCV infection

DC dysfunction has been implicated as a mechanism enabling persistent viral infection, as is well known in patients infected with the measles or human immunodeficiency viruses (HIV). Likewise, monocyte-derived DC generated from hepatitis C patients have an impaired ability to stimulate allogeneic CD4 T cells (Kanto et al., 1999; Bain et al., 2001). Functional impairment of DC diminished when HCV had been eradicated from patients, revealing the evidence of HCV-induced DC disability (Bain et al., 2001). Several reports have been available for functional alterations of DC in HBV infection (Beckebaum et al., 2002). Infection of DC by HBV is still controversial and the described functional defects are minimal when compared with HCV (Lohr et al., 2002).

DC play a decisive role in shaping innate immunity by interacting with NK cells during the primary and secondary immune responses. DC have two means to stimulate NK cells via the production of cytokines (IL-12, IL-18 or IFN-α) and through expression of NK-activating ligands. In response to IFN-α, DC are able to express MHC class-I related chain A/B (MICA/B) and activate NK cells following ligation of the NK receptor, NKG2D (Jinushi et al., 2003). Interestingly, DC from HCV-infected patients are unresponsive to exogenous IFN-α to enhance MICA/B expression and fail to activate NK cells (Jinushi et al., 2003). It is tempting to speculate that the impairment of

DC in NK cell activation is responsible for the failure of HCV control in the early phase of primary HCV infection, where HCV continues to replicate in spite of high-level IFN-α expression in the liver (Thimme et al., 2001, 2002).

Alterations in number and function of blood DC have been reported in HIV infection (Soumelis et al., 2001), suggesting their active participation in the outcomes of the diseases. In HCV infection, MDC and PDC in infected patients were reduced in number and impaired in their ability to promote Th1 polarization (Kanto et al., 2003).

Two plausible explanations exist to explain the mechanisms of DC dysfunction in chronic hepatitis C:

1 direct HCV infection of DC and
2 the presence of circulating HCV proteins which affect DC function and number.

The HCV genome has been reported to be isolated from Mo-DC or blood DC (Bain et al., 2001; Goutagny et al., 2003). These results need to be interpreted carefully, since contamination with free virus in blood cannot be ruled out when amplifying PCR techniques are used. Several studies were conducted to transduce HCV genome into DC to determine whether HCV proteins alter DC function. When HCV core and E1 genes are introduced into Mo-DC recovered from uninfected donors, their capacity to stimulate allogeneic T cell responses was decreased (Sarobe et al., 2002). These reports indicate that expression of HCV structural proteins in infected DC disturbs antigen-presenting function, though the precise mechanisms remain unclear. Several criticisms have been raised recently about DC dysfunction in the setting of chronic HCV infection (Longman et al., 2003), failing to demonstrate any DC defects which may have to do with differences in the populations studied. Cohort studies on chimpanzees following HCV infection showed that functional impairment of DC was observed in some cases but was not a prerequisite of persistent infection (Rollier et al., 2003). Further study needs to be done to clarify whether DC are indeed disabled in the setting of human chronic hepatitis C and, furthermore, whether this contributes to the development of HCV persistence or it is simply a consequence of active HCV infection.

Monitoring immune response during anti-viral therapy

In chronic HBV-infected patients with active viral replication, lamivudine has been used to eradicate HBV (Lok and McMahon, 2001). The reduction of HBV burden by lamivudine improves HBV-specific CD4 as well as CD8 T cell responses (Boni et al., 2001). During IFN-α-based therapy, successful responses are associated with lasting and Th1-type CD4 T cell responses (Rico et al., 2001).

Treatment of patients with chronic hepatitis C most frequently involves a combination of IFN-α and ribavirin (Liang et al., 2000). Currently, HCV-RNA quantity and HCV genotypes are the two major predictors dictating the efficacy of IFN-α-based therapy (Liang et al., 2000). Since both IFN-α and ribavirin potentially exert immunomodulatory capacity *in vivo*, it is conceivable that HCV-specific immune responses play a crucial part in inducing successful outcomes. Earlier studies reported that HCV-specific CD8 T cell response, as examined by CTLpf, was not enhanced after IFN-α monotherapy (Rehermann et al., 1996b). Furthermore, analyses of tetramer positive cells in patients who underwent IFN-α and ribavirin therapy revealed that CD8 T cells did not increase following treatment and were not associated with outcome (Barnes et al., 2002). Combination therapy of IFN-α and ribavirin increases antigen-specific CD4 T cell proliferation and IFN-γ production by CD4 T cells (Cramp et al., 2000; Kamal et al., 2002). The "vigor" of the CD4 T cell response to HCV eradication is reported to be variable, something which is considered quite controversial (Barnes et al., 2002). Sustained and significant CD4 T cell responses with secretion of Th1 type cytokines are characteristic of successful responders to IFN-α and ribavirin therapy. It is plausible that other immune cells, such as NK cells, NKT cells and DC, may play distinct roles during treatment with IFN-α and ribavirin, which needs to be further investigated.

CONCLUSIONS

Studies of patients with viral hepatitis rely on the measurement of antigen-specific immune responses. Owing to the recent development of sensitive techniques performed without *in vitro* modulations, we are now able to monitor directly the existing cells within the liver and the peripheral blood and assess how immunity controls HBV or HCV infections enabling eradication or alleviating virus-induced harmful effects. Several questions remain unresolved with regard to which cells play a predominant role in innate immunity in HCV infection, i.e. NK cells, NKT cells and $\gamma\delta$ T cells. Likewise, limited information is available on the contribution of blood DC subsets, especially the natural interferon-producing PDC. The next steps in evolving innovative approaches to establish HBV- and HCV-specific immunotherapy are to determine the means to direct the magnitude, breadth, quality and duration of antigen-specific immune responses in a desired way.

ACKNOWLEDGEMENT

The author greatly appreciates Dr Michael T. Lotze (University of Pittsburgh) for critical and fruitful discussions.

REFERENCES

Bain, C., Fatmi, A., Zoulim, F., Zarski, J.P., Trepo, C. and Inchauspe, G. (2001). Impaired allostimulatory function of dendritic cells in chronic hepatitis C infection. Gastroenterology *120*, 512–524.

Banchereau, J., Briere, F., Caux, C. et al. (2000). Immunobiology of dendritic cells. Annu Rev Immunol *18*, 767–811.

Barnes, E., Harcourt, G., Brown, D. et al. (2002). The dynamics of T-lymphocyte responses during combination therapy for chronic hepatitis C virus infection. Hepatology *36*, 743–754.

Beckebaum, S., Cicinnati, V.R., Dworacki, G. et al. (2002). Reduction in the circulating pDC1/pDC2 ratio and impaired function of ex vivo-generated DC1 in chronic hepatitis B infection. Clin Immunol *104*, 138–150.

Bertoletti, A. and Ferrari, C. (2003). Kinetics of the immune response during HBV and HCV infection. Hepatology *38*, 4–13.

Boni, C., Penna, A., Ogg, G.S. et al. (2001). Lamivudine treatment can overcome cytotoxic T-cell hyporesponsiveness in chronic hepatitis B: new perspectives for immune therapy. Hepatology *33*, 963–971.

Chang, K.M., Thimme, R., Melpolder, J.J. et al. (2001). Differential CD4(+) and CD8(+) T-cell responsiveness in hepatitis C virus infection. Hepatology *33*, 267–276.

Cooper, S., Erickson, A.L., Adams, E.J. et al. (1999). Analysis of a successful immune response against hepatitis C virus. Immunity *10*, 439–449.

Cramp, M.E., Rossol, S., Chokshi, S., Carucci, P., Williams, R. and Naoumov, N.V. (2000). Hepatitis C virus-specific T-cell reactivity during interferon and ribavirin treatment in chronic hepatitis C. Gastroenterology *118*, 346–355.

Crispe, I.N. (2003). Hepatic T cells and liver tolerance. Nat Rev Immunol 3, 51–62.

Crotta, S., Stilla, A., Wack, A. et al. (2002). Inhibition of natural killer cells through engagement of CD81 by the major hepatitis C virus envelope protein. J Exp Med 195, 35–41.

Day, C.L., Lauer, G.M., Robbins, G.K. et al. (2002). Broad specificity of virus-specific CD4+ T-helper-cell responses in resolved hepatitis C virus infection. J Virol 76, 12584–12595.

Day, C.L., Seth, N.P., Lucas, M. et al. (2003). Ex vivo analysis of human memory CD4 T cells specific for hepatitis C virus using MHC class II tetramers. J Clin Invest 112, 831–842.

Diepolder, H.M., Zachoval, R., Hoffmann, R.M. et al. (1995). Possible mechanism involving T-lymphocyte response to nonstructural protein 3 in viral clearance in acute hepatitis C virus infection. Lancet 346, 1006–1007.

Dzionek, A., Fuchs, A., Schmidt, P. et al. (2000). BDCA-2, BDCA-3, and BDCA-4: three markers for distinct subsets of dendritic cells in human peripheral blood. J Immunol 165, 6037–6046.

Farci, P., Alter, H.J., Wong, D.C. et al. (1994). Prevention of hepatitis C virus infection in chimpanzees after antibody-mediated in vitro neutralization. Proc Natl Acad Sci USA 91, 7792–7796.

Fong, T.L., Di Bisceglie, A.M., Biswas, R. et al. (1994). High levels of viral replication during acute hepatitis B infection predict progression to chronicity. J Med Virol 43, 155–158.

Foy, E., Li, K., Wang, C. et al. (2003). Regulation of interferon regulatory factor-3 by the hepatitis C virus serine protease. Science 300, 1145–1148.

Goutagny, N., Fatmi, A., De Ledinghen, V. et al. (2003). Evidence of viral replication in circulating dendritic cells during hepatitis C virus infection. J Infect Dis 187, 1951–1958.

Grabowska, A.M., Lechner, F., Klenerman, P. et al. (2001). Direct ex vivo comparison of the breadth and specificity of the T cells in the liver and peripheral blood of patients with chronic HCV infection. Eur J Immunol 31, 2388–2394.

Grakoui, A., Shoukry, N.H., Woollard, D.J. et al. (2003). HCV persistence and immune evasion in the absence of memory T cell help. Science 302, 659–662.

Gruener, N.H., Lechner, F., Jung, M.C. et al. (2001). Sustained dysfunction of antiviral CD8+ T lymphocytes after infection with hepatitis C virus. J Virol 75, 5550–5558.

Guidotti, L.G. and Chisari, F.V. (2001). Noncytolytic control of viral infections by the innate and adaptive immune response. Annu Rev Immunol 19, 65–91.

He, X.S., Rehermann, B., Lopez-Labrador, F.X. et al. (1999). Quantitative analysis of hepatitis C virus-specific CD8(+) T cells in peripheral blood and liver using peptide-MHC tetramers. Proc Natl Acad Sci USA 96, 5692–5697.

Heil, F., Ahmad-Nejad, P., Hemmi, H. et al. (2003). The Toll-like receptor 7 (TLR7)-specific stimulus loxoribine uncovers a strong relationship within the TLR7, 8 and 9 subfamily. Eur J Immunol 33, 2987–2997.

Hiroishi, K., Kita, H., Kojima, M. et al. (1997). Cytotoxic T lymphocyte response and viral load in hepatitis C virus infection. Hepatology 25, 705–712.

Jinushi, M., Takehara, T., Kanto, T. et al. (2003). Critical role of MHC class I-related chain A and B expression on IFN-alpha-stimulated dendritic cells in NK cell activation: impairment in chronic hepatitis C virus infection. J Immunol 170, 1249–1256.

Kadowaki, N., Ho, S., Antonenko, S. et al. (2001). Subsets of human dendritic cell precursors express different toll-like receptors and respond to different microbial antigens. J Exp Med 194, 863–869.

Kakimi, K., Guidotti, L.G., Koezuka, Y. and Chisari, F.V. (2000). Natural killer T cell activation inhibits hepatitis B virus replication in vivo. J Exp Med 192, 921–930.

Kamal, S.M., Fehr, J., Roesler, B., Peters, T. and Rasenack, J.W. (2002). Peginterferon alone or with ribavirin enhances HCV-specific CD4 T-helper 1 responses in patients with chronic hepatitis C. Gastroenterology 123, 1070–1083.

Kanto, T., Hayashi, N., Takehara, T. et al. (1999). Impaired allostimulatory capacity of peripheral blood dendritic cells recovered from hepatitis C virus-infected individuals. J Immunol 162, 5584–5591.

Kanto, T., Sato, A., Inoue, M. et al. (2003). IFN-gamma or IL-15 restores the impaired helper T cell polarizing ability of blood dendritic cell subsets in chronic hepatitis C. Hepatology 38 Suppl. 1, 342A.

Kittlesen, D.J., Chianese-Bullock, K.A., Yao, Z.Q., Braciale, T.J. and Hahn, Y.S. (2000). Interaction between complement receptor gC1qR and hepatitis C virus core protein inhibits T-lymphocyte proliferation. J Clin Invest 106, 1239–1249.

Koziel, M.J., Wong, D.K., Dudley, D., Houghton, M. and Walker, B.D. (1997). Hepatitis C virus-specific cytolytic T lymphocyte and T helper cell responses in seronegative persons. J Infect Dis 176, 859–866.

Lau, A.H. and Thomson, A.W. (2003). Dendritic cells and immune regulation in the liver. Gut 52, 307–314.

Lauer, G.M., Ouchi, K., Chung, R.T. et al. (2002). Comprehensive analysis of CD8(+)-T-cell responses against hepatitis C virus reveals multiple unpredicted specificities. J Virol 76, 6104–6113.

Lechner, F., Cuero, A.L., Kantzanou, M. and Klenerman, P. (2001). Studies of human antiviral CD8+ lymphocytes using class I peptide tetramers. Rev Med Virol 11, 11–22.

Lechner, F., Wong, D.K., Dunbar, P.R. et al. (2000). Analysis of successful immune responses in persons infected with hepatitis C virus. J Exp Med 191, 1499–1512.

Leroy, V., Vigan, I., Mosnier, J.F. et al. (2003). Phenotypic and functional characterization of intrahepatic T lymphocytes during chronic hepatitis C. Hepatology 38, 829–841.

Liang, T.J., Rehermann, B., Seeff, L.B. and Hoofnagle, J.H. (2000). Pathogenesis, natural history, treatment, and prevention of hepatitis C. Ann Intern Med 132, 296–305.

Liu, Y.J., Kadowaki, N., Rissoan, M.C. and Soumelis, V. (2000). T cell activation and polarization by DC1 and DC2. Curr Top Microbiol Immunol 251, 149–159.

Lohr, H.F., Pingel, S., Bocher, W.O. et al. (2002). Reduced virus specific T helper cell induction by autologous dendritic cells in patients with chronic hepatitis B-restoration by exogenous interleukin-12. Clin Exp Immunol 130, 107–114.

Lok, A.S. and McMahon, B.J. (2001). Chronic hepatitis B. Hepatology 34, 1225–1241.

Longman, R.S., Talal, A.H., Jacobson, I.M., Albert, M.L. and Rice, C.M. (2003). Patients chronically infected with hepatitis C virus have functional dendritic cells. Blood.

Lyons, A.B. (2000). Analysing cell division in vivo and in vitro using flow cytometric measurement of CFSE dye dilution. J Immunol Methods 243, 147–154.

Maini, M.K., Boni, C., Lee, C.K. et al. (2000). The role of virus-specific CD8(+) cells in liver damage and viral control during persistent hepatitis B virus infection. J Exp Med 191, 1269–1280.

Maini, M.K., Boni, C., Ogg, G.S. et al. (1999). Direct ex vivo analysis of hepatitis B virus-specific CD8(+) T cells associated with the control of infection. Gastroenterology 117, 1386–1396.

Nascimbeni, M., Mizukoshi, E., Bosmann, M. et al. (2003). Kinetics of CD4+ and CD8+ memory T-cell responses during hepatitis C virus rechallenge of previously recovered chimpanzees. J Virol 77, 4781–4793.

Nelson, D.R., Marousis, C.G., Davis, G.L. et al. (1997). The role of hepatitis C virus-specific cytotoxic T lymphocytes in chronic hepatitis C. J Immunol 158, 1473–1481.

Penna, A., Artini, M., Cavalli, A. et al. (1996). Long-lasting memory T cell responses following self-limited acute hepatitis B. J Clin Invest 98, 1185–1194.

Penna, A., Missale, G., Lamonaca, V. et al. (2002). Intrahepatic and circulating HLA class II-restricted, hepatitis C virus-specific T cells: functional characterization in patients with chronic hepatitis C. Hepatology 35, 1225–1236.

Prezzi, C., Casciaro, M.A., Francavilla, V. et al. (2001). Virus-specific CD8(+) T cells with type 1 or type 2 cytokine profile are related to different disease activity in chronic hepatitis C virus infection. Eur J Immunol 31, 894–906.

Rehermann, B., Chang, K.M., McHutchinson, J. et al. (1996a). Differential cytotoxic T-lymphocyte responsiveness to the hepatitis B and C viruses in chronically infected patients. J Virol 70, 7092–7102.

Rehermann, B., Chang, K.M., McHutchison, J.G., Kokka, R., Houghton, M. and Chisari, F.V. (1996b). Quantitative analysis of the peripheral blood cytotoxic T lymphocyte response in patients with chronic hepatitis C virus infection. J Clin Invest 98, 1432–1440.

Rehermann, B., Lau, D., Hoofnagle, J.H. and Chisari, F.V. (1996c). Cytotoxic T lymphocyte responsiveness after resolution of chronic hepatitis B virus infection. J Clin Invest 97, 1655–1665.

Reignat, S., Webster, G.J., Brown, D. et al. (2002). Escaping high viral load exhaustion: CD8 cells with altered tetramer binding in chronic hepatitis B virus infection. J Exp Med 195, 1089–1101.

Rico, M.A., Quiroga, J.A., Subira, D. et al. (2001). Hepatitis B virus-specific T-cell proliferation and cytokine secretion in chronic hepatitis B e antibody-positive patients treated with ribavirin and interferon alpha. Hepatology 33, 295–300.

Rollier, C., Drexhage, J.A., Verstrepen, B.E. et al. (2003). Chronic hepatitis C virus infection established and maintained in chimpanzees independent of dendritic cell impairment. Hepatology 38, 851–858.

Romani, N., Gruner, S., Brang, D. et al. (1994). Proliferating dendritic cell progenitors in human blood. J Exp Med 180, 83–93.

Rubio-Godoy, V., Dutoit, V., Rimoldi, D. et al. (2001). Discrepancy between ELISPOT IFN-gamma secretion and binding of A2/peptide multimers to TCR reveals interclonal dissociation of CTL effector function from TCR-peptide/MHC complexes half-life. Proc Natl Acad Sci USA 98, 10302–10307.

Sarobe, P., Lasarte, J.J., Casares, N. et al. (2002). Abnormal priming of CD4(+) T cells by dendritic cells expressing hepatitis C virus core and E1 proteins. J Virol 76, 5062–5070.

Schirren, C.A., Jung, M.C., Gerlach, J.T. et al. (2000). Liver-derived hepatitis C virus (HCV)-specific CD4(+) T cells recognize multiple HCV epitopes and produce interferon gamma. Hepatology 32, 597–603.

Scognamiglio, P., Accapezzato, D., Casciaro, M.A. et al. (1999). Presence of effector CD8+ T cells in hepatitis C virus-exposed healthy seronegative donors. J Immunol 162, 6681–6689.

Shortman, K. and Liu, Y.J. (2002). Mouse and human dendritic cell subtypes. Nat Rev Immunol 2, 151–161.

Shoukry, N.H., Grakoui, A., Houghton, M. et al. (2003). Memory CD8+ T cells are required for protection from persistent hepatitis C virus infection. J Exp Med 197, 1645–1655.

Soumelis, V., Scott, I., Gheyas, F. et al. (2001). Depletion of circulating natural type 1 interferon-producing cells in HIV-infected AIDS patients. Blood 98, 906–912.

Su, A.I., Pezacki, J.P., Wodicka, L. et al. (2002). Genomic analysis of the host response to hepatitis C virus infection. Proc Natl Acad Sci USA 99, 15669–15674.

Takaki, A., Wiese, M., Maertens, G. et al. (2000). Cellular immune responses persist and humoral responses decrease two decades after recovery from a single-source outbreak of hepatitis C. Nat Med 6, 578–582.

Taylor, D.R., Shi, S.T., Romano, P.R., Barber, G.N. and Lai, M.M. (1999). Inhibition of the interferon-inducible protein kinase PKR by HCV E2 protein. Science 285, 107–110.

Thimme, R., Bukh, J., Spangenberg, H.C. et al. (2002). Viral and immunological determinants of hepatitis C virus clearance, persistence, and disease. Proc Natl Acad Sci USA 99, 15661–15668.

Thimme, R., Oldach, D., Chang, K.M., Steiger, C., Ray, S.C., and Chisari, F.V. (2001). Determinants of viral clearance and persistence during acute hepatitis C virus infection. J Exp Med 194(10), 1395–406.

Thimme, R., Wieland, S., Steiger, C. et al. (2003). CD8(+) T cells mediate viral clearance and disease pathogenesis during acute hepatitis B virus infection. J Virol 77, 68–76.

Ulsenheimer, A., Gerlach, J.T., Gruener, N.H. et al. (2003). Detection of functionally altered hepatitis C virus-specific CD4 T cells in acute and chronic hepatitis C. Hepatology 37, 1189–1198.

Urbani, S., Boni, C., Missale, G. et al. (2002). Virus-specific CD8+ lymphocytes share the same effector-memory phenotype but exhibit functional differences in acute hepatitis B and C. J Virol 76, 12423–12434.

Webster, G.J., Reignat, S., Maini, M.K. et al. (2000). Incubation phase of acute hepatitis B in man: dynamic of cellular immune mechanisms. Hepatology 32, 1117–1124.

Wedemeyer, H., He, X.S., Nascimbeni, M. et al. (2002). Impaired effector function of hepatitis C virus-specific CD8+ T cells in chronic hepatitis C virus infection. J Immunol 169, 3447–3458.

Wertheimer, A.M., Miner, C., Lewinsohn, D.M., Sasaki, A.W., Kaufman, E. and Rosen, H.R. (2003). Novel CD4+ and CD8+ T-cell determinants within the NS3 protein in subjects with spontaneously resolved HCV infection. Hepatology 37, 577–589.

Wong, D.K., Dudley, D.D., Afdhal, N.H. et al. (1998). Liver-derived CTL in hepatitis C virus infection: breadth and specificity of responses in a cohort of persons with chronic infection. J Immunol 160, 1479–1488.

Zhang, J., Randall, G., Higginbottom, A., Monk, P., Rice, C.M. and McKeating, J.A. (2004). CD81 is required for hepatitis C virus glycoprotein-mediated viral infection. J Virol 78, 1448–1455.

Dermatology

Chapter 53

Clemens Esche

Department of Dermatology, The Johns Hopkins University, Baltimore, MD, USA

What if everything is an illusion and nothing exists? In that case, I definitely overpaid for my carpet.

Woody Allen (born 1935)

OVERVIEW

The etiology and pathogenesis of many chronic inflammatory dermatologic diseases are not yet fully understood and therapeutic approaches remain largely symptomatic. Prominent examples include atopic eczema, lupus erythematosus, scleroderma, vasculitis, tumors of skin homing lymphocytes and melanoma. The major skin cancer subtypes include basal cell carcinoma, squamous cell carcinoma, melanoma and cutaneous T cell lymphoma. Skin cancer is actually the most common human malignancy, with more than 1.2 million new cases occurring in Caucasians in the USA annually. This number equals the combined incidence of all other cancers.

Innate immunity is a first line of defense to many exogenous and endogenous danger signals, while adaptive immunity, arising in the setting of chronic inflammation, is associated with primarily an antigen-specific response (Esche and Beck, 2004). We will therefore focus on measuring adaptive immunity, which is capable of recognizing stressed cells through B and T cell receptors. Both *antibody-* and *cell-mediated immunity* are involved in the pathogenesis of many dermatologic conditions. For example, atopic dermatitis is characterized by B cell IgE overproduction and also defective cell-mediated immunity.

Much progress has been made recently in the area of immunobullous diseases. Their classification not only relies on clinicopathological and direct immunofluorescence (DIF) findings, but also can now be refined down to the level of the target antigen, or even the antibody-bound epitope that characterize these disorders. Deposition of immunoglobulins in skin lesions is commonly determined using immunofluorescence and will be discussed below as an example of assessing *antibody-mediated immunity*. Selected aspects of measuring *cell-mediated immunity* are reviewed later.

INTRODUCTION

The skin is the body's largest organ, accounting for approximately 15 per cent of the total weight in adult humans. It is also home to up to three million microbes per cm^2, which feed on its scales and secretions. Therefore, the skin's principal physical function is that of a barrier. The epidermis, the outermost layer, is composed primarily of *keratinocytes* (Figure 53.1). It continuously renews itself through germinative cells, constituents of the basal cell layer. This layer separates the epidermis from the vascularized dermis (Figure 53.1) and also contains mechanoreceptive *Merkel cells* besides *melanocytes* at a frequency of approximately one for every 10 basal keratinocytes (Figure 53.2A). Each melanocyte extends with its dendrites into the upper epidermal layers, transporting pigment-containing melanosomes to approximately 36 keratinocytes, thereby

Measuring Immunity, edited by Michael T. Lotze and Angus W. Thomson
ISBN 0-12-455900-X, London

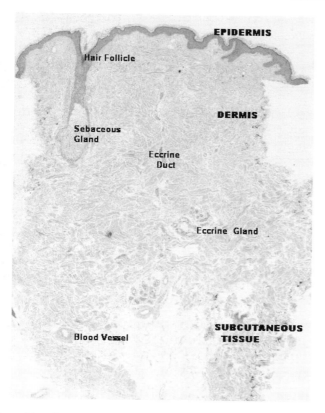

Figure 53.1 Skin is composed of epidermis, dermis and subcutaneous tissue. (Courtesy of Drs P.M. Manolson and T.L. Barrett, Johns Hopkins.) **See colour plate 53.1.**

protecting the skin from ultraviolet radiation (Figure 53.2A). Not the number but rather the activity of melanocytes determines ethnic variations in pigmentation. Cutaneous melanoma is derived from altered epidermal melanocytes and vitiligo is the result of autoantibody-mediated destruction of melanocytes (both conditions are discussed below). Keratinocytes differentiate as they move through spiny, granular and cornified layers towards the skin surface. The epidermal turnover time is about 70 days. The cells take 26–42 days to transit from the basal layer to the granular layer and a further 14 days to pass through the keratin layer. Keratinocytes not only serve a structural function but also actively participate in inflammatory and immunologic processes. This was first appreciated in the early 1970s when keratinocytes were recognized as major factories for IL-1β and GM-CSF. We now know that keratinocytes produce a plethora of biologically active molecules (cytokines, chemokines, growth factors, neuropeptides, antimicrobial peptides, lipid mediators, etc) and respond to a variety of immunological mediators by virtue of their expression of a range of receptors (Esche et al., 2004). In addition to being capable of functioning as antigen-presenting cells (see below), keratinocytes also harbor antigens resulting in autoimmune blistering disease. The pemphigus vulgaris antigen, a desmoglein type of cadherin, is located within keratinocyte desmosomes (see below).

Langerhans cells (LCs) account for up to 4 per cent of all the cells in the epidermis and form a semicontiguous

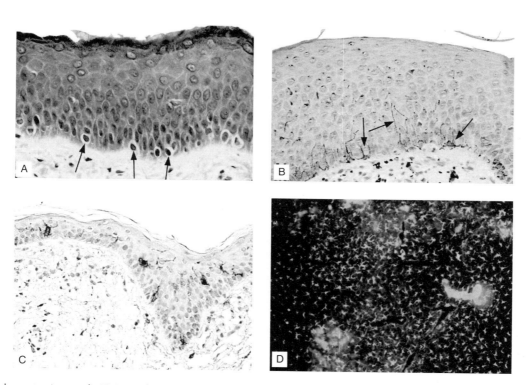

Figure 53.2 (A) Melanocytes (arrowed). (C) Langerhans cells express CD1a protein. (D) Immunofluorescence staining for HLA-DR in an epidermal sheet. (Courtesy of Drs P.M. Manolson and T.L. Barrett, Johns Hopkins (A–C) and N. Romani, University of Innsbruck, Austria (D).) **See colour plate 53.2.**

network (Figure 53.2C,D). They are the prototypic "immature" dendritic cell (DC), specialized for recognition, capturing and processing of exogenous antigen and function as sentinels of the skin immune system by constantly monitoring the local environment and transporting foreign antigen for presentation to responsive T lymphocytes in regional lymph nodes. A classic example is allergic contact hypersensitivity. LCs express CD1a (a feature not observed in other cells of histiocytic origin), Langerin/CD207 (induces the formation of Birbeck granules) and E-cadherin (mediates adhesion to keratinocytes); these are not normally found on dermal DCs. Reciprocally, *dermal DCs* can express DC-SIGN/CD209, the macrophage mannose receptor/CD206 and CD13 (Steinman, 2003). A functional distinction between epidermal and dermal DCs is that the latter stimulate B cells in certain assay systems. In the steady state, LCs are replaced from a local precursor pool, whereas during inflammation, recruitment is largely via a bloodborne bone marrow-derived precursor. LC migration and the transport of antigen from the skin to the lymph nodes may lead to immunity or tolerance, depending on the circumstances.

The interface between the epidermis and the underlying dermis is called the *basement membrane zone*. Electron microscopic examination reveals the following four components:

1 the *basal cell plasma membrane*
2 the *lamina lucida*, a clear zone which is traversed by anchoring filaments that connect the basal cell plasma membrane with

3 the *basal lamina* (an electron dense zone composed primarily of type IV collagen)
4 the *sublamina densa* zone including the *anchoring fibrils* (composed of type VII collagen), that complete the connection with the dermis.

In addition to these structural components there are numerous antigenic epitopes within this region. Specifically, much attention has been focused recently to the involvement of the epidermal basement membrane in bullous diseases. For instance, the bullous pemphigoid antigen constitutes a transmembrane epitope associated with the lamina lucida and the hemidesmosomes of the basal keratinocytes. Binding of autoantibodies to the antigen actually appears to represent the initial pathogenetic event in bullous pemphigoid. Direct immunofluorescence (DIF) staining detects immunoglobulins and complement components within biopsy specimens of blistering and other immune diseases of the skin.

ASSESSMENT OF ANTIBODY-MEDIATED IMMUNITY: IMMUNOFLUORESCENCE TESTING

Immunofluorescence microscopy is the most widely used immunopathology technique and particularly useful in diagnosis and follow-up of bullous and connective tissue diseases (Table 53.1). There are two basic types: *direct immunofluorescence (DIF)* detects molecules such as immunoglobulins and complement components within

Table 53.1 Deposition of immunoglobulins in skin lesions

Disease	Usual direct immunofluorescence
Pemphigus vulgaris	epidermal intercellular IgG, occasionally IgM, IgA and C3
Pemphigus erythematosus	intercellular IgG and/or complement
Pemphigus foliaceus	intercellular IgG and C3
Pemphigus vegetans	epidermal intercellular IgG and C3
Paraneoplastic pemphigus	intercellular and basement membrane IgG and/or C3
Bullous pemphigoid	linear, homogeneous IgG and/or C3 along the basement membrane zone
Cicatricial pemphigoid	linear basement membrane zone IgG and often C3
Pemphigoid gestationis	linear basement membrane zone C3 and sometimes IgG
Dermatitis herpetiformis	papillary dermis stippled IgA, IgM, C3
Linear IgA bullous dermatosis	linear basement membrane zone IgA, sometimes IgG, IgM and/or C3
Erythema multiforme	intraepidermal IgM and sometimes C3
Lichen planus	papillary dermis IgM and complement
Lichen planus pemphigoides	basement membrane zone IgG, C3 and C9
Granuloma anulare	necrobiotic zone fibrinogen, vessel IgM and fibrinogen
Necrobiosis lipoidica	necrobiotic zone fibrinogen, vessel IgM and fibrinogen
Mixed connective tissue disease	epidermal nuclei IgG
Psoriasis	Stratum corneum IgG, C3
Erythropoietic protoporphyria	basement membrane zone IgG
Porphyria cutanea tarda	basement membrane zone IgG
Lepromatous leprosy	dermal—epidermal junction IgM
Epidermolysis bullosa acquisita	IgG, C3b and C5 along the basement membrane zone

(adapted from Dahl).

biopsy specimens. This technique, introduced in 1963, describes immunofluorescent features of lesional skin of lupus erythematosus patients (Burnham et al., 1963). In contrast, *indirect immunofluorescence (IIF)* is a test in which a patient's serum is examined for the presence of antibodies to a defined antigen. This technique, introduced in 1964 by Beutner and Jordan, reported detection of antibodies to the intercellular spaces of stratified squamous epithelia in the sera of patients with pemphigus. Today, IIF is frequently used for detection of antinuclear antibodies (ANA), endomysial antibodies and antibodies against neutrophilic cytoplasm (ANCA).

Blistering autoimmune diseases are a heterogeneous group of conditions that can affect either skin and mucous membrane, or both, varying in presentation, clinical course, histopathology, immunopathology and treatment. Not infrequently the diagnosis is delayed, which may result in severe and sometimes fatal consequences. Pemphigus is a general term for a group of chronic blistering skin diseases in which autoantibodies are directed against the keratinocyte cell surface. *Pemphigus vulgaris*, the most common type of pemphigus, usually starts in the oral mucosa followed by blistering of the skin. The bullae occur intra-epidermally (Figure 53.3B) and therefore rupture easily; leaving denuded and crusted erosions (Figure 53.3A). The hallmark of pemphigus is the finding of IgG autoantibodies against the cell surface of keratinocytes. The target antigen is desmoglein-3, a

130 kD glycoprotein that belongs to the cadherin superfamily of cell adhesion molecules (Amagai et al., 1990). The anti-desmoglein-3 antibodies are bound to lesional epidermis *in vivo* (as illustrated by the DIF test shown in Figure 53.3C) and also circulate in the serum (detectable through IIF), often paralleling disease extent and activity. DIF becomes positive early and demonstrates intercellular IgG throughout the epidermis or the oral epithelium. IgG is found in both involved and clinically normal skin in nearly all patients. In acantholytic areas (acantholysis is loss of cohesion between keratinocytes), C3 deposition is also reliably found. Murine models have identified the autoantibodies as a pathogenic factor. A loss of cell adhesion and blister formation is observed when IgG (Anhalt et al., 1982) or affinity-purified desmoglein 3 specific antibodies (Amagai et al., 1992) from pemphigus vulgaris patients are transferred to neonatal mice. In addition, neonates of mothers with pemphigus vulgaris may have a transient disease caused by maternal IgG that crosses the placenta (Merlob et al., 1986). Frequencies of desmoglein 3 specific IgG producing and memory B cells have been assessed via ELISPOT (Nishifuji et al., 2000). The presence of autoantibodies is actually associated with specific HLA class II alleles (HLA-DRB1*0402 specifically in Jewish patients, while DRB1*14/DQB1*0503 is more prevalent in others), suggesting involvement of a T cell-dependent pathogenesis.

Another condition in which autoreactive CD4+ T cells recognize distinct epitopes is *bullous pemphigoid*, the

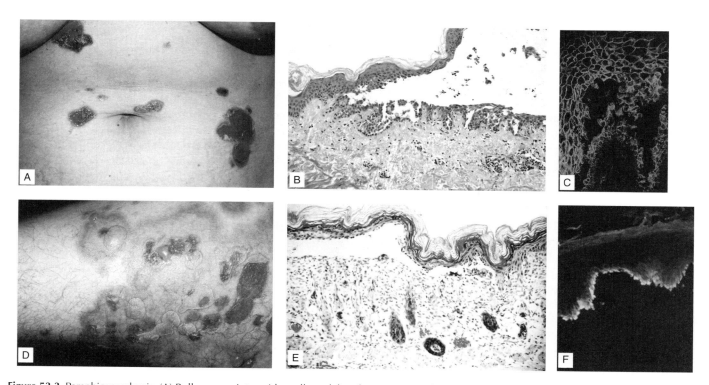

Figure 53.3 Pemphigus vulgaris. (A) Bullae occur intraepidermally and therefore rupture easily, leaving denuded erosions. (B) Suprabasilar blistering. (C) Direct immunofluorescence demonstrates IgG in the intracellular regions of the epidermis. Bullous pemphigoid. (D) Bullae occur on erythematous patches and urticarial plaques. (E) Subepidermal blistering. (F) Direct immunofluorescence staining shows linear deposit of IgG and complement at the dermal-epidermal junction. (Courtesy of Dr G.J. Anhalt, Johns Hopkins.) **See colour plate 53.5.**

most common autoimmune *subepidermal* blistering disease. Known antigens include BP180, also known as BPAG2 or type XVII collagen (Giudice et al., 1992), and BP230, also known as BPAG1 (Stanley et al., 1998). Bullous pemphigoid is characterized by subepidermal bullae (see Figure 53.3E) along with erythematous patches and urticarial plaques (see Figure 53.3d). DIF reveals a linear band of IgG and complement 3 deposited along the basement membrane zone. A positive DIF test result is found in nearly 100 per cent of patients. IIF and also newer techniques such as immunoblot analysis and ELISA are equally sensitive (Chan et al., 2003). Passive transfer of a purified rabbit anti-mouse BP180 IgG antibody into neonatal Balb/c mice induces a blistering disease closely mimicking human bullous pemphigoid (Liu et al., 1993). DIF analysis of the (peri) lesional skin revealed *in vivo* deposition of rabbit IgG and mouse C3 at the basement membrane. This model has proved to be useful in dissecting the anti-BP180 IgG-mediated inflammatory cascade in bullous pemphigoid and could also be used to test experimental therapeutic approaches.

Thus, immunofluorescence testing is indicated for the investigation, diagnosis and follow-up of cutaneous diseases for which an immune mediated pathogenesis is considered (see Table 53.1). This specifically includes blistering disorders such as pemphigus vulgaris and bullous pemphigoid.

ASSESSMENT OF CELL-MEDIATED IMMUNITY

Cell-mediated immunity represents a group of immune reactions mediated by NK cells, NKT cells and especially sensitized T lymphocytes. Intact cell-mediated immunity actually requires a complex interaction between lymphoid effectors, macrophages and dendritic cells, cytokines and chemokines. *In vivo* and *in vitro* measures of antigen-specific cell-mediated immunity can be assessed.

In vivo measures of antigen-specific cell-mediated immunity

Cell-mediated immunity comprises the classic delayed type hypersensitivity (DTH) reaction initiated by CD4+ cells and also direct cytotoxicity mediated by CD8+ cells (Kobayashi et al., 2001). The role of DTH reactions (see Chapter 35) in illustrative dermatologic conditions is summarized in Table 53.2. Even one T cell is capable of mediating a clinical response (Marchal et al., 1982). DTH testing has been commonly used as: (i) anergy screening; (ii) testing for infection with intracellular pathogens and (iii) testing for sensitivity to contact allergens (Rosenstreich, 1993). Anergy screening requires intradermal testing with common recall antigens including *Candida albicans*, tetanus toxoid, mumps and purified protein derivative (PPD). Problems of antigen potency and availability have been addressed by using a multiple tine test-like device that

Table 53.2 Role of delayed type hypersensitivity (DTH) in skin diseases

Disease	DTH
Allergic contact dermatitis	pathogenetic mechanism
Atopic dermatitis	impaired
Chronic actinic dermatitis	pathogenetic mechanism
Erythema induratum	PPD-specific T cells, capable of producing IFN-γ, are likely to be involved in the formation of EI as a type of DTH response to mycobacterial antigens
Erythema nodosum	pathogenetic mechanism
Granulome annulare	DTH to an unknown antigen has been postulated as the precipitating event
Psoriasis	impaired
Photoallergy	pathogenetic mechanism
Wiskott-Aldrich syndrome	usually absent

contains seven different recall antigens (CMI Multitest). Although testing for infection was once common, it is now only recommended for tuberculosis screening because most other antigens are either not predictive of infection or not commercially available. Patch testing remains the standard tool for identifying allergens in patients with contact dermatitis.

Patch testing: gold standard for the diagnosis of allergic contact dermatitis

Contact dermatitis can be either allergic or irritant in etiology. Irritant contact dermatitis (ICD) accounts for approximately 80 per cent of all cases, and allergic contact dermatitis (ACD) accounts for the remaining 20 per cent. ACD is a delayed-type hypersensitivity reaction (Coombs and Gell (1975) type IV) that is elicited when the skin comes in contact with a substance to which an individual has previously been sensitized. The events resulting in allergic contact dermatitis are clearly T cell-dependent, since T cell-deficient mice are unable to mount a contact hypersensitivity (CHS) response. Contact allergens almost invariably represent small-molecule substances of less than 500 daltons. This allows them to penetrate the horny layer. Antigenicity is accomplished by coupling with soluble or cell associated host proteins. The resulting full antigens are called *haptens*. They are captured by epidermal LCs and presented in the regional lymph node (Macatonia et al., 1987). Very low hapten doses result in tolerance mediated by *CD8+ regulatory T cells* (Steinbrink et al., 1996). Otherwise, *effector T cells* are induced. This T cell priming or *sensitization phase* is followed by a clinically relevant *elicitation phase* upon re-exposure to the specific allergen. The elicitation phase actually does not require LCs. Their experimental depletion at this point even enhances CHS responses (Grabbe et al., 1995). Antigens are also presented by keratinocytes, dermal mast cells and macrophages. Primed T cells express the *skin homing* marker *CLA* enabling them to enter the skin (Robert and Kupper, 1999). The eventual result is an inflammatory response clinically recognized as ACD. Both CD4+ and CD8+ T cells can recognize haptenated peptides. Depletion studies have established the importance of CD4+ T cells as the effector cells (Miller and Jenkins, 1985; Gautam *et al.*, 1991) and others have demonstrated the ability of CD8+ T cells to mediate CHS (Gocinski and Tigelaar, 1990; Bour et al., 1995; Xu et al., 1996).

The identification of allergens responsible for ACD is key to the clinical management. *Patch testing* remains the gold standard for establishing the diagnosis (Figure 53.4). It is the oldest and most frequently studied form of *in vivo* T cell-mediated immunity. There is no single patch test panel that will screen all the relevant allergens in a patient's environment. It is generally thought that 20–30 allergens in routine screening tests can identify 50–70 per cent of clinically relevant ACD. The screening series *TRUE test* includes medications, fragrances, preservatives, metals, rubber compounds and miscellaneous chemicals (Fischer et al., 2001). They are applied to patches that are taped on the back of the patient (Figure 53.4A). After 48 h, the patches are removed (Figure 53.4B) and the test site is examined for an eczematous reaction that is graded according to a standard interpretation key: a faint macular erythema indicates a +/− (doubtful) reaction, a *nonvesicular* reaction with erythema, infiltration and papules indicates a +1 reaction, a *vesicular* reaction with erythema, infiltration and papules indicates a +2 reaction (Figure 53.4C) and bullae indicate a +3 reaction (Figure 53.5). There may be no foolproof way to distinguish an irritant from an allergic patch test reaction, but responses suggesting true allergy include increasing inflammation and induration for 48 h after patch test removal, persistence for longer than 1 week, prominent induration, spread beyond the test site, failure to evoke dermatitis in other individuals and flare at patch test site associated with allergen recontact (Dahl, 1996). A more in-depth coverage of all aspects of patch testing is provided by Rietschel and Fowler (2001).

Tuberculin delayed-type hypersensitivity skin testing

The *tuberculin skin test (TST)*, also referred to as *Mantoux test* or *purified protein derivative (PPD)*, detects a cell-mediated immune response to *Mycobacterium tuberculosis*. CD4+ T helper cells sensitized by prior infection are recruited to the test site where they release cytokines that induce induration via local vasodilatation and recruitment of monocytes and other inflammatory cells (Tsicopoulos et al., 1992). Less frequently, CD8+ T cells may mediate a similar response. This is in contrast to CHS reactions that are mediated by both CD4+ and CD8+ T effector cells. The Mantoux test becomes positive between 2 and 10 weeks following infection and remains the most sensitive and specific method of identifying infected individuals (Lee and Holzman, 2002). The test is read 48–72 h after intradermal injection of 0.1 ml PPD solution (5 tuberculin units) using a #27 steel (or #26 platinum) needle attached to a 1.0–1 ml syringe into the volar or dorsal surface of the forearm. Creation of a 6–10–1 mm wheal is essential, subcutaneous administration will result in a false-negative result. The diameter of induration (not erythema) should be measured in millimeters 48–72 h after injection, although positive reactions usually persist for at least 7 days. The interpretation of the TST is based on the risk group a person falls into (Lee and Holzman, 2002). Persons at very high risk of developing active tuberculosis should be considered to have latent tuberculosis infection when the TST measures 5 mm or greater. This group includes:

1 HIV positive persons, regardless of CD4 count
2 Recent contacts to active tuberculosis cases
3 Those with fibrosis on their chest radiograph consistent with prior tuberculosis infection and
4 Patients on immunosuppressive treatment equivalent to 15 mg per day of prednisone or greater.

A TST measuring 10 mm or greater is considered positive in the remainder of the population at high risk of developing tuberculosis. For patients at low risk for the

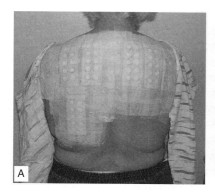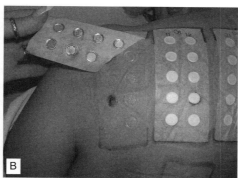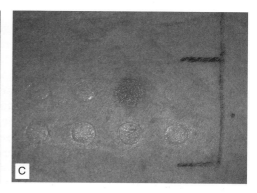

Figure 53.4 Patch testing. (A) Test materials are applied to the skin under occlusive patches (B) that are removed after 48 h. (C) +2 reaction.
See colour plate 53.4.

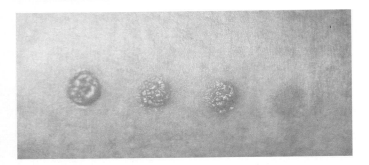

Figure 53.5

development of tuberculosis the TST is considered positive at 15 mm of induration or greater. In addition to identifying immune responses to *Mycobacterium tuberculosis*, DTH testing also remains a useful preliminary screen of the overall immune status, specifically as a monitoring tool for clinical trials. Unfortunately, the cut-off for a positive response has not been standardized yet. In addition, the assay might not be truly antigen-specific (Thurner et al., 1999).

In vitro measures of antigen-specific cellular immunity

Recent developments of measuring cellular immunity *phenotypically* include T cell receptor gene rearrangement as a diagnostic marker of T cell clonality and the detection of antigen-specific cytotoxic T lymphocytes via peptide MHC tetramers (see below). Aspects of *functional* assessment of cellular immunity will be discussed later.

Phenotypic assessment of antigen-specific cellular immunity

There are a variety of strategies to assess the role of T cell-mediated pathology within the skin. These include assessments of T cell clonality and spectratyping, tetramer staining (see Chapter 22), ELISPOT analysis (see Chapter 33), determination of active or activatable signaling pathways/TCR-ζ chain expression and tests for evidence of T cell proliferation (assessment of excision rings) or apoptosis. Some of these are detailed below.

T cell receptor gene rearrangement as a diagnostic marker of T cell clonality in lymphoproliferative skin diseases

The diagnosis of cutaneous T cell lymphoma (CTCL) is notoriously difficult to establish because, in the early stages, histological features may be non-specific. An advance in the molecular immunological features of CTCLs has been the recognition that each normal T and B cell bears a unique antigen receptor on its cell surface that serves as a specific marker for that cell and all of its clonal progeny (Wood, 2001). If the cell should undergo malignant transformation, then this same structure becomes a tumor-specific marker, as well. For B cells, this

marker is the immunoglobulin molecule. For T cells, it is the T cell receptor. A single dominant T cell gene rearrangement can be detected in the majority of T cell neoplasms including mycosis fungoides and used as a marker of monoclonal expansion. Therefore, detection of clonal T cell receptor γ (TCRγ)-chain gene rearrangement has become a widely established approach to distinguish between CTCL and reactive T cell infiltrates. However, the presence of clonality does not necessarily imply malignancy. Cases of pseudolymphomas, lichen planus and pityriasis lichenoides et varioliformis acuta were reported with clonal lymphocytic proliferations. Detection of clonal T cell populations can therefore not be used as an absolute criterion of malignancy, but should always be considered in conjunction with clinical and histological features. Southern blot analysis using probes for the TCR is laborious, has a sensitivity limit of around 5 per cent and requires relatively large quantities of high molecular weight, non-degraded DNA. Therefore, the more sensitive PCR-based amplification has increasingly been used in the diagnosis and staging of CTCL. Amplification products can be detected via polyacrylamide gel electrophoresis (PAGE). Capillary gel electrophoresis provides improved diagnostic sensitivity over conventional methods by producing single nucleotide resolution.

Detection of antigen-specific cytotoxic T lymphocytes via peptide MHC tetramers

A common *phenotypic assay* is the use of *peptide MHC tetramers* for the direct visualization of antigen-specific CD8+ T cells using flow cytometry. Recently, the technique has also been applied to the study of cutaneous disease including melanoma and vitiligo. The use of MHC class I/peptide complexes, which specifically stain CD8+ T cells recognizing melanoma antigens, has become a standard procedure for the monitoring of immunity to *cutaneous melanoma*. The advantages of tetramer assays are that they are more sensitive than ELISPOT, allow for surface and intracellular phenotyping and can be combined readily with functional assays (Klenerman et al., 2002). Very small samples can be evaluated in detail and sorting and cloning from low specific T cell frequencies have been successful. The main disadvantage of tetramers is that only single specificities can be analyzed. Some authors have found correlation of MHC tetramer positivity and cytotoxicity in traditional microcytotoxicity assays and the intensity of staining of CD8+ T cells with peptide MHC tetramers appears to correlate with T cell avidity for the antigen, but tetramer positive cells occasionally fail to kill targets expressing the specific epitope (Clay et al., 2001). The first attempt to immunize against *basal cell carcinoma* has been published recently (Vogt et al., 2004) and immunization with proteins specifically upregulated by hedgehog signaling may hold promise as a preventive option for patients such as those with the basal cell nevus syndrome who are destined to develop large numbers of basal cell carcinomas.

In *vitiligo*, lesional T cells rather than circulating antimelanocytic antibody appear to mediate the supposedly autoimmune but characteristically patchy destruction of cutaneous melanocytes. The use of peptide tetrameric complexes revealed an association between high frequencies of skin-homing melanocyte-specific CD8+ T cells and vitiligo. Furthermore, the frequency of such CD8+ T cells correlates with the extent of disease, suggesting a role for skin-homing melanocyte-specific CD8+ T cells in vitiligo. The ability of such cells to home to sites of potential tissue damage may be a means to control peripheral tolerance *in vivo*. This raises the possibility that CD8-dependent cell-mediated immunity might represent a generalized effector mechanism in autoimmune conditions and as such a potential target for therapeutic intervention. Thus, detection of antigen-specific cytotoxic T lymphocytes via HLA class I tetramers provides new insights into the pathogenesis of cutaneous disease including melanoma and vitiligo. HLA class II tetramers have been relatively slow to follow, but these will also contribute to our understanding of measuring cellular immunity.

Functional assessment of antigen-specific cellular immunity

Functional approaches of assessing antigen-specific cellular immunity in dermatology include *ELISA* and *ELISPOT* for the detection of secreted cytokines, *multiparameter flow cytometry* for the detection of intracellular cytokines and *lymphoproliferation assays*, as discussed in this section on assessing functional cellular immunity to cutaneous melanoma. When identified early, melanoma is one of the most curable of all cancers. If it has spread, it is often deadly. Surgical resection is the treatment of choice for localized melanoma and results in a large number of cures with a long-term survival rate of greater than 90 per cent for AJCC stage I disease. Prognosis worsens with higher stage disease. Patients with AJCC stage IV disease have less than a 5 per cent expected long-term survival rate. Melanoma, however, is considered an immunogenic tumor and many dermatologists believe that spontaneous regressions of melanoma are particularly common. There is extensive evidence indicating that the immune system can recognize and destroy melanoma cells not only *in vitro* but also *in vivo*. Cytotoxic T lymphocyte activity against melanoma antigens, whether endogenous or vaccine-promoted, is now routinely monitored using 'tetramers', cytokine flow cytometry and enzyme-linked immunospot (ELISPOT) assays (antibody-capture-based method for enumerating specific T cells that can secrete a cytokine).

Analysis of intracellular cytokine induction via flow cytometry is more sensitive than the ELISPOT assay and also allows the identification of subsets of reactive cells. In addition, some cytokine flow cytometry studies in melanoma patients have demonstrated correlation with clinical outcome (Maraveyas et al., 1999). The major

drawback of this approach is that the cells detected are no longer viable and thus cells cannot be sorted and cultured to produce clones (Clay et al., 2001). Cytokine flow cytometry, ELISPOT and tetramer staining produce discordant data when applied to the same samples (Whiteside et al., 2003), so it is not clear, which assay, if any, accurately reflects biologically relevant T cell responses. A recent development allows *isolation and ex vivo clonal expansion of viable T cells based on a measurement of their capability to kill melanoma targets* (Rubio et al., 2003). The ability of T cells to proliferate in response to antigen has traditionally been used as an indicator of the presence of antigen-specific CD4+ helper T cells (Clay et al., 2001). However, *lymphoproliferation assays* are imprecise and should not be emphasized in future studies (Keilholz et al., 2002). In contrast, *antibody tests* are simple and accurate and should be incorporated to a greater extent in monitoring plans (Keilholz et al., 2002).

FUTURE PROSPECTS

Even though considerable progress has been made in monitoring antibody- and cell-mediated immunity in dermatology, many issues remain to be solved. Intracellular cytokine analysis, ELISPOT and tetramer based assessment of antigen-specific CD8+ T lymphocytes has allowed a better characterization of their role in dermatologic conditions such as melanoma and vitiligo. HLA class II tetramers have been relatively slow to follow due to technical difficulties in synthesis, but these will also contribute to our understanding of cellular immunity. Future monitoring of clinical trials is expected to include correlates of post-immunization outcomes. The first attempt to immunize against basal cell carcinoma has been published recently and immunization with proteins specifically upregulated by hedgehog signaling may hold promise as a preventive option for patients such as those with the basal cell nevus syndrome who are destined to develop large numbers of basal cell carcinomas. Similar approaches are expected to be developed for squamous cell carcinoma.

The interaction of keratinocytes with T cells, as a non-professional antigen-presenting cell, is just beginning to be studied and is likely to result in new means of assessing immunity in dermatologic conditions. It is becoming increasingly clear that a disturbance in keratinocyte function can induce a variety of diseases such as atopic dermatitis, psoriasis and toxic epidermal necrolysis. In addition, recent evidence of protein expression and functional assays has suggested that TLR1-5 and 9 are either present and/or functional in human keratinocyte host defense. Thus, studying innate immune responses will result in new directions in investigative dermatology. Much work remains to be performed since dermatoses such as atopic dermatitis still await development of a unifying pathogenetic concept.

ACKNOWLEDGMENTS

This work has been supported in part by the 2003 American Skin Association Research Grant for Skin Cancer/Melanoma and a grant from Chiron Corp. Careful review of the manuscript by the editors is appreciated.

REFERENCES

Amagai, M., Klaus-Kovtun, V. and Stanley, J.R. (1991). Autoantibodies against a novel epithelial cadherin in pemphigus vulgaris, a disease of cell adhesion. Cell 67, 869–877.

Amagai, M., Karpati, S., Prussick, R., Klaus-Kovtun, V. and Stanley, J.R. (1992). Autoantibodies against the amino-terminal cadherin-like binding domain of pemphigus vulgaris antigen are pathogenic. J Clin Invest 90, 919–926.

Anhalt, G.J., Labib, R.S., Voorhees, J.J., Beals, T.F. and Diaz, L.A. (1982). Induction of pemphigus in neonatal mice by passive transfer of IgG from patients with the disease. N Engl J Med 306, 1189–1196.

Beutner, E.H. and Jordan, RE. (1964). Demonstration of skin antibodies in sera of pemphigus vulgaris patients by indirect immunofluorescence staining. Proc Soc Exp Biol Med 117, 505–510.

Bour, H., Peyron, E., Gaucherand, M. et al. (1995). Major histocompatibility complex class I-restricted CD8+ T cells and class II-restricted CD4+ T cells, respectively, mediate and regulate contact sensitivity to dinitrofluorobenzene. Eur J Immunol 25, 3006–3010.

Burnham, T.K., Neblett, T.R. and Fine, G. (1963). The application of the fluorescent antibody technic to the investigation of lupus erythematosus and various dermatoses. J Invest Dermatol 41, 451–456.

Chan, Y.C., Sun, Y.J., Ng, P.P. and Tan, S.H. (2003). Comparison of immunofluorescence microscopy, immunoblotting and enzyme-linked immunosorbent assay methods in the laboratory diagnosis of bullous pemphigoid. Clin Exp Dermatol 28, 651–656.

Clay, T.M., Hobeika, A.C., Mosca P.J., Lyerly, H.K. and Morse, M.A. (2001). Assays for monitoring cellular immune responses to active immunotherapy of cancer. Clin Cancer Res 7, 1127–1135.

Coombs, R.R.A. and Gell, P.G.H. (1975). Classification of allergic reactions responsible for clinical hypersensitivity and disease. Clin Aspects Immunol 3.

Dahl, M. (1996). Clinical immunodermatology. Philadelphia: Mosby.

Esche, C. and Beck, L.A. (2004). Chemokines and their receptors: high impact factors of the innate immunity. J Invest Dermatol (in print).

Esche, C., de Benedetto, A. and Beck, L.A. (2004). Keratinocytes in atopic dermatitis: inflammatory signals. Curr Allergy Asthma Rep (in print).

Fischer, T., Kreilgard, B. and Maibach, H.I. (2001). The true value of the TRUE Test for allergic contact dermatitis. Curr Allergy Asthma Rep 1, 316–322.

Gautam, S.C., Matriano, J.A., Chikkala, N.F., Edinger, M.G. and Tubbs, RR. (1991). L3T4 (CD4+) cells that mediate contact sensitivity to trinitrochlorobenzene express I-A determinants. Cell Immunol 135, 27–41.

Giudice, G.J., Emery, D.J. and Diaz, L.A. (1992). Cloning and primary structural analysis of the bullous pemphigoid autoantigen BP180. J Invest Dermatol 99, 243–250.

Gocinski, B.L., Tigelaar, R.E. (1990). Roles of CD4+ and CD8+ T cells in murine contact sensitivity revealed by in vivo monoclonal antibody depletion. J Immunol 144, 4121–4128.

Grabbe, S., Steinbrink, K., Steinert, M., Luger, T.A. and Schwarz, T. (1995). Removal of the majority of epidermal Langerhans cells by topical or systemic steroid application enhances the effector phase of murine contact hypersensitivity. J Immunol 155, 4207–4217.

Keilholz, U., Weber, J., Finke, J.H. et al. (2002). Immunologic monitoring of cancer vaccine therapy: results of a workshop sponsored by the Society for Biological Therapy. J Immunother 25, 97–138.

Klenerman, P., Cerundolo, V. and Dunbar, P.R. (2002). Tracking T cells with tetramers: new tales from new tools. Nat Rev Immunol 2, 263–272.

Kobayashi, K., Kaneda, K. and Kasama, T. (2001). Immunopathogenesis of delayed-type hypersensitivity. Microsc Res Tech 53, 241–245.

Lee, E. and Holzman, R.S. (2002). Evolution and current use of the tuberculin test. Clin Infect Dis 34, 365–370.

Liu, Z., Diaz, L.A., Troy, J.L. et al. (1993). A passive transfer model of the organ-specific autoimmune disease, bullous pemphigoid, using antibodies generated against the hemidesmosomal antigen, BP180. J Clin Invest 92, 2480–2488.

Macatonia, S.E., Knight, S.C., Edwards, A.J., Griffiths, S. and Fryer, P. (1987). Localization of antigen on lymph node dendritic cells after exposure to the contact sensitizer fluorescein isothiocyanate. Functional and morphological studies. J Exp Med 166, 1654–1667.

Marchal, G., Seman, M., Milon, G., Truffa-Bachi, P. and Zilberfarb, V. (1982). Local adoptive transfer of skin delayed-type hypersensitivity initiated by a single T lymphocyte. J Immunol 129, 954–958.

Merlob, P., Metzker, A., Hazaz, B., Rogovin, H. and Reisner, S.H. (1986). Neonatal pemphigus vulgaris. Pediatrics 78, 1102–1105.

Miller, S.D. and Jenkins, M.K. (1985). In vivo effects of GK1.5 (anti-L3T4a) monoclonal antibody on induction and expression of delayed-type hypersensitivity. Cell Immunol 92, 414–426.

Mutasim, D.F. and Adams, B.B. (2001). Immunofluorescence in dermatology. J Am Acad Dermatol 45, 803–822.

Nishifuji, K., Amagai, M., Kuwana, M., Iwasaki, T. and Nishikawa, T. (2000). Detection of antigen-specific B cells in patients with pemphigus vulgaris by enzyme-linked immunospot assay: requirement of T cell collaboration for autoantibody production. J Invest Dermatol 114, 88–94.

Ogg, G.S. (2000). Detection of antigen-specific cytotoxic T lymphocytes: significance for investigative dermatology. Clin Exp Dermatol 25, 312–316.

Ogg, G.S., Rod Dunbar, P., Romero, P., Chen, J.L. and Cerundolo, V. (1998). High frequency of skin-homing melanocyte-specific cytotoxic T lymphocytes in autoimmune vitiligo. J Exp Med 188, 1203–1208.

Rietschel, R.L. and Fowler, J.F. (2001). Fisher's Contact Dermatitis, 5th edn. Baltimore: Lippincott Williams & Wilkins.

Robert, C. and Kupper, T.S. (1999). Inflammatory skin diseases, T cells, and immune surveillance. N Engl J Med 341, 1817–1828.

Rosenstreich, D.L. (1993). Evaluation of delayed hypersensitivity: from PPD to poison ivy. Allergy Proc 14, 395–400.

Rubio, V., Stuge, T.B., Singh, N. et al. (2003). Ex vivo identification, isolation and analysis of tumor-cytolytic T cells. Nat Med 9, 1377–1382.

Steinbrink, K., Sorg, C. and Macher, E. (1996). Low zone tolerance to contact allergens in mice: a functional role for CD8+ T helper type 2 cells. J Exp Med *183*, 759–768.

Steinman, R.M. (2003). Some interfaces of dendritic cell biology. APMIS *111*, 675–697.

Tsicopoulos, A., Hamid, Q., Varney, V. et al. (1992). Preferential messenger RNA expression of Th1-type cells (IFN-gamma+, IL-2+) in classical delayed-type (tuberculin) hypersensitivity reactions in human skin. J Immunol *148*, 2058–2061.

Whiteside, T.L., Zhao, Y., Tsukishiro, T., Elder, E.M., Gooding, W. and Baar, J. (2003). Enzyme-linked immunospot, cytokine flow cytometry, and tetramers in the detection of T-cell responses to a dendritic cell-based multipeptide vaccine in patients with melanoma. Clin Cancer Res *9*, 641–649.

Wood, G.S. (2001). T-cell receptor and immunoglobulin gene rearrangements in diagnosing skin disease. Arch Dermatol *137*, 1503–1506.

Xu, H., DiIulio, N.A. and Fairchild, R.L. (1996). T cell populations primed by hapten sensitization in contact sensitivity are distinguished by polarized patterns of cytokine production: interferon gamma-producing (Tc1) effector CD8+ T cells and interleukin (Il) 4/Il-10-producing (Th2) negative regulatory CD4+ T cells. J Exp Med *183*, 1001–1012.

Zweiman, B. (2003). Cell-mediated immunity in health and disease. In: Middleton's Allergy, Adkinson, N.F et al., eds. Philadelphia: Mosby, pp. 973–995.

Arteriosclerosis

Beatriz Garcia Alvarez and Manuel Matas Docampo

Department of Vascular and Endovascular Surgery, Hospital Universitario Vall d'Hebron, Barcelona, Spain

One of the greatest pains to human nature is the pain of a new idea.

Walter Bagehot (1826–1877)

INTRODUCTION

Observational studies in animals and humans gave rise to the response-to-injury theory to explain the pathophysiology of atherosclerosis (Ross, 1999). According to this idea, the initiation of atherosclerosis is attributed mainly to endothelial denudation in response to aggression by noxious factors. Our knowledge has advanced since then and now it is considered that the initial lesion of atherosclerosis is caused by endothelial dysfunction rather than endothelial denudation. Various stages of a chronic inflammatory process, the host response to a wide range of tissue lesions, have been identified in the different phases of atherosclerosis. Persistence or continuous repetition of the harmful stimulus gives rise to a chronic response that can affect the functionality of the tissue involved. The epidemiological concept of atherosclerosis, i.e. the idea that it is the result of exposure to classic cardiovascular risk factors (smoking, hypercholesterolemia, hypertension, diabetes mellitus) explains less than 50 per cent of the cases (Braunwald, 1997). It is now known that atherosclerosis is a complex process involving several cell types (endothelial cells, smooth muscle cells, monocyte-derived macrophages and specific T lymphocyte subtypes) as well as numerous cytokines and growth factors

and that immune phenomena, mainly those related to cellular immunity, are implicated in the three phases of this condition: initiation, progression and complication. This new focus on a common condition has opened the door to a wide range of diagnostic and therapeutic options and we, as researchers, have the task of further defining the pathophysiologic mechanisms leading to atherosclerosis in order to apply these new approaches.

PATHOPHYSIOLOGIC BASES OF THE ATHEROSCLEROTIC LESION

Initiation of the atherosclerotic lesion

Aggression to the vascular endothelium by many factors provokes a cellular immune response that gives rise to the functional endothelial changes preceding the atherosclerotic lesion. Endothelial dysfunction usually occurs at areas of the vessel walls where there is a bifurcation or elongation that produces blood flow alterations resulting in decreased shear stress and increased turbulence (Gotlieb and Langille, 1996). In physiologic conditions the endothelium maintains the integrity of the cardiovascular system. As a response to aggression it expresses surface adhesion glycoproteins that increase cellular permeability and facilitate immune cell recruitment (mainly monocytes) from the blood to the tissues (Nagel et al., 1994). At the same time secretion of cytokines such as interleukins (IL), mainly IL-1 and IL-6, and vasoactive mediators, such as

Measuring Immunity, edited by Michael T. Lotze and Angus W. Thomson ISBN 0-12-455900-X, London

platelet-derived growth factor, enhance the immune response (Mondy et al., 1997). The adhesion glycoproteins exhibited by the endothelium include those belonging to the family of selectins (E-selectin and P-selectin) and to the superfamily of immunoglobulins (platelet-endothelial cell adhesion molecule-1, PECAM-1), as well as the intercellular adhesion molecules (ICAM-1) and adhesion molecule 1 of the vascular cells (VCAM-1) (Albelda et al., 1994). Once they are expressed on the endothelial surface, the adhesion glycoproteins are recognized by integrins present on the surface of monocytes and T lymphocytes and these cells migrate to the interior of the vessel wall through the spaces between the endothelial cells. Various growth-regulating molecules and chemotactic substances, such as IL-8, leukotrienes, platelet-derived growth factor and monocyte chemoattractant protein-1 (MCP-1), released by the endothelial cells and leukocytes, influence this process by contributing to attract CD4+ and CD8+ lymphocytes to the vascular tissue and by increasing monocyte release of IL-1 and IL-6 (Matsushima and Oppen, 1989). Together with MCP-1, macrophage colony-stimulating factor (M-CSF) facilitates circulating monocyte differentiation into subendothelial macrophages (Qiao et al., 1997).

Progression of the atherosclerotic lesion

The subendothelial macrophages accumulate lipids and release more growth factors and cytokines that attract other macrophages and stimulate smooth muscle cell proliferation. The cytokines increase the production of free radicals, which contribute to low density lipoprotein (LDL) oxidation. The oxidized LDL constitute a ligand for the macrophage scavenger receptor, which internalizes them. The macrophages then become large foam cells characteristic of the initial atherosclerotic lesion: the fatty streak. In these initial phases, migration of smooth muscle cells also occurs, stimulated by platelet-derived growth factor, fibroblast growth factor 2 and transforming growth factor beta and T lymphocyte activation mediated by tumor necrosis factor α (TNF-α), IL-2 and granulocyte-macrophage colony-stimulating factor (Hansson et al., 1989). The activated macrophages, which express human leukocyte antigen-DR (HLA-DR), present antigens to the T lymphocytes, enhancing the immune response (Raines et al., 1996) and release pro-inflammatory cytokines (IL-12, IL-18) that induce T lymphocyte production of interferon gamma (IFN-γ). The macrophages, activated by IFN-γ secrete the pteridine derivative neopterin, which modulates the intracellular redox state, probably through stimulation of NO synthase activity (Schobersberger et al., 1995). As a consequence of the modified redox status, nuclear factor kappa B (NFκB) subunits are translocated toward the nucleus (Wirleitner et al., 1996) and this, in turn, upregulates the pro-inflammatory genes, including IL-1, IL-6, IFN-γ, MCP-1, M-CSF, VCAM, ICAM-1, E-selectin, TNF-α and others. The overall result is increased inflammatory activity in the vessel wall.

The unstable plaque

Advanced atherosclerotic plaques that can cause significant stenosis are characterized by a core consisting of an accumulation of lipids and debris and a fibrous cap that walls off the lesion from the vessel lumen. The lipid core consists of monohydrates and cholesterol esters, phospholipids and, in very advanced lesions, cholesterol crystals. Most of the extracellular lipids seem to be a result of macrophage rupture after apoptosis. The inflammatory phenomena not only promote the initiation and progression of the atheroma, but also actively contribute to complicating the plaque. Certain cytokines and growth factors (e.g. TGF-β) are implicated in the synthesis of collagen in the fibrous areas of the plaques, whereas others (e.g. IFN-γ) alter collagen synthesis and inhibit smooth muscle cell proliferation (Hansson et al., 1988). Since only activated T lymphocytes can produce IFN-γ, maintenance and repair of the collagen matrix is altered in these advanced stages.

Thinning of the fibrous cap is probably due to the production of metalloproteases (MMP) and other proteolytic enzymes by activated macrophages (Galis et al., 1994). These enzymes break down the extracellular matrix and produce fissures on the fibrous surface (ulcerations) or rupture of the vasa vasorum (intraplaque hemorrhage). Anatomical and physiological differences in the vessels make the characteristics of the plaques analogous but not totally comparable: the coronary arteries are muscular and the carotid arteries are flexible; the former receive blood flow in diastole and the latter in systole; and the vasa vasorum network is not so extensive in the coronary arteries. These facts, together with the predominance of certain risk factors in each territory (hypertension in carotid stenosis and dyslipidemia in coronary disease) could explain why the most frequent complication in coronary plaques is thinning and ulceration of the fibrous cap and the common complication in carotid plaques is vasa vasorum rupture and intraplaque hemorrhage caused by systolic hypertension. In any case, the final result is often a sudden increase in the volume of the plaque. Since activated macrophages also produce tissue factor (possibly the only *in vivo* indicator of thrombosis according to Kay and Bach (2001)), thrombosis of the plaque surface sometimes occurs and this can lead to ischemic symptoms related to the affected vascular territory.

Clinical research studies have provided evidence to support these concepts: for example, macrophages are present in greater numbers in unstable plaques than in stable plaques (Moreno et al., 1996; Carr et al., 1997). Our group has corroborated this finding in a study of carotid plaques surgically removed from patients with high-grade stenosis. The number of macrophages, T lymphocytes and activated T lymphocytes was significantly higher in plaques with unstable characteristics (ulceration or recent intraplaque hemorrhage), than in plaques considered stable (fibrous surface or old intraplaque hemorrhage).

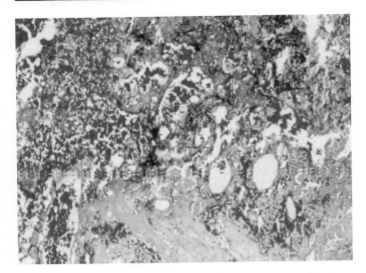

Figure 54.1 Unstable carotid plaque. **See colour plate 54.1.**

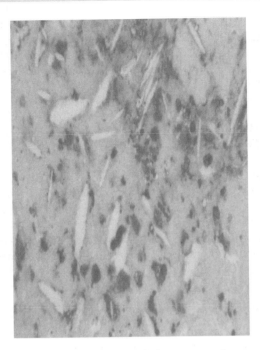

Figure 54.2 Cells in an unstable carotid plaque: macrophages and T lymphocytes. **See colour plate 54.2.**

Moreover unstable plaques were significantly associated with a prior cerebral ischemic event, whereas stable plaques were generally found in asymptomatic patients.

Cells implicated in the atherosclerotic lesion

The presence of macrophages, T lymphocytes and foam cells in all phases of atherogenesis lends support to the idea that immune phenomena are implicated in this entity.

Macrophages

Monocytes, the precursors of macrophages, are involved in all the phases of atherosclerosis. Besides the antigen-presenting function of these cells, they also secrete cytokines, chemokynes, growth-regulating molecules, metalloproteases, tissue factor and other regulating molecules. Replication of these mononuclear cells depends on several factors such as macrophage colony-stimulating factor and granulocyte-macrophage colony-stimulating factor for monocytes. Continuous exposure of the macrophages to these factors allows their survival and, possibly, their multiplication within the atheromatous lesion. Additionally IFN-γ activates macrophages and induces their programmed cell death (apoptosis) only in certain circumstances, as has been seen in the necrotic core of advanced lesions. The capability of these cells to produce cytokines (TNF-α), IL-1, TGF-β and proteolytic enzymes, such as the metalloproteases and tissue factor, seems to make them key elements in remodeling the atherosclerotic lesion. Activated macrophages present HLA-DR to the T lymphocytes and both CD4+ and CD8+ cells are also present in all the phases of atherogenesis. T lymphocytes are activated by the macrophages and secrete cytokines, such as IFN-γ, TNF-α and TNF-β, which amplify the inflammatory response.

T lymphocytes

T lymphocytes are present in the initial phases of atherosclerosis and can be detected in the fatty streak. As the lesion progresses, T lymphocytes secrete IFN-γ, which stimulates the macrophages, cytotoxic T lymphocytes and B lymphocytes, thereby inducing expression of adhesion molecules. T lymphocytes can also inhibit smooth muscle cell proliferation (Davies, 1997).

Smooth muscle cells

Smooth muscle cells are also implicated in atherosclerotic mechanisms. Their proliferation and migration from the media layer to the intima depends on cytokines and growth factors secreted by the endothelial cells, macrophages, lymphocytes and the smooth muscle cells themselves. The contractile genotype of this cell is transformed to a synthetic genotype in the intima and, in these conditions, smooth muscle cells secrete extracellular material, mainly mucopolysaccharides and collagen fibers. This activity, together with their proliferation and elevated vasoconstriction, produces an increase in the volume of the atheromatous plaque and, consequently, an increase in arterial stenosis.

Platelets

Platelets also play a fundamental role in atherogenesis. Activated, dysfunctional endothelium induces platelet adhesion to the subendothelial tissue. Subsequently, the platelets release molecules that affect coagulation and vascular tone and influence proliferation and migration of the smooth muscle cells. Exacerbated mechanisms of platelet aggregation are the final step in the formation of platelet thrombi which, in turn, enhance the inflammatory response (Badimon et al., 1996).

FACTORS THAT INITIATE AND PROMOTE THE ATHEROSCLEROTIC LESION

Potential causes of endothelial dysfunction include elevated levels of modified LDL, free radicals caused by smoking, hypertension, diabetes mellitus, elevated plasma homocysteine concentrations, infections due to microorganisms such as herpesvirus and *Chlamydia pneumoniae*, increased lipoprotein (a) and combinations of several of these factors.

Modified LDL and dyslipidemia

Low density lipoproteins can be modified by oxidation, glycation (in diabetes), aggregation, association with proteoglycans or by the formation of immune complexes. Altered LDL are one of the most important aggressions to the endothelium (Berliner et al., 1997). These lipoproteins are internalized by the macrophages through scavenger receptors on the cell surface, facilitating the accumulation of cholesterol esters and leading to the transformation of macrophages into foam cells. The incorporation of modified LDL into the macrophages is initially a protective mechanism that attempts to minimize the effect of these lipids on the endothelial and smooth muscle cells. However, their incorporation also triggers an inflammatory response. Mediators of inflammation, such as TNF-α, IL-1 and M-CSF increase binding of LDL to the endothelium and smooth muscle and stimulate transcription of the LDL-receptor gene. After binding to the macrophage receptor scavenger, LDL undergo a series of intercellular alterations that include the production of urokinase and pro-inflammatory cytokines (IL-1) that further increase the inflammatory response.

Other lipoproteins, such as very low density lipoproteins (VLDL) are also a cause of endothelial aggression. As in the case of LDL, these lipids also undergo oxidative modifications that trigger inflammatory responses (Dichtl et al., 1999). In contrast, high density lipoproteins (HDL) seem to protect against the atherogenic process because of their transport function. HDL transport cholesterol and anti-oxidating enzymes such as platelet-activating factor, acetylhydrolase and paraoxonase, which downregulate lipid oxidation and partially neutralize the pro-inflammatory effect (Libby et al., 2002).

Hypertension

The main product derived from the renin–angiotensin system is angiotensin II, which has vasoconstrictive properties and is a cause of endothelial injury. Angiotensin II appears to increase smooth muscle cell expression of pro-inflammatory cytokines such as IL-6, MCP-1 and VCAM-1.

Diabetes mellitus

Another highly important risk factor for the development of atherosclerosis is diabetes. The hyperglycemia of this condition favors the formation of advanced glycation end products (AGE), which, through binding with receptors (RAGE), can increase pro-inflammatory cytokine production and lead to an inflammatory response (Schmidt et al., 1999). Additionally, diabetes promotes a state of oxidative stress that triggers an immune response in the same way.

Smoking

Smoking is an independent cardiovascular risk factor. The effect of smoking one cigarette on the cardiovascular system includes immediate alteration of endothelial function. In addition, smoking can produce coronary artery spasms that might lead to coronary plaque rupture and result in an acute coronary event. Nevertheless, the endothelial dysfunction caused by cigarette consumption appears to be reversible. There is a significant decrease in cardiovascular risk after the first year of giving up the habit (Ockene et al., 1990).

Obesity

Excess weight predisposes to diabetes and insulin resistance and this contributes to its atherogenic potential. Additionally, high levels of free fatty acids in the blood can stimulate VLDL production by the hepatocytes and increases the exchange from HDL to VLDL. However, adipose tissue can synthesize TNF-α and IL-6; thus the atherogenic effect of obesity is independent of the hyperglycemia and dyslipidemia it causes (Yudkin et al., 1999).

Homocysteine

Homocysteine is a thiol-containing amino acid, originating from methionine demethylation. It is toxic for the endothelium, prothrombotic, increases collagen production and decreases the availability of nitric oxide. Experimental and clinical studies have demonstrated an association between hyperhomocysteinemia and the development of atherosclerosis. Experimental studies indicate that hyperhomocysteinemia is involved in endothelial dysfunction, lipid peroxidation, altered nitric oxide synthesis and reduced thrombomodulin expression. Auto-oxidation of homocysteine produces cytotoxic, reactive, oxygen-free radicals that initiate the process of lipid peroxidation and activate LDL oxidation, at least *in vitro*. Homocysteine enhances the effect of various coagulation factors and this, together with the reduction in thrombomodulin synthesis, confers its prothrombotic potential. Lastly, it contributes to smooth muscle cell proliferation. A meta-analysis performed by Boushey et al. (1995) demonstrated that increased plasma concentrations of homocysteine are responsible for up to 10 per cent of coronary disease in the general population.

Infectious agents

In the last decade it has been proposed that infectious agents, particularly herpesvirus, *Chlamydia pneumoniae* and *Helicobacter pylori* can have an important role in atherogenesis. However, it seems that infection alone does not suffice, since there is a high prevalence of individuals infected by these microorganisms in the general population and only a small percentage present cardiovascular disease. Actually, infection in these patients may only have marginal importance. *Chlamydia* has been isolated in human atheroma plaques, but its presence could be an epiphenomenon. Monocytes and macrophages can carry internalized fragments of these agents. When the inflammatory cells are attracted to the surface of the plaque during endothelial dysfunction, the infectious fragments would be brought along and their presence detected. Currently the hypothesis that infectious agents may be a direct cause of atherosclerosis has been superseded by two alternative theories. The first proposes that the chronic infection in these cases is always produced by obligated intracellular pathogens and results in elevated antibody titers which would cause increased circulating cytokine concentrations and indirectly enhance cell wall inflammatory phenomena (Zhu et al., 2001). The second theory is based on the cross-reaction produced between antibodies created against certain bacterial antigens and human molecules secreted to protect against specific aggressive situations for the organism (heat shock proteins). In this context, Epstein (2002) proposed that antibodies against chlamydial heat shock protein 65 (HSP65) could cross-react with human HSP60 and produce a deleterious effect on endothelial cells that would contribute to unfavorable evolution of the atherosclerotic lesion.

MARKERS OF INFLAMMATION: DIAGNOSTIC IMPLICATIONS

The pathophysiologic facts described above convert various molecules into potential targets for measuring and, theoretically, for monitoring the inflammatory status. Moreover, these molecules could have an important role in therapeutic strategies for atherosclerosis. The biological markers of inflammation include cytokines such as IL-1, IL-6 and TNF-α, adhesion molecules such as the selectins and ICAM and products dependent on hepatic synthesis, mainly acute-phase reactants such as serum amyloid A (SAA), fibrinogen and C-reactive protein (Table 54.1).

Table 54.1 Inflammatory markers for consideration as predictors of cardiovascular risk

Soluble adhesion molecules	E-selectin
	P-selectin
	Intracellular adhesion molecule-1
	Vascular cell adhesion molecule-1
Cytokines	Interleukin-1, -6, -8 and -10
	Tumor necrosis factor-α
Acute-phase reactants	Fibrinogen
	Serum amyloid A
	Hs-CRP

Cytokines

Cytokines are signal peptides that act as triggers for the production of acute phase reactants; their secretion is a physiological response to aggression. Cytokines generally act through high-affinity receptors on the cell surface (Miller and Krangel, 1992) and exert various actions on the different cells. They generally have local autocrine or paracrine activity, although some, such as IL-6, have endocrine activity. The main function of the cytokines is to prevent hypersensitivity reactions in the organism due to an excessive immune response. They achieve this by coordinating the elimination of invasive microorganisms and injured tissue. Pro-inflammatory cytokines, i.e. those that initiate the immune response, include IL-1, IL-6 and TNF-α. These act together with other families of cytokines such as IL-8, IL-10, IL-12 and IL-18 and their synthesis implies the production of other inflammatory mediators from the complement system (e.g. the fragment C5a) and platelet activator factor. The activity of these mediators and the cytokines is synergistic and results in the induction of other cytokines that increase or decrease the autoregulatory pathways.

Interleukin-1

In inflammation, IL-1 is mainly produced by macrophages and it has several effects. Besides its fundamental role as a stimulator of specific immune responses at the initiation of the inflammatory cascade, it is a potent inducer of acute phase reactant synthesis, as will be discussed later.

Interleukin-6

IL-6 is mainly produced by activated monocytes, fibroblasts and endothelial cells. In monocytes, IL-6 production is stimulated by IL-2 and bacterial endotoxins. The functions of this cytokine include B lymphocyte differentiation, T lymphocyte growth and cytotoxic differentiation and stimulation of blood cell production. In particular, it is a potent stimulator of the acute phase response in liver.

Studies such as the one by Libby et al. (1995) have shown a correlation between plasma cytokine levels and atherosclerosis and it has been suggested that cytokine determination could be useful for identifying patients with an elevated risk of experiencing a cardiovascular event. Bennet et al. (2003) determined inflammatory markers in 1179 survivors of myocardial infarction and 1528 controls and concluded that elevated plasma levels of IL-6 are indeed associated with increased cardiovascular risk.

Nevertheless, it is likely that the cytokines are only an approximate measure of the inflammatory processes occurring in the arterial wall. Analysis of the distribution of plasma levels of these cytokines in patients with and without cardiovascular events has shown considerable overlapping of values between the two groups. Thus, application of these markers in routine clinical practice does not seem practicable at this time.

Tumor necrosis factor-α

Tumor necrosis factor-α is synthesized in monocytes, macrophages and lymphocytes, with induction by bacterial endotoxins, fungal or viral antigens and by other cytokines, such as IL-1. Favored by IFN-γ, TNF-α activity has a wide range, running from hemorrhagic necrosis to the systemic effects of inflammation. Prospective epidemiological studies, such as those by Ridker et al. (2000) have demonstrated that patients presenting elevated concentrations of TNF-α after an acute myocardial infarction have a high risk of experiencing a recurrent coronary event.

Neopterin

The main stimulus for neopterin secretion from activated macrophages is IFN-γ produced by T lymphocytes. This pteridine has also been studied as a potential marker of cardiovascular risk. Some clinical studies have demonstrated an association between neopterin levels and peripheral arterial disease (Tatzber et al., 1991) and carotid atherosclerosis (Weiss et al., 1994). Increased neopterin has been observed in patients with unstable angina and myocardial infarction and it has been suggested that neopterin values may be indicative of the severity of coronary lesions (Garcia-Moll et al., 2000). Among the inflammatory markers, neopterin has received the least attention in the literature.

Adhesion molecules

Adhesion molecules comprise a group of glycoproteins implicated in cell–cell and cell–extracellular matrix interactions. Some are members of the selectin family (e.g. E-selectin and P-selectin) and others of the immunoglobulin family (e.g. PECAM-1, ICAM and VCAM). When these glycoproteins are expressed on the cell surface they are recognized by macrophage and T lymphocyte integrins, which migrate to the subendothelial level through the spaces between the endothelial cells. Additionally, cellular adhesion molecules are involved in thrombus formation through the coagulation cascade, thanks to leukocyte integrins. In the intact vascular endothelium under physiologic conditions, the ligands of the adhesion molecules (von Willebrand factor, fibronectin and collagen) are maintained at a subendothelial level, thereby preventing platelet aggregation. When the endothelium is injured, the adhesion molecules come into contact with von Willebrand factor. This leads to platelet aggregation and binding with extracellular matrix proteins and the formation of a platelet thrombus. Clinical studies have also shown an association between elevated levels of cell adhesion molecules and increased cardiovascular risk. In this line, Hwang et al. (1997) reported positive relationships of VCAM-1, ICAM-1 and selectin-E with carotid and coronary atherosclerosis.

Acute phase reactants

Acute phase reactants (fibrinogen, serum amyloid A and C-reactive protein) are markers of active inflammation with a high sensitivity, but very low specificity. They are comprised of proteins synthesized by the hepatocytes in response to cytokine stimulation. Several studies have demonstrated that these proteins are elevated in patients with ischemic heart disease and are associated with a higher tendency to present adverse effects. The first acute phase reactant studied as a marker of cardiovascular risk was fibrinogen (Wilhelmsen et al., 1984). Considerable epidemiological data have related cardiovascular events with this acute phase reactant. In addition, cardiovascular risk factors such as age, smoking and body mass index show a direct proportional relationship with fibrinogen levels. In the case of serum amyloid A, studies such those of Liuzzo et al. (1994) and Pepys and Baltz (1983) have similarly demonstrated a direct relationship between elevated plasma levels of this protein and increased cardiovascular risk.

However, the acute phase reactant with the most extensive accumulated data is C-reactive protein (CRP). A great deal of research is focused on this protein as a marker of cardiovascular risk. Among other studies, those by Havertake et al. (1997), Ridker et al. (1998) and Sakkinen et al. (2002) have shown that elevated CRP levels have independent prognostic value in patients with atherosclerotic disease. The Multiple Risk Factor Intervention Trial (MRFIT) (Kuller et al., 1991), carried out in 12 866 healthy men followed for 17 years, was the first to associate elevated CRP with increased mortality in ischemic heart disease. Healthy men who had not experienced a cardiac event during 16 years had slightly lower basal CRP levels than apparently healthy men who presented myocardial infarction or who died of cardiac-related causes during this period. A study conducted by Ridker et al. (1997) also demonstrated a direct relationship between this acute phase reactant and cardiac mortality. In a comparison between 543 men who had cardiovascular events and the same number of men without such events, basal CRP levels were significantly lower in the controls than the patients. The first study assessing the prognostic value of CRP as a predictor of cardiovascular risk was published by Ridker et al. (1998). A population of 28 263 apparently healthy postmenopausal women, among whom 122 had had a first cardiovascular event (myocardial infarction, stroke, coronary revascularization surgery or cardiovascular death), were compared with 244 controls adjusted for age and smoking habit. As was seen in men, an independent association was found between increased CRP and elevated incidence of cardiovascular events during follow up. The Cholesterol and Recurrent Events (CARE) study (Ridker et al., 1999) corroborated these findings. Patients were randomized to receive standard treatment with pravastatin or placebo and it was found that survivors of myocardial infarction in the placebo group had higher levels of CRP along the 5-year follow up.

There are fewer studies relating CRP with carotid disease. In this regard, our team demonstrated that patients with high-grade carotid stenosis presenting unstable plaques had significantly higher CRP levels than those with stable plaques (Alvarez et al., 2003). This led us to suggest that CRP could be a risk marker for plaque instability that could be used together with other clinical and paraclinical tests to identify risk populations.

The role of CRP in the inflammatory process related with atherosclerosis is only partially known. It has been suggested that it is not solely a consequence of inflammation occurring in the vascular wall, but that it might be directly implicated in the pathogenesis of atherosclerosis. This protein reacts with receptors on the cell surface and induces opsonization and phagocytosis, activates the classic complement pathway, captures and eliminates chromatin fragments and modulates polymorphonuclear function (Bhadki et al., 1999). It has also been seen that CRP is produced locally in atherosclerotic plaques (Yasojima et al., 2001) and it may be implicated in coronary artery restenosis after interventional treatment (Ishikawa et al., 2003).

The main problem with CRP use as a marker of cardiovascular risk is its low specificity. For this same reason there are still doubts about its use in routine clinical practice as a prognostic marker and as an element for establishing diagnostic or therapeutic decisions. CRP increases in response to many factors such as smoking, hypertension, hypercholesterolemia and excess weight (Danesh et al., 1999) and other pathologies that are generally not related with atherosclerosis also show acute phase reactant alterations, such as psychiatric illnesses (Berk et al., 1997) and respiratory (Yokoe et al., 2003), digestive (Moran et al., 1995), rheumatologic (Wolfe, 1997) and nephrologic (Fink et al., 2002) diseases.

Thus, even though numerous studies report data pointing to CRP as a cardiovascular risk marker, this acute phase reactant shows little precision and wide interindividual variability and the benefit of its determination in cardiovascular diseases is still uncertain. In recent guidelines on the use of clinical markers of inflammation in cardiovascular disease, there is only one class I recommendation for CRP: that it should be expressed in mg/l (evidence level, C) (Pearson et al., 2003).

Metalloproteinases

It has been suggested that destabilization of the atherosclerotic plaque is due to proteolytic enzymes from the metalloprotease family. These gelatinases are secreted by the macrophages and produce collagen degradation in the fibrous cap and extracellular matrix. Several studies have related elevated levels of MMP-9 to atherosclerotic plaque instability. Loftus et al. (2001) demonstrated MMP-9 overexpression in unstable carotid plaques and our studies support this finding. We observed significantly higher MMP-9 concentrations in unstable carotid plaques and a positive correlation between MMP-9 and the presence of macrophages and T lymphocytes in the plaque. Additionally, stable plaques presented lower MMP-9 levels and fewer T lymphocytes. These results support a role for the metalloproteases in plaque complications and for macrophages in atherosclerosis. As in the case of CRP, measurement of metalloproteinase levels could be useful for selecting risk cohorts in patients with high-grade carotid stenosis.

THERAPEUTIC IMPLICATIONS

Advances in our knowledge of the pathophysiologic bases of atherosclerosis have expanded the therapeutic arsenal for treating this pathology. Now some of the molecules involved in this process can be considered therapeutic targets. Antioxidants reduced the size of fatty streaks in a primate model in a study related to the oxidized LDL in atherosclerotic lesions (Chang et al., 1995) and downregulation of monocyte adhesion molecules appeared to produce an anti-inflammatory effect in the lesions (Fruebis et al., 1997). Additionally, elevated vitamin E levels are inversely related with the incidence of myocardial infarction and supplements of this vitamin may reduce coronary events (Stephens et al., 1996). Another candidate molecule for intervention is homocysteine. Folic acid treatment results in homocysteine decreases to normal levels; however, it still must be determined whether this reduction leads to lower cardiovascular morbidity and mortality (Omenn et al., 1998). Since angiotensin II seems to contribute to endothelial dysfunction in hypertensive patients, it is possible that angiotensin-converting enzyme inhibitor therapy may provide clinical benefits. With regard to the potential benefit of antibiotic treatment directed toward pathogens that may affect the atherosclerotic lesion, multicenter studies have yielded negative results in this respect; thus antibiotic treatment is not justified in these patients at this time.

A great deal of investigation has been centered on statins, lipid-lowering drugs that not only regulate cholesterol and triglyceride levels, but also act on the inflammatory process that takes place in atherosclerosis. This is achieved through the so-called pleiotropic effects, including restoration of vasodilatation, antioxidant action, stimulation of vessel neoformation, inhibition of vascular cell apoptosis, decreased expression of adhesion molecules and inhibition of NFκB, which regulates the secretion of several cytokines. All these effects seem to occur regardless of the decrease in cholesterol, as has been seen in experimental animal studies. Statins were found to inhibit the inflammatory process triggered by inoculation of irritants in the foot pads of mice. Moreover, this phenomenon was reproduced in apoE knockout mice, in which these drugs did not lower plasma cholesterol levels (Sparrow et al., 2001). In a subgroup of the CARE study, Ridker et al. (1999) found that patients treated with pravastatin showed a clear reduction in CRP levels. Another potential benefit of this treatment stems from the fact that statins inhibit metalloproteases (Ikeda et al., 2000) and the formation of the neovessels that accompany atherosclerotic lesions (Fuster et al., 2002), which could contribute to plaque stability. A final factor is statin inhibition of smooth muscle cell proliferation and migration of these cells from the arterial media to the intima. It is now believed that the key to the cellular action of the statins resides in modulation of intracellular signaling. Although their exact role is still to be defined, their anti-atherogenic action clearly extends beyond the lowering of cholesterol.

NEW PERSPECTIVES

The new DNA identification techniques can provide important information on which genes are implicated and how they are expressed in atherosclerosis. Advances in molecular genetics can help us elucidate, for example, the exact contribution of the macrophages, the cells with the greatest influence in the complex process leading to atherosclerosis. New diagnostic and therapeutic roads have been opened in the management of cardiovascular disease and there is significant evidence supporting a key role of inflammation in the initiation, progression and complications of atherosclerotic lesions. Experimental, clinical and epidemiological studies have directly related the various inflammatory markers with cardiovascular events in all the vascular structures implicated: coronary, carotid and peripheral arteries. Nevertheless, we are still faced with the challenge of increasing our understanding of the pathophysiological factors involved in the development of arteriosclerosis and improving the precision of inflammatory markers for diagnostic and prognostic purposes.

REFERENCES

Albelda, S.M., Smith, C.W. and Ward, P.A. (1994). Adhesion molecules and inflammatory injury. FASEB J 8, 504–512.

Alvarez, B., Ruiz, C., Chacon, P., Alvarez-Sabin, J. and Matas, M. (2003). High-sensitivity C-reactive protein in high-grade carotid stenosis: risk marker for unstable carotid plaque. J Vasc Surg 38, 1018–1024.

Badimon, L. and Badimon, J.J. (1996). In Atherosclerosis and coronary disease, Fuster V., ed. Philadelphia: Lippincott-Raven, pp. 639–656.

Bennet, A.M., Prince, J.A., Fei, G.Z. et al. (2003). Interleukin-6 serum levels and genotypes influence the risk for myocardial infarction. Atherosclerosis 171, 359–367.

Berk, M., Wadee, A.A., Kuschke, R.H. and O'Neill-Kerr, A. (1997). Acute-phase proteins in major depression. J Psychosom Res 43, 529–534.

Berliner, J., Leitinger, N., Watson, A. et al. (1997). Oxidized lipids in atherogenesis: formation, destruction and action. Thromb Haemost 78, 195–199.

Bhadki, S., Torzewski, M., Klouche, M. and Hemmes, M. (1999). Complement and atherogenesis: binding of CRP to degraded, nonoxidized LDL enhances complement activation. Arterioscler Thromb Vasc Biol 19, 2348–2354.

Boushey, C.J., Beresford, S.A.A., Omenn, G.S. and Motulsky, A.G. (1995). A quantitative assessment of plasma homocysteine as a risk factor for cardiovascular disease. J Am Med Assoc 274, 1049–1057.

Braunwald, E. (1997). Shattuck Lecture – cardiovascular medicine at the turn of the millennium: triumphs, concerns, and opportunities. N Engl J Med 337, 1360–1369.

Carr, S.C., Farb, A., Pearce, W.H., Virmani, R. and Yao, J.S.T. (1997). Activated inflammatory cells are associated with plaque rupture in carotid artery stenosis. Surgery 122, 757–764.

Chang, M.Y., Sasahara, M., Chait Raines, E.W. and Ross, R. (1995). Inhibition of hypercholesterolemia-induced atherosclerosis in the nonhuman primate by probucol. Cellular composition and proliferation. Arterioscler Thromb Vasc Biol 15, 1631–1640.

Danesh, J., Muir, J., Wong, Y.K., Ward, M., Gallimore, J.R. and Pepys, M.B. (1999). Risk factors for coronary heart disease and acute-phase proteins. A population-based study. Eur Heart J 20, 954–999.

Davies, M.J. (1997). The composition of coronary artery plaques. N Engl J Med 336, 1312–1314.

Dichtl, W., Nilsson, L. and Goncalves, I. (1999). Very low-density lipoprotein activates nuclear factor kappa B in endothelial cells. Circ Res 84, 1085–1094.

Epstein, S. (2002). The multiple mechanisms by which infection may contribute to atherosclerosis development and course. Cir Res 90, 2–4.

Fink, J.C., Onuigbo, M.A. and Blahut, S.A. (2002). Pretransplant serum C-reactive protein and the risk of chronic allograft nephropathy in renal transplant recipients: A pilot case-control study. Am J Kidney Dis 39, 10096–10101.

Fruebis, J., Gonzalez, V., Silvestre, M. and Palinski, W. (1997). Effect of probucol treatment on gene expression of VCAM-1, MCP-1 and M-CSF in the aortic wall of LDL receptor-deficient rabbits during early atherogenesis. Arterioscler Thromb Vasc Biol 17, 1289–1302.

Fuster, V., Corti, R. and Badimon J. (2002). Therapeutic targets for the treatment of atherothrombosis in the new millennium.

Clinical frontiers in atherosclerosis research. Circ J 66, 783–790.

Galis, Z.S., Sukhova, G.K., Lark, M.W. and Libby, P. (1994). Increased expression of matrix metalloproteinases and matrix degrading activity in vulnerable regions of human atherosclerotic plaques. J Clin Invest 94, 2493–2503.

Garcia-Moll, X., Coccolo, F., Cole, D. and Kaski, J.C. (2000). Serum neopterin and complex stenosis morphology in patients with unstable angina. J Am Coll Cardiol 35, 956–962.

Gotlieb, A.I. and Langille, B.L. (1996). The role of rheology in atherosclerotic coronary artery disease. In Atherosclerosis and coronary artery disease, Vol.1, Fuster, V., Ross, R. and Topol, E.L., eds. Philadelphia: Lippincott-Raven, pp. 595–606.

Hansson, G.K., Jonasson, L., Holm, J., Clowes, M.K. and Clowes, A. (1988). Gamma interferon regulates vascular smooth muscle proliferation and expression in vivo and in vitro. Circ Res 63, 712–719.

Hansson, G.K., Jonasson, L., Seifert, P.S. and Stemme, S. (1989). Immune mechanisms in atherosclerosis. Arteriosclerosis 9, 567–578.

Havertake, F., Thompsom, S.G., Pyke, S.D.M., Gallimore, J.R. and Pepys, M.B. for the European Concerted Action on Thrombosis and Disabilities Angina Pectoris Study Group. Production of C-reactive protein and risk of coronary events in stable and unstable patients. Lancet 349, 462–466.

Hwang, S.J., Ballantyne, C.M. and Sharrett, A.R. (1997). Circulating adhesion molecules VCAM-1, ICAM-1, and E-selectin in carotid atherosclerosis and incident coronary heart disease cases. The Atherosclerosis Risk in Communities (ARIC) study. Circulation 96, 4219–4225.

Ikeda, U., Shimpo, M., Ohki, R. et al. (2000). Fluvastatin inhibits matrix metalloproteinase-1 expression in human vascular endothelial cells. Hypertension 36, 325–329.

Ishikawa, T., Hatakeyama, K. and Imamura, T. (2003). Involvement of C-reactive protein obtained by directional coronary atherectomy in plaque instability and developing restenosis in patients with stable or unstable angina pectoris. Am J Cardiol 91, 287–292.

Key, N. and Bach, R. (2001). Tissue factor as a therapeutic target. Thromb Haemost 85, 375–376.

Kranzhofer, R., Schmidt, J. and Pfeiffer, C.A. (1999). Angiotensin induces inflammatory activation of human vascular smooth muscle cells. Arterioscler Thromb Vasc Biol. 19, 1623–1629.

Kuller, L.H., Eichner, J.E. and Orchand, T.J. (1991). The relation between serum albumin levels and risk of coronary heart disease in the Multiple Risk Factor Intervention Trial. Am J Epidemiol 134, 1266–1277.

Libby, P., Sukhova, G., Lee, R.T. and Galis, Z.S. (1995). Cytokines regulate vascular functions related to stability of atherosclerotic plaque. J Cardiovasc Pharmacol 25 Suppl 2, S9–S12.

Libby, P., Ridker, P.M. and Maseri, A. (2002). Inflammation and atherosclerosis. Circulation 105, 1135–1143.

Liuzzo, G., Biasucci, L.M. and Gallimore, J.R. (1994). The prognostic value of C-reactive protein and serum amyloid A protein in severe unstable angina. N Engl J Med 331, 417–424.

Loftus, I.M., Naylor, A.R., Bell, P.R. and Thompson, M.M. (2001). Plasma MMP-9 a marker of carotid plaque instability. Eur J Vasc Endovasc Surg 21, 17–21.

Matsushima, K. and Oppen, J.J. (1989). Interleukin 8 and MCAF: novel inflammatory cytokines inducible by IL1 and TNF. Cytokine 1, 2–13.

Miller, M.D. and Krangel, M.S. (1992). Biology and biochemistry of the chemokynes; a family of chemotactic and inflammatory cytokines. Crit Rev Inmmunol 12, 17–46.

Mondy, J.S., Lindner, V., Miyashiro, J.K., Berk, B.C., Dean, R.H. and Geary, R.L. (1997). Platelet-derived growth factor ligand and receptor expression in response to altered blood flow in vivo. Circ Res 81, 320–327.

Moran, A., Jones, A. and Asquith, P. (1995). Laboratory markers of colonoscopy activity in ulcerative colitis and Crohn's colitis. Scand J Gastroenterol 30, 356–360.

Moreno, P.R., Bernardi, V.H., López-Cuellar, J. et al. (1996). Macrophages, smooth muscle cells and tissue factor in unstable angina: implications for cell-mediated thrombogenicity in acute coronary syndromes. Circulation 94, 3090–3097.

Nagel, T., Resnick, N., Atkinson, W.J., Dewey, C.F. Jr and Gimbrone, M.A. Jr (1994). Shear stress selectively upregulates intercellular adhesion molecule-1 expression in cultured human vascular endothelial cells. J Clin Invest 94, 885–891.

Ockene, J.K., Kuller, L.H., Svendsen, K.H. and Meilahn, E. (1990). The relationship of smoking cessation to coronary heart disease and lung cancer in the Multiple Risk Factor Intervention Trial. (MRFIT). Am J Public Health 80, 954–958.

Omenn, G.S., Beresford, S.A.A. and Motulsky, A.G. (1998). Preventing coronary heart disease: B vitamins and homocysteine. Circulation 97, 421–424.

Pearson, Th. A., Mensah, G., Alexander, R. et al. (2003). Markers of inflammation and cardiovascular disease. Application to clinical and public health practice. A statement for healthcare professionals from the Centers for Disease Control and Prevention and the American Heart Association. Circulation 107, 499–511.

Pepys, M.B. and Baltz, M.L. (1983). Acute phase proteins with special reference to C-reactive protein Nd related proteins (pentaxins) and serum amyloid A protein. Adv Immunol 34, 141–212.

Qiao, J.H., Tripathi, J. and Mishra, N.K. (1997). Role of macrophage colony-stimulating factor in atherosclerosis: studies of osteoporotic mice. Am J Pathol 150, 1687–1699.

Raines, E.W., Rosenfeld, M.E. and Ross, R. (1996). The role of macrophages. In Atherosclerosis and coronary artery disease. Vol.1, Fuster, V., Ross, R. and Topol, E.J., eds. Philadelphia: Lippincott-Raven, pp. 539–555.

Ridker, P.M., Cushman, M., Stampfer, M.J., Russell, P.T. and Henekens, C.H. (1997). Inflammation, aspirin, and the risk of cardiovascular disease in apparently healthy men. N Engl J Med 336, 973–999.

Ridker, P.M., Cushman, M., Stampfer, M.J., Tracy, R.P. and Hennekens, C.H. (1998). Plasma concentrations of C-reactive protein and risk of developing peripheral vascular disease. Circulation 97, 425–428.

Ridker, P.M., Rifai, N., Pfeiffer, M.A., Sacks, F. and Braunwald, E. (1999). Long-term effects of pravastatin on plasma concentration of C-reactive protein. The Cholesterol and Recurrent Events (CARE) Investigators. Circulation 100, 230–235.

Ridker, P.M., Rifai, N. and Pfeiffer, M. (2000). Elevation of tumor necrosis factor alpha and increased risk of recurrent coronary events after myocardial infarction. Circulation 101, 2149–2153.

Ross, R. (1999). Atherosclerosis – an inflammatory disease. N Engl J Med. 340, 115–126.

Sakkinen, P., Abbott, R.D., Curb, J.D., Rodriguez, B.L., Yano, K. and Tracy, R.P. (2002). C-reactive protein and myocardial infarction. J Clin Epidemiol 55, 445–451.

Schmidt, A.M., Yan, S.D. and Wautier, J.L. (1999). Activation of receptor for advanced glycation end products: a mechanism for chronic vascular dysfunction in diabetic vasculopathy and atherosclerosis. Cir Res 84, 489–497.

Schobersberger, W., Hoffmann, G. and Grote, J. (1995). Induction of inducible nitric oxide synthase expression by neopterin in vascular smooth muscle cells. FEBS Lett 377, 461–464.

Sparrow, C.P., Burton, Ch. A., Henandez, M., Mundt, S., Hassing, H. and Patel, S. (2001). Simvastatin has anti-inflammatory and anti-atherosclerotic activities independent of plasma cholesterol lowering. Arterioscler Thromb Vasc Biol 21, 122–128.

Stephens, N.G., Parsons, A., Schofield, P.M., Kelly, F., Cheeseman, K. and Mitchinson, M.J. (1996). Randomised controlled trial of vitamin E in patients with coronary disease: Cambridge Heart Antioxidant Study. Lancet 347, 781–786.

Tatzber, F., Rabl, H. and Koriska, K. (1991). Elevated serum neopterin levels in atherosclerosis. Atherosclerosis 89, 203–208.

Weiss, G., Willeit, J. and Kiechl, S. (1994). Increased concentrations of neopterin in carotid atherosclerosis. Atherosclerosis 106, 263–271.

Wilhemsem, L., Svärdsudd, K., Korsan-Bengsten, K., Larsson, B., Welin, L. and Tibblin, G. (1984). Fibrinogen as a risk factor for stroke and myocardial infarction. N Engl J Med 311, 501–505.

Wirleitner, B., Baier-Bitterlich, G. and Hoffmann, G. (1996). Neopterin activates transcription factor nuclear kappa B in vascular smooth muscle cells. FEBS Lett 391, 181–184.

Wolfe, F. (1997). Comparative usefulness of C-reactive protein and erythrocyte sedimentation rate in patients with rheumatoid arthritis. J Rheumatol 24, 1477–1485.

Yasojima, K., Schwab, C., McGeer, E.G. and McGeer, P.L. (2001). Generation of C-reactive protein and complement components in atherosclerotic plaques. Am J Pathol 158, 1039–1051.

Yokoem, T., Minoguchim, K. and Matsuo, H. (2003). Elevated levels of C-reactive protein and interleukin-6 in patients with obstructive sleep apnea syndrome are decreased by nasal continuous positive airway pressure. Circulation 107, 1129–1134.

Yudkin, J.S., Stehouwer, C.D. and Emeis, J.J. (1999). C-reactive protein in healthy subjects: associations with obesity, insulin resistance, and endothelial dysfunction: a potential role of cytokines originating from adipose tissue? Arterioscler Thromb Vasc Biol 19, 972–978.

Zhu, J., Nieto, J., Home, B., Anderson, J., Muhlestein, J. and Epstein, S. (2001). Prospective study of pathogen burden and risk myocardial infarction or death. Circulation 103, 45–51.

Primary Immunodeficiencies

Chapter 55

Robertson Parkman

Division of Research Immunology/Bone Marrow Transplantation and The Saban Research Institute, Childrens Hospital Los Angeles, Los Angeles, CA, USA

Nature fits all her children with something to do, He who would write and can't write, can surely review.

A Fable for Critics James Russell Lowell (1848)

INTRODUCTION

Primary immunodeficiency diseases are genetic diseases that affect the differentiation or function of the immune system. Affected immune defense mechanisms include T lymphocytes, B lymphocytes, natural killer (NK) cells, granulocytes, immunoglobulins and complement. Defects of differentiation usually result in the absence of the effector mechanism whereas in diseases involving dysfunction the effector mechanism is phenotypically present but without function.

ASSESSMENT OF THE IMMUNE SYSTEM

T lymphocytes

T lymphocytes are essential to human defense against infectious organisms and some cancers. Patients with primary T lymphocyte defects are clinically characterized by infections with viral (especially DNA viruses), protozoan (*Pneumocystis carinii*), fungal and bacterial organisms (due to defective antibody synthesis). Patients with clinically presumed defects in their T lymphocyte immunity should be sequentially assayed for the presence of phenotypic T lymphocytes followed by the assessment of T lymphocyte function.

The first phenotypic assessment of T lymphocytes was the formation of E-rosettes by the incubation of peripheral blood leukocytes with sheep red blood cells (E) (Greaves and Brown, 1974). The physical enumeration of T lymphocytes by E rosette formation was rapidly replaced by the immunophenotypic assessment using monoclonal antibodies to differentiation antigens expressed on T lymphocytes (Nagel et al., 1981; Comans-Bitter et al., 1997). Almost universally fluorescence activated cell sorters (FACS) are now used for the enumeration as well as immunophenotypic characterization of T lymphocytes using monoclonal antibodies coupled to fluorescent dyes. CD3 is expressed on all peripheral T lymphocytes. CD2, which was the cell surface receptor initially identified by E-rosette formation, is also present on most T lymphocytes. Normal peripheral blood T lymphocytes express either CD4 or CD8; thus, peripheral blood T lymphocytes can be characterized as CD3+, CD4+ or CD3+, CD8+ leucocytes. The mere presence of CD4 or CD8 is not adequate to characterize a peripheral blood leukocyte as a T lymphocyte since monocytes express low levels of CD4 and some NK cells express CD8. Thus, the co-expression of CD3/CD4 or CD3/CD8 is necessary for the immunophenotypic enumeration of T lymphocytes. Significant numbers of CD3 T lymphocytes are present in cord blood at birth so cord blood can be used for the analysis of newborn infants suspected of having primary T lymphocyte immunodeficiencies. The enumeration of T lymphocytes

Copyright © 2005, Elsevier. All rights reserved.

should be calculated as the number/μl rather than as a percentage of all lymphocytes to control for variation in the number of lymphocytes.

The presence of normal numbers of immunophenotypic T lymphocytes with a normal CD4/CD8 ratio is inadequate to state that a patient has normal T lymphocyte function. Thus, the evaluation of T lymphocyte function is necessary in patients who are clinically suspected of having a defect in T lymphocyte function and who have adequate numbers of immunophenotypic T lymphocytes. The most primitive function of T lymphocytes is their capacity to proliferate in response to stimulation with the mitogen, phytohemagglutinin (PHA), an extract of red kidney beans. The *in vitro* stimulation of peripheral blood T lymphocytes results in maximum cell proliferation after 72 h, which can be measured by either the incorporation of tritiated thymidine into newly synthesized DNA or other measurements of T lymphocyte metabolic activity. The *in vitro* assays are usually performed in the presence of human rather than zenogeneic serum to reduce non-specific stimulation resulting in increased background cell division. In normal individuals, the degree of T lymphocyte proliferation is directly proportional to the percentage of T lymphocytes in the test population. Assays are usually performed in a microtiter culture system where $50–100 \times 10^3$ leukocytes are cultured in each microtiter well. The tests are usually performed in triplicate. The degree of stimulation is compared to the percentage of T lymphocytes in the leukocytes tested. This comparison is necessary since some patients may have a leukocytosis resulting in a reduction in the relative percentage of T lymphocytes in the sample and, therefore, a reduction in the magnitude of the proliferative response induced by the PHA stimulation. Thus, a determination of PHA responsiveness without a correction for the percentage of immunophenotypic T lymphocytes may lead to an overdiagnosis of decreased T lymphocyte function.

A normal proliferative response to PHA stimulation does not always predict protective antigen-specific T lymphocyte function. The only T lymphocyte function that is predictive of protective immunity is the capacity to develop antigen-specific function. Proliferative responses to allogeneic lymphocytes in the mixed lymphocyte culture (MLC) can be performed in newborn infants or individuals who have not been immunized to specific antigens (Bach and Hirschorn, 1964). It is best, however, to measure the antigen-specific response to acquired antigens. Antigenic exposure can be through timed immunizations or exposure to pathogens, as in the case of viral infections. The most widely performed measurement of antigen-specific T lymphocyte function is the determination of the *in vitro* blastogenic response of leucocytes to specific antigenic stimulation. Standard vaccines such as tetanus toxoid (TT) and diphtheria toxoid (DT) can be used for *in vitro* assays as well as lysates of fibroblasts infected with DNA viruses such as varicella zoster virus (VZV), herpes simplex virus (HSV) and cytomegaloviruses (CMV). Viral vaccines, both live and attenuated, used for immunizations, can also be used to determine the presence of antigen-specific T lymphocytes after immunization. The maximum proliferative response of T lymphocytes following *in vitro* antigenic stimulation is at 7 days, which can be measured by tritiated thymidine incorporation or other methods. Since the proportion of T lymphocytes that respond to any single antigen is less than the proportion that respond to polyclonal stimulation with mitogen, the maximal proliferative response to specific antigens is significantly less than the response to mitogen stimulation. Each laboratory needs to identify its own normal values for determining what is a positive proliferative response to antigenic stimulation. Unlike the response to PHA, there is no relationship between the magnitude of the antigen-specific blastogenesis and the proportion of leukocytes that are T lymphocytes. The major factors that determine the magnitude of the T lymphocyte response to specific antigen stimulation are the interval between antigenic stimulation (either vaccination or clinical disease) and the time of the assay. Thus, antigen-specific blastogenic studies are best interpreted on an all or nothing basis with individuals being scored as having antigen-specific blastogenesis either present or absent rather than presenting the results in a quantitative fashion.

The *in vitro* blastogenic response by T lymphocytes to specific antigenic stimulation requires IL-2 production. Only a minority of antigen-specific T lymphocytes (approximately 10 per cent) are capable of producing IL-2 after antigenic stimulation while the other 90 per cent express the IL-2 receptor (CD25) after antigenic-specific stimulation (Greene and Leonard, 1986). The presence of IL-2 producing antigen-specific T lymphocytes is required for the proliferation of the IL-2 receptor expressing antigen-specific T lymphocytes. In some clinical settings, however, there may be deficits in the capacity of antigen-specific T lymphocytes to produce IL-2 even though IL-2 responsive T lymphocytes are present. Therefore, the addition of exogenous IL-2 may be required for the full evaluation of the immunological function of patients with suspected defects in T lymphocyte immunity. A patient, whose peripheral blood leukocytes showed no proliferative response to antigenic stimulation but who did have a proliferative response when exogenous IL-2 was added, would be diagnosed with having antigen-specific IL-2 dependent T lymphocytes but an absence of the antigen-specific subpopulation capable of IL-2 production, i.e. IL-2 deficient (Welte et al., 1984; Weinberg and Parkman, 1990).

Specific defects in the production of other important cytokines after antigen-specific stimulation have also been noted, particularly γ-interferon (γ-inf) which is central to the control of viral infections. The enumeration of antigen-specific T lymphocytes capable of producing cytokines after antigen specific stimulation can be done using assays that enumerate the proportion of T lymphocytes producing cytokines (intracytoplasmic cytokines (ICC), ELISA spot assay). Common to all assays are the stimulation of peripheral blood leukocytes by specific antigen and the enumeration of the proportion of the T lymphocytes capable of producing the specific cytokine by FACS or other methods. Some patients, who have normal proliferative responses to antigen specific stimulation and, therefore, have normal IL-2 production, do not have normal γ-INF production.

One of the most differentiated T lymphocyte functions is the capacity of T lymphocytes to lyse appropriate target cells, either virally infected or tumor cells (Reusser et al., 1991). *In vitro* cytolytic assays can identify cytotoxic T lymphocytes (CTL). In such assays, the leukocytes are stimulated *in vitro* to expand pre-existing antigen-specific T lymphocytes. At the end of 7 days, the capacity of T lymphocytes to lyse the appropriate target cells (usually labeled with chromium) is then determined.

A new assessment of T lymphocyte immunity has focused on the production of T lymphocytes by the thymus. Originally CD4 T lymphocytes that expressed the RA isoform of CD45 were defined as recent thymic immigrants, i.e. cells that had been recently produced by the thymus. Thymic function decreases with age. Thus, the absolute number of new T lymphocytes decreases with age, resulting in an age-dependent decrease in a proportion of CD4 T lymphocytes that express CD45RA (Pilarski et al., 1989). However, a lack of specificity of the immunophenotype led to the development of the T cell receptor excision circle (TREC) assay in which the proportion of T lymphocytes, either CD4 or CD8, which contain TREC are quantified (Douek et al., 1998; 2000). TREC is episomal DNA that represents the excisional DNA product of T cell receptor gene rearrangement. Newly produced T lymphocytes contain TREC as they exit the thymus. As the T lymphocytes undergo peripheral expansion, the proportion of T lymphocytes that contain TREC becomes less since there is no replication of the episomal DNA. Thus, if an individual's T lymphocytes consist primarily of newly produced T lymphocytes, the frequency of TREC containing cells will be relatively high, whereas if T lymphocytes are due to the peripheral expansion of T lymphocytes, the frequency of TREC containing cells will be relatively low.

Thus, the full evaluation of the T lymphocyte immunity of a patient with a possible T lymphocyte defect can be complicated. The most simple assays focused on the enumeration of the presence and distribution of immunophenotypic T lymphocytes followed by a determination of their capacity to respond to mitogen stimulation. If the initial assays demonstrate no defect, but the patient's clinical course is suggestive of defective T lymphocyte immunity, the assays of antigen-specific function are appropriate.

B lymphocytes

It is well established in mice that B lymphocytes are capable of producing antibodies to some antigens, particularly carbohydrate antigens, without interaction with T lymphocytes. Such antigens are termed T lymphocyte independent

antigens. In humans, however, no T lymphocyte-independent antigens exist and all antibody production to carbohydrate as well as protein antigens require interactions between T and B lymphocytes. Thus, patients with profound defects in T lymphocyte function will also have concomitant defects in antibody production, resulting in an increased risk of infection with encapsulated bacterial organisms. The presence of mature B lymphocytes in the peripheral blood can be most readily assayed by the presence of leukocytes with membrane-bound immunoglobulins using monoclonal antibodies to κ and λ light chains as well as the Fab portion of the appropriate heavy chains. Since immunoglobulin molecules can bind to cells like monocytes with Fc receptors, it is important that monoclonal antibodies which react with the Fc portion of the immunoglobulin molecule not be used. B lymphocytes are also characterized by the presence of CD20 and, in most cases, CD19 on their cell surface. The use of monoclonal antibodies to lymphocyte differentiation antigens rather than membrane bound immunoglobulin molecule is less problematic. As in the case of T lymphocytes, results should be expressed as the number of cells/μl rather than a percentage. B lymphocytes undergo a normal differentiation from cells expressing surface IgD to IgM and then IgG and IgA. It is important, therefore, in some clinical setting to enumerate not only the absolute number of circulating B lymphocytes but to determine the distribution of immunoglobulin heavy chain expression by the B lymphocytes by using monoclonal antibodies specific for the immunoglobulin heavy chains. Even though IgG is the most common circulating immunoglobulin, the majority of circulating B lymphocytes do not express membrane IgG since IgG-expressing B lymphocytes migrate into the tissues and become plasma cells.

The levels of serum immunoglobulin are routinely determined by automated machines. At birth, circulating IgG is maternally derived, but both IgM and IgA are of neonatal origin. Thus, the presence of IgM and IgA can be used to determine whether a newborn infant is capable of immunoglobulin production. Maternally derived IgG has a half-life of 22–28 days and, therefore, by 4–6 months it is possible to assess whether an infant is capable of IgG synthesis. However, as in the case of T lymphocytes, the presence of immunoglobulins is inadequate to state with certainty that an individual is capable of normal antibody production. Normal newborn infants are capable of developing normal antibody responses following immunization with protein antigens such as TT and DT (Smith et al., 1964). Greater than 95 per cent of normal infants will have protective antibody levels to protein antigens after two immunizations. The presence of maternal antibody does not interfere with the effectiveness of vaccination with killed vaccines. Therefore, it is possible by 6 months of age to determine whether an infant can develop a normal antibody response to a protein antigen. However, protection against encapsulated respiratory bacteria (*Staphylococcus aureus*, *Streptococcus*,

Pneumococcus, Haemophilus influenzae type b, etc.) requires the ability to make antibodies to bacterial carbohydrate, not to protein antigens. In ontogeny, the capacity of normal individuals to produce antibodies to bacterial carbohydrate antigens does not appear until 18 months (Black et al., 1991). Therefore, it is important when assessing individuals believed to have defects in antibody production to determine their antibody responses to both protein and carbohydrate antigens. Antibodies to *Haemophilus influenzae* type b capsular antigen (polyribosophosphate (PRP)) cross-reacts with the K100 strains of *Escherichia coli*, found in the gastrointestinal tract of normal individuals (Schneerson and Robbins, 1975). Thus, normal individuals are constantly stimulated by PRP antigen, which results in the presence of protective antibodies to PRP after 18 months. Thus, no immunization is necessary to assess in individuals older than 18 months the presence of anti-PRP antibodies, whereas vaccination with TT is required for the assessment of antibodies to TT. Vaccination with conjugated carbohydrate antigens, both PRP and *Pneumococcus*, can confuse the interpretation of antibody responses. The capacity of an individual to respond normally to a conjugated carbohydrate antigen does not predict a capacity to respond to wild type bacterial carbohydrate antigens. In fact, the reason why conjugated carbohydrate vaccines are used in younger individuals is that they cannot respond to the wild type antigen (Black et al., 1991). The increasing use of conjugated PRP vaccines means that normal antibody levels of PRP are no longer adequate documentation in immunized individuals to state conclusively that the individual has a normal capacity to make protective antibodies to wild type respiratory encapsulated bacteria.

Granulocytes

Granulocytes play a central role in protection against encapsulated respiratory bacteria, enteric bacteria, as well as many fungi. Granulocytes can be enumerated by a routine peripheral blood count and the number of granulocytes/μl determined. Although some primary immunodeficiencies are characterized by an absence of granulocytes due to defects in differentiation, the majority of primary immunodeficiences involving granulocytes relate to granulocyte function. The functional defects of granulocytes can be divided into those that affect phagocytosis and those that involve killing. The phagocytosis of bacteria is mediated either through the third component of complement (C3) or properdin. Phagocytic assays can be performed using either lipid droplets containing dye or viable bacteria and then the uptake of the target quantified. After phagocytosis, the oxidative mechanisms of the cells are activated which can be measured by either the reduction of the dye, nitroblue tetrazolium (NBT) or the assessment of bacterial killing (Segal et al., 2000). For the routine screening of oxidative capacity, the NBT test is used. It is important, however, to integrate the results of the phagocytic assays with the oxidative results since decreases in phagocytic function will result in less oxidation and an apparent decrease in oxidative capacity.

Natural killer cells

Natural killer (NK) cells have a poorly defined role in the defense against infectious pathogens and cancer. NK cells can be immunophenotypically enumerated by their expression of surface differentiation antigens, including CD56, CD57 and CD16 (Lanier et al., 1986). Functionally, NK cells are defined by their ability to lyse leukemia cells *in vitro*, particularly the myeloid cell line, K562. Their cytolytic activity is associated with the presence of granzyome and perforin, which can be immunophenotypically detected by appropriate monoclonal antibody staining and FACS analysis (Stepp et al., 1999).

Complement

The complement system represents the complex interaction of nine proteins, each one of which represents a proenzyme which, upon appropriate activation, becomes an active enzyme that activates the next member of the complement system. The complement system has a central role in protection against bacteria. The third component of complement, C3, is essential for the maximal phagocytosis of encapsulated respiratory bacteria. After IgG or IgM antibodies attach to the capsular antigens of bacterial cell wall, the sequential interaction of C1, C2 and C4 with the immunoglobulin molecules results in the binding of C3 and an increased rate of phagocytosis (Colten and Rosen, 1992). Since enteric bacteria have no cell wall-associated carbohydrate antigens, immunoglobulin plays no significant role in protection against enteric bacteria. The primary mediator of the phagocytosis of enteric bacteria is through the properiden system, which binds to the lipoprotein of the enteric bacterial cell wall; C3 then binds to properiden resulting in increased phagocytosis. Disease states, in which there is a decrease in properiden, results in the decreased phagocytosis of enteric bacteria.

EVALUATION OF SPECIFIC PRIMARY DEFICIENCIES

Defects of T lymphocyte differentiation

DiGeorge syndrome

The DiGeorge syndrome is due to the congenital absence/hypoplasia of the third and fourth pharyngeal pouches which can result in the absence or hypoplasia of the thymus in addition to the characteristic facial, auricular and cardiac defects (Di George, 1965; Hong, 1991). A significant reduction in the mass of thymic stroma can result in the decreased differentiation of hematopoietic stem cells into T lymphocytes. Thus, patients with the characteristic anatomic defects should be evaluated for thymic hypoplasia by determining immunophenotypically the number of T lymphocytes. What is of interest is the fact that the T lymphocyes that do exist are functionally normal; therefore, on a per cell basis their blastogenic responses to both mitogen and antigen-specific stimulation are normal. Thus, DiGeorge syndrome represents a quantitative deficit in the number of T lymphocytes, but does not represent a functional defect.

Severe combined immune deficiency (SCID)

SCID is a clinical phenotype characterized by an absence of functional T and B lymphocyte immunity (Hitzig and Willi, 1961; Buckley et al., 1997). Almost 20 genetic defects have now been identified that can produce the clinical phenotype. Among the most common primary genetic defects include the absence of the common gamma (γc) chain (X-linked SCID), the absence of the enzyme adenosine deaminase (ADA deficiency), RAG-1/RAG-2 deficiencies, IL-7/IL-7 receptor deficiencies and JAK3 deficiency.

X-linked SCID

The primary defect in X-linked SCID patients is the absence of a functional γc chain. Since γc is part of the IL-2, IL-4, IL-7, IL-9 and IL-15 receptors, a variety of immunophenotypic and functional defects can exist in X-linked SCID patients (Greene and Leonard, 1986; Noguchi et al., 1993; Nelms et al., 1999). The absence of a functional IL-7 receptor results in a lack of thymic production of T lymphocytes. The defective IL-2 receptor results in a lack of expansion of the few T lymphocytes that are produced. The absence of a functional IL-4 receptor means that no immunoglobulin switching occurs in B cells and the absence of a functional IL-15 receptor results in decreased NK cell production. Thus, X-linked SCID patients have no T lymphocytes or NK cells, but do have dysfunctional B lymphocytes. Patients should be evaluated with a panel of monoclonal antibodies (CD3, CD4, CD8, CD16, CD19, CD20, CD56, CD57), which allows the enumeration of the number of T lymphocytes, B lymphocytes and NK cells. Thus, males, who have no detectable T lymphocytes or NK cells but do have B lymphocytes, have a presumed diagnosis of X-linked SCID. Monoclonal antibodies to the γc chain (CD132) are available. In about half of the X-linked SCID patients, no leukocyte expression of γc is present, while in the other half of the cases, a non-functional γc chain is expressed. Monoclonal staining, therefore, of the B lymphocytes will determine whether γc is expressed. The absence of γc expression by B lymphocytes confirms the diagnosis of X-linked SCID. Positive γc staining of the B lymphocytes requires genomic analysis to confirm the diagnosis of X-linked SCID. In all cases genomic analysis should be done since it will aid in the prenatal testing of future potentially affected fetuses. A compounding

variable in many X linked SCID patients is the presence of transplacentally derived maternal T lymphocytes which may cause graft-versus-host disease. If the diagnosis of X-linked SCID is suspected, but some T lymphocytes are present, the T lymphocytes should be isolated and their HLA type compared to that of the patient's and mother's myeloid cells (granulocytes) to confirm the origin of the T lymphocytes.

Adenosine deaminase (ADA) deficiency

ADA has a central role in purine metabolism. The absence of ADA results in the accumulation of adenosine and deoxyadenosine triphosphate, which results in:

1 the decreased thymic production of T lymphocytes and
2 the decreased survival of the T lymphocytes that are produced (Chen et al., 1974; Hirschorn, 1990).

Patients with ADA deficiency have markedly reduced numbers of T and B lymphocytes and NK cells. The diagnosis of ADA deficiency is confirmed by the analysis of erythrocyte ADA activity as well as increased adenosine and deoxyadenosine metabolites.

IL-7/IL-7α receptor deficiencies

Given the central role of the IL-7/IL-7-receptor axis in thymopoiesis and the peripheral expansion of mature T lymphocytes, it is not surprising that defects in both IL-7 production and the IL-7α chain expression results in T lymphocyte immunodeficiency (Puel et al., 1998). Patients with SCID due to defects in IL-7/IL-7 receptor have an absence of T lymphocytes, but the presence of B lymphocytes and NK cells.

RAG-1/RAG-2 deficiences

Rearrangement of the VDJ genes is central to the generation of TCR diversity. Abnormalities of both the RAG-1 and RAG-2 genes result in the lack of productive VDJ rearrangements. Such patients have no detectable T or B lymphocytes, but do have NK cells (Hansen et al., 1999; Xu et al., 1999). The diagnosis is confirmed by genetic analysis of the genes.

JAK3 deficiency

JAK3 is activated downstream from the γc chain. Therefore, patients with JAK3 deficiency have a similar immunophenotype (no T lymphocytes, but B lymphocytes and NK cells) to X-linked SCID patients, but may be either male or female (Macchi et al., 1995).

Defects in antibody production

Patients with antibody deficiency states are characterized by recurrent infections primarily with encapsulated respiratory bacteria (*Staphyloccocus aureus, Haemophilus influenzae, Streptococcus, Pneumococcus*). Antibody deficiency can occur as part of a more global immunodeficiency involving T lymphocytes in addition to B lymphocytes. However, specific defects in B lymphocyte differentiation/function can lead to a selective inability to produce antibodies in the presence of normal T lymphocyte immunity.

X-linked agammaglobulinemia

The original antibody deficiency syndrome was an X-linked disease, now known to be due to defects in Bruton's tyrosine kinase (BTK) resulting in the absence of circulating B lymphocytes and, therefore, no plasma cells (Hermaszewski and Webster, 1993; Smith et al., 1998). The lack of terminal differentiation of B cell precursors means that no immunoglobulins of any class are produced. The staining of peripheral blood leukocytes with antibodies to differentiate antigens uniquely expressed on B lymphocytes (CD19, CD20) documents the lack of circulating B lymphocytes.

Common variable immune deficiency (CVID)

CVID is a group of diseases characterized by the inability of patients who have circulating B lymphocytes to make protective levels of antibodies. A variety of primary defects have been identified, some of which represent the inability of the B lymphocytes to respond to T lymphocyte cytokines like IL-4 and IL-5, while others represent the inability of the T lymphocytes to produce the cytokines necessary for B cell activation/differentiation (Geha et al., 1974; Pandolfi et al., 1993). CVID patients are characterized by reduced levels of immunoglobulins, particularly when corrected for their history of recurrent infections. In spite of having some immunoglobulins, the patients do not respond to vaccination. Definitive testing is based upon the determination of specific antibody levels after immunization. Response to TT can be used as a prototypic protein antigen and antibodies to PRP as a prototypic carbohydrate antigen.

CD-40/CD40-ligand deficiency (hyper-IgM syndrome)

CD-40/CD-40 ligand interactions are necessary for class switching by B lymphocytes from IgM to IgG antibody production. Patients with defects in either CD40 ligand (expressed by T lymphocytes) or CD40 (expressed by B lymphocytes) have elevated levels of IgM and reduced levels of IgG (Allen et al., 1993; Fuleihan et al., 1993). Although some IgM antibodies are present, they are inadequate to provide protective immunity. The determination of serum immunoglobulin levels is the first step in assessing these patients. The expression of CD40 ligand by T lymphocytes is determined by FACS analysis after the stimulation of peripheral blood leukocytes by mitogens for 48 h. The proportion of T lymphocytes cells expressing CD40 ligand is then determined by FACS analysis. CD40 expression on B lymphocytes is similarly determined.

Defects of T lymphocyte function

Wiskott-Aldrich syndrome

Wiskott-Aldrich syndrome (WAS) is a multi-faceted immunodeficiency characterized by eczema, thrombocytopenia, an inability to make anti-carbohydrate antibodies and a predilection to DNA viral infections. The primary defect in WAS is a defective WAS protein (WASP), a 501 amino protein that has no homologies (Derry et al., 1994). Research has been directed at determining how abnormalities in WASP cause the complex clinical phenotype of the disease. WASP has an important role in the cytoskeletal functioning, but its exact role in producing the thrombocytopenia, the defects in anti-carbohydrate antibody production and eczema is still unclear.

No significant abnormalities in the immunophenotype of T or B lymphocytes are present in WAS patients. Classically, patients are characterized by decreases in their serum IgM levels and an elevation in their other immunoglobulin levels. Scanning EM of the T lymphocytes of WAS patients has shown an absence of the normal microvilli, presumably secondary to their cytoskeletal defects (Kenney et al., 1985). Some patients have no significant immune deficits and their principal clinical manifestation is thrombocytopenia with platelets of reduced size and function. Functionally WAS T lymphocytes are characterized by increased rate of spontaneous apoptosis. The T lymphocytes from some WAS patients show an absence of proliferation to DNA viruses to which the patients have previously been exposed, suggesting that the antigen-specific T lymphocytes do not persist.

X-linked lymphoproliferative syndrome (XLP)

In XLP, affected males succumb to either Epstein-Barr virus (EBV) associated lymphomas or overwhelming EBV infection. The primary defect has now been shown to be due to defects in the SAP protein, which is involved in T lymphocyte activation (Sayos et al., 1998). The definitive diagnosis of XLP is based upon the demonstration of the molecular abnormalities. Functionally, the T lymphocytes of XLP patients are unable to lyse EBV-infected B lymphocytes.

Hereditary lymphohistocytosis (HLH)

Some patients with HLH have perforin deficiency, either functionally or phenotypically. The inability of the patients' T lymphocytes to lyse virally infected cells may result in the excessive stimulation of the immune system and the clinical phenotype of HLH. The absence of perforin can be determined by monoclonal antibody staining and FACS (Stepp et al., 1999).

ZAP-70 deficiency

Deficiency in the lymphocyte kinase, ZAP-70, results in defective TCR signaling and defective thymic selection (Arpaia et al., 1994). Patients have a selective absence of CD8 T lymphocytes but a normal number of CD4 T lymphocytes and reduced proliferation to mitogen stimulation.

Omenn syndrome

Affected patients appear shortly after birth with what appears to be clinically graft-versus-host disease, but no maternal T lymphocyte engraftment can be detected. The circulating T lymphocytes display activation markers (HLA and CD25) and TCR usage reveals a constricted pattern of usage (Kuijpers et al., 1992). Abnormalities in RAG1/RAG2 genes have been reported suggesting defects in negative thymic selection and the presence of autoreactive T lymphocytes.

Defects in granulocyte function

Leukocyte adhesion deficiency

The absence of integrans necessary for granulocyte adhesion to endothelium results in defective chemotaxis, decreased C3 mediated phagocytosis and killing. Patients are characterized by the absence of expression of or the presence of dysfunctional CD11 or CD18. A history of delayed umbilical cord separation and omphalites should be followed by the assessment of CD18 expression (van der Meer et al., 1975; Diacovo et al., 1996).

Phagocytic disorders

Granulocytes from some patients are characterized by a decreased capacity to phagocytose opsinized bacteria due to defects in their cytoskeleton (Boxer et al., 1974). To quantify their phagocytosis, granulocytes are incubated with either viable bacteria or lipid particles, which are incubated in both patient and normal serum to detect opsinizing abnormalities that may lead to decreased phagocytosis. Following ingestion, phagocytosis is quantified and compared to the normal granulocytes. Equal uptake in normal serum by both patient and normal granulocytes indicates an opsonizing defect in the patient serum. Decreased uptake by patient, but not normal granulocytes, indicates an intrinsic defect in the patient cells, requiring further evaluation.

Chronic granulomatous disease (CGD)

Patients with CGD are characterized by recurrent bacterial infections with catalase-positive bacteria (Segal et al., 2000). Although both X-linked and autosomal recessive forms of CGD are known, common to all forms is the decreased capacity of granulocytes to produce superoxide and other oxygen metabolites required for bacterial killing. The presence of catalase in the bacteria (*Serratia*, *Staphylococcus aureus*, etc.) results in the destruction of the small amount of oxygen metabolites that are produced. Thus, although the granulocytes can phagocytose the bacteria, they are unable to kill them. Intracellular bacteria can be seen on blood smears. In screening tests, the defective oxidative metabolisms can be assessed using the NBT test, where the patient's peripheral blood granulocytes are stimulated by PMA and the presence of the precipitated NBT determined. The oxidative burst can now be quantified by FACS (Vowells et al., 1995). In complicated clinical presentations it is important to quantify the amount of phagocytosis in addition to the amount of oxidation.

Complement defects

Although there are nine complement components, there are only two primary clinical syndromes associated with complement deficiencies. First, decreased C3 binding, the central component in the phagocytosis of both encapsulated respiratory and enteric bacteria, leads to reduced phagocytosis by granulocytes and other phagocytic cells, predisposing individuals to recurrent bacterial infections (Colten and Rosen, 1992). Decreased C3 binding can be due to reduced C3 levels or reductions in the earlier complement components (C2, C4). The CH50 test can be used as a screening assay to detect reduced levels of early acting (C1–C4) complement components. Antibody-coated erythrocytes are incubated with the patient's serum and the degree of lysis determined. If a reduced CH50 is present, further assessment of the individual complement components is necessary.

A second clinical syndrome is recurrent infections with *Neisseria* due to defects in the late-acting complement components (C7, C8 and C9). Patients with the clinical syndrome of recurrent *Neisseria* infections should be assessed for the levels of their late-acting complement components.

REFERENCES

Allen, R.C., Armitage, R.J., Conley, M.E. et al. (1993). CD40 ligand gene defects responsible for x-linked hyper IgM syndrome. Science 259, 990–993.

Arpaia, E., Shahar, M., Dadi, H. et al. (1994). Defective T cell receptor signaling and CD8+ thymic section in humans lacking zap-70 kinase. Cell 76, 947–958.

Bach, F.H. and Hirschorn, K. (1964). Lymphocyte interaction, a potential histocompatible test in vitro. Science 143, 813–814.

Black, S.B., Shinefield, H.R., Fireman, B. et al. (1991). Efficacy in infancy of oligosaccharide conjugate Haemophilus influenzae type B (HbOC) vaccine in a United States population of 61 080 children. Pediatr Infect Dis J 10, 92–96.

Boxer, L.A., Hedley-Whyte, E.T. and Stossel, T.P. (1974). Neutrophil action dysfunction and abnormal neutrophil behavior. N Engl J Med 291, 1093–1099.

Buckley, R.H., Schiff, R.I., Schiff, S.E. et al. (1997). Human severe combined immunodeficiency (SCID): genetic, phentoypic and functional diversity in 108 infants. J Pediatr 130, 378–387.

Chen, S.-H., Scott, C.R. and Giblett, E.R. (1974). Adenosine deaminase: demonstration of a 'silent' gene associated with combined immunodeficiency disease. Am J Hum Genet 26, 103–107.

Colten, H.R. and Rosen, F.S. (1992). Complement deficiencies. Annu Rev Immunol 10, 809–834.

Comans-Bitter, W.M., de Groot, R., van den Beemd, R. et al. (1997). Immunophenotyping of blood lymphocytes in childhood. Reference values for lymphocyte populations. J Pediatr 130, 338–393.

Derry, J., Ochs, H. and Francke, U. (1994). Isolation of a novel gene mutated in Wiskott-Aldrich syndrome. Cell 78, 635–644.

Diacovo, T.G., Roth, S.J., Buccola, J.M. et al. (1996). Neutrophil rolling, arrest, and transmigration across activated, surface-adherent platelets via sequential action of P-selectin and the beta 2-integrin CD11b/CD18. Blood 88, 146–157.

DiGeorge, A.M. (1965). A new concept of the cellular basis of immunity. J Pediatr 67, 907–911.

Douek, D.C., McFarland, R.D., Keiser, P.H. et al. (1998). Changes in thymic function with age and during the treatment of HIV infection. Nature 396, 630–631.

Douek D.C, Vescio R.A, Betts M.R, et al. (2000). Assessment of thymic output in adults after haematopoietic stem-cell transplantation and prediction of T-cell reconstitution. Lancet 355, 1875–1881.

Fuleihan, R., Ramesh, N., Loh, R. et al. (1993). Defective expression of the CD40 ligand in X-linked immunoglobulin deficiency with normal or elevated IgM. Proc Natl Acad Sci USA 90, 2170–2173.

Geha, R.S., Schneeberger, E., Merler, E. and Rosen, F.S. (1974). Heterogeneity of 'acquired' or common variable agammaglobulinemia. N Engl J Med 291, 1–6.

Greene, W.C. and Leonard, W.J. (1986). The human interleukin-2 receptor. Annu Rev Immunol 4, 69–95.

Greaves, M.F. and Brown, G. (1974). Purification of human T and B lymphocytes. J Immunol 112, 420–423.

Hansen, R.S., Wijmenga, C., Luo, P. et al. (1999). The DNMT3B DNA methyltransferase gene is mutated in the ICF immunodeficiency syndrome. Proc Natl Acad Sci USA 96, 14412–14417.

Hermaszewski, R.A. and Webster, A.D. (1993). Primary hypogammaglobulinaemia: a survey of clinical manifestations and complications. Q J Med 86, 31–42.

Hirschorn, R. (1990). Adenosine deaminase deficiency. Immunodeficiency Rev 2, 175–195.

Hitzig, W.H. and Willi, H. (1961). Hereditäre lymphoplasmocytäse dysginesie. Schweiz Med Wshchr 91, 1625–1626.

Hong, R. (1991). The DiGeorge anomaly. Immunodeficiency Rev 3, 1–14.

Käyhty, H., Peltola, H., Karanko, V. and Mäkelä, P.H. (1983). The protective level of serum antibodies to the capsular polysaccharide of Haemophilus influenzae type b. J Infect Dis 147, 1100–1106.

Kenney, D.M., Cairns, L., Neustein, H. et al. (1985). Morphological abnormalities in the lymphocytes of patients with the Wiskott-Aldrich syndrome. Blood 68, 1329–1332.

Kuijpers, K.C., van Dongen, J.J., van der Burg, P. et al. (1992). A combined immunodeficiency with oligoclonal CD8+, V beta 3-expressing, cytotoxic T lymphocytes in the peripheral blood. J Immunol 149, 3403–3410.

Lanier, L.L., Le, A.M., Civin, C.I. et al. (1986). The relationship of CD16 (Leu-11) and Leu-19 (NKH-1) antigen expression on human peripheral blood NK cells and cytotoxic T lymphocytes. J Immunol 136, 4480–4486.

Macchi, P., Villa, A., Gillani, S., et al. (1995). Mutations of Jak-3 gene in patients with autosomal severe combined immune deficiency (SCID). Nature 377, 65–68.

Nagel, J.E., Chrest, F.J. and Adler, W.H. (1981). Enumeration of T lymphocyte subsets by monoclonal antibodies in young and aged humans. J Immunol 127, 2086–2088.

Nelms, K., Keegan, A.D., Zamorano, J. et al. (1999). The IL-4 receptor: signaling mechanisms and biologic functions. Annu Rev Immunol 17, 701–738.

Noguchi, M., Yi, H., Rosenblatt, H.M. et al. (1993). Interleukin-2 receptor gamma chain mutation results in X-linked severe combined immunodeficiency in humans. Cell 73, 147–157.

Pandolfi, R., Paganelli, R., Cafaro, A. et al. (1993). Abnormalities of subpopulations in CVI do not correlate with increased p-IL-6. Immunodeficiency 4, 19–23.

Pilarski, L.M., Gillitaer, R., Zola, H. et al. (1989). Definition of the thymic generative lineage by selective expression of high molecular weight isoforms of CD45 (T200). Eur J Immunol 19, 589–595.

Puel, A., Ziegler, S.F., Buckley, R.H. and Leonard, W.J. (1998). Defective IL7R expression in T(−)B(+)NK(+) severe combined immunodeficiency. Nat Genet 20, 394–397.

Reusser, P., Riddell, S.R., Meyers, J.D. and Greenberg, P.D. (1991). Cytotoxic T-lymphocyte response to cytomegalovirus after human allogeneic bone marrow transplantation: pattern of recovery and correlation with cytomegalovirus infection and disease. Blood 78, 1373–1380.

Sayos, J., Wu, C., Morra, M. et al. (1998). The x-linked lymphoproliferative disease gene product SAP regulates signals induced through the co-receptor SLAM. Nature 395, 462.

Schneerson, R. and Robbins, J.B. (1975). Induction of serum Haemophilus influenzae type B capsular antibodies in adult volunteers fed cross-reacting Escherichia coli 075. N Engl J Med 292, 1093–1096.

Segal, B.H., Leto, T.L., Gallin, J.I. et al. (2000). Genetic biochemical and clinical features of chronic granulomatous disease. Medicine (Baltimore) 79, 170–200.

Smith, C.I., Backesjo, C.M., Berglof, A. et al. (1998). X-linked agammaglobulinemia: lack of mature B lineage cells caused by mutations in the Btk kinase. Springer Semin Immunopathol 19, 369–381.

Smith, R.T., Eitzman, D.V., Catlin, M.E. et al. (1964). The development of the immune response. Characterization of the response of the human infant and adult to immunization with salmonella vaccines. Pediatrics 34, 163–171.

Stepp, S.E., Dufourcq-Lagelouse, R., Le Deist, F. et al. (1999). Perforin gene defects in familial hemophagocytic lymphohistiocytosis. Science 286, 1957–1959.

van der Meer, J.W., van Zwet, T.L. and van Furth R. (1975). New familial defect in microbicidal function of polymorphonuclear leucocytes. Lancet 2, 630–632.

Vowells, S.J., Sekhsaria, S., Malech, H.L. et al. (1995). Flow cytometric analysis of the granulocyte respiratory burst: a comparison study of fluorescent probes. J Immunol Methods *178*, 9–97.

Weinberg, K. and Parkman, R. (1990). Severe combined immunodeficiency due to a specific defect in the production of interleukin-2. N Engl J Med *322*, 1718–1723.

Welte, K., Liobanu, N., Moore, M.A.S. et al. (1984). Defective interleukin-2 production in patients after bone marrow transplantation and in vitro restoration of defective T-lymphocyte proliferation by highly purified interleukin 2. Blood *64*, 380–385.

Xu, G., Besto, T., Bourc'his, D. et al. (1999). Chromosome instability and immunodeficiency syndrome caused by mutations in a DNA methyltransferase gene. Nature *402*, 187–191.

Asthma and Allergy

**Chapter
56**

Lanny J. Rosenwasser and Jillian A. Poole

University of Colorado Health Sciences Center and the Division of Allergy and Clinical Immunology, National Jewish Medical and Research Center, Denver, CO, USA

We look forward to the adoption of immunological assays being developed for standardization of proteins and the safety control of vaccines. Slowly but progressively, all these ambitions are being addressed.

Sir Peter Medawar

INTRODUCTION

Allergic diseases are traditionally referred to as immediate or type I hypersensitivity reactions with allergen-specific IgE as an important factor. However, it is also apparent that critical cellular elements such as T lymphocytes constitute a major pathogenesis factor in the development of allergic diseases and, in particular, asthma. Dendritic cells along with molecules such as the T cell receptor, major histocompatibility complex molecules and co-stimulatory molecules are all necessary for inducing an allergic T cell inflammatory response.

Clinical laboratory tools in conjunction with a thorough history and physical examination are used to diagnosis properly and manage patients with allergic disorders. At present there is no *in vitro* test that confirms the presence of clinically relevant allergic disease. Therefore, the immunoassays and tests that will be discussed in this chapter should be viewed as an adjunct to a complete history and physical examination and are not to be used alone in the diagnosis and treatment of allergic disorders.

At present, the gold standard for diagnosing a specific allergen as the cause of disease is by provocation testing to the suspected allergen. Provocation testing involves subjecting the patient to a nasal, oral or bronchial challenge to the specific allergen (pollen, animal dander, food, latex, etc.) in a carefully monitored environment. This can be time consuming and even put the patient in harm by eliciting a severe allergic reaction including anaphylaxis. Therefore, provocation testing is not routinely used and clinical laboratory assessment is commonly used to guide the healthcare provider with useful information.

After a careful history and physical examination is completed and a particular allergic disorder is suspected, various means to detect allergen-specific IgE antibody, either by skin testing or *in vitro* serum assays, are performed to support the initial diagnosis. A simple and easy way to detect allergen-specific IgE antibody is the skin prick/puncture test that was first introduced in 1865 by Dr Blackley (Blackley, 1880). Although modified over the years, the skin prick/puncture test exists as the most routinely used diagnostic tool in the field of allergic diseases. Newer immunologic testing for both research and clinical settings includes quantification of total serum IgE, radioallergosorbent tests, enzyme-linked allergosorbent tests, basophil histamine release assays and allergen-specific lymphocyte proliferation assays.

SKIN PRICK TESTING

The skin prick/puncture test that was first introduced by Dr Blackley in 1865 (Blackley, 1880) still persists today as

Measuring Immunity, edited by Michael T. Lotze and Angus W. Thomson
ISBN 0-12-455900-X, London

the most reliable allergy test to diagnosis specific IgE-mediated allergic reactions in individuals. Briefly, the test is performed by application of a small amount of the test allergen extract on the skin, in addition to histamine (positive) and diluent (negative) controls. Using sterile technique, the epidermal surface of the skin is then pricked or punctured with a needle. In comparison, the intradermal test may be used after obtaining negative results from the skin prick/puncture test by injecting the allergen extract (100- and 1000-fold dilution of concentrated extract) intracutaneously at a volume of 0.01–0.05 ml. Results for both tests are measured after 15–20 minutes and a positive reaction is indicated by a wheal and flare response on the skin at the site of the prick/puncture. A positive reaction is determined by a wheal 3 mm greater than the negative control with surrounding erythema. Limitations in the skin prick/puncture method can occur. For example, not all allergen extracts are standardized and therefore potency and stability of the allergen extract can vary between lots and manufacturers. Use of certain medications (antihistamines, ketotifen and tricyclic antidepressants) by the subject can cause false negative results. Host factors such as the presence of dermatographism or bleeding disorders can cause false positive tests. In addition, operator dependent errors such as improper technique can also lead to false-positive or false-negative results.

Even with these potential limitations, a positive skin prick/puncture reaction does not mean that the symptoms experienced by the subject are caused by an IgE-mediated allergic reaction. Asymptomatic subjects may also have positive skin test results, which only implies the detection of allergen-specific IgE antibody and not the presence of disease. Interpretation of skin tests in conjunction with the clinical history will enhance the positive predictive value of the tests.

TOTAL SERUM IGE

In 1967, two separate groups first identified IgE as a unique serum immunoglobulin isotype (Ishizaka and Ishizaka, 1967; Johansson and Bennich, 1967). Serum IgE will be discussed here for its role in immediate-type hypersensitivity responses, but it is also important in mediating immune defense against parasitic infections. IgE is a 190 kD, four-chain monomeric protein that accounts for approximately 0.0005 per cent of the total serum immunoglobulins in adults. It is commonly reported as kilo international units per liter (kIU/l). Conversion of serum IgE levels to mass per volume (μg/l) units is accomplished by multiplying the kIU/l value by 2.4 (1 kIU/l = 2.4 μg/l). Calibrators for total IgE measurements are set forth by the World Health Organization (WHO) International Reference Preparation for Human IgE, 75/502. The analytical sensitivity of most total serum IgE assays is 0.5–1 μg/l. Total serum IgE should always be

interpreted in comparison to non-atopic age-adjusted reference intervals (Hamilton and Adkinson, 2003).

Although there are a number of assays that are used to determine total serum IgE, the two most commonly used are the two-site, non-competitive immunoenzymetric assays and nephelometric assays. Briefly, the two-site, non-competitive immunoenzymetric assay uses a solid-phase monoclonal antihuman IgE antibody to bind IgE from test serum (capture). Following buffer washes to remove unbound proteins, a second monoclonal antihuman IgE antibody that is labeled (by radionuclide, strepavidin-enzyme or fluorophor) detects bound IgE (detection). Further buffer washes are completed to remove unbound detection antibody. The final step is to quantitate the response signal (counts per minute bound, optical density, fluorescence signal units). The quantity of the response signal measured is proportional to the amount of human IgE that is bound between the capture and detection antibodies (Hamilton and Adkinson, 2003). To ensure specificity while maximizing sensitivity and reproducibility, the two monoclonal antihuman IgE antibody clones used in the assay bind to different epitopes of the Fcϵ region of the human IgE molecule.

A nephelometric assay uses properties of a precipitin reaction in which the test serum is added to a fixed amount of antibody reagent causing antibody:antigen immune complexes. A nephelometer is an instrument designed to measure the extent of incident light scattered. Thus, the nephelometer can monitor and report the amount of light scattered by the increasing amount of immune complexes in the specific assay. Results obtained can be automated and are highly reproducible and rapidly obtained.

QUANTITATIVE SPECIFIC IGE ANTIBODY IMMUNOASSAYS

Since the detection of IgE over 30 years ago, the development of several immunoassays to detect allergen-specific antibodies has arisen. In the same year that IgE was identified, the first immunometric assay was developed and called the radioallergosorbent test (RAST), which detects human IgE antibodies of defined allergen specificity (Wide et al., 1967). Today, several immunoassays for specific IgE antibodies are commercially available to clinicians. The majority of the available tests include different varieties of the modified RAST (A-RAST, L-RAST and C-RAST), the Pharmacia ImmunoCAP system (I-CAP and S-CAP) and the Diagnostic Products AlaSTAT test (A-STAT) (Williams et al., 2000).

Historically, the first RAST assay was similar to the assay used to detect serum IgE (discussed above) except that the allergen was directly coupled to an allergosorbent. The allergosorbent was prepared by covalently coupling specific allergen onto cyanogen bromide-activated cellulose disks. Human test serum was then incubated with the allergosorbent in a test tube allowing allergen-specific antibodies of all isotypes to bind. After a buffer wash to remove unbound serum proteins, bound IgE was detected with a radioiodinated anti-human IgE Fc. After an additional buffer wash, the amount of radioactivity bound to the RAST allergosorbent was detected by a gamma counter which was proportional to the amount of allergen-specific IgE in the test serum. Figure 56.1 provides a schematic of the general principles involved. The first assay used birch allergosorbent and dilutions of a birch-specific human IgE antibody to create a calibration curve for which the assay response could be interpolated. The results were reported in arbitrary Phadebas RAST units per ml of IgE antibirch (Hamilton and Adkinson, 2003).

Modifications since 1967 of the original RAST have improved its overall use in regards to sensitivity, precision, reproducibility and performance. Common to the new preparations is the use of a larger number and higher quality allergen extracts in the making of allergosorbents. The allergosorbent has been altered over the years from the

original use of cyanogen bromide-activated carbohydrate particles to use of various media, including a cellulose sponge (Pharmacia CAP System). In contrast, the AlaSTAT assay utilizes a liquid-allergen method instead of a solid-phase allergen method (AlaSTAT). Additional modifications to the original RAST method include use of non-isotopic labels that has made the reagents last longer and are safer for the technician. The calibration system of these newer assays uses a total serum IgE curve to convert allergen-specific IgE assay response data into quantitative dose estimates of IgE antibody. Lastly, the automation system technology has enhanced the ease, precision and reproducibility of the newer generation of RAST testing, thus making it more diagnostically competitive with the skin prick/puncture test. However, due to the complexities and slight variations between the various commercial assays available, the allergen-specific IgE levels are not equivalent from one test to the next and levels obtained by different methods are not interchangeable (Williams et al., 2000).

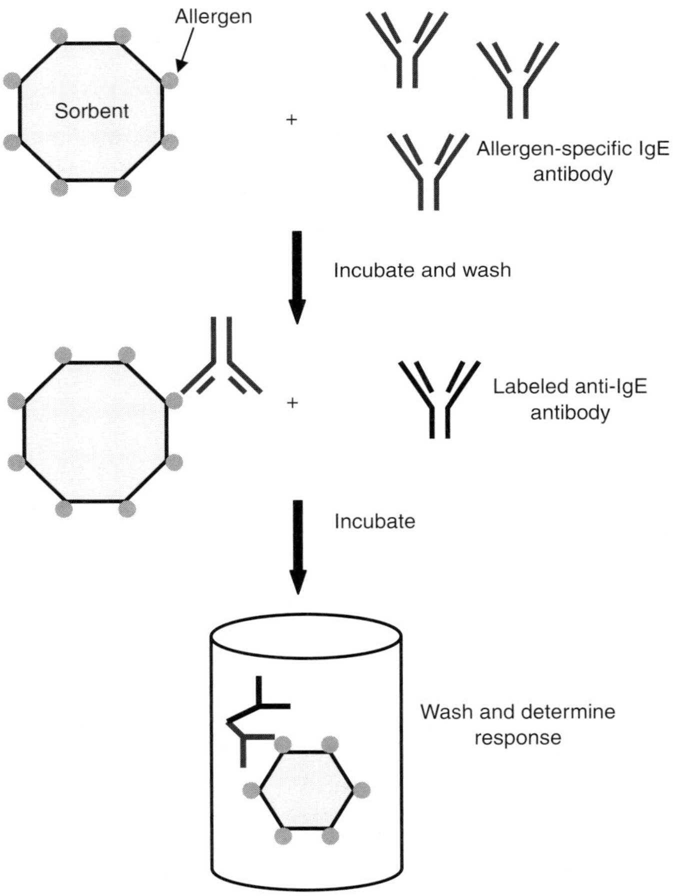

IMMUNOLOGICAL ASSAY ADVANCEMENTS IN DETERMINING CROSS-REACTIVITY VERSUS CO-SENSITIZATION

Advances in immunological techniques have allowed detection of sensitization to important cross-reactive allergens that has clinical applications. For example, the major birch pollen allergen, Bet v1, shares homology with specific food allergens such as apple, or Mal d1. Therefore, a subject who is sensitized to birch pollen may be at risk of developing a significant allergic reaction to certain foods which share similar homology. The early use of RAST inhibition with crude extracts allowed researchers to discover important cross-reactivity, but the RAST technique did not allow identification of the allergens involved. Further advancement in the 1980s with the development of immunoblotting with crude extracts enabled detection of multiple cross-reacting allergens. More recently, the availability and use of purified and/or recombinant allergen has enabled identification of the responsible cross-reactive allergens. Thus with use of high-resolution electrophoresis combined with immuno-blotting, detection of microheterogeneity within allergen groups can be determined (Pauli, 2000). This technology has important application for designing safer recombinant allergens that may ultimately be used to improve allergen immunotherapy.

Figure 56.1 Schematic of the radioallergosorbent test (RAST). Allergen-specific IgE antibodies are incubated with allergosorbent or solid phase allergen, washed and probed with labeled anti-IgE antibody. Response can be determined by counts per minute bound to allergosorbent or residual optical density.

COMPARISONS OF SKIN TESTING VERSUS ALLERGEN SPECIFIC-IGE IMMUNOASSAYS

In clinical practice, the skin prick/puncture test and *in vitro* tests for allergen-specific IgE are commonly used to provide useful adjuncts in diagnosing allergic diseases. The overall positive predictive value of both tests when used with a proper history and physical is adequate. Unfortunately, there is a lack of well-conducted, peer-reviewed publications that compare these assays to the gold standard, an allergen provocation test. However, Crobach and colleagues (Crobach et al., 1998) showed that the positive predictive value of the clinical history alone for the diagnosis of seasonal allergic rhinitis was approximately 85 per cent. This percentage increased when immunological testing was performed to 97 per cent with skin testing and 99 per cent with serum-specific IgE immunoassay measurements. The negative predictive value was assessed in a cat allergen study (Wood et al., 1999) that demonstrated a negative predictive value of 72 per cent with skin testing and 75 per cent with a serum *in vitro* assay in reference to a cat model exposure test. Interestingly, this same study showed that intradermal testing did not add significantly to the evaluation.

In contrast to aeroallergens and animal dander, the newer immunoassays with the ability to quantitate IgE antibodies in mass units (CAP System FEIA) have allowed for healthcare providers to predict which patients with food allergies are highly likely (>95 per cent) to experience clinical reactions (Sampson and Ho, 1997). Cutoff values for IgE antibody concentrations to certain foods (egg, milk, peanut and fish) have been derived to provide a 95 per cent positive and 90 per cent negative predictive value. These cutoff values allows decision points for performing oral food challenges reducing the need for oral challenges by about 50 per cent (Yunginger et al., 2000). At present, due to the labor-intensive regimen of performing double blind, placebo-controlled oral food challenges with comparison to specific IgE antibodies to select foods over a set time period and the cross-reactivity of proteins, determining cutoff values for additional foods has been difficult.

In evaluating other suspected allergens such as hymenoptera sensitivity and drug allergy, a diagnostic test warrants a high sensitivity due to the potential of anaphylactic reactions occurring in subjects. Therefore, it is recommended that intradermal skin testing is performed and *in vitro* IgE antibody serology results are viewed with equal value (Hamilton and Adkinson, 2003). In regards to latex allergen testing, a skin test using a Greer latex reagent has shown adequate sensitivity whereas the current latex-specific IgE antibody assays have not yet shown to be adequate (Hamilton and Adkinson, 2003). For food and respiratory allergy, both serum IgE antibody and skin prick/puncture testing are considered equivalently acceptable and intradermal testing is generally not needed.

BASOPHIL HISTAMINE RELEASE ASSAY

The basophil histamine release (BHR) assay is primarily used in research laboratories and not in the clinical setting. Histamine is a potent mediator of allergic reactions and it is stored in basophils and mast cells. The utility of the BHR assay is in defining the potency of allergen extracts and detecting the presence of allergen-specific IgE on the surface of basophils by direct challenge or passive sensitization. Results of a BHR assay highly correlate with results from skin prick/puncture testing and bronchoprovocation testing (Levy and Osler, 1966).

The BHR direct challenge assay requires obtaining peripheral blood leukocytes from whole blood. Cells are washed and incubated with varying concentrations of allergen extract or antihuman IgE as a positive control. In comparison, a passively sensitized BHR test involves stripping the basophils of their IgE by acid elution and then incubating with serum containing IgE antibody and then subsequently challenging with antigen. In both BHR assays, the assays are completed within 30 minutes and the histamine in the supernatant is subsequently measured by enzymatic, radiometric or spectrophotofluorometric techniques. The concentration of allergen required to induce 50 per cent histamine release is used to define the relative sensitivity of the patient's basophils for a given allergen extract (Hamilton and Adkinson, 2003). The limitations of this immunoassay are secondary to its expense and requirement of fresh whole blood, although anticoagulated whole blood can be used.

Although the BHR assay is used primarily for research, one clinical application is in diagnosing subjects with autoimmune chronic urticaria. In this assay, blood donors whose cells are known to be reactive with anti-IgE antibody are used to test various subjects' serum. In a population of patients with chronic idiopathic urticaria, 30–40 per cent are found to have release of histamine when the serum is incubated with basophils implying the presence of autoantibodies to the high affinity IgE receptor. Currently comparison of histamine release results in this assay to immunoblotting for specific antibody does not correlate (Kikuchi and Kaplan, 2001) and further research is needed.

Limitations in use of human mast cells and human basophils have prompted investigators to seek alternative models for analyzing functional IgE-allergen interactions. One such model is the use of rat basophilic leukemia cells (RBL SX-38) that express the alpha, beta and gamma chains of the human high affinity IgE receptor. Sera from allergic selected subjects who have adequate amounts of total IgE and allergen-specific IgE can effectively sensitize these cells to a specific allergen with high specificity and sensitivity. Although further studies are needed, this type of assay may be useful for detecting functional allergen:IgE interactions and also for standardization of allergens (Dibbern et al., 2003).

LYMPHOCYTE PROLIFERATION ASSAYS

Lymphocyte proliferation assays (LPA) are used to evaluate lymphocyte function *in vitro* by stimulation with a specific antigen/allergen or mitogens (polyclonal activators) such as phytohemagglutinin, pokeweed mitogen, anti-CD3 antibody or concanavalin A. This topic is discussed in detail in a prior chapter (see Chapter 31). The most common clinical application of this assay is to diagnose and monitor patients with primary and secondary immune deficiency disorders (see Chapter 55). In studying allergic diseases, the LPAs provide a correlate to skin testing particularly in assessing delayed-type (type IV) hypersensitivity to recall antigens or in assessing cellular immunity. Use of LPAs in studying allergic disorders is primarily confined to research investigations due to the high degree of individual and interindividual variability (Folds and Schmitz, 2003).

T LYMPHOCYTE FUNCTION IN ALLERGIC DISEASES AND ASTHMA

Although allergen-specific IgE has been traditionally considered the primary mediator of allergic diseases through its interaction with mast cells and basophils, the identification of the T lymphocyte as a major factor in the pathogenesis of allergic diseases and asthma has been well established (Kay, 1991). Research involving differentiating between the helper T lymphocyte type 1 (Th1) and type 2 (Th2) paradigm as it relates to allergic diseases continues to grow and expand. Cytokines predominately considered Th2 and therefore involved in allergic disease, include interleukin-4 (IL-4), IL-5, IL-9, IL-13, IL-25. In contrast, Th1 type cytokines include interferon-gamma (IFN-γ), tumor necrosis factor-β (TNF-β) and IL-18 (Romagnani, 1997). The effects of cytokines in mouse models of allergic asthma have been studied by direct administration of the cytokines, neutralization of them with monoclonal antibodies and gene knock-out and transgenic animals (Leong and Huston, 2001).

Activation of T lymphocytes, however, is dependent on its interaction with professional antigen-presenting cells (APC) such as dendritic cells, macrophages and B cells. APCs process and present the antigen/allergen for T cell recognition in the context of the major histocompatibility complex (MHC) class II molecule. However, in order for T cell activation to occur, a second signal or interaction with co-stimulatory molecules such as CD80 or CD86 (B7-1 or B7-2) and the T cell ligand, CD28, is required. Without this second signal, anergy will occur. The critical importance of MHC class II and co-stimulatory molecule interaction with T cells has been well demonstrated for the development of allergic asthma in mice (Leong and Huston, 2001).

Chemokines, important to allergic inflammation, are predominately the CC chemokine ligand family and include CCL2 (MCP-1), CCL3 (MIP-1α), CCL5 (RANTES), CCL7 (MCP-3), CCL11 (eotaxin-1) and CCL26 (eotaxin-3). At present, the role and importance of these chemokines in the development of allergic disease is not exactly known and further research is ongoing.

IMMUNOLOGICAL MARKERS AND MEDIATORS OF ALLERGY IMMUNOTHERAPY

One example of how the immune system may be modulated is in the study of allergen immunotherapy or allergy shots. Allergen immunotherapy (AIT) is the administration of increasing doses of allergen extract to alleviate symptoms associated with the causative allergen. It was first used by Noon and Freeman (Noon, 1911; Freeman, 1911) to treat hay fever in 1911 and today it is used in the treatment of allergic rhinitis, allergic asthma and stinging-insect hypersensitivity. Although the exact mechanisms of action of AIT are unknown, the various immunological assays discussed in previous chapters have been used to study and understand the immunological mechanisms that are involved. In particular, these assays include T cell production of cytokines, including use of ELISPOTS, intracellular cytokine staining with flow cytometric analysis, specific immunoglobulin production and in vitro lymphocyte responsiveness to allergen.

In previous years research focused on the role of antibody production by B cells demonstrating a long-term reduction in allergen-specific IgE and increases in allergen-specific IgG (IgG1 and IgG4). These initial studies focused on IgG "blocking" antibodies as primarily responsible for the reduction of allergen-specific effects (Lichtenstein et al., 1968; Peng, et al., 1992). However, it is now known that a Th2-driven CD4$^+$ T cell response is critical in the pathogenesis of allergic diseases and asthma. One current hypothesis is that AIT is associated with immune modulation acting by reduction in the function of allergen-specific Th2 cells either by anergy, clonal deletion or T regulatory cell suppression resulting in a predominant Th1 phenotype. Table 56.1 outlines the changes in immunologic mediators occurring with AIT. Using solid-phase enzyme immunoassays for cytokine detection and flow cytometric analysis of peripheral blood mononuclear cells for intracellular staining of cytokines, Lack and colleagues (Lack et al., 1997) demonstrated marked increase in IFN-γ in the serum and increased IFN-γ producing CD4$^+$ cells in subjects treated with rush dust mite allergen immunotherapy. In addition, they demonstrated decrease in allergen-specific lymphocyte proliferation. Further support of this hypothesis by others has shown decreases in IL-4 production in CD4$^+$ T cells in allergic subjects treated with AIT (Secrist et al., 1993) and possibly decreased IL-5 secretion (Jutel et al., 1995).

In addition, AIT may exert its immunoregulatory effects by inducing tolerance to allergen. Rocklin and colleagues (Rocklin et al., 1980) first demonstrated in 1980 that generation of antigen-specific suppressor cells occurred during AIT through use of a suppressor-cell assay. More recently, increased IL-10 production was found in activated allergen-specific CD4$^+$CD25$^+$ T cells (T regulatory cells) during bee venom immunotherapy. Interestingly, neutralization of IL-10 in this study caused restoration of in vitro proliferation and cytokine production (Akdis et al., 1998).

Table 56.1 Evidence for immune modulation with administration of allergen immunotherapy

Mediators of allergen immunotherapy	Immunoassays	References
Change in antibody production Blunting of usual seasonal rise in allergen specific IgE antibodies Increase in serum IgG antibodies, specifically IgG1 (early) and IgG4 (late)	Modification of RAST* Sandwich ELISA**	Lichtenstein et al. (1968) Peng et al. (1992) Akdis et al. (1998)
Downregulation of Th2-type cytokines Decrease in IL-4 production in CD4+ T cells Decrease in IL-5 secretion from PBMCs	Lymphocyte proliferation assay Cytokine quantification by ELISA	Secrist et al. (1993) Jutel et al. (1995)
Upregulation of Th1-type cytokines Increase in IFN-γ production in CD4+ T cells	Lymphocyte proliferation assay Solid-phase enzyme immunoassays Intracellular staining for cytokines using flow cytometry	Lack et al. (1997) Jutel et al. (1995)
T cell anergy Increase IL-10 production in allergen-specific CD4+CD25+ T cells Activation of allergen-specific suppressor cells	Lymphocyte proliferative assay Solid-phase sandwich ELISAs Intracellular staining for cytokines by flow cytometry. Suppressor-cell assay	Akdis et al. (1998) Rocklin et al. (1980)

*RAST: Radioallergosorbent test; **ELISA: Enzyme-linked immunosorbent assay.

FUTURE PROSPECTS

At the present time, researchers can measure cytokine and chemokine profiles in peripheral blood, nasal secretions and bronchial lavages of allergic individuals by the various means discussed in previous chapters including cytokine secretion assays (ELISPOTS) and intracellular cytokine assays. Furthermore, the ability to suppress allergic inflammation or induce peripheral tolerance is being actively investigated with emphasis on T regulatory cells (Th3, Tr1, CD4+/CD25+ cells), the suppressive cytokines such as IL-10 and transforming growth factor-beta (TGF-β) and suppressive enzymes such as indoleamine 2,3-dioxygenase (Levings et al., 2002; Bubnoff et al., 2003). Researching mechanisms that can affect the way antigen presenting cells process and present allergen to T lymphocytes appears to have a critical effect on determining immune stimulation or tolerance.

REFERENCES

Akdis, C.A., Blasken, T., Akdis, M. et al. (1998). Role of interleukin 10 in specific immunotherapy. J Clin Invest 102, 98–106.

Blackley, C. (1880). Hay fever: its causes, treatment and effective prevention; experimental researches, 2nd edn. London: Bailliere, Tindal & Cox.

Bubnoff, D.V., Hanau, D. and Wenzel, J. (2003). Indoleamine 2, 3-dioxygenase-expressing antigen-presenting cells and peripheral T cell tolerance: another piece to the atopic puzzle? J Allergy Clin Immunol 112, 854–860.

Campbell, D., DeKruyff, R.H. and Umetsu, D.T. (2000). Allergen immunotherapy: novel approaches in the management of allergic diseases and asthma. Clin Immunol 97,193–202.

Crobach, M.J., Hermans, J., Kaptein, A.A. et al. (1998). The diagnosis of allergic rhinitis: how to combine the medical history with the results of radioallergosorbent tests and skin prick tests. Scan J Prim Health Care 16, 30–36.

Dibbern, D.A., Palmer G.W., Williams, B. et al. (2003). RBL cells expressing human FcεRI are a sensitive tool for exploring functional IgE-allergen interactions: studies with sera from peanut-sensitive patients. J Immunol Methods 274, 37–45.

Folds, J.D. and Schmitz, J.L. (2003). Clinical and laboratory assessment of immunity. J Allergy Clin Immunol 111, S702–711.

Freeman, J. (1911). Further observations of the treatment of hay fever by hypodermic inoculations of pollen vaccine. Lancet 2, 814–867.

Hamilton, R.G. and Adkinson, N.F. (2003). Clinical laboratory assessment of IgE-dependent hypersensitivity. J Allergy Clin Immunol 111, S687–701.

Ishizaka, K. and Ishizaka, T. (1967). Physiochemical properties of reaginic antibody. 1. Association of reaginic activity with an immunoglobulin other than gammaA- or gammaG-globulin. J Allergy 37, 169–185.

Johansson, S.G. (1967). Raised levels of a new immunoglobulin class in asthma. Lancet 2, 951–953.

Jutel, M. Pilcher, W.J., Skrbic, D. et al. (1995). Bee venom immunotherapy results in decrease of IL-4 and IL-5 and increase of IFN-γ secretion in specific allergen stimulated T cell cultures. J Immunol 95, 4188–4194.

Kay, A.B. (1991). Asthma and inflammation. J Allergy Clin Immunol 87, 893–910.

Kikuchi, Y. and Kaplan, A.P. (2001). Mechanisms of autoimmune activation of basophils in chronic urticaria. J Allergy Clin Immunol 107, 1056–1062.

Leong, K.P. and Huston D.P. (2001). Understanding the pathogenesis of allergic asthma using mouse models. Ann Allergy Asthma Immunol 87, 96–110.

Levings, M.K., Bacchetta, R., Schulz, U. et al. (2002). The role of IL-10 and TGF-beta in the differentiation and effector function of T regulatory cells. Int Arch Allergy Immunol 129, 263–276.

Levy, D.A. and Osler, A.G. (1966). Studies on the mechanisms of hypersensitivity phenomena. XIV. Passive sensitization in vitro of human leukocytes to ragweed pollen antigen. J Immunol 97, 203–212.

Lichtenstein, L.M., Holtzman, N.A. and Burnett, L.S. (1968). A quantitative in vitro study of the chromatographic distribution and immunoglobulin characteristics of human blocking antibody. J Immunol 101, 317–324.

Noon, L. (1911). Prophylactic inoculation against hay fever. Lancet 1, 1572–1573.

Pauli, G. (2000). Evolution in the understanding of cross-reactivities of respiratory allergens: the role of recombinant allergens. Int Arch Allergy Immunol 123, 183–195.

Peng, Z., Naclerio, R.M., Norman, P.S. et al. (1992). Quantitative IgE and IgG subclass responses during and after long-term ragweed immunotherapy. J Allergy Clin Immunol 9, 519–529.

Rocklin, R.E., Sheffer, A.L., Greineder, D.K. et al. (1980). Generation of antigen-specific suppressor cells during allergy desensitization. New Engl J Med 302, 1213–1219.

Romagnani, S. (1997). The Th1/Th2 paradigm. Immunol Today 18, 263–266.

Sampson, H.A. and Ho, D.G. (1997). Relationship between food-specific IgE concentrations and risk of positive food challenges in children and adolescents. J Allergy Clin Immunol 100, 444–451.

Secrist, H., Chelen, C.J., Wen, Y. et al. (1993). Allergen immunotherapy decreases interleukin 4 production in CD4+ T cells from allergic individuals. J Exp Med 178, 2123–2130.

Wide, L., Bennich, H. and Johansson, S.G. (1967). Diagnosis of allergy by an in vitro test for allergen antibodies. Lancet 2, 105–1107.

Williams, P.B., Barnes, J.H., Szeinbach, S.L. et al. (2000). Analytic precision and accuracy of commercial immunoassays for specific IgE: Establishing a standard. J Allergy Clin Immunol 105, 1221–1230.

Wood, R.A., Phipatanakul, W., Hamilton R.G. et al. (1999). A comparison of skin prick tests, intradermal skin tests, and RASTs in the diagnosis of cat allergy. J Allergy Clin Immunol 103, 773–779.

Yunginger, J.W., Ahlstedt, S., Eggleston, P.A. et al. (2000). Quantitative IgE antibody assays in allergic diseases. J Allergy Clin Immunol 105, 1077–1084.

Section VII

New technologies

Serum Proteomic Profiling and Analysis

Chapter 57

Richard Pelikan[1], Michael T. Lotze[2], James Lyons-Weiler[3], David Malehorn[3] and Milos Hauskrecht[1]

[1]Department of Computer Science, University of Pittsburgh;
[2]Translational Research Molecular Medicine Institute,
University of Pittsburgh School of Medicine, Pittsburgh, PA, USA
[3]University of Pittsburgh Cancer Institute, Pittsburgh, PA, USA

They killed him in Sarajevo, Mr Švejk. They shot him with a revolver as he was riding with that archduchess of his in an automobile.

Jaroslav Hašek Fateful Adventures of the Good Soldier Švejk During the World War

Osudy dobrého vojáka Švejka za světové války

INTRODUCTION

The ability to examine serum peptides and proteins using mass spectrometry (MS) has recently become broadly of interest as a novel biomarker and surrogate of disease discovery tool. Just as Švejk's world was transformed by the introduction of modern technology, now, almost a century later, the introduction of modern mass spectrometry strategies, assessing data-dense putative markers associated with inflammatory or immune endpoints, have indeed changed the world of biological investigation. They have become more widely applied, particularly in the setting of cancer diagnostics. Surface-enhanced laser desorption/ionization time-of-flight mass spectrometry (SELDI-TOF-1 MS) proteomic profiling is one of these increasingly popular tools, using 'shooting' of protein mixtures with focused lasers, in the search for known and surrogate biomarkers for disease diagnosis and prognosis. Current diagnostic tests, such as repetitive biopsies done before or after therapy, impose greater costs and risk of injury as opposed to gathering the patient's proteomic profile. The greatest potential promise of proteomic profiling lies in the possibility of the early detection of a malignant or chronic inflammatory condition with simple tests of the serum or urine. In addition, the hope is that different disease types and response to therapy phenotypes might be reproducibly distinguishable using rapid and relatively inexpensive assays.

SELDI-TOF-MS rapidly provides a protein expression profile from a variety of biological and clinical samples. The potential efficacy of this system for serum protein profiling of cancer in human breast (Paweletz et al., 2001), colon (Watkins et al., 2001), head and neck (Wadsworth et al., 2004), lung (Zhukov et al., 2003), ovarian (Petricoin et al., 2002), prostate cancer (Adam et al., 2002; Petricoin and Ornstein, 2002) and hepatoma (Steel et al., 2003; Zeindl-Eberhart et al., 2004) has been recently demonstrated. These studies describe diagnostic features of these profiles and classification algorithms based on these features, which provide at least 80 per cent and, in some cases, >90 per cent classification accuracy between cancer cases and controls. Papers reporting high sensitivity and specificity in class prediction presented promising initial positive results. Efforts to relate the proteomic profiling to changes in known protein factors, including cytokines and chemokines, as well as cellular elements and their signaling capacity, are now being explored, but it is premature to include them in this chapter.

The goal of this chapter is to overview the proteome profiling technology and its potential benefits for identification and clinical assessment of progression of

*Measuring Immunity, edited by Michael T. Lotze and Angus W. Thomson
ISBN 0-12-455900-X, London*

pathological conditions. The initial discussion of the SELDI-TOF technology is followed by a discussion of technical limitations that affect the interpretive analysis of the profiles. Next we focus on the description of some statistical methods used to decipher the profiles and their usage in diagnosing or predicting the condition of patients. We illustrate the potential of these methods on the task of differentiating between individuals with and without cancer. Finally, the review concludes with some insight on the direction of using proteomic data analysis towards the benefit of the medical community.

SELDI-TOF MASS SPECTROMETRY

The ProteinChip© Biology System developed by Ciphergen Biosystems, Inc. uses SELDI-TOF MS to ionize proteins specifically retained on a chromatographic surface, which are then detected by time-of-flight mass spectrometry. The system can be used for the mass analysis of compounds such as proteins, peptides and nucleic acids within a range of 0–200 kD. The procedure begins with the reaction of a biological sample (e.g. bodily fluid, cell lysate or fraction thereof) with the chromatographic surface (or 'spot') of a ProteinChip, which possesses a defined affinity characteristic: anionic/cationic, hydrophobic, metal-binding, or biologically derivatized (e.g. antibody coupled). The ProteinChips, comprised of 8 or 16 of these spots, retain only those analytes that match the surface's physical affinity characteristics – non-binding species are washed away using appropriate conditions. The spots are then overlaid with an energy-absorbing 'matrix' compound, which co-crystallizes around the retained analyte molecules. The spots are 'shot' multiple times by a pulsed nitrogen laser. The laser desorption

process results in ionization of matrix molecules and protonation of intact analyte molecules. The ions produced are differentially accelerated in an electrical field and then detected after passing through a field-free, evacuated 'drift' tube. The time of flight across the tube is converted to provide information on the molecule's mass-to-charge ratio (m/z), since heavier molecules, by Newtonian physics, will take longer to travel the same distance, having acquired less initial velocity from the uniform acceleration force. The detected ions are then represented as a "spectrum" with peaks of varying intensities and molecular weight assignments are made relative to known calibrant species. Figure 57.1 displays a summary of the SELDI-TOF MS process.

Early studies and first applications (Paweletz et al., 2001; Petricoin and Ornstein, 2002; Petricoin et al., 2002) assembled SELDI-TOF MS proteomic profiles of patients with various types of cancer. The primary goal of such studies was to determine whether it is possible to detect peptide markers of the presence of disease by analyzing the profiles, contrasting those with cancer and those without. For, example, Petricoin and coworkers' April 2002 study (Petricoin et al., 2002) compared profiles of 200 patients in order to determine a discriminating pattern between patients with ovarian cancer and those with a variety of non-cancer conditions. A sample profile from this set is shown in Figure 57.2. It consists of intensities measured over 15 154 mass/charge (m/z) values.

LIMITATIONS OF THE SELDI-TOF PROFILES

The profiles obtained by the SELDI-TOF MS system manifest a number of attributes which can complicate analysis. Figure 57.3 compares two unprocessed profiles from the

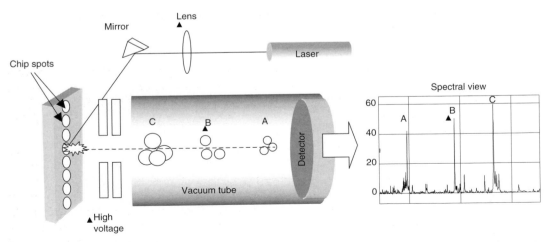

Figure 57.1 Diagram of the Ciphergen SELDI-TOF MS system. Samples are reacted with ProteinChip spots, coated with "matrix" and pulsed with a laser. The ionized species created during this process are differentially accelerated in an electric field, float through the vacuum tube, where their arrival times and quantities (intensity) are measured by a detector. Heavier ions demonstrate longer time-of-flight, which is a unique indicator for each molecular species. The plot of ion intensity versus specific time of flight (or corresponding mass to charge value) constitutes the mass spectrum for a given sample.

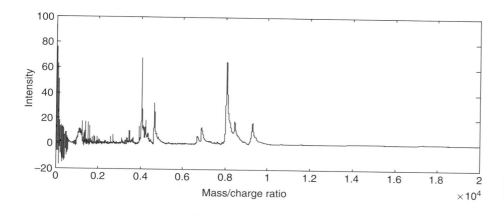

Figure 57.2 A sample SELDI-TOF MS profile. The x-axis plots mass-to-charge ratio. The y-axis plots the relative intensity (flux) of analyte species with the identified mass-to-charge ratio.

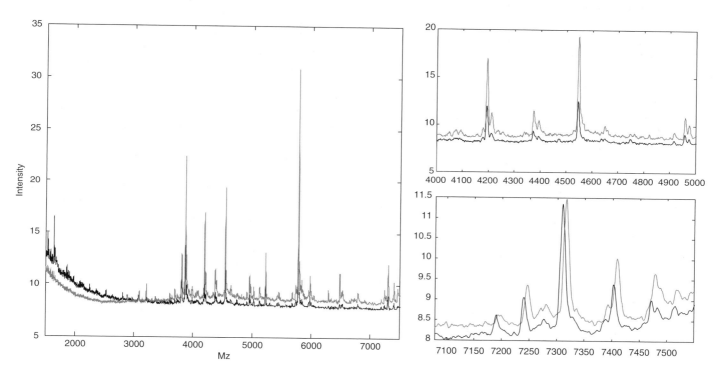

Figure 57.3 Two SELDI-TOF profiles obtained for the same pooled reference serum. The differences in the baseline (left panel), intensity measurements (right top panel) and mass inaccuracies (right bottom panel) are apparent.

same reference serum. Differences are readily visible and illustrate stochastic variations that obscure what would ideally be identical profiles. Many causes may be responsible for the differences: variation in the SELDI-TOF MS instrumentation condition over time, fluctuation in the intensity of the laser and even surface irregularities on the protein chip spots or the matrix crystallization.

All stochastic variations in profiles show up as differences in intensity readings. However, these differences are the result of two intertwined problems: *mass inaccuracy* and *intensity measurement errors*. Mass inaccuracy refers to the misalignment of readings for different *m/z* values. The mass inaccuracy for Ciphergen's SELDI-TOF MS system is reported to be approximately 0.1 per cent for externally calibrated experiments. The intensity measurement error may arise from imperfect performance of

the ion detector in registering the abundance of ions at a given time point (detector saturation). Both types of errors are illustrated in the right panel of Figure 57.3. In addition, the left panel of Figure 57.3 illustrates baseline variation, a systematic intensity measurement error for which the measurements of the profile differ from 0. Note that the baseline shifts between two samples differ despite the fact that the same serum is being analyzed.

The *mass inaccuracy* and *intensity measurement* errors can lead to significant fluctuation in profile readings. In addition, if we analyze samples from multiple individuals a natural biological variation in sera is observed. This can show up as differences in intensity values or as the presence or absence of peaks in the profile. The peaks are believed to indicate the presence of peptides or their fragments. These problems lead to serious challenges in interpretive analysis. Many of the observed variations could be caused by changes in carrier proteins, protein catabolism or the inherent cyclical shifts in relative abundance due to production and release from various tissues. We have considered some of these issues, particularly during nominally chaotic states as represented in patients with various neoplasms reflecting on the notion that an individual analyte may be increased or decreased at any time interval when compared to normal sera, something we have termed the ABA problem (Patel and Lyons-Weiler, 2004).

DATA PREPROCESSING

Despite the problems presented above, there are possible steps one can take before analyzing the data. The cleansing and modifying, or *preprocessing*, of the data are intended to eliminate noise or redundant components in the signal other than true biological variation in the serum. The preprocessing steps include *smoothing, profile alignment, rescaling (normalization)* and *baseline correction*. However, any preprocessing step comes at a risk of loss of useful biological information or introduction of additional errors. Therefore, if any preprocessing is performed, conclusions drawn from an ensuing analysis should be carefully validated.

Smoothing serves to eliminate a high frequency noise component in the signal. Figure 57.4 illustrates the effect of smoothing on a SELDI-TOF profile. High frequency variation is eliminated by local averaging of the signal. Whether smoothing removes useful signal or useless noise is not yet clear.

The mass inaccuracy problem (see Figure 57.3, lower right panel) can be resolved through *profile alignment* methods. A number of strategies for performing profile alignment exist. One option is to define a reference profile in terms of a set of established biomarkers that are easily identifiable in every profile. Another approach is to include indicator peptides in the serum, in order purposely to populate the profile with peaks to be expected at certain *m/z* values. The intensity readings between these peaks could then be stretched or shrunk along the x-axis appropriately. Unfortunately, due to the locality of *m/z* errors, this approach requires the addition of several thousand peptides to the serum in order to recapture properly the information lost through mass inaccuracy. Using alignment algorithms directly on the profiles runs the risk of eliminating important biological variability in the data. Clearly, this challenge is deserving of additional attention; solving the alignment problem entails the possibility of eliminating sample-to-sample variation, which appears to be autocorrelated in terms of temporal (run-to-run) and spatial (spot-to-spot) processing.

A particular profile may suffer from an overall weakness in signal. Variation in the sensitivity of the ion detector or amount of retained molecules on the chip surface may result in profiles which seem to be measured on a different scale (see Figure 57.3, upper right panel). *Rescaling (normalizing)* these profiles allows them to be compared on the same scale. This type of adjustment differs from baseline shifting, which is an additive error, as opposed to scaling, which is a multiplicative error.

Correcting for *baseline shifts* (see Figure 57.3, left panel) involves subtracting a constant intensity value from the profile. The problem is that the baseline shift may vary over the *m/z* range. Figure 57.5 illustrates the process of baseline correction on the reference profile. The method removed the additive component in the signal and brought the baseline to 0. A challenge presented by baseline correction is that the noise from the intensity measurement process appears to be correlated strongly with the magnitude of the measurement. This suggests that any signal rescaling must be performed before the baseline correction.

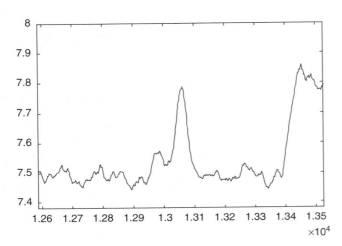 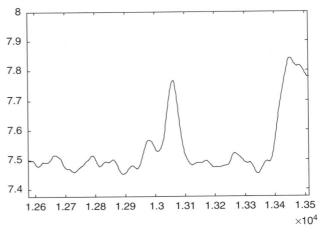

Figure 57.4 An example of smoothing. The original profile (left panel) demonstrates a high-frequency component. By averaging the signal locally, the high-frequency component is removed. Note that this results in a loss of information if this component carries useful content.

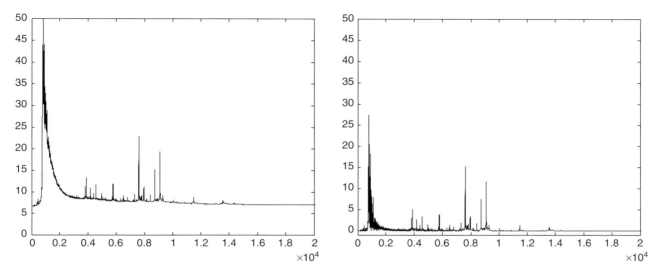

Figure 57.5 An example of baseline correction. Left panel: a profile with a baseline drift. Right panel: the corrected profile. The additive component in the signal is removed and the baseline is shifted to the zero intensity level.

BUILDING A PREDICTIVE MODEL

One of the objectives of SELDI-TOF MS data analysis is to build a predictive model that is able to determine the target condition (case or control, cancer or non-cancer) for a given patient's profile. The predictive model is built from a set of SELDI-TOF profiles (samples) assembled during the study. Each sample in the dataset is associated with a class label determining the target patient condition (case or control, cancer or non-cancer) we would like automatically to recognize. Our objective is to exploit the information in the data and to construct (or learn) a classifier model that is able to predict accurately the label of any new profile. Such a model can be then used to predict labels of new profile samples (diagnosis). The ultimate goal is to build (learn) the best possible classifier, i.e. a model that achieves the highest possible accuracy on future, yet to be seen, proteomic profile samples.

Many types of classification models exist. These include classic statistical models such as logistic regression (Kleinbaum, 1994), linear and quadratic discriminant analysis (Duda et al., 2000; Hastie et al., 2001), or modern statistical approaches such as *support vector machines* (Vapnik, 1995; Burges, 1998; Scholkopf and Smola, 2002). In general, the model defines a decision boundary – a surface in the high dimensional space of profile measurements – that attempts to separate case and control profiles in the best possible way. The left panel of Figure 57.6 illustrates a linear surface (a hyperplane) that lets us separate 193 of the 200 samples from the ovarian study using the intensity information in three profile positions (0.0735, 0.0786, 0.4153 m/z). However, note that in general, the perfect separation of two profiles via a linear surface using just three positions may not be possible. This is illustrated in the right panel of Figure 57.6 where

the linear surface allowing the perfect separation of case and control profiles does not exist. This scenario leads to sample misclassification – the assignment of incorrect profile labels to some samples relative to the decision boundary.

EVALUATION OF A MODEL

To evaluate the quality of a classification model, one must determine the ability of the model to generate accurate predictions of future unseen profile data. Obviously, since such data are unavailable, we can simulate this scenario by splitting the available data (obtained during the study) into a "training" set and a "testing" set. The training set is used to learn/construct the classifier[s]. The learning process adjusts the predictive model (classifier) so that the examples in the training set are classified with a high accuracy. The ability of the model to predict the case and control samples in the future is evaluated on the test set. Figure 57.7 illustrates the basic evaluation setup.

The quality of a binary (case versus control) classification model may be determined among many different metrics. For the purposes of this review, the classification models are evaluated using statistics computed from the confusion matrix, a two-by-two grid that represents the types and percentages of correct and incorrect classifications. A sample confusion matrix is shown in Figure 57.8. The following useful measures can be derived from the confusion matrix:

- Error (misclassification) rate: $E = FP + FN$
- Sensitivity (SN): $\dfrac{TP}{TP + FN}$

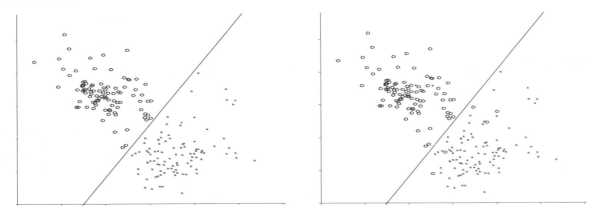

Figure 57.6 (Left panel) An example of a perfect separation of case (X) versus control (O) using a hyperplane in a 2-dimensional projection of the 3-dimensional space defined by *m/z* positions (0.0735, 0.0786, 0.4153) in the ovarian cancer study. Note that all controls samples are above the hyperplane while all cases are below. (Right panel) The perfect separation of the two groups does not exist. Some case and control samples appear on the opposite side of the hyperplane.

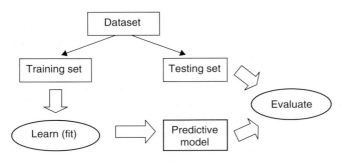

Figure 57.7 The basic evaluation setup. The dataset of samples (case and control profiles) is divided into the training and testing set. The training set is used to learn (fit) the predictive model and testing set serves as a surrogate sample of the future "unseen" examples.

	Actual	
	Case	**Control**
Prediction / Case	TP 0.3	FP 0.1
Prediction / Control	FN 0.2	TN 0.4

Figure 57.8 Diagram of a confusion matrix. The four areas are labeled as follows:

- True positive (TP): the percentage of profiles which the classifier predicts correctly as belonging to the group of cases (cancerous)
- False positive (FP): the percentage of profiles which the classifier predicts as belonging to cases, but truly belong to controls (healthy)
- False negative (FN): the percentage of profiles which the classifier predicts as belonging to controls, but truly belong to cases
- True negatives (TN): the percentage of profiles which the classifier predicts correctly as belonging to the group of controls.

Note that the numbers should always sum to 1. An ideal classifier will have a value of 0 for both false negatives and false positives.

- Specificity (SP): $\dfrac{TN}{TN + FP}$
- Positive predictive value (PPV): $\dfrac{TP}{TP + FN}$
- Negative predictive value (NPV): $\dfrac{TN}{TN + FN}$

A confusion matrix and thus also the above measures can be generated for both the training and testing set. However, the evaluation of the testing set matters more; it is an indicator of how well the classification model generalizes to unseen data. Sensitivity and specificity measures on the testing set are very useful if we consider adopting the classification model for the purpose of clinical screening. Sensitivity reports the percentage of samples with a condition that were correctly classified as having the condition. Specificity, on the other hand, reports the percentage of samples without a condition that were correctly classified as not having the condition. Very high values of these statistics indicate a good screening test. Moreover, one type of error can be often reduced at the expense of the other error. This is very important if we care more about one type of error. For example, we may want to achieve a low number of patients incorrectly classified as suffering from the disease and care a bit less about missing a patient with the disease during screening.

In the simplest evaluation framework, statistics recorded in the confusion matrix are based on a single train/test set split. To eliminate a potential bias due to a lucky or an unlucky train/test split, the average of these statistics over multiple random splits is typically reported.

STRATEGIES FOR LEARNING A CLASSIFICATION MODEL

Classification models come in different guises. They may use a different decision boundary type or optimize slightly different learning criteria. Deeper analyses of many existing

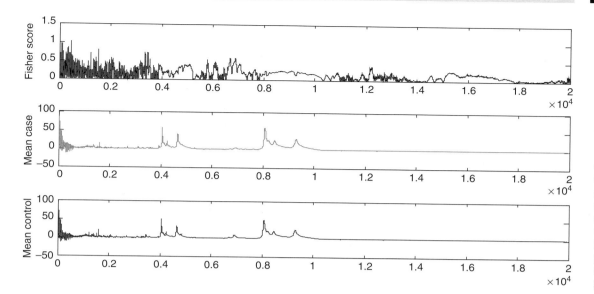

Figure 57.9 Differentially expressed features (profile positions). (Top panel) Fisher score values for each *m/z* position along the profile. (Middle panel) Mean of case profiles. (Lower panel) Mean of control profiles. Higher values of Fisher score indicate areas of the profile which are statistically likely to be good features.

models and their properties are beyond the scope of this work. To illustrate the main steps of the analysis we will focus on one such a model: the linear *support vector machine*. Briefly, the linear support vector machine models a linear decision boundary (a hyperplane) between different classes having the maximum ability to separate the groups of classes as illustrated in Figure 57.6.

Learning and predicting using a classification model is often hampered by the fact that the data are presented with a small number of samples, but have a naturally high dimensionality. In this case, there are only 200 profiles to study, yet the input vector of each profile contains 15 154 *m/z* values, or "features". When the number of features vastly outweighs the number of samples, the parameters of the classifier model are estimated with high variance. This makes it difficult to achieve a model that generalizes well to new examples. To alleviate this problem, we demonstrate the use of several types of *feature selection* approaches to convert the high-dimensional profile data into a low-dimensional dataset consisting of only a small number of *m/z* intensities. A hyperplane dependent on a smaller number of features is a more simplistic boundary and will generalize better to future unseen examples.

The primary goal of feature selection is to obtain a smaller set of features with high discriminative ability from a large set of inputs. To assess an ability of a profile position to discriminate between the case and the control a univariate statistical analysis can be performed. Several methods exist for evaluating the dispersion between cases and controls, including

t-test, Fisher score or AUC score (Fisher, 1936; Hanley and McNeil, 1982; Hastie et al., 2001), etc. Figure 57.9 displays Fisher scores[1] for each position in the profile (top panel). Below, the mean case profile (middle panel) and mean control profile (bottom panel) are shown. Higher values of the Fisher score indicate that the *m/z* position is likely represented differently in all case profiles versus all control profiles. These features can be more commonly referred to as *differentially expressed features*. Features with the highest Fisher score are very likely good feature candidates. These features may be memorized and used as *biomarkers* in screening additional profiles. Thus, selecting features is a short matter of computing the Fisher score of each feature (each *m/z* value) and then eliminating all but the top *k* features, where *k* is the desired quantity of "left-over" features.

A univariate analysis of features ignores possible dependencies between the features. For example, the value of a feature may be highly correlated with values of other features. Because of this, many of the features may be redundant and their inclusion offers very little additional information towards building a predictive model. Figure 57.10 illustrates some of these problems. It shows 30 out of the top 100 positions that would be selected through Fisher score. We see that these 30 features accumulate within two areas related to two peak complexes. These groups of features are highly correlated and the amount of new discriminative information the duplicates add is relatively small. One way to alleviate this problem is by enforcing the maximum-allowed correlation (MAC) threshold on the features selected via univariate analysis (Hauskrecht et al., unpublished observations). This helps to ensure that the feature selection method increases its coverage of the signal and does not miss important information that might otherwise be ignored.

Focusing on individual positions in the profile may narrow the field of view. This is especially concerning if the discriminative signal is weak and noisy. One way to alleviate this problem is to look at aggregate features, or

[1] A particular feature's Fisher score is computed by the following formula $F(i) = \dfrac{(\mu_i^+ - \mu_i^-)^2}{(\sigma_i^+)^2 + (\sigma_i^-)^2}$ where $\mu_i^\pm$ is the mean value for the *i*th feature in the positive or negative profiles, and $\sigma_i^\pm$ is the standard deviation. We utilize a variant of this criterion, the "Fisher the score" (Furey et al., 2000), computed in the following formula: $F(i) = \left| \dfrac{(\mu_i^+ - \mu_i^-)}{(\sigma_i^+ + \sigma_i^-)} \right|$. To avoid confusion, we refer to the second formula above as our "Fisher Score"

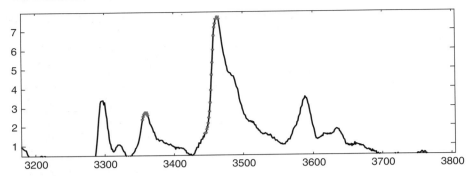

Figure 57.10 Thirty out of the top 100 positions selected by the Fisher score on the mean cancer profile. The positions (defined by the markers) accumulate on only two peak complexes and many features are highly correlated, thus carrying minimum additional discriminative information.

features that combine the information from many profile positions. The intuition is that the useful signal can be amplified over many related positions and thus it is less sensitive to random fluctuations/noise. An example of such a transformation is the principal component analysis (PCA) (Jolliffe, 1986). Intuitively, the PCA identifies orthogonal sets of correlated features and constructs aggregate features (or components) which are uncorrelated, yet are responsible for most of the variance in the original data. Retaining the variance is important; it is often helpful to explore parts of the data where the features spread out across a large space, which gives more room to find a decision boundary between classes. These methods often construct useful features due to their inherent ability to utilize the entire signal, rather than a limited number of positions.

Another popular solution that attempts to alleviate the problem of a noisy signal assumes that all relevant information is carried by peaks (Adam et al., 2002). The subsequent discriminative analysis is restricted to identified peaks only and/or their additional characteristics. Numerous versions of peak selection strategies exist (Adam et al., 2002). However, the utility and advantage of these strategies over other feature selection methods for the purpose of discriminant analysis has not been demonstrated.

RESULTS OF INTERPRETIVE ANALYSIS

The goal of this section is to illustrate the potential of the SELDI-TOF profiling technology on the analysis of the ovarian cancer data from April 2002 (Petricoin et al., 2002). The dataset[2] consists of 200 profile samples: 100 samples exhibit cancer, 100 samples are controls. We rely on concepts and approaches discussed in previous sections and show that it is indeed possible to build predictive models that can classify with high accuracy test samples taken from the SELDI-TOF dataset.

The predictive model used in all of our experiments is the support vector machine (see above). The model builds a linear decision boundary that separates cancer and control samples provided in the training set. In all experiments the model is learned using a limited number of features (5–25). We try different feature selection approaches. The process of finding a good set of features is a highly exploratory process and often remains the bottleneck of the discovery.

[2] The ovarian cancer dataset is available at http://ncifdaproteomics.com/

Table 57.1 Predictive statistics for the linear SVM model on the ovarian cancer dataset. The features are selected according to the Fisher score criterion. The maximum allowed correlation (MAC) threshold is 0.8. Test errors range in between 4 and 2.9 per cent. Sensitivities and specificities are between 94.9 and 97.6 per cent

No. of features	Testing error	Sensitivity	Specificity
5	0.0352	0.9764	0.953
10	0.0402	0.9698	0.9497
15	0.0406	0.9584	0.9604
20	0.0332	0.9641	0.9695
25	0.0299	0.9666	0.9736

Table 57.1 illustrates the quality of the predictive model learned using the top 5–25 m/z positions according to the Fisher score criteria. To remove highly correlated features we used the maximum allowed correlation (MAC) threshold of 0.8. The table shows the test errors (E), sensitivities (SN) and specificities (SP) for a different number of features. All statistics listed are averages over 40 different splits of the data into training and testing sets. This assures that the results are not biased due to a single lucky and unlucky train/test split. The split proportions are 70:30, i.e. 70 per cent of samples are assigned to the training set and 30 per cent to the test set.

Using the univariate statistical analysis approach as discussed above, the results are quite impressive. The best result occurs when the classifier is allowed to use the top 25 features selected by Fisher score. Under this condition, the classification model achieves 96.6 per cent sensitivity and 97.36 per cent specificity. On average, 2.99 per cent of the samples seen during the testing phase were misclassified. A different number of features used can show a tradeoff in the improvement of sensitivity or specificity. Note that sensitivity is highest when using only five features, yet specificity is highest when using 25.

Instead of narrowly examining a small number of individual positions, we can examine the effectiveness of aggregate features. Table 57.2 illustrates the performance statistics of our classification model using features constructed using PCA. The results are included over a range of 5 to 25 principal component features, which amplify patterns found in the profile signal. Again, the resulting statistics are averages over the same

Table 57.2 Predictive statistics for the linear SVM model on the ovarian cancer dataset. The features are constructed using principal component analysis (PCA). Test errors range between 19.9 and 8.9 per cent. Sensitivities and specificities range between 85.3 and 91.1 per cent

No. of features	Testing error	Sensitivity	Specificity
5	0.1992	0.8533	0.7477
10	0.1111	0.9161	0.8615
15	0.1078	0.8998	0.8846
20	0.0926	0.9038	0.911
25	0.0898	0.9087	0.9118

Table 57.3 Performance statistics of the linear SVM classifier after using peak detection. A MAC threshold of 0.8 was enforced before selecting the top 5–25 features using the Fisher score. Testing error ranges from 11.6 to 9.8 per cent, while sensitivity and specificity range from 85 to 93.4 per cent

No. of features	Testing error	Sensitivity	Specificity
5	0.1168	0.9152	0.8508
10	0.1049	0.9169	0.873
15	0.1033	0.9209	0.8722
20	0.0984	0.934	0.8689
25	0.1012	0.934	0.8631

40 train/test splits as used in the univariate analysis, to allow for a more direct comparison of behavior.

The predictive performance of our classifier falls when used in conjunction with principal component features. The reason may be due to too many independencies between positions in the profile. Such a condition causes a problem for PCA, which attempts to find signal-wide relationships between multiple positions. If the signal-wide relationships that do exist are weak, then the benefits from using these features will be minimal. In addition, including many of these features to compensate for their weakness complicates the process of discovering biomarkers.

As a final example of feature selection, we illustrate the behavior of the aforementioned *peak selection* strategy. We refer to a peak as the local maximum over a region in the profile. The signal is smoothed before detecting the maxima on the mean case and control profiles. Peak positions from both mean profiles are then used as the primary set of features. Table 57.3 displays performance statistics of the above model using peak selection prior to selecting the top Fisher score features. Unfortunately, the performance was below what was achieved without the peak selection strategy (see Table 57.1).

Testing error is relatively high considering the results presented earlier in Table 57.1. The likely reason is that informative features are not only found on peaks, but in valleys as well. Another reason is that the particular behavior of the peak detection algorithm is not optimal. As mentioned before, there exist many methods for performing peak selection. Different criteria for selecting peaks will undoubtedly yield differing results.

The results presented above show that it is possible to learn predictive models that can achieve a very low classification error on SELDI-TOF samples. To support the significance of these results, in particular, the fact that the sample profiles carry useful discriminative signals, one may want to perform additional statistical validation. The goal of one such a test, the random class-permutation test, is to verify that the discriminative signal captured by the classifier model is unlikely to be the result of the random case versus control labeling. Figure 57.11 shows the result of the random permutation test for classifiers analyzed in Table 57.1. The figure plots the estimate of the mean test error one would obtain by learning the classifier

on 5–25 features for randomly assigned class labels and estimates of 95 per cent and 99 per cent test error bounds. The estimates are obtained using 100 random class-label permutations of the original ovarian dataset. The results illustrate a large gap between classification errors achieved on the data and classification errors under the null (random class-label) hypothesis. This shows that our achieved error results are not a coincidence.

DISCUSSION

This review deals solely with clinical proteomics, but the analysis techniques reported are typically those that could be used in applications to other domains, including immunologic factors determined in the serum including cytokines, chemokines and antibodies or microarray data/transcription profiling of the peripheral blood. The profiles generated by SELDI-TOF MS are a rich source of information, which floats to the surface after careful analysis. Although there are many ways to analyze and evaluate proteomic profile data, a simple framework such as the one presented above serves as a foothold for future data analysis work.

Using proper feature selection techniques, proteomic profiling can be a valuable discovery tool for locating protein expression patterns in separate case and control populations. As seen above, by comparing expected generalization results on an unseen testing set, one can evaluate the performance of many feature selection strategies. The resulting classification models each contribute knowledge about the profiles, whether there is success or failure with subsequent test sets. In the case explored above, the peak selection strategy used was not effective due to important information being expressed in the "valleys" of the profile. When these were taken into account, the predictive ability of the classification model is higher. When features were found to cluster among one another due to correlation in relation to proximity of *m/z* values, de-correlation became an important step in the process. Ultimately, the classification model was able to obtain a testing error of 3 per cent when using the top 25 *m/z* intensities ranked by Fisher score and having intra-correlation coefficients less than 0.8.

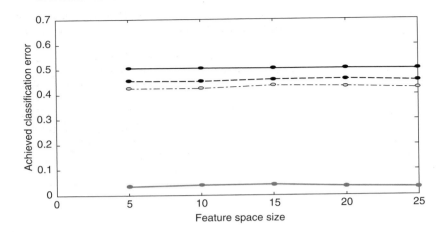

Figure 57.11 Permutation-based validation. The top solid line indicates the mean-achieved classification error (MACE) for the model under the null hypothesis: the class labels in the data are assigned to profiles randomly. The upper dashed line indicates the estimate of the upper 95th percentile of the test error statistic under the null hypothesis. Likewise the lower dashed line indicates the 99th percentile. The bottom solid line indicates the achieved classification error (ACE) using the original data labeling. Only the values for the points marked are computed.

The *m/z* values selected through the favored classifier play the most important role in clinical diagnostics. Databases of peptide masses are easily queried with a list of *m/z* values, which return possible protein sources for those peptide molecules. In this way it is possible to verify the statistically located biomarkers with the support of biological knowledge surrounding these indicators. Even if identifying the protein is not feasible, simply making a note of the *m/z* values is often enough. New patients can have their MS spectra generated and these *m/z* values checked in order to determine the efficacy a treatment will have, the progress a disease has made, or to determine composition of antibodies during an immune response.

Mass spectrometry proteomic profiling is certainly a viable technique for the discovery and detection of biomarkers. Advances in sample preparation and instrumentation are improving the usage of this technology. With continued application and development, the information derived from mass spectrometry studies will contribute substantially to what is currently known about the role, variation and relative abundance of multiple proteins in the setting of normality and disease.

The study of cell biology is, for a large part, dependent on solutions to many structural problems. Accurate structural characterization of protein peptides in femtomole levels is especially important to immunology and the study of proteomics. Surface-enhanced laser desorption/ionization time-of-flight mass spectrometry (SELDI-TOF MS) is a technology which can assist biologists in studying the 'structures' of macromolecules in complex and varying situations; the ultimate goal is to utilize fully this technology for determining the function and abundance of peptides as they relate to health and disease. One important potential application of this technology includes identifying peptides/proteins that are associated with immune responses to diseased cells. Peptide or lipid antigens recognized by T cells in the context of MHC molecules serve as a means to identify relative changes or new proteins or pathogens residing within a cell, serving as a basis for T cell recognition and effector function including the ability to lyse the cell presenting the nominal antigen. These antigens are presented as protein fragments which can be readily identified by the mass spectrometry technology (Castelli et al., 1995).

REFERENCES

Adam, B.L., Qu, Y., Davis, J.W. et al. (2002). Serum protein fingerprinting coupled with a pattern-matching algorithm distinguishes prostate cancer from benign prostate hyperplasia and healthy men. Cancer Res 62, 3609–3614.

Burges, C. (1998). A tutorial on support vector machines for pattern recognition. Data Mining Knowl Discov 2, 121–167.

Castelli, C., Storkus, W.J. et al. (1995). Mass spectrometric identification of a naturally-processed melanoma peptide recognized by CD8+ cytotoxic T lymphocytes. J Exp Med 181, 363–368.

Duda, R.O., Hart, P.E. and Stork, D.G. (2000). Pattern classification, 2nd edn. John Wiley and Sons.

Fisher, R.A. (1936). The use of multiple measurements in taxonomic problems. Ann Eugenics 7, 79–188.

Furey, T.S. and Christianini, N. et al. (2000). Support vector machine classification and validation of cancer tissue samples using microarray expression data. Bioinformatics 16, 906–914.

Hanley, J. and McNeil, B. (1982). The meaning and use of the area under a receiver operating characteristic curve. Diagnost Radiol 143, 29–36.

Hastie, T., Tibshirani, R. and Friedman, J. (2001). The elements of statistical learning. New York: Springer-Verlag.

Jolliffe, I.T. (1986). Principal component analysis. New York: Springer-Verlag.

Kleinbaum, D.G. (1994). Logistic regression: a self-learning text. New York: Springer-Verlag.

Patel, S. and Lyons-Weiler, J. (2004). caGEDA: a web application for the integrated analysis of global gene expression patterns in cancer. Appl Bioinformat, in press.

Paweletz, C., Trock, B., Pennanen, M. et al. (2001). Proteomic patterns of nipple aspirate fluids obtained by SELDI-TOF. Dis Markers 17, 301–307.

Petricoin, E.F., Ardekani, A.M. and Hitt, B.A. (2002). Use of proteomic patterns in serum to identify ovarian cancer. Lancet 359, 572–577.

Petricoin, E.F and Ornstein, D.K. (2002). Serum proteomic patterns for detection of prostate cancer. J Natl Cancer Inst 94, 1576–1578.

Scholkopf, B. and Smola, A. (2002). Learning with kernels. MIT Press.

Steel, L.F., Shumpert, D. and Trotter, M. (2003). A strategy for the comparative analysis of serum proteomes for the discovery of biomarkers for hepatocellular carcinoma. Proteomics 3, 601–609.

Vapnik, V.N. (1995). The nature of statistical learning theory. New York: Springer-Verlag.

Wadsworth, J.T., Somers, K. and Stack, B. (2004). Identification of patients with head and neck cancer using serum protein profiles. Arch Otolaryngol Head Neck Surg 130, 98–104.

Watkins, B., Szaro, R., Shannon, B. et al. (2001). Detection of early stage cancer by serum protein analysis. Am Lab 32–36.

Zeindl-Eberhart, E., Haraida, S. and Liebmann, S. (2004). Detection and identification of tumor-associated protein variants in human hepatocellular carcinomas. Hepatology 39, 540–549.

Zhukov, T.A., Johanson, R.A., Cantor, A.B., Clark, R.A. and Tockman, M.S. (2003). Discovery of distinct protein profiles specific for lung tumors and pre-malignant lung lesions by SELDI mass spectrometry. Lung Cancer 40, 267–279.

Imaging Cytometry: High Content Screening for Large-Scale Cell Research

Michael T. Lotze[1], Lina Lu[2] and D. Lansing Taylor[3]
[1]*Translational Research Molecular Medical Institute,* [2]*Starzl Transplantation Institute,*
University of Pittsburgh School of Medicine; [3]*Cellomics Inc, Pittsburgh, PA, USA*

The use of tools has often been regarded as the defining characteristic of Homo sapiens, that is, as a taxonomically distinctive characteristic of the species … Everyone has observed with more or less wonderment that the tools and instruments devised by human beings undergo an evolution themselves that is strangely analogous to ordinary evolution, almost as if these artifacts propagated themselves as animals do … Some instruments, like spectrophotometers, microscopes and radio-telescopes, are sensory accessories inasmuch as they enormously increase sensibility and the range and quality of the sensory input.

Sir Peter Medawar; *Technology and Evolution*

INTRODUCTION

The information resident in blood samples has been radically expanded during the past few years with the availability of proteomics performed on serum components, likely representing the adherent fraction of proteins and peptides associated with large carrier proteins such as albumin (see Chapters 57 and 59). In addition, microarray analysis of the blood has also brought insights both into the altered function of these cells as well as their ability to reflect pathologic states as migratory biosensors of inflammatory sites. Perhaps the least developed, but one of the most intriguing areas in the identification and development of modern biomarkers and surrogates, is the ability to use signals derived from circulating cells as unstimulated or cytokine/chemokine/agonist stimulated

cells. Activation pathways are altered in cells based on their premature recruitment from the bone marrow or their integration of systemic signals present in the blood during inflammatory states. Most of the signals relate to states of apoptotic death or altered signaling in T cells, likely recirculating from tissues to lymph nodes or hepatic sites, where they are cleared. Little has been done to assess these cells in a systematic fashion.

Imaging cytometry involves the use of plated cells which can be imaged and information captured on a per cell basis of the cell membrane, cytoplasm and intracellular organelles including lysosomes, peroxisomes, mitochondria and nuclei. High content screening has been defined by Cellomics Inc. as the automated method for analyzing cells in arrays containing one or more fluorescent reporter molecules. One of the major strategies for imaging in our hands involves the Cellomics assay system which was pioneered and developed by Cellomics Inc. for the purposes of drug discovery processes. Until recently, it has been mainly used by the pharmaceutical industry to measure the effects of potential drugs on complex molecular events such as signal transduction pathways, as well as effects on cell functions like apoptosis, division, cell adhesion, locomotion, exocytosis and cell–cell communication. The work flow is summarized in Figure 58.1.

We established a Cellomics Core to provide multiplexed functional imaging, screening, analysis and quality control of samples (including the cell products for clinical use) from ongoing research projects. The measurements are based on fluorescence imaging of multiple targets

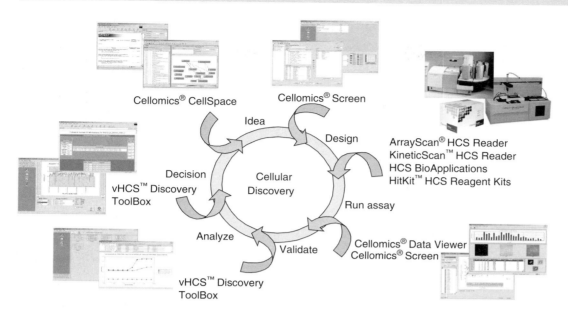

Figure 58.1 Work flow chart.

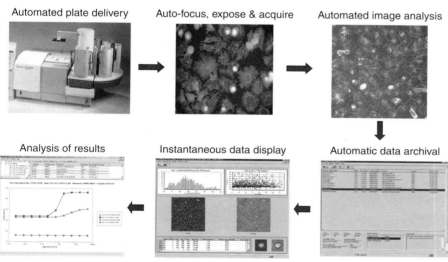

Figure 58.2 High content screening and automated cell analysis.

in the context of intact cells. Up to six different fluorochromes can be used and analyzed separately in one assay. The various assays are performed and screened by an automated instrument, "Array Scan II". Its characteristics include:

1. The instrument accepts various different kind of plates (96-well, 24-well, 12-well, etc.) and rapidly screens the plates and measures in excess of 20 cell measurements from up to four separate cellular targets
2. automatically finds cell fields, sets exposures, focus and thresholds during plate scanning
3. quantifies multiple fluorescent signals on or in cells
4. automatically converts raw image data into signal distribution, area, morphology and activity measurements
5. stores images and all data collected for each cell or cell field measured for later review.

High content screening (HCS) assay systems include fluorescent reagents kits, advanced optical imaging instrumentation and both informatics and bioinformatics software to analyze simultaneously multiple interacting or independent targets on intact cells. In contrast to routine molecular and immunology analysis system, which typically generates only a single read-out per assay, HCS uniquely analyzes mixed cell populations with the following capacities:

1. Extracts high content information on individual cells or fields of cells
2. Measures multiple responses within or on the surface and between individual cells
3. Captures temporal and spatial target activities that typify cell division, communication and apoptosis
4. Measures multiple cellular events, pathways or multiple entities within a single.

By isolating and analyzing subpopulations of cells and cross-correlating activities on a group of individual cells in a well, HCS eliminates potential sources of variability including those associated with pipetting error, cell preparation, transfection efficiency, assay processing and compound stability. More importantly, study of cellular interaction with HCS can be based upon target activity, location (cytoplasm, nuclear, membrane) and kinesis, as well as interacting cellular components and pathway, morphological events and environmental factors that combine to elicit a biologically relevant whole cell response.

This integrated platform provides high content biological information related to a molecule/cytokine candidate's biological impact on specific cellular targets within, on and between cells. HCS technology integrates several elements including video microscopy, robotics, development of modern 2–6 color fluorochromes and advanced data analysis algorithms (Giuliano and Taylor, 1998; Ghosh et al., 2000; Taylor et al., 2001; Kapur, 2002). Many of the changes observed physiologically *in vitro* with lymphoid and myeloid cells have not been routinely examined in peripheral blood mononuclear cells (PMN). These include molecules important for signaling in immune cells including T and NK cells and dendritic cells (DCs), such as p38 MAP kinase (Chini et al., 2000; Trotta et al., 2000; Yu et al., 2000), NFκB (Ye et al., 1995; Grohmann et al., 1998; Liu et al., 1998; Nicolet et al., 1998; Lyakh et al., 2000; Sareneva et al., 2000; David et al., 2001; Jewett, 2001; Tsuyuki et al., 2001; Zhou et al., 2002) and ERK in response to endogenous danger signals (Zhang et al., 2000; Lotze and DeMarco, 2003). Measurement of all of these are now possible in combinations of cells in the peripheral blood and in cell–cell mixtures using HCS strategies. In addition, three measurements of apoptosis can be attained simultaneously:

1 nuclear fragmentation with Hoechst
2 mitochondrial mass using Mitrotracker and
3 F-actin fragments using phylloidin-FITC binding.

This allows evaluation of the status of cells in the peripheral blood or in complex cell mixtures on a cell-by-cell basis.

The limited success in adoptive cell therapy of cancer has primarily been due, in our estimation, to the lack of persistence and proliferation of the functional activated T cells. Integrating DC and NK cells into cancer therapy could elicit an effective adaptive immune response and result in tumor destruction. Testing the coordinate signaling of immune cells including dendritic cells (DCs), T cells and NK cells that effectively initiates optimal Th1 polarization and subsequently drives an effective anti-tumor T cell response is difficult outside of murine model systems. New, whole cell-based screening and cell-cell screening approaches generate information-rich data regarding the effects of potential molecules on cell surface (TNF, TRAIL, cytokine receptors, etc) and intracellular transcription factors (JAK/Tyk, NF-κB, STATs) on multiple

Table 58.1 T cell parameters in peripheral blood which are frequently present or altered in tumor patients

Low T cell frequencies
T cell subset changes (CD4+, naive T cells decreased)
Decreased zeta-chain expression
Increased apoptosis (CD95, Annexin V)
Cytokine profiles
Memory T cell function
Treg (CD4+CD25+)
Tumor-specific T cell responses

cellular targets (activation/differentiation/apoptosis) on a cell-by-cell or population basis.

TRANSCRIPTION FACTOR ACTIVATION

By this application, it is possible to measure the spatial translocation of molecules and proteins from the cell cytoplasm to the nucleus. Typical target molecules are transcription factors (e.g. NFκB, STATs, c-Jun, c-Fos, CREB, NFAT), various kinases (p38 MAP kinase, Jun-kinase) and proteases (caspases). Cells and cell nuclei are first detected by Hoechst dye and the studied molecules are detected, e.g. by FITC-conjugated antibodies. The redistribution of target molecules is quantified by calculating the fluorescent intensity difference between cytoplasmic and nuclear areas (Figure 58.3A and B). The ArrayScan II system is capable of simultaneously measuring multiple cytoplasm to nucleus translocations within individual cells. The transcription factors and kinases, either alone or in various combinations can be detected (Figure 58.3C).

RECEPTOR ACTIVATION AND TRAFFICKING

Hormones and cytokines typically induce the internalization of their ligand-receptor complexes from the cell membrane into the cytoplasmic compartment. The internalization and translocation of the ligand-receptor complex can be followed and measured using fluorescent markers for the articular receptors. Cells and cell nuclei are detected by Hoechst dye (Figure 58.4). Examples of the analyzed receptors include: PTH-receptor, transferrin receptor, P2Y1 receptor, bradykinin B2 receptor and adrenergic receptors $\beta1, -\beta2 -\alpha2a$.

APOPTOSIS

Apoptosis pathways involve many biochemical, morphological and physiological events that are highly orchestrated in tome and space within living cells. The Cellomics technology has assembled an array of assays including changes in nuclear morphology, cytoskeleton organization, mitochondrial physiology and enzyme activation

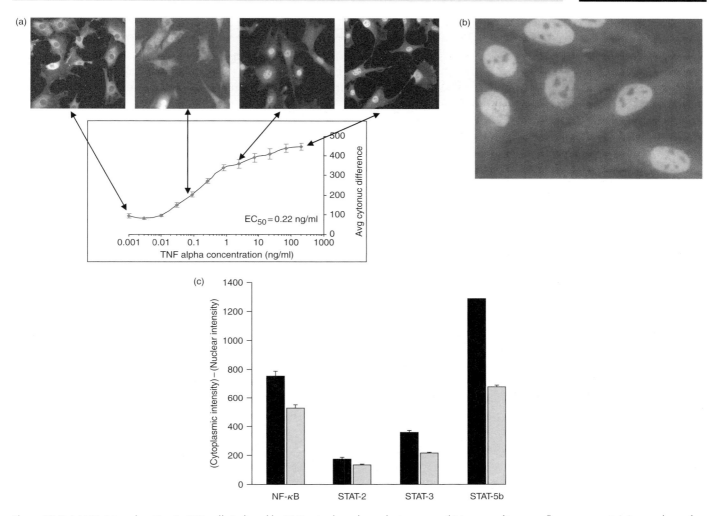

Figure 58.3 (a) NFκB translocation in 3T3 cells induced by TNF-α in dose-dependent manner. (b) Images of immunofluorescence staining nucleus of Hela cells after activation of NFκB by IL-1a. (c) Quantitative analysis of multiple transcription factors from scanning in treated and untreated cells ($P < 0.0001$).

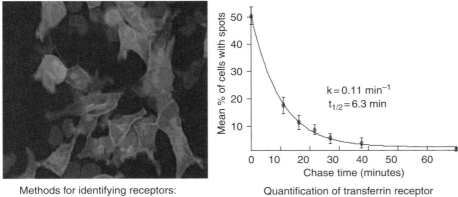

Methods for identifying receptors:
• Receptor chimeras
• Fluorescent ligands
• Receptor specific antibodies

Quantification of transferrin receptor recycling rate in HEK293 cells

Figure 58.4 Receptor internalization and trafficking.

and has combined them into a multiparameter HCS assay. The array of targets include: caspase activation and DNA fragmentation, nuclear fragmentation and condensation, cytoskeleton, PARP, mitochondrial mass/potential,

ssDNA detection, phosphatidylserine externalization and BAX. The screening can be optimized for various cell types, cancers, temporal events, or signaling pathways (Figure 58. 5).

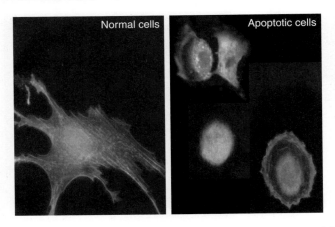

Figure 58.5 Multiple apoptosis analysis. F-actin appears in green, nuclei in blue and mitochondria in red. **See colour plate 58.5.**

CELL MORPHOLOGY

Morphology-based assay relies on cell size or shape determinations, in addition to cytoskeletal organization and/or other parameters. Both exogenous (i.e. cytokines, cell contact) and endogenous (i.e. cytokines, signaling protein) factors can alter cell morphology in predictable and quantifiable ways. Cell morphology can be used as an indicator of cell health, metastatic potential of cancer cells, angiogenic potential of endothelial cells, cell–cell contact, cell dispersion, cell adhesion, cell motility and migration and activation of lymphocytes. HCS-generated cell morphology measurements have been performed on human and rodent lymphocytes, endothelial cells and tumor cells for angiogenesis, neurite outgrowth and cancer. These morphological applications can incorporate additional screening criteria to live cells or to a specific subtype of cells within a mixed cell culture.

CELL VIABILITY

The cell viability screen images a cell population and then identifies which cells in the population are alive or dead, based upon the uptake or retention of respective fluorescent dyes. The quality of screen is enhanced by distinguishing live cells from dead cell measurements with the associated software. Figure 58.6 shows the application that determines the actual number of cells in the live and dead fluorescent channels, as well as a total cell count. Functional fluorescence dyes and subpopulation and target-specific dyes allow the analysis of dead cells in cell subpopulations, independent cell type, or conditions that affect only a fraction of cells within a mixed cell cultures.

MITOTIC INDEX

HCS-based approach to mitotic index measurements, as compared to flow cytometric methods, includes the

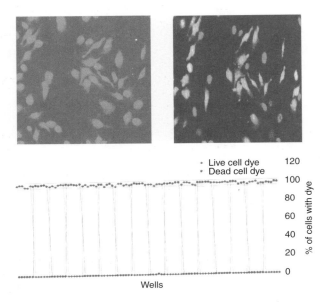

Figure 58.6 Cell viability assay by ArrayScan II. **See colour plate 58.6.**

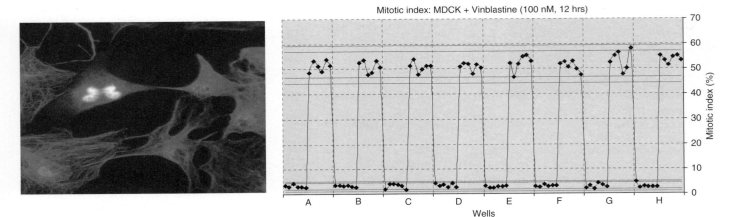

Figure 58.7 Mitotic index to quantify curacin A antimitotic effect. **See colour plate 58.7.**

ability to multiplex several targets in the same cells and to distinguish the fraction of '2n' (DNA content) cells that are mitotic from those that are in interphase (Figure 58.7). Furthermore, since indices of cell proliferation or cell cycle are integral to cell apotosis, in conjunction with cell viability and morphology measurements imaging cytometry provides substantial information simultaneously about activation, cytotoxicity and survival of a variety of immune (T cells, NK cells, DCs) or non-immune (e.g. cancer) cells in the setting of developing novel biomarkers and surrogates (Lotze, 2003; Lotze and Papamichail, 2004; Lotze and Rees, 2004). Its integration with more conventional assays of cellular function by flow cytometry, in particular the use of fluorophores coupled to activated kinases would represent important next steps for development of cell-based biomarkers (Maino and Picker, 1998; Bleesing and Fleisher, 2001; Krutzik and Nolan, 2003; Krutzik et al., 2004; Maino and Maecker, 2004; Perez et al., 2004).

REFERENCES

Bleesing, J.J. and Fleisher, T.A. (2001). Cell function-based flow cytometry. Review. Semin Hematol *38*, 169–178.

Chini, C.C., Boos, M.D., Dick, C.J., Schoon, R.A. and Leibson, P.J. (2000). Regulation of p38 mitogen-activated protein kinase during NK cell activation. Eur J Immunol *30*, 2791–2798.

David, M., Ford, D., Bertoglio, J., Maizel, A.L. and Pierre, J. (2001). Induction of the IL-13 receptor alpha2-chain by IL-4 and IL-13 in human keratinocytes: involvement of STAT6, ERK and p38 MAPK pathways. Oncogene *20*, 6660–6668.

Ghosh, R.N., Chen, Y.T., DeBiasio, R. et al. (2000). Cell-based, high-content screen for receptor internalization, recycling and intracellular trafficking. Biotechniques *29*, 170–175.

Giuliano, K.A. and Taylor, D.L. (1998). Fluorescent-protein biosensors: new tools for drug discovery. Trends Biotechnol, *16*, 135–140.

Grohmann, U., Belladonna, M.L., Bianchi, R.C. et al. (1998). IL-12 acts directly on DC to promote nuclear localization of NF-kappaB and primes DC for IL-12 production. Immunity 9, 315–323.

Jewett, A. (2001). Activation of c-Jun N-terminal kinase in the absence of NFkappaB function prior to induction of NK cell death triggered by a combination of anti-class I and anti-CD16 antibodies. Hum Immunol *62*, 320–331.

Kapur, R. (2002). Fluorescence imaging and engineered biosensors: functional and activity-based sensing using high content screening. Ann NY Acad Sci *961*, 196–197.

Krutzik, P.O., Irish, J.M., Nolan, G.P. and Perez, O.D. (2004). Analysis of protein phosphorylation and cellular signaling events by flow cytometry: techniques and clinical applications. Clin Immunol *110*, 206–221.

Krutzik, P.O. and Nolan, G.P. (2003). Intracellular phospho-protein staining techniques for flow cytometry: monitoring single cell signaling events. Cytometry *55A*, 61–70.

Liu, J., Finke, J., Krauss, J.C., Shu, S. and Plautz, G.E. (1998). Ex vivo activation of tumor-draining lymph node T cells reverses defects in signal transduction molecules. Cancer Immunol Immunother *46*, 268–276.

Lotze, M.T. (2003). The critical need for cancer biometrics: quantitative, reproducible measures of cancer to define response to therapy. Review. Curr Opin Investig Drugs 4, 649–651.

Lotze, M.T. and DeMarco, R.A. (2003). Dealing with death: HMGB1 as a novel target for cancer therapy. Review. Curr Opin Investig Drugs 4, 1405–1409.

Lotze, M.T. and Papamichail, M. (2004). A primer on cancer immunology and immunotherapy. Cancer Immunol Immunother 53, 135–138.

Lotze, M.T. and Rees, R.C. (2004). Identifying biomarkers and surrogates of tumors (cancer biometrics): correlation with immunotherapies and immune cells. Review. Cancer Immunol Immunother 53, 256–261.

Lyakh, L.A., Koski, G.K., Telford, W., Gress, R.E., Cohen, P.A. and Rice, N.R. (2000). Bacterial lipopolysaccharide, TNF-alpha, and calcium ionophore under serum-free conditions promote rapid dendritic cell-like differentiation in CD14+ monocytes through distinct pathways that activate NK-kappa B.PG-. J Immunol 165.

Maino, V.C. and Picker, L.J. (1998). Identification of functional subsets by flow cytometry: intracellular detection of cytokine expression. Review. Cytometry 34, 207–215.

Maino, V.C. and Maecker, H.T. (2004). Cytokine flow cytometry: a multiparametric approach for assessing cellular immune responses to viral antigens. Clin Immunol *110*, 222–231.

Nicolet, C.M., Surfus, J.M., Hank, J.A. and Sondel, P.M. (1998). Transcription factor activation in lymphokine activated killer cells and lymphocytes from patients receiving IL-2 immunotherapy. Cancer Immunol Immunother 46, 327–337.

Perez, O.D., Krutzik, P.O. and Nolan, G.P. (2004). Flow cytometric analysis of kinase signaling cascades. Methods Mol Biol. *263*, 67–94.

Sareneva, T., Julkunen, I. and Matikainen, S. (2000). IFN-alpha and IL-12 induce IL-18 receptor gene expression in human NK and T cells. J Immunol 165, 1933–1938.

Taylor, D.L., Woo, E.S. and Giuliano, K.A. (2001). Real-time molecular and cellular analysis: the new frontier of drug discovery. Curr Opin Biotechnol *12*, 75–81.

Trotta, R., Fettucciari, K., Azzoni, L. et al. (2000). Differential role of p38 and c-Jun N-terminal kinase 1 mitogen-activated protein kinases in NK cell cytotoxicity. J Immunol *165*, 1782–1789.

Tsuyuki, S., Horvath-Arcidiacono, J.A. and Bloom, E.T. (2001). Effect of redox modulation on xenogeneic target cells: the combination of nitric oxide and thiol deprivation protects porcine endothelial cells from lysis by IL-2-activated human NK cells. J Immunol *166*, 4106–4114.

Ye, J., Ortaldo, J.R., Conlon, K., Winkler-Pickett, R. and Young, H.A. (1995). Cellular and molecular mechanisms of IFN-gamma production induced by IL-2 and IL-12 in a human NK cell line. J Leukoc Biol 58, 225–233.

Yu, T.K., Caudell, E.G., Smid, C. and Grimm, E.A. (2000). IL-2 activation of NK cells: involvement of MKK1/2/ERK but not p38 kinase pathway. J Immunol 164, 6244–6251.

Zhang, W., Chen, T., Wan, T. et al. (2000). Cloning of DPK, a novel dendritic cell-derived protein kinase activating the ERK1/ERK2 and JNK/SAPK pathways. Biochem Biophys Res Commun 274, 872–879.

Zhou, J., Zhang, J., Lichtenheld, M.G. and Meadows, G.G. (2002). A role for NF-kappa B activation in perforin expression of NK cells upon IL-2 receptor signaling. J Immunol 169, 1319–1325.

Cancer Biometrics

Chapter
59

Monica C. Panelli and Francesco M. Marincola

Immunogenetics Section, Department of Transfusion Medicine, Clinical Center, National Institutes of Health, Bethesda, MD, USA

Everything should be made as simple as possible, but not one bit simpler.

Albert Einstein 1879–1955

INTRODUCTION

Perhaps in the world of 'omics' where sceince is measured and measures in terms of thousands of elements the key to a deeper understanding is to maintain a simplified global view. Traditional protein biochemistry and the modern science of proteomics are, in the year 2004, still facing the challenging tasks of identifying proteins. Proteomic technologies are in rapid evolution and are branching into a multitude of different areas of research beyond the advances brought by state of the art genomics technologies (see Chapter 60). Yet, the process of identifying proteins and characterizing their expression and function, whether employing classical or implementing new technologies, remains very complex due to obstacles related to the structure and biochemical diversity of proteins. Once these obstacles are overcome the science of proteomics will have the power of identifying a biomarker which is in itself a functional endpoint and thus a true signature of a physiological or pathological state.

The complexity of protein identification becomes apparent when the following is considered: while genomics analysis is based on amplifiable material such as RNA or DNA, no amplification technology exists for proteomics. To complicate protein analysis further, the detection limits for measurement of proteins spans up to eight log orders of magnitude between the most and the least expressed proteins. In addition, proteins exhibit a wide range of biochemical properties dependent on the 3D structure of the folded peptides, their biochemical stability at different pH and a series of post-translational modifications and biochemical protein–protein interactions. Furthermore, proteins may be expressed in various truncated or proteolytically-modified forms. Finally, proteins, unlike RNA or DNA, do not display distinct high-affinity/high-specificity binding partners and, in most instances, specific capture reagents must be developed for individual protein identification and quantitation (Panelli and Burns, 2004).

This chapter will discuss the new challenges introduced by proteomic technology and will address how protein arrays, one of the most exciting proteomic technologies to date, are contributing to protein identification and characterization of biomarkers. These solid, semisolid, or liquid platforms feature multiplexing of capture reagents (usually antibodies or combinations of antibody and anchoring molecules) capable of binding different protein analytes or can present substrates (tissue, lysates, cells) to be probed for *ex vivo* protein quantification and identification.

The impact of proteomic technologies and discoveries in the context of translational medicine will be discussed, presenting their application in the study of immunological responses and disease.

Measuring Immunity, edited by Michael T. Lotze and Angus W. Thomson
ISBN 0-12-455900-X, London

PRINCIPLES OF PROTEOMIC TECHNOLOGIES AND PROTEIN ARRAYS

High throughput genomic analysis has identified the need to complement genetic or transcriptional information with technologies for large scale screening of protein expression for confirmation or interpretation of results.

Although traditional biochemical methods have uncovered an extraordinary number of protein functions, they cannot realistically be applied to the study of every protein in a cell, tissue or organism. As MacBeth and Schreiber (2000) suggest, "if we hope to assign function on a broader level we must turn to miniaturized assays that can be performed in a highly parallel format". State of the art proteomic strategies aimed at characterizing proteins in various states (modified and unmodified) are characterized by medium to high throughput (when automated) and currently comprise two-dimensional gel electrophoresis (2D-GE), liquid chromatography-mass spectrometry (LC-MS/MS), isotope coded affinity tag (ICAT) and multidimensional protein identification technology (Mud PIT which couples 2D-LC to MS/MS). An increasing variety of protein and tissue arrays, quantitative protein array surface enhanced laser desorption time of flight mass spectrometry (SELDI-TOF-MS) and surface plasmon resonance platforms (SPR), complete the assortment of available tools for profiling proteins in abundance. For review of traditional and state of the art technologies in proteomics research refer to *Trends in Biotechnology 20* no.12 Supplement, A Trends Guide to Proteomics.

A series of exciting reports over the past few years exemplified the utilization of protein microarray technologies in various configurations as a tool for the miniaturized assays suggested by MacBeth and Schreiber (2000). In addition, they offer the fascinating possibility to study protein interactions in parallel including protein–protein, enzyme–substrate, protein–DNA, protein–oligosaccharide, protein–drug interaction (Schwenk et al., 2002).

Several pioneer studies have established the usefulness of protein chips and brought important advances in developing protein arrays (Lee and Mrksich, 2002). On this note the impact of protein arrays for protein characterization and clinical diagnostics is indeed reflected by the increasing awareness of the commercial potential of this technology. It is in fact predicted that business will grow in this area from US $963 million spent in 2000 to approximately $5.6 billion in 2006 (http://www. genomeweb.com/Articles/view-article.asp? Article=20018156158). Furthermore, the protein array market is estimated to increase 10-fold reaching $500 million in 2006 (Kusnezow and Hoheisel, 2002).

This booming technology is in constant development. However, many challenges remain ahead in the manufacturing and application of protein arrays. We will discuss here the principles of miniaturized multiplexed assays and the four major challenges in the design of protein arrays:

1 implementation of well characterized surface chemistries
2 immobilization strategies
3 prevention of non-specific adsorption and denaturation of immobilized proteins and
4 signal amplification.

For a summary of the technologies based on protein array principles refer to Table 59.1.

Pioneer work in protein arrays

MacBeth and Schreiber were the first to report that proteins could be printed and assayed in a microarray platform (MacBeth and Schreiber, 2000). Proteins were immobilized at high spatial densities by reacting lysine side chain amino groups with aldehyde modified glass slides. In this fashion, proteins were attached covalently to the glass surface and were capable of retaining the ability to interact with other proteins. MacBeth and Schreiber validated their arrays by demonstrating their application in three different areas: screening of protein–protein interaction (binding of protein G and immunoglobulin G among others), identification of substrates of protein kinases (protein kinase-PKA and Kemptide as an example) and identification of proteins targeted by small molecules (DIG) (Figure 59.1).

Zhu and coworkers (2001) demonstrated the construction of a protein array consisting of 6566 yeast proteins obtained from overexpression of open reading frames (ORFs) cloned into a yeast high copy expression vector. The yeast proteins were fused to glutathione S-transferase polyhistidine (GST-hisX6) at their NH_2 termini and spotted on either aldehyde-treated or nickel-coated microscope slides (Figure 59.2a and b). Proteins were bound to the aldehyde slide through the primary amine at the NH_2 termini while the HisX6 tags constituted the binding site for the nickel-coated slides. Although both types of slides were successful, the nickel-coated slides gave superior signal and presumably had proteins uniformly oriented away from the surface. Testing of this protein chip effectively identified new classes of calmodulin and phospholipid binding proteins. Although powerful, Zhu and co-workers' protein array featured intrinsic limitations anticipating critical problems related to array development. Properly folded extracellular domains and secreted proteins were likely under-represented in these chips because GST and HisX6 Tags were fused at the NH_2 terminus. Another limitation was that not all proteins were readily overproduced and purified in this high throughput approach, therefore not all possible interactions could be detected.

Concomitant to this work was the development of antibody arrays. de Wildt and Tomlinson (de Wildt et al.,

Table 59.1 Summary of proteomic technologies utilizing protein arrays

Technology	Sensitivity	Protein/marker identification	Utilization	Throughput	Advantages and disadvantages
Antibody arrays 1 Chemiluminescence Multi ELISA platforms 2 Glass fluorescence based arrays (Cy3-Cy5)	Medium to highest (depending on detection system)	Possible when coupled to MS technologies; or probable, if antibodies have been highly defined by epitope mapping and neutralization	Multiparametric analysis of many analytes simultaneously	High	1 Format is flexible Can be used to assay for multiple analytes in a single specimen or a single analyte in a number of specimens 2 Requires prior knowledge of analyte being measured 3 Limited by antibody sensitivity and specificity 4 Requires extensive cross-validation for antibody cross-reactivity 5 Requires use of an amplified tag detection system 6 Requires more sample to measure low abundant proteins, needs to be measured undiluted
Tissue arrays	Medium	Yes	FISH, *in situ* hybridization, immunofluorescence (including confocal), immunohistochemistry and in traditional histochemical staining methods	High	The majority of the tissue used to construct the TARP arrays is obtained from the Cooperative Human Tissue Network (CHTN). Other sources are also used to supplement this material which is formalin-fixed, paraffin-embedded tissue. Limited history, from surgical pathology reports is available, more than 10% of cases have neither age or sex available
Inductively coupled plasma MS immunoassay I CP-MS Antibody array with element tagged antibodies	High	Yes with - secondary MS	Multiparametric analysis (limited protein number to date) with MS detection	N/A	New technology Very early stage 1 Non-amplified, analysis of element allows for direct measurement without background or contamination 2 Acidification of sample allows archiving 3 May require too much sample
MALDI SELDI-TOF-MS SELDI-QqTOF	Medium-to-high . sensitivity SELDI-TOF-MS and MALDI are both capable of analyzing a wide mw range of proteins with generally diminishing signal at higher masses. Compact MS systems typically yield a sensitivity benefit as a trade-off for	Molecular mass of intact proteins or peptides yields a very tentative ID while the principle of SELDI pattern diagnostics conveniently defines a path to rapid marker enrichment for the purposes of ID (Nakamura et al., 2002) SELDI-QqTOF platform provides a more direct	Diagnostic pattern analysis in body fluids (serum, urine, CSF, feces, etc.) and tissue (with or without LCM) Potential biomarker identification SELDI protein interaction mapping for functional studies as well as biomarker assays (with specific	High	SELDI 1 Protein ID not necessary for biomarker pattern analysis, but patterns narrow down the relevant proteins for ID studies while the SELDI process is useful to defining a rapid isolation and ID protocol 2 Reproducibility and quantitative performance better than MALDI; debate exists over current reproducibility achieved

Table 59.1 Continued

Technology	Sensitivity	Protein/marker identification	Utilization	Throughput	Advantages and disadvantages
	resolution; shorter drift tubes allow more ions to reliably reach the detector SELDI-QqTOF technology with distinct resolution advantages has been shown to have comparable sensitivity in low mass range, but has an effective cut-off in analysis at fairly low masses	route to protein ID by enabling on-chip tandem MS for peptide sequencing. Some complete protocols for on-chip - marker purification, proteolysis and MS/MS ID have been shown (Caputo et al., 2003) Rapid, on-chip immunoaffinity identification protocols for SELDI when antibodies exist to tentatively identified markers	bait protein coupled to chip)		from site-to-site 3 Rapid analysis and parallel processing of large sample populations possible 4 Revolutionary tool; as little as 1–2 µl amount of material required; slightly more (20 µl) with prefractionation procedures 5 As with other technologies, SELDI works synergistically with upfront fractionation of serum and other complex samples – fractionation increases the number of proteins detected at a cost of time and amount of sample; downstream purification methods necessary to obtain absolute protein identification MALDI 1 Commonly available equipment can be employed to combine off-line LC with MALDI for proteomic pattern generation 2 Matrix crystallization procedure is a large source of irreproducibility and can be matrix and sample dependent 3 High mw proteins often not directly detectable requiring global digestion and shot-gun MS/MS approaches
Sensor chips Surface Plasmon Resonance (SPR) SELDI antibody treated chip	High	Yes	Protein–protein interaction analysis Identification of disease markers in clinical samples Quantitative measurement of binding interaction and specificity between molecules, ligand fishing	High	New technology 1 Can be used to assay for a single analyte in a number of specimens 2 SELDI chip limited by antibody sensitivity and specificity 3 Hardware limitation with the PBS II versus the QqTOF 4 Promising combined strategy of protein array chip and MS

(modified from Panelli and Burns, 2004)

Abbreviations: 2D GE 2 dimensional gel electrophoresis; DIGE differential in gel electrophoresis; SDS-PAGE sodium dodecyl sulfate-polyacrylamide gel electrophoresis; PAGE polyacrylamide gel electrophoresis; SERPA serological proteome analysis; ICAT isotope coded affinity tag; MudPIT multidimensional protein identification technology; MALDI matrix assisted laser desorption ionization; SELDI-qTOF surface enhanced laser desorption ionization quadrupole time of flight; ESI electrospray ionization; ESI FTICR electrospray ionization fourier transform cyclotron resonance; LC-MS/MS liquid chromatography- tandem mass spectrometry; SRP sensor chip surface plasmon resonance; LCM laser capture microdissection; ICH immunoaffinity subtraction chromatography; IHC immunohistochemistry; TARP arrays Tissue Array Research Program; UMSA unified maximum separability analysis.

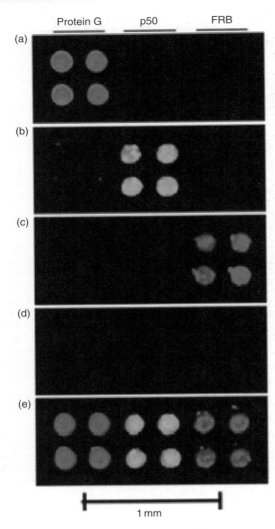

Figure 59.1 Detecting protein-protein interactions on glass slides. (a) Slide probed with BODIPY-FL-IgG (0.5 μg/ml). (b) Slide probed with Cy3-IkBα (0.1 μg/ml). (c) Slide probed with Cy5-FKBP12(0.5 μg/ml) and 100nM rapamycin. (d) Slide probed with Cy5-FKBP12 (0.5 μg/ml) and no rapamycin. (e) Slide probed with BODIPY-FL-IgG (0.5 μg/ml)), Cy3-IkBα (0.1 μg/ml), Cy5-FKBP12 (0.5 μg/ml), and 100 nM rapamycin. In all panels, BODIPY-FL, Cy3, and Cy5 fluorescence were false-colored blue, green, and red, respectively. **See colour plate 59.1.**

slides. Protein mixtures were labelled with Cy3 or Cy5 dyes (Amersham Bioscience, Piscataway, NJ) allowing antibody–antigen detection to be measured by fluorescence intensity signal. Of the 115 tested antibody–antigen pairs, only 50 per cent of the antigens and 20 per cent of the arrayed antibodies provided sufficient affinity and specificity. The results of this study revealed that although the antibody chip in itself could be assembled in a fairly simple manner, selection of the appropriate (with minimal or no cross-reactivity) antibodies constituted a foremost challenge for protein array manufacturing. de Wildt and Haab's work not only represented a major breakthrough in protein array science but pointed out crucial requirements of array technology. Most importantly, it indicated that mass production of antibodies with minimal cross-reactivity represented the most critical bottleneck for antibody microarrays. In addition, they substantiated the hypothesis that antibody display libraries (phage, ribosome and mRNA display libraries) (Schaffitzel et al., 1999; Hanes et al., 2000) were probably the most practical and promising solution for the success of protein chip technology.

MAJOR CHALLENGES IN PROTEIN ARRAY TECHNOLOGY

Independently of which molecule served as capture reagent (protein fused to GST-hisX6, single scFvs or any other type of protein as we have seen in the previous studies), it soon became apparent that positive hits in a multiplexed protein array had to be validated and quantified with subsequent experiments. Proteins often immobilized in various orientations and underwent partial denaturation on the chip surface. Furthermore, non-specific adsorption of protein to the chip occurred, resulting in the obstruction of immobilized proteins. These still common problems are summarized by Figure 59.3.

Four aspects of protein chip manufacturing portray the major challenges of this technology:

1 implementation of well characterized surface chemistries
2 immobilization strategies
3 prevention of non-specific adsorption and denaturation of immobilized proteins (Lee and Mrksich, 2002)
4 signal amplification.

1 The choice of surface chemistry is critical for proper conformation and orientation of proteins because, unlike DNA, proteins are chemically and physically heterogeneous, have 3D structure and cannot be amplified (Lee et al., 2000). Several different surface chemistries include aldehyde, epoxy, amine (poly-L-lysine coating), active esters, maleimide, histidine-tag-nickel chelates, organic surfaces/derivative of collagen, dextran, nitrocellulose, hydrogel-aldehyde monolayers of alkanethiolates

2000) developed a technique for high throughput screening of recombinant antibodies by immobilizing up to 18 342 phage libraries presenting single chain antibody variable region fragments (scFvs) on filter paper to select for specific antigens in a complex mixture. This method used robotic picking and high-density gridding of bacteria containing antibody genes followed by filter-based enzyme-linked immunosorbent assay (ELISA) screening to identify clones that expressed binding antibody fragments. The study clearly demonstrated the power of high throughput screening and suggested that antibody arrays could be used to identify differentially expressed antigens/proteins. Haab et al. (2001) expanded this idea generating a multiplexed array where 115 different antibodies were linked to poly-lysine-coated glass

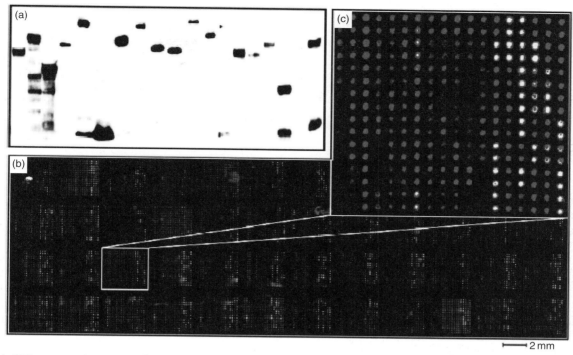

Figure 59.2(a) GST yeast proteins were purified in a 96-well format. (a) Sixty samples were examined by immunoblot analysis using anti-GST; 19 representative examples are shown. Greater than 80% of the preparations produce high yields of fusion protein. (b) 6566 protein samples representing 5800 unique proteins were spotted in duplicate on a single nickel-coated microscope slide. The slide was probed with anti-GST (10). (c) An enlarged image of one of the 48 blocks is depicted to the right of the proteome chip.

on gold (Lee et al., 2000; Kusnezow and Hoheisel, 2002). Each type of surface has its own advantages and disadvantages and may be best suited, for example, for antibody binding (maleimide derivatized surface covalently binds sulfydryl groups that become available in biomolecules after the reduction of disulfide bonds) or His-tag fusion proteins (nickel-coated slides) (Zhu et al., 2001). It remains, however, unresolved whether three-dimensional matrices are better than two-dimensional surface chemistries in binding capture molecules without affecting the original protein conformation.

2 Development of immobilization strategies as anticipated in 1 (above) is directly correlated to the method used to obtain proteins printed on chips and, more importantly, to the protein 2D structure and/or 3D conformation. In theory, oriented attachment is preferable to immobilization strategies (Kusnezow and Hoheisel, 2002). Methods that rely on common reactions to bind proteins to their substrate (lysine amino groups to aldehydes or adsorption of protein without chemical bonding) do not allow for proper orientation and density of immobilized proteins (Lee and Mrksich, 2002). An interesting immobilization strategy has been reported by Weng et al. (2002) who developed mRNA fusion proteins consisting of a polypeptide covalently linked to its corresponding mRNA. Weng and coworkers exploited the nucleic acid component of the mRNA protein fusion (PROfusion) to create an addressable protein microarray

that self assembles via hybridization to surface-bound DNA capture probes and allows strong anchoring of the protein in a uniform orientation. This platform successfully detected sub-attomole quantities of displayed protein without signal amplification.

3 Development of inert surfaces that prevent non-specific adsorption and denaturation is also a critical aspect for protein arrays. Methods presented earlier have made use of blocking reagents such as bovine serum albumin (BSA) or detergents to eliminate background signal due to non-specific binding and adsorption of unwanted protein to the array. It is now widely recognized that BSA may interfere with the immobilized proteins and that detergents can downregulate protein activity. A possible solution to this problem may be the implementation of capture reagent in suspension instead of bound to a solid surface (Houseman and Mrksich, 2002a,b; Houseman et al., 2002); also refer to LiquidChip™ Protein Suspension Array System, eTag Assay System, Table 59.2).

4 Achievement of adequate sensitivity and multiplexing in protein chips has been difficult to attain. Conventional signal amplification procedures such as enzyme catalyzed chemiluminescence have restricted multiplexing capability because of signal diffusion. Isothermal rolling circle amplification (RCA) is an example of a useful alternative for on chip signal amplification. Schweitzer et al. (2002) described coupling of RCA to universal antibodies to achieve improved sensitivity

(a)

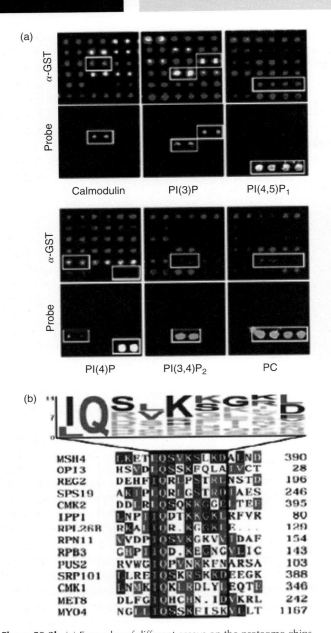

Calmodulin PI(3)P PI(4,5)P₁

PI(4)P PI(3,4)P₂ PC

(b)

MSH4	LRET IQSVKSLKDAI ND	390
OPI3	HSVDI QSSNFQLAT VCT	28
REG2	DEHF IQRI PSTRLNST D	196
SPS19	AKIP IQRIGSTRD AES	246
CMK2	DDIR IQSQNKGG LTE I	395
IPP1	LNP I IQDTKKGKLRFVK	80
RPL26B	RKAL IQR. KGKIE...	129
RPN11	KVDP IQSVNGKVLIDAF	154
RPB3	GIP IIQD. NEGNGYLIC	143
PUS2	RVWG IQPVNKKFNARSA	103
SRP101	ILRE IQSKRSKKD EEGK	388
CMK1	LNVKIQKLRDLYLEQT H	346
MET8	DLFGIQHCIN. IDVKRL	242
MYO4	NGIIIQSSFEISKVILT	1167

Figure 59.2b (a) Examples of different assays on the proteome chips. Proteome chips containing 6566 yeast proteins were spotted in duplicate and incubated with the biotinylated probes indicated. The positive signals in duplicate (green) are in the bottom row of each panel; the top row of each panel shows the same yeast protein preparations of a control proteome chip probed with anti-GST (red). The upper panel shows the amounts of GST fusion proteins as detected by the anti-GST (red). (b) A putative calmodulin-binding motif (32) is shown, which was identified by searching for amino acid sequences that are shared by the different calmodulin targets (10). Fourteen of 39 positive proteins share a motif whose consensus is (I/L)QXK(K/X)GB. where X is any residue and B is a basic residue. The size of the letter indicates the relative frequency of the amino acid indicated.

(femtomolar range) and high specificity in multiplexed assays performed on antibody microarrays. This technology uses the 5′ end of an oligonucleotide primer attached to an antibody. The antibody–DNA conjugate (antibiotin

(a) 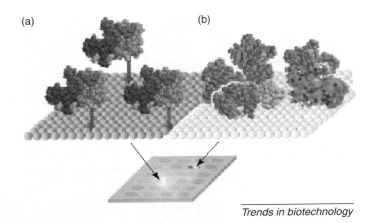 (b)

Trends in biotechnology

Figure 59.3 An illustration of the presentation of immobilized proteins in an array. (a) An idealized illustration of the presentation of immobilized proteins in an array. The proteins are all uniformly oriented, properly folded and optimally spaced to allow protein-protein interactions. (b) Current technologies present proteins in a range of orientations, with varying degrees of denaturation and with the presence of non-specifically absorbed proteins. **See colour plate 59.3.**

antibody) binds to a specific target molecule (biotinilated secondary antibody). A circular DNA molecule hybridizes to its complementary primer on the conjugate and, in the presence of DNA polymerase and nucleotides, RCA occurs. This generates a long complement of the circular DNA which remains bound to the antibody and it is detected by hybridization of complementary fluorescent probes. The amount of specific protein in the original sample is proportional to the fluorescence detected by a microarray scanner. This type of microarray could accommodate up to 1000 sandwich immunoassays of this type (Figure 59.4). Schweitzer et al. (2002) used a 51-feature RCA cytokine glass array successfully to measure secretion from human dendritic cells induced by lipopolisaccharide (LPS) or tumor necrosis factor (TNF-α).

Although academic science has largely contributed to protein chip developments, industry is currently playing a pivotal role in making advances and meeting the challenges discussed so far. Since the success of proteomics is ultimately dependent on contributions from both academia and industry, we present below significant advances brought to the field by biotech-companies. These are state of the art protein array applications approaching issues **1–4** (see also Table 59.2).

In addition to the profiling of protein levels by antibody microarrays, many other applications may help the study of immunological responses.

Living arrays

Living arrays make peptides or proteins available for assays in the cellular milieu as opposed to non-living arrays where synthetic peptides and proteins are arrayed on plastic, glass or cellulose filter paper and are used to search for biochemical activities in a defined environ-

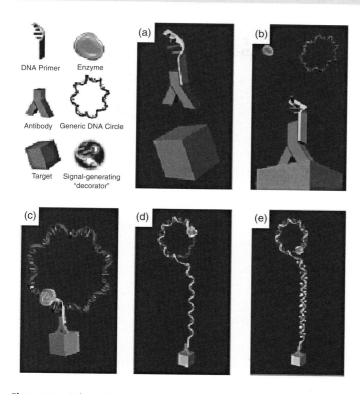

DNA Primer   Enzyme

Antibody   Generic DNA Circle

Target   Signal-generating "decorator"

Figure 59.4 Schematic representation of immunoassays with RCA signal amplification. (a) In the adaptation of RCA used for protein signal amplification, the 5′ end of an oligonucleotide primer is attached to an antibody. (b) The antibody–DNA conjugate binds to its specific target molecule; in the multiplexed microarray immunoassay, the targets are biotinylated secondary antibodies and the conjugate is an anti-biotin antibody. (c) A circular DNA molecule hybridizes to its complementary primer on the conjugate, and in the presence of DNA polymerase and nucleotides, rolling-circle replication occurs. (d) A long single DNA molecule that represents a concatamer of complements of the circle DNA sequence is generated that remains attached to the antibody. (e) This RCA product is detected by hybridization of multiple fluorescent, complementary oligonucleotide probes. RCA product fluorescence is measured with a conventional microaray scanning device. The amount of fluorescence at each spot is directly proportional to the amount of specific protein in the original sample. **See colour plate 59.4.**

ment (described earlier and reviewed by Emili and Cagney, 2000). Among the living arrays, *cell microarrays* are of great importance in high throughput antibody–antigen/receptor-ligand binding studies. Ziauddin and Sabatini (2001) developed a microarray-driven gene expression system that can be used as an alternative to protein microarray for the identification of drug targets and as an expression cloning system for the discovery of gene products that alter cellular physiology and immunological responses. Mammalian cells are cultured on a glass slide printed in defined location with different DNAs (Figure 59.5). Cells growing on the printed area took up the DNA (transfection) creating spots of living microarrays of cell clusters expressing a gene product. The approach of converting microarrays of DNA which are stables for months into live-protein arrays when

needed, was an obvious advantage and challenged the potential instability of immobilized protein arrays. The authors used transfected cell microarrays to screen a collection, enriched for signaling molecules, of 192 epitope-tagged cDNA cloned in expression vectors. Ziauddin and Sabatini examined gene products that increase the activity of kinase signaling pathways, induce apoptosis or are involved in cell adhesion. Utilizing phosphospecific antibodies they identified cell clusters with increased levels of phosphotyrosine or activated phosphorylated forms of mitogen-activated protein kinases (MAPKs). Five clusters expressed known tyrosine kinases and one encoded a protein of unknown function, demonstrating the power of this technique in detecting not only new target molecules for specific antibodies but possibly new roles for proteins. To identify gene products that could have a function in apoptosis or cell adhesion, it was possible to screen directly microarray cell clusters for abnormal morphology and for DNA fragmentation by TdT-mediated dUTP nick end-labeling reaction. A positive apoptotic cluster was found to express CD36, a cell surface protein with functions in cell-to-cell recognition and adhesion. A major advantage of the living arrays is that screening of live cells allows the detection of transient phenotypes such as change in intracellular calcium concentration or the movement of GFP tagged protein.

A different approach in generating living-cell microarrays was reported by Schwenk and coworkers (2002). Several cell lines (monocytic, B cell, lymphoma, neuroblastoma, embryonic kidney cell, hamster ovary, rat adrenal cell) with a known cell surface protein panel were spotted on poly-lysine coated microscope slides at a density on average of 18 cells/spot and used to generate cell microarrays. These arrays were in turn utilized to characterize successfully a panel of membrane protein specific-antibodies (CD45, CD3, MCH class I and II, epidermal growth factor receptor (EGFR)). A clear advantage of this system is not only the multiplexing capacity but also the extraordinary small amount of antibody that needed to be used for binding studies. Although the quality of this system only allowed the discrimination of binding versus non-binding, currently ongoing advances in array performance will help to make cell arrays useful tools in the multiplex profiling of the level of surface receptor expression.

Membrane biochips G proteins coupled receptors (GPCR) microarrays

Fang et al. (2002) recently described the fabrication of microarrays of GPCR, key mediators of many cellular functions, on surfaces coated with γ-aminopropylsilane (GAPS). They described their use for ligand screening assays across different families of GPCR (adrenergic, neurotensin and dopamine receptors). These arrays not only detected GPCR coupling but presented the possibility to screen potential ligand of orphan GPCR.

Table 59.2 State of the art protein arrays

Protein chip/array platform type	Multiplexed protein assay	Detection of known/unknown proteins	Size/sample	Sensitivity/limit of detection	Reference/website
Living arrays	Synthetic peptides on plastic or paper Affinity purified proteins	Protein interactions epitope mapping Biochemical activities			Emili and Cagney (2000)
Reverse phase antigen array	Total cellular lysate is spotted, probed with specific antibodies, sera or antigen labeled with fluorochromes			As low as 10^{-1} mol of spotted antigen	Paweletz et al. (2000) Shreekumar and Chinnaiyan (2000)
Membrane biochips G proteins coupled receptors (GPCR) microarrays	GPCR printed on surfaces coated with y-aminopropylsilane (GAPS)	Ligand screening assay across different families of GPCR (adrenergic, neurotensin and dopamine receptors) and presented the possibility to screen potential ligand of orphan GPCR	Variable 0.5 nl/microspot and µM soluconcentration of potential ligand	Variable	Fang et al. (2000)
Cell microarrays	1 Mammalian cells cultured on a glass slide printed in defined location with different DNAs. Cells growing on the printed area take up the DNA (by transfection) creating spots of living microarrays of cell clusters expressing a gene product 2 Monocytic, B cell, lymphoma, neuroblastoma, embryonic kidney cell, hamster ovary, rat adrenal cell with a known cell surface protein panel are spotted on poly-lysine coated microscope slides at a density on average	1 Identification of drug targets and as an expression cloning system for the discovery of gene products that alter cellular physiology and immunological responses Detection of possibly new role for proteins Direct screening of microarray cell clusters for abnormal morphology Detection of transient phenotypes such as change in intracellular calcium concentration or the movement of GFP tagged protein 2 Characterization of panels of membrane protein specific-antibodies (CD45, CD3, MCH class I and II, EGFR)	Extraordinary small amount of antibody that needed to be used for binding studies Efficient conversion of DNA microarrays which are stables for months into live-protein arrays when needed	Rapid characterization of different binding molecules against strongly expressed cell surface antigens not quantitative assay	1 Ziauddin and Sabatini (2000) 2 Schwenk et al. (2000)

TARP tissue arrys	of 18 cells/spot and used to generate cell microarrays TARP5 T-BO-1-TARP Breast and ovarian cancer array T-Pr-1TARP Prostate cancer array T-CL-1-TARP Colon and lung cancer array T-MT-1-Tarp Mixed tumor array (coming soon)	FISH, _in situ_ hybridization, immunofluorescence (including confocal), immunohistochemistry and in traditional histo-chemical staining methods Additional methodologies are being developed There are limitations – laser capture micro-dissection cannot be used on tissue array slides	Variable upon type of assay	http://ccr.cancer.gov/tech_initiatives/tarp/faq.asp
Frozen protein arrays	Wells made in a frozen block of embedding material are filled with biological samples, which freeze and bond to the surrounding block The loaded block is cut in a cryostat and sections are transferred to nitrocellulose slides Frozen protein arrays can also detect native tissue proteins	Detection of protein using antibodies for Western blotting or other types of biological assays	>10 µl/well protein lysates, tissue homogenates	Fluorescence intensity	Miyaji et al. (2000) http://www.niddk.nih.gov/intram/people/rstar.htm
SearchLight™	The SearchLight array utilizes a special plate pre-spotted with up to 16 different capture antibodies per well. Following a simple ELISA procedure, the array generates a chemiluminescent signal that is imaged using a commercially-available 12-bit or 16-bit cooled CCD camera. Using array software, the intensity of the spots for each unknown sample are	70 known cytokines, chemokines and soluble factors GMCSF, IFN alpha, IFN gamma, IL-1 alpha, IL-1 beta, IL-2, IL-4, IL-5, IL-6, IL-7, IL-8, IL-9, IL-10, IL-12p70, IL-13, IL-15, IL-16, IL-18, TNF alpha, ENA-78, Eotaxin, Exodus II, GRO alpha, I-309, IP-10, I-TAC, Lymphotactin, MCP-1, MCP-2, MCP-3, MCP-4, MDC, MIG, MIP-1 alpha, MIP-1 beta, MIP-3 alpha, MIP-3 beta, NAP-2, SDF-1 beta, RANTES, Tarc, ANG-2, FGF-basic, KGF, HGF, HB-EGF, PDGF-BB, TIMP-1, TIMP-2, Tpo,	Serum, plasma, tumor tissue lysates, lavage fluids broncoalveolar lavage (BAL), nipple aspirate fluid (NAF), cerebrospinal fluid, nasopharingeal fluid, gyneco/cervical lavage, ascites of peritoneal lavage, culture media	10–50 µl	pg/ml	http://www.piercenet.com/ www.searchlightonline.com

Table 59.2 *Continued*

Protein chip/array platform type	Multiplexed protein assay	Detection of known/unknown proteins	Size/sample	Sensitivity/limit of detection	Reference/website
SearchLight™ (cont.)	compared with standard curves and exact values of each cytokine (pg/ml) are calculated	VEGF, MMP-1, MMP-2, MMP-3, MMP-8, MMP-9, MMP-10, MMP-13, BDNF, CNTF, LIF, E-Selectin, L-Selectin, ICAM-1, VCAM, IL-12p40, IL-6R, TNFaR1, TNFaR2, and lactoferrin			
ProVision™	Monoclonal antibodies bound to 3D-nitrocellulose coated glass (FAST™ slide surface). Each slide contains eight identical arrays of 16 monoclonal capture antibodies in triplicate. The antibody pairs the cytokine antigen in a 'sandwich type' assay. Cytokine detection is fluorescence based (streptavidin-linked) fluorophore (Cy3-Cy5) binds biotin labeled secondary antibody. Fluorescence can be detected by standard microarray scanner	16 known cytokines, Chemokines and soluble Factors simultaneously: Angiogenin, IL-2, IL-10, TNF RII, ICAM-1, IL-4, IL-12 p40, TGF-β1, IFN-γ, IL-6, IL-12 p70, TNF-α, IL-1β, IL-8, IP-10, VEGF	20–30 μl serum, plasma, tissue lysate, cerebrospinal fluid	pg/ml intensity values	http://www.schleicher-schuell.com/icm11be.nsf/(html)/FramesetBioScience
Zyomyx Protein Profiling Biochip™ System	The Zyomyx protein biochip platform consists of a micro-fabricated silicon microarray containing 1200 addressable features partitioned into six individually assayable flowcells. Each biochip supports the analysis of up to six 40 μl samples assayed with up to 200 distinct	30 known cytokines, chemokines and soluble factors simultaneously: IL-1α, IL-3, IL-6, IL-10, IL-12 (p70), TNF-α, MCP-1, CD95 (sFas), IP-10, GM-CSF, IL-1β, IL-4, IL-7, IL-12 (p40), IL-13, TNF-β, MCP-3, MIG, CD23, GCSF, IL-2, IL-5, IL-8, IL-12 (p40/p70), IL-15, Eotaxin, TRAIL, sICAM-1, TGF-β, IFN-γ	Up to 40 μl synovial fluid, cell lysates, serum, plasma and tissue culture supernatants	Intensity value/ transformed in pg/ml high-density analyte binding, high assay sensitivity and reduced non-specific binding	http://www.zyomyx.com/products/cytokine.html

Zyomyx Protein (cont.)	maximizing the amount of biological information gained from valuable biological samples Each array feature is printed with capture molecules of a single specificity, each specificity is printed in 5-fold redundancy in order to provide statistical information. Twelve microliters of sample are loaded in each flowcell and processed in a workstation capable of processing up to 12 biochips in parallel. The signal output is fluorescence which can be read in Zyomyx fluorescent scanner.				immunoassays,	
RayBio™ Human Cytokine Array I-IV	Monoclonal antibodies embedded in membrane array	124 known cytokines, chemokines and soluble factors 4-1BB/TNFRSF9, adiponectin/Acrp30, AgRP(ART), Angiogenin Angiopoietin-2, AR (amphiregulin) Axl, BDNF, bFGF, BLC, BMP-4, BMP-6, b-NGF, BTC CCL28/VIC, CK b 8-1, CNTF CTACK/CCL27, Dtk, EGF, EGF R,ENA-78, Eotaxin, Eotaxin-2, Eotaxin-3, Fas/TNFRSF6, FGF-4, FGF-6, FGF-7, FGF-9, Flt-3L, Fractalkine, GCP-2, GCSF, GDNF, GITR Ligand/TNFSF18, GITR/TNFRF18, GM-CSF, GRO, GRO-a, HCC-4/ CCL16, HGF, I-309,	100 µl	pg/ml Intensity signal measured by densitometry (x-ray film) or by chemiluminescence		http://www.raybiotech.com/product.htm

Table 59.2 *Continued*

Protein chip/array platform type	Multiplexed protein assay	Detection of known/unknown proteins	Size/sample	Sensitivity/limit of detection	Reference/website
		ICAM-1, ICAM-3, IFN-g, IGFBP-1, IGFBP-2, IGFBP-3, IGFBP-4, IGFBP-6, IGF-I, IGF-I SR, IL-1 R4/ST2, IL-1sRI, IL-1sRII, IL-10, IL-12 p40p70, IL-12 p40, IL-12 p70, IL-13, IL-15, IL-16, IL-17, IL-1a, IL-1b, IL-1ra, IL-2, IL-2 sRa, IL-3, IL-4, IL-5, IL-6, IL-6 sR, IL-7, IL-8, IP-10, I-TAC/CXCL11, LEPTIN(OB), LIF, LIGHT, Lymphotactin, MCP-1, MCP-2, MCP-3, MCP-4, MCSF, MDC, MIF, MIG, MIP-1a, MIP-1b, MIP-1d, MIP-3 alpha, MIP-3b, MSPa, NAP-2, NT-3, NT-4, Osteoprotegerin, oncostatin M, PARC, PDGF-BB, PlGF, RANTES, SCF, SDF-1, sgp130, sTNF RII/TNFRS1B, sTNT RI/TNFRS1A, TARC, TECK/CCL25, TGF-β1, TGF-β2, TGF-β3, TIMP-1, TIMP-2, TNF-α, TNF-β, Thrombopoietin, TRAILs R3/TNFRS10C, TRAIL s R4/TNFRS10D, uPAR, VEGF, VEGF-D			
The ProteinChip® Biomarker System	Cyphergen proteinChip system analyzes proteins captured on protein chip arrays by means of surface enhanced laser desorption ionization (SELDI) technology. Chemical surfaces (reverse phase, cation	Pattern profiling\n\nOn biochemical surfaces single protein capture (see Table 59.1)	1–2 μl amount of material required; slightly more (20 μl) with prefractionation procedures	The SELDI-QqTOF platform provides a more direct route to protein ID by enabling on-chip tandem MS for peptide sequencing\nRapid, on-chip immunoaffinity identification protocols for SELDI when antibodies exist to tentatively identified markers	http://www.ciphergen.com/

Name	Description	Analytes	Sample	Sensitivity	Website
The ProteinChip (cont.)	exchange/WCX2, anion exchange/SAX2, immobilized metal affinity capture/IMAC, hydrophobic/C16, normal phase/SiO₂) Biochemical surface (PS-1, PS-2, antibody- antigen, receptor ligand, DNA- protein)				
LiquidChip™ Protein Suspension Array System Qiaexpress	Analytes bind to capture molecules immobilized in bead suspension and are quantified using fluorescence detection reagent. Capture molecules are bound to beads by 6xHis-tag technology, biotin avidin interaction or covalent coupling chemistry	10 cytokines and 7 kinases: IL-1b, IL-2, IL-4,IL-6, IL-8, IL-10, IL-12(p70), GMCSF, IFN-g, TNF-α, JNK, P38-MAKP, SPK 4, PKB-α, PKC, ErK-2, GSKb	Cell lysate, supernatant	Fluorescence intensity pg/ml	http://www1.qiagen.com/
eTAG™	The eTag Assay System uses eTag reporters, low molecular weight fluorescent proteins bound to a specific antibody or protein recognition element and high performance, solution-phase chemistries to multiplex the analysis of genes and proteins from the same sample and directly from cell lysates The molecular binding events that occur during a reaction between an analyte and its binding partner	eTag Cytokine 7-Plex Assay quantifying cytokine expression in cell-based or soluble samples IL1a, IL2, IL4, IL6, IL8, IFNg, and TNF-α Cell based binding assays. In this context a lipophilic molecular scissor reagent is intercalated into the cell membrane of most cell types, including primary human cells. Recognition elements or cognate receptor ligands (such as CD40L, CD47, CD81, CD82, HLA-A, B, C, CD69) are labeled differentially with unique eTag reporters eTag Multiplex Cytochrome P450 Protein Assay for	10 µl supernatants, cell lysates	1 pM	http://www.aclara.com/gene_protein_assays.asp

Table 59.2 *Continued*

Protein chip/array platform type	Multiplexed protein assay	Detection of known/unknown proteins	Size/sample	Sensitivity/limit of detection	Reference/website
	(antibody or protein recognition element) result in the release of electrophoretically distinct eTag reporters, which are then resolved by capillary electrophoresis to provide very sensitive quantification of multipe analytes The eTag Informer software identifies and quantifies eTag reporter molecules The signals from the eTag reporters are proportional to the concentrations of cytokines present.	toxicoproteomic analysis following stimulation of cells or tissues by lead compounds (in development)			

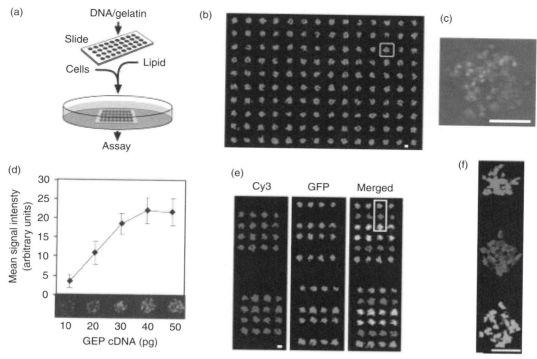

Figure 59.5 Well-less transfection of plasmid DNAs in defined areas of a lawn of mammalian cells. (a) Protocol for making microarrays of transfected cells. (b) Laser scan image of a GFP-expressing microarray made from a slide printed in a 14 10 pattern with a GFP expression construct . (c) Higher magnification image obtained with fluorescence microscopy of the cell cluster boxed in b. Scale bar, 100 μm. (d) Expression levels of cell clusters in a microarray are proportional, over a fourfold range, to the amount of plasmid DNA printed on the slide. Indicated amounts of the GFP construct assume a 1-nl printing volume. The graph shows the mean s.d. of the fluorescence intensities of the cell clusters ($n = 6$). The fluorescent image is from a representative expirement. (e) Co-transfection is possible with transfected cell microarrays. Arrays with elements containing expression constructs for HA-GST, GFP or both were transfected and processed for immunofluorescence and imaged with a laser scanner. Cy3, cell clusters expressing HA-GST; GFP, cell clusters expressing GFP; merged, superimposition of Cy3 and GFP signals. Yellow colour indicates co-expression. Scale bar, 100 μm. (f) Enlarged view of boxed area of scan image from (e). **See colour plate 59.5.**

Tissue arrays/example of TARP arrays

The Tissue Array Research Program (TARP) is a collaborative effort between The National Cancer Institute and The National Human Genome Research Institute. TARP has been developing and distributing Multi-tumor Tissue Microarray slides and the related technology to cancer research investigators. TARP 5 are the currently available arrays and spot breast, ovarian, prostate and colon tissues. This technology is very promising and can provide a tool for high throughput screening of multiple tumor tissues using immunohistochemical, *in situ* and FISH analyses. The majority of the tissue used to construct the TARP arrays is obtained from the Cooperative Human Tissue Network (CHTN). This material is formalin-fixed, paraffin-embedded tissue. The tissue is anonymous and de-linked and is obtained with the understanding that it will be used to depletion. Any of the following can be performed on these arrays: FISH, *in situ* hybridization, immunofluorescence (including confocal), immunohistochemistry and traditional histochemical staining methods. Additional methodologies are being developed. There are, however, limitations: for instance, laser capture micro-dissection cannot be performed on tissue array slides (see Table 59.2).

Reverse phase antigen arrays

Paweletz et al. (2001) and Shreekumar and Chinnaiyan (2002) have recently described reverse phase protein arrays that immobilize the whole repertoire of patient proteins or tumor cell lines in the form of lysate arrayed onto nitrocellulose slides (see below). A high degree of sensitivity, precision and linearity was achieved, making it possible to quantify the phosphorylated status of signal proteins in human tissue cell subpopulations (Paweletz) or tumor antigens (Shreekumar and Chinnaiyan). Slides containing the arrayed lysate were probed with Cy3/Cy5 labeled antibodies and normalized to actin.

Frozen protein arrays

This is an economical method of arraying liquid samples (protein lysates, tissue homogenates) and detecting proteins using antibodies developed for Western blotting or other types of biological assays. Wells made in a frozen block of histologic embedding compound (Miyaji et al., 2002) are filled with biological samples, which freeze and bond to the surrounding block. The loaded block is cut in a cryostat and sections are transferred to nitrocellulose-coated slides. The reproducibility, linearity and sensitivity have been tested using protein arrays filled with prostate specific antigen (PSA) and reported to be excellent. Frozen protein arrays could also detect native tissue proteins Nak-ATPase, with good correlation with Western blotting. Thus, frozen protein arrays are a low cost, moderate size platform for arraying samples. Production of many identical frozen protein arrays is easy, inexpensive and requires only small sample volumes (see Table 59.2).

REPRESENTATIVE COMMERCIAL PROTEIN ARRAY TECHNOLOGIES

A constantly increasing number of proteomic platforms is reaching the benchside, transforming not only the way many immunological and biological assays are conducted but enormously increasing the amount of output data and critical information obtainable at once. Furthermore, these high-throughput technologies are making their appearance in clinical diagnostics laboratories allowing rapid and simultaneous screening of multiple biomarkers of immune responses and disease. Representative protein array technologies are summarized here and in Table 59.1. Features and protein-specificity of the associated arrays are presented in Table 59.2.

Searchlight™ Proteome Arrays

SearchLight™ Proteome Arrays (Pierce-Endogen, Boston, MA) are multiplexed assays that measure up to 16 proteins per well. They are produced by spotting up to 16 different monoclonal antibodies into each well of a 96-well plate. Following a typical sandwich ELISA procedure, signal is generated using a chemiluminescent substrate. The light produced at each spot in the array is captured by imaging the entire plate with a commercially available cooled CCD camera (Alpha Immunotech corporation Fluorchem™). The data are reduced using image analysis software that calculates the exact values (pg/ml) for unknowns from standard curves.

This type of platform has the power of analyzing 70 different chemokines, cytokines and soluble factors in a variety of physiological fluids and culture media (see Table 59.2.). We have employed Searchlight™ arrays in several studies analyzing the effect of IL-2 stimulation of peripheral blood mononuclear cells (PBMC) in vitro (Panelli et al., 2003), the effect of maturing dendritic cells with cytokines (Nagorsen et al., 2003) and the level of chemokines cytokines and soluble factors in the serum of patients undergoing high dose IL-2 therapy (manuscript in preparation).

Provision™ arrays

Another very powerful technology in glass slides based protein arrays is ProVision™ (Schleicher and Schuell Bioscience, Keene, NH). Capture monoclonal antibodies are bound to 3D-nitrocellulose-coated glass (FAST™ slide surface). FAST™ slides are glass slides coated with a proprietary nitrocellulose polymer which binds proteins in a non-covalent, irreversible manner and can be probed using the same method as in traditional blots. One visible advantage of this surface is that it is usable with fluorescent, chemiluminescent or radiographic detection systems and is compatible with microarray scanners and robots. Another major advantage of FAST slides over modified glass surfaces is that the matrix retains arrayed proteins in near-quantitative manner. This property allows for the manufacturing of antibody arrays with very high sensitivity. Each slide contains eight identical arrays of 16 monoclonal capture antibodies in triplicate. The antibody pairs the unknown antigen in a sandwich type assay. The nitrocellulose binding surface makes the array very versatile and suitable for binding multiple types of chemokines, cytokines and soluble factors (16) to capture reagents simultaneously (see Table 59.2). This platform has been used successfully by the authors to measure the amount of chemokines, cytokines and soluble factors in the serum of patients undergoing high dose IL-2 therapy (manuscript in preparation).

Zyomyx Protein Profiling Biochip™ System

Protein Profiling Biochip™ supports the analysis of up to six 40 μl samples assayed with up to 200 distinct immunoassays. Zyomyx Biochips are compatible with diverse sample types (see Table 59.2). The Zyomyx protein profiling biochip™ (Zyomyx, CA) platform consists of a micro-fabricated silicon microarray containing 1200 addressable features (3D pillar structures) partitioned into six individually assayable flowcells. The array possesses a unique surface chemistry consisting of a well-defined thin film that enables immobilization of directionally oriented capture agents such as antibodies. Each array feature is printed with capture molecules of a single specificity, each specificity is printed in 5-fold redundancy in order to provide statistical information. Direct liquid transfer protein dispensing technology allows simultaneous deposition of capture agents across the entire biochip. Twelve microliters (and up to 40 μl) of sample is loaded in each flowcell and processed in a workstation capable of running up to 12 biochips in parallel. The signal output is fluorescence, which can be read in a Zyomyx fluorescent scanner. This immobilization of capture agents allows for high-density analyte binding, high assay sensitivity and reduced non-specific binding. We have utilized the human cytokine biochip to screen for 30 proteins potentially secreted by immature and mature dendritic cells (DC) (Nagorsen et al., 2003) and to analyze the effect of IL-2 stimulation of PBMC in vitro (Panelli et al., 2003).

RayBio™ Human Cytokine Array I–IV

Surfaces other than glass or plastic have been used to generate multiplex protein arrays. The RayBio™ Human Cytokine Array I–IV (www.Raybiotech.com) consists of a proprietary membrane in which captured monoclonal antibodies specific for multiple antigens (124 cytokines, chemokines and soluble factors) are embedded. The analyte is incubated on the membrane with a cocktail of biotin-labeled antibodies and subsequently with streptavidin-HRP. Intensity of signal is measured by chemiluminescence or by densitometry (x-ray film).

LiquidChip™ Protein Suspension Array System Qiaexpress

LiquidChip™ Protein Suspension Array System Qiaexpress (Qiagen, San Diego, Ca) is based on the XMAP™ technology. Capture molecules are immobilized in bead suspension by 6xHis-tag technology, biotin avidin interaction or covalent coupling chemistry. Analytes bind to capture molecules immobilized in bead suspension and are quantified using fluorescence detection reagents that carry fluorosphores whose emission wavelength and high fluorescence make detection very sensitive. This bead-based platform offers the potential to assay up to 100 different analytes in a single sample. Several platforms have been constructed and are available for various cytokines and kinases (see Table 59.2).

Surface enhanced laser desorption ionization (SELDI) technology

Ciphergen ProteinChip system (Ciphergen, Fremont, CA) analyzes proteins captured on protein chip arrays by means of surface enhanced laser desorption ionization (SELDI) technology (see Tables 59.1, 59.2 and 59.4). A protein chip reader is integrated with protein chip software. This technology is based on specific capture of proteins through chemical interaction (chemical surfaces) or protein–protein interaction (biochemical surfaces). Chemical surfaces include reverse phase, cation exchange/WCX2, anion exchange/SAX2, immobilized metal affinity capture/IMAC, hydrophobic/C16, normal phase/SiO2. Biochemical surfaces include PS-1, PS-2, antibody–antigen, receptor ligand, DNA–protein. Processing of sample and chip preparation can be automated and consists essentially of three steps:

1 application of crude sample: proteins within the sample bind to chemical or biological 'docking sites' on the ProteinChip surface through an affinity interaction
2 protein chip wash: proteins that bind non-specifically or buffer contaminants are washed away, eliminating sample 'noise'
3 addition of energy absorbing material (EAM): after sample processing the chip is dried and EAM is applied to each spot to facilitate desorption and ionization in the ProteinChip Reader (Figure 59.6).

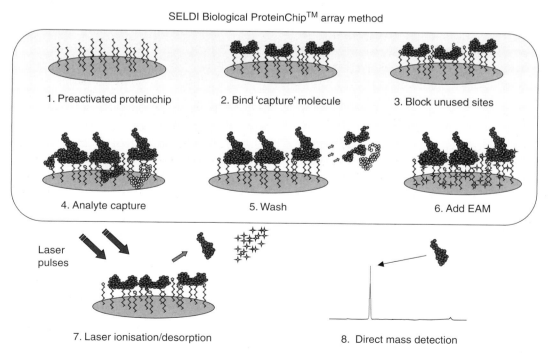

SELDI Biological ProteinChip™ array method

1. Preactivated proteinchip   2. Bind 'capture' molecule   3. Block unused sites

4. Analyte capture   5. Wash   6. Add EAM

Laser pulses

7. Laser ionisation/desorption   8. Direct mass detection

Figure 59.6 SELDI Biological PoteinChip™ Array Method. **See colour plate 59.6.**

This technology has been widely implemented in the discovery and detection of biomarker and surrogate of diseases and cancer (see Figure 59.6).

eTag Assay System

The eTag Assay System (ACLARA, Mountain View, CA) uses eTag reporters, low molecular weight fluorescent proteins bound to a specific antibody or protein recognition element and high performance, solution-phase chemistries to multiplex the analysis of genes and proteins from the same sample and directly from cell lysates. A critical feature of these types of proteomic assays is that the affinity agents (e.g. antibodies, peptides, small molecules, aptamers, etc.) are not immobilized on surfaces. Solution-based binding eliminates surface-induced denaturation and non-specific binding and improves sensitivity and reaction kinetics. The molecular binding events that occur during a reaction between an analyte and its binding partner (antibody or protein recognition element) results in the release of electrophoretically distinct eTag reporters, which are then resolved by capillary electrophoresis to provide very sensitive quantification of multiple analytes. The eTag Informer software is then capable of identifying and quantifying eTag reporter molecules. Standard or custom reports can also be exported for further data analysis. A large number of eTag reporters and a broad menu of assay chemistries (intracellular and secreted proteins, cell surface proteins, protein modifications, protein–protein interactions) have been developed. eTag Multiplex Protein Proximity Assays uses a sandwich format and can quantify cytokine expression in cell-based or soluble samples (eTag Cytokine 7-Plex Assay). The signals from the eTag reporters are proportional to the concentrations of cytokines present. eTag Multiplex Cytochrome P450 Protein Assay can be used for toxicoproteomic analysis following stimulation of cells or tissues by lead compounds (assay in development). The eTag technology can also be applied for cell-based binding assays. In this context a lipophilic molecular scissor reagent is intercalated into the cell membrane of most cell types, including primary human cells. Recognition elements or cognate receptor ligands (such as CD40L, CD47, CD81, CD82, HLA-A, B, C, CD69) are labeled differentially with unique eTag reporters. Upon specific binding and subsequent exposure of the assay to the proper light wavelength, eTag reporters attached to proteins bound to cells are released into solution (see Table 59.2)

Sensor chips surface plasmon resonance (SPR)

This a new technology with high sensitivity that can be used to assay for a single analyte in a number of specimens, protein–protein interaction analysis, identification of disease markers in clinical samples, quantitative measurement of binding interaction and specificity between molecules, ligand fishing. Surface plasmon resonance (SPR) (Biacore-USA) arises when light is reflected under certain conditions from a conducting film at the interface between two media of different refractive index. In Biacore systems the media are the sample and the glass of the sensor chip and the conducting film is a thin layer of gold on the chip surface. SPR causes a reduction in the intensity of reflected light at a specific angle of reflection. This angle varies with the refractive index close to the surface on the side opposite from the reflected light (the sample side in Biacore). Binding of the sample molecule to the sensor surface, causes the concentration and therefore the refractive index at the surface to change which, in turn, allows detection of an SPR response. Plotting the response against time during the course of an interaction provides a quantitative measure of the progress of the interaction (sensorgram plot). What Biacore actually measures is the angle of minimum reflected light intensity. The light is not absorbed by the sample: instead the light energy is dissipated through SPR in the gold film.

Other technologies supporting protein arrays manufacturing and automated high throughput protein analysis

Accelr8 technology

OptArray™-Protein slides and OptiPlate™-Protein arraying microplates have OptiChem™ and are an example of activated microarraying surfaces whose coatings are optimized for immobilizing peptides and proteins by covalent binding to available amine groups. A long hydrophilic linking tether extends from the no-block inert matrix to provide probe mobility in the solution phase and to help preserve protein activity. Optimized contact angle helps keep spot size small and morphology uniform. These surfaces can be used in multiplex protein arrays and in micro ELISA type assays (Table 59.3).

Protein array workstation™

Protein array workstations can be used to automate fully the processing of multiple protein microarrays using the desired capture molecules. Several complete systems are now available and new developments promise to soon match high throughput DNA technologies. One such example is the PerkinElmer set of equipment designed to take the process of protein array assays from start to finish: from slide making, sample loading, incubation, detection and data evaluation. Proteins can be spotted on special substrates such as HydroGel™-coated slides using protein microarray printing technologies such as Piezo Tipnology™, a non-contact ink-jet technology that does not heat samples during dispensing. Protein array workstation™ can automatically load multiple samples onto slides and perform the appropriate analyte binding protocol. Finally, intensities of fluorochrome-labeled protein bound to arrays are detected by scanners (Scan Array™

Table 59.3 State of the art equipment for protein arrays

Technology	Sensitivity	Utilization	Advantages and disadvantages
OptArray™-Protein slides and OptiPlate™-Protein arraying microplates	OptArray™-Protein slides and OptiPlate™-Protein arraying microplates have OptiChem™ activated microarraying surfaces whose coatings are optimized for immobilizing peptides and proteins by covalent binding to available amine groups	Variable depending on the the desired amount of capture molecule Surfaces can be used for custom protein microarrays	http://www.accelr8.com/pagegen.php?key = products-optarray_protein
HydroGel™	Coated slides with 3D substrate which accommodates high probe capacity and allows for preservation of protein function	Surfaces can be used for custom protein microarrays	http://las.perkinelmer.com/
FAST™ slide surface	FAST™ Slides are glass slides coated with a proprietary nitrocellulose polymer which binds proteins in a non-covalent, irreversible manner and can be probed using the same method as in traditional blots	Custom protein microarrays Usable with fluorescent, chemiluminescent or radiographic detection systems compatible with DNAmicroarray scanners and robots Matrix retains arrayed proteins in near-quantitative manner	http://www.schleicher-schuell.com/icm11be.nsf/(html)/FramesetBioScience
Biochip or Spot array™ Enterprise arrayers	Non-contact ink-jet technology no heating of samples during dispensing	Arrayer for protein chips	http://las.perkinelmer.com/

Express) and analyzed by specific software packages (Quantarrays). Array-based multiplex screening and quantitation of 43 human chemokines and cytokines using this system has been recently reported (Wang et al., 2002).

LiquidChip™ Protein Suspension Array System Qiaexpress

Another fully automated system capable of providing high throughput protein analysis is the LiquidChip™ Protein Suspension Array System (Qiagen, San Diego, Ca) based on the XMAP™ technology (see description above). This bead-based platform offers the potential to assay up to 100 different analytes in a single sample. Platforms have been constructed and are available for various cytokines and kinases (see Tables 59.2 and 59.3) and are now designed to accommodate any type of compound to any type of bead set (Activated bead set). The process of array preparation and liquid handling is provided by a robotic unit (Biorobot 3000), while chip processing and reading is conducted by the LiquidChip™ workstation which includes chip reader, microplate handler and fluid module. Data are analyzed using an integrated system software.

UTILITY OF PROTEIN ARRAYS IN EVALUATING DISEASE STATES AND IMMUNE RESPONSES

The applications of proteomics technologies and, in particular, protein arrays, has been the basis of several clinical studies and are beginning to be employed to characterize a wide range of pathological states: autoimmune diseases, allergy, host immune responses against pathogenic organisms and cancer. Each of these diseases features thousands of biological variables that ultimately are expressed by proteins or peptides derived from host peripheral circulation, different organs, tissues and tumor microenvironment. Most often the object of analysis is represented by fragments resulting from the metabolism, enzymatic degradation or protein–protein interactions of host cells. Serum, plasma, saliva, urine, cerebrospinal fluid (CSF), skin blister fluids, stools, peripheral blood mononuclear cells, organs or tumor tissue (excisional biopsies or fine needle aspirates), lavage fluids (bronchoalveolar lavage, nipple aspirate fluids, gyneco-cervical lavage and ascites) represent the major sources of biological material accessible for immunological studies and biomarker discovery.

The following reports reflect the current status of the utilization of protein arrays.

Autoimmune disease/chronic inflammatory disease

In spite of significant research efforts, the etiology of the majority of autoimmune diseases such as rheumatoid arthritis (RA), multiple sclerosis (MS), autoimmune diabetes, insulin dependent diabetes mellitus (IDDM), remains poorly understood. Current research suggests that autoimmunity arises in genetically predisposed individuals possibly following exposure to environmental triggers. Proteomic technologies represent a powerful and promising strategy to identify pathogens and self-proteins involved in the initiation and progression of autoimmune diseases (Robinson et al., 2002a). Robinson and coworkers (2002b) recently constructed miniaturized *autoantigen arrays* to perform large-scale multiplex characterization of autoantibody responses directed against distinct autoantigens, utilizing only submicroliter quantities of clinical serum samples. Autoantigen microarrays were generated by attaching hundreds of proteins, peptides and other biomolecules to the surface of derivatized glass slides using a robotic arrayer. Spectrally resolvable fluorescent labels were used to detect autoantibody–autoantigens binding on the array. The major autoantigens in eight distinct human autoimmune diseases, including systemic lupus erythematosus and rheumatoid arthritis were included in the autoantigen array. Autoantigen arrays represent a platform for future validation and detection of antibodies recognizing autoantigens including proteins, peptides, enzyme complexes, ribonucleoprotein complexes, DNA and post-translationally modified antigens. Although there is debate upon the relevance of autoantibodies directed against linear epitopes, antigen arrays enable simultaneous profiling of autoantibodies specific for both conformational epitopes contained in recombinant proteins as well as linear epitopes represented by peptides (Robinson et al., 2002a). Monitoring of immunotherapies of children with autoimmune diseases is particularly difficult due to small samples volume (sera) obtainable from this patient population. de Jager et al. (2003) were able to overcome this limitation by using protein arrays (Bioplex from BioRad Laboratories) to detect simultaneously 15 human cytokines in cell culture supernatant. This multiplex system, combining the principle of a sandwich immunoassay with the Luminex-fluorescent bead technology, was able to detect and quantify cytokines from both autoimmune (juvenile idiopathic arthritis) and healthy individuals.

Immune responses against pathogenic organisms

Microbial diseases remain the most common cause of worldwide mortality. Progress in understanding how the immune response ultimately succumbs to or controls infection and growth of microbial organisms is of vital importance. A number of genomes of microbial organisms (*Plasmodium, Toxoplasma, Mycobacterium, Streptococcus, Neisseria, Salmonella, Borrelia* and *Rickettsia*) have already been sequenced and high throughput proteomic technologies, such as antigen arrays, offer the opportunity to identify the microbial antigens that either alone or in combination are the target of natural acquired immunity against infectious diseases. The only limiting step for the development of arrays containing the entire parasitic and bacterial proteome is the high throughput production and purification of microbial proteins (Bacarese-Hamilton et al., 2002). However, Bacarese-Hamilton and coworkers

are currently developing the first protein chip that will contain most of the *P. falciparum* antigens.

Microarrays consisting of printed spots of microbial antigens have been recently employed for determination of the presence of specific IgG or IgM antibodies directed against other parasitic and viral antigens (*Toxoplasma,* cytomegalovirus, rubella and herpesvirus) in human sera. These microbial arrays incorporate internal calibration curves for each Ig subclass, which is a crucial advantage over current immunoassay protocols (Mezzasoma et al., 2002). Furthermore, rolling circle amplification (RCA described above) has very much increased the sensitivity of detection of this array type (Schweitzer et al., 2002).

In yet another report, Robinson and coworkers (Neuman et al., 2003) developed antigen microarrays to profile the breadth, strength and kinetics of epitope specific antiviral antibody responses in vaccine trials with a simian-immunodeficiency virus (SHIV).These arrays contained 430 distinct proteins and overlapping peptides spanning the SHIV proteome. Loaded with sera, these arrays were able to distinguish vaccinated (with vaccines encoding Gag-Pol, Gag-Pol-Env) from challenged macaques, identified three novel viral epitopes and predicted survival.

Allergy

Allergen microarrays have also been developed based on the principle of antigen arrays. High sensitivity arrays capable of revealing the presence of allergen-specific IgE in human sera have been described by Bacarese-Hamilton et al. (2002). Multiplexed allergen arrays consisting of 24 recombinant and purified allergens have successfully discriminated between patients with and without elevated levels of allergen-specific IgE (Fall et al., 2003).

Cancer/immunotherapy monitoring

We recently summarized current achievements in biomarker detection and the related proteomic technology (Panelli and Burns, 2004) for several different types of cancer. We refer the reader to the summary in Table 59.4. Protein chip SELDI technology has been widely implemented in many of these studies. However, a combination of several different proteomic approaches usually resulted in the final identification of a specific biomarker or pattern profiling that could segregate among normal, early stages or progressing disease samples.

Antibody arrays can be very useful for monitoring and assessing the effects of immune or drug-therapy in cancer patients. We have used protein arrays for high throughput detection of cytokines, chemokines and soluble factors in the serum of patients with renal cell cancer receiving the systemic administration of high dose IL-2 (Panelli et al., 2003; Panelli et al. 2004). A Searchlight™ (see Table 59.2) custom made (antibody–based platform including 70 different cytokines, chemokines and soluble factors) was commercially developed to measure crude serum levels of

Table 59.4 State of the art achievements in cancer biomarker detection

Reference	Type of cancer/clinical study	Source of biological material	Proteomic technology of choice	Biomarker/ surrogate	Significance and potential
Petricoin et al. (2002a)	Ovarian	Crude serum	SELDI-TOF C16 chip Bioinformatics/pattern generation: use of genetic algorithm to obtain a pattern that best segregates between training sets of spectra from sera of ovarian cancer and normal New recent development; High resolution mass spec ABI Hybrid Pulsar QqTOF (Q-Star) fitted with Ciphergen SELDI	Cluster pattern	Identification of Finding justifies prospective population-based assessment of proteomic pattern technology as a screening tool for all stages of ovarian cancer in high risk and general population Problems with spectra alignment machine-to-machine variance and reproducibility. New adjustment to the configuration of SELDI introduced an enormous increase in resolution and increase in mass accuracy. Introduction of the Q-star has the potential to allow for sequence analysis and identification of the ions that comprise the diagnostic information
Kim et al. (2002)	Epithelial ovarian	Preoperative plasma, tumor tissue, control normal ovarian tissue	MICROMAX RNA arrays Immunohistochemistry (IHC) Laser capture microdissection (LCM) ELISA	Osteopontin	Invasive ovarian cancer tissue and borderline ovarian tumors higher levels of osteopontin than benign tumors. Osteopontin level in plasma of epithelial ovarian cancer significantly higher than controls, benign ovarian disease and other gynecological cancers Potential useful screening marker for early asymptomatic disease
Nishizuka et al. (2003)	Ovarian, colon Multistep protocol NCI*	Ovarian and colon cell lines	Multistep protocol: 1 cDNA microarrays 2 clone verification by resequencing 3 Affimetrix oligo chips 4 Reverse protein lysate microarrays 5 Validation on candidate markers by TARP tissue microarrays	Villin (colon cancer) Moiesin (ovarian cancer)	Potential for differential diagnosis of colon and ovarian malignancies, discrimination of colon from ovarian carcinoma in ovarian masses, peritoneal carcinomatosis and metastasis to distant lymph nodes Multistep process potential to produce additional markers for cancer diagnosis, prognosis and therapy
Kozak et al. (2003)	Ovarian	Unfractionated serum	SELDI-TOF-MS; SAX2 Protein Chip Arrays	Three recursively partitioned pattern models generated comprised of a total of 13 protein peaks	Both the potential for early detection screening and differentiation of benign versus malignant disease is presented. ROC areas under the curve were in the range of 0.90 to 0.94 Contrary to other reports of SELDI and MALDI having limited utility in a relatively low mass range of detection, the 13 protein peaks uncovered in this study ranged up to 106.7 kDa
Ye et al. (2003)	Ovarian	Unfractionated serum Ovarian cell lines	SELDI- TOF-MS IMAC-3 chip Affinity chromatography SDS-PAGE LC-MS/ MS for aa sequence	Pattern profiling + identification of protein in discriminatory patterns	Elevated levels of Hp-α in ovarian cancer patients seen. As a single marker, the predictive power of Hp- α appeared lower than CA-125, but may be complementary to it in a multi-marker profile

Table 59.4 *Continued*

Reference	Type of cancer/clinical study	Source of biological material	Proteomic technology of choice	Biomarker/ surrogate	Significance and potential
Ye et al. (cont.)			Peptide synthesis and specific development PCR and western blot testing for over expression in tumor cells	A serum biomarker at ~11 700 Da was identified as the α chain of haptoglobin	A candidate biomarker of 11.7 kDa was rapidly picked up in this study using the SELDI platform; ID was accomplished with a combination of affinity column enrichment, SELDI monitoring of fractions, digestion and LC-MS/MS Protein profiling valuable tool for screening potential biomarkers but confirmation of protein identity with specific antibodies and classical immune assays is crucial for clinical application and functional studies Proteolytic cleavage of Hp a from b detected in the presence of cancer serum only and not in cancer cells, Hp a subunit elevation caused by specific enzymatic cleavage and abnormal protein–protein interaction in the circulation of cancer patients rather then in the tumor Evidence for potential detection of metabolic peptide biomarkers and post-translational modifications by proteomics technologies
Rai et al. (2002)	Ovarian	Plasma	SELDI-TOF-MS, H4, NP, IMAC3 Arrays, SELDI-QqTOF, Biomarker Patterns analysis	7 biomarkers: 8.6, 9.2, 19.8, 39.8, 54, 60, 79 kDa. Only the three peaks at 9.2, 54, and 79 kDa could be identified; the 79 kDa peak corresponded to transferrin, the 9.2 kDa peak corresponded to a fragment of the haptoglobin precursor protein, and the 54 kDa peak was identified as immunoglobulin heavy chain	The combined use of bioinformatics tools and proteomic profiling provides an effective approach to screen for potential tumor markers Comparison of plasma profiles from patients with and without known ovarian cancer uncovered a limited panel of potential biomarkers These biomarkers, in combination with CA125, provide significant discriminatory power for the detection of ovarian cancer
Jones et al. (2002)	Ovarian	Invasive ovarian cancer and non-invasive low malignant potential (LMP)	LCM 2D-PAGE Reverse phase array technology	FK506, RhoG protein dissociation inhibitor Gyoxalase I	Direct comparison of LCM generated profiles of invasive versus LMP cancer, directly generated important markers for early detection and/or therapeutic targets unique to the invasive phenotype
Li et al. (2002)	Breast	Serum	SELDI-TOF IMAC3chip Bioinformatics to	Three distinct pattern profiles Putative	Identification of potential biomarkers that can detect breast cancer at

Table 59.4 *Continued*

Reference	Type of cancer/clinical study	Source of biological material	Proteomic technology of choice	Biomarker/ surrogate	Significance and potential
			achieve best pattern selection: unified maximum separability analysis (UMSA) algorithm + Bootstrap cross-validation with introduction of random perturbations ProPeak	biomarkers BC1 = 4.3 kDa, BC2 = 8.1 kDa, BC3 = 8.9 kDa	early stages: separation between stage 0–1 and non-cancer control AUC AUC composite index for the three marker panel was 0.972 The best single marker (BC3) showed an AUC of 0.934
Caputo et al. (2003)	Breast	Breast cyst fluid	SELDI-TOF-MS, H4, PS10 Arrays	Pathological differences between similar proteins GCDFP-15/PIP and physiological gp17/SABP shown	SELDI used to investigate interaction with these proteins and CD4 and FN. It was determined that the physiological form was involved with the binding to CD4 Depending on its conformational state, GCDFP-15/gp17 could differentially bind to its various binding molecules and change its function(s) in the microenvironments where it is expressed
Vlahou et al. (2003)	Breast	In press	In press	In press	In press
Yousef et al. (2003)	Breast, ovarian	Serum	Recombinant protein ELISA	Human kallikrein 5 (hK5)	Development of first fluorimetric assay for hK5, distribution of hK5 in biological fluids and tissue extracts Potential valuable diagnostic and prognostic marker for ovarian and other cancers
Sauter et al. (2002)	Breast	Nipple aspirate	SELDI-TOF-MS, H4, NP1, SAX2 Arrays	Five differentially expressed proteins were identified. The most sensitive and specific proteins were at 6500 and 15940 Da	Analysis of nipple aspirate fluid proteins by SELDI may predict the presence of breast cancer
Govorukhina et al. (2003)	Squamous cervical cancer	Serum depleted of albumin and γ-globulin	LC/MS ELISA	SCCA1	SCCA1 is low abundance protein although ELISA is commercially available, this study shows that this type of protein can be successfully detected by LC-MS following depletion of albumin and γ globulin LC-MS promising technique for biomarker discovery
Lehrer et al. (2003)	Prostatic neoplasm	Crude serum	SELDI-TOF	Novel 3 proteins 15.2, 15.9, 17.5 kDa	15.9 kDa molecule may be used for diagnosis of PC versus benign prostatic hyperplasia (BPH). Potential for antibody based chip SELDI -TOF
Hlavaty et al. (2003)	Prostatic intraepithelial neoplasia (PIN)	Serum purified of lipids, IgG, human serum albumin (HSA) and fractionated by HPLC/anion exchange column	SELDI-TOF (WCX2 chip) SDS-PAGE, tryptic digest Peptide mass fingerprinting	Novel 50.8 kDa protein NMP48	Detection in PIN not in BPH or controls Assay for NMP48 maybe useful for early detection of prostate cancer

Table 59.4 *Continued*

Reference	Type of cancer/clinical study	Source of biological material	Proteomic technology of choice	Biomarker/ surrogate	Significance and potential
Banez et al. (2003)	Prostate cancer (CaP)	Crude serum	SELDI-TOF Combination of IMAC3-Cu and WCX2 chips Biomarker Pattern Software (BPS)	Combination of pattern profiles from two different chips	Combined effect of using two array types enhances the ability of using protein profile patterns for CaP detection
Cazares et al. (2002)	Prostate cancer (PCA)	LCM BPH, PIN, PCA Cell lysate	SELDI-TOF-MS	Several small molecular mass peptides and protein (3000–5000 D) a) more abundant in PIN and PCA 5000 Da peak upregualted in 86% of BPH	Protein profiles from prostate cells with different disease states have discriminating differences Pioneer study in pattern profiling
Adam et al. (2002)	Prostate cancer (CaP)	Serum samples BPH, PCA and normal	SELDI-MS coupled with artificial intelligence learning algorithm using a nine protein mass pattern		Algorithm correctly classified 96% of the samples with 83% sensitivity and 97% specificity and 96% predictive value. Classification system highly accurate and innovative approach for early diagnosis of PCA
Petricoin and Liotta (2002)	Prostate	Serum	SELDI-TOF-MS, H4 Array	The proteomic pattern correctly predicted 36 of 38 patients with prostate cancer while 177 of 228 patients were correctly classified as having benign conditions	Serum proteomic pattern analysis may be used in the future to aid clinicians so that fewer men are subjected to unnecessary biopsies
Petricoin et al. (2002b)	Prostate CaP screening (Chile clinical trial)*	Blinded serum LCM prostate cells	SELDI-TOF-MS C16 chip Bioinformatics/pattern generation: use of genetic algorithm to obtain a pattern that best segregates between training sets of spectra from sera of BPH and CaP	Best proteomic pattern obtained from bioinformatic algorithm	Evaluated the ability to detect and discriminate BPH and CaP in men with normal or elevated PSA levels Algorithm from training sets correctly classified prostate cancer patients in 95% of cases Potential secondary screen for men who have marginally elevated PSA serum levels. Patients classified as BPH by biopsy and as BPH by biopsy and as CaP+by serum proteomics pattern in a follow-up study subsequently developed cancer
Qu et al. (2002)	Prostate	Serum	SELDI-TOF-MS, IMAC Array	Boosted decision tree classification was used to find 12 protein peaks ranging from 3 to 10 kDa to differentiate prostate cancer versus non-cancer; 9 different proteins ranging in size from 3	Boosted decision tree analysis employed to reduce problem of overfitting the classification model and have an easy to interpret model as an outcome In one part of the study, 100% sensitivity and specificity was achieved in classifying 197 cancer patients versus 96 healthy individuals Greater than 90% sensitivity and specificity was also achieved in the test set for the more difficult problem of distinguishing BPH

Table 59.4 *Continued*

Reference	Type of cancer/clinical study	Source of biological material	Proteomic technology of choice	Biomarker/ surrogate	Significance and potential
Qu et al. (Cont.)				to 9 kDa were similarly selected to differentiate healthy versus benign prostatic hyperplasia (BPH) patients	
Adam et al. (2001)	Prostate cancer (CaP)	LCM cell lysate and serum from BPH, PIN, PCA	SELDI–MS	Pattern profile different in PIN PCA BPH and normal	Pioneer study in SELDI-MS Importance of pattern profiling for biomarker discovery
Howard et al. (2003)	Lung	Serum Small lung cancer tissue sample and non-small lung cancer	Isoelectric focusing (IEF) MALDI-TOF-MS genetic algorithm analysis Protein identification by RP-HPLC/C18 column and SDS-PAGE In gel tryptic digestion Peptide mapping AntiSAA immunoblot ELISA quantitation of SAA in lung cancer versus normal	Protein expression profile Identification of serum amyloid A (SAA)	MALDI-TOF MS powerful tool in the search of serum biomarkers of lung cancer and in discriminating between serum from lung cancer patients from that of normal individuals Potential alternative strategy and non invasive diagnostic tool for lung cancer
Yanigisawa et al. (2003)	Lung tumors	Fresh frozen lung tumor tissue	MALDI TOF Training algorithm	1600 protein picks, class prediction models able to classify lung cancer histologies, distinguish primary tumors from metastasis and classify nodal involvement	Proteomic patterns obtained directly from small amounts of fresh frozen lung tumor tissues accurately classified and predicted histological groups as well as nodal involvements and survival in resected non-small cell lung cancer
Steel et al. (2003)	Hepatocellular carcinoma (HCC)	Fractionated serum from clinically defined diagnostic groups: Active, inactive, chronic HBV and controls	2 dimensional gel electrophoresis (2D GE) tryptic fragment mass fingerprinting	Identification of C3 and isoform apolipoprotein A1	Proteomic methodologies can be used for the identification of serum biomarkers in HCC
Poon et al. (2003)	Hepatocellular carcinomas	Serum	SELDI-TOF-MS, Anion Exchange Fractionation, IMAC and WCX Arrays	250 differentially regulated protein peaks detected in a 20 × 38 study were narrowed down by an Artificial Neural Network (ANN) and Significant Analysis of Microarray (SAM) data approach to 10 most significant differentiators ranging from 4.6 to 51.2 kDa.	A potential diagnostic model was rapidly created showing good differentiation of hepatocellular carcinoma from chronic liver disease regardless of input AFP levels ROC areas under the curve were 0.91 for all cases tested and 0.954 for cases also differentiated by AFP < 500 μg/l

Table 59.4 *Continued*

Reference	Type of cancer/clinical study	Source of biological material	Proteomic technology of choice	Biomarker/ surrogate	Significance and potential
Zhou et al. (2002)	Esophageal carcinoma	LCM esophageal carcinoma cells and normal epithelial cells	2D Differential in gel electrophoresis (2D-DIGE) Bioinformatic Quantitation of protein expression by 3D simulation of protein spot Protein identification by capillary HPLC/MS/MS	Annexin I (gp96) unregulated in esophageal carcinoma	DIGE new approach in comparative differential display proteomics Global quantification of protein expression between LCM patient matched cancer cells and normal cells using 2D-DIGE in combination with MS is a powerful tool for the molecular characterization of cancer progression and identification for cancer specific protein markers
Melle et al. (2003)	Head and neck	LCM procured cells	SELDI-TOF-MS and SELDI-QqTOF; H4, SAX2 Arrays	Annexin V found differentially expressed ($P = 0.000029$) in 57×44 study of tumors versus adjacent mucosa procured by LCM	Looking for a better understanding of molecular mechanisms behind tumorigenesis and tumor progression in head and neck cancer Protein expression changes between microdissected normal pharyngeal epithelium and tumor tissue (3000–5000 cells in each sampling– a reasonable number for the pathologist to excise) were analyzed by SELDI Both the mass and a rough estimate of pI of a putative marker at 35.9 kDa were determined by SELDI and this information was used to guide isolation of the marker by 2D-PAGE; following isolation, in-gel digestion and peptide mapping was performed by SELDI-TOF-MS and a high confidence ID score for annexin V was obtained showing a rapid pathway from marker discovery to ID. Further ID verification was performed by a SELDI immunodepletion assay as well as SELDI-QqTOF partial sequencing
Wadsworth et al. (2003)	Head and neck cancer	In press	In press	In press	In press
Review by Le Naour (2001)	Neuroblastoma (NB) Breast	Autologous tumor cells and serum	Serological proteome analysis (SERPA) 2D-GE and serum immunoblotting	b-tubulin I and III isoform (NB) RNA binding protein regulatory subunit RS-DJ1 (breast cancer)	Occurrence of autoantibody and proteomic screening in different cancers may be useful in cancer screening and diagnosis Potential of SERPA to detect new biomarkers
Klade et al. (2001)	Renal cell carcinoma (RCC)	Autologous tumor cells and serum	Serological proteome analysis SERPA 2D-GE and serum immunoblotting	SM22a, CAI	
Shiwa et al. (2003)	Colon	Cell culture	SELDI-TOF-MS, H4, NP1, WCX2, SAX2, IMAC3 Arrays	One biomarker of 12 kDa. Identified as prothymosin-α by SELDI-TOF-MS and confirmed by SELDI-QqTOF	Prothymosin-α could be a potential biomarker for colon cancer adding to existing markers (CEA and CA19-9) that show relatively poor predictive value Expression screening by SELDI-TOF-MS and on-chip 'retentate chromatography' were used to rapidly develop a mini-column

Table 59.4 *Continued*

Reference	Type of cancer/clinical study	Source of biological material	Proteomic technology of choice	Biomarker/ surrogate	Significance and potential
Shiwa et al. (Cont.)					purification scheme to isolate enough enriched candidate 12 kDa for positive identification by SELDI peptide mapping and confirmatory SELDI-QqTOF analysis
Nakamura et al. (2002)	Acute leukemia	Cell cultures	Combination of column chromatography, 1D SDS-PAGE and SELDI-TOF-MS peptide mapping	27 interactors of ALL-1 protein, a histone methyl-transferase, were identified	The ALL-1 supercomplex of proteins is believed to be a significant player in transcriptional regulation and is involved in acute leukemia. As a functional study, 27 of more than 29 interactors believed to exist were rapidly isolated and identified. Studies of this nature may lead to the creation of diagnostically relevant Interaction assays

(Panelli and Burns, 2004)

Abbreviations: 2D GE 2 dimensional gel electrophoresis; DIGE differential in gel electrophoresis; SDS-PAGE sodium dodecyl sulfate-polyacrylamide gel electrophoresis; PAGE polyacrylamide gel electrophoresis; SERPA serological proteome analysis; ICAT isotope coded affinity tag; MudPIT multidimensional protein identification technology; MALDI matrix assisted laser desorption ionization; SELDI-qTOF surface enhanced laser desorption ionization quadrupole time of flight; ESI electrospray ionization; ESI FTICR electrospray ionization fourier transform cyclotron resonance; LC-MS/MS liquid chromatography-tandem mass spectrometry; SRP sensor chip surface plasmon resonance; LCM laser capture microdissection; ICH immunoaffinity subtraction chromatography; IHC immunohistochemistry; TARP arrays Tissue Array Research Program; UMSA unified maximum separability analysis.

various cytokines. A first step diagnostic screening of this type allows the rapid exclusion of factors irrelevant to the diagnosis of the disease, its progression or response to therapy. More importantly, these high-throughput screenings may identify clusters of proteins (signatures) descriptive of various biological states such as response to therapy or therapy-induced toxicity.

Reverse phage arrays (see above) also represent a valuable tool that has been effectively used to represent the state of individual tissue cell populations undergoing disease transitions (Paweletz et al, 2001). Using this novel protein microarray, Paweletz et al. longitudinally analyzed the state of pro-survival checkpoint proteins (EKT, ERK) at the microscopic transition stage from patient matched histologically normal prostate epithelium to prostate intraepithelial neoplasia (PIN) and then to invasive prostate cancer. Cancer progression was associated with increased phosphorylation of Akt ($P < 0.04$), suppression of apoptosis pathways, as well as decreased phosphorylation of ERK. At the transition from histologically normal epithelium to PIN, the authors observed a statistically significant surge in phosphorylated Akt and a concomitant suppression of downstream apoptosis pathways which proceeds the transition into invasive carcinoma.

FUTURE PROSPECT OF PROTEIN ARRAYS

Multiplex proteomic technologies have initiated a revolutionary approach to disease analysis, which is only at its infancy. We anticipate that in the future the progress will be exponential and a massive output of information will

be accumulated in several areas of basic and clinical research. Although the technologies that we presented in this report are already changing the way we make biological observations, further validation and optimization will be required. With specific reference to protein arrays several aspects will need to be considered:

1 rapid characterization of new ligand-antibody pairs for sample enrichment and array analysis
2 enhancing cross-reactivity testing and epitope mapping to increase specificity and sensitivity
3 generation of highly defined binding partners (antibodies, peptides, single-chain antibodies, aptamers) developed for new classes of proteins
4 increasing density of proteins to address sample volume limitations, and
5 increasing surface capacity to extend range of measurement.

In broader terms, validation and optimization will be an integral part of identification of biomarkers and surrogates for routine clinical use (early detection of disease, disease progression). As we have emphasized in a recent report (Panelli and Burns, 2003), three main issues need to be resolved before a novel biomarker can be introduced in clinical trials with the purpose of early detection, diagnosis, monitoring of therapy and prevention or risk assessment of cancer or other disease:

1 *Feasibility* (sensitivity, specificity and selectivity for measuring natural protein and its post-translationally modified forms

2 *Reproducibility* (using established controls, day-to-day variability, precision, matrix effects, etc.

3 *Standardization* (calibration of instrument and standards (recombinant or natural) of the selected technology).

In fact, to our knowledge, none of the state of the art technologies summarized in Table 59.1 utilized in the studies that we outlined (see also Table 59.4) has fully satisfied these three criteria and can be convincingly applied in clinical trials. The closest to obtaining approval by the FDA is high resolution protein pattern profiling (Petricoin et al., 2002a, b; Petricoin and Liotta, 2002).

A combination of several traditional and modern strategies simultaneously (protein arrays, SELDI, 2D gels LC/MS/MS and MudPIT technologies) (Smith, 2002; Petricoin et al., 2002b) will probably be the best approach for biomarker discovery in the clinical settings.

Furthermore, future prospects for the identification of specific biomarkers that could discriminate patients with early stage or minimal disease from healthy individuals will have to include:

1 multi-center collections of plasma/serum/tissue for individuals at risk of developing recurrence of malignant disease

2 registry studies (extensive patient history correlated with transcriptional and proteomic profiling)

3 single or multi-center clinical trials prospectively designed to collect materials relevant to the interpretations of the disease and its response to treatment

4 normal range databases for distinct demographic populations.

Possibly, the success of proteomics will not only depend on the application of a combination of traditional and modern biochemical approaches but on collaborations with clinicians through initiatives such as the ones outlined below (see Reference/ Website) aimed at accelerating and simultaneously regulating the process of protein identification in translational research:

- NCI/Cancer Diagnosis Program (CDP)
- Cancer Molecular Analysis Project C-MAP
- Academic Public/Private Partnership project (AP4)
- NCI/ The Early Detection Research Network: Biomarkers Developmental Laboratories (EDRN)
- NIH/NCI-FDA/CBER Clinical proteomics program databank
- SBIR and non-SBIR cooperative grants to accelerate clinical applications
- HUPO human proteome organization.

Finally, bioinformatics and data interpretation tools will need to be refined (refer to the comprehensive reviews by Fenyo and Beavis (2002) and Hancock et al. (2002)) to parallel new developments in proteomics strategies and automation in protein identification. Hopefully these tools will ease the mechanization of high throughput proteomics and at the same time will assist in the interpretation of the complicated and extensive output results.

REFERENCES

Adam, B.-L., Vlahou, A., Semmes. O.J. and Wright, G.L. (2001). Proteomic approaches to biomarker discovery in prostate and bladder cancers. Proteomics 1, 1264.

Adam, B.-L., Davis, J.W., Ward, M.D. et al. (2002). Serum protein fingerprinting coupled with a pattern matching algorithm that distinguishes prostate cancer from benign prostate hyperplasia and healthy men. Cancer Research 62, 3609–3614.

Bacarese-Hamilton, T., Bistoni, F. and Crisanti, A. (2002). Protein microarrays: from serodiagnosis to whole proteome scale analysis of the immune response against pathogenic microorganisms. Biotechniques 33, S24–S29.

Baley, S.N., Wu, R.Z. and Sabatini, D.M. (2002). Application of transfected cells microarrays in high throughput drug discovery. Drug Discov Today 7, S13–S18.

Banez, L.L., Prasanna, P., Sun, L. et al. (2003). Diagnostic potential of serum proteomic patterns in prostate cancer. J Urol 170, 442–446.

Bye, D.W., Cramer, S.J., Skates, S.P. et al. (2003). Mok haptoglobin – α subunit as potential serum biomarker in ovarian cancer: identification and characterization using proteomic profiling and mass spectrometry. Clin Cancer Res 9, 2904–2911.

Caputo, E., Moharram, R. and Martin, B.M. (2003). Methods for on-chip protein analysis. Analyt Biochem 321, 116–124.

Cazares, L.H., Adam, B.-L., Ward, M. D. et al. (2002). Normal, benign, pre-neoplastic and malignant prostate cells have distinct protein expression profiles resolved by SELDI mass spectrometry. Clinical Cancer Res 8, 2541–2552.

de Jager, W., te Velthuis, H., Prakken, B.J., Kuis, W. and Rijkers, G.T. (2003). Simultaneous detection of 15 human cytokines in a single sample of stimulated peripheral blood mononuclear cells. Clin Diagn Lab Immunol 10, 133–139.

de Wildt, R.M., Mundy, C.R., Gorick, B.D. and Tomlinson, I.M. (2000). Antibody arrays for high-throughput screening of antibody-antigen interactions. Nat Biotechnol 18, 989–994.

Emili, A.Q. and Cagney, G. (2000). Large scale functional analysis using peptide or protein arrays. Nature Biotech 18, 393–397.

Fall, B.I., Eberlein-Konig, B., Behrendt, H., Niessner, R., Ring, J. and Weller, M.G. (2003). Microarrays for the screening of allergen-specific IgE in human serum. Anal Chem 1 75, 556–562.

Fang, Y., Frutos, A.G., Webb, B. et al. (2002). Membrane biochips. Biotechniques 33, S62–S65.

Fenyo, D. and Beavis, R.C. (2002). Informatics and data management in proteomics. Trends Biotech 20, S35–S38.

Govorukhina, N.I., Keizer-Gunnink, A., van der Zee, A.G., de Jong, S., de Bruijn, H.W. and Bischoff, R. (2003). Sample preparation of human serum for the analysis of tumor markers. Comparison of different approaches for albumin and gamma-globulin depletion. J Chromatogr A 15, 171–178.

Haab, B.B., Dunham, M.J. and Brown, P.O. (2001). Protein microarrays for highly parallel detection and quantitation of specific proteins and antibodies in complex solutions'. Genome Biology 2.

Hancock, W.S., Wu, S.L., Stanley, R.R. and Gombocz, E.A. (2002). Publishing large proteome data set: scientific policy meets emerging technologies. Trends Biotech 20, S39–S44.

Hanes, J., Schaffitzel, C., Knappik, A. and Pluckthun, A. (2000). Picomolar affinity antibodies from a fully synthetic naive library selected and evolved by ribosome display. Nat Biotechnol 18, 1287–1292.

Hlavaty, J.J., Partin, A.W., Shue, M.J. et al. (2003). Identification and preliminary clinical evaluation of a 50.8-kDa serum marker for prostate cancer. Urology 61, 1261–1265.

Houseman, B.T. and Mrksich, M. (2002a). Carbohydrate arrays for the evaluation of protein binding and enzymatic modification. Chem Biol 9, 443–454.

Houseman, B.T. and Mrksich, M. (2002b). Towards quantitative assays with peptide chips: a surface engineering approach. Trends Biotechnol 20, 279–281.

Houseman, B.T., Huh, J.H., Kron, S.J. and Mrksich, M. (2002). Peptide chips for the quantitative evaluation of protein kinase activity. Nat Biotechnol 20, 270–274.

Howard, B.A., Wang, M.Z., Campa, M.J., Corro, C., Fitzgerald, M.C. and Patz, E.F. Jr (2003). Identification and validation of a potential lung cancer serum biomarker detected by matrix-assisted laser desorption/ionization-time of flight spectra analysis. Proteomics 3, 1720–1724.

Kim, J.H., Skates, S.J., Uede, T. et al. (2002). Osteopontin as a potential diagnostic biomarker for ovarian cancer. J Am Med Assoc 287, 1671–1679.

Klade, C.S., Voss, T., Krystek, E. et al. (2001). Identification of tumor antigens in renal cell carcinoma by serological proteome analysis. Proteomics 1, 890–898.

Kusnezow, W. and Heheisel, D. (2002). Antibody microarrays: promises and problems. Biotechnique 33, S14–S23.

Kozak, K.R., Amneus, M.W., Pusey, S.M. et al. (2003). Identification of biomarkers for ovarian cancer using strong anion-exchange ProteinChips: Potential use in diagnosis and prognosis. Proc Natl Acad Sci 100, 12343–12348.

Lee, Y., Lee, E.K., Cho, Y.W. et al. (2003). Proteochip: a highly sensitive protein microarray prepared by a novel method of protein immobilization for application of protein-protein interaction studies. Proteomics 3, 2289–2304.

Lee, Y.S. and Mrksich, M. (2002). Protein chip from concept to practice. Trends Biotech 20 (Suppl.), 14–18.

Lehrer, S., Roboz, J., Ding, H. et al. (2003). Putative protein markers in the sera of men with prostatic neoplasms. BJU International 92, 223.

Li, J., Zhang, Z., Rosenzweig, J., Wang, Y.Y. and Chan, D.W. (2002). Proteomics and bioinformatics approaches for identification of serum biomarkers to detect breast cancer. Clin Chem 48, 1296–1304.

MacBeath, G. and. Schreiber, S.L. (2000). Printing proteins as microarrays for high-throughput function determination. Science 1760–1763.

Melle, C., Ernst, G., Schimmel, B. et al. (2003). Biomarker discovery and identification in laser microdissected head and neck squamous cell carcinoma with ProteinChip® Technology, two-dimensional gel electrophoresis, tandem mass spectrometry, and immunohistochemistry. Molec Cell Proteomics 2, 443–452.

Mezzasoma, L., Bacarese-Hamilton, T., Di Cristina, M., Rossi, R., Bistoni, F. and Crisanti A. (2002). Antigen microarrays for serodiagnosis of infectious diseases. Clin Chem 48, 121–130.

Miyaji, T., Hewitt, S.M, Liotta, L.A. and Star, R.A. (2002). Frozen protein arrays: a new method for arraying and detecting recombinant and native tissue proteins. Proteomics 2, 1489–1493.

Nagorsen, D., Marincola, F.M., Panelli, M.C. et al. (2003). Cytokine and chemokine expression profiles of maturing dendritic cells using multiprotein platform arrays. Cytokines.

Neuman de Vegvar, H.E., Amara, R.R., Steinman, L., Utz, P.J., Robinson, H.L. and Robinson, W.H. (2003). Microarray profiling of antibody responses against simian-human immunodeficiency virus: postchallenge convergence of reactivities independent of host histocompatibility type and vaccine regimen. J Virol 77, 11125–11138.

Nishizuka, S., Chen, S.T., Gwadry, F.G. et al. (2003). Diagnostic markers that distinguish colon and ovarian adenocarcinomas: identification by genomic, proteomic, and tissue array profiling. Cancer Res 63, 5243–5250.

Panelli, M.C. and Burn, C.A. (2003). Serum and plasma, tumor proteomics/ protein-protein interaction workshop document. International Society of Biological Therapy of Cancer Workshop on Cancer Biometrics: Identifying Biomarkers and Surrogates of Tumor in Patients, October 30, 2003 NIH, Bethesda, MD. J Immunother (in press).

Panelli, M.C., Martin B., Nagorsen D. et al. (2003). A genomic and proteomic-based hypothesis on the eclectic effects of systemic interleukin-2 administration in the context of melanoma-specific immunization. J Invest Dermatol (in press).

Paweletz, C.P., Charboneau, L., Bichsel, V.E. et al. (2001). Reverse phase protein microarrays which capture disease progression show activation of pro-survival pathways at the cancer invasion front. Oncogene 12, 1981–1989.

Petricoin, E.F. III, Ardekani, A.M., Hitt, B.A et al. (2002a). Use of proteomic patterns in serum to identify ovarian cancer. Lancet 359.

Petricoin, E. and Liotta, L.A. (2002). Proteomics analysis at the bedside: early detection of cancer. Trends Biotech 20 (Suppl.), 30–34.

Petricoin, E.F. III, Onstein, D.K., Pawletz, C.P. et al. (2002b). Serum proteomic pattern for detection of prostate cancer. J Natl Cancer Inst 94.

Poon, T.C.W., Yip, T.-T., Chan, A.T.C. et al. (2003). Comprehensive proteomic profiling identifies serum proteomic signatures for detection of hepatocellular carcinoma and its subtypes. Clin Chem 49, 752–760.

Qu, Y., Adam, B.-L., Yasui, Y. et al. (2002). Boosted decision tree analysis of SELDI mass spectral serum profiles discriminates prostate cancer from non-cancer patients. Clin Chem 48, 1835–1843.

Rai, A.J., Zhang, Z., Rosenzweig, J. et al. (2002). Proteomic approaches to tumor marker discovery. Arch Pathol Lab Med 126, 1518–1526.

Robinson, W.H., Steinman, L. and Utz, P.J. (2002a). Protein and peptide array analysis of autoimmune disease. Biotechniques 33, S66–S69.

Robinson, W.H., DiGennaro, C., Hueber, W. et al. (2002b). Autoantigen microarrays for multiplex characterization of autoantibody responses. Nat Med 8, 295–301.

Sauter, E.R., Zhu, W., Fan, X-J, Wassell, R.P., Chervoneva, I. and Du Bois, G.C. (2002). Proteomic analysis of nipple aspirate fluid to detect biologic markers of breast cancer. Br J Cancer 86, 1440–1443.

Schaffitzel, C., Hanes, J., Jermutus, L. and Pluckthun, A. (1999). Ribosome display: an in vitro method for selection and evolution of antibodies from libraries. J Immunol Methods *231*, 119–135.

Schwenk, J.M., Stoll, D., Templin, M.F. and Joos, T.O. (2002). Cell microarrays: an emerging technology for the characterization of antibodies. Biotechnique *33*, S54–S61.

Schweitzer, B., Roberts, S., Grimwade, B. et al. (2002). Multiplexed protein profiling on microarrays by rolling-circle amplification. Nat Biotechnol *20*, 359–365.

Shiwa, M., Nishimura, Y., Wakatabe, R. et al. (2003). Rapid discovery and identification of a tissue-specific tumor biomarker from 39 human cancer cell lines using the SELDI ProteinChip platform. Biochem Biophys Res Commun *309*, 18–25.

Shreekumar, A. and Chinnaiyan, A. M. (2002). Using protein arrays to study cancer. Biotechniques *33*, S46–S53.

Smith, R.D. (2002). Trends in mass spectrometry instrumentation for proteomics. Trends Biotechnol *20*, S3–S7.

Steel, L.F., Shumpert, D., Trotter, M. et al. (2003). A strategy for the comparative analysis of serum proteomes for the discovery of biomarkers for hepatocellular carcinoma. Proteomics *3*, 601–609.

Trends in Biotechnology (2002). Trends Guide to Proteomics. *20* Supplement.

Vlahou, A., Laronga, C., Wilson, L. et al. (2003). A novel approach towards development of a rapid blood test for breast cancer. Clin Breast Cancer (in press).

Wadsworth, J.T., Somers, K.D., Cazeres, L.H. et al. (2003). Distinguishing healthy smokers from head and neck cancer. Arch Otolaryngol HN Surg (in press).

Wang, C.C, Huang, R.P, Sommer, M. et al. (2002). Array-based multiplexed screening and quantitation of human cytokines and chemokines. J Proteome Res *1*, 337–343.

Weng, S., Gu, K., Hammond, P.W. et al. (2002). Generating addressable protein microarrays with PROfusionTM covalent mRNA-protein fusion technology. Proteomics *2*, 48–57.

Yanagisawa, K., Shyr, Y., Xu, B.J. et al. (2003). Proteomic patterns of tumour subsets in non-small-cell lung cancer. Lancet *362*, 433–439.

Yousef, G.M., Polymeris, M.E., Grass, L. et al. (2003). Human kallikrein 5: a potential novel serum biomarker for breast and ovarian cancer. Cancer Res *63*, 3958–3965.

Zhou, G., Li, H., DeCamp, D. et al. (2002). 2D differential in-gel electrophoresis for the identification of esophageal scans cell cancer-specific protein markers. Mol Cell Proteomics *1*, 117–124.

Zhu, H., Bilgin, M., Bangham, R. et al. (2001). Global analysis of protein activities using proteome chips. Science 2101–2105.

Ziauddin, J. and. Sabatini, D.M. (2001). Microarrays of cells expressing defined cDNAs. Nature *411*, 107–110.

REFERENCES/WEBSITES

NCI/Cancer Diagnosis Program (CDP)
Advice and resources for cancer diagnostics researchers
http://www.cancerdiagnosis.nci.nih.gov/assessment/index.html
Cancer Molecular Analysis Project C-MAP
http://cmap.nci.nih.gov/
Academic Public/Private Partnership project (AP4)
http://grants.nih.gov/grants/guide/rfa-files/RFA-CA-04–005.html
http://deainfo.nci.nih.gov/concepts/AP4conceptU54.htm
NCI/ The Early Detection Research Network: Biomarkers Developmental Laboratories (EDRN)
National network that has responsibility for the development, evaluation and validation of biomarkers for earlier cancer detection and risk assessment
http://www3.cancer.gov/prevention/cbrg/edrn/
http://grants1.nih.gov/grants/guide/rfa-files/RFA-CA-99–007.html
NIH/NCI-FDA/CBER Clinical proteomics program databank
http://clinicalproteomics.steem.com
SBIR and non-SBIR cooperative grants to accelerate clinical applications
http://www.nsbdc.org/assistance/sbir_sttr/
Human proteome organization HUPO
http://www.hupo.org/

Genomics and Microarrays

Chapter 60

Minnie Sarwal and Farzad Alemi

Lucile Salter Packard Children's Hospital Nephrology, Stanford, CA, USA

By convention there is color, by convention sweetness, by convention bitterness, but in reality there are atoms and space.

Democritus (c. 460–400 BC), Greek philosopher

INTRODUCTION

The past few decades can truly be described as a golden age in the disciplines of biology and medicine. Beginning with the decoding of the genome itself to the gradual characterization of the structures, functions and interactions of genes and proteins, the rate of increase of what is known about biological systems can truly be described as exponential. In spite of these breakthroughs, however, much is still left to be discovered and understood. Fields such as immunology and neurology are still in their infancy and while their basic tenets are beginning to unravel, their molecular details are yet to be finalized. Nevertheless, the recent merging of powerful computing technology with fundamental research methodologies promises to revolutionize our understanding of genes, proteins and indeed life itself.

The 1990s heralded large-scale DNA sequencing endeavors to codify the entire genomes of multiple organisms, including man. It had been estimated that a human being was comprised of more than tens of thousands of distinct genes, their protein products coding for both the physical and biochemical components necessary for life. When an international consortium of research groups,

The Human Genome Project, announced in June 2000 that a working draft of the genetic code had been completed (Pennisi, 2000), a new age in biomedical research was born: the era of genomics. Functionally understood as the simultaneous study of the structure and function of very large numbers of genes (Staudt and Brown 2000), genomics carries the potential of uncovering not only structural–functional relationships among genes, but more importantly their expression profiles and roles in development.

The Human Genome Project eventually identified between 30 000 and 35 000 genes that code for human life (Ewing and Green, 2000); however, only a small fraction of those genes have had their functions deciphered. From a scientific perspective, then, June 2000 represented a fundamental shift in research objectives: no longer was gene discovery of particular interest, but rather decoding *what* genes did and *when* they did it. To facet an understanding of the function and expression patterns of the large volume of genetic data, researchers have since employed techniques such as comparative genomics and functional genomics. Using comparative genomics, for instance, scientists infer the function of an unknown human gene by comparing it to a homologous gene with a known function in a different, but related, species. Because much is already known about genetic mechanisms in a variety of different species such as *Escherichia coli*, *Saccharomyces cerevisiae* and *Caenorhabditis elegans*, comparative genomics has proven to be an invaluable tool in the initial analysis of the function of human genes.

Measuring Immunity, edited by Michael T. Lotze and Angus W. Thomson
ISBN 0-12-455900-X, London

The use of comparative techniques to discern functionality, while straightforward, at best gives a limited glimpse into the inherent complexity of biological systems. Recently, more powerful techniques have been developed to study large numbers of genes, concomitantly giving insights into their functions, interrelationships and expression patterns. This fundamental principle of functional genomics – namely large-scale analysis of expression and function – seeks to transcend viewing biologic behavior as 'one gene/one protein' modalities, but rather as a complex web of processes working together to produce a physiologic effect, normal or otherwise (Nagorsen et al., 2003). Such approaches are especially important to the field of immunology, where the complex interaction of lymphocytes, macrophages and cytokines dictate both protective responses against pathogens, as well as harmful responses against normal cells in the context of autoimmune diseases or allograft rejection. As stated by Louis Staudt and Patrick Brown in 2000:

> The established, model-driven field of immunology is about to collide with the upstart, discovery-driven field of genomics. Traditional research in molecular biology and molecular immunology can be likened to trying to understand a movie by successively examining a few pixels (genes) at a time from each frame. Genomic approaches allow the scientist to view the entire movie in one sitting and discover complex interrelationships among the plot, characters and recurring themes.

This novel concept of "Immunogenomics", as named by Wang and Falus, in 2004, therefore reflects a genuine paradigm shift from the age-old dogma of Scientific Method. The new strategy of complementing hypothesis-driven research with genomics-based 'fishing expeditions' of large data sets has already produced surprising insights into diverse biological phenomena, especially in the field of immunology, but also in pharmacology, oncology and cardiology (Wang and Falus, 2004). In essence, the application of immunogenomics to focus and guide traditional hypothesis-based experiments will revolutionize research outcomes as well as the rate at which they are achieved.

TOOLS OF THE TRADE: HIGH THROUGHPUT MICROARRAYS

Array generation

The DNA microarray is the principal technology driving the advances in functional genomics. Systematically developed in the 1990s with technical contributions from a number of researchers in academia and industry, the microarray allows for high throughput genomic analysis that is simultaneously relatively inexpensive, comprehensive and systematic (Schena, 1995). The technology is based on the simple principles of DNA binding and specificity: a given DNA strand will preferentially bind to its complement. It logically follows, then, that in order to qualify genes expressed in a given cellular sample at a given time, one can hybridize a collection of sample genetic material to a reference sample containing all the known, possible complements. The expressed genes will bind to their reference counterparts and, utilizing schemes for visualization, it is possible to glimpse into the spatial and temporal genetic profile of a biologic sample.

In practice, microarray technology is significantly more complex. A tangible "microarray" is a high-density collection of discrete DNA molecules photolithographically printed by a robotic arrayer onto a structural support, such as a microscope glass slide (Brown and Botstein, 1999). The printed DNA sequences tend to be either oligonucleotides – 20 or 25 nucleotide sequences of single-stranded DNA – or complementary DNA – 500–600 nucleotide sequences of DNA derived from a reverse-transcribed mRNA template – and represent known genes or subsets of genes from a given cell culture or tissue (Mansfield et al., 2003). With the capacity to spot more than 50 000 genes onto a single slide, microarrays can be customized for specific uses and investigations (Chua and Sarwal, 2003). For example, microarrays can be created to contain all the known and predicted genes for certain organisms, such as S. cerevisiae; they can also be customized for immunological research in the form of a 'lymphochip', a microarray which consists of genes thought to be expressed in the normal immune system and preferentially expressed in lymphoid cells (Alizadeh et al., 1999). The last few years have witnessed developments in printing technology and lowered printing costs, which has led to the creation of novel arrays and a new-found ability to study processes in a variety of organisms and tissues.

With microarray analyses, the most common strategy for data generation is the use of a two-color hybridization system. Because gene expression is the desired variable in most experiments, mRNA is extracted from the test sample and reference sample and transcribed into DNA using the enzyme reverse transcriptase. During this process the DNA sequences are labeled with fluorescent tags for visualization, with green (Cy3/fluorescein) the standard color for reference samples and red (Cy5/rhodamine) the color for test samples. The reference sample itself is usually a collection of mRNAs derived from a variety of cellular sources that contains most of the genes present on the microarray at standardized levels. In most laboratories a common reference sample is used for all microarray experiments for consistency purposes and also to allow for comparison of test samples from different experiments (Chua and Sarwal, 2002).

The next step in analysis involves competitive overnight hybridization of labeled test and reference samples onto the array itself. After the wash and fluorescent visualization, the relative abundance of test versus reference mRNA is indicated by color intensity of individual

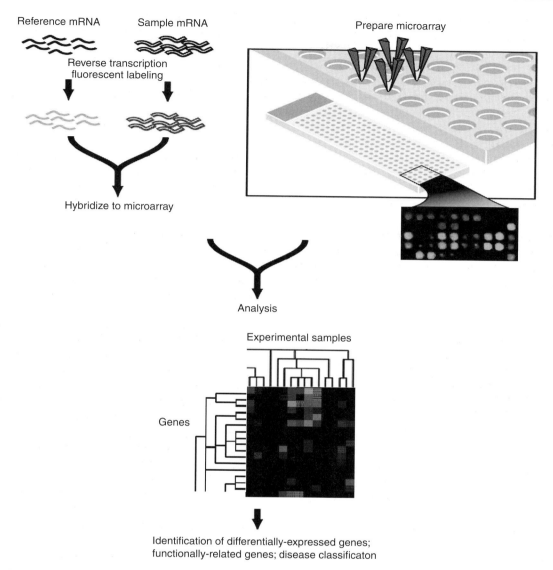

Figure 60.1 The generation of a microarray experiment begins with the labeling and reverse transcription of sample and reference mRNA. After competitive hybridization to a pre-formed cDNA or oligonucleotide microarray, data are scanned and subsequently analyzed according to a variety of protocols. Among the most popular is "clustering" of data, or organizing genes and experimental samples according to their expression patterns and relatedness (adapted from Chua and Sarwal, 2002). **See colour plate 60.1.**

spots. If test mRNA is more abundant than reference mRNA, a red spot will show; likewise, if reference mRNA is more abundant than test mRNA, a green spot will appear. If test and reference mRNA are present in equal proportions, a yellow spot will materialize. A ratio of red to green fluorescence, in addition, will give a relative expression level for a particular gene. Out of a mesmerizing palette of reds, greens and yellows, then, a microarray experiment can give a quantitative readout of genes which are up- or down-regulated vis-à-vis a standard reference.

Data analysis

The creation of a microarray is a relatively simple process when compared to the requisite interpretation of tens of

thousands of genes and subsequent inference into their biochemical significance. In general, analysis of microarray output data differentiates into two approaches: first, a systematic search for differentially-expressed levels of single genes related to particular biologic phenomena, or second, the generation of gene-expression profiles to examine signatures across multiple genes (Wang and Falus, 2004). With both approaches, the sheer amount of data generated per experiment necessitates the use of powerful statistical tools and computational analysis. In general, three steps are required for scrutiny of data: normalization for effective expression comparison, filtering to remove genes expressed below acceptable thresholds of significance and pattern identification to make biological sense of data sets (Chan et al., 2000).

Whereas normalization and filtering are relatively straightforward computer-assisted processes, a certain amount of finesse is required for pattern identification. Conceptually, the most common analysis tool is clustering, whereby genes are grouped according to expression level and function and from which insights with respect to biologic function can be derived (Eisen et al., 1998). There are a variety of protocols, but in general, clustering can be divided into unsupervised or supervised techniques. While their common intent is the creation of maps of expression data, each is suited toward particular applications and their use is determined by the intent of the experiment itself.

Unsupervised clustering methods

With unsupervised clustering, no previous knowledge of gene functional classes is presumed and data are organized according to computational algorithms. This method is generally employed as a survey technique in order to determine if patterns exist within the data. Hierarchical clustering, a common and reliable method of unsupervised clustering, groups genes with similar expression profiles across a set of experimental samples along the vertical axis (Chua and Sarwal, 2002). Likewise, experimental samples are grouped together on the horizontal axis depending on the degree of expression similarity across a specified set of genes. A dendrogram is used to display the degree of relatedness – the closer samples are to one another, the greater the similarity between them. This format has the added advantage of showing fold-deviation from average expression levels graphically via color intensity, with red representing upregulation of gene expression, black representing average expression and green denoting downregulation of gene expression. One trouble with hierarchical clustering is the number of inherent biases in the algorithm, but this dilemma can be overcome by the integration of self-organizing maps (SOMs) (Tamayo et al., 1999). Unlike rigid hierarchical clustering, SOMs allow the creation of partially structured clusters to allow for better visualization and interpretation. Their speed, adaptability to large data sets and ease of implementation make them a powerful complement to the hierarchical cluster.

Another form of unsupervised clustering involves singular value decomposition (SVD), a useful algorithm used to process and model data (Alter et al., 2000). In this methodology, the gene and array expression data is transformed to "eigengenes" and "eigenarrays". Data can be normalized by filtering the eigengenes and corresponding eigenarrays that are presumed to represent noise or experimental artifact, thereby enabling comparison of the expression of genes across different arrays in different experiments. SVD improves analysis of the expression data by eliminating systematic biases, allowing for the discovery of genes that appear to be classified by regulation and function.

Supervised clustering methods

Supervised clustering, on the other hand, requires a general sense of data patterns and prior knowledge of the data which should cluster together. This method requires first the selection of a subset of informative genes for analysis followed by the assignment of relative weights according to the predictive strengths of the genes of interest. Classical statistical tools that can be used for analysis include non-parametric statistical tests such as t tests, Wilcoxon tests and ANOVA. The applicability of these statistical tools is somewhat limited, though, in that they fail to give array-wide representations of statistical significance of expression differences. To this end, algorithms such as significance analysis of microarrays (SAM) have been developed specifically for use with microarray data and are utilized to provide statistical strength to data investigation (Tusher et al., 2001). With SAM, each gene is scored with respect to gene expression changes relative to the standard deviation of repeated measurements of that gene; significance thresholds are user-determined and modifiable according to the experiment. In addition to providing statistical power to microarray analysis, one of the benefits of SAM includes calculation of false discovery rate, an estimation of the degree of false positives among the final analysis of differentially-expressed genes (Chua et al., 2003).

One of the most novel applications of microarray experiments is the ability to classify and predict the diagnostic category of a sample based on its gene expression profile. For instance, classification of different subsets of tumors and leukemias has been achieved by such methods and this success can be attributable to analytic tools such as prediction analysis of microarrays (PAM). This method

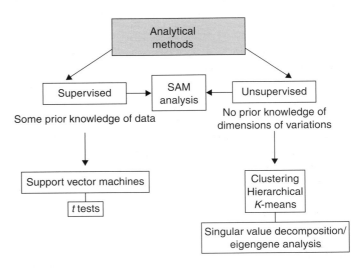

Figure 60.2 Making sense of microarray data using two widely-accepted patterns of analysis: supervised and unsupervised clustering. Both make different assumptions about the data prior to analysis and utilize a variety of statistical tools to draw conclusions about the significance of expression differences within data sets (adapted from Chua and Sarwal, 2002).

Table 60.1 On-line resources for microarray data analysis

Useful websites for array analysis	URL
SAM Significance analysis of microarrays	http://www-stat.stanford.edu/~tibs/ElemStatLearn/
PAM Prediction analysis of microarrays	http://www-stat.stanford.edu/%7Etibs/PAM/Rdist/index.html
R: Statistics for microarray analysis	http://ihome.cuhk.eduhk/~b400559/arraysoft_rpackages.html
Cluster and Treeview (Eisen Lab)	http://rana.lbl.gov/EisenSoflware.htm
Xcluster (Sherlock lab, Stanford)	http://genetics.stanford.edu/~sherlock/c luster .html#formats
BRB Array Tools (NIH informatics tools)	http://linus nci.nih.gov/BRB- ArrayTools.html
KEGG Kyoto gene classification database	http://www.genome.ad.jp/kegg/
GoMiner gene classification	http://disc over.nci.nihgov/gominer/index .jsp
Argon Laboratories metabolic pathways	http://wit.mcs.anl gov/WIT2/
Gene Ontology(GO) Consortium	http://www.geneontology.org/
ExP AS biochemical pathways	http://www.expasy.org/cgi-bin/search-biochem-index
GenMAPP metabolic pathways	http://www.genmapp.org/
GeneCards human gene database	http://bioinformatics.weizmann.ac.il/cards/
Stanford Microarray Database (SMD)	http://genome-www5.stanford.edu/
SOURCE clone & gene information database	http://genome-www5.stanford.edu/cgi-bin/source/sourceSearch
DRAGON microarray bioinformatics tools	http://pevsnerlab.kennedykrieger.org/dragon.htm
NCBI Entrez tutorials	http://www.ncbi.nlm.nih.gov/Education/index.html
The Wellcome Trust Sanger Institute	http://www.sanger.ac.uk/
European Molecular Biology Lab	http://www.ebi.ac.uk/embl
Swiss Institute of Bioinformatics	http://www.expasy.ch/
Protein Information Resource (PIR)	http://pir.georgetown.edu
EMBL Genome Browser	http://www.ensembl.org/
NIH list of genome sites	http://linus.nci.nih.gov/pilot/links.htm
UK list of genome sites	http://www.hgmp.mrc.ac.uk/Genome Web/ UK genome sites

Adapted from Mansfield et al., 2004

circumvents the typical classification problems inherent with microarrays: a large number of genes from which to predict classes and the relatively small number of samples (Tibshirani et al., 2002). PAM also allows for identification of expression profiles and genes that are most characteristic of, and therefore contribute most to, the classification. This method can be applied to both supervised as well as unsupervised analyses and can help identify the minimal subsets of genes that characterize each cluster.

ADVANTAGES AND DISADVANTAGES OF MICROARRAY ANALYSIS

Although a powerful technology which enables novel analysis, there are a number of drawbacks to the integrity of microarray data. Because of this, additional research procedures and controls are undertaken to maximize the data significance and eliminate bias. Of note, many microarray experiments today are designed to minimize sources of error and most results are validated using conventional techniques.

Variability

A frequent criticism of microarray analysis is the lack of data reproducibility arising from either introduced errors in experimental techniques or biological variations within samples (Wu, 2001). As with all experiments, it is advisable to repeat microarray batches whenever possible in order to reduce variability between sample runs. Repetition with similar experimental cell types controls not only for fluctuations between the samples themselves, but also for variations due to microarray printing and hybridization (Chua and Sarwal, 2003). Published results have supported the integrity of the microarray as a research tool and experiments performed in replicate demonstrate tight reproducibility and similar clustering patterns among samples (Sarwal et al., 2003b).

Variations between biologic specimens must be tightly controlled for as well. For instance, microarray examination of biopsied tissue might be misleading if tissue sampling differences exist (Chua and Sarwal, 2003), or if examined cellular samples differ in cell cycle or age. Nevertheless, these differences can be remedied by using stringent filtering practices as well as newer, more precise techniques of tissue laser dissection (Ohyama et al., 2000; Kitahara et al., 2001).

Amplification bias

Another cause of concern with respect to the integrity of microarray genomic analysis is the bias introduced as a result of multiple rounds of sample amplification. In many applications, generation of the requisite 50 µg of total RNA required for investigation cannot be achieved. In these instances, the extracted RNA must be amplified according to various protocols; usually this is done by reverse transcription followed by one or two successive rounds of amplification, yielding up to five to fifty orders of magnitude of starting material. Fortunately, the bias introduced during amplification procedures has been demonstrated to be insignificant (Wang et al., 2000) and such protocols are in wide use today (Chua et al., 2003).

Independent verification

The generation of experimental data for microarray analysis can further be compounded by technical difficulties such as unequal efficiency of dye labeling during reverse transcription, generation of unwanted secondary structures which prevent adequate hybridization and even cross-hybridization of genetic material (Chua and Sarwal, 2002). Therefore, because microarrays are prone to experimental error as a result of multiple experimental procedures, the results are generally viewed as semi-quantitative and independent verification of the expression levels are indicated using conventional techniques such as PCR, RT-PCR and quantitative PCR.

RNA/protein correlation

Extrapolation of microarray results carries an additional pitfall in that the generation of expression differences among mRNA samples may or may not correlate with actual protein expression levels and subsequent biological function (Ewton et al., 2003). Results from microarray experiments may therefore only provide a partial or exaggerated view into ongoing biochemical processes. To counter this problem, additional assays such as immunohistochemistry, Western blotting, 2-D Gel electrophoresis and mass spectrometry may be required to evaluate cellular localization, quantify protein expression and determine protein function (Goodstadt and Ponting, 2001; Sarwal et al., 2003a).

Oligonucleotide versus cDNA arrays

A final limitation of microarray technology is the platform to which sample genetic material will bind – oligonucleotides or cDNA clones. Each platform has its particular advantages as well as disadvantages and the final usage decision is dictated by a variety of factors including, among others, experimental techniques and cost. Oligonucleotide arrays offer the advantages of increased binding specificity due to shorter lengths (and concomitant ability to detect nucleotide polymorphisms in samples), as well as the ability to be synthesized *in situ* (Nagorsen et al., 2003). Drawbacks of oligonucleotide arrays include increased cost as a result of requisite purification and printing schemes, as well as errors in synthesis of oligonucleotide sequences. cDNA arrays are advantageous because of increased binding sensitivity due to longer lengths (and often presence of the full gene sequence), easier printing techniques and versatility of use. The major disadvantage of cDNA-based arrays is the increased possibility of cross-hybridization on account of

Table 60.2 Comparison of various microarry formats

Array format Comparison	cDNA	Oligoncleotide	Long Oligonucleotide
Probe length on the array	0.5–3 kB	15–25 bases	45–70 bases
Use in mRNA profiling	++	++	++
Genotyping	−	+++	+
Detect splice variants	−	++	+++
Spot consistency	−	++	+++
Current availability	+	+++	++
Manufacturability	−	++	+++
Batch consistency	−	++	++++
Ability to customize	++	−	+++
Template required	5 μg	16 μg	5 μg
Cost per array	Moderate	Highest	Lowest
Base system cost	$50K	$15K	$50K

Adapted from Mansfield et al., 2004

repeated and homologous sequences on different clones. The advent of longer length oligonucleotide arrays will circumvent some of the issues noted with the short oligonucleotide and cDNA arrays. Consequently, it is beneficial to consider a combination of issues when deciding on a platform and factors such as availability, cost and time must be considered in addition to the criteria above (Mansfield and Sarwal, 2004).

USES OF MICROARRAY TECHNOLOGY: EARLY SUCCESSES

Although still a relatively novel technology in terms of its concept and application to research, genomics has already achieved fundamental breakthroughs in what is known about a variety of pathophysiological processes. Initially viewed with hesitancy and skepticism, the microarray is rapidly gaining acceptance by the scientific community as an invaluable tool for studying the genetic signatures of disease. The field of oncology has already accepted the microarray as a diagnostic and prognostic tool and applications to other areas such as immunology, drug discovery and cardiology are not far behind. The power of microarray technology truly lies in the types of experiments performed and examination of its early contributions to science gives a full sense of its diverse and groundbreaking uses.

Cancer biology

The investigation of tumors is particularly amenable to study with microarrays due to the diversity in their behavior. Most neoplasms result from multiple insults to the integrity of the genome and while many of the causative mutations are known, their impact on the rest of the cell and organism remains a mystery. With the help of the microarray, tumors have been successfully classified based on their genomic signatures and with this information clinicians have been able to define prognostic markers of clinical outcome and, in some cancers, give a more accurate predictive ability regarding the course of the disease.

In the case of breast cancers, for instance, which are frequently differentiated using biochemical markers such as estrogen receptors, microarray analysis of dozens of patients has generated original classification schemes. Six categories of breast cancers have been identified using a genomic approach (Perou et al., 2000) and correlating patient survival analysis with the different categories demonstrates that some types are more prone to a favorable prognosis as compared to others. In other studies, investigators have used microarrays to identify patterns of gene expression which correlate to the metastatic spread of the disease, thereby allowing for predictive insights into tumor behavior. Of particular note is the demonstration that microarray profiling actually predicts tumor outcome more reliably as compared to traditional, receptor-based methods (van de Vijver et al., 2002).

The success with breast cancers is not an isolated example but rather one of many instances where microarrays are aiding tumor classification and prognostic outcomes. Lymphochips have been used to study and classify successfully B cell lymphoma and acute lymphoblastic leukemia (Alizadeh et al., 2000) and ongoing studies are investigating Hodgkin's lymphoma and a variety of other tumors including prostate and carcinomas of the bladder (Nagorsen et al., 2003). Microarray technology used in this manner has resulted in numerous discoveries that can be used to identify the genetic mutations common to all tumors as well as genomic profiles characteristic of tumor subcategories. As the technology and subsequent knowledge about cancers develops, microarrays will become an invaluable tool in diagnosis and therapeutic decision making for oncologists.

Pharmacogenomics

The ability to survey a large number of genes simultaneously makes the microarray particularly suited for a role in drug discovery and pharmacogenomics, or the recent trend of tailoring drugs to patients and predicting drug response depending on their genetic profile. Microarrays allow for examination of gene expression and molecular response of multiple cells and tissues after exposure to putative pharmacological therapies. The advantages of microarrays in this process include the ability for high throughput analysis of many different tissues and the examination of multiple drugs simultaneously. Already this approach has produced results; in the field of cancer therapy, Okutsu et al. (2002) used microarrays to predict the response of leukemia patients to different chemotherapy regimens. Analysis of 44 patients yielded 28 genes which were significantly different between patients who responded to chemotherapy and those who did not. Using these data, a drug response algorithm was developed and used to predict individual responses to chemotherapy in additional patients; predicted outcomes were confirmed in 85 per cent of cases.

In the field of immunology and pharmacogenomics, microarrays are being widely appreciated as a tool for analyzing the efficacy of immunosuppressive treatment (Diehn et al., 2002). After organ transplantation, for instance, immunosuppression achieved with corticosteroids has been the benchmark therapy for prevention of organ rejection, despite side-effects such as Cushing's syndrome, hypertension, diabetes mellitus and stunted growth. A recent trial by Sarwal et al. (2003b) substituted a steroid-free regimen in lieu of traditional corticosteroids and results demonstrated better graft function coupled with fewer incidents of rejection. Microarray analysis has identified T cell activation differences in patient responses to the therapies (Satterwhite et al., 2003) and further comparison of the two will shed light on the biochemistry of transplants and immunotherapies. The aim of such techniques is prospective identification of patients who are likely to benefit from current treatment strategies versus those who should be treated with alternative therapies. Microarray analysis of the patient's genetic signature holds great promise for the customization of therapy in the coming years.

Immunology

The application of genomics to the field of immunology has already provided key insights into the composition and function of the immune response. Early expression studies of the differences between B and T lymphocytes showed that both lineages express a very similar subset of genes, but when differences in gene expression do arise, they are definitive of the role and function of the cells (Kondo et al., 1997). As a result of these early insights, experiments have been conducted examining everything from animal and human models of immune disease to the study of immune response activation. For instance, studies into B cell activation have demonstrated the timeframe of immune response induction and the discovery of dozens of early response genes which are upregulated only 1 h post-activation (Glynne and Watson, 2001).

Other experiments have demonstrated the effect of immunosuppression on lymphocyte activation and its relationship to immune system tolerance (Diehn et al., 2002). Practical application of such studies is particularly important in fields such as solid organ transplantation, where the immune system often dictates graft function and survival. Acute rejection is one phenomenon that has been studied extensively at a biochemical level with the aid of microarrays. Oligonucleotide arrays have been used to screen for genetic mechanisms underlying rejection phenomena and interestingly different molecular forms of acute rejection have been identified (Sarwal et al., 2003a). This is important not only for immunological research purposes, but also because of its implications to patient survival: patients with certain genetic characteristics as identified

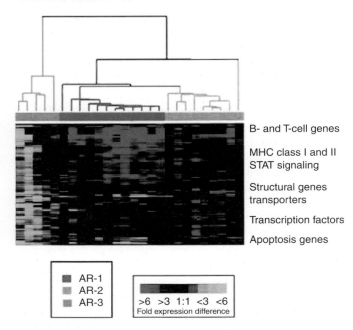

B- and T-cell genes

MHC class I and II
STAT signaling

Structural genes
transporters

Transcription factors

Apoptosis genes

AR-1
AR-2
AR-3

>6 >3 1:1 <3 <6
Fold expression difference

Figure 60.3 Classification of renal allograft acute rejection samples into three categories based on microarray clustering. Each rejection subtype demonstrates differential expression of genes involved in biological processes such as apoptosis and cell signaling. With this information, novel therapies can be developed and tailored according to patient subtype (adapted from Sarwal et al., 2003a). **See colour plate 60.3.**

by microarrays require increased therapeutic vigilance and surveillance. Moreover, comparison of acute rejection samples with normal samples and those undergoing chronic rejection demonstrate the expression of different subsets of genes and the identification and study of those genes is being undertaken to understand the mechanisms of rejection and immune system function.

Likewise, microarrays are being utilized to understand long-term sequelae of organ transplantation in the form of immune-mediated organ injury. Chronic allograft nephropathy (CAN), a post-transplant manifestation of renal pathology, is under investigation to understand its causes and develop prevention strategies. Animal models of vascular injury (Aavik et al., 2001; Du Toit et al., 2001) have identified a number of pathways resulting in CAN and correlation studies with human subjects will hopefully corroborate findings and lead to strategies of prevention. Interestingly, in the case of CAN, "many of the pathways involved in chronic injury and fibrosis are regulated very early in the course of the injury … when the downstream effects of these alterations are still not evident by pathology" (Chua et al., 2003) suggesting an additional role of microarray technology as markers for disease progression.

Indeed, the use of microarrays for surveillance purposes is another success in the application of the technology. In the case of transplant rejection for instance, it is helpful to utilize non-invasive techniques of graft monitoring to prevent rejection and modify immunosuppressive therapy when appropriate. Recently, peripheral blood and urine

markers such as granulysin have been validated using microarrays as successful monitors of post-transplant renal function (Sarwal et al., 2001). Bench-to-bedside approaches therefore validate the microarray as a legitimate tool in clinical and research practice. Other recently developed applications promise to expand the scope of applications. One example is the detection of unknown single nucleotide polymorphisms (SNPs) using a novel technique of fluorescent detection by hybridization to oligonucleotide microarrays (Wang et al., 2003). This technology promises to become a powerful tool for HLA typing studies as well as examination of cytokines, receptors and other components of the immune system.

BEYOND THE DNA ARRAY: PROTEIN AND TISSUE ARRAYS

Addressing an inherent problem of DNA-based arrays, namely the questionable correlation between mRNA levels and protein expression, protein arrays operate on the principle of identifying proteins themselves or the molecules that bind them. Similar to DNA microarrays, large numbers of different proteins are spotted on a solid support and to them bind ligands or other molecules. On the basis of these interactions, insights can be made into not only the binding of protein and substrate, but also global views of protein expression and function. Already protein array technology is proving useful, as researchers have used them to investigate carcinogenesis, markers of tumor progression, enzymatic expression and determination of biochemical signaling pathways (Russo et al., 2003). In the field of immunology, protein arrays are of particular importance in the study of immune response to antigens in the form of cytokine and antibody expression (Wilson and Nock, 2003). Robinson et al. (2002) have used protein arrays to study autoimmune disorders by screening hundreds of known autoantigens against serum from patients with different diseases and have determined that accurate differentiation of syndromes could be ascertained. Results were verified using standard assays such as ELISA, demonstrating the validity of tissue microarrays as a research tool. In some instances, autoantigens were detected at lower thresholds than conventional techniques, suggesting that protein arrays are more powerful than their conventional counterparts.

Another exciting development in array technology is the advent of tissue arrays. In this application, biological specimens are first fixed in formalin and later embedded in paraffin to create a solid block from which cylinders of tissue are removed and analyzed. One advantage of this method is the ability simultaneously to analyze DNA, RNA and protein, using immunohistochemistry, immunofluorescence, or other hybridization assays. Moreover, tissue arrays have the additional benefit of allowing samples from multiple patients to be visualized on the same slide, thereby allowing for identical reagent concentrations, incubation times and experimental techniques. As with other array formats, tissue arrays allow for large-scale amplification of results, decreased sample volume and experimental uniformity. Their uses include typical applications such as tumor typing and progression and they have been used for staging of breast, prostate and renal neoplasms (Kononen et al., 1998; Bubendorf et al., 1999; Moch et al., 1999). The technology has also been used to screen for oncogenic amplification by fluorescence *in situ* hybridization (Schraml et al., 1999), as well as to validate and discover markers for tumor expression and growth. Despite their growing role in cancer research, though, tissue arrays are still primarily a screening tool and not designed to provide in-depth molecular analysis of tumors. Nevertheless, they hold great promise in assisting with new insights into a wide variety of tissue-based phenomena.

THE FUTURE OF IMMUNOGENOMICS

The process of scientific inquiry has truly transformed with the advent of the microarray. Amenable for large-scale, hypothesis-generating experiments or for targeted examination of molecular pathways, genomic study into the immune system has already produced dramatic discoveries. Furthermore, the future of immunogenomics looks favorable as the utilization of technologies such as the protein array and tissue array promises to provide key insights into the fundamentals of the immune system. The promise of the microarray – DNA, protein, tissue or otherwise – rests in a combination of factors, including speed, high throughput, large data production and small amount of required starting material. Together these technologies promise to revolutionize and accelerate scientific study as we know it and to advance our understanding, monitoring and therapy for a variety of disease processes.

REFERENCES

Aavik, E., du Toit, D., Myburgh, E., Frosen, J. and Hayry, P. (2001). Estrogen receptor beta dominates in baboon carotid after endothelial denudation injury. Mol Cell Endocrinol 20, 91–98.

Alizadeh, A., Eisen, M., Davis, R.E. et al. (1999). The lymphochip: a specialized cDNA microarray for the genomic-scale analysis of gene expression in normal and malignant lymphocytes. Cold Spring Harb Symp Quant Biol 64, 71–78.

Alizadeh, A.A., Eisen, M.B., Davis, R.E. et al. (2000). Distinct types of diffuse large B-cell lymphoma identified by gene expression profiling. Nature 403, 503–511.

Alter, O., Brown, P.O. and Botstein, D. (2000). Singular value decomposition for genome-wide expression data processing, and modeling. Proc Natl Acad Sci USA 97, 10101–10106.

Alter, O., Brown, P.O. and Botstein, D. (2003). Generalized singular value decomposition for comparative analysis of genome-scale expression data sets of two different organisms. Proc Natl Acad Sci 100, 3351–3356.

Brown, P.O. and Botstein, D. (1999). Exploring the new world of the genome with DNA microarrays. Nat Genet 21, 33–37.

Bubendorf, L., Kononen, J., Koivisto, P. et al. (1999). Survey of gene amplifications during prostate cancer progression by high-throughout fluorescence in situ hybridization on tissue microarrays. Cancer Res 59, 803–806.

Chan, V., Hontzeas, N. and Park, V. (2000). Gene expression. http://citeseer.nj.nec.com/cache/papers/cs/19764/http:zSzzSzmonod.uwaterloo.cazSzpaperszSz00798ggeneexpression.pdf/chan00gene.pdf

Chua, M.S. and Sarwal, M.M. (2002). Exploiting DNA microarrays in renal transplantation. Graft 5, 223–231.

Chua, M.S. and Sarwal, M.M. (2003). Microarrays: new tools for transplantation research. Pediatr Nephrol 18, 319–327.

Chua, M.S., Mansfield, E. and Sarwal, M.M. (2003). Applications of microarrays to renal transplantation: progress and possibilities. Frontiers Biosci 8, 913–923.

Diehn, M., Alizadeh, A.A., Rando, O.J. et al. (2002). Genomic expression programs and the integration of the CD28 costimulatory signal in T cell activation. Proc Natl Acad Sci 99, 11796–11801.

Du Toit, D., Aavik, E., Taskinen, E. et al. (2001). Structure of carotid artery in baboon and rat and differences in their response to endothelial denudation angioplasty. Ann Med 33, 63–78.

Eisen, M.B., Spellman, P.T., Brown, P.O. and Botstein, D. (1998). Cluster analysis and display of genome-wide expression patterns. Proc Natl Acad Sci 95, 14863–14868.

Ewing, B. and Green, P. (2000). Analysis of expressed sequence tags indicates 35,000 human genes. Nat Genet 25, 232–234.

Ewton, D.Z., Lee, K., Deng, X., Lim, S. and Friedman, E. (2003). Rapid turnover of cell-cycle regulators found in Mirk/dyrk1B transfectants. Int J Cancer 103, 21–28.

Glynne, R.J. and Watson, S.R. (2001). The immune system and gene expression microarrays – new answers to old questions. J Pathol 195, 20–30.

Goodstadt, L. and Ponting, C.P. (2001). Sequence variation and disease in the wake of the draft human genome. Hum Mol Genet 10, 2209–2214.

Kitahara, O., Furukawa, Y., Tanaka, T. et al. (2001). Alterations of gene expression during colorectal carcinogenesis revealed by cDNA microarrays after laser-capture microdissection of tumor tissues and normal epithelia. Cancer Res 61, 3544–3549.

Kondo, M., Weissman, I.L. and Akashi, K.(1997). Identification of clonogenic common lymphoid progenitors in mouse bone marrow. Cell 91, 661–672.

Kononen, J., Bubendorf, L., Kallioniemi, A. et al. (1998). Tissue microarrays for high-throughput molecular profiling of tumor specimens. Nat Med 4, 844–847.

Mansfield, E.S., Hernandez-Boussard, T. and Sarwal, M.M. (2003). Arrays amaze: unraveling the transcriptsome in transplantation. ASHI Q 27, 11–15.

Mansfield, E.S. and Sarwal, M.M. (2004). Arraying the orchestration of allograft pathology. Am J Transplant 4, 853–862.

Moch, H., Schraml, P., Bubendorf, L. et al. (1999). High-throughput tissue microarray analysis to evaluate genes uncovered by cDNA microarray screening in renal cell carcinoma. Am J Pathol 154, 981–986.

Nagorsen, D., Wang, E. and Panelli, M.C. (2003). High-throughput genomics: an emerging tool in biology and immunology. ASHI Q 27, 96–99.

Ohyama, H., Zhang, X., Kohno, Y. et al. (2000). Laser capture microdissection-generated target sample for high-density oligonucleotide array hybridization. Biotechniques 29, 530–536.

Okutsu, J., Tsunoda, T., Kaneta, Y. et al. (2002). Prediction of chemosensitivity for patients with acute myeloid leukemia, according to expression levels of 28 genes selected by genome-wide complementary DNA microarray analysis. Mol Cancer Ther 1, 1035–1042.

Pennisi, E. (2000). Human genome: finally, the book of life and instructions for navigating it. Science 288, 2304–2307.

Perou, C.M., Sorlie, T., Eisen, M.B et al. (2000). Molecular portraits of human breast tumours. Nature 406, 747–752.

Robinson, W.H., DiGennaro, C., Hueber W. et al. (2002). Autoantigen microarrays for multiplex characterization of autoantibody responses. Nat. Med 8, 295–301.

Russo, G., Zegar, C. and Giordano, A. (2003). Advantages and limitations of microarray technology in human cancer. Oncogene 22, 6497–6507.

Sarwal, M.M., Jani, A., Chang, S. et al. (2001). Granulysin expression is a marker for acute rejection and steroid resistance in human renal transplantation. Hum Immunol 62, 21–31.

Sarwal, M.M., Chen, X., Chua, M.-S. et al. (2003a). Molecular heterogeneity in acute renal allograft rejection identified by DNA micrarray profiling. New Engl J Med 349, 125–138.

Sarwal, M.M., Vidhun, J.R., Alexander, S.R., Satterwhite, T., Millan, M. and Salvatierra, O. Jr (2003b). Continued superior outcomes with modification and lengthened follow-up of a steroid-avoidance pilot with extended daclizumab induction in pediatric renal transplantation. Transplantation 76, 1331–1339.

Satterwhite, T., Chua, M.S., Hsieh, S.C. (2003). Increased expression of cytotoxic effector molecules: different interpretations for steroid-based and steroid-free immunosuppression. Pediatr Transplant 7, 53–58.

Schena, M. (1995). Quantitative monitoring of gene expression patterns with a cDNA microarray. Science 270, 467–470.

Schraml, P., Kononen, J., Bubendorf, L. et al. (1999). Tissue microarrays for gene amplification surveys in many different tumor types. Clin Cancer Res 5, 1966–1975.

Staudt, L.M. and Brown, P.O. (2000). Genomic views of the immune system. Annu Rev Immunol. 18, 829–859.

Tamayo, P., Slonim, D., Mesirov, J. et al. (1999). Interpreting patterns of gene expression with self-organizing maps: methods and application to hematopoietic differentiation. Proc Natl Acad Sci 96, 2907–2912.

Tibshirani, R., Hastie, T., Narasimhan, B. and Chu, G. (2002). Diagnosis of multiple cancer types by shrunken centroids of gene expression. Proc Natl Acad Sci 99, 6567–6572.

Tusher, V.G., Tibshirani, R. and Chu, G. (2001). Significance analysis of microarrays applied to the ionizing radiation response. Proc Natl Acad Sci 98, 5116–5121.

van de Vijver, M.J., He, Y.D., van't Veer, L.J. et al. (2002). A gene-expression signature as a predictor of survival in breast cancer. N Engl J Med 347, 1999–2009.

Wang, E., Miller, L.D., Ohnmacht, G.A., Liu, E.T. and Marincola, F.M. (2000). High-fidelity mRNA amplification for gene profiling. Nat Biotechnol 8, 457–459.

Wang, E., Adams, S., Zhao, Y. et al. (2003). A strategy for detection of known and unknown SNP using a minimum number of oligonucleotides applicable in the clinical settings. J Transl Med 1, 4.

Wang, E. and Falus, A. (2004). Changing paradigm through a genome-based approach to clinical and basic immunology. J Transl Med 2, 2.

Wilson, D.S. and Nock, S. (2003). Recent developments in protein microarray technology. Angewandte Chem Internatl Edn 42, 494–500.

Wu, T.D. (2001). Analysing gene expression data from DNA microarrays to identify candidate genes. J Pathol 195, 53–65.

Image Informatics

Andres Kriete

*School of Biomedical Engineering, Science and Health Systems,
Drexel University, Philadelphia, PA, USA*

There is no one who can return from there, To describe their
nature, to describe their dissolution, That he may still our
desires, Until we reach the Place where they have gone.

The Song of the Harper; 2600 BC

INTRODUCTION

Like in other areas of biomedical sciences, progress in the
understanding of tissues, their structure, function and
dynamics and role in immunity critically relies on the precision and quality of information available. Improvements
to obtain more structural information are not only critical
to carry out a sensitive and reproducible phenotyping
suitable for diagnosis of inflammation, but are also
increasingly valuable to elucidate the downstream effects
of gene function and gene products. Moreover, quantitative tissue information helps to model and understand
the structure–functional relationships of cellular assem-
blies in normal and disease tissues and transplants. An
automated morphometry in conjunction with image informatics, which includes computer assisted imaging, data
storage, analysis and correlation of tissue images serves
this emerging requirement.

Despite the enormous progress in digital microscopy
and automated applications in cytology and molecular
screening techniques, the prevailing method for analyzing histological tissue sections in medical research, pharmacology and clinical diagnostics remains visual inspection.
However, visual pathological assessment of tissues lacks

sufficient quantification to enable accurate discrimination
between samples and/or experimental groups, it is tedious
and time consuming for new tissue preparation techniques like tissue microarrays and when a large numbers
of tissue slides have to be screened, like in drug safety
and investigative toxicological studies.

A number of technical barriers for a fully automated
tissue analysis, such as the lack of time-efficient data
acquisition of complete tissue sections, robust machine
vision and handling and mining of large image datasets,
have long prevented digital tissue analysis to be applied
routinely. However, recent technological progress has
allowed the development of systems that carry out a
comprehensive structural profiling of normal and disease
tissue specimens fully automatically, in a high-content
and high throughput fashion. In the following the technical components for image acquisition, image handling,
analysis and interpretation are described and applications in immunology are given.

HIGH THROUGHPUT IMAGE ACQUISITION AND DIGITAL TISSUE REPOSITORIES

Imaging modalities in light microscopy include bright-
field, multispectral, fluorescence, confocal and non-linear
methods that provide an always increasing variety of new
insights into form and function of cells and tissues (Arndt-
Jovin et al., 1985; Denk et al., 1990; Pawley, 1995; Herman,
1998; Kriete and Gundlach, 2001). For digital image

Measuring Immunity, edited by Michael T. Lotze and Angus W. Thomson
ISBN 0-12-455900-X, London

acquisition, TV-tube–type cameras were first used, which were later replaced by more sensitive and higher-resolving CCD cameras. The relationship between the resolution of the optics, the resolution of the camera and the ability to detect and measure structures is well understood (Young, 1996). Concomitantly, new image informatics solutions were developed to deal with the acquisition, analysis and distribution of the digital image information. One example is in telepathology (Weinstein et al., 1997) where remote control of a distant microscope and the distribution of the digital images over the Internet can be performed to support image-guided decision support. These methods have stimulated the development of more automated robotic microscopes that encompass automated slide loading devices, automated focusing, tissue detection and scanning methodologies. The individual image captures, or tiles, can be assembled to image montages to review the image information of the complete tissue section at different resolutions. These types of automation, if joined with machine vision analysis, are the necessary prerequisites to execute a tissue morphometry in a fully automated fashion.

The prevailing tissue diagnostic methods use histological staining protocols, which are the basis of most pathological assessments including the diagnosis of inflammation. Specimens prepared from tissue blocks or biopsies are embedded in paraffin, cut in 5–7 μm thick sections, placed on glass slides sized 20 × 50 mm and stained with hematoxilyn-eosin (H&E). Complete imaging of such a glass slide at 20 × microscopic magnification would generate about 3000 individual digital color images. Research microscopes equipped with scanning stages and autofocus mechanisms require acquisition times around 1 s for each one image or tile. Consequently, the total scanning time for a complete slide is approximately 1 h, which is not suited for the screening of a large number of slides. In contrast, specialized robotic microscopes scan a complete slide within minutes (Aperio, Trestle), one example of such a device is shown in Figure 61.1. These solutions have implemented a continuous stage movement to deliver sharp images over the entire slide. The information about focus levels to guide the auto-focusing mechanism is generated either prior to the scanning process by probing and interpolating randomly selected points on the slide or by a parallel detection path that is looking ahead and continuously determines focal position information. These systems have been automated further by robotic slide–loading mechanisms that allow the scanning of hundreds of slides without any user interaction. The images are digitized, automatically assembled into montages and saved to disk.

Since the amount of data to be handled can reach several GB of data per slide, depending on resolution and size of tissue, more advanced solutions use databases with automated data entry. Associated clinical

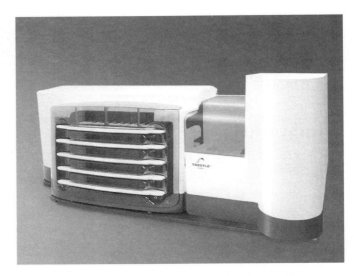

Figure 61.1 Robotic light microscopes with slide loading devices allow automated workflows for screening a large number of slides (with permission of Trestle Corporation, Newport Beach, CA).

information can also be stored automatically if these data are provided by a bar code on the slide. Since conventional databases only deal with textual and numerical information and are no longer adequate for diagnostic purposes, instead more powerful digital image management systems (DIMS) are used. All tissues from a study or project can be placed in such a system to form a digital tissue repository and both the images and associated data can be reviewed, queried and shared. Based on clinical information standards, tissue image data can also be integrated into clinical imaging networks. One example is the visible light DICOM-VL standard, an extension of the Digital Imaging and Communication in Medicine (DICOM) protocol, which is the most used form of image storage and distribution in the clinic.

MACHINE VISION ANALYSIS OF INFLAMMATION

Currently available solutions in automated image analysis use a pixel-by-pixel processing for the identification and quantification of features (Furness, 1997; Sun and Horng, 1997) and the main steps in such a process are image enhancement, image segmentation based on histograms and identification of image objects. Measured features, such as object related geometrical, field specific and intensity parameters are subsequently derived to establish classification of the objects segmented. As the segmentation process is the critical bottleneck in many applications and may lead to inconsistent objects, the handling of pixels in a context-related or object-related fashion has gained interest.

Object segmentation

Objects like larger tissue areas, cells and cell nuclei are mainly characterized by using color information. For a correct segmentation of color in a digital image a physical model of stain absorption that relates the amount of stain present in an image area with the color and intensity of light transmitted through the tissue specimen is of advantage. This allows for improved detection of stained tissue areas as well as determinations of the amount of stain (color) present in each tissue area. These improvements, in turn, are required for other automated processes such as the accurate detection of areas of tissue on slides. Since the relative absorption of different stains is the means by which tissue structures are made visible, the computer-assisted detection of these structures is also facilitated.

The classical approach of processing an image pixel-by-pixel has several drawbacks. First, the computational process is difficult to automate since it is extremely sensitive to variations introduced by histological procedures and imaging parameters, such as stain, section thickness, intensity and color variations and subtle general differences in histopathology between similar tissues. Second, the process of correct object classification can be very tedious, since a wide range of parameters like thresholds, geometrical ranges must be constantly varied to achieve an optimal result.

Once initial areas of objects are defined, textures (Kriete et al., 1985) or other high-level information can be used to provide stronger discriminative power. Improvements also include the definition of objects at different levels of resolution and the relational analysis of these components to improve the definition of objects (object oriented image analysis). The definition of relationships between structures that exist both within the same range of resolution (local neighborhoods), or on different levels of resolution, help to establish a very robust

and stable identification process. As an example, in liver, dark Kupffer cells are always located adjacent to unstained sinusoid spaces. The accurate identification of a Kupffer cell can, therefore, be enhanced through its coincident local association to a different tissue structure, namely a sinusoid. Building these types of relationships can be a recursive process with feedback loops, which is a typical property of an image understanding system (Kanade, 1980).

High-content morphometrical analysis

Once the classification of the objects is completed, a comprehensive, high-content assessment can be carried out for the geometric, intensity and field specific properties. In particular the following features are available:

1 For cell layers and areas: size, form, orientation, thickness, variation in thickness, relative orientation, tissue substructures and functional building blocks, such as lobuli, acini, may be in different functional states such as inflammatory or necrotic areas
2 For cells (20–40 μm): size, shape, density, orientation, distributions, can be in different functional states such as in differentiation, mitosis and apoptosis
3 For cell nuclei (3–14 μm): size, shape, orientation, nucleolus and chromatin

Typically 30–100 features can be extracted that are descriptors for the 'expression' of structural elements of the tissue. In practical applications, when a time component is involved, these qualifiers can be visualized as tissue feature expression profiles. Inflammation can cause quite a number of different features to be expressed differentially, since inflammatory reaction involves hyperemia, edema, fibrin deposition, cell degeneration and necrosis, neutrophil proliferation followed by an influx of monocytes and macrophages. In severe damage, tissue repair by granulation may occur to form a collagenous scar.

A high-content analysis typically reveals many features to be regulated differentially in inflamed tissues. In many cases, quantitative features can describe pathological observations; the example given in Figure 61.3 demonstrates different distance distributions of monocytes of an acute inflamed area and a normal liver. The introduction of precise and sensitive machine vision may also reveal significant diagnostic tissue features that have not been described previously as visual pathological markers.

Classification

The classification of high-content data may serve very different needs, such as the detailed grouping of cells or grouping of slides and diseases. Integration of a priori expert knowledge, provided by a pathologist, can greatly support the training of such a system. Classification of

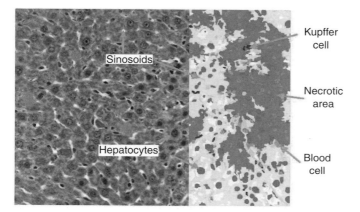

Figure 61.2 Image segmentation in liver. The right hand side displays an overlay that shows how the image can be broken down and classified into different tissue objects. These components are a prerequisite for a high-content morphometric quantification. **See colour plate 61.2.**

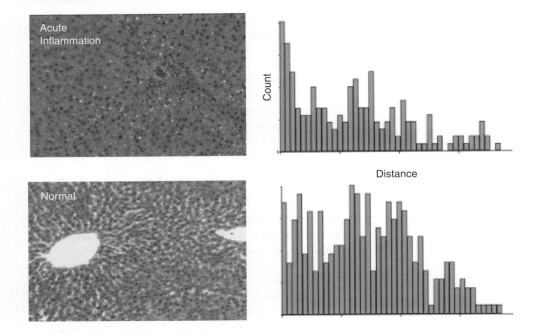

Figure 61.3 Distance distribution of monocytes (marked) in normal and acute inflamed liver. Assessments like these are consistent with pathological diagnosis. **See colour plate 61.3.**

comprehensive datasets can also be achieved by the use of advanced classifiers like multivariate analysis (Lachenbruch, 1975) or neural nets. One example for the application of neural nets has been reported for the automated differentiation of apoptotic and necrotic cells stained for DNA (Weisser et al., 1998) in the absence of visually identifiable necrotic or lytic cell death criteria. Despite the many biochemical markers that exist to identify apoptosis, it appears that morphological features remain indispensable criteria useful for screening applications.

ANALYSIS OF TISSUE MICROARRAYS

The tissue microarray (TMA) is a new form of tissue preparation composed of hundreds of tissue cores on one slide. Such preparations can substantially increase the throughput of many investigations, specifically in those areas where tissues of many donors have to be compared for testing antibodies or biomarker identification. Visual inspection of these slides are particularly time consuming, therefore the application of automated analysis appears to be particularly useful. A TMA is constructed by taking needle core tissue biopsies from hundreds of different "donor" paraffin embedded tissue blocks. These core biopsies are then precisely arrayed into a "recipient" paraffin block (35×20 mm) using a standard tissue-arrayer (such as Beecher Instruments). These cores are neatly arranged in identifiable positions in rows and columns (hence the name "microarrays"). The location of each tissue in the donor block is cataloged. It is recommended that at least 2–6 replicate tissue samples from the same block be inserted in the array to compensate for losses during processing as well as to ensure redundancy.

Paraffin tissue microarrays (TMA) have been used extensively for evaluation of the clinical significance of markers in a variety of different tumor types and immunological applications (Kononen et al., 1998; Moch et al., 1999; Wang et al., 2004). The evaluation of markers can be accomplished using a variety of different techniques, including immunohistochemistry (for protein detection), fluorescent in-situ hybridization or FISH (for detection of DNA changes) and mRNA ISH/HC (for detection of mRNA). The tissue microarray technology is a powerful tool for studying the multifocal and heterogeneous nature of diseases. So-called progression arrays, for example, based on multiple biopsies, can help to monitor efficiently the progression of inflammation or disease.

Complete TMAs can be imaged and analyzed using robotic imaging platform and machine vision software described above, reporting results for each core within the TMA. The general steps for automated TMA imaging and core detection include the following:

1 Digital images of the complete TMA slide are automatically captured using a $10\times$ objective at 0.5 μm/pixel resolution using the above mentioned robotic imaging platform
2 Tissue detection algorithms are applied to the resulting complete TMA slide image, providing the area and location for each tissue core
3 A flexible grid (or grids) is fitted to the TMA slide in order to identify individual tissue cores within the TMA (see Figure 61.4). Grids can be derived from a template or drawn manually. Grids can also be of arbitrary shape and orientation, with the only spatial constraint being that the grid object contains four sides. Each grid contains user entered label characteristics (or derived

automatically from barcode information at time of capture) that define individual indexes for each grid cell, allowing for externally associated data to be linked to the TMA structure

4 The detected tissue cores from step 2 above are then placed into each respective grid cell based on the center of the tissue area. Quality assurance is performed at this stage by measuring the goodness of fit of the tissue cores to the grid cells via a number of different metrics (e.g. tissue area inside/outside cell ratios, etc.). Manual review can be performed by navigating to each grid cell; the system will highlight the tissue areas via the cell boundaries for visual confirmation and inclusion within a grid square. This information can be saved for later recall, review and modification

5 As the grids and their respective cells are organized in a parent-child hierarchy, additional parametric information can be assigned to each grid for use in the analysis processing. For example, each grid on the slide may derive a reference threshold for background staining from a set of cells denoted as negative controls.

Immunoperoxidase DAB stain is frequently used in developmental and comparative immunology. The analysis of stain intensity is difficult but is greatly enhanced by using image informatics. First, each tissue area is located with respect to the grid to which it belongs, parameters are collected from the parent-child relationship defining the analysis method and the tissue is sampled to determine the chromatic content. Once all tissues have been pre-processed in this fashion, the chromatic distribution is analyzed and a transformation is created to relate specific RGB colors to their respective stain intensities (Figure 61.5).

Tissue masks are created for each tissue core for the determination of tissue area per core contained within the TMA. These masks are derived via a number of parameters and can represent the entire area of the core, areas that differ from background (tissue area) and areas that differ from a set spatial distribution (e.g. location of adipose tissue via structure). In addition, non-tissue artifacts can be automatically subtracted from the tissue via spatial and chromatic processing.

Once the basic parameters regarding stain intensity and tissue area have been defined for a core, the software can then apply statistical methods for core comparison based on tissue pixels expressing stain, mean/median stain values, min/max stain values. The TMA technique is most informative and reliable for evaluating the prognostic value of homogeneously expressed biomarkers (Kallioniemi et al., 2001).

OUTLOOK

Image informatics applied to microscopy is a comprehensive approach in biomedical research that covers imaging of tissues with automated devices, the computer analysis of these images and associated information, the storage and mining of this information in tissue repositories and the comparison of image information in health and disease. Recent progress in machine vision now provides detailed phenotypic tissue information through the rapid delivery of quantitative analysis of all structural components within tissue that can be made visible.

In particular the inclusion of tissue profiles as co-variants in transcriptomics opens a new way for both discovery and diagnostic purposes on a broader scale that brings

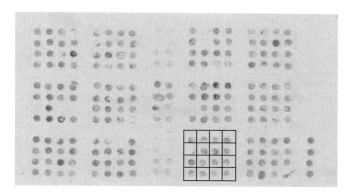

Figure 61.4 Montage of a tissue microarray acquired using an automated microscope. Grids can be automatically fitted to separate cores.

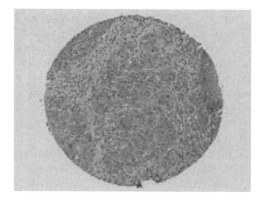 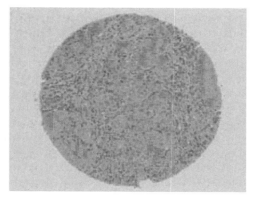

Figure 61.5 Displayed is an immunoperoxidase stained tissue core and the computer processed false color image that gives the concentration of the stain. Colors are graded from green to red, with red representing the highest intensity staining. The automated stain analysis allows efficient high-throughput evaluation of expressions in TMAs. **See colour plate 61.5.**

along new aspects to the identification of genes and their role in disease. Current biological research in tissues centers on comparison of visual observations with gene expressions (Hamadeh et al., 2002), or toolsets that establish direct relationships between the visual appearance of microstructures and their genetic profiles, like laser microdissection (Best and Emmert-Buck, 2001). Most methodologies in transcriptomics are tuned towards identification of the most up- or downregulated genes, without consideration of individual responses. Individual responses revealed by tissue co-variants, as demonstrated in toxicogenomics (Kriete et al., 2003), are likely more relevant in a personalized medicine approach, not only for computational, e-diagnostic applications but also for optimization of treatment regimens. Such methods will help to realize a highly personalized biomedical informatics, but the challenge will remain to establish long-term consistency for any phenotypical analysis (Nadkarni, 2003).

ACKNOWLEDGEMENTS

I would like to thank Ron Stone, Drew Lesniak, Mark Braughler and Peter Johnson from Tissueinformatics.Inc., Icoria, Pittsburgh, for contributions and many elucidating discussions.

REFERENCES

Arndt-Jovin, D.J. et al. (1985). Fluorescence digital imaging microscopy in cell biology. Science 230, 247–256.

Best, C.J. and Emmert-Buck, M.R. (2001). Molecular profiling of tissue samples using laser capture microdissection. Expert Rev Mol Diagn 1, 53–60.

Denk, W., Strickler, H.J. and Webb, W.W. (1990). Two-photon laser scanning fluorescence microscopy. Science 248, 73–76.

Furness, P.N. (1997). The use of digital images in pathology. J Pathol 183, 253–263.

Hamadeh, H.K., Knight, B.L., Haugen, A.C. et al. (2002). Methapyrilene toxicity: anchorage of pathologic observations to gene expression alterations. Toxicol Pathol 30, 470–482.

Herman, B. (1998). Fluorescence microscopy. Oxford: BIOS Scientific Publisher.

Kallioniemi, O.P., Wagner, U., Kononen, J. and Sauter, G. (2001). Tissue microarray technology for high–throughput molecular profiling of cancer. Hum Mol Genat, 10, 657–662.

Kanade, T. (1980). Region segmentation: signal vs semantics. Comp Graphics Image Process 13, 279–297.

Kriete, A. and Gundlach, G. (2002). Modern microscopy. Ullmann's encyclopedia of industrial chemistry, sixth edition, Vol. 33. Wiley-VCH.

Kriete, A., Schäffer, R., Harms, H. and Aus, H.M. (1985). Computer based cytophotometry analysis of thyroid tumors in imprint. J Cancer Res Clin Oncol 109, 252–256.

Kriete, A., Anderson, M., Love, B. et al. (2003). Combined histomorphometric and gene expression profiling applied to toxicology. Genome Biol 4, R32.

Kononen, J., Bubendorf, L., Kallioniemi, A. et al. (1998). Tissue microarrays for high-throughput molecular profiling of tumor specimens. Nat Med 4, 844–847.

Lachenbruch, P.A. (1975): Discriminant analysis. New York: Hafner Press.

Moch, H., Schraml, P., Bubendorf, L. et al. (1999). High-throughput tissue microarray analysis to evaluate genes uncovered by cDNA microarray screening in renal cell carcinoma. Am J Pathol 154, 981–986.

Nadkarni, P.M. (2003). The challenges of recording phenotype in a generalizable and computable form. Pharmacogenomics J 3, 8–10.

Pawley, J. (1995). Handbook of biological confocal microscopy, 2nd edn. New York: Plenum Press.

Sun, Y.N. and Horng, M.H. (1997). Assessing liver tissue fibrosis with an automatic computer morphometry system. IEEE Eng Med Biol 5/6, 66–73.

Wang, T., Wang, Y., Wu, M.C., Guan, X.Y. and Yin, Z.F. (2004). Activating mechanism of transcriptor NF-kappaB regulate by hepatitis B virus X protein in hepatocellular carcinoma. World J Gastroenterol 10, 356–360.

Weinstein, R.S., Bhattacharyya, A.K. and Graham, A.R. (1997). Telepathology: A ten year progress report. Hum Pathol 28, 1–7.

Weisser, M., Tiegs, G., Wendel, A. and Uhlig, S. (1998). Quantification of apoptotic and lytic cell death by video microscopy in combination with artificial neural networks. Cytometry 31, 20–28.

Young, Y. (1996). Quantitative microscopy. IEEE Eng Med Biol Jan/Feb, 59–66.

Index

complement, 215–16
DNA antibodies, 211–12
histone antibodies, 213
lupus anticoagulant and antiphospholipid
    antibodies, 213–15
Smoking, 623
Smooth muscle cells, in atherosclerosis, 622
SOCS, 72
Solid tumors, 465–72
    antigen-specific cytokine production,
        466–8
        cytokine flow cytometry, 467–8
        ELISPOT, 466–7
    T lymphocyte response to tumor
        antigens, 468–9
Soluble receptor activator of nuclear factor κB
    ligand (sRANKL), 487
STATs, 66, 68–9
Streptococcus faecalis, 528
Subacute bacterial endocarditis, 300
Subacute cutaneous lupus, 506
Sublamina densa, 612
Sulfoxidation status, rheumatoid
    arthritis, 486
Suppression assay, 326
Suppressor cells, 322–35
Suppressors of cytokine signaling see SOCS
Surface enhanced laser desorption ionization
    see SELDI
Surface phenotyping, 260–1, 262
Surgery, monocyte changes during, 302
Synovial fluid, 124
Synovium-specific markers, 487–8
Systemic lupus erythematosus see SLE

T lymphocytes, 630–2
    allergy and asthma, 643
    antigen-driven activation/proliferation,
        249–51, 252
    apoptosis, 248–9, 250
    atherosclerosis, 622
    cytotoxic, 580–1
    hepatitis, 599–604
        cell division assay, 600
        CTL precursor frequency, 603
        cytotoxicity assay, 600, 603
        ELISA and ELISPOT, 603
        intracellular cytokine staining, 600
        proliferation assay, 599–600
        tetramers, 603
    immunity, 380–1
    recognition of transplant antigens, 386–7
    regulatory see regulatory cells
    selection, 18
    signal transduction, 63
    tumor-specific immunity, 465–72
        cytokine flow cytometry, 467–8
        ELISPOT, 466–7
    see also NKT lymphocytes
T lymphocyte differentiation defects
    antibody production defects, 634–5
    DiGeorge syndrome, 633–4
    severe combined immune deficiency
        (SCID), 634
T lymphocyte function defects
    hereditary lymphohistocytosis, 635
    Omenn syndrome, 636
    Wiskott-Aldrich syndrome, 635

X-linked lymphoproliferative syndrome, 635
ZAP-70 deficiency, 636
T lymphocyte receptor V analysis, 582
T lymphocyte receptors
    gene rearrangement, 616
    pMHC interactions, 16, 268–9
        MHCII rearrangement, 17
T lymphocyte subsets, 337–8
    antigen specificity and T lymphocyte
        receptor repertoire, 246–7, 248
    identification of, 240–2
    multiple drug resistance transporter
        P-gp, 247–8, 249
TAB1, 65
TAB2, 65
TAK1, 65
Takayasu's arteritis, 560, 561
TAP1 proteins, 5
TAP2 proteins, 5
Tapasin, 5
TARP arrays, 681
TATA binding protein, 91
Temporal arteritis, 560, 561
Terminal complement complex, 149
Tetrachoroethane, 300
Tetramer analysis, 268–76
    advanced uses, 271–4
        analysis of 'structural avidity', 274
        functional analysis, 274
        intracellular staining, 273–4
        isolation by sorting and cloning, 272–3
        phenotypic analysis by multi-color flow
            cytometry, 273, 274
        in situ hybridization, 274
    anti-CD8 antibodies, 271
    clinical trials and future prospects, 275
    comparison with other assays, 269
    data interpretation, 271, 272, 273
    dermatology, 616–17
    hepatitis, 603
    HIV-1, 581
    production of, 269–70
    quality and number of cells, 270–1
    staining volume, temperature and
        time, 271
    T lymphocyte tumor-specific immunity,
        468–9
    TCR-pMHC interactions, 268–9
    tetramer concentration, 271
    validation and titration, 270
TGF-β1 gene polymorphisms, 571
Thoracentesis, 124
Thymopoiesis, 101–2
Thyroglobulin, 547
Thyroid disease, autoimmune, 545–51
    autoimmune hyperthyroidism, 167, 168,
        549–50
    chronic autoimmune thyroiditis, 550–1
    histopathology, 544–7
    thyroid autoantibodies, 547–9
        thyroglobulin, 547
        thyroid stimulating hormone receptor,
            548–9
        thyroperoxidase, 548
Thyroid stimulating hormone receptor, 548–9
Thyroperoxidase, 548
TIR-domain-containing adaptor inducing IFNβ
    see TRIP

TNF see tumor necrosis factor
Toll-like receptors, 62
    direction of adaptive immunity, 83
    gene expression, 66
    innate immunity, 80–90
        murine models of infection, 83–6
        susceptibility to human infection, 86–8
    ligands for, 81
    macrophage activation, 103
    polymorphism, and susceptibility to
        infection, 86–7
    response to pathogens, 63–6
        IκB and IKK and NF-κB activation, 65–6
        IRAKS, 64–5
        Mal/TIRAP, 64
        MyD88, 63–4
        TRAF6/TAB1/TAB2/TAK1, 65
        TRIF and TRAM, 64
    signal transduction, 80–3
Total serum IgE, 640
Toxoplasma gondii, immunocompromised
    patients, 281
TR cells see Regulatory cells
TRAF6, 65
TRAF6-regulated IKK activator 1 see TRIKA1
TRAM, 64
Transcription factor activation, 98, 662, 663
Transferrin, 126
Transplant antigens, immunity to, 386–91
    clinical utility of ELISPOT, 388
    defining and monitoring immune tolerance,
        390–1
    measurement of transplant reactive
        immunity in humans, 387–8
    measurement of transplant reactive
        T lymphocytes, 387
    prediction of chronic graft dysfunction,
        389–90
    prediction/evaluation of acute rejection,
        388–9
    T lymphocyte recognition of transplant
        antigens, 386–7
    withdrawal of immunosuppressants, 390
Transplant rejection, 388–9
Transplantation, 18, 569–77
    adaptive immunity, 569
    allograft recognition, 570
    anti-allograft repertoire, 570
    cellular and humoral alloimmunity,
        413–14
    dendritic cells in, 295
    DTH reactivity
        post-transplant, 412–13
        pre-transplant, 412
        tolerant patients, 414
    innate immunity, 569
    measurement of immunity, 570–5
        cellular immunity, 573–4
        genomic factors, 571–2
        humoral immunity, 572–3
        molecular characterization of solid organ
            graft recipients, 574
        non-invasive and molecular biomarkers,
            574–5
    NK receptor variation in, 115
    regulatory cells in, 330–1
    see also Post-transplant lymphoproliferative
        disease